evolve

•• *To access your Learning Resources, visit:*
http://evolve.elsevier.com/Dental/drug/

New Evolve® Learning Resources for *Mosby's Dental Drug Reference,*
Eighth Edition, offer the following features:

Learning Resources

- **Color Pill Atlas**
  Full-color photos of the most commonly prescribed drugs.

- **Expanded Coverage on Drugs of Abuse and Alternative Medicine**
  Tables and text for further understanding of these subjects
  and how they relate to dentistry.

- **Glossary of Terms**
  A glossary of terms frequently used in the pharmacy and
  clinical setting.

- **Appendices From the Book**
  All of the appendices presented in full, searchable form.

- **Patient Teaching Guides**
  Handouts in Spanish and English to educate patients about
  the medications they are taking.

- **Update Section**
  Content updates posted periodically to help keep students
  informed of new developments in the pharmacy world.

MOSBY'S
DENTAL
DRUG
REFERENCE

Eighth Edition

Editor-in-Chief
Arthur H. Jeske, DMD, PhD
Chair, Professor
Restorative Dentistry and Biomaterials
The University of Texas
Dental Branch at Houston
Houston, Texas

MOSBY

ELSEVIER

11830 Westline Industrial Drive
St. Louis, Missouri 63146

MOSBY'S DENTAL DRUG REFERENCE,
EIGHTH EDITION

ISBN: 978-0-323-05266-5

Notice

Knowledge and best practice in this field are constantly changing. As new research and experience broaden our knowledge, changes in practice, treatment and drug therapy may become necessary or appropriate. Readers are advised to check the most current information provided (i) on procedures featured or (ii) by the manufacturer of each product to be administered, to verify the recommended dose or formula, the method and duration of administration, and contraindications. It is the responsibility of the practitioner, relying on their own experience and knowledge of the patient, to make diagnoses, to determine dosages and the best treatment for each individual patient, and to take all appropriate safety precautions. To the fullest extent of the law, neither the Publisher nor the Editor assumes any liability for any injury and/or damage to persons or property arising out of or related to any use of the material contained in this book.

The Publisher

Library of Congress Control Number: 2007928961

Publishing Director: Linda Duncan
Acquisitions Editor: John Dolan
Developmental Editor: Elizabeth Clark
Editorial Assistant: Joslyn Dumas
Publishing Services Manager: Melissa Lastarria
Senior Project Manager: Joy Moore
Design Direction: Kimberly Denando
Cover Designer: Elaine Rickles

Working together to grow
libraries in developing countries
www.elsevier.com | www.bookaid.org | www.sabre.org

ELSEVIER   BOOK AID International   Sabre Foundation

Printed in the United States of America

Last digit is the print number: 9 8 7 6 5 4 3 2 1

DRUG MONOGRAPH
CONTENT CONTRIBUTORS

Catherine Ulbricht, PharmD
Massachusetts General Hospital
Natural Standard Research Collaboration
Cambridge, Massachusetts

Erica Seamon, PharmD
Natural Standard Research Collaboration
Cambridge, Massachusetts

PREFACE

Members of the dental care team are being increasingly challenged to deal with the vast array of prescription drugs now available. New medications, and new classes of medications, introduce complexity into the dental care of patients who have systemic diseases and require that new and up-to-date drug information resources be readily available in the dental office. This new edition of *Mosby's Dental Drug Reference* is designed to address this need for rapid access to accurate drug information and to focus on issues that directly affect dental management of medically compromised patients.

This edition of *Mosby's Dental Drug Reference* contains many useful features, including:

1. *Practice-oriented precautions, dental considerations and recommended medical consultations for every drug entry, and essential drug facts that are directly placed into the context of the dentist's and dental hygienist's care.*
2. *Highlights of serious adverse reactions and contraindications.* In each drug entry, the book calls attention to dangerous or life-threatening reactions so that you can identify them easily and deal with them promptly.
3. *Specialized dental care guidelines, including the most recent AHA recommendations for the prevention of infective endocarditis.* Suggested protocols for the treatment of medically compromised patients and the therapeutic management of common oral lesions are also included.
4. *Combination drug guide.* Detailed index of combination drugs arranged by trade name.
5. *Herbal and nonherbal remedies.* Extensive clinical data and dental considerations for commonly used alternative remedies.
6. *Comprehensive appendices.* Ten ready-reference appendixes give you easy access to additional vital drug-related information and detailed sections concerning anesthetics, controlled substances, disorders and conditions, pregnancy and pediatrics, and sample prescriptions for drugs more commonly prescribed in dental practice.

A detailed guide to *Mosby's Dental Drug Reference,* **Eighth Edition:**

Mosby's Dental Drug Reference provides essential drug information in a user-friendly format. The bulk of this handbook contains an alphabetical listing of drug entries by generic name. Drug entries include the following:

Generic and Brand Names. Drug entries begin with the generic drug name, followed by its pronunciation and its U.S., Canadian, and Australian brand names.

Category and Schedule. This section lists the drug's pregnancy risk category and, when appropriate, its controlled substance schedule or over-the-counter (OTC) status.

Mechanism of Action. This section clearly and concisely describes the drug's mechanism of action and therapeutic effects.

Pharmacokinetics. Under this heading, a quick-reference chart outlines the drug's route, onset, peak, and duration, when known. This information is followed by a brief description of the drug's absorption, distribution, metabolism, excretion, and half-life.

Indications and Dosages. Here you'll find the approved indications and routes, along with age-appropriate dosage information and, for selected agents, dosage adjustments for preexisting conditions, such as liver or kidney disease.

Precautions/Contraindications. Using a practice-oriented format and written specifically for dentistry, this section presents precautions and considerations for each drug entry. Each entry lists conditions in which use of the generic drug is contraindicated.

Interactions. For drugs, herbal supplements, and food, this section supplies vital information about adverse interactions of the medical drug with drugs prescribed in dentistry.

Adverse Effects. Unlike other handbooks that mix more common adverse effects with rare, minor ones in a long, undifferentiated list, this book ranks side effects by frequency of occurrence, indicating expected, frequent, occasional, and rare.

Serious Reactions. Because serious adverse reactions can be life-threatening emergencies that require prompt intervention, this section highlights them, separate from other side effects, for easy identification.

Mosby's Dental Drug Reference, **Eighth Edition,** is an easy-to-use source of current drug information for a wide spectrum of dental care providers. When it comes to providing quality patient care, all members of the dental team can rely on the eighth edition of *Mosby's Dental Drug Reference* for current, dentally relevant information, presented in an easy-to-use format.

CONTENTS

Based on Material from AAOM Clinician's Guide to Treatment of Common Oral Conditions and Appendix B from Dental Management of the Medically Compromised Patient

This is a summary of the etiologic factors, clinical description, currently accepted therapeutic management, and patient education of the more common oral conditions. Some of the recommended treatments have been investigated more thoroughly than others, but all have been reported to be of clinical value.

Many oral conditions described here have no cure, but treatment modalities are available that can relieve discomfort, shorten their clinical duration and frequency, and minimize recurrences.

Clinicians are reminded that an accurate diagnosis is imperative for clinical success. Every effort should be made to determine the diagnosis before initiating treatment. Infection and malignancy must be ruled out. When signs, symptoms, and microscopic and other laboratory evidence do not support a definitive diagnosis, empirical treatment may be initiated and evaluated on a therapeutic, trial basis.

Patient management should be governed by the natural history of the oral condition and whether a palliative, supportive, or curative treatment exists. Referral of patients should be made when the patient's problems are beyond the scope of the clinician trial. Further treatment can be determined by the patient's response. However, when healing of a lesion or an expected response to treatment is not achieved within an expected period of time, a biopsy is recommended.

All drugs require a prescription unless identified as over-the-counter (OTC) drugs. Please note that in recent years, the Food and Drug Administration (FDA) has been active in allowing OTC status for drugs formerly available by prescription only. Be sure to check the dosages of the newly released OTC drugs because they usually are of a different strength than those available by prescription.

SUPPORTIVE CARE

Management of oral mucosal conditions may require topical and systemic interventions. Therapy should address patient nutrition and hydration, oral discomfort, oral hygiene, management of secondary infection, and local control of the disease process. Depending on the extent, severity, and location of oral lesions, consideration should be given to obtaining a consultation from a dentist who specializes in oral medicine, oral pathology, or oral surgery. When a question arises involving a medical condition, a physician should be consulted.

Symptomatic relief of painful conditions can be provided with topical preparations, such as 2% viscous lidocaine hydrochloride or 0.5% dyclonine hydrochloride. Topical anesthetics can be used as a rinse in adults but should be applied with a cotton swab in a child so that the child does not swallow the medication. Swallowing these anesthetics is contraindicated, in part, because they may interfere with the patient's gag reflex. Symptomatic relief also can be obtained by mixing equal parts of diphenhydramine hydrochloride elixir and magnesium hydroxide/aluminum hydroxide. Children's formula diphenhydramine hydrochloride elixir does not contain alcohol. Sucralfate suspension also can be used before meals. The diphenhydramine mixture and the sucralfate coat the ulcerated lesions and may allow the patient to eat more comfortably.

Meticulous oral hygiene is absolutely mandatory for these patients. Mucosal lesions contacting bacterial plaque present on the dentition are more likely to become secondarily infected. Patients should be seen by the dentist or hygienist for scaling and root planing, under local anesthesia when necessary, in all cases in which oral hygiene is suboptimal. Patients must be encouraged to brush and floss their teeth after meals in a gentle yet efficient manner. This may be enhanced by placing a soft toothbrush under hot water to further soften the bristles. Tartar control toothpastes containing calcium pyrophosphate should be avoided because of their caustic nature and reported involvement in circumoral dermatitis.

HERPES SIMPLEX

Infection with the herpes simplex virus produces a disease that has a primary, or acute, phase and a secondary, or recurrent, phase.

Primary Herpetic Gingivostomatitis

Etiology:
A transmissible infection with herpes simplex virus, usually type I or, less commonly, type II.

Clinical description:
Clear, then yellowish, vesicles develop intraorally and extraorally. These vesicles rupture within hr and form shallow, painful ulcers.

The gingivae often are red, enlarged, and painful. The patient may have systemic signs and symptoms including regional lymphadenitis, fever, and malaise. Usually it is self-limiting, with healing in 7–10 days.

Rationale for treatment:
Relieve symptoms, prevent secondary infection, and support general health. Supportive therapy includes forced fluids, protein, vitamin and mineral food supplements, and rest. Systemic acyclovir is effective in treating herpes in immunocompromised patients. Topical steroids should be avoided because they tend to permit spread of the viral infection on mucous membranes, particularly ocular membranes. Patients should be cautioned to avoid touching the herpetic lesions and then touching the eyes, genitals, or other body areas because of the possibility of self-inoculation.

Topical Anesthetics and Coating Agents

Rx
Diphenhydramine (Benadryl) elixir 12.5 mg/5 ml (Note: Elixir is Rx and syrup [Benylin] is OTC) 4 oz mixed with Kaopectate OTC 4 oz (to make a 50% mixture by volume).
Disp: 8 oz
Sig: Rinse with 1 teaspoonful every 2 hr and spit out.
Maalox OTC can be used in place of Kaopectate.

Rx
Diphenhydramine (Benadryl) elixir 12.5 mg/5 ml
Disp: 4 oz bottle
Sig: Rinse with 1 teaspoonful for 2 min every 2 hr and before each meal and spit out.

Systemic Antiviral Therapy
Acyclovir oral capsules may relieve and decrease the duration of symptoms.

Rx
Acyclovir (Zovirax) capsules 200 mg
Disp: 50 (or 60) capsules
Sig: Take 1 capsule 5 times a day for
10 days (or 2 capsules 3 times a day
for 10 days).

(Current FDA-approved indication
is that systemic acyclovir be used
to treat oral herpes only in
immunocompromised patients.)
Systemic Antibiotics
(For secondary bacterial infection in
susceptible individuals. Do not use
routinely.)
Rx
Penicillin V tablets 500 mg
Disp: 40 tablets
Sig: Take 1 tablet 4 times a day.
For patients allergic to penicillin:
Rx
Erythromycin tablets 250 mg
Disp: 40 tablets
Sig: Take 1 tablet 4 times a day.
If nausea or stomach cramps occur,
prescribe enteric-coated preparations
(e.g., E-Mycin, ERYC, PCE, etc.)
or a second-generation erythromycin
(e.g., clarithromycin [Biaxin]).
Nutritional Supplements
Rx
Meritene (protein-vitamin-mineral
food supplement) OTC
Disp: 1-lb can (plain vanilla,
chocolate, and eggnog flavors)
Sig: Take 3 servings per day. Prepare
as indicated on the label. Serve cold.
Rx
Ensure Plus (protein-vitamin-mineral
food supplement) OTC
Disp: 20 cans
Sig: Drink 3–5 cans in divided doses
throughout the day as tolerated.
Serve cold.
Analgesic
Rx
Acetaminophen tablets 325 mg OTC
Sig: Take 2–3 tablets q4h PRN for
pain and fever. Limit 4 g/24 hr.

For Moderate Pain
Acetaminophen 300 mg with codeine
30 mg (Tylenol no. 3)
Sig: Take 1 or 2 tablets q4h for pain
(requires Drug Enforcement Agency
[DEA] number).
**Recurrent (Orofacial) Herpes
Simplex**
Etiology:
Reactivation of the latent virus that
resides in the sensory ganglion of the
trigeminal nerve. Precipitating
factors include fever, stress, exposure
to sunlight, trauma, and hormonal
alterations.
Clinical description:
Intraoral—single or small clusters of
vesicles that quickly rupture, forming
painful ulcers. The lesions usually
occur on the keratinized tissue of the
hard palate and gingiva.

Labial—clusters of vesicles on
the lips that rupture within hr and
then crust.
Rationale for treatment:
Should be initiated as early as
possible in the prodromal stage, with
the objective of reducing the duration
and symptoms of the lesion. Oral
acyclovir, prophylactically and
therapeutically, can be considered
when frequent recurrent herpetic
episodes interfere with daily function
and nutrition. (Current FDA-approved
indication is that systemic acyclovir
be used to treat oral herpes only in
immunocompromised patients.)
Prevention
Rx
PreSun 15-sunscreen lotion (OTC)
Disp: 4 fl oz
Sig: Apply to susceptible area
1 hr before sun exposure and
every hr thereafter.
Rx
PreSun 15-lip gel (OTC)
Disp: 15 oz

Sig: Apply to lips 1 hr before sun exposure and every hr thereafter. If a recurrence on the lips usually is precipitated by exposure to sunlight, the lesion may be prevented by applying a sunscreen with a high skin protection factor (SPF 15 or greater) to the area.

Topical Antiviral Agents

Antiviral creams and ointments are of minimal efficacy for recurrent herpes simplex. Their value may be attributable to coating of the lesion by the petrolatum vehicle, which reduces the possibility of self-inoculation. Constant or intermittent application of ice to the area for 90 min during the prodromal phase may result in aborting the lesion. Cocoa butter ointment, lanolin-based lip preparations, or petrolatum (Vaseline) as an emollient may be palliative.

Rx
Penciclovir (Denavir) topical ointment 5%
Disp: 15-g tube
Sig: Apply to area q2h during waking hours, beginning when symptoms first occur.

Rx
Docosanol (Abreva) cream (OTC)
Disp: 2-g tube
Sig: Dab on lesion 5 times a day during waking hours for 4 days, beginning when symptoms first occur.

VARICELLA ZOSTER (SHINGLES)

Etiology:
Reactivation of latent herpes varicella virus present since an original varicella infection through chickenpox. Precipitating factors include thermal, inflammatory, radiologic, or mechanical trauma.
Clinical description:
Usually painful segmental eruption of small vesicles that later rupture to form punctate or confluent ulcers. Acute zoster follows a portion of the trigeminal nerve distribution in approximately 20% of cases. It is rare in the young, more common in the elderly.
Rationale for treatment:
Promptly initiate antiviral therapy to reduce duration and symptoms of the lesions. Patients older than 60 yr are particularly prone to postherpetic neuralgia. In the absence of specific contraindications, consideration should be given to prescribing short-term, high-dose corticosteroid prophylaxis for postherpetic neuralgia, in conjunction with oral acyclovir.
Rx
Acyclovir (Zovirax) capsules 200 mg
Disp: 200 capsules
Sig: Take 4 capsules 5 times a day for 10 days.
Rx
Valacyclovir (Valtrex) HCl caplets 500 mg
Disp: 42 capsules
Sig: Take 2 capsules 3 times a day for 7 days.
Use with caution in immunocompromised patients.

RECURRENT APHTHOUS STOMATITIS

Etiology:
An altered local immune response is the predisposing factor. Patients with frequent recurrences should be screened for diseases, such as anemia, diabetes mellitus, vitamin deficiency, inflammatory bowel disease, and immunosuppression.

Precipitating factors include stress, trauma, allergies, endocrine alterations, dietary components, such as acidic foods and juices, and foods that contain gluten. Inspect the oral cavity closely for sources of trauma.

Clinical description:

Minor aphthae (canker sore), smaller than 0.6 cm, small, shallow, painful ulceration covered by a gray membrane and surrounded by a narrow erythematous halo. They usually occur on nonkeratinized (moveable) oral mucosa.

Major aphthae, larger than 0.6 cm, large painful ulcers. A more severe form of aphthae that may last weeks or months. They may mimic other diseases, such as granulomatous or malignant lesions.

Herpetiform ulcers, crops of small, shallow, painful ulcers, may occur anywhere on nonkeratinized oral mucosa and resemble recurrent intraoral herpes simplex clinically but are of unknown etiology.

Rationale for treatment:

Effective treatment involves barriers, amlexanox, topical or systemic corticosteroids, and immunosuppressants or combination therapy, when indicated. Treatment should be initiated as early as possible in the course of lesions. Identification and elimination of precipitating factors may minimize recurrent episodes. Medications such as mycophenolate mofetil, pentoxifylline, and thalidomide are used to treat patients with severe, persistent, recurrent aphthous ulcers but should not be routinely used.

Nonsteroidal

Rx

Amlexanox oral paste 5%

Disp: 5-g tube

Sig: Apply to affected area 4 times a day until healed.

Rx

Orabase Soothe-N-Seal Protective Barrier (OTC)

Disp: 1 package

Sig: Apply as per the package directions every 6 hr when necessary.

Therapies with steroids and immunomodulating drugs are presented to inform the clinician that such modalities are available. Because of the potential for side effects, close collaboration with the patient's physician is recommended if these medications are prescribed. These modalities may be beyond the scope of clinical experience of general dentists, and referral to a specialist in oral medicine or to an appropriate physician may be necessary.

Topical Steroids

Prolonged use of topical steroids (longer than 2 wk of continuous use) may result in mucosal atrophy or secondary candidiasis and may increase the potential for systemic absorption. It may be necessary to prescribe antifungal therapy with steroids.

Rx

Triamcinolone acetonide (Kenalog) in Orabase 0.1%

Disp: 5-g tube

Sig: Coat the lesion with a thin film after each meal and at bedtime.

Other topical steroid preparations (cream, gel rinse, ointment) include:

Ultra-Potent:

Clobetasol propionate (Temovate) 0.05%

Halobetasol propionate (Ultravate) 0.05%

Potent:

Dexamethasone (Decadron) 0.5 mg/5 ml

Intermediate:

Betamethasone valerate (Valisone) 0.1%

Triamcinolone acetonide (Kenalog) 0.1%

Low:

Hydrocortisone 1%

(Mixing ointments with equal parts of Orabase B paste promotes adhesion.)

Rx
Dexamethasone (Decadron) elixir
0.5 mg/5 ml
Disp: 100 ml
Sig: Rinse with 1 teaspoon for 2 min
4 times a day and expectorate.
Discontinue when lesions become
asymptomatic.

Oral candidiasis may result from
topical steroid therapy. The oral
cavity should be monitored for
emergence of fungal infection in
patients who are placed on therapy.
Prophylactic antifungal therapy
should be initiated in patients with a
history of fungal infections with
previous steroid administration
(see Candidiasis/Candidosis).

System Steroids and
Immunosuppressants for Severe
Cases
Rx
Dexamethasone (Decadron) elixir
0.5 mg/5 ml
Disp: 320 ml
Sig:
1. For 3 days, rinse with 1 tablespoon
   (15 ml) 4 times a day and swallow.
   Then
2. For 3 days, rinse with
   1 teaspoonful (5 ml) 4 times a day
   and swallow. Then
3. For 3 days, rinse with
   1 teaspoonful (5 ml) 4 times a
   day and swallow every other time.
   Then
4. Rinse with 1 teaspoonful
   (5 ml) 4 times a day and spit out.
   Discontinue medication when
   mouth becomes comfortable.

If mouth discomfort recurs, restart
treatment at step 3. Rinsing should
be done after meals and at bedtime.
Refill one time.
Rx
Prednisone tablets 5 mg
Disp: 40 tablets

Sig: Take 5 tablets in the morning for
5 days, then 5 tablets in the morning
every other day until gone.
For Very Severe Cases
Rx
Prednisone tablets 10 mg
Disp: 26 tablets
Sig: Take 4 tablets in the morning for
5 days, then decrease by 1 tablet on
each successive day.

Therapy with medications, such
as systemic steroids,
immunosuppressants, and
immunomodulators are presented to
inform the clinician that such
modalities have been reported
effective for patients suffering from
severe, persistent, recurrent aphthous
stomatitis. Medications such as
azathioprine, pentoxifylline,
levamisole, colchicine, dapsone, and
thalidomide are used to treat patients
with severe, persistent recurrent
aphthous stomatitis but should not be
routinely used because of the
potential for serious adverse effects.
Close collaboration with the patient's
physician is recommended when
these medications are prescribed.

CANDIDIASIS

Etiology:
Candida albicans, a yeastlike fungus.
Candida is an opportunistic organism
that tends to proliferate with the use
of broad-spectrum antibiotics,
corticosteroids, medicines that
reduce salivary output, and cytotoxic
agents. Conditions that contribute to
candidiasis include xerostomia,
diabetes mellitus, poor oral hygiene,
prosthetic appliances, and
suppression of the immune system
(i.e., AIDS or the side effects of
some medications). It is important to
determine the predisposing
factors.

Clinical description:
The disease is characterized by soft, white, slightly elevated plaques that usually can be wiped away, leaving an erythematous area (pseudomembranous type). Candidiasis also may appear as generalized erythematous, sensitive areas (atrophic or erythematous type) or as confluent white areas (hypertrophic form). When the clinical diagnosis is questionable, it is advisable to culture for *C. albicans* concurrent with starting medication.
Rationale for treatment:
To reestablish a normal balance of oral flora and improve oral hygiene. Medication should be continued for 48 hr after disappearance of clinical signs to prevent immediate recurrence.
Topical Antifungal Agents
Rx
Nystatin (Mycostatin, Nilstat) oral suspension 100,000 units/ml
Disp: 60 ml
Sig: Take 2–5 ml 4 times a day. Rinse for 2 min and swallow. Nystatin suspension has a high sugar content; therefore good oral hygiene should be reinforced. A few drops of nystatin oral suspension can be added to the water used for soaking acrylic prostheses.
Rx
Nystatin ointment
Disp: 15-g tube
Sig: Apply a thin coat to inner surface of denture and to the affected area after each meal.
Rx
Nystatin topical powder
Disp: 15 g
Sig: Apply a thin layer under the prosthesis after each meal.
Rx (Mycostatin)
Nystatin pastilles 200,000 units
Disp: 50 pastilles

Sig: Let 1 pastille dissolve in mouth 5 times a day.
Rx
Nystatin vaginal suppositories 100,000 units
Sig: Let suppository dissolve in mouth 4 times a day. Do not rinse for 30 min.
Rx
Clotrimazole (Mycelex) troches 10 mg
Disp: 70 troches
Sig: Let 1 troche dissolve in mouth 5 times a day. If concern exists about sugar content of the nystatin and clotrimazole troches, vaginal tablets can be substituted.
Rx
Ketoconazole (Nizoral) cream 2%
Disp: 15-g tube
Sig: Apply thin coat to inner surface of denture and affected areas after meal.
Rx
Clotrimazole (Gyne-Lotrimin, Mycelex-G) Vaginal Cream 1% (OTC)
Disp: 1 tube
Sig: Apply small dab to tissue side of denture or to the infected oral mucosa 4 times a day.
Rx
Miconazole (Monistat 7) Vaginal Cream 2% (OTC)
Disp: 1 tube
Sig: Apply small dab to tissue side of denture or to the infected oral mucosa 4 times a day.
Systemic Antifungal Agents
Note: In many cases, combinations of these antifungal preparations (liquids, troches, and ointments) can be used depending upon clinical considerations and response to therapy.
When topical therapy is not practical or is ineffective, ketoconazole (Nizoral) and

fluconazole (Diflucan) are effective, well-tolerated, systemic drugs for mucocutaneous candidiasis. They should be used with caution in patients with impaired liver function (i.e., with history of alcoholism or hepatitis) and in patients taking drugs metabolized by the cytochrome P450 isoenzyme CYP3A4. Liver function tests should be performed initially and conducted monthly when ketoconazole is prescribed for an extended period. Several drug interactions have been reported with ketoconazole.

Rx
Ketoconazole (Nizoral) tablets 200 mg
Disp: 20 tablets
Sig: Take 1 tablet a day with a meal or orange juice.

Rx
Fluconazole (Diflucan) tablets 100 mg
Disp: 20 tablets
Sig: Take 2 tablets stat, then 1 tablet a day.

Rx
Itraconazole (Sporanox) tablets 100 mg
Disp: 28 tablets
Sig: Take 1 tablet twice a day or 2 tablets a day with meal or orange juice.

Rx
Amphotericin B (Fungizone) oral suspension 100 mg/ml
Disp: 48 ml
Sig: 1 ml 4 times a day. Swish in mouth 3–4 min then swallow.

CHEILITIS AND CHEILOSIS

Angular Cheilitis and Cheilosis
Etiology:
Fissured lesions in the corners of the mouth are caused by a mixed infection of the microorganisms *C. albicans, Staphylococcus,* and *Streptococcus.* Predisposing factors include local habits, drooling, a decrease in intermaxillary space,

anemia, immunosuppression, and an extension of oral infections.
Clinical description:
The commissures may appear wrinkled, red, fissured, cracked, or crusted.
Rationale for treatment:
Identification and correction of predisposing factors and elimination of the secondary infection and inflammation.

Rx
Nystatin plus triamcinolone acetonide (Mycolog II) ointment
Disp: 15-g tube
Sig: Apply to affected area after each meal and at bedtime. Concomitant intraoral antifungal treatment may be indicated.

Rx
Ketoconazole (Nizoral) cream 2%
Disp: 15-g tube
Sig: Apply a small dab to corners of mouth daily at bedtime.

Rx
Clotrimazole (Gyne-Lotrimin, Mycelex-G) vaginal cream 1% (OTC)
Disp: 1 tube
Sig: Apply small dab to corner of mouth 4 times a day.

Rx
Miconazole (Monistat 7) nitrate vaginal cream 2% (OTC)
Disp: 1 tube
Sig: Apply small dab to corner of mouth 4 times a day.

Actinic Cheilitis and Solar Cheilosis
Etiology:
Prolonged exposure to sunlight results in irreversible degenerative changes in the vermilion of the lips, especially the everted lower lip.
Clinical description:
The normal red translucent vermilion with regular vertical fissuring of a smooth surface is replaced by a white

flat surface that may exhibit periodic ulceration.

Rationale for treatment:

If exposure to the ultraviolet light in the sun's rays is allowed to continue, the degenerative changes may progress to a malignancy. Sunscreens with a high skin protection factor (SPF greater than 15) should be used constantly.

Rx

Several OTC sunscreen preparations are available (e.g., PreSun 15 lotion and lip gel). For those patients allergic to paraaminobenzoic acid, non–paraaminobenzoic acid sunscreens should be prescribed.

GEOGRAPHIC TONGUE (BENIGN MIGRATORY GLOSSITIS; ERYTHEMA MIGRANS)

Etiology:

The etiology is unknown. Because its histologic appearance is similar to psoriasis, some have associated it with psoriasis. This may be purely coincidental. Oral lesions should not be associated with psoriasis if no cutaneous signs exist of this disorder. It has been associated with Reiter's syndrome and atopy.

Clinical description:

A benign inflammatory condition caused by desquamation of superficial keratin and filiform papillae. It is characterized by both red, denuded, irregularly shaped patches of the tongue dorsum and lateral borders surrounded by a raised white-yellow border.

Rationale for treatment:

Generally, no treatment is necessary as most patients are asymptomatic. When symptoms are present, they may be associated with secondary infection with *C. albicans* (see Supportive Care). Topical steroids, especially in combination with topical antifungal agents, are the treatment modality of choice. Patients must be told that this condition does not suggest a more serious disease and is not contagious. In most cases, biopsy is not indicated because of the pathognomonic clinical appearance.

Rx

Nystatin-triamcinolone acetonide (Mycolog II, Mytrex) ointment

Disp: 15-g tube

Sig: Apply to affected areas after meals and at bedtime.

Rx

Clotrimazole-betamethasone dipropionate (Lotrisone) cream

Disp: 15-g tube

Sig: Apply to affected area after each meal and at bedtime.

Rx

Betamethasone Valerate ointment, 0.1%

Disp: 15-g tube

Sig: Apply to affected areas after meals and at bedtime.

Rx

Nystatin ointment

Disp: 15-g tube

Sig: Apply to affected areas after meals and at bedtime.

XEROSTOMIA

Etiology:

Acute or chronic reduced salivary flow may result from drug therapy, mechanical blockage, dehydration, emotional stress, infection of the salivary glands, local surgery, avitaminosis, diabetes, anemia, connective tissue diseases, Sjögren's syndrome, radiation therapy, and congenital factors (e.g., ectodermal dysplasia) (see Box 21-9).

Clinical description:

The tissues may be dry, pale, or red and atrophic. The tongue may be devoid of papillae, atrophic, fissured, and inflamed. Multiple carious lesions may be present, especially at the gingival margin and on exposed root surfaces.

Rationale for treatment:
Salivary stimulation or replacement therapy to keep mouth moist, prevention of caries and candidal infection, and palliative relief.

Saliva Substitutes

Rx
Sodium carboxymethyl cellulose 0.5% aqueous solution (OTC)
Disp: 8 fl oz
Sig: Use as a rinse as frequently as needed.

Saliva substitutes (OTC): Optimoist, MouthKote, Sage Moist Plus, Xero-Lube, Salivart, Moi-Stir, Orex

Commercial oral moisturizing gels (OTC): Sage Mouth Moisturizer, Oral Balance

Relief from oral dryness and accompanying discomfort can be achieved conservatively by sipping water frequently all day long, letting ice melt in the mouth, restricting caffeine intake, not using mouth rinses that contain alcohol, humidifying sleeping area, and coating lips with Blistex or Vaseline

Saliva Stimulants

Chewing sugarless gum and sucking sugarless mints are conservative methods to temporarily stimulate salivary flow in patients with medication xerostomia or with salivary gland dysfunction. Patients should be cautioned against using products that contain sugar.

Rx
Pilocarpine HCl solution 1 mg/ml
Disp: 100 ml
Sig: Take 1 teaspoonful 4 times a day. (The dosage should be adjusted to increase saliva while minimizing the adverse side effects [sweating, stomach upset].)

Rx
Pilocarpine HCl (Salagen) tablets 5 mg
Disp: 100 tablets
Sig: Take 1 tablet 3 times a day. An extra tablet (10 mg) may be taken at bedtime.

Rx
Cevimeline HCl (Evoxac) tablets 30 mg
Disp: 100 tablets
Sig: Take 1 tablet PO 3 or 4 times a day

Rx
Bethanechol (Urecholine) 25 mg
Disp: 21 tablets
Sig: Take 1 tablet 3 times a day.

Caries Prevention

Rx
Stannous fluoride gel 0.4%
Disp: 4.3 oz
Sig: Apply to teeth daily for 5 min; 5–10 drops in a custom tray. Do not swallow the gel.

SnF_2 gels available include IDP Gel-Oh, Stan-Gard, Perfect Choice, Flo-Gel, True Gel, Nova Gel, Omni-Gel, Control, Gel-Pro, Perfect Choice, Basic Gel, Gel-Tin, IDP Gel-Oh, Gel-Kam, Stan-Gard, Easy-Gel, Thera-Flur

When the taste of acidulated SnF_2 gels is poorly tolerated or where there is etching of ceramic restorations, neutral pH sodium fluoride gel 1% (Thera-Flur-N) should be considered.

Rx
Neutral NaF gel (Thera-Flur-N) 1.0% or PreviDent (Colgate) 1.1% neutral NaF
Disp: 24 ml
Sig: Place 1 drop per tooth in custom tray; apply for 5 min daily. Avoid rinsing or eating for 30 min following treatment.

FDA regulations have limited the size of bottles of fluoride because of toxicity if ingested by infants. Because most preparations do not come in childproof bottles, the sizes of topical fluoride preparations vary; 24 ml is an approximately 2-wk supply for application to a full dentition in custom carriers. Xerostomia provides an excellent environment for overgrowth of *C. albicans.* The patient is likely to require treatment for candidiasis along with treatment for dry mouth. In a dry oral environment, plaque control becomes more difficult. Scrupulous oral hygiene is essential.

LICHEN PLANUS

Etiology:

Postulated to be a chronic mucocutaneous autoimmune disorder with a genetic predisposition that is initiated by a variety of factors, including emotional stress, hypersensitivity to drugs, dental products, or foods.

Clinical description:

Lichen planus varies in clinical appearance. Oral forms of this disorder include lacy white lines representing Wickham's striae (reticular), an erythematous form (atrophic), and an ulcerating form that often is accompanied by striae peripheral to the ulceration (ulcerative).

The lesions are commonly found on the buccal mucosa, gingiva, and tongue, but they can be found on the lips and palate. Lichen planus lesions are chronic and also may affect the skin.

Any refractory lesion should be considered for biopsy to establish a diagnosis and to rule out a malignancy.

Rationale for treatment:

To provide oral comfort if the lesions are symptomatic. No known cure exists. Systemic and local relief with

antiinflammatory and immunosuppressant agents is indicated. Identification of any dietary component, dental product, or medication (lichenoid drug reaction) should be undertaken to ensure against a hypersensitivity reaction. Treatment or prevention of a secondary fungal infection with a systemic antifungal agent also should be considered.

Therapies with steroids and immunomodulating drugs are presented to inform the clinician that such modalities are available. Because of the potential for side effects, close collaboration with the patient's physician is recommended when these medications are prescribed. These modalities may be beyond the scope of clinical experience of general dentists, and referral to a specialist in oral medicine or to an appropriate physician may be necessary.

Topical Steroids

Prolonged use of topical steroids (for a period longer than 2 wk of continuous use) may result in mucosal atrophy and secondary candidiasis and may increase the potential for systemic absorption. The prescribing of antifungal therapy with steroids may be necessary. Therapy with topical steroids, once the lichen planus is under control, should be tapered to alternate day therapy or less depending on control of the disease and the tendency for recurrence.

Rx

Fluocinonide (Lidex) gel 0.05%
Disp: 30-g tube
Sig: Coat the lesion with a thin film after each meal and at bedtime.

Rx

Dexamethasone (Decadron) elixir
0.5 mg/5 ml

Disp: 100 ml
Sig: Rinse with 1 teaspoonful for
2 min 4 times a day and spit out.
Discontinue when lesions become
asymptomatic.

Other topical steroid preparations
(cream, gel ointment) include:
Ultra-Potent:
Clobetasol propionate
(Temovate) 0.05%
Halobetasol propionate
(Ultravate) 0.05%
Potent:
Dexamethasone (Decadron)
0.5 mg/5 ml
Fluocinonide (Lidex) 0.05%
Intermediate:
Betamethasone valerate
(Valisone) 0.1%
Triamcinolone acetonide
(Kenalog) 0.1%
Low:
Hydrocortisone 1%

Oral candidiasis may result from
topical steroid therapy. The oral
cavity should be monitored for
emergence of fungal infection in
patients who are placed on therapy.
Prophylactic antifungal therapy
should be initiated in patients with a
history of fungal infection with prior
steroid administration (see
Candidiasis/Candidosis).

**Systemic Steroids and
Immunosuppressants
for Severe Cases**

Rx
Dexamethasone (Decadron) elixir
0.5 mg/5 ml
Disp: 320 ml
Sig:
1. For 3 days, rinse with
1 tablespoonful (15 ml) 4 times a
day and swallow. Then
2. For 3 days rinse with 1 teaspoonful
(5 ml) 4 times a day and swallow.
Then
3. For 3 days, rinse with 1 teaspoonful

(5 ml) 4 times a day and swallow
every other time. Then
4. Rinse with 1 teaspoonful (5 ml)
4 times a day and expectorate.
Rx
Prednisone tablets 10 mg
Disp: 26 tablets
Sig: Take 4 tablets in the morning for
5 days, then decrease by 1 tablet on
each successive day.
Rx
Prednisone tablets 5 mg
Disp: 40 tablets
Sig: Take 5 tablets in the morning for
5 days, then 5 tablets in the morning
every other day until gone.

If oral discomfort recurs, the
patient should return to the clinician
for reevaluation.

Many studies suggest that oral
lichen planus has an intrinsic
property predisposing to malignant
transformation. However, the
etiology is complex, with interaction
among genetic, infectious agents,
environmental, and lifestyle factors.
Prospective studies have
demonstrated that lichen planus
patients have a slightly increased risk
to develop oral squamous cell
carcinoma. All patients exhibiting
lichen planus intraorally, particularly
those who have had the ulcerative
form, should receive periodic
follow up.

Therapy with medications such
as systemic steroids,
immunosuppressants, and
immunomodulators is presented to
inform the clinician that such
modalities have been reported
effective for patients suffering from
ulcerative lichen planus. Medications
such as azathioprine, mycophenolate
mofetil, tacrolimus
hydroxychloroquine sulfate, acitretin,
and cyclosporin A are used to treat
patients with severe persistent

ulcerative lichen planus, but should not be routinely used because of the potential for side effects. Close collaboration with the patient's physician is recommended when these medications are prescribed.

Pemphigus and Mucous Membrane Pemphigoid

Pemphigus and mucous membrane pemphigoid are relatively uncommon lesions. They should be suspected when chronic, multiple oral ulcerations and a history of oral and skin blisters exist. Often they may occur only in the mouth. Diagnosis is based on history and on histologic and immunofluorescent characteristics of a biopsy specimen of the primary lesion.

Etiology:

Both are autoimmune diseases with autoantibodies against antigens appearing in different portions of the epithelium (mucosa). In pemphigus the antigens are within the epithelium (desmosomes), whereas in pemphigoid the antigens are located at the base of the epithelium in the hemidesmosomes.

Clinical description:

In pemphigus the lesion may stay in one location for a long period of time with small placid bullae. The bullae may rupture, leaving an ulcer. Approximately 80%–90% of patients have oral lesions. The oral manifestations are the first signs of the disease in approximately two-thirds of patients. All parts of the mouth may be involved. The bullae rupture almost immediately in the mouth but may stay intact for some time on the skin. One of the classic signs, the Nikolsky's sign (blister formation induced with gentle rubbing of an affected mucosal site), is positive in pemphigus but is not pathognomonic because it also has

been found positive in other disorders. Because the vesicles or bullae are intraepithelial, they often are filled with clear fluid. Histologically, a cleavage (Tzanck cells, acantholytic cells) exists within the spinous layer of the epithelium.

In pemphigoid the cleavage or split is beneath the epithelium, resulting in bullae that usually are blood filled. Mucous membrane pemphigoid often is limited to the oral cavity, but some patients have ocular lesions (symblepharon, ankyloblepharon) that must be evaluated by an ophthalmologist. Gingiva is the most common oral site involved. Pemphigoid may appear clinically as a red, nonulcerated gingival lesion.

Rationale for treatment:

Because both pemphigus and pemphigoid are autoimmune disorders, the primary treatment is topical or systemic steroids or other immunomodulating drugs. Custom trays can be used to localize topical steroid medications on the gingival tissues (occlusive therapy). Because they can resemble other ulcerative bullous diseases, a biopsy is necessary for a definitive diagnosis. Specimens should be submitted for light microscopic, immunofluorescent, and immunologic testing. Because of the potential serious nature, referral to a specialist in oral medicine, dermatology, and ophthalmology must be considered. When eye lesions are present, an ophthalmologist must be consulted immediately to prevent blindness.

Therapy with medications such as systemic steroids, immunosuppressants, and immunomodulators are presented to inform the clinician that such modalities have been reported effective for patients suffering from vesiculobullous disorders such as pemphigus vulgaris and mucous membrane pemphigoid. Therapies such as dapsone, methotrexate, mycophenolate mofetil, cyclosporine A, niacinamide with tetracycline, and plasmapheresis are used to treat patients with vesiculobullous disorders such as pemphigus vulgaris and mucous membrane pemphigoid but should not be routinely used because of the potential for serious adverse effects. Close collaboration with the patient's physician is recommended when these medications are prescribed.

Injectable Steroids

Dexamethasone phosphate injectable, 1 ampule (4 mg/ml), can be used in the following manner. After anesthetizing the area with lidocaine, inject 0.5 to 1 ml around margins of ulcer with a 25-gauge needle twice a wk until ulcer heals. Therapy with systemic or injectable steroids should be coordinated with the patient's physician because of side effects and potential systemic complications.

ORAL ERYTHEMA MULTIFORME

Etiology:
Oral erythema multiforme is believed to be an autoimmune condition. It can occur at any age. Drug reactions to medications such as penicillin and sulfonamides may play a role in some cases. In a few patients who developed oral erythema multiforme, a herpetic infection occurred immediately before the onset of clinical signs.
Clinical description:
Signs of oral erythema multiforme include "blood-crusted" lips, "targetoid" or "bull's-eye" skin lesions, and a nonspecific mucosal slough.

The name multiforme is used because its appearance may take multiple different forms.

A severe form of erythema multiforme is called Stevens-Johnson syndrome, or erythema multiforme major. Erythema multiforme as a skin disease occurs most frequently because of an allergic reaction.
Rationale for treatment:
Treatment is primarily antiinflammatory in nature. Steroids are initiated then tapered. Because of the possible relationship of oral erythema multiforme with herpes simplex virus, suppressive antiviral therapy may be necessary before initiation of steroid therapy. Patients should be questioned carefully about a previous history of recurrent herpetic infections and prodromal symptoms that might have preceded the onset of erythema multiforme.

Dosing must be titrated to specific situations.

Steroid Therapy

Rx
Prednisone tablets 10 mg
Disp: 100 tablets
Sig: Take 6 tablets in the morning until lesions recede, then decrease by 1 tablet on each successive day.

Suppressive Antiviral Therapy

Renew as needed to the following:
Rx
Acyclovir (Zovirax) capsules 400 mg
Disp: 90 capsules
Sig: Take 1 tablet 3 times a day.
Rx
Valacyclovir (Valtrex) capsules 500 mg
Disp: 30 capsules
Sig: Take 1 tablet a day.

DENTURE SORE MOUTH

Etiology:
Discomfort under oral prosthetic appliances may result from

combinations of candidal infections, poor denture hygiene, an occlusive syndrome, overextension, or excessive movement of the appliance. This condition may be erroneously attributed to an allergy to denture material, which is a rare occurrence. The retention and fit of the denture should be idealized, and mechanical irritation should be ruled out.

Clinical description:

The tissue covered by the appliance, especially one made of acrylic, is erythematous and smooth or granular, and it may be asymptomatic or associated with burning.

Rationale for treatment:

Therapy is directed toward controlling all possible etiologies and improving oral comfort. If therapy is ineffective, consider underlying systemic conditions such as diabetes mellitus and poor nutrition.

Treatment:

1. Institute appropriate antifungal medication (see Candidiasis/ Candidosis).
2. Improve oral and appliance hygiene. The patient may have to leave the appliance out for extended periods of time and should be instructed to leave the denture out overnight. The appliance should be soaked in a commercially available denture cleanser or soaked in a 1% sodium hypochlorite solution (1 teaspoon of sodium hypochlorite in a denture cup of water) for 15 min and thoroughly rinsed for at least 2 min under running water.
3. Reline, rebase, or construct a new appliance.
4. Apply an artificial saliva or oral lubricant gel, such as Laclede Oral Balance or Sage gel, to the tissue contact surface of the denture to reduce frictional trauma.

If all the above actions fail to control symptoms, a biopsy or short trial of topical steroid therapy can be used to rule out contact mucositis (an allergic reaction to denture materials). If a therapeutic trial fails to resolve the condition, a biopsy should be performed to establish the diagnosis.

BURNING MOUTH SYNDROME

Etiology:

Multiple conditions have been implicated in the causation of burning mouth syndrome. Current literature suggests neurogenic, vascular, and psychogenic etiologies. However, other conditions, such as xerostomia, candidiasis, referred pain from the tongue musculature, chronic infections, reflux of gastric acid, medications, blood dyscrasias, nutritional deficiencies, hormonal imbalances, and allergic and inflammatory disorders, must also be considered.

Clinical description:

Burning mouth syndrome is characterized by the absence of clinical signs.

Rationale for treatment:

To reduce discomfort by addressing possible etiologic factors.

Treatment:

On the basis of the history, physical evaluation, and specific laboratory studies, rule out all possible organic etiologies. Minimal blood studies should include CBC and differential, fasting glucose, iron, ferritin, folic acid, and B_{12} levels, and thyroid profile (TSH, T3, T4).

Rx

Diphenhydramine (Children's Benadryl) elixir 12.5 mg/5 ml (OTC)

Disp: 1 bottle

Sig: Rinse with 1 teaspoon for 2 min before each meal and swallow.

Children's Benadryl is alcohol free.

When the burning mouth is considered psychogenic or idiopathic, a tricyclic antidepressant or benzodiazepine in low doses exhibits the properties of analgesia and sedation and frequently is successful in reducing or eliminating the symptoms after several wk or mo. The dosage is adjusted according to patient reaction and clinical symptomatology, and the potential for serious adverse effects (e.g., anticholinergic) should be considered.

Rx

Clonazepam (Klonopin) tablets 0.5 mg

Disp: 100 tablets

Sig: Take 1 tablet 3 times a day, then adjust dose after 3-day intervals.

This therapy probably is best managed by an appropriate specialist or the patient's physician at this time.

Rx

Amitriptyline (Elavil) tablets 25 mg

Disp: 50 tablets

Sig: Take 1 tablet at bedtime for 1 wk, then 2 tablets HS. Increase to 3 tablets HS after 2 wk and maintain at that dosage or titrate as appropriate.

Rx

Chlordiazepoxide (Librium) tablets 5 mg

Disp: 50 tablets

Sig: Take 1 or 2 tablets 3 times a day.

Rx

Alprazolam (Xanax) tablets 0.25 mg

Disp: 50 tablets

Sig: Take 1 tablet 3 times a day.

Rx

Diazepam (Valium) tablets 2 mg

Disp: 50 tablets

Sig: Take 1 or 2 tablets.

The dosage should be adjusted according to the patient's response.

Anticipated side effects are dry mouth and morning drowsiness. The rationale for use of tricyclic antidepressants and other psychotropic drugs should be thoroughly explained to the patient, and the patient's physician should be made aware of the therapy. Those medications have a potential for addiction and dependence.

Rx

Capsaicin (Zostrix) cream 0.025% (OTC)

Disp: 1 tube

Sig: Apply sparingly to affected site(s) 4 times a day.

Wash hands after each application and do not use near the eyes.

Topical capsaicin may improve the burning sensation in some individuals. As with topical capsaicin, an increase in discomfort for a 2- to 3-wk period should be anticipated.

CHAPPED OR CRACKED LIPS

Etiology:

Alternate wetting and drying, resulting in inflammation and possible secondary infection.

Clinical description:

The surface of the vermilion is rough and peeling and may be ulcerated with crusting. The normal vertical fissuring may be lost.

Rationale for treatment:

An interrupted and chronically inflamed surface invites secondary infection. An antiinflammatory agent in a petrolatum or adhesive base will interrupt the irritating factors and allow healing.

Rx

Betamethasone valerate (Valisone) ointment 0.1%

Disp: 15-g tube

Sig: Apply to lips after each meal and at bedtime.

Prolonged use of corticosteroids can result in thinning of the tissue. Their use should be closely monitored.

For maintenance, the frequent application of lip care products (e.g., Blistex, Chapstick, Vaseline, or cocoa butter) should be suggested.

If the lesions do not resolve with treatment, consider biopsy to rule out dysplasia or malignancy.

GINGIVAL ENLARGEMENT
Etiology:
Phenytoin sodium (Dilantin), calcium channel-blocking agents (nifedipine and others), and cyclosporine therapy are drugs known to predispose some patients to gingival enlargement. Blood dyscrasias and hereditary fibromatosis should be ruled out by history and indicated laboratory tests.
Clinical description:
The gingival tissues, especially in the anterior region, are dense, resilient, insensitive, and enlarged but essentially of normal color.
Rationale for treatment:
Local factors, such as plaque and calculus accumulation, contribute to secondary inflammation and the hyperplastic process. This further interferes with plaque control. Specific drugs tend to deplete serum folic acid levels, which result in compromised tissue integrity. Folic acid and drug serum levels should be determined every 6 mo. This should be coordinated with the patient's physician.
Treatment:
Consists of (1) meticulous plaque control, (2) gingivectomy when indicated, and (3) folic acid oral rinse.

Rx
Folic acid oral rinse 1 mg/ml
Disp: 16 oz
Sig: Rinse with 1 teaspoonful for 2 min twice a day and spit out.
Rx
Chlorhexidine gluconate (Peridex) 0.12%
Disp: 16 oz
Sig: Rinse with $1/_2$ oz twice a day for 30 sec and spit out.

TASTE DISORDERS
Etiology:
Taste acuity may be affected by neurologic and physiologic changes and by drugs. Diagnostic procedures should first rule out a neurologic deficiency, olfactory deficit, and systemic influences such as malnutrition, metabolic disturbances, drugs, chemical and physical trauma, and radiation sequelae. Blood tests for trace elements should be conducted to identify any deficiencies.
Rationale for treatment:
A reduction in salivary flow may concentrate the electrolytes in the saliva, resulting in a salty or metallic taste (see treatment for xerostomia). A deficiency of zinc has been associated with a loss of taste (and smell) sensation.
For Zinc Replacement (in Patients with Proven Zinc Deficiency)
Rx
Orazinc capsules 220 mg (OTC)
Disp: 100 capsules
Sig: Take 1 capsule with milk 3 times a day for at least 1 mo.
Rx
Z-Bec tablets (OTC)
Disp: 60 tablets
Sig: Take 1 tablet a day with food or after meals.

MANAGEMENT OF PATIENTS RECEIVING ANTINEOPLASTIC AGENTS AND RADIATION THERAPY

Etiology:

Cancer chemotherapy and radiation to the head and neck tend to reduce the volume and alter the character of the saliva. The balance of the oral flora is disrupted, allowing overgrowth of opportunistic organisms (e.g., *C. albicans*). Anticancer therapy damages fast-growing tissues, especially the oral mucosa.

Clinical description:

The oral mucosa becomes red and inflamed. The saliva is viscous or absent.

Rationale for treatment:

The treatment of these patients is symptomatic and supportive. Patient education, frequent monitoring, and close cooperation with the patient's physician are important. The oral discomfort may be relieved with topical anesthetics, such as diphenhydramine elixir (Benadryl) and dyclonine (Dyclone). Artificial salivas (i.e., Sage Moist Plus, Moi-Stir, Salivart, Xero-Lube) will reduce oral dryness. Mouth moisturizing gels (i.e., Sage Mouth Moisturizer or Oral Balance gel) may be helpful. Nystatin and clotrimazole preparations will control fungal overgrowth. Chlorhexidine rinses help control plaque and candidiasis. Fluorides are applied for caries control. The patient information sheet that follows this topic can be reproduced and given to the patient.

Mouth Rinses

Rx

Alkaline saline (salt/bicarbonate) mouth rinse. (Mix $1/_2$ teaspoonful each of salt and baking soda in a glass of water.)

Sig: Rinse with copious amounts 4 times a day.

Commercially available as Sage Salt and Soda Rinse.

Gingivitis Control

Rx

Chlorhexidine gluconate mouthwash (Peridex) 0.12%

Disp: 32 oz

Sig: Rinse with $1/_2$ oz twice a day for 30 sec and spit out. Avoid rinsing or eating for 30 min following treatment. (Rinse after breakfast and at bedtime.)

In xerostomic patients, chlorhexidine (Peridex) should be used concurrently with artificial saliva to provide the needed protein-binding agent for efficacy and substantivity.

Caries Control

(See Xerostomia)

Rx

Neutral NaF gel (Thera-Flur-N) 1.0%

Disp: 24 ml

Sig: Place 1 drop per tooth in the custom tray; apply for 5 min daily. Avoid rinsing or eating for 30 min after treatment.

Topical Anesthetics

Rx

Diphenhydramine (Benadryl) elixir 12.5 mg/5 ml, 4 oz, mixed with Kaopectate (OTC) 4 oz (to make a 50% mixture by volume).

Disp: 8 oz

Sig: Rinse with 1 teaspoonful every 2 hr and spit out.

Maalox (OTC) can be used in place of Kaopectate. Dyclonine (Dyclone) HCl 0.5% 1 oz can be added to the above for greater anesthetic efficacy.

Rx

Diphenhydramine (Benadryl) elixir 12.5 mg/5 ml. (Note: Elixir is Rx and syrup [Benylin] is OTC.)

Disp: 4-oz bottle

Sig: Rinse with 1 teaspoonful for 2 min before each meal and spit out.
Rx
Clotrimazole (Mycelex) troches 10 mg
Disp: 70 troches
Sig: Let 1 troche dissolve in the mouth 5 times a day.
Rx
Nystatin pastilles 200,000 units
Disp: 50 pastilles
Sig: Let 1 pastille dissolve in the mouth 5 times a day.
(See Candidiasis for additional antifungal therapy.)

KEY POINTS TO REMEMBER

• When topical anesthetics are used, patients should be warned about a reduced gag reflex and the need for caution while eating and drinking to avoid possible airway compromise. Allergies are rare but may occur.
• In immunocompromised patients, herpes virus lesions can occur on any mucosal surface and may have atypical appearances. They can resemble major aphthae and allergic responses.
• Mixing ointments with equal parts of Orabase promotes adhesion.
• Therapy with systemic steroids and immunosuppressants is presented to inform the clinician that such modalities are available. Because of the potential for side effects, close collaboration with the patient's physician is recommended when these medications are prescribed.
• Although some consultants disagree with the use of vaginal creams intraorally, the efficacy of the creams has been observed clinically in selected cases in which other topical antifungal agents have failed.
• Generic carboxymethyl cellulose solutions may be prepared by a pharmacist.
• The rationale for use of tricyclic antidepressants and other psychotropic drugs should be thoroughly explained to patients, and their physician also should be made aware of the therapy. These medications have a potential for addiction and dependency. These anticholinergics should be prescribed in consultation with a physician because of significant adverse effects.
• When testing for serum folate level, it is judicious to also check for the vitamin B_{12} level because a B_{12} deficiency can be masked by the patient's use of folic acid supplement. The phenytoin level also should be assessed for future reference.

Patient Information Sheet

The oral regimen for patients receiving chemotherapy and radiotherapy is outlined earlier in this chapter. The following are general guidelines to be individualized by your doctor. Follow your doctor's advice or discuss any questions with your doctor if these guidelines differ from what you have been told or have heard.

A. Rinses

1. Rinse with warm, dilute solution of sodium bicarbonate (baking soda) or salt and bicarbonate every 2 hr to bathe the tissues and control oral acidity. Take 2 teaspoonfuls of bicarbonate (or 1 teaspoonful of table salt plus 1 teaspoonful of bicarbonate) per quart of water.

Continued

Patient Information Sheet—cont'd

2. If you are experiencing pain, rinse with 1 teaspoonful of elixir of Benadryl before each meal. Be careful when eating while your mouth is numb to avoid choking.
3. If your mouth is dry, sip cool water frequently (every 10 min) all day long. Allowing ice chips to melt in the mouth is comforting. Artificial salivas (e.g., Moi-Stir, Salivart, Xero-Lube, Orex) can be used as frequently as needed to make the mouth moist and "slick." Keep the lips lubricated with petrolatum or a lanolin-containing lip preparation. Commercial mouth rinses containing alcohol or coffee, tea, and colas should be avoided because they tend to dry the mouth.
4. If an oral yeast infection develops, antifungal medications can be prescribed.
   a. Nystatin pastille,* let one dissolve in mouth 5 times a day, or
   b. Let a 10-mg clotrimazole (Mycelex)* troche dissolve in the mouth 5 times a day.

B. Care of teeth and gums
1. Floss your teeth after each meal. Be careful not to cut the gums.
2. Brush your teeth after each meal. Use a soft even-bristle brush and a bland toothpaste containing fluoride (e.g., Aim, Crest, Colgate). Brushing with a sodium bicarbonate–water paste is also helpful. Arm & Hammer Dental Care toothpaste and tooth powder are bicarbonate based. If a toothbrush is too irritating, cotton-tip swabs (Q-Tips) or foam sticks (Toothettes) can provide some mechanical cleaning.
3. A pulsating water device (e.g., Water-Pik) will remove loose debris. Use warm water with a half teaspoonful of salt and baking soda and low pressure to prevent damage to tissue.
4. Have custom, flexible trays made by your dentist to self-apply fluoride gel to the teeth for 5 min once a day after brushing.
5. Rinse with an antiplaque solution (Peridex) (if prescribed by your dentist) 2 or 3 times a day when you cannot follow other oral hygiene procedures.
6. Follow any alternative oral hygiene instructions prescribed by your dentist.

C. Nutrition
Adequate nutrition and fluid intake are very important for oral and general health. Use diet supplements (e.g., Carnation Instant Breakfast, Meritene, Ensure). If your mouth is sore, a blender can be used to soften food.

D. Maintenance
Have your oral health status reevaluated at regularly scheduled intervals by your dentist.

E. Supportive
A humidifier in the sleeping area will alleviate or reduce nighttime oral dryness.

*Drugs that must be prescribed by your dentist or physician.
The above regimen is also applicable to patients with AIDS.

Suggested Readings

1. Boger J, Araujo O, Flowers F: Sunscreens: efficacy, use and misuse, South Med J 77:1421–1427, 1984.
2. Brooke RI, Sapp JP: Herpetiform ulceration, Oral Surg Oral Med Oral Pathol 42:182–188, 1976.
3. Brown RS, Bottomley WK: Combination immunosuppressant and topical steroid therapy for treatment of recurrent major aphthae, Oral Surg Oral Med Oral Pathol 69:42–44, 1990.
4. Browning S, et al: The association between burning mouth syndrome and psychosocial disorders, Oral Surg Oral Med Oral Pathol 64:171–174, 1987.
5. Burns RA, Davis WJ: Recurrent aphthous stomatitis, Am Fam Physician 32:99–104, 1988.
6. Bystryn JC: Adjuvant therapy of pemphigus, Arch Dermatol 120:941–951, 1984.
7. Dilley D, Blozis G: Common oral lesions and oral manifestations of systemic illnesses and therapies, Pediatr Clin North Am 29:585–611, 1982.
8. Drew H, et al: Effect of folate on phenytoin hyperplasia, J Clin Periodontol 14:350–356, 1987.
9. Duxbury AJ, et al: Clinical trial of a mucin-containing artificial saliva, IRCS Med Sci 13:1197–1198, 1985.
10. Fardal O, Turnbull RS: A review of the literature on use of chlorhexidine in dentistry, J Am Dent Assoc 112:863–869, 1986.
11. Feinmann C: Pain relief by antidepressants: possible modes of action, Pain 23:1–8, 1985.
12. Fenske NA, Greenberg SS: Solar-induced skin changes, Am Fam Physician 25:109–117, 1982.
13. Fharav V, et al: The analgesic effect of amitriptyline on chronic facial pain, Pain 31:199–207, 1987.
14. Fox PC, et al: Systemic therapy of salivary gland hypofunction, J Dent Res 66:689–692, 1987 (special issue).
15. Gabriel SA, et al: Lichen planus: possible mechanisms of pathogenesis, J Oral Med 40:56–59, 1985.
16. Gorsku M, Silverman S, Chinn H: Clinical characteristics and management outcome in the burning mouth syndrome, Oral Surg Oral Med Oral Pathol 72:192–195, 1991.
17. Gorsline J, Bradlow HL, Sherman MR: Triamcinolone acetonide 21-oic acid methyl ester: a potent local anti-inflammatory steroid without detectable systemic effects, Endocrinology 116:263–273, 1985.
18. Greenberg MS: Oral herpes simplex infections in immunosuppressed patients, Compendium 9(suppl):289–291, 1988.
19. Grushka M: Clinical features of burning mouth syndrome, Oral Surg Oral Med Oral Pathol 63:30–36, 1987.
20. Hay KD, Reade PC: The use of an elimination diet in the treatment of recurrent aphthous ulceration of the oral cavity, Oral Surg Oral Med Oral Pathol 57:504–507, 1984.
21. Holst E: Natamycin and nystatin for treatment of oral candidiasis during and after radiotherapy, J Prosthet Dent 51:226–231, 1984.
22. Huff JC, et al: Therapy of herpes zoster with oral acyclovir, Am J Med 85:85–89, 1988.
23. Hughes WT, et al: Ketoconazole and candidiasis: a controlled study, J Infect Dis 147:1060–1063, 1983.
24. Katz S: The use of fluoride and chlorhexidine for the prevention of radiation caries, J Am Dent Assoc 104:164–169, 1982.
25. Lamey PJ, et al: Vitamin status of patients with burning mouth syndrome and the response to replacement therapy, Br Dent J 160:81–84, 1986.
26. Lang NP, Brecx MC: Chlorhexidine digluconate—an agent for chemical plaque control and prevention of gingival inflammation, J Periodont Res 43(suppl):74–89, 1986.
27. Lever WF, Schaumburg-Lever G: Treatment of pemphigus vulgaris: results obtained in 84 patients between 1961 and 1982, Arch Dermatol 120:44–47, 1984.
28. Lozada F, Silverman S Jr, Migliorati C: Adverse side effects associated with prednisone in the treatment of patients with oral inflammatory ulcerative

diseases, J Am Dent Assoc 109:
269–270, 1984.

29. Lucatorto FM, et al: Treatment of
refractory oral candidiasis with
fluconazole: A case report, Oral Surg
Oral Med Oral Pathol 71:42–44, 1991.

30. Lundeen RC, Langlais RP, Terezhalmy
GT: Sunscreen protection for lip
mucosa: a review and update, J Am
Dent Assoc 111:617–621, 1985.

31. O'Neil T, Figures K: The effects of
chlorhexidine and mechanical
methods of plaque control on the
recurrence of gingival hyperplasia in
young patients taking phenytoin, Br
Dent J 152:130–133, 1982.

32. Owens NJ, et al: Prophylaxis of oral
candidiasis with clotrimazole troches,
Arch Intern Med 144:290–293, 1984.

33. Poland JM: The spectrum of HSV-1
infections in nonimmunosuppressed
patients, Compendium 9(suppl):310–
312, 1988.

34. Porter SR, Sculy C, Flint S:
Hematologic status in recurrent
aphthous stomatitis compared with
other oral disease, Oral Surg Oral
Med Oral Pathol 66:41–44, 1988.

35. Raborn GW, et al: Oral acyclovir and
herpes labialis: a randomized, double-
blind, placebo-controlled study, J Am
Dent Assoc 11:38–42, 1987.

36. Rhodus NL, et al: Candia albicans
levels in patients with Sjögren's
syndrome before and after long-term
use of pilocarpine hydrochloride,
Quintessence Int 29:705–710, 1998.

37. Rhodus, NL, Schuh, MJ: The effects
of pilocarpine on salivary flow in
patients with Sjögren's syndrome,
Oral Surg Oral Med Oral Pathol
72:545–549.36, 1991

38. Rowe NJ: Diagnosis and treatment of
herpes simplex virus disease,
Compendium 9(suppl):292–295, 1988.

39. Schiffman SS: Taste and smell in
disease (pts a and b), N Engl
J Med 308:1275–1279, 1337–1343,
1983.

40. Scully C, Mason DK: Therapeutic
measures in oral medicine. In Jones JH,
Mason DK, editors: Oral
manifestations of systemic disease,
London, 1980, WB Saunders.

41. Silverman S, et al: A prospective of
findings and management in 214
patients with oral lichen planus, Oral
Surg Oral Med Oral Pathol 72:
665–670, 1991.

42. Silverman S Jr, et al: Oral mucous
membrane pemphigoid, Oral Surg
Oral Med Oral Pathol 61:233–237,
1986.

43. Sonis ST, Sonis AL, Lieberman A:
Oral complications in patients
receiving treatment for malignancies
other than of the head and neck,
JAMA 97:468–471, 1978.

44. Straus SE, moderator: Herpes simplex
virus infection: biology, treatment,
and prevention, Ann Intern Med
103:404–419, 1985.

45. Thompson PJ, et al: Assessment of
oral candidiasis in patients with
respiratory disease and efficacy of a
new nystatin formulation, Br Med J
292:699–700, 1986.

46. Vincent SD, et al: Oral lichen
planus: the clinical, historical and
therapeutic features of 100 cases,
Oral Surg Oral Med Oral Pathol
70:165–171, 1990.

47. Wood MJ, et al: Efficacy of
oral acyclovir treatment of acute
herpes zoster, Am J Med 85:
79–83, 1988.

48. Wright WE, et al: An oral disease
prevention program for patients
receiving radiation and chemotherapy,
J Am Dent Assoc 110:43–47, 1985.

Medically Compromised Patients

ENDOCARDITIS AND ENDARTERITIS PREVENTION

In 2007, the American Heart Association (AHA) updated its recommendations for antibiotic prophylaxis prior to dental procedures to prevent infective endocarditis (Wilson W. et al., Prevention of Infective Endocarditis. Guidelines from the American Heart Association. *Circulation* April, 2007). These guidelines recommend antibiotic prophylaxis only in patients with cardiac conditions that are associated with the highest risk of adverse outcomes from infective endocarditis, including (1) patients with a **prosthetic heart valve,** (2) patients who have **previously had infective endocarditits,** (3) patients with **congenital heart disease** (unrepaired cyanotic heart disease; completely repaired congenital heart defects with prosthetic material or device, whether placed by surgery or catheter intervention, during the first 6 mo after the procedure; or repaired congenital heart disease with residual defects at the site or adjacent to the site of a prosthetic patch or prosthetic device), and (4) **cardiac transplant recipients** who develop cardiac **valvulopathy.** The list of dental procedures for which prophylaxis is recommended has been expanded and now includes *all dental procedures* that involve manipulation of gingival tissue or the periapical region of teeth or perforation of the oral mucosa (except for routine anesthetic injections through noninfected tissue, taking dental radiographs, placement of removable prosthodontic or orthodontic appliances, adjustment of orthodontic appliances, placement of orthdontic brackets, shedding of deciduous teeth, and bleeding from trauma to the lips or oral mucosa).

The antibiotic regimens recommended for prophylaxis in patients at risk of adverse outcomes of infective endocarditis are to be administered as a *single dose* and *30 min to 1 hr before the dental procedure*:

Oral: Amoxicillin 2 g (children 50 mg/kg)

Patients unable to take/absorb oral medications:

- Ampicillin 2 g IM or IV (children 50 mg/kg IM or IV)

OR

- Cefazolin or Ceftriaxone 1 g IM or IV (children 50 mg/kg IM or IV)

Patients allergic to penicillins or ampicillin—oral:

- Cephalexin 2 g (children 50 mg/kg) or
- Clindamycin 600 mg orally (children 20 mg/kg)

OR

- Azithromycin or clarithromycin 500 mg (children 15 mg/kg)
- Patients allergic to penicillins or ampicillin and unable to take/absorb oral medications:-Cefazolin or Ceftriaxone 1 g IM or IV (children 50 mg/kg IM or IV)

OR

- Clindamycin 600 mg IM or IV (children 20 mg/kg IM or IV).

If the antibiotic was *inadvertently* not administered prior to the procedure, the antibiotic dosage should be administered within 2 hr after the procedure. Practitioners should be cautious of coincidental infective endocarditis in patients at risk who present with a fever or other signs and symptoms of a systemic infection. Patients should also be monitored following the dental procedure for such signs and symptoms, which may be the initial indicators of infective endocarditis. In patients receiving anticoagulant therapy, intramuscular (IM) injections should be avoided and preference given to the oral route of adminstration if possible.

NONVALVULAR CARDIOVASCULAR DEVICE-RELATED INFECTIONS

In 2003, the AHA published guidelines regarding the use of antibiotic prophylaxis for patients with nonvalvular cardiovascular devices undergoing dental, respiratory, GI, or GU procedures. The devices considered included pacemakers, defibrillators, total artificial hearts, ventriculoatrial shunts, patent ductus arteriosus occlusion devices (plugs, umbrellas, buttons, discs, embolization coils), atrial septal defect and ventricular septal defect closure devices (Bard clamshell occluders, discs, buttons, double umbrellas), conduits, patches, peripheral vascular stents, vascular grafts (including hemodialysis), coronary artery stents, and vena caval filters.

Antibiotic prophylaxis is not routinely recommended after device placement for patients undergoing these dental procedures. It is recommended, however, for dental patients having such devices prior to incision and drainage of oral abscesses. Antibiotic prophylaxis is also recommended for patients with residual leak after device placement for attempted closure of the leak associated with patent ductus arteriosus, atrial septal defect, or ventricular septal defect. In these patients, prophylaxis is indicated for the dental procedures listed in the endocarditis section, and the same antibiotic regimens listed in that section can be used.

Other Surgically-Implanted Prosthetic Devices

At this time, there are no guidelines formally promulagated by any professional organizations for antibiotic prophylaxis prior to dental procedures in patients with noncardiac, nonorthopedic implanted devices, such as breast implants. The dental practitioner should consult the patient's physician in cases involving such devices in whom implant infection may be a concern as a result of dental procedures and, with the informed consent of the patient, make a decision regarding the use of antibiotic prophylaxis.

ORTHOPEDIC DEVICES: SCREWS, PLATES, PINS, AND PROSTHETIC JOINTS

In 1997 and 2002, the American Dental Association (ADA) and the American Academy of Orthopedic Surgeons (AAOS) jointly published an advisory on antibiotic prophylaxis for dental patients with total joint replacements. Antibiotic prophylaxis was not indicated for patients with plates or pins. Antibiotic prophylaxis was not suggested for most patients with total joint replacements. However, they do suggest that prophylaxis **be considered** for patients who may be at "high risk" for hematogenous infection, including patients with inflammatory arthropathies, immunosuppression, type 1 diabetes mellitus, joint replacement within 2 years, previous prosthetic joint infection (PJI), malnourishment, or hemophilia. (Of note, there is no evidence that even these "higher-risk" patients are at increased risk from dentally induced bacteremias. In fact, the microbiology of PJI in these "higher-risk" patients is the same as for other patients with PJI. A more appropriate interpretation is that these patients are at increased risk for PJI from the usual sources, such as wound contamination and acute infection from distant sites.)

The advisory statement also makes clear that the final decision as to whether to provide antibiotic prophylaxis lies with the dentist, who must weigh perceived potential benefits against the risks. The advisory statement provides suggested antibiotic regimens should the practitioner elect to provide antibiotic prophylaxis. If prophylaxis is selected, it should be used only for the dental procedures listed in the Endocarditis section.

Nonallergic (penicillin) patients:
Amoxicillin 2 g orally, 1 hr before dental procedure
Cephalexin 2 g orally, 1 hr before dental procedure

Patients allergic to penicillin:
Clindamycin 600 mg orally,
   1 hr before dental procedure
* Note that macrolide antibiotics (azithromycin clarithromycin) are not included in the ADA/AAOS guidelines

ADRENAL INSUFFICIENCY (PRIMARY AND SECONDARY): PREVENTION OF ADRENAL CRISIS

Patients with primary (Addison's disease) or secondary (exogenous corticosteroid induced) adrenal insufficiency may be at risk for adrenal crisis during or following surgical procedures performed in dentistry. Adrenal crisis is a medical emergency that requires prompt intervention to save the patient's life. In order to prevent adrenal crisis, supplemental steroids in rather large doses have been recommended since the mid 1950s for patients with adrenal insufficiency. Adrenal crisis is a rare event in dentistry, especially in patients with secondary adrenal insufficiency. Four factors appear to be associated with the risk for adrenal crisis: (1) magnitude of surgery, (2) general anesthesia,

(3) health status and stability of the patient, and (4) degree of pain control.

The most significant acute adverse outcome of adrenal insufficiency is adrenal crisis. This event can occur when a patient with adrenal insufficiency, most commonly Addison's disease, is challenged by stress (e.g., illness, infection, or surgery) and in response is unable to synthesize adequate amounts of cortisol and aldosterone. This potentially life-threatening emergency usually evolves slowly over a few hr and then is manifested by severe exacerbation of the condition, including profuse sweating, hypotension, weak pulse, cyanosis, nausea, vomiting, weakness, headache, dehydration, fever, sunken eyes, dyspnea, myalgias, arthralgia, hyponatremia, and eosinophilia. If not treated rapidly, the patient may develop hypothermia, severe hypotension, hypoglycemia, confusion, and circulatory collapse that can culminate in death.

Four factors appear to contribute to the risk of "adrenal crisis" during the perioperative period of oral surgery: (1) magnitude of surgery, (2) general anesthesia, (3) overall health of the patient (e.g., stable vs. ongoing infection), and (4) degree of pain control.

Negligible Risk: Nonsurgical Dental Procedures

The vast majority of patients with adrenal insufficiency can undergo routine, nonsurgical dental treatment *without* the need for supplemental glucocorticoids. This is supported by the fact that routine, nonsurgical dental procedures do not stimulate cortisol production at levels comparable to oral surgery, and local anesthesia blocks neural stress pathways required for adrenocorticotropic hormone

(ACTH) secretion. This guideline does not advocate dental treatment on patients whose adrenal insufficiency is uncontrolled or undiagnosed. However, stable patients with adrenal insufficiency and those with a history of steroid use in whom glucocorticoid medication was discontinued prior to surgery have withstood general surgical procedures without developing adrenal crisis.

Low-Risk Regimen

For minor oral and periodontal surgery (e.g., few simple extractions, soft tissue surgery), evidence suggests that adrenal insufficiency is prevented when **circulating levels of glucocorticoids are approximately 25 mg hydrocortisone equivalent per day.** This is equivalent to a dose of **approximately 5 mg prednisone.** The clinician should confirm that the patient has taken the recommended amount of steroid within 2 hr of the surgical procedure and schedule the surgery in the morning when normal cortisol levels are highest. Stress reduction measures should be implemented. Benefits can be gained from use of (1) oral, inhalation, or intravenous sedation, which provides stress reduction; (2) intravenous fluids (i.e., 5% dextrose), which can prevent hypovolemia and hypoglycemia; (3) long-acting local anesthetics; and (4) adequate postoperative analgesics.

Moderate-Risk to Major-Risk Regimen

Patients with adrenocortical suppression undergoing major oral surgery are at increased risk for adrenal crisis when compared with minor surgery. Major surgical procedures are more stressful than minor surgical procedures. They increase the demand for cortisol because of postoperative pain. Blood loss is

greater, thus increasing the risk for hypovolemia and hypotension.

For major oral surgical stress (multiple extractions, quadrant periodontal surgery, extraction of bony impactions, osseous surgery, osteotomy, bone resections, cancer surgery), surgical procedures involving use of general anesthesia, procedures lasting more than 1 hr, or procedures associated with significant blood loss, the **glucocorticoid target is approximately 50–100 mg/day hydrocortisone equivalent for the day of surgery and at least 1 postoperative day.** Higher doses may be necessary if excessive bleeding or complications are encountered. Patients should take their normal steroid dose prior to the procedure and be provided supplemental intravenous hydrocortisone intraoperatively to achieve a total of 100 mg. Hospitalization should be considered for these patients because blood pressure can be more closely monitored postoperatively in this setting. Hydrocortisone 25 mg usually is prescribed every 8 hr following surgery for 24–48 hr, depending on the procedure and anticipated level of postoperative pain.

Following the recommendations listed will further minimize the risk of adrenal crisis associated with surgical stress in adrenally insufficient individuals:

• Define the risk for adrenal insufficiency with a thorough medical history and clinical examination. Patients with a past or present history of tuberculosis or HIV infection are at increased risk for adrenal insufficiency because opportunistic infectious agents can attack the adrenal glands.

- Ensure that adrenally insufficient patients take their glucocorticoid prior to a stressful surgery.
- Schedule surgery in the morning when cortisol levels normally are highest.
- Provide proper stress reduction because anxiety can increase cortisol demand.
- Minor surgeries require minimal steroid coverage. The patient's customary daily dose usually is sufficient.
- Major surgeries and those procedures lasting more than 1 hour or requiring use of general anesthesia should be performed in a hospital with steroid supplementation.
- Use of nitrous oxide-oxygen or intravenous or oral benzodiazepine sedation is helpful, as plasma cortisol levels are not reduced by these agents.
- Avoid outpatient general anesthesia, as general anesthesia increases glucocorticoid demand. Also, avoid use of barbiturates, which increase the metabolism of cortisol and reduce blood levels of cortisol.

SUMMARY OF NEED FOR SUPPLEMENTATION
Negligible-Risk Category
Nonsurgical dental procedures
Regimen: No supplementation required.
Low-Risk Category
Minor oral surgery
Few simple extractions, biopsy
Minor periodontal surgery
Regimen: Target 25 mg hydrocortisone equivalent (5 mg prednisone), day of surgery
Moderate-Risk to Major-Risk Category
Major oral surgery
Multiple extractions
Quadrant periodontal surgery
Extraction of bony impactions

Osseous surgery
Osteotomy
Bone resections
Cancer surgery
Surgical procedures involving use of general anesthesia
Procedures lasting more than 1 hr
Procedures associated with significant blood loss
Regimen: Target glucocorticoid target is approximately 50–100 mg/day hydrocortisone equivalent, day of surgery and at least 1 postoperative day.

CONTROL OF BLEEDING IN PATIENTS ON ANTICOAGULANT THERAPY
Oral Anticoagulants
In patients taking oral anticoagulant drugs (e.g., warfarin, Coumadin®) to prevent thromboembolic complications (e.g., stroke), the dentist should consult the patient's physician regarding the patient's reason for taking the drug and determine the level of anticoagulation reported as the international normalized ratio (INR). In most patients, the therapeutic range of the INR is approximately 2 to 3, whereas patients with prosthetic heart valves are maintained at an INR of 2.5 to 3.5. The AMA and the ADA suggest that an INR value 2 and 3 before a surgical procedure is attempted. Local measures should be used to control bleeding if it occurs.

In patients with INR > 3, the dentist should consult with the patient's physician regarding possible reduction of the anticoagulant dosage before surgery. Minor surgery usually can be performed safely in patients with an INR up to 3.5. In general, treating these patients without reducing the anticoagulant dose is safer than stopping the anticoagulant. Current information does not support stopping the drug, which increases the risk for thrombotic events. If the physician desires a reduced dosage, he or she will direct the patient to reduce the anticoagulant dosage. At least 3–4 days must pass before the effect of the reduced dosage will be reflected in a decreased INR. The INR value should be checked on the scheduled day of surgery to be certain that the desired reduction of anticoagulation effect has occurred.

If acute infection is present, surgery should be delayed until the infection has been treated. When the patient is free of acute infection and the INR is 3.5 or lower, the procedure can be performed. The procedure should be done with as little trauma as possible. If excessive postoperative bleeding (slow blood flow and oozing) occurs, one or more of the following measures can be used to control it:

Use a splint constructed before surgery (in cases with multiple extractions)

Pressure using gauze pack

Absorbable gelatin sponge (Gelfoam)
  Dental packing blocks:
    20 × 20 × 7 mm, can be cut to fit and applied to bleeding site.
  Powder: Apply to bleeding site.

Gelfoam with thrombin
  Thrombogen: Powder with isotonic saline diluent (5,000-unit container with isotonic saline). For bleeding from skin or mucosa, use solution of 100 units/ml. Do not use with Oxycel, Surgicel, or microfibrillar collagen because they inactivate the thrombin.

Oxidized cellulose (Oxycel)
  Pad: 3 × 3 inch; pledget: 2 × 1 × 1 inch; strip: 18 × 2, 5 × $\frac{1}{2}$, 36 × $\frac{1}{2}$ inch. Cut to appropriate size and apply dry.

Tranexamic acid (Cyklokapron)
  Solution: 100 mg/ml in 10-ml vials; tablets: 500 mg, after surgery 25 mg/kg orally 3 times a day.

Oxidized regenerated cellulose (Surgicel absorbable hemostat)
  Surgicel sheets: 2 × 14, 4 × 8, 2 × 3, $\frac{1}{2}$ × 2 inch; Surgicel Nu-Knit sheets: 1 × 1, 3 × 4, 6 × 9 inch. Pick appropriate size and lay over extraction site to control bleeding.

Microfibrillar collagen hemostat (Avitene, CollaTape, Instat MCH)
  Avitene sheets: 35 × 35, 70 × 35, 70 × 70 mm; CollaTape: 1 × 3, 3/4 × 1$\frac{1}{2}$, $\frac{3}{8}$ × $\frac{3}{4}$ inch.
  Instat MCH: Coherent fibers packaged in 0.5- and 1.0-g containers. Apply topically, and it adheres firmly to bleeding surfaces.

Collagen hemostat
  Pads: 1 × 2, 3 × 4 inch. Apply directly to bleeding surface with pressure. It is more effective when applied dry.

Antiplatelet Therapy

Patients with drug-eluting stents for treatment of coronary artery disease take a combination of aspirin and another antiplatelet drug from the thienopyridine group (clopidogrel, Plavix®; ticlopidine, Ticlid) for at least one year following placement of the stent. Abrupt discontinuation of this dual antiplatelet therapy in patients prior to routine dental procedures is not recommended. In 2007, the American Heart Association issued an advisory statement that strongly advised against the common practice of discontinuing these agents, which included references to very high mortality rates in at-risk patients who develop thromboemboli.

MANAGEMENT OF ANXIETY
IN THE DENTAL PATIENT
Anxiety

The dentist may detect anxiety in a patient on the basis of his or her physical appearance, speech, dress, and presence of certain signs and symptoms. The anxious person looks overalert, displayed in ways such as sitting forward in a chair; moving fingers, arms, or legs; getting up and moving; pacing around the room; checking certain parts of clothing; and straightening ties or scarves. On the other hand, sloppy dress habits and other signs, just the opposite of a concern with perfection, may also be seen. An anxious person may show signs of being watchful of possessions, always trying to keep them in sight.

The anxious person may speak mechanically and rapidly and at times may seem to block out or not connect thoughts together. The anxious person may respond to questions quickly, often not allowing the dentist to finish a question.

Signs of sweating, tension in muscles, increased breathing, and rapid heart rate may be seen. The patient may complain of an inability to sleep, may wake at an early hour, and may not be able to go back to sleep. Attacks of diarrhea and increased frequency of urination may occur. In general, anxious persons are overalert and tense, feel apprehensive, and have a sense of impending disaster that has no apparent cause. Insomnia, tension, and apprehension lead to fatigue, which makes it even more difficult for the individual to deal with anxiety.

The dentist should talk with the patient and show personal interest. Verbal and nonverbal communication must be consistent. The dentist should confront the patient with the observation that the patient appears anxious, then ask if the individual would like to talk about feelings, which may include the person's attitude toward the dentist. During these discussions, tension-free pauses should be allowed to develop between ideas, as a temporary state of regression will help the patient return to a more anxiety-free state. Some patients may respond well to this approach without ever indicating why they were anxious.

If the patient remains anxious in the dental situation, the dentist can plan to use hypnosis, oral or parenteral sedation agents or nitrous oxide, and oxygen to better manage the dental treatment.

Patients with uncontrolled hyperthyroidism may have associated anxiety. Epinephrine must not be used in these patients, including even the small amounts that are used in local anesthetics. Patients with signs and symptoms of hyperthyroidism should be referred for medical evaluation and treatment.

Dental Management of the Anxious Patient

1. Preoperative
   A. Behavioral
      Establish effective communication with the patient
      Be open and honest; let the patient see who you are
      Consistent verbal and nonverbal communication
      Explain procedures and answer any questions
      Explain possible discomfort associated with a procedure
      Explain what you will do to make procedures "pain free"
      Possibly confront patient who appears anxious: "You seem tense today. Would you like to talk about it?"

B. *Pharmacologic*
  Oral sedation: benzodiazepines
  Night before appointment: aid
    patient in getting a good
    night's sleep
  Day of appointment: reduce
    anxiety prior to appointment
  Select a fast-acting drug, at the
    lowest dosage that will be
    effective

2. Operative
  A. *Behavioral*
    Allow patient to ask questions
      about what is happening
    Let patient know if any
      discomfort is about to be felt
    Reassure patient that the
      procedure is going well
  B. *Pharmacologic*
    Effective local anesthesia
    Oral sedation*: benzodiazepines
    Inhalation sedation*: nitrous oxide
    Intramuscular sedation*:
      midazolam, promethazine,
      meperidine
    Intravenous sedation*: diazepam,
      midazolam, fentanyl
  *NOTE: Many states require
    that dentists have special permits
    for the use of various sedation
    modalities; appropriate emergency
    and monitoring equipment is
    recommended whenever sedative
    agents are employed.

3. Postoperative
  A. *Behavioral*
    Explain what usually occurs
      after the procedure
    Explain what the patient needs
      to do
    Explain what the patient needs
      to avoid
    Describe complications that
      can occur:
        Pain
        Bleeding
        Infection
        Allergic reaction to medication

    Tell patient to inform you if any
      complications develop
  B. *Pharmacologic*
    Effective postoperative pain
      control is essential
    Select the most appropriate
      medication for pain control
    Analgesics: nonsteroidal
      antiinflammatory drugs
      (NSAIDs) or acetaminophen
      (in patients who cannot
      take aspirin/NSAIDs) with
      codeine, hydrocodone, or
      oxycodone
    Adjunctive medications:
      antidepressants, muscle
      relaxants, steroids,
      anticonvulsants, antibiotics

Specific Drugs and Dosage for Anxiety Control (Dosage for Older Adults and Children Must Be Reduced):
Nitrous oxide, inhalation, titrated to
  20%–50%
Diazepam (Valium), oral (2-, 5-, or
  10-mg tablets)
Triazolam (Halcion), oral (0.125- or
  0.25-mg tablets)
Lorazepam (Ativan), oral (1- or 3-mg
  tablets)

DEPRESSION IN DENTAL PATIENTS
Signs of low-grade chronic
depression include fatigue (even
after adequate sleep); difficulty
getting up in the morning;
restlessness; loss of interest in
family, work, and sex; inability to
make decisions; anger and
resentment; chronic complaining;
self-criticism; feelings of inferiority;
and excessive daydreaming. Signs of
more severe depression include
excessive crying, change in sleeping
habits, thoughts of food making one
sick, weight loss without dieting,
strong feelings of guilt, nightmares,
thoughts about suicide, feeling unreal

or in a "fog," and an inability to concentrate.

Patients with major depression are depressed most of the day, show a marked decrease in interest or pleasure in most activities, have a marked gain or loss in weight, and manifest insomnia or hypersomnia. These symptoms must be present for at least 2 weeks before major depression can be diagnosed.

Dental Management

Significant impairment of all personal hygiene may occur during the depth of a depressive episode, including a total lack of oral hygiene. Salivary flow may be reduced, and patients may complain of xerostomia (dry mouth), an increased rate of dental caries, and periodontal disease. The xerostomia may be compounded by the side effects of the medications used to treat depression. Complaints of glossodynia and various facial pain syndromes are common.

The dentist should provide an aggressive preventive dental education program for depressed patients, including the use of artificial salivary products, antiseptic mouthwash, and daily fluoride mouth rinses. Xerostomia provides an excellent environment for overgrowth of *Candida albicans;* as a result, patients are likely to require treatment for candidiasis along with treatment for dry mouth.

Small amounts of epinephrine (0.04 mg or 2 cartridges of a 1:100,000 concentration) can be used in patients taking tricyclic or heterocyclic antidepressants, provided the dentist aspirates before injecting and injects the anesthetic slowly. In general, no more than two cartridges should be injected at any appointment. Excessive amounts of epinephrine can result in hypertension. Levonordefrin is contraindicated in patients taking tricyclics or heterocyclics because of the possibility of an exaggerated hypertensive response. A lower dosage of sedative medications may be necessary to avoid excessive CNS depression.

Patients taking tricyclic or heterocyclic antidepressant drugs may be prone to orthostatic hypotension. Dentists should avoid rapid changes in chair position for these patients and provide support when patients first get out of the dental chair. Atropine should be used with care because increased intraocular pressure can result. Acetaminophen should be used with care because it can decrease the metabolic rate of the heterocyclics, which could lead to toxic levels of the tricyclic antidepressant. Phenobarbital increases the metabolism of tricyclic antidepressants, which can attenuate their antidepressant effects.

No medical contraindication exists for dental treatment during a depressive episode; however, most depressed patients may be best managed by dealing with their immediate dental needs only during the depression. More complex dental procedures can be performed once the patient has responded to medical treatment.

Patients with signs and symptoms of severe depression must be referred for medical evaluation and treatment. If the patient is not responsive to this recommendation, the problem should be shared with a family member and every attempt made to get the individual to medical attention. During severe depression, suicide is always a possibility; however, medical treatment currently is able to reduce this possibility.

Suicidal Patients

Studies have shown that questions about suicide do not prompt these patients to act. The dentist should ask the very depressed patient if he or she has had any thoughts about suicide. Patients who state they have had these thoughts must be referred for immediate medical care; members of the family need to be involved if possible.

Bisphosphonate-Associated Osteonecrosis of the Jaw (Osteochemonecrosis)

With the increased frequency of bisphosphonate use for the treatment of osteoporosis (e.g., alendronate, Fosamax), dentists have been alerted to the possibility of osteonecrosis of the jaw related to these drugs. These medications are also used in other resorptive bone diseases, including breast and prostate cancer metastatic to the bones, Paget's disease, and cases of bone fragility related to chronic renal failure. This group of drugs currently includes aminobisphosphonates (alendronate, Fosamax; ibandronate, Boniva; pamidronate, Aredia; risedronate, Actonel; and zolendronate, Zometa) and non-aminobisphosphonates (clodronate, Bonefos; etidronate, Didronel; and tiludronate, Skelid). These agents are used both orally and intravenously, the latter appearing to place the patient at highest risk for osteonecrosis of the jaw. There are no prospective, randomized scientific studies on which to base dental management algorithms for these patients, but guidelines presently exist, based on retrospective studies and case reports.

Clinically, osteonecrosis of the jaw usually presents as exposed bone in the maxillofacial area, reportedly more frequently in the mandible, spontaneously or following oral surgery, that does not heal within 6 wk (confirmed when other possible causes have been ruled out [e.g. osteoradionecrosis]). Signs and symptoms may include one or more of the following: mucosal ulceration with exposed bone; infection (with or without purulence); pain or swelling in the affected jaw, and/or paresthesia or other sensory alterations.

This condition occurs only rarely in patients taking oral bisphosphonates, but a higher risk has been determined for the intravenous agents in this group. The dental management of patients at-risk for osteonecrosis include identification of at-risk patients and the following:

• Patients should have a comprehensive dental exam prior to starting bisphosphonate therapy and should be reevaluated every 6 mo or more frequently, as appropriate;

• Oral surgical procedures should be completed before starting bisphosphonate therapy;

• The dental team should emphasize excellent oral hygiene for patients on bisphosphonate therapy;

• If dental treatment is necessary after bisphosphonate therapy has been started, the least invasive (nonsurgical) technique is recommended, although routine restorative and dental hygiene procedures may be performed;

• The risks and potential benefits of withholding bisphosphonate therapy should be discussed with the patient and the patient's treating physician(s) prior to tooth extraction or other oral

surgical procedures (NOTE: there are no prospective studies at this time on which to base this decision);
• In patients with oral osteonecrosis, conservative management is recommended and includes the use of antibiotics, antibacterial mouthrinses, limited debridement of the site, and analgesic medications to control pain associated with the osteonecrosis. Steroid drugs may increase the risk for development of osteonecrosis. (NOTE: there are no data at the present time on which to base the use of surgery or hyperbaric oxygen to manage this condition).

COMPLEMENTARY MEDICINES AND DENTISTRY

The term alternative medicine is used to describe practices that are used instead of mainstream medical practice. Complementary medicine refers to practices that are used as adjuncts to conventional medicine. These systems are divided into five major categories: alternative medical systems (traditional Chinese medicine, Ayurveda medicine of India, and Native-American healing approaches), biologically based therapies (natural products), manipulative and body-based methods (chiropractic and osteopathic manipulation), mind–body interventions (hypnosis, cognitive therapies and biofeedback), and energy therapies (use of magnets and acupuncture). Both of these systems use treatments that often have no established efficacy. An estimated 42% of Americans use alternative and complementary medicine therapies.

Complementary medicines are defined as herbal medicines, homeopathic remedies, and essential oils. The basic principle of homeopathy is selection of a remedy, which, if given to a healthy individual, will produce a range of symptoms similar to those observed in the ill patient (like cures like). Only minute amounts are given to avoid toxicity. Only one remedy is used at any one time. Dilute tinctures are used rather than concentrated ones. In homeopathic practice, medication in tablet form is commonly used.

The standard tinctures used in Western tradition herbal medicine are very different from those used in homoeopathy. Alcohol is used to dissolve the plant, and the final product is not diluted. Thus these remedies are concentrated, highly potent preparations and usually are taken as the unmodified liquid tincture. Other preparations used in herbal remedies include lotions and creams for topical application. Tablet form of medication is not used very often (less than 5%).

Efficacy of Herbal Medicines

Many herbal remedies have been used for hundreds of years. However, traditional use is not a good indication of efficacy. The gold standard for testing efficacy is the randomized clinical trial (RCT). This standard should apply as much to herbal medicines as for conventional medicines. A number of RCTs of herbal medical products have been conducted. However, many of these studies differ with regard to how they were conducted and in their findings. Ernst suggests that the best way to evaluate a number of RCTs on the efficacy of a specific herbal medicine is to do a systematic review or meta-analysis of all RCTs for that product. Herbal medicines with proven efficacy: Several herbal remedies have been repeatedly tested in placebo-controlled RCTs. Systematic reviews of these

TABLE 1
Drug Interactions of Significance to Dentistry

Dental Drug	Interacting Drug	Medical Condition/Situation	Effect
Antibiotics			
Antibiotics	Oral contraceptives (birth control pills)	Contraception	Decreased effectiveness of oral contraceptives has been suggested for several antibiotic classes because of elimination of gut bacteria responsible for second round cleavage and activation of contraceptive. However, most well-designed studies do not show any reduction in estrogen serum levels in patients taking antibiotics (except rifampin). **Recommendation:** Okay to use dental antibiotics, advise patient of possible but rare interactions.
β-Lactams (penicillins, cephalosporins)	Allopurinol (Lopurin, Zyloprim)	Gout	Incidence of minor allergic reactions to ampicillin is increased. Other penicillins have not been implicated. **Recommendation:** Avoid ampicillin.
	β-blockers (Tenormin, Lopressor, Inderal, Corgard)	Hypertension	Serum levels of atenolol are reduced after prolonged use of ampicillin. Anaphylactic reactions to penicillins or other drugs may be more severe in patients taking β-blockers because of increased mediator release from mast cells. **Recommendation:** Use ampicillin cautiously, advise patient of potential reaction.
	Tetracyclines and other bacteriostatic antibiotics	Infection, acne, periodontal disease	Effectiveness of penicillins and cephalosporins may be reduced by bacteriostatic agents. **Recommendation:** Avoid interaction.
Tetracyclines	Antacids	Dyspepsia, gastroesophageal reflux, peptic ulcer	Antacids, dairy products, and other agents containing divalent and trivalent cations will chelate tetracyclines and limit their absorption in the gut. Doxycycline is least influenced by this interaction. **Recommendation:** Avoid interaction.

	Insulin	Diabetes mellitus	Doxycycline and oxytetracycline have been documented as enhancing the hypoglycemic effects of exogenously administered insulin. **Recommendation:** Select different antibiotic or increase carbohydrate intake.
Metronidazole	Ethanol	Alcohol use or abuse	Severe disulfiramlike reactions are well documented. **Recommendation:** Avoid interaction.
	Lithium	Manic depression	Inhibits renal excretion of lithium, leading to elevated/toxic levels of lithium. Lithium toxicity produces confusion, ataxia, and kidney damage. **Recommendation:** Avoid interaction.
	Benzodiazepines	Anxiety	Delayed metabolism of benzodiazepine, increasing the pharmacologic effects can result in excessive sedation and irrational behavior. **Recommendation:** Reduce dose of benzodiazepine.
	Carbamazepine (Tegretol)	Seizure disorder	Increased blood levels of carbamazepine leading to toxicity (symptoms include drowsiness, dizziness, nausea, headache, and blurred vision). Hospitalization has been required. **Recommendation:** Avoid interaction.
	Cyclosporine	Organ transplant	Enhanced immunosuppression and nephrotoxicity. **Recommendation:** Avoid interaction, monitor patient.
	Lovastatin, pravastatin, simvastatin, other statins	Hyperlipidemia	Muscle (eosinophilia) myalgia and rhabdomyolysis **Recommendation:** Avoid interaction.
	Prednisone, methylprednisolone	Autoimmune disorders, organ transplant	Increased risk of Cushing's syndrome and immunosuppression. **Recommendation:** Monitor patient, shorten duration of antibiotic administration if possible.

Continued

TABLE 1
Drug Interactions of Significance to Dentistry—cont'd

Dental Drug	Interacting Drug	Medical Condition/Situation	Effect
	Theophylline (Theo-Dur)	Asthma	Some macrolide antibiotics (erythromycin, clarithromycin) inhibit metabolism of theophylline, leading to toxic serum levels (symptoms of toxicity: headache, nausea, vomiting, confusion, thirst, cardiac arrhythmias, convulsions). Conversely, theophylline reduces serum levels of erythromycin. **Recommendation:** Avoid prescribing these antibiotics in such patients.
Antibiotics (especially erythromycin and tetracycline)	Digoxin (Lanoxin)	Congestive heart failure	Alters gastrointestinal flora and retards metabolism of digoxin in approximately 10% of patients, resulting in dangerously high digoxin serum levels that may persist for several weeks after discontinuation of antibiotic. Strongest documentation for erythromycin and tetracycline. Patients should be cautioned to report any signs of digitalis toxicity (salivation, visual disturbances, arrhythmias) during antibiotic therapy. **Recommendation:** Avoid interaction by using noninteractive antibiotic.
Antibiotics (cephalosporins, erythromycin, clarithromycin, metronidazole)	Warfarin (Coumadin)	Atrial fibrillation, MI, post major surgery, stroke prevention	Anticoagulant effect of warfarin may be increased by several antibiotic classes. Reduced synthesis of vitamin K by gut flora is a putative mechanism, but several antibiotics have antiplatelet and anticoagulant activity.

Macrolide antibiotics (erythromycin, clarithromycin)	Infection	Most convincing documentation for cephalosporins, macrolide antibiotics, and metronidazole. **Recommendation:** Penicillins, tetracyclines, and clindamycin are preferred choices but must be used cautiously.
Benzodiazepines with high oral bioavailability (triazolam, midazolam)	Infection	Reduced hepatic first-pass metabolism of benzodiazepine with increased blood level and unpredictably increased levels of CNS depression **Recommendation:** Avoid interaction with alternative sedative or reduce dose of interacting benzodiazepine
Azole antifungal agents (e.g., ketoconazole, Nizoral®)	Systemic fungal infection	Reduced hepatic metabolism (CYP 3A4 inhibition) of benzodiazepine results in unpredictably increased CNS depression. **Recommendation:** Avoid interaction with alternative sedative agent or reduce dose of interacting benzodiazepine
Analgesics Acetaminophen	Alcohol use and abuse	Increased risk of liver toxicity, especially during fasting state or at least 4 g/day acetaminophen, exacerbated by abrupt discontinuation of alcohol use. **Recommendation:** Use lower dose of acetaminophen, allow patient to continue alcohol use. (NOTE: alcohol-related liver damage may absolutely contraindicate use of acetaminophen.)
Aspirin	Diabetes type 2	Increased hypoglycemic effects. **Recommendation:** Avoid interaction.
Aspirin, NSAIDs	Atrial fibrillation, myocardial infarction, postsurgery	Increased risk of gastrointestinal bleeding. **Recommendation:** Avoid interaction.

Continued

TABLE 1
Drug Interactions of Significance to Dentistry— cont'd

Dental Drug	Interacting Drug	Medical Condition/ Situation	Effect
Aspirin, NSAIDs	Alcohol	Alcohol use and abuse	Increases risk of GI bleeding. **Recommendation:** Lower dose, encourage discontinuation of alcohol use.
NSAIDs	β-Blocker angiotensin-converting enzyme inhibitor	Hypertension, postmyocardial infarction	Decreased antihypertensive effect. **Recommendation:** Limit duration of NSAID dosage to approximaately 4 days.
NSAIDs	Lithium	Manic depression	Produces symptoms of lithium toxicity, including nausea, vomiting, slurred speech, and mental confusion. **Recommendation:** NSAIDs should not be prescribed to patients with manic depression who take lithium. It can result in toxic levels of lithium.
NSAIDs	Methotrexate (MTX)	Connective tissue disease, cancer therapy	Toxic levels of MTX may accumulate. **Recommendation:** Avoid interaction if patient on high-dose MTX for cancer therapy. Low-dose MTX for arthritis is not a concern.
Anesthetics			
Lidocaine	Bupivacaine		Additive effect of these two local anesthetics increases risk. **Recommendation:** Limit dose of each.
Mepivacaine	Meperidine (Demerol)		Sedation with opioids may increase risk of local anesthetic toxicity, especially in children. **Recommendation:** Reduce anesthetic dose.

Sedatives			
Barbiturates	Digoxin, theophylline, corticosteroids, oral anticoagulants	CHF, asthma, autoimmune disease, atrial fibrillation	Barbiturates bind cytochrome P450 system in liver, enhance metabolism of many drugs. **Recommendation:** Limit dose, observe for adverse effects.
	Benzodiazepines, alcohol, antihistamines	Anxiety, alcohol use and abuse, seasonal allergies	Additive effects for sedation and respiratory depression. **Recommendation:** Reduce dose, administer combination of sedatives with extreme caution.
Benzodiazepines (BZDP; e.g., alprazolam, chlordiazepoxide, diazepam)	Cimetidine, oral contraceptives, fluoxetine, isoniazid (INH), alcohol	Peptic ulcer disease, depression, tuberculosis, alcohol use and abuse	Delayed metabolism of BZDP, increasing pharmacologic effects can result in excessive sedation and irrational behavior. **Recommendation:** Reduce dose of BZDP. Delayed metabolism of BZDP, increasing pharmacologic effects can result in excessive sedation and irrational behavior. **Recommendation:** Reduce dose of BZDP.
	Digoxin (Lanoxin), phenytoin, theophylline (Theo-Dur)	CHF, epilepsy, asthma	Serum concentrations of digoxin, phenytoin may be increased, resulting in toxicity. Antagonize sedative effects of BZDP. **Recommendation:** Avoid interaction.
	Protease inhibitors (Indinavir, Nelfinavir)	HIV, AIDS	Increased bioavailability and effects of BZDP, especially triazolam and oral midazolam. **Recommendation:** Avoid interaction.

Continued

TABLE 1
Drug Interactions of Significance to Dentistry—cont'd

Dental Drug	Interacting Drug	Medical Condition/Situation	Effect
Vasoconstrictor			
Epinephrine and levonordephrine (Neo-Cobefrin)	Nonselective β-blockers: propranolol (Inderal), nadolol (Corgard), penbutolol (Levatol), pindolol (Visken), sotalol (Betapace), timolol (Blocadren)	Angina pectoris, hypertension, glaucoma, migraine, headache, hyperthyroidism, panic syndromes	Unopposed effects: increased B/P with secondary bradycardia. **Recommendation:** Initial dose is 1/2 cartridge containing 1:100,000 epinephrine, aspirate to avoid intravascular injection, inject slowly. Monitor vital signs; if no adverse cardiovascular change, up to two cartridges containing a vasoconstrictor can be administered at 5-min intervals with continual monitoring. Avoid epinephrine-containing retraction cord and higher concentrations of epinephrine in the dental anesthetic.
	Cocaine	Illicit use, topical anesthetic for mucous membrane procedures	Blocks reuptake of norepinephrine and intensifies postsynaptic response to epinephrine-like drugs. This potentiates the adrenergic effects on the heart, with potential for a heart attack. **Recommendation:** Recognize signs and symptoms of cocaine abuse. Avoid use of vasoconstrictors in these patients until cocaine has been withheld for at least 24 hr.

Halothane	General anesthetic for surgical procedures	Stimulation of 1 and receptors resulting in arrhythmia at doses greater than 2 g/kg. **Recommendation:** Limit dose to remain below 2 g/kg threshold, aspirate to avoid intravascular injection. Monitor vital signs. Avoid epinephrine-containing retraction cord and concentrations of epinephrine greater than 1:100,000.
Tricyclic antidepressants (amitriptyline [Elavil], doxepin [Sinequan], imipramine [Tofranil])	Depression, severe anxiety, neuropathic pain, attention deficit disorder	Blocks reuptake of norepinephrine resulting in unopposed effects (increased B/P, increased heart rate), potential cardiac arrhythmias; effect is greater with levonordefrin. **Recommendation:** Avoid levonordephrin. Limit dose to 2 cartridges containing 1:100,000 epinephrine (36 g), aspirate to avoid intravascular injection. Monitor vital signs. Avoid epinephrine-containing retraction cord and higher concentrations of epinephrine in the dental anesthetic.

Continued

TABLE 1
Drug Interactions of Significance to Dentistry—cont'd

Dental Drug	Interacting Drug	Medical Condition/Situation	Effect
	Peripheral adrenergic antagonists (reserpine [Serpasil], guanethidine [Ismelin], guanadrel [Hylorel])	Hypertension	Potential for increased sensitivity of adrenergic receptors to epinephrine and levonordefrin. **Recommendation:** Administer cautiously. Monitor vital signs during and following administration of first cartridge. Limit dose to 2 cartridges containing 1:100,000 epinephrine (36 g) or less depending on vital signs and patient response. Aspirate to avoid intravascular injection. Avoid epinephrine-containing retraction cord and higher concentrations of epinephrine in the dental anesthetic.
	Catechol-O-methyltransferase inhibitors (tolcapone [Tasmar], entacapone [Comtan])	Parkinson's disease	Potential for increased sensitivity of adrenergic receptors to epinephrine and levonordefrin, resulting in increased heart rate and B/P and arrhythmias. **Recommendation:** Administer cautiously. Monitor vital signs during and after administration of first cartridge. Limit dose to 2 cartridges containing 1:100,000 epinephrine (36 g) or less depending on vital signs and patient response. Aspirate to avoid intravascular injection. Avoid epinephrine-containing retraction cord and higher concentrations of epinephrine in the dental anesthetic.

studies have shown that some herbal medicines are effective for certain conditions. For example, ginkgo biloba has been shown to be effective for symptomatic treatment of dementia and intermittent claudication. Table 2 lists the more commonly used herbal medicines that have proved to be effective for the condition(s) listed.

Herbal medicines with doubtful or no efficacy:

TABLE 2

Claims for Herbal Actions Supported by Clinical Trials

Herb	Claimed Action	Effectiveness Supported by Clinical Trials
Kava	Used to treat anxiety.	Clinical trials have shown it reduces anxiety significantly more than placebo.
Artichoke	Used to lower the lipid levels in blood.	Only one randomized clinical study shows it moderately lowers elevated total cholesterol levels when given orally for several weeks.
Feverfew	Used for women's ailments and inflammatory diseases. Recently has been suggested for headache and migraine.	Three studies showed greater effect than placebo in alleviating symptoms of headache or migraine.
Garlic	Used to reduce blood pressure and lower blood lipid levels.	Data show a small but statistically significant reduction in systolic and diastolic blood pressures. No data support claims for lipid-lowering properties of garlic.
Ginger	Used to treat nausea and vomiting.	Several studies support the antiemetic use for ginger. Used to treat or prevent nausea or vomiting.
Ginkgo biloba	Used to treat cerebral insufficiency, prevent loss of cognitive function, and tinnitus.	Studies have shown it is effective in the treatment of cerebral insufficiency when given for 4–6 weeks. Data show that regular oral intake of ginkgo biloba slows the loss of cognitive function in patients with dementia.
Hawthorn	Used to treat heart failure.	Various studies show it is effective for the early signs of congestive heart failure.
Horse chestnut	Used to treat venous congestion.	Studies have shown it is effective in reducing signs and symptoms of chronic venous insufficiency.

Continued

TABLE 2
Claims for Herbal Actions Supported by Clinical Trials—cont'd

Herb	Claimed Action	Effectiveness Supported by Clinical Trials
Saw palmetto	Used in Europe to treat prostate enlargement.	Clinical trials support its use for symptoms of benign prostatic hypertrophy.
St. John's wort	Used to treat depression.	Studies show that it is effective for treating mild to moderate depression. The question of its effectiveness for severe depression remains to be answered.

Asian ginseng, one of the most popular herbal medicines in the United States, showed no convincing evidence for efficacy as a general tonic or in enhancing mental and physical performance. A review of studies regarding the use of valerian as a hypnotic agent was inconclusive because of flaws in the study designs. A systematic review of RCTs found no evidence that evening primrose was effective for treatment of premenstrual syndrome in women. Garlic was not found to be effective as a cholesterol-lowering drug. Table 3 lists some of the more common herbal medicines that were found not to be effective for the conditions listed.

Side Effects and Adverse Reactions
Recent increased use of herbal remedies seems to come from the public's view that natural products are harmless or at least have fewer side effects than regular drugs. The assumption that phytomedicines (herbal medicines)

have only beneficial effects has proved to be incorrect.

Toxicity can be associated with use of herbal remedies. These reactions can be caused by accidental or deliberate contamination of the product. For example, lead, mercury, cadmium, pesticides, microorganisms, and fumigants have been found to contaminate some herbal products. Substitution of animal substances such as enzymes, hormones, or organ extracts and synthetic drugs has accounted for some of the toxic reactions to herbal products. Adulteration by accidental or deliberate substitution of the original plant material by other plant species has been reported to be a source of toxic reactions to herbal products.

Other sources of adverse reactions to herbal products are intrinsic or plant associated. In some cases, the manufacturer ignored the known toxicity of a plant

TABLE 3
Claims for Herbal Actions Unsupported by Clinical Trials

Herb	Claimed Action	Effectiveness Unsupported by Clinical Trials
Aloe vera	Used as an adjunct oral treatment for diabetes and skin conditions such as herpes and psoriasis.	Currently, compelling data support none of the claims made for aloe vera.

TABLE 3

Claims for Herbal Actions Unsupported by Clinical Trials—cont'd

Herb	Claimed Action	Effectiveness Unsupported by Clinical Trials
Echinacea	Used to prevent and treat the common cold.	Overall there is insufficient evidence that Echinacea extracts are effective for treatment or prevention of the common cold.
Evening primrose	Used for treatment of premenstrual syndrome.	Current evidence suggests uncertain value when it is used to treat premenstrual syndrome.
Ginseng	Used to treat type 2 diabetes and herpes simplex infections. Also has been used to increase physical and psychomotor performance and enhance cognitive function.	None of the 16 double-blinded, randomized clinical trials support any effective action on physical performance, psychomotor performance, or cognitive function, type 2 diabetes, or herpes simplex infections.
Guar Gum	Used to treat obesity and overweight.	Clinical trials have not supported these claims.
Mistletoe	Has been suggested for treatment of cancer.	Current studies do not support these claims.
Peppermint	Used to treat irritable bowel syndrome.	Studies show that it alleviates the symptoms of irritable bowel syndrome. However, many of the trials had flaws.
Valerian	Used to promote sleep.	Randomized clinical trials are necessary to demonstrate effectiveness. Studies to date have been flawed.

or constituent in the herbal product. In other cases, the product contains plants for which no or insufficient data regarding safety are available. If a highly concentrated or specifically processed extract is used, toxic reactions may occur. If a plant contains constituents known to affect the bioavailability and/or pharmacokinetics of other drugs, serious drug interactions can occur.

Long-term users, consumers of large amounts of phytomedicines, or people who use many different medicinal products may be prone to side effects. Pregnant or nursing women, babies, and the elderly, sick, and undernourished are at higher risk for side effects. Some of the more common side effects associated with herbal remedies include bleeding with ginkgo biloba; upset stomach, fatigue, dizziness, confusion, dry mouth, and photosensitivity with St. John's wort; high blood pressure, arrhythmias, nervousness, headaches, heart attack, or stroke with ephedra; and sleepiness, rash, and motor dysfunction of skeletal muscles with kava kava. Table 4 lists some of the serious adverse reactions that can occur with use of natural products.

TABLE 4
Selected Herbal Medicines with Potentially Serious Adverse Effects

Product	Effect
Aristolochia	Nephrotoxicity Carcinogenicity
Chaparral	Cholestatic hepatitis
Comfrey	Acute and chronic hepatitis
Digitalis leaf	Arrhythmias
Ephedra	Hypertension Stroke MI
Germander	Acute and chronic hepatitis
Kava kava	Hepatitis
Khat	Tachycardia Psychosis
Kombucha	Hepatotoxicity Lactic acidosis
Mistletoe	Anaphylaxis
Skullcap	Seizures Acute and chronic hepatitis
St. John's wort	Photosensitivity Possible hypertension with tyramine-containing foods

Medical Problems

Certain medical problems can make consumption of herbal medicines unsafe. Individuals with high blood pressure, thyroid disease, psychiatric disorders, Parkinson's disease, enlarged prostate gland, diabetes mellitus, heart disease, epilepsy, glaucoma, blood clotting problems, and a history of stroke should check with their physician before taking any herbal remedies. Patients with a history of aspirin allergy can be at risk if they take an herb containing willow bark.

Drug Interactions

Important drug interactions can occur between certain herbal products and conventional medications (Table 5). The most common drug involved with drug–herb interactions is warfarin. The most common herb involved with these interactions is St. John's wort. Long-term administration of St. John's wort may result in diminished clinical effectiveness or increased dosage requirements for all CYP3A4 substrates, which represent approximately 50% of all prescription medications. Garlic extracts alter the disposition of coadministered medications metabolized by the CYP3A4 pathway.

TABLE 5
Selected Natural Medicines That Potentiate or Interfere with Approved
Prescription and Over-the-Counter Drugs

Natural Medicine	Drug
Ephedra	Theophylline (P) Antihypertensives (I) Corticosteroids (I)
Evening primrose	Anticoagulants (P) Antiplatelet agents (P) Low-molecular-weight heparins (P) Anticonvulsants (I)
Garlic	Aspirin (P) Clopidogrel (P) Ticlopidine (P)
Ginkgo leaf extract	Anticoagulants (P) Antiplatelet (P) Anticonvulsants (I)
Glucosamine	Antidiabetic drugs (I)
Panax ginseng	Anticoagulants (P) Diabetic agents (possible P) Nifedipine (P)
Saw palmetto	Hormone replacement therapies (P)
Soy	Estrogenic drugs (P)
St. John's wort	Antidepressants (P) HIV protease inhibitors (I) Cyclosporine (I)
Valerian	Sedatives (P)
Yohimbe	Antihypertensives (I)

I = interferes; P = potentiates.

Patients taking aspirin, warfarin, ticlopidine, clopidogrel, or dipyridamole should not take ginkgo biloba because bleeding may occur. Patients taking an antidepressant should not take St. John's wort. Patients taking a decongestant, a stimulant drug, or who drink caffeinated beverages should not take ephedra. Individuals taking a benzodiazepine, a barbiturate, an antipsychotic medication, or any medicine used to treat Parkinson's disease should not take kava kava products. It is important that patients notify their general practitioner if they are taking phytomedicines concurrently with conventional drugs, especially those with cardiac, diuretic, sedative, hypotensive or other properties. Individuals taking a prescription medicine should check with their physician before taking any herbal health product.

Dental Implications

A limited number of papers describe the use of complementary and alternative medical systems for dental problems. Dentists should accept and encompass science-based advances and reject unproved or disproved methods. Selected unconventional treatments can be incorporated into conventional dentistry in certain patients for specific purposes that will be beneficial to the patient.

Information for Dentists

Herbal remedies have the potential to affect on the safety of invasive or prolonged dental procedures. Excessive bleeding can occur with some of these medications. Other herbal medicines may affect the cardiovascular system and render the patient more susceptible to cardiac arrhythmias and other cardiovascular complications. Ginseng may cause hypoglycemia. Chinese cancer patients undergoing chemotherapy who were users of Chinese herbal medicine were found to have higher scores of mucositis. It is important for the dentist to include a section in the patient's medical history on the consumption of herbal medications and over-the-counter drugs. Because most U.S. dental schools teach very little on the use, side effects, toxicity, and drug interactions associated with herbal remedies, the dentist must find a way to become informed regarding these issues.

Important references for dentists are Mosby's Medical Drug Reference 2007, by Allan J. Ellsworth, and Natural Standard Herb and Supplement Reference, Mosby, 2005. Dentists should use only treatment procedures that have been established to be effective and with minimal risks involved. As clinical trials demonstrate certain alternative and complementary treatments to be effective and safe, they can be incorporated into conventional medicine and dentistry. The dentist may find a medically compromised patient is taking an herbal remedy that is potentially harmful. This should be discussed with the patient and the patient referred to his or her physician for evaluation and management.

Sources for Major Topics Covered in Parts I and II

1. ADA: ADA guide to dental therapeutics, ed 3, Chicago, 2003, ADA Publishing Division.
2. ADA and AAOS: Advisory statement for dental patients with total joint replacements, JADA 128:1004, 1997.
3. American Heart Association Science Advisory, Prevention of premature discontinuation of dual antiplatelet therapy in patients with coronary artery stents. *Circulation* 2007;115(6):813–818.
4. Baddour LM, et al: AHA scientific statement: nonvalvular cardiovascular device-related infections, Circulation 108:2015, 2003.
5. Jeske AH, Suchko GD. Lack of a scientific basis for routine discontinuation of anticoagulant therapy prior to dental therapy. *JADA* 2003;134:1492–1497.
6. Little JW: Behavioral and psychiatric disorders. In Little JW, Falace DA, Miller CS, Rhodus NL. editors: Dental management of the medically compromised patient, ed 6, St. Louis, 2002, Mosby.
7. Little, JW: Anxiety disorders: dental implications, J Gen Dent 51:562–570, 2003.
8. Little JW: Dental implication of mood disorders, J Gen Dent 52:442, 2004.
9. Little JW: Complementary and alternative medicine: impact on dentistry, Oral Surg Oral Med Oral Path Oral Radiol Endod 98:137, 2004.
10. Little JW: Drugs, drugs, and more drugs: their impact on dentistry, J Northwest Dent July-August:23, 2005.

11. Little JW, et al: Antithrombotic agents: implications in dentistry, Oral Surg Oral Med Oral Path Oral Radiol Endod 93:544, 2002.

12. Miller CS: Drug interactions of significance to dentistry. In Little JW, Falace DA, Miller CS, Rhodus NL, editors: Dental management of the medically compromised patient, ed 6, St. Louis, 2002, Mosby.

13. Miller CS, Little JW, Falace DA: Need of supplemental corticosteroids for dental patients with adrenal insufficiency: reconsideration of the problem, JADA 132:1570, 2001.

14. Rhodus NL: Therapeutic management of common oral lesions. In Little JW, Falace DA, Miller CS, Rhodus NL, editors: Dental management of the medically compromised patient, ed 6, St. Louis, 2002, Mosby.

15. Ruggiero S, Gralow J, Marx RE et al. Practice guidelines for the prevention, diagnosis and treatment of osteonecrosis of the jaw in patients with cancer. *J. Oncol. Prac.* 2006;2(1):7–14.

16. Siegel MA, Silverman S, Sollecato TP, editors: American Academy of Oral Medicine: clinician's guide to treatment of common oral conditions, ed 6, Baltimore, 2005, B.C. Decker.

17. Wilson, W, Taubert KA, Gewitz M, Lockhart PB, Baddour LM et al. Prevention of infective endocarditis. Guidelines from the American Heart Association. *Circulation* 2007;April 23.

abacavir
ah-bah´-cah-veer
(Ziagen)

CATEGORY AND SCHEDULE
Pregnancy Risk Category: C

Drug Class: Antiviral, nucleoside analog

MECHANISM OF ACTION
An antiretroviral that inhibits the activity of HIV-1 reverse transcriptase by competing with the natural substrate deoxyguanosine-5´-triphosphate (dGTP) and by its incorporation into viral DNA. *Therapeutic Effect:* Inhibits viral DNA growth.

USES
Used in combination with other antiviral drugs for treatment of HIV-1 infection

PHARMACOKINETICS
Rapidly and extensively absorbed after PO administration. Protein binding: 50%. Widely distributed, including to CSF and erythrocytes. Metabolized in the liver to inactive metabolites. Primarily excreted in urine. Unknown if removed by hemodialysis. *Half-life:* 1.5 hr.

INDICATIONS AND DOSAGES
▶ **HIV Infection (in combination with other antiretrovirals)**
PO
Adults. 300 mg twice a day.
Children (3 mo–16 yr). 8 mg/kg twice a day. Maximum: 300 mg twice a day.
▶ **Dosage in Hepatic Impairment**
Mild impairment: 200 mg twice a day.

Moderate to severe impairment: Not recommended.

SIDE EFFECTS/ADVERSE REACTIONS
Adults
Frequent
Nausea, nausea with vomiting, diarrhea, decreased appetite
Occasional
Insomnia

Children
Frequent
Nausea with vomiting, fever, headache, diarrhea, rash
Occasional
Decreased appetite

PRECAUTIONS AND CONTRAINDICATIONS
Hypersensitivity to abacavir or its components
Caution
Breast-feeding, bone marrow depression, renal or hepatic impairment, use with other antivirals to avoid emergence of resistant viruses, avoid alcohol use

DRUG INTERACTIONS OF CONCERN TO DENTISTRY
None reported

SERIOUS REACTIONS
! A hypersensitivity reaction may be life threatening. Signs and symptoms include fever, rash, fatigue, intractable nausea and vomiting, severe diarrhea, abdominal pain, cough, pharyngitis, and dyspnea.
! Life-threatening hypotension may occur.
! Lactic acidosis and severe hepatomegaly may occur.

DENTAL CONSIDERATIONS
General:
• Examine for oral manifestation of opportunistic infection.
• Patient on chronic drug therapy may rarely have symptoms of blood dyscrasias, which include infection, bleeding, and poor healing.
• Avoid dental light in patient's eyes; offer dark glasses for patient comfort.
• Place on frequent recall because of oral side effects.
• Consider semisupine chair position for patient comfort if GI side effects occur.
Consultations:
• In a patient with symptoms of blood dyscrasias, request a medical consultation for blood studies and postpone treatment until normal values are reestablished.
• Medical consultation may be required to assess disease control.
Teach Patient/Family to:
• Use effective oral hygiene to prevent soft tissue inflammation
• Prevent trauma when using oral hygiene aids
• Be alert for the possibility of secondary oral infection and the need to see dentist immediately if signs of infection occur

abarelix
ah-bar´-eh-lex
(Plenaxis)

CATEGORY AND SCHEDULE
Pregnancy Risk Category: X

Drug Class: Antineoplastics

MECHANISM OF ACTION
A luteinizing hormone-releasing hormone (LHRH) antagonist that inhibits gonadotropin and androgen production by blocking gonadotropin releasing-hormone receptors in the pituitary. **Therapeutic Effect:** Suppresses luteinizing hormone, follicle-stimulating hormone secretion, reducing the secretion of testosterone by the testes.

USES
Treatment of cancer of the breasts, endometrium, and prostate

PHARMACOKINETICS
Slowly absorbed following intramuscular administration. Distributed extensively. Protein binding: 96%–99%. **Half-life:** 13.2 days.

INDICATIONS AND DOSAGES
▸ **Prostate Cancer**
IM
Adults, Elderly. 100 mg on days 1, 15, 29 and every 4 wk thereafter. Treatment failure can be detected by obtaining serum testosterone concentration prior to abarelix administration, day 19 and every 8 wk thereafter.

SIDE EFFECTS/ADVERSE REACTIONS
Frequent
Hot flashes, sleep disturbances, breast enlargement
Occasional
Breast pain, nipple tenderness, back pain, constipation, peripheral edema, dizziness, upper respiratory tract infection, diarrhea
Rare
Fatigue, nausea, dysuria, micturition frequency, urinary retention, UTI

PRECAUTIONS AND CONTRAINDICATIONS
This drug should not be used in women and children.

DRUG INTERACTIONS OF CONCERN TO DENTISTRY

Dental drug interactions have not been studied.

SERIOUS REACTIONS

! Immediate-onset systemic allergic reaction characterized by hypotension, urticaria, pruritus, periorbital and/or circumoral edema, shortness of breath, wheezing, and syncope may occur.

! Prolongation of the QT interval may occur. Tightening of throat, tongue swelling, wheezing, shortness of breath, and low blood pressure occur rarely.

DENTAL CONSIDERATIONS

General:

• If additional analgesia is required for dental pain, consider alternative analgesics (NSAIDs) in patients taking narcotics for acute or chronic pain.

• This drug may be used in the hospital or on an outpatient basis. Confirm the patient's disease and treatment status.

Consultations:

• Medical consultation may be required to assess disease control and patient's ability to tolerate stress.

Teach Patient/Family to:

• Use effective oral hygiene to prevent soft tissue inflammation

• Prevent trauma when using oral hygiene aids

• Update health and medication history if physician makes any changes in evaluation or drug regimens; include OTC, herbal, and nonherbal remedies in the update

abciximab

ab-six´-ih-mab
(c7E3 Fab, ReoPro)

CATEGORY AND SCHEDULE

Pregnancy Risk Category: C

Drug Class: Glycoprotein IIb/IIIa receptor inhibitor

MECHANISM OF ACTION

A glycoprotein IIb/IIIa receptor inhibitor that rapidly inhibits platelet aggregation by preventing the binding of fibrinogen to GP IIb/IIIa receptor sites on platelets.

Therapeutic Effect: Prevents closure of treated coronary arteries. Prevents acute cardiac ischemic complications.

USES

Adjunct to aspirin and heparin therapy to prevent cardiac ischemic complications in patients undergoing percutaneous cornary intervention and those with unstable angina not responding to conventional medical therapy.

PHARMACOKINETICS

Rapidly cleared from plasma. Initial-phase half-life is less than 10 min; second-phase half-life is 30 min. Platelet function generally returns within 48 hr.

INDICATIONS AND DOSAGES

▶ Percutaneous Coronary Intervention (PCI)

IV Bolus

Adults. 0.25 mg/kg 10–60 min before angioplasty or atherectomy, then 12-hr IV infusion of 0.125 mcg/kg/min. Maximum: 10 mcg/min.

▶ **PCI (unstable angina)**
IV Bolus
Adults. 0.25 mg/kg, followed by
18- to 24-hr infusion of
10 mcg/min, ending 1 hr after
procedure.

SIDE EFFECTS/ADVERSE REACTIONS
Frequent
Nausea, hypotension
Occasional
Vomiting
Rare
Bradycardia, confusion, dizziness,
pain, peripheral edema, UTI

PRECAUTIONS AND CONTRAINDICATIONS
Active internal bleeding,
arteriovenous malformation or
aneurysm, cerebrovascular accident
(CVA) with residual neurologic
defect, history of CVA (within the
past 2 yr) or oral anticoagulant use
within the past 7 days unless PT is
less than 1.2 times control,
history of vasculitis, intracranial
neoplasm, prior IV dextran use
before or during PTCA, recent
surgery or trauma (within the past
6 wk), recent (within the past 6 wk
or less) GI or GU bleeding,
thrombocytopenia (less than
100,000 cells/mcl), and severe
uncontrolled hypertension.

DRUG INTERACTIONS OF CONCERN TO DENTISTRY
• Increased risk of bleeding: drugs
that interfere with coagulation or
platelet function, such as NSAIDs
and aspirin.

SERIOUS REACTIONS
❗ Major bleeding complications may
occur. If complications occur, stop
the infusion immediately.

❗ Hypersensitivity reaction may
occur.
❗ Atrial fibrillation or flutter,
pulmonary edema, and complete
atrioventricular block occur
occasionally.

DENTAL CONSIDERATIONS
General:
• Monitor vital signs at every
appointment due to cardiovascular
side effects.
• For use in hospitals or emergency
rooms.
• Review patient's medical and drug
history.
• Provide palliative emergency
dental care only during drug use.
• Patients may be at risk of bleeding,
check for oral signs.
Consultations:
• Medical consultation may be
required to assess disease control
and patient's ability to tolerate
stress.
• Medical consultation should
include routine blood counts
including platelet counts and
bleeding time.
• Avoid products that affect platelet
function, such as aspirin and
NSAIDs.
Teach Patient/Family to:
• Use effective oral hygiene to
prevent soft tissue inflammation
• Prevent trauma when using oral
hygiene aids
• Report oral lesions, soreness, or
bleeding to dentist
• Update health and medication
history if physician makes any
changes in evaluation
or drug regimens; include OTC,
herbal, and nonherbal remedies in
the update
• Use soft tooth brush to reduce risk
of bleeding

absorbable gelatin sponge
(Gelfoam)

CATEGORY AND SCHEDULE
Hemostatic

Drug Class: Hemostatic, purified gelatin sponge

MECHANISM OF ACTION
Absorbs blood, provides area for clot formation

USES
Hemostasis adjunct in dental surgery

PHARMACOKINETICS
IMPLANT: Absorbed in 4–6 wk

INDICATIONS AND DOSAGES
▶ **Dental use**
Adult. Top can be applied dry or moistened with normal saline solution; blot on sterile gauze to remove excess solution, shape to fit with light finger compression; hold pressure until dry. Apply to bleeding surfaces. Material may be cut to appropriate size or secured in extraction sites with sutures.

SIDE EFFECTS/ADVERSE REACTIONS
None reported.

PRECAUTIONS AND CONTRAINDICATIONS
Hypersensitivity, frank infection
Caution
Avoid use in presence of infection, potential nidus of infection, do not resterilize product.

DENTAL CONSIDERATIONS
Teach Patient/Family to:
• Immediately report any sign of infection to the dentist

acamprosate calcium
(ah-kam-PROE-sate)
(Campral)

CATEGORY AND SCHEDULE
Pregnancy Risk Category: C

Drug Class: Alcohol-abuse deterrent

MECHANISMS OF ACTIONS
Actual mechanism unknown, may facilitate balance between GABA and glutamate neurotransmitter systems in the CNS to decrease alcohol craving

USES
Alcohol-abuse deterrent

PHARMACOKINETICS
Partially absorbed from GI tract, steady-state levels reached within 5 days of dosing; Protein binding negligible. *Half-life:* 20-33 hr. Does not undergo metabolism, excreted unchanged in urine.

INDICATIONS AND DOSAGES
▶ **Maintenance of Alcohol Abstinence**
PO
Adult. 666 mg 3 times a day with or without food.

SIDE EFFECTS/ADVERSE REACTIONS
ORAL: Dry mouth

CNS: Headache, somnolence, decreased libido, amnesia, abnormal thinking, tremor
CV: Palpitation, syncope, vasodilation, changes in B/P
GI: Vomiting, dyspepsia, constipation, increased appetite
RESP: Rhinitis, cough, dyspnea, pharyngitis, bronchitis
GU: Impotence
EENT: Abnormal vision, taste alterations
INTEG: Rash
MS: Myalgia, arthralgia
SYST: Back pain, infection, flu syndrome, chest pain, chills, attempts at suicide
(see Precautions)

PRECAUTIONS AND CONTRAINDICATIONS
Hypersensitivity, severe renal impairment
Caution
Renal impairment, depression/suicidal tendency

DRUG INTERACTIONS OF CONCERN TO DENTISTRY
None reported

DENTAL CONSIDERATIONS
General:
• Assess salivary flow as a factor in caries, periodontal disease, and candidiasis
• After supine positioning, allow patient to sit upright for 2 min to avoid orthostatic hypotension
• Avoid alcohol-containing products (elixirs, mouth rinses) to assist maintenance of alcohol abstinence
Consultations:
• Consult physician to assess disease control

Teach Patient/Family to:
• Use effective oral hygiene to prevent caries and periodontal disease
• Use sugarless gum, frequent sips of water, and saliva substitutes if dry mouth occurs
• Use home fluoride products for anticaries effect
• Avoid mouth rinses with high alcohol content because of drying effects

acarbose
ah-car´-bose
(Glucobay[AUS], Prandase[CAN], Precose)
Do not confuse Precose with PreCare.

CATEGORY AND SCHEDULE
Pregnancy Risk Category: B

Drug Class: Oral antidiabetic

MECHANISM OF ACTION
An alpha glucosidase inhibitor that delays glucose absorption and digestion of carbohydrates, resulting in a smaller rise in blood glucose concentration after meals.
Therapeutic Effect: Lowers postprandial hyperglycemia.

USES
Use as single drug or in combination with insulin or oral hypoglycemics (sulfonylureas, metformin) in type 2 diabetes (non–insulin-dependent diabetes mellitus [NIDDM]) when diet control is ineffective in controlling blood glucose levels

PHARMACOKINETICS
PO: Limited oral absorption, absorbed dose excreted in urine,

metabolized in the GI tract and major portion of dose excreted in feces

INDICATIONS AND DOSAGES
▶ **Diabetes Mellitus**
PO
Adults, Elderly. Initially, 25 mg 3 times a day with first bite of each main meal. Increase at 4- to 8-wk intervals. Maximum: For patients weighing more than 60 kg, 100 mg 3 times a day; for patients weighing 60 kg or less, 50 mg 3 times a day.

SIDE EFFECTS/ADVERSE REACTIONS
Side effects diminish in frequency and intensity over time.
Frequent
Transient GI disturbances: flatulence, diarrhea, abdominal pain

PRECAUTIONS AND CONTRAINDICATIONS
Chronic intestinal diseases associated with marked disorders of digestion or absorption, cirrhosis, colonic ulceration, conditions that may deteriorate as a result of increased gas formation in the intestine, diabetic ketoacidosis, hypersensitivity to acarbose, inflammatory bowel disease, partial intestinal obstruction or predisposition to intestinal obstruction, significant renal dysfunction (serum creatinine level greater than 2 mg/dl)
Caution
Use glucose for hypoglycemia, monitor blood glucose levels, pregnancy category B, avoid use in lactation, children.

DRUG INTERACTIONS OF CONCERN TO DENTISTRY
None reported

SERIOUS REACTIONS
None known.

DENTAL CONSIDERATIONS
General:
• Ensure that patient is following prescribed diet and takes medication regularly.
• Type 2 patients may also be using insulin. If symptomatic hypoglycemia occurs while taking this drug, use dextrose rather than sucrose because of interference with sucrose metabolism.
• Place on frequent recall to evaluate healing response.
• Patients with diabetes may be more susceptible to infection and have delayed wound healing.
• Question the patient about self-monitoring the drug's antidiabetic effect.
• Consider semisupine chair position for patient comfort if GI side effects occur.
Consultations:
• Medical consultation may be required to assess disease control and patient's ability to tolerate stress.
Teach Patient/Family to:
• Use effective oral hygiene to prevent soft tissue inflammation

acetaminophen
ah-seet´-ah-min-oh-fen
(Abenol[CAN], Apo-Acetaminophen[CAN], Atasol[CAN], Dymadon[AUS], Feverall, Panadol[AUS], Panamax[AUS], Paralgin[AUS], Setamol[AUS], Tempra, Tylenol)
Do not confuse with Fiorinal, Hycodan, Indocin, Percodan, or Tuinal.

CATEGORY AND SCHEDULE
Pregnancy Risk Category: B

Drug Class: Nonnarcotic analgesic

MECHANISM OF ACTION

A central analgesic whose exact mechanism is unknown, but appears to inhibit prostaglandin synthesis in the CNS and, to a lesser extent, block pain impulses through peripheral action. Acetaminophen acts centrally on hypothalamic heat-regulating center, producing peripheral vasodilation (heat loss, skin erythema, sweating). *Therapeutic Effect:* Results in antipyresis. Produces analgesic effect. Results in antipyresis.

USES

Mild-to-moderate pain, fever; also used in combination with other ingredients, including opioids

PHARMACOKINETICS

Route	Onset	Peak	Duration
PO	15–30 mins	1–1.5 hr	4–6 hr

Rapidly, completely absorbed from GI tract; rectal absorption variable. Protein binding: 20%–50%. Widely distributed to most body tissues. Metabolized in liver; excreted in urine. Removed by hemodialysis. *Half-life:* 1–4 hr (half-life is increased in those with liver disease, elderly, neonates; decreased in children).

INDICATIONS AND DOSAGES

▶ **Analgesia and Antipyresis**

PO

Adults, Elderly. 325–650 mg q4–6h or 1 g 3–4 times a day. Maximum: 4 g/day.
Children. 10–15 mg/kg/dose q4–6h as needed. Maximum: 5 doses/24 hr.
Neonates. 10–15 mg/kg/dose q6–8h as needed.

Rectal
Adults. 650 mg q4–6h. Maximum: 6 doses/24 hr.
Children. 10–20 mg/kg/dose q4–6h as needed.
Neonates. 10–15 mg/kg/dose q6–8h as needed.
Dosage in Renal Impairment

Creatinine Clearance	Frequency
10–50 ml/min	q6h
Less than 10 ml/min	q8h

SIDE EFFECTS/ADVERSE REACTIONS

Rare
Hypersensitivity reaction

PRECAUTIONS AND CONTRAINDICATIONS

Active alcoholism, liver disease, or viral hepatitis, all of which increase the risk of hepatotoxicity
Caution
Anemia, hepatic disease, renal disease, chronic alcoholism

DRUG INTERACTIONS OF CONCERN TO DENTISTRY

• Decreased effects: barbiturates, oral contraceptives, loop diuretics
• Nephrotoxicity: NSAIDs, salicylates (chronic, high-dose, concurrent use)
• Liver toxicity: chronic use of hydantoins, chronic alcohol use, high-dose carbamazepine
• Possible increased effects of zidovudine
• Possible increased effects of acetaminophen: β-blockers, probenecid
• Increased bleeding: warfarin

SERIOUS REACTIONS
! Acetaminophen toxicity is the primary serious reaction.
! Early signs and symptoms of acetaminophen toxicity include anorexia, nausea, diaphoresis, and generalized weakness within the first 12–24 hr.
! Later signs of acetaminophen toxicity include vomiting, right upper quadrant tenderness, and elevated liver function tests within 48–72 hr after ingestion.
! The antidote to acetaminophen toxicity is acetylcysteine (Mucomyst), but it should be administered as soon as possible following toxic dose.

DENTAL CONSIDERATIONS
General:
• Reports regarding the concomitant use of acetaminophen and warfarin seem to suggest a possible increase in anticoagulant effects, especially in patients with other diseases or contributing factors, diarrhea, age, debilitation, etc. Patients taking warfarin should be questioned about recent use of acetaminophen and current international normalized ratio (INR) values. Acetaminophen has been shown to increase the INR depending on the amount and duration of acetaminophen use. A new PT or INR value may be required if surgical procedures are planned. Data from one study (JAMA 279:657–662, 1998) indicated that use of four regular-strength acetaminophen tablets (325 mg) qd for 1 wk can increase the INR values. It is important to closely monitor INR values with use of acetaminophen over a long duration and in higher doses.
• Avoid prolonged use with aspirin-containing products or NSAIDs.
• Determine why the patient is taking the drug.

• Patients on chronic drug therapy may rarely have symptoms of blood dyscrasias, which can include infection, bleeding, and poor healing.
• Question patient about the use of other drug products, including OTC products, that contain acetaminophen because of risk of acetaminophen overdose
Consultations:
• For a patient with symptoms of blood dyscrasias, request a medical consult for blood studies and postpone dental treatment until normal values are reestablished.

acetazolamide
ah-seet-ah-zole'-ah-mide
(Apo-Acetazolamide[CAN], Dazamide, Diamox, Diamox Sequels)
Do not confuse with acetohexamide.

CATEGORY AND SCHEDULE
Pregnancy Risk Category: C

Drug Class: Diuretic, carbonic anhydrase inhibitor

MECHANISM OF ACTION
A carbonic anhydrase inhibitor that reduces formation of hydrogen and bicarbonate ions from carbon dioxide and water by inhibiting, in proximal renal tubule, the enzyme carbonic anhydrase, thereby promoting renal excretion of sodium, potassium, bicarbonate, water. Ocular: Reduces rate of aqueous humor formation, lowers intraocular pressure.
Therapeutic Effect: Produces anticonvulsant activity.

A

USES

Treatment of open-angle glaucoma, narrow-angle glaucoma (preoperatively, if surgery delayed), epilepsy (petit mal, grand mal, mixed), edema in CHF, drug-induced edema, acute mountain sickness in climbers, drug-induced edema

PHARMACOKINETICS

Rapidly absorbed. Protein binding: 95%. Widely distributed throughout body tissues including erythrocytes, kidneys, and blood-brain barrier. Not metabolized. Excreted unchanged in urine. Removed by hemodialysis.
Half-life: 2.4–5.8 hr.

INDICATIONS AND DOSAGES

▸ **Glaucoma**
PO
Adults. 250 mg 1–4 times a day.
Extended-Release: 500 mg 1–2 times a day usually given in morning and evening.
▸ **Secondary Glaucoma, Preoperative Treatment of Acute Congestive Glaucoma**
PO/IV
Adults. 250 mg q4h, 250 mg q12h; or 500 mg, then 125–250 mg q4h.
PO
Children. 10–15 mg/kg/day in divided doses.
IV
Children. 5–10 mg/kg q6h.
▸ **Edema**
IV
Adults. 25–375 mg once daily.
Children. 5 mg/kg or 150 mg/m^2 once daily.
▸ **Epilepsy**
PO
Adults, Children. 375–1000 mg/day in 1–4 divided doses.
▸ **Acute Mountain Sickness**
PO
Adults. 500–1000 mg/day in divided doses. If possible, begin 24–48 hr before ascent; continue at least 48 hr at high altitude.
▸ **Usual Elderly Dosage**
PO
Initially, 250 mg 2 times a day; use lowest effective dose.
▸ **Dosage in Renal Impairment**

Creatinine Clearance	Dosage Interval
10–50 ml/min	q12h
Less than 10 ml/min	Avoid use

SIDE EFFECTS/ADVERSE REACTIONS

Frequent
Unusually tired/weak, diarrhea, increased urination/frequency, decreased appetite/weight, altered taste (metallic), nausea, vomiting, numbness in extremities, lips, mouth
Occasional
Depression, drowsiness
Rare
Headache, photosensitivity, confusion, tinnitus, severe muscle weakness, loss of taste

PRECAUTIONS AND CONTRAINDICATIONS

Severe renal disease, adrenal insufficiency, hypochloremic acidosis, hypersensitivity to acetazolamide, to any component of the formulation, or to sulfonamides
Caution
Hypercalciuria, chronic use of oral sulfonylureas has been associated with increased risk of cardiovascular mortality; risk is controversial.

DRUG INTERACTIONS OF CONCERN TO DENTISTRY

• Toxicity: salicylates (large doses)
• Hypokalemia: corticosteroids (systemic use)
• Crystalluria: ciprofloxacin

SERIOUS REACTIONS

! Long-term therapy may result in acidotic state.

! Nephrotoxicity/hepatotoxicity occurs occasionally, manifested as dark urine/stools, pain in lower back, jaundice, dysuria, crystalluria, renal colic/calculi.

! Bone marrow depression may be manifested as aplastic anemia, thrombocytopenia, thrombocytopenic purpura, leukopenia, agranulocytosis, hemolytic anemia.

DENTAL CONSIDERATIONS

General:
• Patients on chronic drug therapy may rarely have symptoms of blood dyscrasias, which can include infection, bleeding, and poor healing.
• Assess salivary flow as a factor in caries, periodontal disease, and candidiasis.
• Avoid drugs that may exacerbate glaucoma (e.g., anticholinergics).
Consultations:
• In a patient with symptoms of blood dyscrasias, request a medical consultation for blood studies and postpone dental treatment until normal values are reestablished.
• Consultation may be required to assess disease control.
Teach Patient/Family to:
• Use effective oral hygiene to prevent soft tissue inflammation
• Prevent injury when using oral hygiene aids
• When chronic dry mouth occurs, advise patient to:
  • Avoid mouth rinses with high alcohol content because of drying effects
  • Use daily home fluoride products for anticaries effect
  • Use sugarless gum, frequent sips of water, or saliva substitutes

acetohexamide
ah-seet-oh-hex´-ah-mide
(Dymelor)
Do not confuse with acetazolamide.

CATEGORY AND SCHEDULE
Pregnancy Risk Category: D

Drug Class: Sulfonylurea (first generation), antidiabetic

MECHANISM OF ACTION
An intermediate-acting sulfonylurea that promotes the release of insulin from beta cells of pancreas, increases insulin sensitivity at peripheral sites. *Therapeutic Effect:* Lowers blood glucose concentration.

USES
Treatment of stable adult-onset diabetes mellitus (type 2)

PHARMACOKINETICS
Well absorbed from the GI tract. Protein binding: 65%–90%. Metabolized in liver. Excreted in urine. Not removed by hemodialysis. *Half-life:* 1.3 hr.

INDICATIONS AND DOSAGES
▶ Diabetes Mellitus
PO
Adults, Elderly. Initially, 250 mg/day. Adjust dosage in 250- to 500-mg increments at intervals of 5–7 days. Maximum daily dose: 1.5 g. Elderly patients may be more sensitive and should be started at a lower dosage initially.

SIDE EFFECTS/ADVERSE REACTIONS
Frequent
Altered taste sensation, dizziness, drowsiness, weight gain, constipation, diarrhea, heartburn,

nausea, vomiting, stomach fullness, headache.
Occasional
Increased sensitivity of skin to sunlight, peeling of skin, itching, rash.

PRECAUTIONS AND CONTRAINDICATIONS

Diabetic ketoacidosis with or without coma, Type 1 diabetes mellitus, hypersensitivity to acetohexamide or any component of the formulation
Caution
Elderly, cardiac disease, renal disease, hepatic disease, thyroid disease, severe hypoglycemic reactions

DRUG INTERACTIONS OF CONCERN TO DENTISTRY

- Increased hypoglycemic effects: salicylates (large doses)
- Decreased action: corticosteroids
- Disulfiram-like reaction: alcohol

SERIOUS REACTIONS

! Hypoglycemia may occur because of overdosage or insufficient food intake, especially with increased glucose demands.
! GI hemorrhage, cholestatic hepatic jaundice, leukopenia, thrombocytopenia, pancytopenia, agranulocytosis, aplastic or hemolytic anemia occurs rarely.

DENTAL CONSIDERATIONS

General:
- Monitor vital signs at every appointment because of cardiovascular effects of diabetes.
- Patients on chronic drug therapy may rarely have symptoms of blood dyscrasias, which can include infection, bleeding, and poor healing.
- Place on frequent recall to evaluate healing response.

- Ensure that patient is following prescribed diet and takes medication regularly.
- Question patient about self-monitoring of drug's antidiabetic effect, including self-monitored blood glucose (SMBG) values or finger-stick records.
- Avoid prescribing aspirin-containing products.
- Early-morning appointments and a stress reduction protocol may be required for anxious patients.
- Patients with diabetes may be more susceptible to infection and have delayed wound healing.
Consultations:
- In a patient with symptoms of blood dyscrasias, request a medical consultation for blood studies and postpone dental treatment until normal values are reestablished.
- Medical consultation may include data from patient's blood glucose monitoring, including glycosylated hemoglobin or hemoglobin A1c (HbA1c) testing.
Teach Patient/Family to:
- Use effective oral hygiene to prevent soft tissue inflammation
- Prevent injury when using oral hygiene aids
- Avoid mouth rinses with high alcohol content

acetylcholine chloride

ah-seh-teel-koe′-leen
(Miochol-E, Miochol-E/Steri-Tags, Miochol-E System Pak)

CATEGORY AND SCHEDULE

Pregnancy Risk Category: C

Drug Class: Cholinergics

MECHANISM OF ACTION
A cholinergic agonist that causes contraction of the sphincter muscles of the iris. *Therapeutic Effect:* Results in miosis and contraction of ciliary muscle, leading to accommodation spasm.

USES
To produce miosis for selected types of eye surgery.

PHARMACOKINETICS
Rapid miosis of short duration.

INDICATIONS AND DOSAGES
▶ Production of Miosis
Intraocular
Adults, Elderly. 0.5–2 ml instilled into anterior chamber before or after securing one or more sutures.

SIDE EFFECTS/ADVERSE REACTIONS
Rare
Corneal clouding, corneal decompensation

PRECAUTIONS AND CONTRAINDICATIONS
Acute iritis and acute inflammatory disease of the anterior chamber, hypersensitivity to acetylcholine chloride or any component of the formulation

DRUG INTERACTIONS OF CONCERN TO DENTISTRY
None reported

SERIOUS REACTIONS
❗ Systemic effects rarely occur. These effects include bradycardia, hypotension, flushing, breathing difficulties, and sweating.

General:
• Acute-use drug in selected types of eye surgery.
• Avoid dental light in patient's eyes; offer dark glasses for patient comfort.

acetylcysteine
ah-see-til-sis´-tay-een
(Acetadote, Mucomyst, Parvolex[CAN])
Do not confuse acetylcysteine with acetylcholine.

CATEGORY AND SCHEDULE
Pregnancy Risk Category: B

Drug Class: Antidotes; Mucolytics

MECHANISM OF ACTION
An intratracheal respiratory inhalant that splits the linkage of mucoproteins, reducing the viscosity of pulmonary secretions. *Therapeutic Effect:* Facilitates the removal of pulmonary secretions by coughing, postural drainage, mechanical means. Protects against acetaminophen overdose-induced hepatotoxicity.

USES
Adjuvant therapy for patients with abnormal, viscid, or inspissated mucous secretions

PHARMACOKINETICS
INH/INSTILL: Onset 1 min, duration 5–10 min, metabolized by liver, excreted in urine. *Half-life:* 5.6 hr (adult); 11 hr (newborn).

INDICATIONS AND DOSAGES

▶ **Adjunctive Treatment of Viscid Mucus Secretions from Chronic Bronchopulmonary Disease and for Pulmonary Complications of Cystic Fibrosis**

Nebulization

Adults, Elderly, Children. 3–5 ml (20% solution) 3–4 times a day or 6–10 ml (10% solution) 3–4 times a day. Range: 1–10 ml (20% solution) q2–6h or 2–20 ml (10% solution) q2–6h.

Infants. 1–2 ml (20%) or 2–4 ml (10%) 3–4 times a day.

▶ **Treatment of Viscid Mucus Secretions in Patients with a Tracheostomy**

Intratracheal

Adults, Children. 1–2 ml of 10% or 20% solution instilled into tracheostomy q1–4h.

▶ **Acetaminophen Overdose**

PO (Oral solution 5%)

Adults, Elderly, Children. Loading dose of 140 mg/kg, followed in 4 hr by maintenance dose of 70 mg/kg q4h for 17 additional doses (unless acetaminophen assay reveals nontoxic level).

IV

Adults, Elderly, Children. 150 mg/kg infused over 15 min, then 50 mg/kg infused over 4 hr, then 100 mg/kg infused over 16 hr. See administration and handling. Repeat dose if emesis occurs within 1 hr of administration. Continue until all doses are given, even if acetaminophen plasma level drops below toxic range.

▶ **Prevention of Renal Damage from Dyes Used During Certain Diagnostic Tests**

PO (Oral solution 5%)

Adults, Elderly. 600 mg twice a day for 4 doses starting the day before the procedure.

SIDE EFFECTS/ADVERSE REACTIONS

Frequent

Inhalation: Stickiness on face, transient unpleasant odor

Occasional

Inhalation: Increased bronchial secretions, throat irritation, nausea, vomiting, rhinorrhea

Rare

Inhalation: Rash

PRECAUTIONS AND CONTRAINDICATIONS

None known

DRUG INTERACTIONS OF CONCERN TO DENTISTRY

None reported

SERIOUS REACTIONS

! Large doses may produce severe nausea and vomiting.

DENTAL CONSIDERATIONS

General:

• Be aware that aspirin and/or sulfite preservatives in vasoconstrictor-containing products may exacerbate asthma.

• Acute asthmatic episodes may be precipitated in the dental office. A rapid-acting sympathomimetic inhalant (rescue inhaler) should be available for emergency use. Many patients may already have a prescribed rescue inhaler they normally use for acute asthmatic events.

• Consider semisupine chair position for patients with respiratory disease.

• Determine dose and duration of glucocorticoid therapy to assess for risk of stress tolerance and immunosuppression. Patients on chronic glucocorticoid therapy may require supplemental doses for dental treatment.

• Examine for oral manifestation of opportunistic infection.
• Evaluate respiration characteristics and rate.
• Short appointments and a stress reduction protocol may be required for anxious patients.
• Inquire about other drugs patients are using for respiratory disease.
Consultations:
• Consultation with physician may be necessary if sedation or general anesthesia is required.
• Consultation may be required to confirm glucocorticoid dose and duration of use.
• Medical consultation may be required to assess disease control and patient's ability to tolerate stress
Teach Patient/Family to:
• Use effective oral hygiene to prevent soft tissue inflammation
• Update health and medication history if physician makes any changes in evaluation or drug regimens; include OTC, herbal, and nonherbal remedies in the update
• Gargle, rinse mouth with water, and expectorate after each aerosol dose

acitretin
ah-sih-tre´-tin
(Soriatane)

CATEGORY AND SCHEDULE
Pregnancy Risk Category: X

Drug Class: Systemic retinoid

MECHANISM OF ACTION
A second-generation retinoid that adjusts factors influencing epidermal proliferation, RNA/DNA synthesis, controls glycoprotein, and governs immune response.

Therapeutic Effect: Regulates keratinocyte growth and differentiation.

USES
Severe psoriasis; unlabeled uses: nonpsoriatic dermatoses, keratinization disorders, palmoplantar keratoses, lichen planus, Darier's disease, Sjögren-Larrson syndrome; should be prescribed only by physicians knowledgeable in the use of systemic retinoids

PHARMACOKINETICS
Well absorbed from the GI tract. Food increases rate of absorption. Protein binding: greater than 99%. Metabolized in liver. Excreted in bile and urine. Not removed by hemodialysis.
Half-life: 49 hr.

INDICATIONS AND DOSAGES
▶ **Psoriasis**
PO
Adults, Elderly. 25–50 mg/day as a single dose with main meal. May increase to 75 mg/day if necessary and dose tolerated. Maintenance: 25–50 mg/day after the initial response is noted. Continue until lesions have resolved.

SIDE EFFECTS/ADVERSE REACTIONS
Frequent
Lip inflammation, alopecia, skin peeling, shakiness, dry eyes, rash, hyperesthesia, paresthesia, sticky skin, dry mouth, epistaxis, dryness/thickening of conjunctiva
Occasional
Eye irritation, brow and lash loss, sweating, chills, sensation of cold, flushing, edema, blurred vision, diarrhea, nausea, thirst

PRECAUTIONS AND CONTRAINDICATIONS

Women who are pregnant or those who intend to become pregnant within 3 yr following discontinuation of therapy; severely impaired liver or kidney function; chronic abnormal elevated lipid levels; concomitant use of methotrexate or tetracyclines, ingestion of alcohol (in females of reproductive potential); hypersensitivity to acitretin, etretinate, or other retinoids; sensitivity to parabenz (used as preservative in gelatin capsule)
Caution
Women are advised to use effective contraception during use and for 3 yr after use, renal impairment, lactation, hyperlipidemia, cardiovascular disease

DRUG INTERACTIONS OF CONCERN TO DENTISTRY

• Avoid vitamin preparations containing vitamin A
• Avoid tetracyclines and other drugs that cause photosensitivity

SERIOUS REACTIONS

! Benign intracranial hypertension (pseudotumor cerebri) occurs rarely.

DENTAL CONSIDERATIONS
General:
• Determine why patient is taking the drug.
• Apply lubricant to dry lips for patient comfort before dental procedures.
• Assess salivary flow as factor in caries, periodontal disease, and candidiasis.
• Palliative medication may be required for management of oral side effects.

• Place on frequent recall because of oral side effects.
• Consider semisupine chair position for patient comfort if GI side effects occur.
• Avoid dental light in patient's eyes; offer dark glasses for patient comfort.
Consultations:
• Medical consultation may be required to assess disease control.
Teach Patient/Family to:
• Use effective oral hygiene to prevent soft tissue inflammation
• Prevent trauma when using oral hygiene aids
• Report oral lesions, soreness, or bleeding to dentist
• When chronic dry mouth occurs, advise patient to:
  • Avoid mouth rinses with high alcohol content because of drying effects
  • Use daily home fluoride products for anticaries effect
  • Use sugarless gum, frequent sips of water, or saliva substitutes

acyclovir
ay-sye´-kloe-ver
(Aciclovir-BC IV[AUS], Acihexal[AUS], Acyclo-V[AUS], Avirax[CAN], Lovir[AUS], Zovirax, Zyclir[AUS])
Do not confuse with Zostrix, Zyvox.

CATEGORY AND SCHEDULE
Pregnancy Risk Category: B

Drug Class: Antiviral

MECHANISM OF ACTION
A synthetic nucleoside that converts to acyclovir triphosphate, becoming part of the DNA chain. *Therapeutic Effect:* Interferes with DNA synthesis and viral replication. Virustatic.

USES
Management of initial genital herpes and in limited non–life-threatening mucocutaneous herpes simplex infection in immunocompromised patients

PHARMACOKINETICS
Poorly absorbed from the GI tract; minimal absorption following topical application. Protein binding: 9%–36%. Widely distributed. Partially metabolized in liver. Excreted primarily in urine. Removed by hemodialysis. *Half-life:* 2.5 hr (increased in impaired renal function).

INDICATIONS AND DOSAGES
▶ **Genital Herpes (initial episode)**
IV
Adults, Elderly, Children 12 yr and older. 5 mg/kg q8h for 5 days.
PO
Adults, Elderly, Children 12 yr and older. 200 mg q4h 5 times a day.
▶ **Genital Herpes (recurrent)**
▶ **Fewer Than 6 Episodes Per Yr:**
PO
Adults, Elderly, Children 12 yr and older. 200 mg q4h 5 times a day for 5 days.
▶ **6 Episodes or More Per Yr:**
PO
Adults, Elderly, Children 12 yr and older. 400 mg 2 times a day or 200 mg 3–5 times a day for up to 12 mo.
▶ **Herpes Simplex Mucocutaneous**
IV
Adults, Elderly, Children 12 yr and older. 5 mg/kg/dose q8h for 7 days.

Children younger than 12 yr. 10 mg/kg q8h for 7 days.
▶ **Herpes Simplex Neonatal**
IV
Children younger than 4 mo. 10 mg/kg q8h for 10 days.
▶ **Herpes Simplex Encephalitis**
IV
Adults, Elderly, Children 12 yr and older. 10 mg/kg q8h for 10 days.
Children younger than 12 yr. 20 mg/kg q8h for 10 days.
▶ **Herpes Zoster (caused by varicella)**
IV
Adults, Elderly, Children 12 yr and older. 10 mg/kg q8h for 7 days.
Children younger than 12 yr. 20 mg/kg q8h for 7 days.
▶ **Herpes Zoster (shingles)**
PO
Adults, Elderly, Children 12 yr and older. 800 mg q4h 5 times a day for 7–10 days.
Topical
Adults, Elderly. Apply to affected area 3–6 times a day for 7 days.
▶ **Varicella (chickenpox)**
PO
Adults, Elderly, Children older than 12 yr or children 2–12 yr, weighing 40 kg or more. 800 mg 4 times a day for 5 days.
Children 2–12 yr, weighing less than 40 kg. 20 mg/kg 4 times a day for 5 days. Maximum: 800 mg/dose.
Children younger than 2 yr. 80 mg/kg/day.
▶ **Dosage in Renal Impairment**
Dosage and frequency are modified on the basis of severity of infection and degree of renal impairment.
PO
For creatinine clearance of 10 ml/min or less, dosage is 200 mg q12h.

IV

Creatinine Clearance	Dosage Percent	Dosage Interval
Greater 50 ml/min	100	8 hr
25–50 ml/min	100	12 hr
10–25 ml/min	100	24 hr
Less than 10 ml/min	50	24 hr

SIDE EFFECTS/ADVERSE REACTIONS

Frequent
Parenteral: Phlebitis or inflammation at IV site, nausea, vomiting
Topical: Burning, stinging
Occasional
Parenteral: Pruritus, rash, urticaria
Oral: Malaise, nausea
Topical: Pruritus
Rare
Oral: Vomiting, rash, diarrhea, headache
Parenteral: Confusion, hallucinations, seizures, tremors
Topical: Rash

PRECAUTIONS AND CONTRAINDICATIONS

Use in neonates when acyclovir is reconstituted with bacteriostatic water containing benzyl alcohol
Caution
Modify dose with acute or chronic renal impairment, safety of oral doses in pediatric patients less than 2 yr old not established, lactation, hepatic disease, renal disease, electrolyte imbalance, dehydration.

SERIOUS REACTIONS

! Rapid parenteral administration, excessively high doses, or fluid and electrolyte imbalance may produce renal failure exhibited by such signs and symptoms as abdominal pain, decreased urination, decreased appetite, increased thirst, nausea, and vomiting.
! Toxicity has not been reported with oral or topical use.

DENTAL CONSIDERATIONS

General:
• Postpone dental treatment when oral herpetic lesions are present.
Teach Patient/Family to:
• Dispose of toothbrush or other contaminated oral hygiene devices used during period of infection to prevent reinoculation of herpetic infection
• Apply with a finger cot or latex glove to prevent herpes infection on fingers
• Avoid mouth rinses with high alcohol content because of irritating effects

adalimumab
ah-dah-lim´-you-mab
(Humira)

CATEGORY AND SCHEDULE
Pregnancy Risk Category: B

Drug Class: Monoclonal antibody, antiinflammatory, immunosuppressant

MECHANISM OF ACTION

A monoclonal antibody that binds specifically to tumor necrosis factor (TNF) alpha, blocking its interaction with cell surface TNF receptors.

Therapeutic Effect: Reduces inflammation, tenderness, and swelling of joints; slows or prevents progressive destruction of joints in rheumatoid arthritis.

USES

Treatment of signs and symptoms and inhibition of structural damage in moderately to severely active rheumatoid arthritis in adults who have an inadequate response to one or more disease-modifying antirheumatic drugs (DMARDs)

PHARMACOKINETICS
Half-life: 10–20 days.

INDICATIONS AND DOSAGES
▶ **Rheumatoid Arthritis**
Subcutaneous
Adults, Elderly. 40 mg every other wk. Dose may be increased to 40 mg/wk in those not taking methotrexate.

SIDE EFFECTS/ADVERSE REACTIONS
Frequent
Injection site, erythema, pruritus, pain, and swelling
Occasional
Headache, rash, sinusitis, nausea
Rare
Abdominal or back pain, hypertension

PRECAUTIONS AND CONTRAINDICATIONS
Active infections
Caution
Appearance of new infection with use; risk of exacerbation of demyelinating diseases; risk of malignancies; risk of TB reactivation; lactation; elderly; safety and effectiveness in children not established

DRUG INTERACTIONS OF CONCERN TO DENTISTRY
None known

SERIOUS REACTIONS
❗ Rare reactions include hypersensitivity reactions, malignancies, respiratory tract infections, bronchitis, UTIs, and more serious infections (such as pneumonia, tuberculosis, cellulitis, pyelonephritis, and septic arthritis).

DENTAL CONSIDERATIONS
General:
• Patient may need assistance in getting into and out of dental chair.
• Adjust chair position for patient comfort.
• Determine why patient is taking the drug.
• Question patient about other drugs being taken.
• Examine for oral manifestation of opportunistic infection.
• Report oral infections to patient's physician; treat infections aggressively.
• Consider semisupine chair position for patient comfort if GI side effects occur.
Consultations:
• Medical consultation may be required to assess disease control and patient's ability to tolerate stress.
Teach Patient/Family to:
• Use effective oral hygiene to prevent soft tissue inflammation
• Immediately report any signs or symptoms of oral infection

adapalene
a-dap´-ah-leen
(Differin)

CATEGORY AND SCHEDULE
Pregnancy Risk category: C

Drug Class: Dermatologics, retinoids

MECHANISM OF ACTION
Binds to retinoic acid receptors in cell nuclei modulating cell differentiation, keratinization. Possesses antiinflammatory properties. *Therapeutic effect:* Normalizes differentiation of follicular epithelial cells.

USES
Treatment of acne

PHARMACOKINETICS
Absorption through the skin is low. Trace amount found in plasma following topical application. Excreted primarily by biliary route.

INDICATIONS AND DOSAGES
▶ Acne Vulgaris
Topical
Adults, Elderly, Children Older Than 12 years. Apply to affected area once daily at bedtime after washing.

SIDE EFFECTS/ADVERSE REACTIONS
Frequent
Erythema, scaling, dryness, pruritus, burning (likely to occur first 2–4 wk, lessens with continued use)
Occasional
Skin irritation, stinging, sunburn, acne flares, erythema, photosensitivity, pruritus, xerosis

PRECAUTIONS AND CONTRAINDICATIONS
Hypersensitivity to adapalene, vitamin A or any one of its components

DRUG INTERACTIONS OF CONCERN TO DENTISTRY
• Avoid use of topical antiinfectives on same skin application site

SERIOUS REACTIONS
❗ Concurrent use of other potentially irritating topical products (soaps, cleansers, aftershave, cosmetics) may produce severe topical irritation.

DENTAL CONSIDERATIONS
General:
• Advise patient if dental drugs prescribed have a potential for photosensitivity.
• Apply lubricant to dry lips for patient comfort prior to dental procedures
• Limit systemic vitamin A doses to no more than the RDA
Teach Patient/Family to:
• Avoid getting in eyes or mouth, or on other mucous membranes.

adefovir
ah-deff´-oh-veer
(Hepsera)

CATEGORY AND SCHEDULE
Pregnancy Risk Category: C

Drug Class: Antiviral

MECHANISM OF ACTION
An antiviral that inhibits the enzyme DNA polymerase, causing DNA chain termination after its incorporation into viral DNA. *Therapeutic Effect:* Prevents cell replication of viral DNA.

USES

Treatment of chronic hepatitis B in adults showing evidence of active viral replication and with persistent elevations of ALT or AST or histologically active disease

PHARMACOKINETICS

Binds to proteins after PO administration. Excreted in urine. *Half-life:* 7 hr (increased in impaired renal function).

INDICATIONS AND DOSAGES

▶ **Chronic Hepatitis B in Patients with Normal Renal Function**
PO
Adults, Elderly. 10 mg once a day.
▶ **Chronic Hepatitis B in Patients with Impaired Renal Function**
PO
Adults, Elderly with creatinine clearance 20–49 ml/min.
10 mg q48h.
Adults, Elderly with creatinine clearance 10–19 ml/min. 10 mg q72h.
Adults, Elderly on hemodialysis. 10 mg every 7 days following dialysis.

SIDE EFFECTS/ADVERSE REACTIONS

Frequent
Asthenia
Occasional
Headache, abdominal pain, nausea, flatulence
Rare
Diarrhea, dyspepsia

PRECAUTIONS AND CONTRAINDICATIONS

Hypersensitivity
Caution
Severe acute exacerbations of hepatitis in patients who have discontinued drug, renal dysfunction with chronic use, HIV resistance, lactic acidosis, severe hepatomegaly with steatosis, monitor renal and hepatic function, safety and effectiveness in children and lactation not established

DRUG INTERACTIONS OF CONCERN TO DENTISTRY

None reported

SERIOUS REACTIONS

❗ Nephrotoxicity (characterized by increased serum creatinine and decreased serum phosphorus levels) is a treatment-limiting toxicity of adefovir therapy.
❗ Lactic acidosis and severe hepatomegaly occur rarely, particularly in female patients.

DENTAL CONSIDERATIONS
General:
• Examine for oral manifestation of opportunistic infection.
• Determine why patient is taking the drug.
• Consider semisupine chair position for patient comfort if GI side effects occur.
• Do not provide treatment if clinician does not have seroconversion to protective antibodies to hepatitis B.
Consultations:
• Medical consultation may be required to assess disease control and patient's ability to tolerate stress.
• Patients who report feeling symptoms of lactic acidosis, such as weakness, malaise, with unusual muscle pain, difficulty breathing, stomach pain with nausea, cold feeling in arms or legs, dizziness or light-headedness, and irregular heartbeat, should be immediately referred to their physician.

Teach Patient/Family to:
• Use effective oral hygiene to prevent soft tissue inflammation
• Prevent trauma when using oral hygiene aids
• Update health and drug history if physician makes any changes in evaluation or drug regimens

adenosine
ah-den´-oh-seen
(Adenocard, Adenocor[AUS], Adenoscan)

CATEGORY AND SCHEDULE
Pregnancy Risk Category: C

Drug Class: Antiarrhythmics

MECHANISM OF ACTION
A cardiac agent that slows impulse formation in the SA node and conduction time through the AV node. Adenosine also acts as a diagnostic aid in myocardial perfusion imaging or stress echocardiography. *Therapeutic Effect:* Depresses left ventricular function and restores normal sinus rhythm.

USES
Treatment of paroxysmal supraventriculoar tachycardia

PHARMACOKINETICS
Rapidly cleared from blood after IV administration, metabolized to cyclic AMP and inosine primarily by red blood cells and vascular endothelial cells.

INDICATIONS AND DOSAGES
▶ **Paroxysmal Supraventricular Tachycardia (PSVT)**
Rapid IV bolus

Adults, Elderly. Initially, 6 mg given over 1–2 sec. If first dose does not convert within 1–2 min, give 12 mg; may repeat 12-mg dose in 1–2 min if no response has occurred.
Children. Initially 0.1 mg/kg (maximum: 6 mg). If ineffective, may give 0.2 mg/kg (maximum: 12 mg).
▶ **Diagnostic Testing**
IV infusion
Adults. 140 mcg/kg/min for 6 min.

SIDE EFFECTS/ADVERSE REACTIONS
Frequent
Facial flushing, dyspnea
Occasional
Headache, nausea, light-headedness, chest pressure
Rare
Numbness or tingling in arms; dizziness; diaphoresis; hypotension; palpitations; chest, jaw, or neck pain

PRECAUTIONS AND CONTRAINDICATIONS
Atrial fibrillation or flutter, second- or third-degree AV block or sick sinus syndrome (with functioning pacemaker), ventricular tachycardia

DRUG INTERACTIONS OF CONCERN TO DENTISTRY
• Increased risk of heart block: carbamazepine

SERIOUS REACTIONS
! May produce short-lasting heart block.

DENTAL CONSIDERATIONS
General:
• Acute-use drug for use in emergency rooms, hospitals, or cardiac testing labs. If a patient reports use of this drug in his or her medical history, question about

cardiovascular disease and drugs he or she may be taking.
• Provide palliative emergency dental care only during drug use.
Consultations:
• Medical consultation may be required to assess disease control and patient's ability to tolerate stress.

albendazole
all-ben´-dah-zole
(Albenza)

CATEGORY AND SCHEDULE
Pregnancy Risk Category: C

Drug Class: Anthelmintic, systemic

MECHANISM OF ACTION
A benzimidazole carbamate anthelmintic that degrades parasite cytoplasmic microtubules, irreversibly blocks cholinesterase secretion, glucose uptake in helminth and larvae (depletes glycogen, decreases ATP production, depletes energy). Vermicidal. ***Therapeutic Effect:*** Immobilizes and kills worms.

USES
Treatment of infections caused by worms

PHARMACOKINETICS
Poorly and variable absorbed GI tract. Widely distributed, cyst fluid and including CSF. Protein binding: 70%. Extensively metabolized in liver. Primarily excreted in urine and bile. Not removed by hemodialysis. ***Half-life:*** 8–12 hr.

INDICATIONS AND DOSAGES
▶ **Neurocysticercosis**
PO

Adults, Elderly weighing more than 60 kg. 400 mg 2 times a day. Continue for 28 days, rest 14 days, repeat cycle 3 times.
Adults, Elderly weighing less than 60 kg. 15 mg/kg/day. Continue for 28 days, rest 14 days, repeat cycle 3 times.
▶ **Cystic Hydatid**
PO
Adults, Elderly weighing more than 60 kg. 400 mg 2 times a day. Continue for 8–30 days.
Adults, Elderly weighing less than 60 kg. 15 mg/kg/day. Continue for 8–30 days.

SIDE EFFECTS/ADVERSE REACTIONS
Frequent
Neurocysticerosis: Nausea, vomiting, headache
Hydatid: Abnormal liver function tests, abdominal pain, nausea, vomiting
Occasional
Neurocysticerosis: Increased intracranial pressure, meningeal signs
Hydatid: Headache, dizziness, alopecia, fever

PRECAUTIONS AND CONTRAINDICATIONS
Hypersensitivity to albendazole or any component of the formulation, pregnancy

DRUG INTERACTIONS OF CONCERN TO DENTISTRY
• Possible increase in blood levels: glucocorticoids, cimetidine

SERIOUS REACTIONS
❗ Pancytopenia occurs rarely.
❗ In presence of cysticerosis, drug may produce retinal damage in presence of retinal lesions.

<table>
<tr><td>DENTAL CONSIDERATIONS</td></tr>
</table>

General:

- Determine why patient is taking the drug.
- Patient on chronic drug therapy may rarely present with symptoms of blood dyscrasias, which can include infection, bleeding, and poor healing. If dyscrasia is present, caution patient to prevent oral tissue trauma when using oral hygiene aids.
- Question patients about other drugs they may be taking

Consultations:

- In a patient with symptoms of blood dyscrasias, request a medical consultation for blood studies and postpone treatment until normal values are reestablished

albuterol

al-byoo´-ter-ole
(AccuNeb, Airomir[AUS], Asmol CFC-Free[AUS], Epaq Inhaler[AUS], Novosalmol[CAN], Proventil, Proventil Repetabs, Respax[AUS], Ventolin, Ventolin CFC-Free[AUS], Volmax, Vospire ER)
Do not confuse albuterol with Albutein or atenolol, or Proventil with Prinivil.

CATEGORY AND SCHEDULE

Pregnancy Risk Category: C

Drug Class: Adrenergic β2-agonist

MECHANISM OF ACTION

A sympathomimetic that stimulates β_2-adrenergic receptors in the lungs, resulting in relaxation of bronchial smooth muscle.
Therapeutic Effect: Relieves bronchospasm and reduces airway resistance.

USES

Prevention and relief of bronchospasm in reversible obstructive airway disease, exercise-induced bronchospasm; unlabeled use acute, serious hyperkalemia in hemodialysis patients

PHARMACOKINETICS

Route	Onset	Peak	Duration
PO	15–30 min	2–3 hr	4–6 hr
PO (extended-release)	30 min	2–4 hr	12 hr
Inhalation	5–15 min	0.5–2 hr	2–5 hr

Rapidly, well absorbed from the GI tract; gradually absorbed from the bronchi after inhalation. Metabolized in the liver. Primarily excreted in urine. **Half-life:** 2.7–5 hr (PO); 3.8 hr (inhalation).

INDICATIONS AND DOSAGES

▶ **Bronchospasm**

PO
Adults, Children older than 12 yr.
2–4 mg 3–4 times a day. Maximum: 8 mg 4 times a day.
Elderly. 2 mg 3–4 times a day. Maximum: 8 mg 4 times a day.
Children 6–12 yr. 2 mg 3–4 times a day. Maximum: 24 mg/day.
PO (Extended-Release)
Adults, Children older than 12 yr.
4–8 mg q12h.
Inhalation
Adults, Elderly, Children older than 12 yr. 1–2 puffs by metered dose inhaler q4–6h as needed.
Children 4–12 yr. 1–2 puffs 4 times a day.
Nebulization
Adults, Elderly, Children older than 12 yr. 2.5 mg 3–4 times a day.

Children 2–12 yr. 0.63–1.25 mg 3–4 times a day.
▶ **Exercise-Induced Bronchospasm**
Inhalation
Adults, Elderly, Children 4 yr and older. 2 puffs 15–30 min before exercise.

SIDE EFFECTS/ADVERSE REACTIONS
Frequent
Headache; restlessness, nervousness, tremors; nausea; dizziness; throat dryness and irritation, pharyngitis; B/P changes, including hypertension; heartburn, transient wheezing
Occasional
Insomnia, asthenia, altered taste Inhalation: Dry, irritated mouth or throat; cough; bronchial irritation
Rare
Somnolence, diarrhea, dry mouth, flushing, diaphoresis, anorexia

PRECAUTIONS AND CONTRAINDICATIONS
History of hypersensitivity to sympathomimetics
Caution
Lactation, cardiac disorders, hyperthyroidism, diabetes mellitus, hypertension, prostatic hypertrophy, narrow-angle glaucoma, seizures, paradoxic bronchospasm

DRUG INTERACTIONS OF CONCERN TO DENTISTRY
None reported

SERIOUS REACTIONS
❗ Excessive sympathomimetic stimulation may produce palpitations, extrasystole, tachycardia, chest pain, a slight increase in B/P followed by a substantial decrease, chills, diaphoresis, and blanching of skin.
❗ Too-frequent or excessive use may lead to decreased bronchodilating effectiveness and severe, paradoxical bronchoconstriction.

DENTAL CONSIDERATIONS
General:
• Monitor vital signs at every appointment because of cardiovascular and respiratory side effects.
• Assess salivary flow as a factor in caries, periodontal disease, and candidiasis.
• Consider semisupine chair position for patients with respiratory disease.
• Midday appointments and a stress reduction protocol may be required for anxious patients.
• Be aware that aspirin or sulfite preservatives in vasoconstrictor-containing products can exacerbate asthma.
• Acute asthmatic episodes may be precipitated in the dental office. Sympathomimetic inhalants should be available for emergency use.
Consultations:
• Medical consultation may be required to assess disease control and patient's ability to tolerate stress.
Teach Patient/Family to:
• Rinse mouth with water after each dose to prevent dryness (for inhalation dosage forms)
• When chronic dry mouth occurs, advise patient to:
  • Avoid mouth rinses with high alcohol content because of drying effects
  • Use daily home fluoride products for anticaries effect

• To use sugarless gum, frequent sips of water, or saliva substitutes

alclometasone
al-kloe-met´-ah-sone
(Aclovate)

CATEGORY AND SCHEDULE
Pregnancy Risk Category: C

Drug Class: Antiinflammatory, steroidal

MECHANISM OF ACTION
Topical corticosteroids exhibit antiinflammatory, antipruritic, and vasoconstrictive properties. Clinically, these actions correspond to decreased edema, erythema, pruritus, plaque formation, and scaling of the affected skin.

USES
Provide relief of inflammation/pruritus associated with contact dermatitis, eczema, insect bite reactions

PHARMACOKINETICS
Approximately 3% is absorbed during an 8-hr period. Metabolized in the liver. Excreted in urine.

INDICATIONS AND DOSAGES
▶ **Atopic Dermatitis, Contact Dermatitis, Dermatitis, Discoid Lupus Erythematosus, Eczema, Exfoliative Dermatitis, Granuloma Annulare, Lichen Planus, Lichen Simplex, Polymorphous Light Eruption, Pruritus, Psoriasis, Rhus Dermatitis, Seborrheic Dermatitis, Xerosis**
Topical
Adults, Adolescents, Children 1 yr and older. Apply a thin film to the affected area 2–3 times a day.

SIDE EFFECTS/ADVERSE REACTIONS
Frequent
Burning, erythema, maculopapular rash, pruritus, skin irritation, xerosis
Occasional
Acneiform rash, contact dermatitis, folliculitis, glycosuria, growth inhibition, headache, hyperglycemia, infection, miliaria, papilledema, skin atrophy, skin hypopigmentation, skin ulcer, striae, telangiectasia
Rare
Adrenalcortical insufficiency, increased intracranial pressure, pseudotumor cerebri, impaired wound healing, Cushing's syndrome, HPA suppression, skin ulcers, tolerance, withdrawal, visual impairment, ocular hypertension, cataracts

PRECAUTIONS AND CONTRAINDICATIONS
Hypersensitivity to alclometasone, other corticosteroids, or any of its components

DRUG INTERACTIONS OF CONCERN TO DENTISTRY
None reported

SERIOUS REACTIONS
None listed

DENTAL CONSIDERATIONS
General:
• Determine why patient is taking the drug.
Teach Patient/Family to:
• Avoid use on herpetic lesions

Interleukin-2 (aldesleukin)

in-tur-lew´-kin
(IL-2, Proleukin)
Do not confuse interleukin-2 with interferon 2.

CATEGORY AND SCHEDULE
Pregnancy Risk Category: C

Drug Class: Antineoplastics

MECHANISM OF ACTION
A biological response modifier that acts like human recombinant interleukin-2, promoting proliferation, differentiation, and recruitment of T and B cells, lymphokine-activated and natural cells, and thymocytes. *Therapeutic Effect:* Enhances cytolytic activity in lymphocytes.

USES
Treatment of metastatic renal cell cancer

PHARMACOKINETICS
Primarily distributed into plasma, lymphocytes, lungs, liver, kidney, and spleen. Metabolized to amino acids in the cell lining the kidneys. *Half-life:* 85 min.

INDICATIONS AND DOSAGES
▶ **Metastatic Melanoma, Metastatic Renal Cell Carcinoma**
IV
Adults 18 yr and older.
600,000 units/kg q8h for 14 doses; followed by 9 days of rest, then another 14 doses for a total of 28 doses per course. Course may be repeated after rest period of at least 7 wk from date of hospital discharge.

SIDE EFFECTS/ADVERSE REACTIONS
Side effects are generally self-limiting and reversible within 2–3 days after discontinuing therapy.
Frequent
Fever, chills, nausea, vomiting, hypotension, diarrhea, oliguria or anuria, mental status changes, irritability, confusion, depression, sinus tachycardia, pain (abdominal, chest, back), fatigue, dyspnea, pruritus
Occasional
Edema, erythema, rash, stomatitis, anorexia, weight gain, infection (UTI, injection site, catheter tip), dizziness
Rare
Dry skin, sensory disorders (vision, speech, taste), dermatitis, headache, arthralgia, myalgia, weight loss, hematuria, conjunctivitis, proteinuria

PRECAUTIONS AND CONTRAINDICATIONS
Abnormal pulmonary function or thallium stress test results, bowel ischemia or perforation, coma or toxic psychosis lasting longer than 48 hr, GI bleeding requiring surgery, intubation lasting more than 72 hr, organ allografts, pericardial tamponade, renal dysfunction requiring dialysis for longer than 72 hr, repetitive or difficult-to-control seizures; retreatment in those who experience any of the following toxicities: angina, MI, recurrent chest pain with EKG changes, sustained ventricular tachycardia, uncontrolled or unresponsive cardiac rhythm disturbances

DRUG INTERACTIONS OF CONCERN TO DENTISTRY

Possible reduction in antitumor efficacy: glucocorticoids

SERIOUS REACTIONS

! Anemia, thrombocytopenia, and leukopenia occur commonly.

! GI bleeding and pulmonary edema occur occasionally.

! Capillary leak syndrome results in hypotension (systolic pressure less than 90 mm Hg or a 20-mm Hg drop from baseline systolic pressure), extravasation of plasma proteins and fluid into extravascular space, and loss of vascular tone. It may result in cardiac arrhythmias, angina, MI, and respiratory insufficiency.

! Other rare reactions include fatal malignant hyperthermia, cardiac arrest, CVA, pulmonary emboli, bowel perforation, gangrene, and severe depression leading to suicide.

DENTAL CONSIDERATIONS

General:

• Monitor vital signs at every appointment due to cardiovascular side effects.

• If additional analgesia is required for dental pain, consider alternative analgesics (NSAIDs) in patients taking narcotics for acute or chronic pain.

• Examine for oral manifestation of opportunistic infection.

• Avoid products that affect platelet function, such as aspirin and NSAIDs.

• Chlorhexidine mouth rinse prior to and during chemotherapy may reduce severity of mucositis.

• Patient on chronic drug therapy may rarely present with symptoms of blood dyscrasias, which can include infection, bleeding, and poor healing. If dyscrasia is present, caution patient to prevent oral tissue trauma when using oral hygiene aids.

• Palliative medication may be required for management of oral side effects.

• Short appointments and a stress reduction protocol may be required for anxious patients.

• Provide emergency dental care only during drug use.

• Patients may be at risk of bleeding, check for oral signs.

• Oral infections should be eliminated and/or treated aggressively.

Consultations:

• Medical consultation should include routine blood counts including platelet counts and bleeding time.

• Consult physician; prophylactic or therapeutic antiinfectives may be indicated if surgery or periodontal treatment is required.

• Medical consultation may be required to assess immunologic status during cancer chemotherapy and determine safety risk, if any, posed by the required dental treatment.

• Medical consultation may be required to assess disease control and patient's ability to tolerate stress.

Teach Patient/Family to:

• See dentist immediately if secondary oral infection occurs

• Be aware of oral side effects

• Use effective oral hygiene to prevent soft tissue inflammation

• Report oral lesions, soreness, or bleeding to dentist

• Prevent trauma when using oral hygiene aids

• Update health and medication history if physician makes any changes in evaluation or drug regimens; include OTC, herbal, and nonherbal remedies in the update

alefacept
ale´-fah-sept
(Amevive)

CATEGORY AND SCHEDULE
Pregnancy Risk Category: B

Drug Class: Biologic response modifier, immunosuppressant

MECHANISM OF ACTION
An immunologic agent that interferes with the activation of T lymphocytes by binding to the lymphocyte antigen, thus reducing the number of circulating T lymphocytes.
Therapeutic Effect: Prevents T cells from becoming overactive, which may help reduce symptoms of chronic plaque psoriasis.

USES
Treatment of moderate to severe chronic plaque psoriasis in adults who are candidates for systemic therapy or phototherapy

PHARMACOKINETICS
Half-life: 270 hr.

INDICATIONS AND DOSAGES
▶ Plaque Psoriasis
IV
Adults, Elderly. 7.5 mg once weekly for 12 wk.
IM
Adults, Elderly. 15 mg once weekly for 12 wk.

SIDE EFFECTS/ADVERSE REACTIONS
Frequent
Injection site pain and inflammation (with IM administration)
Occasional
Chills

Rare
Pharyngitis, dizziness, cough, nausea, myalgia

PRECAUTIONS AND CONTRAINDICATIONS
History of systemic malignancy, concurrent use of immunosuppressive agents or phototherapy
Caution
Live or live-attenuated vaccines require regular monitoring of lymphocyte counts; lactation data not available (caution), elderly, safety and efficacy in pediatric patients not known

DRUG INTERACTIONS OF CONCERN TO DENTISTRY
None reported

SERIOUS REACTIONS
❗ Rare reactions include hypersensitivity reactions, lymphopenia, malignancies, and serious infections requiring hospitalization (such as abscess, pneumonia, and postoperative wound infection).
❗ Coronary artery disease and MI occur in less than 1% of patients.

DENTAL CONSIDERATIONS
None reported

alemtuzumab
al-em-two´-zoo-mab
(Campath)

CATEGORY AND SCHEDULE
Pregnancy Risk Category: C

Drug Class: Antineoplastics

MECHANISM OF ACTION

Binds to CD52, a cell surface glycoprotein, found on the surface of all B and T lymphocytes, most monocytes, macrophages, natural killer cells, and granulocytes. *Therapeutic Effect:* Produces cytotoxicity reducing tumor size.

USES

Treatment of B-cell chronic lymphocytic leukemia in patients who have been treated with alkylating agents and who have failed fludarabine therapy

PHARMACOKINETICS

Half-life: About 12 days. Peak and trough levels rise during first few weeks of therapy and approach steady state by about week 6.

INDICATIONS AND DOSAGES

▶ Chronic Lymphocytic Leukemia
IV

Adults, Elderly. Initially, 3 mg/day as a 2-hr infusion. When the 3-mg daily dose is tolerated (with only low-grade or no infusion-related toxicities), increase daily dose to 10 mg. When the 10 mg/day dose is tolerated, maintenance dose may be initiated. Maintenance: 30 mg/day 3 times a wk on alternate days (such as Monday, Wednesday, and Friday or Tuesday, Thursday, and Saturday) for up to 12 wk. The increase to 30 mg/day is usually achieved in 3–7 days.

SIDE EFFECTS/ADVERSE REACTIONS

Frequent

Rigors, tremors, fever, nausea, vomiting, rash, fatigue, hypotension, urticaria, pruritus, skeletal pain, headache, diarrhea, anorexia

Occasional

Myalgia, dizziness, abdominal pain, throat irritation, vomiting, neutropenia, rhinitis, bronchospasm, urticaria

PRECAUTIONS AND CONTRAINDICATIONS

Active systemic infections, history of hypersensitivity or anaphylactic reaction to the drug, immunosuppression

DRUG INTERACTIONS OF CONCERN TO DENTISTRY

None reported

SERIOUS REACTIONS

❗ Neutropenia occurs in 85% of patients, anemia occurs in 80% of patients, and thrombocytopenia occurs in 72% of patients.
❗ A rash occurs in 40% of patients.
❗ Respiratory toxicity, manifested as dyspnea, cough, bronchitis, pneumonitis, and pneumonia, occurs in 26%–16% of patients.

DENTAL CONSIDERATIONS

General:
• Monitor vital signs at every appointment due to cardiovascular side effects.
• Examine for oral manifestation of opportunistic infection.
• Avoid products that affect platelet function, such as aspirin and NSAIDs.
• This drug may be used in the hospital or on an outpatient basis. Confirm the patient's disease and treatment status.
• Chlorhexidine mouth rinse prior to and during chemotherapy may reduce severity of mucositis.
• Patient on chronic drug therapy may rarely present with symptoms of blood dyscrasias, which can include infection, bleeding, and poor healing.

If dyscrasia is present, caution patient to prevent oral tissue trauma when using oral hygiene aids.
- Palliative medication may be required for management of oral side effects.
- Short appointments and a stress reduction protocol may be required for anxious patients.
- Patients may be taking a prophylactic antiinfective.
- Patients are at risk of bleeding, check for oral signs.
- Place on frequent recall due to oral side effects.

Consultations:
- Medical consultation should include routine blood counts including platelet counts and bleeding time.
- Consult physician; prophylactic or therapeutic antiinfectives may be indicated if surgery or periodontal treatment is required.
- Medical consultation may be required to assess immunologic status during cancer chemotherapy and determine safety risk, if any, posed by the required dental treatment.
- Medical consultation may be required to assess disease control and patient's ability to tolerate stress.

Teach Patient/Family to:
- Inform dentist of unusual bleeding episodes following dental treatment
- See dentist immediately if secondary oral infection occurs
- Be aware of oral side effects
- Use effective oral hygiene to prevent soft tissue inflammation
- Report oral lesions, soreness, or bleeding to dentist
- Prevent trauma when using oral hygiene aids
- Update health and medication history if physician makes any changes in evaluation or drug regimens; include OTC, herbal, and nonherbal remedies in the update

alendronate sodium
ah-len´-dro-nate
(Fosamax)
Do not confuse Fosamax with Flomax.

CATEGORY AND SCHEDULE
Pregnancy Risk Category: C

Drug Class: Amino bisphosphonate

MECHANISM OF ACTION
A bisphosphonate that inhibits normal and abnormal bone resorption, without retarding mineralization. *Therapeutic Effect:* Leads to significantly increased bone mineral density; reverses the progression of osteoporosis.

USES
Osteoporosis treatment and prevention in men and postmenopausal women, glucocorticoid-induced osteoporosis in men and women receiving glucocorticoids at daily dose of 7.5 mg prednisone, Paget's disease of bone

PHARMACOKINETICS
Poorly absorbed after oral administration. Protein binding: 78%. After oral administration, rapidly taken into bone, with uptake greatest at sites of active bone turnover. Excreted in urine. *Terminal Half-life:* Greater than 10 yr (reflects release from skeleton as bone is resorbed).

INDICATIONS AND DOSAGES

▶ **Osteoporosis (in men)**
PO
Adults, Elderly. 10 mg once a day in the morning.

▶ **Glucocorticoid-Induced Osteoporosis**
PO
Adults, Elderly. 5 mg once a day in the morning.
Postmenopausal women not receiving estrogen. 10 mg once a day in the morning.
Postmenopausal Osteoporosis
PO (treatment)
Adults, Elderly. 10 mg once a day in the morning or 70 mg weekly.
PO (prevention)
Adults, Elderly. 5 mg once a day in the morning or 35 mg weekly.

▶ **Paget's Disease**
PO
Adults, Elderly. 40 mg once a day in the morning.

SIDE EFFECTS/ADVERSE REACTIONS

Frequent
Back pain, abdominal pain
Occasional
Nausea, abdominal distention, constipation, diarrhea, flatulence
Rare
Rash

PRECAUTIONS AND CONTRAINDICATIONS

GI disease, including dysphagia, frequent heartburn, GI reflux disease, hiatal hernia, and ulcers, inability to stand or sit upright for at least 30 min; renal impairment; sensitivity to alendronate. Carefully evaluate patients when considering the use of dental implants. Osteonecrosis of the jaw has been reported in patients following oral surgical procedures and who are also taking bisphosphonates.
Caution
Renal insufficiency, active upper GI disease, may see decrease in serum calcium/phosphate, ensure adequate calcium and vitamin D intake, lactation

DRUG INTERACTIONS OF CONCERN TO DENTISTRY

• Increased risk of GI side effects in doses greater than 10 mg/day: Use NSAIDs, acetylsalicylic acid (ASA) with caution
• After administration, must wait at least 30 min before taking any other drug

SERIOUS REACTIONS

❗ Overdose causes hypocalcemia, hypophosphatemia, and significant GI disturbances.
❗ Esophageal irritation occurs if alendronate is not given with 6–8 oz of plain water or if the patient lies down within 30 min of drug administration.

DENTAL CONSIDERATIONS
General:
• Be aware of oral manifestations of Paget's disease (macrognathia, alveolar pain).
• Consider semisupine chair position for patient comfort because of pain experienced in osteoporosis and GI side effects of drug.
• Consider short appointments for patient comfort.
Consultations:
• Medical consultation may be required to assess disease control and patient's ability to tolerate stress.

alfuzosin hydrochloride
ale-few´-zoe-sin hi-droh-klor´-ide
(Uroxatral)

CATEGORY AND SCHEDULE
Pregnancy Risk Category: B

Drug Class: Adrenoreceptor antagonist

MECHANISM OF ACTION
An alpha1 antagonist that targets receptors around bladder neck and prostate capsule. *Therapeutic Effect:* Relaxes smooth muscle and improves urinary flow and symptoms of prostatic hyperplasia.

USES
Signs and symptoms of benign prostatic hyperplasia (BPH)

PHARMACOKINETICS
Rapidly absorbed and widely distributed. Protein binding: 90%. Extensively metabolized in the liver. Primarily excreted in urine. *Half-life:* 3–9 hr.

INDICATIONS AND DOSAGES
▶ **Benign Prostatic Hyperplasia**
PO
Adults. 10 mg once a day, approximately 30 min after same meal each day.

SIDE EFFECTS/ADVERSE REACTIONS
Frequent
Dizziness, headache, malaise
Occasional
Dry mouth
Rare
Nausea, dyspepsia (such as heartburn, and epigastric discomfort), diarrhea, orthostatic hypotension, tachycardia, drowsiness

PRECAUTIONS AND CONTRAINDICATIONS
History of hypersensitivity to alfuzosin
Caution
Increase in angina pectoris symptoms, severe renal impairment, known history of QT-interval prolongation, caution in use of drugs that prolong the QT interval, not for use in women or children

DRUG INTERACTIONS OF CONCERN TO DENTISTRY
• Potential for hypotension: antihypertensive drugs, other adrenergic antagonists
• Contraindicated with ketoconazole, itraconazole
• Possible risk of orthostatic hypotension may be increased with conscious sedation techniques
• Opioids and anticholinergic drugs may enhance urinary retention in BPH; use alternative analgesics (NSAIDs)
• Erythromycin is an inhibitor of CYP3A4, but no data reported for possible interaction: use with caution

SERIOUS REACTIONS
! Ischemia-related chest pain may occur rarely.

DENTAL CONSIDERATIONS
General:
• Monitor vital signs at every appointment because of cardiovascular side effects.
• Consider semisupine chair position for patient comfort if GI side effects occur.

• After supine positioning, have patient sit upright for at least 2 min before standing to avoid orthostatic hypotension.

alglucosidase alfa
al-gloo-ko-sy´-dase al´-fa
(Myozyme)

CATEGORY AND SCHEDULE
Pregnancy Risk Category: B

Drug Class: Enzyme

MECHANISM OF ACTION
Alglucosidase alfa is a recombinant form of the enzyme acid alpha-glucosidase (GAA), produced in a Chinese hamster ovary cell line. Alglucosidase alfa binds to mannose-6-phosphate receptors on the cell surface and is internalized and transported to lysosomes, resulting in increased enzymatic activity and glycogen cleavage. *Therapeutic Effect:* Provides an exogenous source of GAA which is the enzyme deficient or absent in Pompe disease.

USES
Used as replacement therapy for Pompe disease (GAA deficiency)

PHARMACOKINETICS
Half-life: 2.3 hr.

INDICATIONS AND DOSAGES
▶ **Replacement Therapy for Pompe Disease**
IV infusion
Adults. 20 mg/kg over 4 hr, every 2 wk.
Children (1 mo–3.5 yr. at first infusion). 20 mg/kg over 4 hr, every 2 wk.

SIDE EFFECTS/ADVERSE REACTIONS:
Frequent
Fever, diarrhea, rash, infusion reaction, vomiting, cough, pneumonia, upper respiratory tract infection, otitis media, oxygen saturation decreased, gastroenteritis, diaper dermatitis, pharyngitis, respiratory distress, oral candidiasis, anemia, respiratory failure, catheter-related infections, pain (postprocedural), gastroesophageal reflux, rhinorrhea, constipation, tachycardia, bronchiolitis, nasopharyngitis, tachypnea, bradycardia, flushing, urticaria.
Less frequent adverse effects were not mentioned.

PRECAUTIONS AND CONTRAINDICATIONS
Hypersensitivity to alglucosidase alfa or its components
Caution
Cardiovascular disease, respiratory impairment, acute underlying illness (increased risk of infusion reactions)

DRUG INTERACTIONS OF CONCERN TO DENTISTRY
None reported

SERIOUS REACTIONS
! Severe hypersensitivity reactions, including anaphylactic reactions and anaphylactic shock, have been reported during infusion. Infusion-related reactions are common—discontinue immediately for severe hypersensitivity or anaphylactic reaction.
! Cardiac arrhythmia, including ventricular fibrillation, ventricular tachycardia, and bradycardia,

resulting in cardiac arrest or death, have been reported.

DENTAL CONSIDERATIONS
General:
• Monitor vital signs at every appointment because of cardiovascular side effects.
• Evaluate carefully for drug-related candidiasis and treat in consultation with patient's physician.
• Place patient on frequent recall and use multiple preventive measures to assist with patient's oral hygiene.
• Consult physician to determine disease control and ability of patient to tolerate dental procedures.
Teach Patient/Family to:
• Use atraumatic, effective oral hygiene measures and assist patient with oral care.

alitretinoin
ah-lee-tret´-ih-noyn
(Panretin)

CATEGORY AND SCHEDULE
Pregnancy Risk Category: D

Drug Class: Topical retinoid

MECHANISM OF ACTION
Binds to and activates all known retinoid receptors. Once activated, receptors act as transcription factors, regulating genes that control cellular differentiation and proliferation. *Therapeutic Effect:* Inhibits growth of Kaposi's sarcoma cells.

USES
Topical treatment of cutaneous lesions in patients with AIDS-related Kaposi's sarcoma (KS)

PHARMACOKINETICS
Minimally absorbed following topical administration.

INDICATIONS AND DOSAGES
▸ **KS Skin Lesions**
Topical
Adults. Initially, apply 2 times a day to lesions. May increase to 3–4 times a day.

SIDE EFFECTS/ADVERSE REACTIONS
Frequent
Rash (erythema, scaling, irritation, redness, dermatitis), itching, exfoliative dermatitis (flaking, peeling, desquamation, exfolliation), stinging, tingling, edema skin disorders (scabbing, crusting, drainage)

PRECAUTIONS AND CONTRAINDICATIONS
When systemic therapy is required (more than 10 new KS lesions in previous mo, symptomatic pulmonary KS, symptomatic visceral involvement, symptomatic lymphedema, hypersensitivity to retinoids or alitretinoin ingredients)
Caution
Avoid pregnancy, discontinue breast-feeding when used, safety in children unknown, patients older than 65 yr, occlusive dressings; do not use products containing DEET

DRUG INTERACTIONS OF CONCERN TO DENTISTRY
• Risk of photosensitivity reaction: tetracyclines, fluoroquinolones, other photosensitizing drugs

SERIOUS REACTIONS
! Severe local skin reaction (intense erythema, edema, vesiculation) may limit treatment.

DENTAL CONSIDERATIONS
General:
• Patients will be taking antiviral drugs; note which drugs are being used because some have potential for significant drug interactions.
• Take a complete medical history, including a current drug history with doses and duration of therapy.

allopurinol
al-oh-pure′-ih-nole
(Aloprim, Allohexal[AUS], Allosig[AUS], Apo-Allopurinol[CAN], Capurate[AUS], Progout[AUS] Purinol[CAN], Zyloprim)
Do not confuse Zyloprim with ZORprin.

CATEGORY AND SCHEDULE
Pregnancy Risk Category: C

Drug Class: Antigout drug, antihyperuricemic

MECHANISM OF ACTION
A xanthine oxidase inhibitor that decreases uric acid production by inhibiting xanthine oxidase, an enzyme. ***Therapeutic Effect:*** Reduces uric acid concentrations in both serum and urine.

USES
Chronic gout, hyperuricemia associated with malignancies, recurrent calcium oxalate calculi, uric acid nephropathy

PHARMACOKINETICS

Route	Onset	Peak	Duration
PO/IV	2–3 days	1–3 wk	1–2 wk

Well absorbed from the GI tract. Widely distributed. Metabolized in the liver to active metabolite. Excreted primarily in urine. Removed by hemodialysis. ***Half-life:*** 1–3 hr; metabolite, 12–30 hr.

INDICATIONS AND DOSAGES
▸ **Chronic Gouty Arthritis**
PO
Adults, Children older than 10 yr. Initially, 100 mg/day; may increase by 100 mg/day at weekly intervals. Maximum: 800 mg/day. Maintenance: 100–200 mg 2–3 times a day or 300 mg/day.
▸ **To Prevent Uric Acid Nephropathy During Chemotherapy**
PO
Adults. Initially, 600–800 mg/day starting 2–3 days before initiation of chemotherapy or radiation therapy.
Children 6–10 yr. 100 mg 3 times a day or 300 mg once a day.
Children younger than 6 yr. 50 mg 3 times a day.
IV
Adults. 200–400 mg/m^2/day beginning 24–48 hr before initiation of chemotherapy.
Children. 200 mg/m^2/day. Maximum: 600 mg/day.
▸ **Prevention of Uric Acid Calculi**
PO
Adults. 100–200 mg 1–4 times a day or 300 mg once a day.
▸ **Recurrent Calcium Oxalate Calculi**
PO
Adults. 200–300 mg/day.
Elderly. Initially, 100 mg/day, gradually increased until optimal uric acid level is reached.

DOSAGE IN RENAL IMPAIRMENT
Dosage is modified on the basis of creatinine clearance.

Creatinine Clearance	Dosage Adjustment
10–20 ml/min	200 mg/day
3–9 ml/min	100 mg/day
Less than 3 ml/min	100 mg at extended intervals

SIDE EFFECTS/ADVERSE REACTIONS

Occasional
Oral: Somnolence, unusual hair loss
IV: Rash, nausea, vomiting
Rare
Diarrhea, headache

PRECAUTIONS AND CONTRAINDICATIONS

Asymptomatic hyperuricemia
Caution
Lactation, renal disease, hepatic disease, children

DRUG INTERACTIONS OF CONCERN TO DENTISTRY

• Increased risk of rash: ampicillin, amoxicillin, bacampicillin, hetacillin

SERIOUS REACTIONS

❗ Pruritic maculopapular rash possibly accompanied by malaise, fever, chills, joint pain, nausea, and vomiting should be considered a toxic reaction.
❗ Severe hypersensitivity may follow appearance of rash.
❗ Bone marrow depression, hepatic toxicity, peripheral neuritis, and acute renal failure occur rarely.

DENTAL CONSIDERATIONS

General:
• Patients on chronic drug therapy may rarely have symptoms of blood dyscrasias, which can include infection, bleeding, and poor healing.

Consultations:
• In a patient with symptoms of blood dyscrasias, request a medical consultation for blood studies and postpone dental treatment until normal values are reestablished.
• Medical consultation may be required to assess disease control.
Teach Patient/Family to:
• Use effective oral hygiene to prevent soft tissue inflammation
• Avoid mouth rinses with high alcohol content because of drying effects

almotriptan malate
al-moe-trip´-tan
(Axert)
Do not confuse Axert with Antivert.

CATEGORY AND SCHEDULE
Pregnancy Risk Category: C

Drug Class: Selective serotonin agonist

MECHANISM OF ACTION

A serotonin receptor agonist that binds selectively to vascular receptors, producing a vasoconstrictive effect on cranial blood vessels. ***Therapeutic Effect:*** Produces relief of migraine headache.

USES

Acute treatment of migraine with or without aura in adults

PHARMACOKINETICS

Well absorbed after PO administration. Metabolized by the liver, excreted in urine. ***Half-life:*** 3–4 hr.

INDICATIONS AND DOSAGES
▶ **Migraine Headache**
PO
Adults, Elderly. 6.25–12.5 mg. If
headache improves but then returns,
dose may be repeated after 2 hr.
Maximum: 2 doses/24 hr.
▶ **Dosage in Renal Impairment**
For adult and elderly patients,
recommended initial dose is 6.25 mg,
and maximum daily dose is 12.5 mg.

SIDE EFFECTS/ADVERSE REACTIONS
Frequent
Nausea, dry mouth, paresthesia,
flushing
Occasional
Changes in temperature sensation,
asthenia, dizziness

PRECAUTIONS AND CONTRAINDICATIONS
Arrhythmias associated with
conduction disorders, hemiplegic or
basilar migraine, ischemic heart
disease (including angina pectoris,
history of MI, silent ischemia, and
Prinzmetal's angina), uncontrolled
hypertension, use within 24 hr of
ergotamine-containing preparation
or another serotonin receptor
antagonist, use within 14 days of
MAOIs, Wolff-Parkinson-White
syndrome
Caution
Hypertension, diabetes, hepatitis,
renal impairment, elevated
cholesterol, obesity, smoking,
postmenopause, men older than
40 yr, preexisting heart disease,
elderly, lactation, safety/efficacy for
pediatric patients not evaluated

DRUG INTERACTIONS OF CONCERN TO DENTISTRY
• Avoid concurrent use of
ketoconazole, itraconazole,
erythromycin

SERIOUS REACTIONS
❗ Excessive dosage may produce
tremor, red extremities, reduced
respirations, cyanosis, seizures, and
chest pain.
❗ Serious arrhythmias occur rarely,
particularly in patients with
hypertension or diabetes, obese
patients, smokers, and those with a
strong family history of coronary
artery disease.

DENTAL CONSIDERATIONS
General:
• This is an acute-use drug; it is
doubtful that patients will undergo
dental treatment during acute
migraine attacks.
• Be aware of patient's disease, its
severity, and frequency.
Consultations:
• If treating chronic orofacial pain,
consult with physician of record.
• Medical consultation may be
required to assess disease control and
patient's ability to tolerate stress.
Teach Patient/Family to:
• Avoid mouth rinses with high
alcohol content because of drying
effects
• Update health and drug history if
physician makes any changes in
evaluation or drug regimens

alosetron
al-ohs´-eh-tron
(Lotronex)
Do not confuse Lotronex with
Lovenox.

CATEGORY AND SCHEDULE
Pregnancy Risk Category: B

Drug Class: Selective serotonin
antagonist, neuroenteric modulator

MECHANISM OF ACTION

A serotonin (5-HT3) receptor antagonist that mediates abdominal pain, bloating, nausea, vomiting, peristalsis, and secretory reflexes. *Therapeutic Effect:* Alleviates diarrhea, reduces gastric pain.

USES

Treatment of women with diarrhea-predominant irritable bowel syndrome (IBS) failing to respond to conventional therapy

PHARMACOKINETICS

Rapidly absorbed after PO administration. Extensively metabolized in liver. Excreted primarily in urine and, to a lesser extent, in feces. *Half-life:* 1.5 hr.

INDICATIONS AND DOSAGES

IBS
PO
Adults (Women older than 18 yr). 1 mg twice a day. Maximum: 2 mg/day.

SIDE EFFECTS/ADVERSE REACTIONS

Frequent
Constipation
Occasional
Nausea, GI or abdominal discomfort or pain, dyspepsia, flatulence, hypertension, clinical depression
Rare
Sedation, abnormal dreams, anxiety

PRECAUTIONS AND CONTRAINDICATIONS

Breast-feeding; constipation; diverticulitis (active or history of); GI bleeding, obstruction, or perforation; history of ischemic colitis, ulcerative colitis, or Crohn's disease; thrombophlebitis

Caution
Food retards absorption, elderly, reduced hepatic or renal function, notify physician immediately if severe constipation or worse occurs, lactation, children; physicians prescribing this drug must be enrolled in the manufacturer's prescribing program

DRUG INTERACTIONS OF CONCERN TO DENTISTRY

• Does not appear to induce CYP450 isoenzymes; no interactions are documented
• Avoid use of drugs (opioids) that could lead to increased risk of constipation
• Use NSAIDs or acetaminophen for mild-to-moderate dental pain

SERIOUS REACTIONS

! Acute ischemic colitis and serious complications of constipation have resulted in the need for blood transfusions and surgery.

DENTAL CONSIDERATIONS

General:
• Short appointments and a stress reduction protocol may be required for anxious patients.
• Consider semisupine chair position for patient comfort because of GI side effects of disease.
• Avoid drugs with anticholinergic activity, such as antihistamines, opioids, benzodiazepines, propantheline, atropine, and scopolamine.
• Question patient about tolerance of NSAIDs or aspirin related to GI disease.
Consultations:
• Consider consulting with physician before prescribing drugs that can cause constipation (opioids).

• Consultation with physician may be necessary if sedation or general anesthesia is required.
• Medical consultation may be required to assess disease control and patient's ability to tolerate stress.

Teach Patient/Family:
• Importance of updating health and drug history if physician makes any changes in evaluation or drug regimens

alprazolam
al-praz´-oe-lam
Schedule IV
(Apo-Alpraz[CAN], Kalma[AUS], Niravam, Novo-Alprazol[CAN], Xanax, Xanax XR)
Do not confuse alprazolam with lorazepam, or Xanax with Tenex or Zantac.

CATEGORY AND SCHEDULE
Pregnancy Risk Category: D
Controlled Substance: Schedule IV

Drug Class: Benzodiazepine

MECHANISM OF ACTION
A benzodiazepine that enhances the action of the inhibitory neurotransmitter gamma-aminobutyric acid in the brain. *Therapeutic Effect:* Produces anxiolytic effect from its CNS depressant action.

USES
Treatment of generalized anxiety disorder, panic disorders, anxiety with depressive symptoms; unapproved: agoraphobia

PHARMACOKINETICS
Well absorbed from GI tract. Protein binding: 80%. Metabolized in the liver. Primarily excreted in urine.

Minimal removal by hemodialysis. *Half-life:* 11–16 hr.

INDICATIONS AND DOSAGES
▸ **Anxiety Disorders**
PO (Immediate-Release)
Adults. Initially, 0.25–0.5 mg 3 times a day. May titrate q3–4 days. Maximum: 4 mg/day in divided doses.
Elderly, Debilitated patients, Patients with hepatic disease or low serum albumin. Initially, 0.25 mg 2–3 times a day. Gradually increase to optimum therapeutic response.
PO (Orally Disintegrating)
Adults. 0.25–0.5 mg 3 times a day. Maximum: 4 mg/day in divided doses.
▸ **Anxiety with Depression**
PO
Adults. 2.5–3 mg/day in divided doses.
▸ **Panic Disorder**
PO (Immediate-Release)
Adults. Initially, 0.5 mg 3 times a day. May increase at 3- to 4-day intervals. Range: 5–6 mg/day. Maximum: 10 mg/day.
Elderly. Initially, 0.125–0.25 mg twice a day. May increase in 0.125-mg increments until desired effect attained.
PO (Extended-Release)
ALERT
To switch from immediate-release to extended-release form, give total daily dose (immediate release) as a single daily dose of extended-release form.
Adults. Initially, 0.5–1 mg once a day. May titrate at 3- to 4-day intervals. Range: 3–6 mg/day. Maximum: 10 mg/day.
Elderly. Initially, 0.5 mg once a day.
PO (Orally Disintegrating)

Adults. Initially, 0.5 mg 3 times a day. May increase at 3- to 4-day intervals. Range: 5–6 mg/day. Maximum: 10 mg/day.
▶ **Premenstrual Syndrome**
PO
Adults. 0.25 mg 3 times a day.

SIDE EFFECTS/ADVERSE REACTIONS
Frequent
Ataxia; lightheadedness; transient, mild somnolence; slurred speech (particularly in elderly or debilitated patients)
Occasional
Confusion, depression, blurred vision, constipation, diarrhea, dry mouth, headache, nausea
Rare
Behavioral problems such as anger, impaired memory, paradoxical reactions such as insomnia, nervousness, or irritability

PRECAUTIONS AND CONTRAINDICATIONS
Acute alcohol intoxication with depressed vital signs, acute angle-closure glaucoma, concurrent use of itraconazole or ketoconazole, myasthenia gravis, severe COPD
Caution
Elderly, debilitated, hepatic disease, renal disease; dependence, potential for abuse; avoid in lactation, safety and efficacy in patients younger than 18 yr not established

DRUG INTERACTIONS OF CONCERN TO DENTISTRY
• Increased CNS depression: alcohol, other CNS depressants, clarithromycin, erythromycin, fluconazole, miconazole, fluoxetine, isoniazid, fluvoxamine, nefazodone, rifamycin; St. John's wort (herb), kava (herb)

• Contraindicated with ketoconazole, itraconazole, ritonavir, indinavir, saquinavir

SERIOUS REACTIONS
! Abrupt or too-rapid withdrawal may result in pronounced restlessness, irritability, insomnia, hand tremors, abdominal and muscle cramps, diaphoresis, vomiting, and seizures.
! Overdose results in somnolence, confusion, diminished reflexes, and coma.
! Blood dyscrasias have been reported rarely.

DENTAL CONSIDERATIONS
General:
• Monitor vital signs at every appointment because of cardiovascular side effects.
• After supine positioning, have patient sit upright for at least 2 min to avoid orthostatic hypotension.
• Assess salivary flow as a factor in caries, periodontal disease, and candidiasis.
• Psychologic and physical dependence may occur with chronic administration.
Consultations:
• Medical consultation may be required to assess disease control.
Teach Patient/Family:
• When chronic dry mouth occurs, advise patient to:
  • Avoid mouth rinses with high alcohol content because of drying effects
  • Use daily home fluoride products for anticaries effect
  • Use sugarless gum, frequent sips of water, or saliva substitutes

alprostadil (prostaglandin E1, PGE1)

al-pros´-ta-dil
(Caverject, Edex, Muse, Prostin VR Pediatric)

CATEGORY AND SCHEDULE
Pregnancy Risk Category: C

Drug Class: Naturally occurring prostaglandin (E1, PGE1)

MECHANISM OF ACTION
A prostaglandin that directly affects vascular and ductus arteriosus smooth muscle and relaxes trabecular smooth muscle. *Therapeutic Effect:* Causes vasodilation; dilates cavernosal arteries, allowing blood flow to and entrapment in the lacunar spaces of the penis.

USES
Treatment of erectile dysfunction due to neurogenic, vasculogenic, psychogenic, or mixed causes

PHARMACOKINETICS
Rapidly metabolized and cleared from body by urinary excretion

INDICATIONS AND DOSAGES
▸ **Maintain Patency of Ductus Arteriosus**
IV infusion
Neonates. Initially, 0.05–0.1 mcg/kg/min. Maintenance: 0.01–0.4 mcg/kg/min. Maximum: 0.4 mcg/kg/min.
▸ **Impotence**
Pellet, Intracavernosal
Adults. Dosage is individualized.

SIDE EFFECTS/ADVERSE REACTIONS
Frequent
Intracavernosal: Penile pain, prolonged erection, hypertension, localized pain, penile fibrosis, injection site hematoma or ecchymosis, headache, respiratory infection, flu-like symptoms
Intraurethral: Penile pain, urethral pain or burning, testicular pain, urethral bleeding, headache, dizziness, respiratory infection, flu-like symptoms
Systemic: Fever, seizures, flushing, bradycardia, hypotension, tachycardia, apnea, diarrhea, sepsis
Occasional
Intracavernosal: Hypotension, pelvic pain, back pain, dizziness, cough, nasal congestion
Intraurethral: Fainting, sinusitis, back and pelvic pain
Systemic: Anxiety, lethargy, myalgia, arrhythmias, respiratory depression, anemia, bleeding, thrombocytopenia, hematuria

PRECAUTIONS AND CONTRAINDICATIONS
Conditions predisposing to anatomic deformation of penis, hyaline membrane disease, penile implants, priapism, respiratory distress syndrome
Caution
Patients on anticoagulant therapy, use of sterile technique, care of syringe, physician instruction in use required, sexually transmitted disease

DRUG INTERACTIONS OF CONCERN TO DENTISTRY
None reported

SERIOUS REACTIONS
! Overdose is manifested as apnea, flushing of the face and arms, and bradycardia.
! Cardiac arrest and sepsis occur rarely.

DENTAL CONSIDERATIONS

DENTAL CONSIDERATIONS
None reported

alteplase, recombinant
al-teep´-lase
(Activase, Actilyse[AUS], Cathflo Activase)
Do not confuse alteplase or Activase with Altace.

CATEGORY AND SCHEDULE
Pregnancy Risk Category: C

Drug Class: Tissue plasminogen activator

MECHANISM OF ACTION
A tissue plasminogen activator that acts as a thrombolytic by binding to the fibrin in a thrombus and converting entrapped plasminogen to plasmin. This process initiates fibrinolysis. *Therapeutic Effect:* Degrades fibrin clots, fibrinogen, and other plasma proteins.

USES
Treatment of acute MI, acute ischemic stroke, acute massive pulmonary embolism; treatment of occluded central venous catheters

PHARMACOKINETICS
Rapidly metabolized in the liver. Primarily excreted in urine. *Half-life:* 35 min.

INDICATIONS AND DOSAGES
▸ **Acute MI**
IV Infusion
Adults weighing greater than 67 kg. 100 mg over 90 min, starting with 15-mg bolus over 1–2 min, then 50 mg over 30 min, then 35 mg over 60 min. Or a 3-hour infusion, giving 60 mg over first hr (6–10 mg as bolus over 1–2 min), 20 mg over second hr, and 20 mg over third hr.
Adults weighing 67 kg or less. 100 mg over 90 min, starting with 15-mg bolus, then 0.75 mg/kg over 30 min (maximum: 50 mg), then 0.5 mg/kg over 60 min (maximum: 35 mg). Or 3-hr infusion of 1.25 mg/kg giving 60% of dose over first hr (6%–10% as 1- to 2-min bolus), 20% over second hr, and 20% over third hr.
▸ **Acute Pulmonary Emboli**
IV Infusion
Adults. 100 mg over 2 hr. Institute or reinstitute heparin near end or immediately after infusion when aPTT or TT returns to twice normal or less.
▸ **Acute Ischemic Stroke**
IV Infusion
Adults. 0.9 mg/kg over 60 min (10% total dose as initial IV bolus over 1 min).
▸ **Central Venous Catheter Clearance**
IV
Adults, Elderly. 2 mg; may repeat after 2 hr.

SIDE EFFECTS/ADVERSE REACTIONS
Frequent
Superficial bleeding at puncture sites, decreased B/P
Occasional
Allergic reaction, such as rash or wheezing; bruising

PRECAUTIONS AND CONTRAINDICATIONS
Active internal bleeding, AV malformation or aneurysm, bleeding diathesis, intracranial neoplasm, intracranial or intraspinal surgery or trauma, recent (within past 2 mo) cerebrovascular accident, severe uncontrolled hypertension

DRUG INTERACTIONS OF CONCERN TO DENTISTRY
• Increased risk of bleeding: drugs that interfere with coagulation or platelet function, such as NSAIDs and aspirin

SERIOUS REACTIONS
! Severe internal hemorrhage may occur.
! Lysis of coronary thrombi may produce atrial or ventricular arrhythmias or stroke.

DENTAL CONSIDERATIONS
General:
• An acute use drug for use in hospitals or emergency rooms.
• Patients are at risk of bleeding; check for oral signs.
• Avoid products that affect platelet function, such as aspirin and NSAIDs.
• Monitor vital signs every appointment due to cardiovascular side effects.
• Patients who have been treated with drug may present with cardiovascular disease or stroke; review medical and drug history.
Consultations:
• Consultation should include data on bleeding time.
• Medical consultation should include routine blood counts including platelet counts and bleeding time.
• In a patient with symptoms of blood dyscrasias, request a medical consultation for blood studies and postpone treatment until normal values are reestablished.
• Medical consultation may be required to assess disease control and patient's ability to tolerate stress.
Teach Patient/Family to:
• Use soft tooth brush to reduce risk of bleeding

• Use effective oral hygiene to prevent soft tissue inflammation
• Report oral lesions, soreness, or bleeding to dentist
• Prevent trauma when using oral hygiene aids
• Update health and medication history if physician makes any changes in evaluation/drug regimens; include OTC, herbal, and nonherbal remedies in the update

amantadine hydrochloride
ah-man´-ta-deen hi-droh-klor´-ide (Endantadine[CAN], PMS-Amantadine[CAN], Symmetrel)

CATEGORY AND SCHEDULE
Pregnancy Risk Category: C

Drug Class: Antiviral, antiparkinsonian agent

MECHANISM OF ACTION
A dopaminergic agonist that blocks the uncoating of influenza A virus, preventing penetration into the host and inhibiting M2 protein in the assembly of progeny virions. Amantadine also blocks the reuptake of dopamine into presynaptic neurons and causes direct stimulation of postsynaptic receptors.
Therapeutic Effect: Antiviral and antiparkinsonian activity.

USES
Prophylaxis or treatment of respiratory tract illness caused by influenza type A; drug-induced extrapyramidal reactions; parkinsonism

PHARMACOKINETICS
Rapidly and completely absorbed from the GI tract. Protein binding: 67%. Widely distributed. Primarily excreted in urine. Minimally removed by hemodialysis. *Half-life:* 11–15 hr (increased in the elderly, decreased in impaired renal function).

INDICATIONS AND DOSAGES
▶ **Prevention and Symptomatic Treatment of Respiratory Illness Due to Influenza A Virus**
PO
Adults older than 64 yr. 100 mg/day.
Adults 13–64 yr. 200 mg/day.
Children 10–12 yr. 5 kg/kg/day up to 200 mg/day.
Children 1–9 yr. 5 kg/kg/day (up to 150 mg/day).
▶ **Parkinson's Disease, Extrapyramidal Symptoms**
PO
Adults, Elderly. 100 mg twice a day. May increase up to 300 mg/day in divided doses.
▶ **Dosage in Renal Impairment**
Dose and frequency are modified on the basis of creatinine clearance.

Creatinine Clearance	Dosage
30–50 ml/min	200 mg first day; 100 mg/day thereafter
15–29 ml/min	200 mg first day; 100 mg on alternate days
Less than 15 ml/min	200 mg every 7 days

SIDE EFFECTS/ADVERSE REACTIONS
Frequent
Nausea, dizziness, poor concentration, insomnia, nervousness

Occasional
Orthostatic hypotension, anorexia, headache, livedo reticularis (reddish blue, netlike blotching of skin), blurred vision, urine retention, dry mouth or nose
Rare
Vomiting, depression, irritation or swelling of eyes, rash

PRECAUTIONS AND CONTRAINDICATIONS
Hypersensitivity, lactation, child younger than 1 yr
Caution
Epilepsy, CHF, orthostatic hypotension, psychiatric disorders, hepatic disease, renal disease (necessitates dose adjustment)

DRUG INTERACTIONS OF CONCERN TO DENTISTRY
• Increased anticholinergic response: anticholinergic drugs
• Increased CNS depression: alcohol, other CNS depressants

SERIOUS REACTIONS
❗ CHF, leukopenia, and neutropenia occur rarely.
❗ Hyperexcitability, seizures, and ventricular arrhythmias may occur.

DENTAL CONSIDERATIONS
General:
• Monitor vital signs at every appointment because of cardiovascular side effects.
• Assess salivary flow as a factor in caries, periodontal disease, and candidiasis.
• After supine positioning, have patient sit upright for at least 2 min to avoid orthostatic hypotension.
• Avoid dental light in patient's eyes; offer dark glasses for patient comfort.

- Short appointments and stress reduction protocol may be required for anxious patients.
- Consider semisupine chair position for patients with respiratory distress.

Teach Patient/Family to:
- Avoid mouth rinses with high alcohol content because of drying effects
- Use electric toothbrush if patient has difficulty holding conventional devices

ambenonium
am-be-noe´-nee-um
(Mytelase)

CATEGORY AND SCHEDULE
Pregnancy Risk Category: C

Drug Class: Cholinesterase inhibitor

MECHANISM OF ACTION
A cholinesterase inhibitor that enhances and prolongs cholinergic function by increasing the concentration of acetylcholine through inhibition of the hydrolysis of acetylcholine. **Therapeutic Effect:** Increases muscle strength in myasthenia gravis.

USES
Treatment of myasthenia gravis, when other drugs cannot be used

PHARMACOKINETICS
Poorly absorbed after PO administration.

INDICATIONS AND DOSAGES
▶ **Myasthenia Gravis**
PO
Adults. 5–25 mg 3 or 4 times a day. If well tolerated, after 1 or 2 days, may increase to 50–75 mg 3 times

a day. Range: 5–200 mg/day in divided doses.

SIDE EFFECTS/ADVERSE REACTIONS
Frequent
Abdominal pain, diarrhea, increased salivation, miosis, sweating, and vomiting
Occasional
Anxiety, blurred vision, and urinary urgency
Rare
Trembling, difficulty moving or controlling movement of the tongue, neck, or arms

PRECAUTIONS AND CONTRAINDICATIONS
Not recommended in patients receiving routine administration of atropine or other belladonna derivatives. Not recommended in patients receiving mecamylamine
Caution
Seizure disorders, bronchial asthma, coronary occlusion, hyperthyroidism, dysrhythmias, peptic ulcer, megacolon, poor GI motility, bradycardia, hypotension, lactation, children

DRUG INTERACTIONS OF CONCERN TO DENTISTRY
- Avoid drugs with anticholinergic activity and neuromuscular blocking agents
- Avoid systemic use of ester-type local anesthetics because of reduced plasma cholinesterase activity
- Use glucocorticoids with caution

SERIOUS REACTIONS
! Overdosage may result in cholinergic crisis, characterized by severe nausea, vomiting, diarrhea, increased salivation, diaphoresis, bradycardia, hypotension,

flushed skin, stomach pain, respiratory depression, seizures, and paralysis of muscles.
! Increasing muscle weakness of myasthenia gravis may occur. Antidote: 0.5-1mg IV atropine sulfate with other supportive treatment.

DENTAL CONSIDERATIONS

General:
• Control excessive salivary flow with rubber dam and suction.
• Avoid drugs that reduce salivary flow because they will antagonize this drug.
• Patient may be unable to keep mouth open for long periods because of disease; short appointments may be necessary.
• Monitor vital signs at every appointment because of cardiovascular side effects.
• Evaluate respiration characteristics and rate.
• Consider semisupine chair position for patient comfort if GI side effects occur.
• After supine positioning, have patient sit upright for at least 2 min to avoid orthostatic hypotension.
Consultations:
• Consultation with physician may be necessary if sedation or general anesthesia is required.
• Medical consultation may be required to assess disease control and patient's ability to tolerate stress.
Teach Patient/Family to:
• Use electric tooth brush if patient has difficulty holding conventional devices
• Update health and drug history, reporting changes in health status, drug regimen changes, or disease/treatment status

amcinonide
am-sin´-oh-nide
(Cylocort)

CATEGORY AND SCHEDULE
Pregnancy Risk Category: C

Drug Class: Antiinflammatory, steroidal, topical

MECHANISM OF ACTION
Topical corticosteroids have antiinflammatory, antipruritic, and vasoconstrictive properties. The exact mechanism of the antiinflammatory process is unclear. *Therapeutic Effect:* Reduces or prevents tissue response to inflammatory process.

USES
Relief of redness, swelling, itching, and discomfort of many skin problems

PHARMACOKINETICS
Well absorbed systemically. Large variation in absorption among sites: forearm 1%; scalp 4%, forehead 7%, scrotum 36%. Greatest penetration occurs at groin, axillae, and face. Protein binding in varying degrees. Metabolized in liver. Primarily excreted in urine.

INDICATIONS AND DOSAGES
▶ **Dermatoses**
Topical
Adults, Elderly. Apply sparingly 2–3 times a day.

SIDE EFFECTS/ADVERSE REACTIONS
Frequent
Itching, redness, irritation, burning

Occasional
Dryness, folliculitis, hypertrichosis, acneiform eruptions, hypopigmentation, perioral dermatitis
Rare
Allergic contact dermatitis, maceration of the skin, secondary infection, skin atrophy.
Systemic: Absorption more likely with occlusive dressings or extensive application in young children.

PRECAUTIONS AND CONTRAINDICATIONS
History of hypersensitivity to amcinonide or other corticosteroids

DRUG INTERACTIONS OF CONCERN TO DENTISTRY
None reported

SERIOUS REACTIONS
! The serious reactions of long-term therapy and the addition of occlusive dressings are reversible hypothalamic-pituitary-adrenal (HPA) axis suppression, manifestations of Cushing's syndrome, hyperglycemia and glucosuria.
! Abruptly withdrawing the drug after long-term therapy may require supplemental systemic corticosteroids.

DENTAL CONSIDERATIONS
General:
• Determine why patient is taking the drug.
• Side effects include a variety of skin lesions.
Teach Patient/Family to:
• Avoid use on oral herpetic ulcerations

amifostine
am-ih-fos´-teen
(Ethyol)
Do not confuse Ethyol with ethanol.

CATEGORY AND SCHEDULE
Pregnancy Risk Category: C

Drug Class: Cytoprotective, radioprotective

MECHANISM OF ACTION
An antineoplastic adjunct and cytoprotective agent that is converted to an active metabolite by alkaline phosphatase in tissues. The active metabolite binds to and detoxifies metabolites of cisplatin. These actions occur more readily in normal tissues than in tumor tissue.
Therapeutic Effect: Reduces the toxic effect of the chemotherapeutic agent cisplatin.

USES
(1) Incidence reduction in moderate to severe xerostomia in patients undergoing postoperative head and neck radiation for cancer where the radiation port includes a substantial part of the parotid gland; (2) reduction in cumulative renal toxicity associated with repeated cisplatin use in patients with advanced ovarian or non–small cell lung cancers

PHARMACOKINETICS
Rapidly cleared from plasma. Converted in tissue to active free thiol metabolite. Tissue uptake highest in bone marrow, skin, GI mucosa, salivary glands.
Half-life: less than 1 min. Less than 10% remains in plasma 6 min after drug administration.

INDICATIONS AND DOSAGES
▶ **To Reduce Cumulative Renal
Toxicity from Repeated
Administration of Cisplatin in
Patients with Advanced Ovarian
Cancer**
IV
Adults. 910 mg/m^2 once a day as
15-min infusion, beginning 30 min
before chemotherapy. A 15-min
infusion is better tolerated than
extended infusions. If the full dose
can't be administered, dose for
subsequent cycles should be
740 mg/m^2.
▶ **Treatment of Postoperative
Radiation-Induced Xerostomia in
Patients with Head and Neck Cancer**
IV
Adults. 200 mg/m^2 once a day as
3-min infusion, starting 15–30 min
before radiation therapy.
Subcutaneous
Adults. 500 mg/day during radiation
therapy.

SIDE EFFECTS/ADVERSE REACTIONS
Frequent
Transient reduction in B/P (usually
starts 14 min into infusion, lasts
about 6 min and returns to normal in
5–15 min); severe nausea, vomiting
Occasional
Flushing or feeling of warmth or
chills or feeling of coldness;
dizziness, hiccups, sneezing,
somnolence
Rare
Clinically relevant hypocalcemia,
mild rash

PRECAUTIONS AND CONTRAINDICATIONS
Sensitivity to aminothiol compounds
or mannitol
Caution
Patients should be well hydrated,
monitor blood pressure, safety not
established in CV disease; elderly,
cerebrovascular disease, lactation,
children

DRUG INTERACTIONS OF CONCERN TO DENTISTRY
None reported

SERIOUS REACTIONS
❗ A pronounced drop in B/P may
require temporary cessation of
amifostine and fluid resuscitation.

DENTAL CONSIDERATIONS
General:
• This is an in-hospital or outpatient
chemotherapy drug. Confirm the
patient's disease and treatment
status.
• Dental treatment may be provided
if necessary during treatment.
• Monitor vital signs at every
appointment because of
cardiovascular side effects.
• Consider semisupine chair position
for patient comfort if GI side effects
occur.
• Patients taking opioids for acute or
chronic pain should be given
alternative analgesics for dental pain.
• Short appointments and a stress
reduction protocol may be required
for anxious patients.
• Palliative medication may be
required for management of oral side
effects caused by chemotherapeutic
drugs.
• Assess salivary flow as a factor in
caries, periodontal disease, and
candidiasis.
• Chlorhexidine mouth rinse before
and during chemotherapy may
reduce severity of mucositis.
• Apply lubricant to dry lips for
patient comfort before dental
procedures.
• Examine for oral manifestation of
opportunistic infection.

Consultations:
• Medical consultation may be required to assess immunologic status during cancer therapy and determine safety risks posed by dental treatment.
• Consultation with physician may be necessary if sedation or general anesthesia is required.
Teach Patient/Family to:
• Prevent trauma when using oral hygiene aids
• Use effective oral hygiene to prevent soft tissue inflammation, infection
• Report oral lesions, soreness, or bleeding to dentist
• When chronic dry mouth occurs, advise patient to:
  • Avoid mouth rinses with high alcohol content because of drying effects
  • Use daily home fluoride products for anticaries effect
  • Use sugarless gum, frequent sips of water, or saliva substitutes
  • Update health and drug history, reporting changes in health status, drug regimen changes, or disease/treatment status

amiloride hydrochloride
a-mill´-oh-ride hi-droh-klor´-ide
(Kaluril[AUS], Midamor)
Do not confuse amiloride with amiodarone or amlodipine.

CATEGORY AND SCHEDULE
Pregnancy Risk Category: B (D if used in pregnancy-induced hypertension)

Drug Class: Potassium-sparing diuretic

MECHANISM OF ACTION
A guanidine derivative that acts as a potassium-sparing diuretic, antihypertensive, and antihypokalemic by directly interfering with sodium reabsorption in the distal tubule. ***Therapeutic Effect:*** Increases sodium and water excretion and decreases potassium excretion.

USES
Edema in CHF in combination with other diuretics, for hypertension as an adjunct with other diuretics to maintain potassium

PHARMACOKINETICS

Route	Onset	Peak	Duration
PO	2 hr	6–10 hr	24 hr

Incompletely absorbed from the GI tract. Protein binding: Minimal. Primarily excreted in urine; partially eliminated in feces. ***Half-life:*** 6–9 hr.

INDICATIONS AND DOSAGES
▶ **To Counteract Potassium Loss Induced by Other Diuretics**
PO
Adults, Children weighing more than 20 kg. 5–10 mg/day up to 20 mg.
Elderly. Initially, 5 mg/day or every other day.
Children weighing 6–20 kg. 0.625 mg/kg/day. Maximum: 10 mg/day.
▶ **Dosage in Renal Impairment**

Creatinine Clearance	Dosage
10–50 ml/min	50% of normal
Less than 10 ml/min	Avoid use

SIDE EFFECTS/ADVERSE REACTIONS
Frequent
Headache, nausea, diarrhea, vomiting, decreased appetite

Occasional
Dizziness, constipation, abdominal pain, weakness, fatigue, cough, impotence
Rare
Tremors, vertigo, confusion, nervousness, insomnia, thirst, dry mouth, heartburn, shortness of breath, increased urination, hypotension, rash

PRECAUTIONS AND CONTRAINDICATIONS

Acute or chronic renal insufficiency, anuria, diabetic nephropathy, patients on other potassium-sparing diuretics, serum potassium greater than 5.5 mEq/L
Caution
Dehydration, diabetes, acidosis, lactation

DRUG INTERACTIONS OF CONCERN TO DENTISTRY

• Decreased effects: corticosteroids, NSAIDs, indomethacin

SERIOUS REACTIONS

! Severe hyperkalemia may produce irritability; anxiety; a feeling of heaviness in the legs; paresthesia of hands, face, and lips; hypotension; bradycardia; tented T waves; widening of QRS, and ST depression.

DENTAL CONSIDERATIONS

General:
• Monitor vital signs at every appointment because of cardiovascular side effects.
• Assess salivary flow as a factor in caries, periodontal disease, and candidiasis.
• After supine positioning, have patient sit upright for at least 2 min to avoid orthostatic hypotension.

• Patients on chronic drug therapy may rarely have symptoms of blood dyscrasias, which can include infection, bleeding, and poor healing.
• Limit use of sodium-containing products, such as saline IV fluids, for those patients with a dietary salt restriction.
Consultations:
• Medical consultation may be required to assess patient's ability to tolerate stress.
• Medical consultation may be required to assess disease control.
• In a patient with symptoms of blood dyscrasias, request a medical consultation for blood studies and postpone dental treatment until normal values are reestablished.
Teach Patient/Family to:
• Use effective oral hygiene to prevent soft tissue inflammation
• Prevent injury when using oral hygiene aids
• When chronic dry mouth occurs, advise patient to:
  • Avoid mouth rinses with high alcohol content because of drying effects
  • Use daily home fluoride products for anticaries effect
  • Use sugarless gum, frequent sips of water, or saliva substitutes

aminocaproic acid
ah-mee-noe-ka-proe´-ik
(Amicar)
Do not confuse Amicar with amikacin or Amikin.

CATEGORY AND SCHEDULE
Pregnancy Risk Category: C

Drug Class: Hemostatic

MECHANISM OF ACTION

A systemic hemostatic that acts as an antifibrinolytic and antihemorrhagic by inhibiting the activation of plasminogen activator substances. *Therapeutic Effect:* Prevents formation of fibrin clots.

USES

Treatment of hemorrhage from hyperfibrinolysis; adjunctive therapy in hemophilia, postsurgical hemorrhage

PHARMACOKINETICS

PO: Protect granules by giving with acidic foods, mean peak serum levels 6 hr, 50%–60% protein bound; acetylated form excreted mostly in urine.

INDICATIONS AND DOSAGES

▶ **Acute Bleeding**
PO, IV Infusion
Adults, Elderly. 4–5 g over first hr; then 1–1.25 g/hr. Continue for 8 hr or until bleeding is controlled. Maximum: 30 g/24 hr.
Children. 3 g/m^2 over first hr; then 1 g/m^2/hr. Maximum: 18 g/m^2/24 hr.
▶ **Dosage in Renal Impairment**
Decrease dose to 25% of normal.

SIDE EFFECTS/ADVERSE REACTIONS

Occasional
Nausea, diarrhea, cramps, decreased urination, decreased B/P, dizziness, headache, muscle fatigue and weakness, myopathy, bloodshot eyes

PRECAUTIONS AND CONTRAINDICATIONS

Evidence of active intravascular clotting process, disseminated intravascular coagulation without concurrent heparin therapy, hematuria of upper urinary tract origin (unless benefit outweighs risk); newborns (parenteral form)
Caution
Neonates/infants, mild or moderate renal disease, hepatic disease, thrombophlebitis, cardiac disease, lactation

DRUG INTERACTIONS OF CONCERN TO DENTISTRY

None reported

SERIOUS REACTIONS

❗ Too-rapid IV administration produces tinnitus, rash, arrhythmias, unusual fatigue, and weakness.
❗ Rarely, a grand mal seizure occurs, generally preceded by weakness, dizziness, and headache.

DENTAL CONSIDERATIONS

General:
• Monitor vital signs at every appointment because of cardiovascular side effects.
• After supine positioning, have patient sit upright for at least 2 min to avoid orthostatic hypotension.
• Consider additional local hemostasis measures to prevent excessive bleeding in patients with hemophilia.
• Determine why the patient is taking the drug.
• Avoid drugs such as aspirin; NSAIDs may have the potential to prolong bleeding.
Consultations:
• Medical consultation may be required to assess disease control.
• Medical consultation may be required to assess patient's ability to tolerate stress.
Teach Patient/Family to:
• Use effective oral hygiene to prevent soft tissue inflammation

• Prevent injury when using oral hygiene aids

aminoglutethimide
ah-mee-noe-gloo-teth´-ih-mide
(Cytadren)

CATEGORY AND SCHEDULE
Pregnancy Risk Category: D

Drug Class: Antineoplastic, antiadrenal

MECHANISM OF ACTION
An antiadrenal agent that partially inhibits the conversion of cholesterol to pregnenolone in the adrenal glands and blocks the conversion of androstenedione to estrone and estradiol in peripheral tissues. *Therapeutic Effect:* Suppresses adrenal function.

USES
Treatment of some kinds of tumors that affect the adrenal cortex

PHARMACOKINETICS
Rapidly and completely absorbed from the GI tract. Protein binding: Low (20%–25%). Metabolized in the liver by acetylation. Primarily excreted in urine. *Half-life:* 12.5 hours.

INDICATIONS AND DOSAGES
▶ **Cushing's Syndrome**
PO
Adults. Initially, 250 mg q6h. May increase by 250 mg daily every 1 to 2 wk. Maximum: 2 g/day.

SIDE EFFECTS/ADVERSE REACTIONS
Frequent
Drowsiness, rash, loss of appetite, nausea

Occasional
Dizziness, headache, fever, myalgia, hypotension, tachycardia, pruritus, depression
Rare
Neck tenderness, swelling, increased hair growth in females

PRECAUTIONS AND CONTRAINDICATIONS
Hypersensitivity to glutethimide or aminoglutethimide

DRUG INTERACTIONS OF CONCERN TO DENTISTRY
None reported

SERIOUS REACTIONS
! Adrenal insufficiency, agranulocytosis, leukopenia, neutropenia, and pancytopenia may occur.

DENTAL CONSIDERATIONS
General:
• Determine why patient is taking the drug.
• Monitor vital signs at every appointment due to cardiovascular side effects.
• Determine dose and duration of glucocorticoid therapy to assess for risk of stress tolerance and immunosuppression. Patients on chronic glucocorticoid therapy may require supplemental doses for dental treatment.
• Precaution if dental surgery is anticipated or general anesthesia is required.
• Patient on chronic drug therapy may rarely present with symptoms of blood dyscrasias, which can include infection, bleeding and poor healing. If dyscrasia is present, caution patient to prevent oral tissue trauma when using oral hygiene aids.

• After supine positioning, have patient sit upright for at least 2 min before standing to avoid orthostatic hypotension.

• Patient may need assistance in getting into and out of dental chair. Adjust chair position for patient comfort.

• Examine for oral manifestation of opportunistic infection.

• Caution: use of additional CNS depressants.

• If cancer is present, evaluate surgical, radiation, and chemotherapy history.

Consultations:

• Consultation may be required to confirm glucocorticoid dose and duration of use.

• Medical consultation may be required to assess disease control and patient's ability to tolerate stress.

• In a patient with symptoms of blood dyscrasias, request a medical consultation for blood studies and postpone treatment until normal values are reestablished.

Teach Patient/Family to:

• Update health and medication history if physician makes any changes in evaluation or drug regimens; include OTC, herbal, and nonherbal remedies in the update

• Report oral lesions, soreness, or bleeding to dentist

• Avoid driving or performing other tasks requiring mental alertness while taking aminoglutethimide

• Use effective oral hygiene to prevent soft tissue inflammation

• Prevent trauma when using oral hygiene aids

aminophylline/ theophylline
am-in-off´-ih-lin
(aminophylline) Phyllocontin,
(theophylline) Elixophyllin,
Quibron-T, Quibron-T/SR,
Nuelin[AUS], Nuelin SR[AUS], Slo-
Bid Gyrocaps, Theo-24, Thoechron,
Theodur, Theolair, T-Phyl, Uniphyl
Do not confuse aminophylline
with amitriptyline or ampicillin, or
Slo-Bid with Dolobid.

CATEGORY AND SCHEDULE
Pregnancy Risk Category: C

Drug Class: Xanthine

MECHANISM OF ACTION
A xanthine derivative that acts as a bronchodilator by directly relaxing smooth muscle of the bronchial airways and pulmonary blood vessels. *Therapeutic Effect:* Relieves bronchospasm and increases vital capacity.

USES
Treatment of bronchial asthma, bronchospasm, Cheyne-Stokes respirations

PHARMACOKINETICS
PO: Peak 1 hr; metabolized in liver; excreted in urine, breast milk; crosses placenta.

INDICATIONS AND DOSAGES
▸ **Chronic Bronchospasm**
PO
Adults, Elderly, Children. 16 mg/kg or 400 mg/day (whichever is less) in 3–4 divided doses (8-hr intervals); may increase by 25% every 2–3 days. Maximum: 13 mg/kg/day (children 13–16 yr); 18 mg/kg/day

(children 9–12 yr); 20 mg/kg/day (children 1–8 yr). Maximum dosages are based on serum theophylline concentrations, clinical condition, and presence of toxicity.

▶ **Acute Bronchospasm in Patients not Currently Taking Theophylline**
PO
Adults, Children older than 1 yr.
Initially, loading dose of 5 mg/kg (theophylline); then maintenance dosage of theophylline based on patient group (shown below).

Patient Group	Maintenance Theophylline Dosage
Healthy, nonsmoking adults	3 mg/kg q8h
Elderly patients, patients with cor pulmonale	2 mg/kg q8h
Patients with CHF or hepatic disease	1–2 mg/kg q12h
Children 9–16 yr, young adult smokers	3 mg/kg q6h
Children 1–8 yr	4 mg/kg q6h

IV
Adults, Children older than 1 yr.
Initially, loading dose of 6 mg/kg (aminophylline); maintenance dosage of aminophylline based on patient group (shown below).

Patient Group	Maintenance Aminophylline Dosage
Healthy, nonsmoking adults	0.7 mg/kg/hr
Elderly patients, patients with cor pulmonale, CHF, or hepatic impairment	0.25 mg/kg/hr
Children 13–16 yr	0.7 mg/kg/hr

Children 9–12 yr, young adult smokers	0.9 mg/kg/hr
Children 1–8 yr	1–1.2 mg/kg/hr
Children 6 mo–1 yr	0.6–0.7 mg/kg/hr
Children 6 wk–6 mo	0.5 mg/kg/hr
Neonates	5 mg/kg q12h

▶ **Acute Bronchospasm in Patients Currently Taking Theophylline**
PO, IV
Adults, Children older than 1 yr.
Obtain serum theophylline level. If not possible and patient is in respiratory distress and not experiencing toxic effects, may give 2.5 mg/kg dose. Maintenance: Dosage based on peak serum theophylline concentration, clinical condition, and presence of toxicity.

SIDE EFFECTS/ADVERSE REACTIONS
Frequent
Altered smell (during IV administration), restlessness, tachycardia, tremor
Occasional
Heartburn, vomiting, headache, mild diuresis, insomnia, nausea

PRECAUTIONS AND CONTRAINDICATIONS
History of hypersensitivity to caffeine or xanthine
Caution
Elderly, CHF, cor pulmonale, hepatic disease, active peptic ulcer disease, diabetes mellitus, hyperthyroidism, hypertension, children, glaucoma, prostatic hypertrophy

DRUG INTERACTIONS OF CONCERN TO DENTISTRY
• Increased action: erythromycin (macrolides), ciprofloxacin

• Cardiac dysrhythmia:
CNS stimulants, hydrocarbon
inhalation anesthetics
• Decreased effects: barbiturates,
carbamazepine
• Decreased effects of
benzodiazepines

SERIOUS REACTIONS

! Too-rapid IV administration
may produce marked hypotension
with accompanying faintness,
light-headedness, palpitations,
tachycardia, hyperventilation,
nausea, vomiting, angina-like pain,
seizures, ventricular fibrillation, and
cardiac standstill.

DENTAL CONSIDERATIONS

General:
• Monitor vital signs at every
appointment because of
cardiovascular and respiratory
side effects.
• Consider semisupine chair
position for patient comfort
because of respiratory
disease and GI side effects
of drug.
• Midday appointments and a
stress reduction protocol
may be required for anxious
patients.
• Be aware that aspirin or sulfite
preservatives in vasoconstrictor-
containing products can exacerbate
asthma.
• Acute asthmatic episodes
may be precipitated in the
dental office. Sympathomimetic
inhalants should be available for
emergency use.
Consultations:
• Medical consultation may be
required to assess disease
control.

aminosalicylic acid

ah-mee-noe-sal-ih-sil-ik as-id
(Nemasol[CAN], Paser)

CATEGORY AND SCHEDULE
Pregnancy Risk Category: C

Drug Class: Antitubercular
antiinfective

MECHANISM OF ACTION
An antitubercular agent active
against *M. tuberculosis.* Thought to
exhibit competitive antagonism of
folic acid synthesis. ***Therapeutic
Effect:*** Bacteriostatic activity in
susceptible microorganisms.

USES
Tuberculosis, in combination with
other *M. tuberculosis* antiinfectives

PHARMACOKINETICS
Readily absorbed from the GI tract.
Protein binding: 50%–60%. Widely
distributed (including CSF).
Metabolized in liver. Primarily
excreted in urine. Removed by
hemodialysis. ***Half-life:*** 1.1–1.62 hr.

INDICATIONS AND DOSAGES
▶ **Tuberculosis**
PO
Adults, Elderly. 4 g in divided doses
3 times a day.
Children. 150 mg/kg/day in divided
doses
3 times a day. Maximum: 12 g/day.

SIDE EFFECTS/ADVERSE REACTIONS
Occasional
Abdominal pain, diarrhea, nausea,
vomiting

Rare
Hypersensitivity reactions, hepatotoxicity, thrombocytopenia

PRECAUTIONS AND CONTRAINDICATIONS

End-stage renal disease, hypersensitivity to aminosalicylic acid products

Caution
Hepatic dysfunction, refrigeration required for storage, malabsorption of vitamin B_{12}, no data on safe use in children or lactation

DRUG INTERACTIONS OF CONCERN TO DENTISTRY

None reported

SERIOUS REACTIONS

! Liver toxicity and hepatitis, blood dyscrasias occur rarely.
! Agranulocytosis, methemoglobinemia, thrombocytopenia have been reported.

DENTAL CONSIDERATIONS

General:
• Determine that noninfectious status exists by ensuring that (1) anti-tuberculosis (TB) drugs have been taken for more than 3 wk, (2) culture confirmed TB susceptibility to antiinfectives, (3) patient has had three consecutive negative sputum smears, and (4) patient is not in the coughing stage.
• Determine why patient is taking drug (i.e., for prophylaxis or active therapy).
• Explain importance of taking medication for full length of regimen to ensure effectiveness of treatment and to prevent the emergence of resistant strains.
• Patients on chronic drug therapy may rarely have symptoms of blood

dyscrasias, which can include infection, bleeding, and poor healing.
• Consider semisupine chair position for patient comfort if GI side effects occur.

Consultations:
• Medical consultation may be required to assess disease control and patient's ability to tolerate stress.
• In a patient with symptoms of blood dyscrasias, request a medical consultation for blood studies and postpone treatment until normal values are reestablished.

Teach Patient/Family to:
• Update health and drug history if physician makes any changes in evaluation or drug regimens
• Prevent trauma when using oral hygiene aids

amiodarone hydrochloride

ay´-mee-oh-da-rone
hi-droh-klor´-ide
(Aratac[AUS], Cordarone, Cordarone X[AUS], Pacerone)
Do not confuse amiodarone with amiloride or Cordarone with Cardura.

CATEGORY AND SCHEDULE

Pregnancy Risk Category: D

Drug Class: Antidysrhythmic (class III)

MECHANISM OF ACTION

A cardiac agent that prolongs duration of myocardial cell action potential and refractory period by acting directly on all cardiac tissue. Decreases AV and SN function.
Therapeutic Effect: Suppresses arrhythmias.

USES
Documented life-threatening ventricular tachycardia; unapproved: ventricular fibrillation not controlled by first-line agents

PHARMACOKINETICS

Route	Onset	Peak	Duration
PO	3 days–3 wk	1 wk–5 mo	7–50 days after discontinuation

Slowly, variably absorbed from GI tract. Protein binding: 96%. Extensively metabolized in the liver to active metabolite. Excreted via bile; not removed by hemodialysis. *Half-life:* 26–107 days; metabolite, 61 days.

INDICATIONS AND DOSAGES
▶ **Life-Threatening Recurrent Ventricular Fibrillation or Hemodynamically Unstable Ventricular Tachycardia**
PO
Adults, Elderly. Initially, 800–1600 mg/day in 2–4 divided doses for 1–3 wk. After arrhythmia is controlled or side effects occur, reduce to 600–800 mg/day for about 4 wk. Maintenance: 200–600 mg/day.
Children. Initially, 10–15 mg/kg/day for 4–14 days, then 5 mg/kg/day for several wk. Maintenance: 2.5 mg/kg or lowest effective maintenance dose for 5 of 7 days/wk.
IV Infusion
Adults. Initially, 1050 mg over 24 hr; 150 mg over 10 min, then 360 mg over 6 hr; then 540 mg over 18 hr. May continue at 0.5 mg/min for up to 2–3 wk regardless of age or renal or left ventricular function.

SIDE EFFECTS/ADVERSE REACTIONS
Expected
Corneal microdeposits are noted in almost all patients treated for more than 6 mo (can lead to blurry vision).
Frequent
Parenteral: Hypotension, nausea, fever, bradycardia.
Oral: Constipation, headache, decreased appetite, nausea, vomiting, paresthesias, photosensitivity, muscular incoordination.
Occasional
Oral: Bitter or metallic taste; decreased libido; dizziness; facial flushing; blue-gray coloring of skin (face, arms, and neck); blurred vision; bradycardia; asymptomatic corneal deposits.
Rare
Oral: Rash, vision loss, blindness.

PRECAUTIONS AND CONTRAINDICATIONS
Bradycardia-induced syncope (except in the presence of a pacemaker), second- and third-degree AV block, severe hepatic disease, severe SN dysfunction
Caution
Goiter, Hashimoto's thyroiditis, SN dysfunction, second- or third-degree AV block, electrolyte imbalances, bradycardia; lactation, not recommended for children

DRUG INTERACTIONS OF CONCERN TO DENTISTRY
• Bradycardia, hypotension: inhalation anesthetics, lidocaine, anticholinergics, vasoconstrictors
• Increased photosensitization: tetracyclines
• Do not use with grapefruit juice, gatifloxacin, moxifloxacin, or sparfloxacin

17

• Amiodarone is both a substrate and an inhibitor of CYP3A4; potential interactions with strong inhibitors of CYP3A4 isoenzymes

SERIOUS REACTIONS

! Serious, potentially fatal pulmonary toxicity (alveolitis, pulmonary fibrosis, pneumonitis, acute respiratory distress syndrome) may begin with progressive dyspnea and cough with crackles, decreased breath sounds, pleurisy, CHF, or hepatotoxicity.

! Amiodarone may worsen existing arrhythmias or produce new arrhythmias (called proarrhythmias).

DENTAL CONSIDERATIONS

General:
• Monitor vital signs at every appointment because of cardiovascular and respiratory side effects.
• Assess salivary flow as a factor in caries, periodontal disease, and candidiasis.
• Avoid dental light in patient's eyes; offer dark glasses for patient comfort.
• After supine positioning, have patient sit upright for at least 2 min before standing to avoid orthostatic hypotension.
• Use vasoconstrictors with caution, in low doses, and with careful aspiration. Avoid gingival retraction cord with epinephrine.
• Stress from dental procedures may compromise cardiovascular function; determine patient risk.
• Delay or avoid dental treatment if patient shows signs of cardiac symptoms or respiratory distress.
Consultations:
• Medical consultation may be required to assess patient's ability to tolerate stress.

• Medical consultation may be required to assess disease control.
Teach Patient/Family to:
• Update health and drug history, reporting changes in health status, drug regimen changes, or disease/treatment status
• When chronic dry mouth occurs, advise patient to:
  • Avoid mouth rinses with high alcohol content because of drying effects
  • Use daily home fluoride products for anticaries effect
  • Use sugarless gum, frequent sips of water, or saliva substitutes

amitriptyline hydrochloride

ah-mee-trip´-ti-leen hi-droh-klor´-ide
(Apo-Amitriptyline[CAN], Elavil, Endep[AUS], Levate[CAN], Novo-Triptyn[CAN], Tryptanol[AUS])
Do not confuse amitriptyline with aminophylline or nortriptyline, or Elavil with Equanil or Mellaril.

CATEGORY AND SCHEDULE
Pregnancy Risk Category: C

Drug Class:
Antidepressant-tricyclic

MECHANISM OF ACTION
A tricyclic antidepressant that blocks the reuptake of neurotransmitters, including norepinephrine and serotonin, at presynaptic membranes, thus increasing their availability at postsynaptic receptor sites. Also has strong anticholinergic activity.
Therapeutic Effect: Relieves depression.

USES
Treatment of major depression; unapproved: treatment of enuresis and neurogenic pain

PHARMACOKINETICS
Rapidly and well absorbed from the GI tract. Protein binding: 90%. Undergoes first-pass metabolism in the liver. Primarily excreted in urine. Minimal removal by hemodialysis. *Half-life:* 10–26 hr.

INDICATIONS AND DOSAGES
▶ **Depression**
PO
Adults. 30–100 mg/day as a single dose at bedtime or in divided doses. May gradually increase up to 300 mg/day. Titrate to lowest effective dosage.
Elderly. Initially, 10–25 mg at bedtime. May increase by 10–25 mg at weekly intervals. Range: 25–150 mg/day.
Children 6–12 yr. 1–5 mg/kg/day in 2 divided doses.
IM
Adults. 20–30 mg 4 times a day.
▶ **Pain Management**
PO
Adults, Elderly. 25–100 mg at bedtime.

SIDE EFFECTS/ADVERSE REACTIONS
Frequent
Dizziness, somnolence, dry mouth, orthostatic hypotension, headache, increased appetite, weight gain, nausea, unusual fatigue, unpleasant taste
Occasional
Blurred vision, confusion, constipation, hallucinations, delayed micturition, eye pain, arrhythmias, fine muscle tremors, parkinsonian syndrome, anxiety, diarrhea, diaphoresis, heartburn, insomnia

Rare
Hypersensitivity, alopecia, tinnitus, breast enlargement, photosensitivity

PRECAUTIONS AND CONTRAINDICATIONS
Acute recovery period after MI, use within 14 days of MAOIs
Caution
Suicidal patients, convulsive disorders, prostatic hypertrophy, asthma, schizophrenia, psychotic disorders, severe depression, increased intraocular pressure, narrow-angle glaucoma, urinary retention, cardiac disease, hepatic disease, renal disease, hyperthyroidism, electroshock therapy, elective surgery, children younger than 12 yr, elderly, MAOIs, St. John's wort

DRUG INTERACTIONS OF CONCERN TO DENTISTRY
• Increased anticholinergic effects: muscarinic blockers, antihistamines, phenothiazines
• Increased effects of direct-acting sympathomimetics (epinephrine, levonordefrin)
• Possible risk of increased CNS depression: alcohol, barbiturates, benzodiazepines, CNS depressants, antidepressants
• Possible increase in serum levels: fluconazole, ketoconazole, bupropion, fluvoxamine, paroxetine, sertraline
• Decreased antihypertensive effect: clonidine, guanadrel, guanethidine
• Possible decrease in serum levels: barbiturates, St. John's wort (herb)

SERIOUS REACTIONS
! Overdose may produce confusion, seizures, severe somnolence, arrhythmias, fever, hallucinations, agitation, dyspnea, vomiting, and unusual fatigue or weakness.

! Abrupt discontinuation after prolonged therapy may produce headache, malaise, nausea, vomiting, and vivid dreams.
! Blood dyscrasias and cholestatic jaundice occur rarely.

DENTAL CONSIDERATIONS
General:
• Take vital signs every appointment because of cardiovascular side effects.
• Assess salivary flow as a factor in caries, periodontal disease, and candidiasis.
• Patients on chronic drug therapy may rarely have symptoms of blood dyscrasias, which can include infection, bleeding, and poor healing.
• After supine positioning, have patient sit upright for at least 2 min to avoid orthostatic hypotension.
• Use vasoconstrictors with caution, in low doses, and with careful aspiration. Avoid use of gingival retraction cord with epinephrine.
• Place on frequent recall because of oral side effects.
Consultations:
• In a patient with symptoms of blood dyscrasias, request a medical consultation for blood studies and postpone dental treatment until normal values are reestablished.
• Medical consultation may be required to assess disease control.
• Physician should be informed if significant xerostomic side effects occur (e.g., increased caries, sore tongue, problems eating or swallowing, difficulty wearing prosthesis) so that a medication change can be considered.
Teach Patient/Family to:
• Use effective oral hygiene to prevent soft tissue inflammation
• Prevent injury when using oral hygiene aids

• When chronic dry mouth occurs, advise patient to:
  • Avoid mouth rinses with high alcohol content because of drying effects
  • Use daily home fluoride products for anticaries effect
  • Use sugarless gum, frequent sips of water, or saliva substitutes

amlexanox
am-lecks´-ah-knocks
(Apthasol)
Do not confuse with Ambesol.

CATEGORY AND SCHEDULE
Pregnancy Risk Category: B

Drug Class: Topical antiinflammatory

MECHANISM OF ACTION
A mouth agent that has anti-allergic and antiinflammatory properties. Appears to inhibit formation and/or release of inflammatory mediators (e.g., histamine) from mast cells, neutrophils, mononuclear cells.
Therapeutic Effect: Alleviates signs and symptoms of aphthous ulcers.

USES
Treatment of aphthous ulcers in patients with normal immune systems

PHARMACOKINETICS
After topical application, most systemic absorption occurs from the GI tract. Metabolized to inactive metabolite. Excreted in urine.
Half-life: 3.5 hr.

INDICATIONS AND DOSAGES
▶ **Aphthous Ulcers**
Topical
Adults, Elderly. Administer ¼ inch directly to ulcers 4 times a day (after meals and at bedtime) following oral hygiene.

SIDE EFFECTS/ADVERSE REACTIONS
Rare
Stinging, burning at administration site, transient pain, rash

PRECAUTIONS AND CONTRAINDICATIONS
Hypersensitivity
Caution
Wash hands immediately before and after each use; discontinue if mucositis appears, lactation, children

DRUG INTERACTIONS OF CONCERN TO DENTISTRY
None reported

SERIOUS REACTIONS
! Ingestion of a full tube would result in nausea, vomiting, and diarrhea.

DENTAL CONSIDERATIONS
General:
• Recurrent aphthous ulcers may be associated with systemic conditions; evaluate as needed if healing has not occurred after 10 days.
Teach Patient/Family to:
• Apply paste as directed and wash hands immediately before and after each use
• Report oral lesions or soreness to dentist

amoxapine
ah-moks-ah-peen
(Ascendin)
Do not confuse amoxapine with atomoxetine or atropine.

CATEGORY AND SCHEDULE
Pregnancy Risk Category: C

Drug Class: Antidepressant, tricyclic

MECHANISM OF ACTION
A tricyclic antidepressant that blocks the reuptake of neurotransmitters, such as norepinephrine and serotonin, at CNS presynaptic membranes, increasing their availability at postsynaptic receptor sites. The metabolite 7-OH-amoxapine has significant dopamine receptor blocking activity similar to haloperidol. *Therapeutic Effect:* Produces antidepressant effects.

USES
Treatment of depression

PHARMACOKINETICS
Rapidly, well absorbed from the GI tract. Protein binding: 90%. Metabolized in liver. Excreted in urine and feces. *Half-life:* 8 hr.

INDICATIONS AND DOSAGES
▶ **Depression**
PO
Adults. 25 mg 2–3 times a day. May increase to 100 mg 2–3 times a day.
Adolescents. Initially, 25–50 mg/day as single or divided doses. May increase to 100 mg/day.
Elderly. Initially, 25 mg at bedtime. May increase by 25 mg/day q3–7 days. Maximum: 400 mg/day (outpatient), 600 mg/day (inpatient).

SIDE EFFECTS/ADVERSE REACTIONS
Frequent
Drowsiness, fatigue, xerostomia, constipation, weight gain
Occasional
Nausea, dizziness, headache, confusion, nervousness, restlessness, insomnia, edema, tremor, blurred vision, aggressiveness, muscle weakness
Rare
Paradoxical reactions (agitation, restlessness, nightmares, insomnia, extrapyramidal symptoms, particularly fine hand tremor), laryngitis, seizures

PRECAUTIONS AND CONTRAINDICATIONS
Acute recovery period following MI, within 14 days of MAOI ingestion, hypersensitivity to dibenzoxazepine compounds
Caution
Suicidal patients, severe depression, increased intraocular pressure, narrow-angle glaucoma, urinary retention, cardiac disease, hepatic disease, hyperthyroidism, electroshock therapy, elective surgery, elderly, MAOIs

DRUG INTERACTIONS OF CONCERN TO DENTISTRY
• Increased anticholinergic effects: muscarinic blockers, antihistamines, phenothiazines
• Increased effects of direct-acting sympathomimetics (epinephrine, levonordefrin)
• Potential risk of increased CNS depression: alcohol, barbiturates, benzodiazepines, CNS depressants
• Decreased antihypertensive effect: clonidine, guanadrel, guanethidine
• Avoid concurrent use with St. John's wort (herb)

SERIOUS REACTIONS
❗ High dosage may produce cardiovascular effects, including severe postural hypotension, dizziness, tachycardia, palpitations, arrhythmias, and seizures. High dosage may also result in altered temperature regulation, such as hyperpyrexia or hypothermia.
❗ Abrupt withdrawal from prolonged therapy may produce headache, malaise, nausea, vomiting, and vivid dreams.

DENTAL CONSIDERATIONS
General:
• Take vital signs every appointment because of cardiovascular side effects.
• Assess salivary flow as a factor in caries, periodontal disease, and candidiasis.
• Patients on chronic drug therapy may rarely have symptoms of blood dyscrasias, which can include infection, bleeding, and poor healing.
• After supine positioning, have patient sit upright for at least 2 min to avoid orthostatic hypotension.
• Use vasoconstrictors with caution, in low doses, and with careful aspiration. Avoid use of gingival retraction cord with epinephrine.
• Place on frequent recall because of oral side effects.
Consultations:
• In a patient with symptoms of blood dyscrasias, request a medical consultation for blood studies and postpone dental treatment until normal values are reestablished.
• Medical consultation may be required to assess disease control.
• Physician should be informed if significant xerostomic side effects occur (e.g., increased caries, sore tongue, problems eating or

swallowing, difficulty wearing prosthesis) so that a medication change can be considered.

Teach Patient/Family to:
• Use effective oral hygiene to prevent soft tissue inflammation
• Prevent injury when using oral hygiene aids
• When chronic dry mouth occurs, advise patient to:
  • Avoid mouth rinses with high alcohol content because of drying effects
  • Use daily home fluoride products for anticaries effect
  • Use sugarless gum, frequent sips of water, or saliva substitutes

amoxicillin/ clavulanate potassium

ah-mox´-ih-sill-in /clav-u-lan´-ate poh-tass´-ee-um
(Augmentin, Augmentin ES 600, Augmentin XR, Ausclay[AUS], Ausclay Duo Forte[AUS], Ausclay Duo 400[AUS], Clamoxyl[AUS], Clamoxyl Duo 400[AUS], Clamoxyl Duo Forte[AUS], Clavulin[CAN], Clavulin Duo Forte[AUS])
Do not confuse amoxicillin with amoxapine.

CATEGORY AND SCHEDULE
Pregnancy Risk Category: B

Drug Class: Aminopenicillin with a β-lactamase inhibitor

MECHANISM OF ACTION
Amoxicillin inhibits bacterial cell wall synthesis, while clavulanate inhibits bacterial β-lactamase.
Therapeutic Effect: Amoxicillin is bactericidal in susceptible

microorganisms. Clavulanate protects amoxicillin from enzymatic degradation.

USES
For treatment of infections caused by susceptible β-lactamase–producing strains of microorganisms as listed: lower respiratory tract infections, otitis media, and sinusitis caused by *H. influenzae, M. catarrhalis;* skin and skin structure infections caused by *S. aureus, E. coli, Klebsiella* species; UTIs caused by *E. coli, Klebsiella, Enterobacter* species; Augmentin ES-600: treatment of recurrent or persistent otitis media, *S. pneumoniae,* and β-lactamase–producing strains of *H. influenzae* or *M. catarrhalis*

PHARMACOKINETICS
Well absorbed from the GI tract. Protein binding: 20%. Partially metabolized in the liver. Primarily excreted in urine. Removed by hemodialysis. *Half-life:* 1–1.3 hr (increased in impaired renal function).

INDICATIONS AND DOSAGES
▶ **Mild-to-Moderate Infections**
PO
Adults, Elderly. 500 mg q12h or 250 mg q8h.
▶ **Severe Infections, Respiratory Tract Infections**
PO
Adults, Elderly. 875 mg q12h or 500 mg q8h.
▶ **Community-Acquired Pneumonia, Sinusitis**
PO
Adults, Elderly. 2 g (extended-release tablets) q12h for 7–10 days.
▶ **Usual Pediatric Dosage**
PO
Children weighing 40 kg and less. 25–45 mg/kg/day (200 or 400 mg/5 ml

powder or 200 or 400 mg chewable tablets) in 2 divided doses or 20–40 mg/kg/day (125 or 250 mg/5 ml powder or 125 or 250 mg/5 ml chewable tablets) in 3 divided doses.

▸ **Otitis Media**
PO
Children. 90 mg/kg/day (600 mg/5 ml suspension) in divided doses q12h for 10 days.

▸ **Usual Neonate Dosage**
PO
Neonates, Children younger than 3 mo. 30 mg/kg/day (125 mg/5 ml suspension) in divided doses q12h.

▸ **Dosage in Renal Impairment**
Dosage and frequency are modified on the basis of creatinine clearance.
Creatinine clearance 10–30 ml/min. 250–500 mg q12h.
Creatinine clearance less than 10 ml/min. 250–500 mg q24h.

SIDE EFFECTS/ADVERSE REACTIONS
Frequent
GI disturbances (mild diarrhea, nausea, vomiting), headache, oral or vaginal candidiasis
Occasional
Generalized rash, urticaria

PRECAUTIONS AND CONTRAINDICATIONS
Hypersensitivity to any penicillins, infectious mononucleosis
Caution
Hypersensitivity to cephalosporins, hepatic function impairment

DRUG INTERACTIONS OF CONCERN TO DENTISTRY
• Decreased antimicrobial effectiveness: tetracyclines, erythromycins, lincomycins

• Increased amoxicillin concentrations: probenecid
• Increased risk of skin rashes: allopurinol
• When used for dental infection:
• Oral contraceptives: advise patient of a potential risk for decreased contraceptive action, to maintain compliance with oral contraceptive use while using antibiotics, and to consider the use of additional nonhormonal contraception

SERIOUS REACTIONS
❗ Antibiotic-associated colitis and other superinfections may result from altered bacterial balance.
❗ Severe hypersensitivity reactions including anaphylaxis and acute interstitial nephritis occur rarely.

DENTAL CONSIDERATIONS
General:
• Take precautions regarding allergy to medication.
• Determine why the patient is taking the drug.
Consultations:
• Medical consultation may be required to assess disease control.
Teach Patient/Family:
• Importance of good oral hygiene to prevent soft tissue inflammation
• Caution to prevent injury when using oral hygiene aids
• When used for dental infection, advise patient:
  • To report sore throat, oral burning sensation, fever, and fatigue, any of which could indicate superinfection
  • To take at prescribed intervals and complete dosage regimen
  • To immediately notify the dentist if signs or symptoms of infection increase

amphetamine
am-fet´-ah-meen

CATEGORY AND SCHEDULE
Pregnancy Risk Category: C
Controlled substance: Schedule II

Drug Class: Amphetamine

MECHANISM OF ACTION
A sympathomimetic amine that produces CNS and respiratory stimulation, mydriasis, bronchodilation, a pressor response, and contraction of the urinary sphincter. Directly affects α and β receptor sites in peripheral system. Enhances release of norepinephrine by blocking reuptake, inhibiting monoamine oxidase. *Therapeutic Effect:* Increases motor activity, mental alertness; decreases drowsiness, fatigue.

USES
Narcolepsy, attention deficit disorder with hyperactivity (ADHD)

PHARMACOKINETICS
Well absorbed from the GI tract. Protein binding: 20%. Widely distributed (including CSF). Metabolized in liver. Excreted in urine. Unknown if removed by hemodialysis. *Half-life:* 7–31 hr.

INDICATIONS AND DOSAGES
▸ ADHD
PO
Adults. 5–20 mg 1–3 times a day.
Adults, Children older than 12 yr.
Initially, 5 mg twice a day. Increase by 10 mg at weekly intervals until therapeutic response achieved.
Children 6–12 yr. Initially, 2.5 mg twice a day. Increase by 5 mg/day at weekly intervals until therapeutic response achieved.
Children 3–6 yr. Initially, 2.5 mg twice a day. Increase by 2.5 mg/day at weekly intervals until therapeutic response achieved.
▸ Narcolepsy
PO
Adults. 5–20 mg 1–3 times a day.
Adults, Children older than 12 yr.
Initially, 5 mg twice a day. Increase by 10 mg at weekly intervals until therapeutic response achieved.
Children 6–12 yr. Initially, 2.5 mg twice a day. Increase by 5 mg/day at weekly intervals until therapeutic response achieved.

SIDE EFFECTS/ADVERSE REACTIONS
Frequent
Irregular pulse, increased motor activity, talkativeness, nervousness, mild euphoria, insomnia
Occasional
Headache, chills, dry mouth, GI distress, worsening depression in patients who are clinically depressed, tachycardia, palpitations, chest pain

PRECAUTIONS AND CONTRAINDICATIONS
Advanced arteriosclerosis, agitated states, glaucoma, history of drug abuse, history of hypersensitivity to sympathomimetic amines, hyperthyroidism, moderate to severe hypertension, symptomatic cardiovascular disease, within 14 days following discontinuation of an MAOI
Caution
Gilles de la Tourette's syndrome, lactation, children younger than 3 yr

DRUG INTERACTIONS OF CONCERN TO DENTISTRY
• Increased sensitivity to effects of sympathomimetics; increased risk of serotonin syndrome with selective serotonin reuptake inhibitors (SSRIs)
• Increased pressor response: tricyclic antidepressants

SERIOUS REACTIONS
❗ Overdose may produce skin pallor or flushing, arrhythmias, and psychosis.
❗ Abrupt withdrawal following prolonged administration of high dosage may produce lethargy (may last for weeks).
❗ Prolonged administration to children with ADHD may produce a temporary suppression of normal weight and height patterns.

DENTAL CONSIDERATIONS
General:
• Monitor vital signs at every appointment because of cardiovascular side effects.
• Assess salivary flow as a factor in caries, periodontal disease, and candidiasis.
• Psychologic and physical dependence may occur with chronic use.
• Consider short appointments, frequent recall if patient becomes restless during a dental appointment.
Consultations:
• Medical consultation may be required to assess disease control and patient's ability to tolerate stress.
Teach Patient/Family to:
• Update health and drug history, reporting changes in health status, drug regimen changes, or disease/treatment status
• Use effective oral hygiene to prevent soft tissue inflammation, infection

• To prevent trauma when using oral hygiene aids
• When chronic dry mouth occurs, advise patient to:
  • Avoid mouth rinses with high alcohol content because of drying effects
  • Use daily home fluoride products for anticaries effect
  • Use sugarless gum, frequent sips of water, or saliva substitutes

amphotericin B
am-foe-ter´-ih-sin bee
(Abelcet, AmBisome, Amphocin, Amphotec, Fungizone)

CATEGORY AND SCHEDULE
Pregnancy Risk Category: B

Drug Class: Polyene antifungal

MECHANISM OF ACTION
An antifungal and antiprotozoal that is generally fungistatic but may become fungicidal with high dosages or very susceptible microorganisms. This drug binds to sterols in the fungal cell membrane. *Therapeutic Effect:* Increases fungal cell-membrane permeability, allowing loss of potassium and other cellular components.

USES
Oral mucocutaneous infections caused by Candida species

PHARMACOKINETICS
Protein binding: 90%. Widely distributed. Metabolic fate unknown. Cleared by nonrenal pathways. Minimal removal by hemodialysis. Amphotec and Abelcet are not dialyzable. *Half-life:* Fungizone, 24 hr (increased in neonates and

children); Amphotec, 26–28 hr; Abelcet, 7.2 days; AmBisome, 100–153 hr.

INDICATIONS AND DOSAGES

▶ **Cryptococcosis; Blastomycosis; Systemic Candidiasis; Disseminated Forms of Moniliasis, Coccidioidomycosis, and Histoplasmosis; Zygomycosis; Sporotrichosis; Aspergillosis**
IV Infusion (Fungizone)
Adults, Elderly. Dosage based on patient tolerance and severity of infection. Initially, 1-mg test dose is given over 20–30 min. If test dose is tolerated, 5-mg dose may be given the same day. Subsequently, dosage is increased by 5 mg q12–24h until desired daily dose is reached. Alternatively, if test dose is tolerated, 0.25 mg/kg is given on same day and 0.5 mg/kg on second day; then dosage is increased until desired daily dose reached. Total daily dose: 1 mg/kg/day up to 1.5 mg/kg every other day. Maximum: 1.5 mg/kg/day.
Children. Test dose of 0.1 mg/kg/dose (maximum 1 mg) is infused over 20–60 min. If test dose is tolerated, initial dose of 0.4 mg/kg may be given on same day; dosage is then increased in 0.25-mg/kg increments as needed. Maintenance dose: 0.25–1 mg/kg/day.
▶ **Invasive Fungal Infections Unresponsive to or Intolerant of Fungizone**
IV Infusion (Abelcet)
Adults, Children. 5 mg/kg at rate of 2.5 mg/kg/hr.
▶ **Empiric Treatment of Fungal Infections in Patients with Febrile Neutropenia; Aspergillosis, Candidiasis, or Cryptococcosis in Patients with Renal Impairment and Those Who Have Experienced Toxicity or Treatment Failure with Fungizone**

IV Infusion (AmBisome)
Adults, Children. 3–5 mg/kg over 1 hr.
▶ **Invasive Aspergillosis in Patients with Renal Impairment and Those Who Have Experienced Toxicity or Treatment Failure with Fungizone**
IV Infusion (Amphotec)
Adults, Children. 3–4 mg/kg over 2–4 hr.
▶ **Cutaneous and Mucocutaneous Infections Caused by Candida Albicans, such as Paronychia, Oral Thrush, Perléche, Diaper Rash, and Intertriginous Candidiasis**
Topical
Adults, Elderly, Children. Apply liberally to affected area and rub in 2–4 times a day.

SIDE EFFECTS/ADVERSE REACTIONS

Frequent
Abelcet: Chills, fever, increased serum creatinine level, multiple organ failure
AmBisome: Hypokalemia, hypomagnesemia, hyperglycemia, hypocalcemia, edema, abdominal pain, back pain, chills, chest pain, hypotension, diarrhea, nausea, vomiting, headache, fever, rigors, insomnia, dyspnea, epistaxis, increased hepatic or renal function test results
Amphotec: Chills, fever, hypotension, tachycardia, increased serum creatinine level, hypokalemia, bilirubinemia
Fungizone: Fever, chills, headache, anemia, hypokalemia, hypomagnesemia, anorexia, malaise, generalized pain, nephrotoxicity
Topical: Local irritation, dry skin
Rare
Topical: Rash

PRECAUTIONS AND CONTRAINDICATIONS
Hypersensitivity to amphotericin B or sulfites
Caution
Lactation; not for systemic fungal infections

DRUG INTERACTIONS OF CONCERN TO DENTISTRY
None reported

SERIOUS REACTIONS
! Cardiovascular toxicity (as evidenced by hypotension, ventricular fibrillation, and anaphylaxis) occurs rarely.
! Altered vision and hearing, seizures, hepatic failure, coagulation defects, multiple organ failure, and sepsis may be noted.

DENTAL CONSIDERATIONS
General:
• Determine why the patient is taking the drug.
• Broad-spectrum antibiotics may contribute to oral *Candida* infections.
Teach Patient/Family to:
• Complete entire course of medication
• Not use commercial mouthwashes for mouth infection unless prescribed by dentist
• Soak removable appliance in antifungal agent overnight
• Prevent reinoculation of *Candida* infection by disposing of tooth brush or other contaminated oral hygiene devices used during period of infection

amphotericin B, lipid-based
am-foe-ter-ih-sin bee
(Abelcet, Amphotec, AmBisome)

CATEGORY AND SCHEDULE
Pregnancy Risk Category: B

Drug Class: Antifungal

MECHANISM OF ACTION
An antifungal and antiprotozoal that is generally fungistatic but may become fungicidal with high dosages or very susceptible microorganisms. This drug binds to sterols in the fungal cell membrane. *Therapeutic Effect:* Increases fungal cell-membrane permeability, allowing loss of potassium and loss of other cellular components.

USES
Treatment of infections caused by fungus

PHARMACOKINETICS
Protein binding: 90%. Widely distributed. Metabolic fate unknown. Cleared by nonrenal pathways. Minimal removal by hemodialysis. Not dialyzable. *Half-life:* 7.2 days.

INDICATIONS AND DOSAGES
▸ **Invasive fungal infections unresponsive to, or intolerant of, Fungizone.**
IV Infusion
Adults, Children. 5 mg/kg at rate of 2.5 mg/kg/hr.

SIDE EFFECTS/ADVERSE REACTIONS
Frequent
Chills, fever, increased serum creatinine, multiple organ failure

Occasional
Nausea, hypotension, vomiting,
dyspnea, diarrhea, headache,
hypokalemia, abdominal pain, rash

PRECAUTIONS AND CONTRAINDICATIONS
Hypersensitivity to amphotericin B
or sulfites

DRUG INTERACTIONS OF CONCERN TO DENTISTRY
• Risk of hypokalemia:
glucocorticoids and
mineralocorticoids

SERIOUS REACTIONS
! Cardiovascular toxicity
(as evidenced by hypotension,
ventricular fibrillation, and
anaphylaxis) occurs rarely.
! Altered vision and hearing,
seizures, hepatic failure, coagulation
defects, multiple organ failure, and
sepsis may be noted.

DENTAL CONSIDERATIONS
General:
• Intended for serious systemic
fungal infections; palliative
emergency dental care only.
• Determine why patient is taking
the drug.
• Patient on chronic drug therapy
may rarely present with symptoms of
blood dyscrasias, which can include
infection, bleeding, and poor healing.
If dyscrasia is present, caution
patient to prevent oral tissue trauma
when using oral hygiene aids.
• Monitor vital signs at every
appointment due to cardiovascular
side effects.
• Avoid prescribing aspirin-
containing products.
Consultations:
• In a patient with symptoms of
blood dyscrasias, request a medical

consultation for blood studies and
postpone treatment until normal
values are reestablished.
• Medical consultation may be
required to assess disease control and
patient's ability to tolerate stress.
Teach Patient/Family to:
• Use effective oral hygiene to
prevent soft tissue inflammation
• Report oral lesions, soreness, or
bleeding to dentist
• Prevent trauma when using oral
hygiene aids

ampicillin
am´-pi-sill-in
(Alpovex[AUS], Amficot, Apo-
Ampi[CAN], Novo-Ampicillin[CAN],
Nu-Ampi[CAN], Omnipen,
Omnipen-N, Polycillin,
Polycillin-N, Principen, Totacillin,
Totacillin-N)
Do not confuse with aminophylline,
Imipenem, or Unipen.

CATEGORY AND SCHEDULE
Pregnancy Risk Category: B

Drug Class: Aminopenicillin

MECHANISM OF ACTION
A penicillin that inhibits cell wall
synthesis in susceptible
microorganisms. ***Therapeutic Effect:***
Produces bactericidal effect.

USES
Treatment of sinus infections,
pneumonia, otitis media, skin
infections, UTIs; effective for
susceptible strains of β-lactamase
negative *E. coli, P. mirabilis,*
H. influenzae, S. faecalis,
S. pneumoniae, S. typhosa,
N. gonorrhoeae, N. meningitidis,
L. monocytogenes, shigella, enterococci

PHARMACOKINETICS

Moderately absorbed from the GI tract. Protein binding: 28%. Widely distributed. Partially metabolized in liver. Primarily excreted in urine. Removed by hemodialysis. *Half-life:* 1–1.9 hr (half-life increased in impaired renal function).

INDICATIONS AND DOSAGES

▶ **Respiratory Tract, Skin/Skin-Structure Infections**
PO
Adults, Elderly, Children weighing more than 20 kg. 250–500 mg q6h.
Children weighing less than 20 kg. 50 mg/kg/day in divided doses q6h.
IM/IV
Adults, Elderly, Children weighing more than 40 kg. 250–500 mg q6h.
Children weighing less than 40 kg. 25–50 mg/kg/day in divided doses q6–8h.

▶ **Bacterial Meningitis, Septicemia**
IM/IV
Adults, Elderly. 2 g q4h or 3 g q6h.
Children. 100–200 mg/kg/day in divided doses q4h.

▶ **Gonococcal Infections**
PO
Adults. 3.5 g one time with 1 g probenecid.

▶ **Perioperative Prophylaxis**
IM/IV
Adults, Elderly. 2 g 30 min before procedure. May repeat in 8 hr.
Children. 50 mg/kg using same dosage regimen.

▶ **Usual Neonate Dosage**
IM/IV
Neonates 7–28 days old. 75 mg/kg/day in divided doses q8h up to 200 mg/kg/day in divided doses q6h.
Neonates 0–7 days old. 50 mg/kg/day in divided doses q12h up to 150 mg/kg/day in divided doses q8h.

SIDE EFFECTS/ADVERSE REACTIONS

Frequent

Pain at IM injection site, GI disturbances, including mild diarrhea, nausea, or vomiting, oral or vaginal candidiasis

Occasional

Generalized rash, urticaria, phlebitis, thrombophlebitis with IV administration, headache

Rare

Dizziness, seizures, especially with IV therapy

PRECAUTIONS AND CONTRAINDICATIONS

Hypersensitivity to any penicillin, infectious mononucleosis

DRUG INTERACTIONS OF CONCERN TO DENTISTRY

* Decreased antimicrobial effectiveness: tetracyclines, erythromycins, lincomycins
* Increased ampicillin concentrations: probenecid
* Increased skin rash: allopurinol
* Decreased effects of atenolol
* Suspected increased risk of methotrexate toxicity
* When used for dental infection:
  * Oral contraceptives: advise patient of a potential risk for decreased contraceptive action, to maintain compliance with oral contraceptive use while using antibiotics, and to consider the use of additional nonhormonal contraception

SERIOUS REACTIONS

! Altered bacterial balance may result in potentially fatal superinfections and antibiotic-associated colitis as evidenced by abdominal cramps, watery or severe diarrhea, and fever.

! Severe hypersensitivity reactions including anaphylaxis and acute interstitial nephritis occur rarely.

DENTAL CONSIDERATIONS

General:
- Take precautions regarding allergy to medication.
- Determine why the patient is taking the drug.

Consultations:
- Medical consultation may be required to assess disease control.

Teach Patient/Family to:
- Use effective oral hygiene to prevent soft tissue inflammation
- Prevent injury when using oral hygiene aids
- When used for dental infection, advise patient to:
  - Report sore throat, oral burning sensation, fever, and fatigue, any of which could indicate superinfection
  - Take at prescribed intervals and complete dosage regimen
  - Immediately notify the dentist if signs or symptoms of infection increase

ampicillin sodium
am-pi-sill´-in soe´-dee-um
(Alphacin[AUS], Apo-Ampi[CAN], Novo-Ampicillin[CAN], Nu-Ampi[CAN], Polycillin, Principen)
Do not confuse ampicillin with aminophylline, Imipenem, or Unipen.

CATEGORY AND SCHEDULE
Pregnancy Risk Category: B

Drug Class: Aminopenicillin

MECHANISM OF ACTION
A penicillin that inhibits cell wall synthesis in susceptible microorganisms. ***Therapeutic Effect:*** Bactericidal.

USES
Sinus infections, pneumonia, otitis media, skin infections, UTIs; effective for susceptible strains of β-lactamase negative) *E. coli, P. mirabilis, H. influenzae, S. faecalis, S. pneumoniae, S. typhosa, N. gonorrhoeae, N. meningitidis, L. monocytogenes,* shigella, enterococci

PHARMACOKINETICS
Moderately absorbed from the GI tract. Protein binding: 28%. Widely distributed. Partially metabolized in the liver. Primarily excreted in urine. Removed by hemodialysis. ***Half-life:*** 1–1.5 hr (increased in impaired renal function).

INDICATIONS AND DOSAGES
▸ **Respiratory Tract, Skin and Skin-Structure Infections**
PO
Adults, Elderly. 250–500 mg q6h.
Children. 50–100 mg/kg/day in divided doses q6h.
Maximum: 3 g/day.
IV, IM
Adults, Elderly. 500 mg to 3 g q6h.
Maximum: 14 g/day.
Children. 100–200 mg/kg/day in divided doses q6h
Neonates. 50–100 mg/kg/day in divided doses q6–12h.
▸ **Meningitis**
IV
Children. 200–400 mg/kg/day in divided doses q6h.
Maximum: 12 g/day
Neonates. 100–200 mg/kg/day in divided doses q6–12h.

▸ **Gonococcal Infections**
PO
Adults. 3.5 g one time with
1 g probenecid.
▸ **Perioperative Prophylaxis**
IV, IM
Adults, Elderly. 2 g 30 min
before procedure. May repeat
in 8 hr.
Children. 50 mg/kg 30 min before
procedure. May repeat in 8 hr.
▸ **Dosage in Renal Impairment**

Creatinine Clearance	% of Normal Dosage
10–30 ml/min	Give q6–12h
Less than 10 ml/min	Give q12h

SIDE EFFECTS/ADVERSE REACTIONS

Frequent
Pain at IM injection site, GI
disturbances (mild diarrhea,
nausea, vomiting), oral or vaginal
candidiasis

Occasional
Generalized rash, urticaria, phlebitis
or thrombophlebitis (with IV
administration), headache

Rare
Dizziness, seizures (especially with
IV therapy)

PRECAUTIONS AND CONTRAINDICATIONS

Hypersensitivity to any penicillin,
infectious mononucleosis

DRUG INTERACTIONS OF CONCERN TO DENTISTRY

● Decreased antimicrobial
effectiveness: tetracyclines,
erythromycins, lincomycins
● Increased ampicillin
concentrations: probenecid
● Increased skin rash: allopurinol
● Decreased effects of atenolol

● Suspected increased risk of
methotrexate toxicity
● When used for dental infection:
  ● Oral contraceptives: advise
  patient of a potential risk for
  decreased contraceptive action, to
  maintain compliance with oral
  contraceptive use while using
  antibiotics, and to consider the use
  of additional nonhormonal
  contraception

SERIOUS REACTIONS

❗ Antibiotic-associated colitis and
other superinfections may result from
altered bacterial balance.
❗ Severe hypersensitivity reactions,
including anaphylaxis and acute
interstitial nephritis, occur rarely.

DENTAL CONSIDERATIONS

General:
● Take precautions regarding allergy
to medication.
● Determine why the patient is taking
the drug.

Consultations:
● Medical consultation may be
required to assess disease control.

Teach Patient/Family to:
● Use effective oral hygiene
to prevent soft tissue
inflammation
● Prevent injury when using oral
hygiene aids
● When used for dental infection,
advise patient to:
  ● Report sore throat, oral
  burning sensation, fever, and
  fatigue, any of which could
  indicate superinfection
  ● Take at prescribed
  intervals and complete dosage
  regimen
  ● Immediately notify the dentist
  if signs or symptoms of infection
  increase

ampicillin/sulbactam sodium
am´-pi-sill-in/sul-bac´-tam
so´-dee-um
(Unasyn)

CATEGORY AND SCHEDULE
Pregnancy Risk Category: B

Drug Class: Aminopenicillin

MECHANISM OF ACTION
Ampicillin inhibits bacterial cell wall synthesis, while sulbactam inhibits bacterial β-lactamase. *Therapeutic Effect:* Ampicillin is bactericidal in susceptible microorganisms. Sulbactam protects ampicillin from enzymatic degradation

USES
Elimination of bacteria

PHARMACOKINETICS
Protein binding: 28%–38%. Widely distributed. Partially metabolized in the liver. Primarily excreted in urine. Removed by hemodialysis. *Half-life:* 1 hr (increased in impaired renal function).

INDICATIONS AND DOSAGES
▸ **Skin and Skin-Structure, Intra-Abdominal, and Gynecologic Infections**
IV, IM
Adults, Elderly. 1.5 g (1 g ampicillin/500 mg sulbactam) to 3 g (2 g ampicillin/1 g sulbactam) q6h.
▸ **Skin and Skin-Structure Infections**
IV
Children 1–12 yr. 150–300 mg/kg/day in divided doses q6h.
▸ **Dosage in Renal Impairment**
Dosage and frequency are modified based on creatinine clearance and the severity of the infection.

Creatinine Clearance	Dosage
Greater than 30 ml/min	0.5–3 g q6–8h
15–29 ml/min	1.5–3 g q12h
5–14 ml/min	1.5–3 g q24h
Less than 5 ml/min	Not recommended

SIDE EFFECTS/ADVERSE REACTIONS
Frequent
Diarrhea and rash (most common), urticaria, pain at IM injection site, thrombophlebitis with IV administration, oral or vaginal candidiasis

Occasional
Nausea, vomiting, headache, malaise, urine retention

PRECAUTIONS AND CONTRAINDICATIONS
Hypersensitivity to any penicillin, infectious mononucleosis

DRUG INTERACTIONS OF CONCERN TO DENTISTRY
• Decreased antimicrobial effectiveness: tetracyclines, erythromycins, lincomycins
• Increased ampicillin concentration: probenecid
• Increased skin rash: allpurinol
• Decreased effects of atenolol
• Suspected increased risk of methotrexate toxicity
• Increased risk of bleeding with anticoagulants: large IV doses of penicillins
• When used for dental infection:
  • Oral contraceptives: advise patient of a low potential risk for decreased contraceptive action, to maintain compliance with oral contraceptive use while using antibiotics, and to consider the use of additional nonhormonal contraception

SERIOUS REACTIONS

❗ Severe hypersensitivity reactions including anaphylaxis, acute interstitial nephritis, and blood dyscrasias may occur.

❗ Antibiotic-associated colitis and other superinfections may result from altered bacterial balance.

❗ Overdose may produce seizures.

DENTAL CONSIDERATIONS

General:
● For selected infections in the hospital setting; provide emergency dental treatment only.
● Caution regarding allergy to medication.
● Examine for oral manifestation of opportunistic infection.
● Determine why patient is taking the drug.

Consultations:
● Medical consultation may be required to assess disease control.
● Consult patient's physician if an acute dental infection occurs and another antiinfective is required.

Teach Patient/Family to:
● Use effective oral hygiene to prevent soft tissue inflammation
● Report oral lesions, soreness, or bleeding to dentist
● Prevent trauma when using oral hygiene aids
● See dentist immediately if secondary oral infection occurs
● When antibiotics are used for dental infection:
  ● Oral contraceptives: advise patient of a low potential risk for decreased contraceptive action, to maintain compliance with oral contraceptive use while using antibiotics, and to consider the use of additional nonhormonal contraception

● When used for dental infection, advise patient to:
  ● Report sore throat, oral burning sensation, fever, or fatigue, any of which could indicate superinfection
  ● Take at prescribed intervals and complete dosage regimen
  ● Immediately notify the dentist if signs or symptoms of infection increase

amprenavir
am-pren -eh-veer
(Agenerase)
Do not confuse Agenerase with asparaginase.

CATEGORY AND SCHEDULE
Pregnancy Risk Category: C

Drug Class: Antiviral

MECHANISM OF ACTION
An antiretroviral that inhibits HIV-1 protease by binding to the enzyme's active site, thus preventing processing of viral precursors and resulting in the formation of immature, noninfectious viral particles. *Therapeutic Effect:* Impairs HIV replication and proliferation.

USES
HIV-1 infection, in combination with other antiretroviral agents

PHARMACOKINETICS
Rapidly absorbed after PO administration. Protein binding: 90%. Metabolized in the liver. Primarily excreted in feces. *Half-life:* 7.1–10.6 hr.

INDICATIONS AND DOSAGES
▸ **HIV-1 Infection (in combination with other antiretrovirals)**
PO
Adults, Children 13–16 yr. 1200 mg capsules twice a day.
Children 4–12 yr, and children 13–16 yr weighing less than 50 kg. 20 mg/kg twice a day or 15 mg/kg 3 times a day.
Maximum: 2400 mg/day.
Oral solution
Adults. 1400 mg 2 times/day.
Children 4–12 yr, and children 13–16 yr weighing less than 50 kg. 22.5 mg/kg/day (1.5 ml/kg) oral solution twice a day or 17 mg/kg/day (1.1 ml/kg) 3 times a day. Maximum: 2800 mg/day.
▸ **Dosage in Hepatic Impairment**
Dosage and frequency are modified on the basis of the Child-Pugh score.

Child-Pugh Score	Capsules	Oral Solution
5–8	450 mg bid	513 mg bid
9–12	300 mg bid	342 mg bid

SIDE EFFECTS/ADVERSE REACTIONS
Frequent
Diarrhea or loose stools, nausea, oral paresthesia, rash, vomiting
Occasional
Peripheral paresthesia, depression

PRECAUTIONS AND CONTRAINDICATIONS
Concurrent use with midazolam, triazolam, bepridil, disulfiram, metronidazole, pimozide, and ergot-like drugs; hypersensitivity; serious reactions could occur with lidocaine (systemic) or other antiarrhythmics and tricyclic antidepressants; avoid use of drugs metabolized by CYP3A4 enzymes; lactation
Caution
Exacerbation of diabetes, hyperglycemia, use of additional vitamin E, hemophilia, viral resistance, risk of cross allergy with sulfonamides, fat redistribution, hepatic disease, patients on oral contraceptives, sildenafil; oral solution contains propylene glycol with risk of toxicity to children younger than 4 yr

DRUG INTERACTIONS OF CONCERN TO DENTISTRY
● Contraindicated with midazolam, triazolam, tricyclic antidepressants
● Increased plasma levels of erythromycin, clarithromycin, itraconazole, alprazolam, clorazepate, diazepam, carbamazepine, loratadine, flurazepam, ketoconazole, itraconazole; lidocaine (systemic use for cardiac arrhythmias)
● Decreased effectiveness: dexamethasone, St. John's wort (herb)
● Use with caution: sildenafil, vardenafil, todalafil

SERIOUS REACTIONS
❗ Severe hypersensitivity reactions or Stevens-Johnson syndrome as evidenced by blisters, peeling of the skin, loosening of skin and mucous membranes, and fever may occur.

DENTAL CONSIDERATIONS
General:
● Palliative medication may be required for management of oral side effects.
● Examine for oral manifestation of opportunistic infection.
● Patients on chronic drug therapy may rarely have symptoms of blood

dyscrasias, which can include infection, bleeding, and poor healing.
• Consider semisupine chair position for patient comfort if GI side effects occur.
Consultations:
• In a patient with symptoms of blood dyscrasias, request a medical consultation for blood studies and postpone treatment until normal values are reestablished.
• Medical consultation may be required to assess disease control and patient's ability to tolerate stress.
Teach Patient/Family to:
• Use effective oral hygiene to prevent soft tissue inflammation
• Prevent trauma when using oral hygiene aids
• Update health and drug history if physician makes any changes in evaluation or drug regimens
• See dentist immediately if secondary oral infection occurs

amyl nitrite
am´-il nye´-trate
(Amyl Nitrite)
Do not confuse with Nicobid, Nicoderm, Nilstat, nitroprusside, Nizoral, or Nystatin.

CATEGORY AND SCHEDULE
Pregnancy Risk Category: C

Drug Class: Antianginal

MECHANISM OF ACTION
A nitrite vasodilator that relaxes smooth muscles. Reduces afterload and improves vascular supply to the myocardium. *Therapeutic Effect:* Dilates coronary arteries, improves

blood flow to ischemic areas within myocardium. Following inhalation, systemic vasodilation occurs.

USES
Pain relief of anginal attacks

PHARMACOKINETICS
The vapors are absorbed rapidly through the pulmonary alveoli and metabolized rapidly. Partially excreted in the urine.

INDICATIONS AND DOSAGES
▸ **Acute Relief of Angina Pectoris**
Nasal inhalation
Adults, Elderly. Place crushed capsule to nostrils for 0.18–0.3 ml inhalation of vapors. Repeat at 5–10 min intervals. No more than 3 doses in a 15–30 min period.

SIDE EFFECTS/ADVERSE REACTIONS
Frequent
Headache (may be severe) occurs mostly in early therapy, diminishes rapidly in intensity, usually disappears during continued treatment; transient flushing of face and neck; dizziness (especially if patient is standing immobile or is in a warm environment); weakness; postural hypotension
Occasional
Nausea, rash vomiting
Rare
Involuntary passage of urine and feces, restlessness, weakness

PRECAUTIONS AND CONTRAINDICATIONS
Closed-angle glaucoma, severe anemia, head injury, postural hypotension, pregnancy, hypersensitivity to nitrates

DRUG INTERACTIONS OF CONCERN TO DENTISTRY
None reported

SERIOUS REACTIONS
! Large doses may produce hemolytic anemia or methemoglobinemia.
! Severe postural hypotension manifested by fainting, pulselessness, cold or clammy skin, and profuse sweating may occur.
! Tolerance may occur with repeated, prolonged therapy.
! High dose tends to produce severe headache.

DENTAL CONSIDERATIONS
General:
* For emergency relief of acute angina; if angina is not relieved call 911 for transfer of patient to a medical emergency facility.
* Prior to treatment, inquire about disease control and frequency of angina episodes.
* Ensure that patient's rescue antianginal drug is available for use.
* Monitor vital signs at every appointment due to cardiovascular side effects.
* Postpone elective dental treatment if patient shows signs of cardiac symptoms or respiratory distress.
* After supine positioning, have patient sit upright for at least 2 min before standing to avoid orthostatic hypotension.
Consultations:
* Medical consultation may be required to assess disease control and patient's ability to tolerate stress.
Teach Patient/Family to:
* Report angina symptoms to physician
* Update health and medication history if physician makes any changes in evaluation or drug

regimens; include OTC, herbal, and nonherbal remedies in the update
* Use effective oral hygiene to prevent soft tissue inflammation

anagrelide
ah-na´-greh-lide
(Agrylin)

CATEGORY AND SCHEDULE
Pregnancy Risk Category: C

Drug Class: Platelet count–reducing agent

MECHANISM OF ACTION
A hematologic agent that reduces platelet production and prevents platelet shape changes caused by platelet aggregating agents. *Therapeutic Effect:* Inhibits platelet aggregation.

USES
Decreases the risk of blood clots in patients who have too many platelet cells

PHARMACOKINETICS
After oral administration, plasma concentration peak within 1 hr. Extensively metabolized. Primarily excreted in urine. *Half-life:* About 3 days.

INDICATIONS AND DOSAGES
▶ Thrombocythemia
PO
Adults, Elderly. Initially, 0.5 mg 4 times a day or 1 mg twice a day. Adjust to lowest effective dosage, increasing by up to 0.5 mg/day or less in any 1 wk. Maximum: 10 mg/day or 2.5 mg/dose.

SIDE EFFECTS/ADVERSE REACTIONS

Frequent
Headache, palpitations, diarrhea, abdominal pain, nausea, flatulence, bloating, asthenia, pain, dizziness

Occasional
Tachycardia, chest pain, vomiting, paresthesia, peripheral edema, anorexia, dyspepsia, rash

Rare
Confusion, insomnia

PRECAUTIONS AND CONTRAINDICATIONS

Caution
Cardiac disease, renal impairment, hepatic impairment, monitor reduction in platelets, risk of thrombocytopenia especially while correct dose is being found, sudden discontinuance of use, lactation, children younger than 16 yr

DRUG INTERACTIONS OF CONCERN TO DENTISTRY

• Possible risk of hemorrhage: NSAIDs, aspirin

SERIOUS REACTIONS

! Angina, heart failure, and arrhythmias occur rarely.

DENTAL CONSIDERATIONS

General:
• Laboratory studies should include routine complete blood counts (CBCs).
• Patients have risk of thrombohemorrhagic complications; prolonged bleeding time, anemia, or splenomegaly may occur in some patients with this disease. However, thrombosis may also occur in some patients.
• Mucosal bleeding can be a symptom of disease.

• Patients with severe symptoms may be taking chemotherapy.
• Monitor vital signs at every appointment because of cardiovascular side effects.
• Consider semisupine chair position for patient comfort if GI side effects occur.

Consultations:
• Medical consultation with hematologist or physician directing therapy is essential before dental treatment.

Teach Patient/Family to:
• Inform dentist of unusual bleeding episodes following dental treatment
• Update health and drug history if physician makes any changes in evaluation or drug regimens

anakinra
an-ah-kin´-ra
(Kineret)

CATEGORY AND SCHEDULE
Pregnancy Risk Category: B

Drug Class: Antirheumatic

MECHANISM OF ACTION

An interleukin-1 (IL-1) receptor antagonist that blocks the binding of IL-1, a protein that is a major mediator of joint disease and is present in excess amounts in patients with rheumatoid arthritis.
Therapeutic Effect: Inhibits the inflammatory response.

USES

Treatment of moderate to severe symptoms of rheumatoid arthritis

PHARMACOKINETICS

No accumulation of anakinra in tissues or organs was observed after daily subcutaneous doses. Excreted in urine. *Half-life:* 4–6 hr.

INDICATIONS AND DOSAGES

▸ **Rheumatoid Arthritis**

Subcutaneous

Adults, Children older than 18 yr, Elderly. 100 mg/day, given at same time each day.

SIDE EFFECTS/ADVERSE REACTIONS

Occasional

Injection site ecchymosis, erythema, and inflammation

Rare

Headache, nausea, diarrhea, abdominal pain

PRECAUTIONS AND CONTRAINDICATIONS

Known hypersensitivity to Escherichia coli-derived proteins, serious infection

DRUG INTERACTIONS OF CONCERN TO DENTISTRY

None reported

SERIOUS REACTIONS

! Infections, including upper respiratory tract infection, sinusitis, flu-like symptoms, and cellulitis, have been noted.

! Neutropenia may occur, particularly when anakinra is used in combination with tumor necrosis factor-blocking agents.

DENTAL CONSIDERATIONS

General:

• Question patient about other drugs or products he or she may be taking for arthritis.

• Patient may be at risk for infection.

• Oral infections should be eliminated and/or treated aggressively.

• Evaluate efficacy of oral hygiene home care; preventive instruction appointment may be necessary.

• Patient on chronic drug therapy may rarely present with symptoms of blood dyscrasias, which can include infection, bleeding, and poor healing. If dyscrasia is present, caution patient to prevent oral tissue trauma when using oral hygiene aids.

• Patient may need assistance in getting into and out of dental chair. Adjust chair position for patient comfort.

Consultations:

• Medical consultation may be required to assess disease control.

• In a patient with symptoms of blood dyscrasias, request a medical consultation for blood studies and postpone treatment until normal values are reestablished.

Teach Patient/Family to:

• Use electric tooth brush if patient has difficulty holding conventional devices

• Prevent trauma when using oral hygiene aids

• Use effective oral hygiene to prevent soft tissue inflammation

• Update health and medication history if physician makes any changes in evaluation or drug regimens; include OTC, herbal, and nonherbal remedies in the update

anastrozole

ah-nas´-trow-zole
(Arimidex)
Do not confuse Arimidex with Imitrex.

CATEGORY AND SCHEDULE

Pregnancy Risk Category: D

Drug Class: Antineoplastic

MECHANISM OF ACTION

Decreases the circulating estrogen level by inhibiting aromatase, the enzyme that catalyzes the final step in estrogen production. *Therapeutic Effect:* Inhibits the growth of breast cancers that are stimulated by estrogens.

USES

Treatment of breast cancer

PHARMACOKINETICS

Well absorbed into systemic circulation (absorption not affected by food). Protein binding: 40%. Extensively metabolized in the liver. Eliminated by biliary system and, to a lesser extent, kidneys. Mean *Half-life:* 50 hr in postmenopausal women. Steady-state plasma levels reached in about 7 days.

INDICATIONS AND DOSAGES
▶ **Breast Cancer**
PO
Adults, Elderly. 1 mg once a day.

SIDE EFFECTS/ADVERSE REACTIONS
Frequent

Asthenia, nausea, headache, hot flashes, back pain, vomiting, cough, diarrhea
Occasional

Constipation, abdominal pain, anorexia, bone pain, pharyngitis, dizziness, rash, dry mouth, peripheral edema, pelvic pain, depression, chest pain, paresthesia
Rare

Weight gain, diaphoresis

PRECAUTIONS AND CONTRAINDICATIONS

None known

DRUG INTERACTIONS OF CONCERN TO DENTISTRY

None reported

SERIOUS REACTIONS

❗ Thrombophlebitis, anemia, leukopenia, and vaginal hemorrhage occur rarely.
❗ Vaginal hemorrhage occurs rarely (2%).

DENTAL CONSIDERATIONS
General:

* Monitor vital signs at every appointment due to cardiovascular side effects.
* If additional analgesia is required for dental pain, consider alternative analgesics (NSAIDs) in patients taking narcotics for acute or chronic pain.
* Avoid products that affect platelet function, such as aspirin and NSAIDs.
* Consider semisupine chair position for patient comfort if GI side effects occur.
* Examine for oral manifestation of opportunistic infection.
* Patient on chronic drug therapy may rarely present with symptoms of blood dyscrasias, which can include infection, bleeding, and poor healing. If dyscrasia is present, caution patient to prevent oral tissue trauma when using oral hygiene aids.
* Assess salivary flow as a factor in caries, periodontal disease, and candidiasis
Consultations:

* Consider consulting with physician before prescribing drugs that may cause constipation (narcotics).
* Consultation with physician may be necessary if sedation or general anesthesia is required.
* In a patient with symptoms of blood dyscrasias, request a medical

consultation for blood studies and postpone treatment until normal values are reestablished.

* Medical consultation may be required to assess disease control and patient's ability to tolerate stress.

Teach Patient/Family to:

* Use effective oral hygiene to prevent soft tissue inflammation
* Prevent trauma when using oral hygiene aids
* Update health and medication history if physician makes any changes in evaluation or drug regimens; include OTC, herbal, and nonherbal remedies in the update
* When chronic dry mouth occurs, advise patient to:
    * Avoid mouth rinses with high alcohol content due to drying effects
    * Use daily home fluoride products for anticaries effect
    * Use sugarless gum, frequent sips of water, or saliva substitutes

anidulafungin
ann-id-yoo-la-fun´-jin
(Eraxis)

CATEGORY AND SCHEDULE
Pregnancy Risk Category: C

Drug Class: Antifungal

MECHANISM OF ACTION
An antifungal that inhibits the synthesis of 1,3-β-D-glucan, an essential component of the fungal cell wall. *Therapeutic Effect:* Fungistatic.

USES
Treatment of fungal infections including candidemia and esophageal candidiasis.

PHARMACOKENETICS
Protein binding: 84%. Metabolism in the liver has not been observed. Approximately 30% eliminated in feces; less than 1% excreted in the urine. *Half-life:* 26.5 hr.

INDICATIONS AND DOSAGES
▶ **Candidemia**
IV
Adults. 200 mg loading dose on day 1, followed by 100 mg daily thereafter. Continue for at least 14 days after the last positive culture.
▶ **Esophageal Candidiasis**
IV
Adult. 100 mg loading dose on day 1, followed by 50 mg daily for a minimum of 14 days and for at least 7 days following resolution of symptoms.
Children. Safety and efficacy have not been established.

SIDE EFFECTS/ADVERSE REACTIONS
Rare

Diarrhea, hypokalemia, abnormal liver function, rash, urticaria, flushing, pruritus, dyspnea, hypotension, deep vein thrombosis

PRECAUTIONS AND CONTRAINDICATIONS
Hypersensitivity to anidulafungin or its components
Caution

Do not breast-feed, hepatic impairment

DRUG INTERACTIONS OF CONCERN TO DENTISTRY
None reported

SERIOUS REACTIONS
! Histamine-mediated symptoms including rash, urticaria, flushing,

pruritus, dyspnea, and hypotension
have been reported.

DENTAL CONSIDERATIONS

General:

* Determine why the patient is taking
the drug
* Examine oral mucous membranes
for signs of residual fungal infection
* Monitor vital signs at each
appointment because of
cardiovascular side effects
* Consult physician to determine
control of disease
* Consider removable prostheses as
source of residual source of candidal
organisms

Teach Patient/Family to:

* Soak full or partial dentures in an
antifungal solution at night until
lesions are absent; prolonged
infections may require fabrication of
new prosthesis
* Dispose of tooth brush used during
oral infection after oral lesions are
absent to prevent reinoculation
* Comply with antifungal therapy
completely to eliminate infection and
complete entire course of medication

---

anthralin

anth-rah´-lin
(A-Fil, Anthra-Derm,
Anthraforte[CAN], Anthranol[CAN],
Anthrascalp[CAN],
Dithrocream[AUS], Drithocreme,
Dritho-Scalp, Micanol, Psoriatec)
(capsules, tablets, chewable tablets,
syrup, elixir, cream, spray)
Do not confuse with Antagon,
Antabuse, or Andriol.

CATEGORY AND SCHEDULE

Pregnancy Risk Category: C

Drug Class: Antipsoriatic

MECHANISM OF ACTION

A topical agent that binds DNA,
inhibiting synthesis of nucleic
protein, and reduces mitotic activity.
Therapeutic Effect: Results in
damage to DNA sugar and enhances
membrane lipid peroxidation, which
may play a critical role in the
antipsoriatic action.

USES

Treatment of psoriasis

PHARMACOKINETICS

Poorly absorbed systemically, but
excellent epidermal absorption.
Auto-oxidized to inactive
metabolites—danthrone and
dianthrone. Rapid urinary excretion,
so significant levels do not
accumulate in the blood or other
tissues. *Half-life:* 6 hr.

INDICATIONS AND DOSAGES

▸ **Psoriasis**

Topical
Adults, Elderly. Apply in a thin
layer to affected areas q12h
or q24h.

**SIDE EFFECTS/ADVERSE
REACTIONS**

Frequent

Irritation

Rare

Neutrophilia, proteinuria, staining of
the skin

**PRECAUTIONS AND
CONTRAINDICATIONS**

Acute psoriasis where
inflammation is present,
erythroderma, hypersensitivity
to anthralin

**DRUG INTERACTIONS OF
CONCERN TO DENTISTRY**

None reported

SERIOUS REACTIONS

! Patients with renal disease should have routine urine tests for albuminuria.
! Hypersensitivity reaction, such as burning, erythema, and dermatitis, may occur.

DENTAL CONSIDERATIONS

General:

* Determine why patient is taking the drug.
* Arthritic symptoms may occur in some patients; inquire about use of other medications.

apomorphine

ah-poe-more´-feen
(Apokyn)

CATEGORY AND SCHEDULE

Pregnancy Risk Category: C

Drug class: Anti-Parkinson's agent

MECHANISM OF ACTION

Stimulation of postsynaptic dopamine receptors in the brain, counteracting the excess cholinergic activity responsible for striatal excitation and involuntary movements.

USES

Control of acute loss of control of body movements in advanced Parkinson's disease

PHARMACOKINETICS

Rapidly absorbed after subcutaneous injection. Protein binding: 99.9%. Widely distributed. **Half-life:** 45 min; rapidly metabolized, not detectable in urine or bodily secretions in unchanged form.

INDICATIONS AND DOSAGES

▶ **Acute, Intermittent Treatment of Hypomobility ("Off Episodes") Asscociated with Advanced Parkinson's Disease:**
Injection pen for subcutaneous administration
Adult, Elderly. Subcutaneous, 0.2 ml (2 mg) initially; may be increased in 0.1-ml (1-mg) increments every few days, up to a maximum of 0.6 ml (6 mg)

SIDE EFFECTS/ADVERSE REACTIONS

ORAL: Stomatitis, taste alterations
CNS: Somnolence, dizziness, headache, depression, hallucinations (rare)
CV: Chest pain, tachycardia, shortness of breath
GI: Nausea, vomiting
RESP: Respiratory depression, tachypnea
INTEG: Injection site discomfort
MS: May exacerbate preexisting dyskinesias

PRECAUTIONS AND CONTRAINDICATIONS

Hypersensitivity, irritable bowel or antiemetic therapy with 5-HT3 antagonists (e.g., ondansetron)
Do not administer with antiemetics other than 5-HT3 antagonists. Use with caution in patients with cardiac decompensation or impaired hepatic or renal function. Do not use if solution is cloudy, contains particulates or is discolored.

DRUG INTERACTIONS OF CONCERN TO DENTISTRY:

* CNS depressants may intensify adverse effects of therapy (e.g., dizziness)
* Phenothiazines may reduce effectiveness of apomorphine

DENTAL CONSIDERATIONS

General:
- Monitor vital signs due to possible cardiovascular and respiratory effects
- Understand limitations of Parkinson's disease on dental treatment
- After supine positioning, have patient sit upright for 2 min before standing to avoid orthostatic hypotension
- Assist patient with ambulation if dizziness or loss of coordination occurs
- Differentiate taste alterations due to drug from those associated with restorative materials

Consultations:
- Consult physician to determine degree of disease control and patient's ability to tolerate dental treatment

Teach Patient/Family to:
- Use effective oral hygiene measures to prevent soft-tissue inflammation
- Help patient with effective dental home care to minimize oral diseases if patient lacks adequate motor coordination

---

apraclonidine hydrochloride

ap-ra-kloe´-ni-deen
hi-droh-klor´-ide
(Iopidine)
Do not confuse with Cetapred, clomiphene, Klonopin, or quinidine.

CATEGORY AND SCHEDULE

Pregnancy Risk Category: C

Drug Class: Selective
α_2-adrenergic agonist

MECHANISM OF ACTION

An ocular α-adrenergic agent that is relatively selective for α_2 receptor agonist. ***Therapeutic Effect:*** Reduces intraocular pressure.

USES

Control or prevention of increases in intraocular pressure related to laser surgery of eye; short-term control of increased intraocular pressure as an adjunctive drug

PHARMACOKINETICS

Onset of action occurs within 1 hr. The duration of a single dose is about 12 hr. ***Half-life:*** 8 hr.

INDICATIONS AND DOSAGES

▸ **Glaucoma**
Ophthalmic
Adults, Elderly. Instill 1 drop of 0.5% solution to affected eye(s) 3 times a day.

▸ **Intraocular Hypertension, Post Laser Surgery**
Ophthalmic
Adults, Elderly. Instill 1 drop of 1% solution in operative eye(s) 1 hr before surgery and 1 drop postoperatively.

SIDE EFFECTS/ADVERSE REACTIONS

Frequent
Eye discomfort, dry mouth.
Occasional
Headache, constipation, redness around eye, conjunctivitis, changes in visual acuity, mydriasis, ocular inflammation.
Rare
Nasal decongestion.

PRECAUTIONS AND CONTRAINDICATIONS

Hypersensitivity to apraclonidine or clonidine or any component of the formulation

Caution
Tachyphylaxis, impaired renal or liver function, depression, lactation, children, cardiovascular disease, cardiovascular drugs

DRUG INTERACTIONS OF CONCERN TO DENTISTRY
• No drug interactions have been reported; this is a new drug and data are lacking
• Avoid using drugs that can exacerbate glaucoma: anticholinergic drugs

SERIOUS REACTIONS
❗ Allergic reaction occurs rarely.
❗ Peripheral edema and arrhythmias have been reported

DENTAL CONSIDERATIONS
General:
• Protect patient's eyes from accidental spatter during dental treatment.
• Avoid dental light in patient's eyes; offer dark glasses for patient comfort.
• Determine why the patient is taking the drug.
• Assess salivary flow as a factor in caries, periodontal disease, and candidiasis.
Consultations:
• Medical consultation may be required to assess disease control.
Teach Patient/Family:
• When chronic dry mouth occurs, advise patient to:
  • Avoid mouth rinses with high alcohol content because of drying effects
  • Use daily home fluoride to prevent caries
  • Use sugarless gum,
frequent sips of water, or saliva substitutes

aprepitant
ah-prep´-ih-tant
(Emend)

CATEGORY AND SCHEDULE
Pregnancy Risk Category: B

Drug Class: Antiemetic

MECHANISM OF ACTION
A selective human substance P and neurokinin-1 (NK1) receptor antagonist that inhibits chemotherapy-induced nausea and vomiting centrally in the chemoreceptor trigger zone.
Therapeutic Effect: Prevents the acute and delayed phases of chemotherapy-induced emesis, including vomiting caused by high-dose cisplatin.

USES
Prevention of acute and delayed nausea/vomiting associated with cancer chemotherapy including high-dose cisplatin; for acute use only

PHARMACOKINETICS
Crosses the blood-brain barrier. Extensively metabolized in the liver. Eliminated primarily by liver metabolism (not excreted renally).
Half-life: 9–13 hr.

INDICATIONS AND DOSAGES
▸ **Prevention of Chemotherapy-Induced Nausea and Vomiting**
PO
Adults, Elderly. 125 mg 1 hr before chemotherapy on day 1 and 80 mg once a day in the morning on days 2 and 3.

SIDE EFFECTS/ADVERSE REACTIONS

Frequent
Fatigue, nausea, hiccups, diarrhea, constipation, anorexia

Occasional
Headache, vomiting, dizziness, dehydration, heartburn

Rare
Abdominal pain, epigastric discomfort, gastritis, tinnitus, insomnia

PRECAUTIONS AND CONTRAINDICATIONS

Breast-feeding, concurrent use of pimozide (Orap)

Caution
Patients taking drugs metabolized by CYP3A4 enzymes; not for chronic use; acts as a moderate inhibitor of CYP3A4 and an inducer of CYP3A4 and CYP2C9; use with caution in lactation, safety and efficacy in pediatric patients not established

DRUG INTERACTIONS OF CONCERN TO DENTISTRY

● Increased plasma concentrations of midazolam and other benzodiazepines metabolized by CYP3A4
● Increased plasma levels: concurrent use of drugs that inhibit CYP3A4 enzymes (fluconazole, itraconazole, ketoconazole, erythromycin, and clarithromycin)
● Decreased plasma levels: concurrent use of drugs that induce CYP3A4 enzymes (carbamazepine)

SERIOUS REACTIONS

! Neutropenia and mucous membrane disorders occur rarely.

DENTAL CONSIDERATIONS

General:
● Patients using this drug are also undergoing or have recently undergone cancer chemotherapy; take a complete health history.
● Chemotherapy patients may show stomatitis and ulceration; palliative therapy may be required.
● Consider semisupine chair position for patient comfort if GI side effects occur.
● Examine for oral manifestation of opportunistic infection.
● Short appointments and a stress reduction protocol may be required for anxious patients.
● Patients taking opioids for acute or chronic pain should be given alternative analgesics for dental pain.
● Patients on chronic drug therapy may rarely have symptoms of blood dyscrasias, which can include infection, bleeding, and poor healing.
● Consult physician; prophylactic or therapeutic antibiotics may be indicated to prevent or treat infection if surgery or periodontal debridement is required for patients undergoing chemotherapy.

Consultations:
● Medical consultation may be required to assess immunologic status during cancer therapy and determine safety risks posed by dental treatment.
● Consultation with physician may be necessary if sedation or general anesthesia is required.
● Medical consultation may be required to assess disease control and patient's ability to tolerate stress.

Teach Patient/Family to:
● Use effective oral hygiene to prevent soft tissue inflammation
● Prevent trauma when using oral hygiene aids

• Importance of updating health and drug history if physician makes any changes in evaluation or drug regimens

arformoterol tartrate
ar-for-moe´-ter-ole tar´-trate
(Brovana)

CATEGORY AND SCHEDULE
Pregnancy Risk Category: C

Drug Class: β-2 agonist

MECHANISM OF ACTION
A long-acting β-2 agonist that stimulates adrenergic receptors in bronchial smooth muscle causing relaxation of smooth muscle. *Therapeutic Effect:* Produces bronchodilation.

USES
Used for chronic obstructive pulmonary disease (COPD)

PHARMACOKENETICS
Primarily absorbed by the pulmonary system following inhalation. Protein binding: 52%–65%. Primarily metabolized by glucuronidation. Primarily excreted in urine; partial elimination in feces. *Half-life:* 26 hr.

INDICATIONS AND DOSAGES
▸ COPD
Oral inhalation
Adults. 15 mcg (2 ml) twice a day by nebulization.
Children. Safety and efficacy have not been established in children.

SIDE EFFECTS/ADVERSE REACTIONS
Occasional
Pain, chest pain, back pain, sinusitis, rash, leg cramps, dyspnea, peripheral edema
Rare
Oral candidiasis, pulmonary congestion

PRECAUTIONS AND CONTRAINDICATIONS
Hypersensitivity to arformoterol or its components
Caution
Acutely deteriorating COPD, cardiovascular disorders, convulsive disorders, diabetes mellitus, thyrotoxicosis, coadministration with other long-acting β-2 agonists

DRUG INTERACTIONS OF CONCERN TO DENTISTRY
• Methylxanthines (e.g., aminophylline, theophylline), steroids, diuretics: May potentiate hypokalemic effects.
• Tricyclic antidepressants, drugs that prolong QT interval: May potentiate cardiovascular effects

SERIOUS REACTIONS
! May increase the risk of asthma-related death.
! May exacerbate cardiovascular conditions including arrhythmias and hypertension
! Hypersensitivity reactions including urticaria, angioedema, rash, bronchospasm, and anaphylaxis may occur.

DENTAL CONSIDERATIONS
• Monitor vital signs at every appointment due to

cardiovascular and respiratory side effects
* Evaluate oral mucous membranes for signs of candidiasis
* Consider semisupine chair position for patients with respiratory disease
* Midday appointments and stress-reduction protocol may be required for anxious patients
* Aspirin, NSAIDs, and bisulfites in local anesthetics may exacerbate asthma
* Acute asthmatic episodes may be precipitated in the dental office. Sympathomimetic/bronchodilator inhalants should be available for emergency use
Consultations:
* Consult physician to determine control of disease and ability of patient to tolerate dental procedures
Teach Patient/Family to:
* Rinse mouth with water after each dose of drug to prevent dryness

argatroban

ar-gat´-tro-ban
(Acova)
Do not confuse argatroban with Aggrestat or Organan.

CATEGORY AND SCHEDULE
Pregnancy Risk Category: B

Drug Class: Anticoagulants

MECHANISM OF ACTION
A direct thrombin inhibitor that reversibly binds to thrombin-active sites. Inhibits thrombin-catalyzed or thrombin-induced reactions, including fibrin formation, activation of coagulant factors V, VIII, and XIII; also inhibits protein C

formation; and platelet aggregation. ***Therapeutic Effect:*** Produces anticoagulation.

USES
An anticoagulant for prophylaxis or treatment of thrombosis in patients with heparin-induced thrombocytopenia

PHARMACOKINETICS
Following IV administration, distributed primarily in extracellular fluid. Protein binding: 54%. Metabolized in the liver. Primarily excreted in the feces, presumably through biliary secretion. ***Half-life:*** 39–51 min.

INDICATIONS AND DOSAGES
▶ **To Prevent and Treat Heparin-Induced Thrombocytopenia**
IV Infusion
Adults, Elderly. Initially, 2 mcg/kg/min administered as a continuous infusion. After initial infusion, dose may be adjusted until steady state aPTT is 1.5–3 times initial baseline value, not to exceed 100 sec.
▶ **Percutaneous Coronary Intervention**
IV Infusion
Adults, Elderly. Initially, 25 mcg/kg/min and administer bolus of 350 mcg/kg over 3–5 min. ACT (activated clotting time) checked in 5–10 min following bolus. If ACT is less than 300 sec, give additional bolus 150 mcg/kg, increase infusion to 30 mcg/kg/min. If ACT is greater than 450 sec, decrease infusion to 15 mcg/kg/min. Once ACT of 300–450 sec achieved, proceed with procedure.
▶ **Dosage in Hepatic Impairment**
Adults, Elderly. Initially, 0.5 mcg/kg/min.

SIDE EFFECTS/ADVERSE REACTIONS
Frequent

Dyspnea, hypotension, fever, diarrhea, nausea, pain, vomiting, infection, cough

PRECAUTIONS AND CONTRAINDICATIONS
Overt major bleeding

DRUG INTERACTIONS OF CONCERN TO DENTISTRY
* Increased risk of bleeding: drugs that interfere with coagulation or platelet function, such as NSAIDs and aspirin

SERIOUS REACTIONS
! Ventricular tachycardia and atrial fibrillation occur occasionally.
! Major bleeding and sepsis occur rarely.

DENTAL CONSIDERATIONS
General:

* Patients are at risk of bleeding, check for oral signs.
* Delay elective dental treatment until patient completes parenteral anticoagulant therapy.
* Determine why patient is taking the drug.
* Avoid products that affect platelet function, such as aspirin and NSAIDs.
* Consider local hemostasis measures to prevent excessive bleeding.
Consultations:

* Medical consultation should include partial prothrombin time, prothrombin time, or INR
* Medical consultation should include routine blood counts including platelet counts and bleeding time.

Teach Patient/Family to:
* Use soft tooth brush to reduce risk of bleeding
* Use effective oral hygiene to prevent soft tissue inflammation
* Report oral lesions, soreness, or bleeding to dentist
* Prevent trauma when using oral hygiene aids
* Update health and medication history if physician makes any changes in evaluation or drug regimens; include OTC, herbal, and nonherbal remedies in the update
* Inform dentist of unusual bleeding episodes following dental treatment

---

aripiprazole
ar-ah-pip´-rah-zole
(Abilify)

CATEGORY AND SCHEDULE
Pregnancy Risk Category: C

Drug Class: Antipsychotic

MECHANISM OF ACTION
An antipsychotic agent that provides partial agonist activity at dopamine and serotonin (5-HT1A) receptors and antagonist activity at serotonin (5-HT2A) receptors. *Therapeutic Effect:* Diminishes schizophrenic behavior.

USES
Treatment of schizophrenia

PHARMACOKINETICS
Well absorbed through the GI tract. Protein binding: 99% (primarily albumin). Reaches steady levels in 2 wk. Metabolized in the liver. Eliminated primarily in feces and,

to a lesser extent, in urine. Not removed by hemodialysis.
Half-life: 75 hr.

INDICATIONS AND DOSAGES
▶ **Schizophrenia, Bipolar Disorder**
PO
Adults, Elderly. Initially, 10–15 mg once a day. May increase up to 30 mg/day.

SIDE EFFECTS/ADVERSE REACTIONS
Frequent

Weight gain, headache, insomnia, vomiting
Occasional

Light-headedness, nausea, akathisia, somnolence
Rare

Blurred vision, constipation, asthenia or loss of energy and strength, anxiety, fever, rash, cough, rhinitis, orthostatic hypotension

PRECAUTIONS AND CONTRAINDICATIONS
Hypersensitivity
Caution

Known cardiovascular diseases, cerebrovascular disease, or other conditions predisposing the patient to hypotension; seizures, may impair judgement or motor skills, elevated body temperature, suicide, dysphagia, dehydration, severe renal or hepatic impairment, avoid breast-feeding and use in children

DRUG INTERACTIONS OF CONCERN TO DENTISTRY
* Possible lowering of blood levels: carbamazepine and other inducers of CYP3A4 isoenzymes
* Increased blood levels: ketoconazole and other inhibitors of CYP3A4 or CYP2D6 isoenzymes
* Caution with CNS depressants and alcohol

SERIOUS REACTIONS
! Extrapyramidal symptoms and neuroleptic malignant syndrome occur rarely.

DENTAL CONSIDERATIONS
General:
* Assess for presence of extrapyramidal motor symptoms, such as tardive dyskinesia and akathisia. Extrapyramidal motor activity may complicate dental treatment.
* Consider semisupine chair position for patient comfort if GI side effects occur.
Consultations:
* Consultation with physician may be necessary if sedation or general anesthesia is required.
* Medical consultation may be required to assess disease control and patient's ability to tolerate stress.
Teach Patient/Family to:
* Consult physician if signs of tardive dyskinesia or akathisia are present
* Use effective oral hygiene to prevent soft tissue inflammation
* Use electric tooth brush if patient has difficulty holding conventional devices
* Update health and drug history if physician makes any changes in evaluation or drug regimens

articaine hydrochloride
ar-ti-kane hi-droh-klor´-ide
(Astracaine[CAN], Astracaine Forte[CAN], Septocaine)

CATEGORY AND SCHEDULE
Pregnancy Risk Category: C

Drug Class: Amide local anesthetic with vasoconstrictor (epinephrine)

MECHANISM OF ACTION
An amide anesthetic that inhibits conduction of nerve impulses. *Therapeutic Effect:* Causes temporary loss of feeling and sensation.

USES
Local, infiltrative, or conductive anesthesia in both simple and complex dental and periodontal procedures

PHARMACOKINETICS
Onset of action occurs within 1–6 min depending on route of administration. Complete anesthesia lasts approximately 1 hr. Well absorbed. Protein binding: 60%–80%. Rapidly metabolized by plasma carboxyesterase to its primary metabolite, articainic acid, which is inactive. Excreted in urine. *Half-life:* 20–120 min.

INDICATIONS AND DOSAGES
These recommended doses serve only as a guide to the amount of anesthetic required for most routine procedures. The actual volumes to be used depend on a number of factors, such as type and extent of surgical procedure, depth of anesthesia, degree of muscular relaxation, and condition of the patient.

Local, Infiltrative, or Conductive Anesthesia in Both Simple and Complex Dental or Periodontal Procedures
Infiltration
Adults, Elderly, Children older than 4 yr. 0.5–2.5 ml of a 4% solution, which corresponds to 20–100 mg. Maximum dose administered should not exceed 7 mg/kg (0.175 ml/kg) or 3.2 mg/lb (0.0795 ml/lb) of body weight (up to 500 mg).

SIDE EFFECTS/ADVERSE REACTIONS
Rare

Drowsiness, dizziness, disorientation, light-headedness, tremors, blurred or double vision, nausea, sensation of heat, cold, numbness

PRECAUTIONS AND CONTRAINDICATIONS
History of hypersensitivity to local anesthetics of the amide type or sodium metabisulfite
Caution

Accidental intravascular injections may be associated with convulsions, CNS depression, or cardiorespiratory depression; reduce dose for elderly, debilitated, or pediatric patients; exaggerated response to intravascular epinephrine, severe hepatic impairment, lactation

DRUG INTERACTIONS OF CONCERN TO DENTISTRY
* CNS depressants: increased risk of CNS depression with all CNS depressants, especially in children and when larger doses are used
* Avoid placing dental cartridges in disinfectant solutions with heavy metals or surface-active agents; may see release of metal ions into local anesthetic solutions with tissue irritation following injection
* Risk of cardiovascular side effects; rapid intravascular administration of local anesthetic containing vasoconstrictor, either alone or in patients taking tricyclic antidepressants, MAOIs, digitalis drugs, cocaine, phenothiazines, β-blockers, and in presence of halogenated hydrocarbon general anesthetics; use smallest effective vasoconstrictor dose and careful aspiration technique

• Avoid use of vasoconstrictors in patients with uncontrolled hyperthyroidism, diabetes, angina, or hypertension; refer these patients for medical treatment before elective dental procedures

SERIOUS REACTIONS

! Tachycardia or bradycardia, B/P changes, syncope, cardiac arrest, and seizures have been observed in some patients during dental procedures.

DENTAL CONSIDERATIONS
General:
• Monitor vital signs at every appointment because of cardiovascular side effects.
• Apply lubricant to dry lips for patient comfort before dental procedures.
• Use vasoconstrictor with caution, in low doses, and with careful aspiration.
Teach Patient/Family to:
• Use care to prevent injury while numbness exists and to not chew gum or eat following dental anesthesia
• Report any signs of infection, muscle pain, or fever to dentist when feeling returns
• Report any unusual soft tissue reactions

ascorbic acid (vitamin C)
ah-skor´-bic as´-id
(Apo-C[CAN], Cecon, Cenolate, Pro-C[AUS], Redoxon[CAN])

CATEGORY AND SCHEDULE
Pregnancy Risk Category: C
OTC

Drug Class: Vitamin C, water-soluble vitamin

MECHANISM OF ACTION
Assists in collagen formation and tissue repair and is involved in oxidation reduction reactions and other metabolic reactions.
Therapeutic Effect: Involved in carbohydrate use and metabolism, as well as synthesis of carnitine, lipids, and proteins. Preserves blood vessel integrity.

USES
Vitamin C deficiency, scurvy, urine acidification, and supplemental use in a variety of debilitated patients with poor vitamin C intake

PHARMACOKINETICS
Readily absorbed from the GI tract. Protein binding: 25%. Metabolized in the liver. Excreted in urine. Removed by hemodialysis.

INDICATIONS AND DOSAGES
▶ **Dietary Supplement**
PO
Adults, Elderly. 50–200 mg/day.
Children. 35–100 mg/day.
▶ **Acidification of Urine**
PO
Adults, Elderly. 4–12 g/day in 3–4 divided doses.
Children. 500 mg q6–8h.
▶ **Scurvy**
PO
Adults, Elderly. 100–250 mg 1–2 times a day.
Children. 100–300 mg/day in divided doses.
▶ **Prevention and Reduction of Severity of Colds**
PO
Adults, Elderly. 1–3 g/day in divided doses.

SIDE EFFECTS/ADVERSE REACTIONS

Rare
Abdominal cramps, nausea, vomiting, diarrhea, increased urination with doses exceeding 1 g
Parenteral: Flushing, headache, dizziness, sleepiness or insomnia, soreness at injection site

PRECAUTIONS AND CONTRAINDICATIONS

Caution
Gout

DRUG INTERACTIONS OF CONCERN TO DENTISTRY

● Increased urinary excretion: salicylates, barbiturates

SERIOUS REACTIONS

❗ Ascorbic acid may acidify urine, leading to crystalluria.
❗ Large doses of IV ascorbic acid may lead to deep vein thrombosis.
❗ Abrupt discontinuation after prolonged use of large doses may produce rebound ascorbic acid deficiency.

DENTAL CONSIDERATIONS

General:
● An increased incidence of caries and soft tissue injury has been reported with excessive use of chewable ascorbic acid tablets.

aspirin/ acetylsalicylic acid

as´-pir-in/ah-seet´-il-sill-ic as´-id
(Ascriptin, Aspro[AUS], Bayer, Bex[AUS], Bufferin, Disprin[AUS], Ecotrin, Entrophen[CAN], Halfprin, Novasen[CAN], Solprin[AUS], Spren[AUS])
Do not confuse aspirin or Ascriptin with Aricept, Afrin, or Asendin, or Ecotrin with Edecrin.

CATEGORY AND SCHEDULE

Pregnancy Risk Category: D
OTC

Drug Class: Nonnarcotic analgesic salicylate

MECHANISM OF ACTION

A nonsteroidal salicylate that inhibits prostaglandin synthesis, acts on the hypothalamus heat-regulating center, and interferes with the production of thromboxane A_2, a substance that stimulates platelet aggregation.
Therapeutic Effect: Reduces inflammatory response and intensity of pain; decreases fever; inhibits platelet aggregation.

USES

Treatment of mild-to-moderate pain or fever, including arthritis, thromboembolic disorders, transient ischemic attacks in men, rheumatic fever, post–MI

PHARMACOKINETICS

Route	Onset	Peak	Duration
PO	1 hr	2–4 hr	24 hr

Rapidly and completely absorbed from GI tract; enteric-coated absorption delayed; rectal absorption delayed and incomplete. Protein binding: High. Widely distributed. Rapidly hydrolyzed to salicylate. *Half-life:* 15–20 min (aspirin); 2–3 hr (salicylate at low dose); more than 20 hr (salicylate at high dose).

INDICATIONS AND DOSAGES
▶ **Analgesia, Fever**
PO, Rectal
Adults, Elderly. 325–1,000 mg q4–6h
Children. 10–15 mg/kg/dose q4–6h.
Maximum: 4 g/day.
▶ **Antiinflammatory**
PO
Adults, Elderly. Initially, 2.4–3.6 g/day in divided doses; then 3.6–5.4 g/day.
Children. Initially, 60–90 mg/kg/day in divided doses; then 80–100 mg/kg/day.
▶ **Suspected MI**
PO
Adults, Elderly. 162 mg as soon as the MI is suspected, then daily for 30 days after the MI.
▶ **Prevention of MI**
PO
Adults, Elderly. 75–325 mg/day.
▶ **Prevention of Stroke after Transient Ischemic Attack**
PO
Adults, Elderly. 50–325 mg/day.
▶ **Kawasaki Disease**
PO
Children. 80–100 mg/kg/day in divided doses.

SIDE EFFECTS/ADVERSE REACTIONS
Occasional

GI distress (including abdominal distention, cramping, heartburn, and mild nausea); allergic reaction (including bronchospasm, pruritus, and urticaria)

PRECAUTIONS AND CONTRAINDICATIONS
Allergy to tartrazine dye, bleeding disorders, chickenpox or flu in children and teenagers, GI bleeding or ulceration, hepatic impairment, history of hypersensitivity to aspirin or NSAIDs
Caution

Anemia, hepatic disease, renal disease, Hodgkin's disease, preoperative, postoperative

DRUG INTERACTIONS OF CONCERN TO DENTISTRY
* Increased risk of GI complaints and occult blood loss: alcohol, NSAIDs, corticosteroids
* Buffered aspirin: Decreased absorption of tetracycline
* Recent report indicated ibuprofen may block clot-preventing effects of aspirin
* Interactions when used as a dental drug:
    * Increased risk of bleeding: oral anticoagulants, valproic acid, dipyridamole
    * Increased risk of hypoglycemia: sulfonylureas
    * Increased risk of toxicity: methotrexate, lithium, zidovudine
    * Decreased effects of probenecid, sulfinpyrazone
* Avoid prolonged or concurrent use with NSAIDs, corticosteroids, acetaminophen
* Suspected reduction in antihypertensives and vasodilator effects of angiotensin-converting enzyme (ACE) inhibitors; monitor blood pressure if used concurrently

SERIOUS REACTIONS
! High doses of aspirin may produce GI bleeding and gastric mucosal lesions.

! Dehydrated, febrile children may experience aspirin toxicity quickly. Reye's syndrome may occur in children with the chickenpox or the flu.

! Low-grade toxicity is characterized by tinnitus, generalized pruritus (possibly severe), headache, dizziness, flushing, tachycardia, hyperventilation, diaphoresis, and thirst.

! Market toxicity is characterized by hyperthermia, restlessness, seizures, abnormal breathing patterns, respiratory failure, and coma.

DENTAL CONSIDERATIONS

General:
• Patients on chronic drug therapy may rarely have symptoms of blood dyscrasias, which can include infection, bleeding, and poor healing.
• Avoid prescribing buffered aspirin-containing products if patient is on a sodium-restricted diet.
• Chewable forms of aspirin should not be used for 7 days following oral surgery because of possible soft tissue injury.
• Evaluate allergic reactions: rash, urticaria; patients with allergy to salicylates may not be able to take NSAIDs; drug may need to be discontinued.

Consultations:
• In a patient with symptoms of blood dyscrasias, request a medical consultation for blood studies and postpone dental treatment until normal values are reestablished.
• Take precautions if dental surgery is anticipated because of risk of increased bleeding; avoid prescribing aspirin before dental surgery.
• Tinnitus, ringing, roaring in ears after high-dose and long-term therapy necessitates referral for salicylism.

Teach Patient/Family to:
• Not place aspirin or buffered aspirin tablets directly on a tooth or mucosal surface because of the risk of chemical burn
• Read label on other OTC drugs; may contain aspirin
• Avoid alcohol ingestion; GI bleeding may occur

atazanavir sulfate

ah-tah-zan´-ah-veer sul´-fate
(Reyataz)
Do not confuse Reyataz with Retavase.

CATEGORY AND SCHEDULE
Pregnancy Risk Category: B

Drug Class: Antiviral, HIV-1 protease inhibitor

MECHANISM OF ACTION
An antiviral that acts as an HIV-1 protease inhibitor, selectively preventing the processing of viral precursors found in cells infected with HIV-1. *Therapeutic Effect:* Prevents the formation of mature HIV cells.

USES
HIV-1 infection in combination with other antiretroviral medications

PHARMACOKINETICS
Rapidly absorbed after PO administration. Protein binding: 86%. Extensively metabolized in the liver. Excreted primarily in urine and, to a lesser extent, in feces. *Half-life:* 5–8 hr.

INDICATIONS AND DOSAGES
▸ **HIV-1 Infection**
PO
Adults, Elderly (antiretroviral-naive).
400 mg (2 capsules) once a day with
food.
Adults, Elderly (antiretroviral-experienced). 300 mg and
ritonavir (Norvir) 100 mg
once a day.
▸ **HIV-1 Infection (concurrent
therapy with efavirenz)**
PO
Adults, Elderly. 300 mg atazanavir,
100 mg ritonavir, and 600 mg
efavirenz as a single daily dose
with food.
▸ **HIV-1 Infection (concurrent
therapy with didanosine)**
PO
Adults, Elderly. Give atazanavir
with food 2 hr before or 1 hr after
didanosine.
▸ **HIV-1 Infection (concurrent
therapy with tenofovir)**
PO
Adults, Elderly. 300 mg atazanavir
and 100 mg ritonavir and 300 mg
tenofovir given as a single daily dose
with food.
▸ **HIV-1 Infection in Patients with
Mild-to-Moderate Hepatic
Impairment**
PO
Adults, Elderly. 300 mg once a day
with food.

SIDE EFFECTS/ADVERSE
REACTIONS

Frequent
Nausea, headache

Occasional
Rash, vomiting, depression, diarrhea,
abdominal pain, fever

Rare
Dizziness, insomnia, cough, fatigue,
back pain

PRECAUTIONS AND
CONTRAINDICATIONS
Concurrent use with ergot
derivatives, midazolam, pimozide,
or triazolam; severe hepatic
insufficiency

Caution
Prolongs PR interval, use with
caution in preexisting conduction
disorders; diabetes mellitus,
hyperglycemia, hepatic impairment;
monitor liver function, HBV
infection, redistribution of body fat,
do not breast-feed infants, safety and
efficacy in children not established

DRUG INTERACTIONS OF
CONCERN TO DENTISTRY
● Avoid drugs metabolized by
CYP3A4 isoenzymes; however, the
package insert notes that significant
drug interactions are not expected
with azithromycin, erythromycin,
itraconazole, or ketoconazole; use
with caution and monitor

SERIOUS REACTIONS
❗ A severe hypersensitivity reaction
(marked by angioedema and chest
pain) and jaundice may occur.

DENTAL CONSIDERATIONS
General:
● Short appointments and a stress
reduction protocol may be required
for anxious patients.
● Use precaution if sedation or
general anesthesia is required; risk of
hypotensive episode.
● Consider semisupine chair position
for patient comfort if GI side effects
occur.
● Patient history should include all
medications and herbal or nonherbal
remedies taken by the patient.
● Assess salivary flow as a factor in
caries, periodontal disease, and
candidiasis.

• Examine for oral manifestation of opportunistic infection.

• Palliative medication may be required for management of oral side effects.

• Advise patient if dental drugs prescribed have a potential for photosensitivity.

• Take precautions if dental surgery is anticipated and general anesthesia required.

• Patients on chronic drug therapy may rarely have symptoms of blood dyscrasias, which can include infection, bleeding, and poor healing.

Consultations:
• Consultation with physician may be necessary if sedation or general anesthesia is required.

• Medical consultation may be required to assess disease control and patient's ability to tolerate stress.

Teach Patient/Family to:
• Be aware of oral side effects and potential sequelae

• Update health and drug history, reporting changes in health status, drug regimen changes, or disease/ treatment status

• Use effective oral hygiene to prevent soft tissue inflammation, infection

• Prevent trauma when using oral hygiene aids

atenolol
ah-ten´-oh-lol
(Apo-Atenol[CAN], AteHexal[AUS], Noten[AUS], Tenolin[CAN], Tenormin, Tensig[AUS])
Do not confuse atenolol with albuterol or timolol.

CATEGORY AND SCHEDULE
Pregnancy Risk Category: D

Drug Class: Antihypertensive, selective β1-blocker

MECHANISM OF ACTION
A β1-adrenergic blocker that acts as an antianginal, antiarrhythmic, and antihypertensive agent by blocking β1-adrenergic receptors in cardiac tissue. **Therapeutic Effect:** Slows SN heart rate, decreasing cardiac output and B/P. Decreases myocardial oxygen demand.

USES
Treatment of mild-to-moderate hypertension, treatment and prophylaxis of angina pectoris, arrhythmia, adjunct therapy in hypertrophic cardiomyopathy, MI therapy and prophylaxis, adjunct therapy in pheochromocytoma, prophylaxis for vascular headache, adjunct therapy in thyrotoxicosis, mitral valve prolapse syndrome

PHARMACOKINETICS

Route	Onset	Peak	Duration
PO	1 hr	2–4 hr	24 hr

Incompletely absorbed from the GI tract. Protein binding: 6%–16%. Minimal liver metabolism. Primarily excreted unchanged in urine. Removed by hemodialysis. **Half-life:** 6–7 hr (increased in impaired renal function).

INDICATIONS AND DOSAGES
▸ **Hypertension**
PO
Adults. Initially, 25–50 mg once a day. May increase dose up to 100 mg once a day.
Elderly. Usual initial dose, 25 mg a day.
Children. Initially, 0.8–1 mg/kg/dose given once a day. Range: 0.8–1.5 mg/ kg/day. Maxiumum: 2 mg/kg/day or 100 mg/day.

▸ **Angina Pectoris**
PO
Adults. Initially, 50 mg once a day.
May increase dose up to 200 mg
once a day.
Elderly. Usual initial dose,
25 mg a day.
▸ **Acute MI**
IV
Adults. Give 5 mg over 5 min; may
repeat in 10 min. In those who
tolerate full 10-mg IV dose, begin
50-mg tablets 10 min after last IV
dose followed by another 50-mg oral
dose 12 hr later. Thereafter, give
100 mg once a day or 50 mg twice a
day for 6–9 days. Or, for those who
do not tolerate full IV dose, give
50 mg orally twice a day or 100 mg
once a day for at least 7 days.

DOSAGE IN RENAL IMPAIRMENT
Dosage interval is modified on the
basis of creatinine clearance.

Creatinine Clearance	Dosage Interval
15–35 ml/min	50 mg a day
less than 15 ml/min	50 mg every other day

SIDE EFFECTS/ADVERSE REACTIONS
Atenolol is generally well tolerated,
with mild and transient side effects.
Frequent
Hypotension manifested as cold
extremities, constipation or diarrhea,
diaphoresis, dizziness, fatigue,
headache, and nausea
Occasional
Insomnia, flatulence, urinary
frequency, impotence or decreased
libido, depression
Rare
Rash, arthralgia, myalgia, confusion
(especially in the elderly), altered
taste

PRECAUTIONS AND CONTRAINDICATIONS
Cardiogenic shock, overt heart
failure, second- or third-degree heart
block, severe bradycardia
Caution
Major surgery, lactation, diabetes
mellitus, severe renal disease, thyroid
disease, COPD, asthma, well-
compensated heart failure

DRUG INTERACTIONS OF CONCERN TO DENTISTRY
● Decreased antihypertensive effects:
NSAIDs, indomethacin, salicylates
● May slow metabolism of lidocaine
● Decreased β-blocking effects (or
decreased β-adrenergic effects) of
epinephrine, levonordefrin,
isoproterenol, and other
sympathomimetics
● Reduced bioavailability suspected
with ampicillin

SERIOUS REACTIONS
❗ Overdose may produce profound
bradycardia and hypotension.
❗ Abrupt atenolol withdrawal may
result in diaphoresis, palpitations,
headache, and tremors.
❗ Atenolol administration may
precipitate CHF or MI in patients
with cardiac disease; thyroid storm
in those with thyrotoxicosis; and
peripheral ischemia in those with
existing peripheral vascular disease.
❗ Hypoglycemia may occur in patients
with previously controlled diabetes.
❗ Thrombocytopenia, manifested as
unusual bruising or bleeding, occurs
rarely.

DENTAL CONSIDERATIONS
General:
● Monitor vital signs at every
appointment because of cardiovascular
and respiratory side effects.

• After supine positioning, have patient sit upright for at least 2 min before standing to avoid orthostatic hypotension.

• Patients on chronic drug therapy may rarely have symptoms of blood dyscrasias, which can include infection, bleeding, and poor healing.

• Assess salivary flow as a factor in caries, periodontal disease, and candidiasis.

• Stress from dental procedures may compromise cardiovascular function; determine patient risk.

• Short appointments and a stress reduction protocol may be required for anxious patients.

• Use vasoconstrictors with caution, in low doses, and with careful aspiration. Avoid use of gingival retraction cord with epinephrine.

Consultations:
• In a patient with symptoms of blood dyscrasias, request a medical consultation for blood studies and postpone dental treatment until normal values are reestablished.

• Medical consultation may be required to assess disease control and stress tolerance of patient.

• Use precautions if general anesthesia is required for dental surgery.

Teach Patient/Family to:
• Use effective oral hygiene to prevent soft tissue inflammation

• Use caution to prevent injury when using oral hygiene aids

• When chronic dry mouth occurs, advise patient to:

  • Avoid mouth rinses with high alcohol content because of drying effects

  • Use daily home fluoride products for anticaries effect

  • Use sugarless gum, frequent sips of water, or saliva substitutes

atomoxetine
aw-toh-mox´-eh-teen
(Strattera)

CATEGORY AND SCHEDULE
Pregnancy Risk Category: C

Drug Class: Selective norepinephrine reuptake inhibitor

MECHANISM OF ACTION
A norepinephrine reuptake inhibitor that enhances noradrenergic function by selective inhibition of the presynaptic norepinephrine transporter. **Therapeutic Effect:** Improves symptoms of attention-deficit hyperactivity disorder (ADHD).

USES
Treatment of ADHD

PHARMACOKINETICS
Rapidly absorbed after PO administration. Protein binding: 98% (primarily to albumin). Eliminated primarily in urine and, to a lesser extent, in feces. Not removed by hemodialysis. **Half-life:** 4–5 hr in general population, 22 hr in 7% of Caucasians and 2% of African-Americans (increased in moderate to severe hepatic insufficiency).

INDICATIONS AND DOSAGES
▸ **ADHD**
PO
Adults, Children weighing 70 kg and more. 40 mg once a day. May increase after at least 3 days to 80 mg as a single daily dose or in divided doses. Maximum: 100 mg.
Children weighing less than 70 kg. Initially, 0.5 mg/kg/day. May increase after at least 3 days to 1.2 mg/kg/day. Maximum: 1.4 mg/kg/day or 100 mg.

▶ **Dosage in Hepatic Impairment**
Expect to administer 50% of normal
atomoxetine dosage to patients with
moderate hepatic impairment and
25% of normal dosage to those with
severe hepatic impairment.

SIDE EFFECTS/ADVERSE REACTIONS
Frequent
Headache, dyspepsia, nausea,
vomiting, fatigue, decreased appetite,
dizziness, altered mood
Occasional
Tachycardia, hypertension, weight
loss, delayed growth in children,
irritability
Rare
Insomnia, sexual dysfunction in
adults, fever

PRECAUTIONS AND CONTRAINDICATIONS
Angle-closure glaucoma, use within
14 days of MAOIs
Caution
Hypertension, tachycardia, CV
disease, urinary retention, nursing,
use of herbs, poor metabolizers of
CYP2D6 drugs, hepatic impairment,
monitor weight and growth changes,
use in geriatric patients not
established

DRUG INTERACTIONS OF CONCERN TO DENTISTRY
* No dental drug interactions
reported; however, drugs that inhibit
CYP2D6 enzymes (paroxetine,
fluoxetine) can increase plasma
levels
* Albuterol and other β2-agonists
should be used with caution because
of potential effects on the
cardiovascular system

SERIOUS REACTIONS
! Urine retention or urinary
hesitance may occur.

! In overdose, gastric emptying and
repeated use of activated charcoal
may prevent systemic absorption.

DENTAL CONSIDERATIONS
General:
* Assess salivary flow as a factor
in caries, periodontal disease, and
candidiasis.
* Monitor vital signs at every
appointment because of
cardiovascular side effects.
* Consider semisupine chair position
for patient comfort if GI side effects
occur.
* Use vasoconstrictor with caution, in
low doses, and with careful aspiration.
Consultations:
* Medical consultation may be
required to assess disease control and
patient's ability to tolerate stress.
Teach Patient/Family to:
* Use effective oral hygiene
to prevent soft tissue inflammation,
infection
* When chronic dry mouth occurs,
advise patient to:
  * Avoid mouth rinses with high
  alcohol content because of drying
  effects
  * Use daily home fluoride products
  for anticaries effect
  * Use sugarless gum, frequent sips
  of water, or saliva substitutes

atorvastatin
ah-tore-vah´-stah-tin
(Lipitor)
Do not confuse Lipitor with
Levatol.

CATEGORY AND SCHEDULE
Pregnancy Risk Category: X

Drug Class: Cholesterol-
lowering agent

MECHANISM OF ACTION
An antihyperlipidemic that inhibits HMG-CoA reductase, the enzyme that catalyzes the early step in cholesterol synthesis. *Therapeutic Effect:* Decreases LDL and VLDL cholesterol, and plasma triglyceride levels; increases HDL cholesterol concentration.

USES
An adjunct in homozygous familial hypercholesterolemia, mixed lipidemia, elevated serum triglyceride levels, and type IV hyperproteinemia, also reduces total cholesterol, LDL-C, apo B, and triglyceride levels; patient should first be placed on cholesterol-lowering diet; familial hypercholesterolemia age 10–17 yr

PHARMACOKINETICS
Poorly absorbed from the GI tract. Protein binding: greater than 98%. Metabolized in the liver. Minimally eliminated in urine. Plasma levels are markedly increased in chronic alcoholic hepatic disease but are unaffected by renal disease.
Half-life: 14 hr.

INDICATIONS AND DOSAGES
▶ **Hyperlipidemia, Reduction of Risk of MI, Angina Revascularization Procedures**
PO
Adults, Elderly. Initially, 10–40 mg a day given as a single dose. Dose range: Increase at 2- to 4-wk intervals to maximum of 80 mg/day.
Children 10–17 yr. Initially, 10 mg/day, may increase to 20 mg/day.
▶ **Familial Hypercholesterolemia**
PO
Children 10–17 yr. Initially, 10 mg/day. May increase to 20 mg/day.

SIDE EFFECTS/ADVERSE REACTIONS
Atorvastatin is generally well tolerated. Side effects are usually mild and transient.
Frequent
Headache
Occasional
Myalgia, rash or pruritus, allergy
Rare
Flatulence, dyspepsia

PRECAUTIONS AND CONTRAINDICATIONS
Active hepatic disease, lactation, pregnancy, unexplained elevated hepatic function test results.
Caution
Chronic alcohol liver disease, pregnancy risk category X, monitor liver function and lipid levels.

DRUG INTERACTIONS OF CONCERN TO DENTISTRY
* Severe myopathy or rhabdomyolysis: erythromycin, niacin, itraconazole, ketoconazole
* Increase in plasma levels: erythromycin, itraconazole, alcohol, ketoconazole
* Suspected increase in midazolam effects when used in general anesthesia (Anesthesia 58:899–904, 2003)

SERIOUS REACTIONS
! Cataracts may develop, and photosensitivity may occur.

DENTAL CONSIDERATIONS
General:
* Consider semisupine chair position for patient comfort if GI side effects occur.

atropine sulfate
a´-troe-peen
(Atropine Sulfate, Atropt[AUS])
Do not confuse atropine sulfate
with Akarpine or Aplisol.

CATEGORY AND SCHEDULE
Pregnancy Risk Category: C

Drug Class: Anticholinergic

MECHANISM OF ACTION
An acetylcholine antagonist that
inhibits the action of acetylcholine
by competing with acetylcholine for
common binding sites on muscarinic
receptors, which are located on
exocrine glands, cardiac and smooth-
muscle ganglia, and intramural
neurons. This action blocks all
muscarinic effects. *Therapeutic
Effect:* Decreases GI motility and
secretory activity, and GU muscle
tone (ureter, bladder); produces
ophthalmic cycloplegia and
mydriasis.

USES
Reduction of salivary and bronchial
secretions

PHARMACOKINETICS
Onset 0.5–1 hr, moderate protein
binding, duration of action 4–6 hr,
renal excretion.

INDICATIONS AND DOSAGES
▶ **Asystole, Slow, Pulseless
Electrical Activity**
IV
Adults, Elderly. 1 mg; may repeat
q3–5 min up to total dose of 0.04
mg/kg.
▶ **Preanesthetic**
IV/IM/Subcutaneous
Adults, Elderly. 0.4–0.6 mg
30–60 min preoperatively.

Children weighing 5 kg and more.
0.01–0.02 mg/kg/dose to maximum
of 0.4 mg/dose.
*Children weighing less than
5 kg.* 0.02 mg/kg/dose 30–60 min
pre-op.
▶ **Bradycardia**
IV
Adults, Elderly. 0.5–1 mg q5min not
to exceed 2 mg or 0.04 mg/kg.
Children. 0.02 mg/kg with a
minimum of 0.1 mg to a
maximum of 0.5 mg in children
and 1 mg in adolescents. May
repeat in 5 min. Maximum total
dose: 1 mg in children, 2 mg in
adolescents.

SIDE EFFECTS/ADVERSE REACTIONS
Frequent
Dry mouth, nose, and throat that
may be severe; decreased sweating,
constipation, irritation at
subcutaneous or IM injection site
Occasional
Swallowing difficulty, blurred vision,
bloated feeling, impotence, urinary
hesitancy
Rare
Allergic reaction, including rash and
urticaria; mental confusion or
excitement, particularly in children,
fatigue

PRECAUTIONS AND CONTRAINDICATIONS
Bladder neck obstruction due to
prostatic hypertrophy, cardiospasm,
intestinal atony, myasthenia gravis in
those not treated with neostigmine,
narrow-angle glaucoma, obstructive
disease of the GI tract, paralytic
ileus, severe ulcerative colitis,
tachycardia secondary to cardiac
insufficiency or thyrotoxicosis, toxic
megacolon, unstable cardiovascular
status in acute hemorrhage

DRUG INTERACTIONS OF CONCERN TO DENTISTRY
- Increased anticholinergic effects: tricyclic antidepressants, antihistamines, opioid analgesics, antipsychotic medications, or other drugs with anticholinergic activity
- Decreased absorption of ketoconazole

SERIOUS REACTIONS
! Overdosage may produce tachycardia, palpitations, hot, dry or flushed skin, absence of bowel sounds, increased respiratory rate, nausea, vomiting, confusion, somnolence, slurred speech, dizziness, and CNS stimulation.
! Overdosage may also produce psychosis as evidenced by agitation, restlessness, rambling speech, visual hallucinations, paranoid behavior, and delusions, followed by depression.

DENTAL CONSIDERATIONS

General:
- Give PO dose 30–60 min before drying effects are required for dental procedures.
- Request that patient remove contact lenses before using drug because of possible drying effects in the eyes.
- Caution patients that they may feel a dry, burning sensation in the throat and experience blurred vision.
- This drug is intended for acute use, usually in single doses only; therefore chronic dry mouth should not be a concern.
- Avoid dental light in patient's eyes; offer dark glasses for patient comfort.

Consultations:
- Medical consultation is advisable before using this drug in patients

with a history of GI disease, cardiac disease, or glaucoma.

---

aurothioglucose/ gold sodium thiomalate
(Gold-50[AUS], Solganal); (Myochrysine, Myocrisin[AUS])

CATEGORY AND SCHEDULE
Pregnancy Risk Category: C

Drug Class: Antiinflammatory gold compound

MECHANISM OF ACTION
Aurothioglucose: A gold compound that alters cellular mechanisms, collagen biosynthesis, enzyme systems, and immune responses. *Therapeutic Effect:* Suppresses synovitis of the active stage of rheumatoid arthritis.
Gold sodium thiomalate: A gold compound whose mechanism of action is unknown. May decrease prostaglandin synthesis or alter cellular mechanisms by inhibiting sulfhydryl systems. *Therapeutic Effect:* Decreases synovial inflammation, retards cartilage and bone destruction, suppresses or prevents but does not cure, arthritis, synovitis.

USES
Treatment of rheumatoid arthritis; juvenile arthritis; unapproved: psoriatic arthritis, Felty's syndrome

PHARMACOKINETICS
Aurothioglucose (50% gold): Slow, erratic absorption after IM administration. Protein binding: 95%–99%. Primarily excreted in

urine. *Half-life:* 3–27 days (half-life increased with increased number of doses).

Gold sodium thiomalate: Well absorbed. Protein binding: 95%. Widely distributed. Metabolized in liver. Excreted in urine and feces. Not removed by hemodialysis. *Half-life:* 5 days.

INDICATIONS AND DOSAGES
▶ **Rheumatoid Arthritis (Aurothioglucose)**
IM
Adults, Elderly. Initially, 10 mg, then 25 mg for 2 doses, then 50 mg weekly thereafter until total dose of 0.8–1 g given. If patient is improved and there are no signs of toxicity, may give 50 mg at 3- to 4-wk intervals for many months.
Children. 0.25 mg/kg, may increase by 0.25 mg/kg each week. Maintenance: 0.75–1 mg/kg/dose. Maximum: 25-mg dose for total of 20 doses, then q2–4wk.
▶ **Rheumatoid Arthritis (Gold Sodium Thiomalate)**
IM
Adults, Elderly. Initially, 10 mg, then 25 mg for second dose. Follow with 25–50 mg/wk until improvement noted or total of 1 g administered. Maintenance: 25–50 mg q2wk for 2–20 wk; if stable, may increase to q3–4wk intervals.
Children. Initially, 10 mg, then 1 mg/kg/wk. Maximum single dose: 50 mg. Maintenance: 1 mg/kg/dose at 2- to 4-wk intervals.
▶ **Dosage in Renal Impairment**

Creatinine Clearance	Dosage
50–80 ml/min	50% of usual dosage
Less than 50 ml/min	Not recommended

SIDE EFFECTS/ADVERSE REACTIONS
Frequent
Aurothioglucose: Rash, stomatitis, diarrhea
Gold sodium thiomalate: Pruritic dermatitis, stomatitis, marked by erythema, redness, shallow ulcers of oral mucous membranes, sore throat, and difficulty swallowing, diarrhea or loose stools, abdominal pain, nausea
Occasional
Aurothioglucose: Nausea, vomiting, anorexia, abdominal cramps
Gold sodium thiomalate: Vomiting, anorexia, flatulence, dyspepsia, conjunctivitis, photosensitivity
Rare
Gold sodium thiomalate: Constipation, urticaria, rash

PRECAUTIONS AND CONTRAINDICATIONS
Aurothioglucose. Bone marrow aplasia, history of gold-induced pathologies, including blood dyscrasias, exfoliative dermatitis, necrotizing enterocolitis, and pulmonary fibrosis, serious adverse effects with previous gold therapy, severe blood dyscrasias
Gold sodium thiomalate. Colitis, concurrent use of antimalarials, immunosuppressive agents, penicillamine, or phenylbutazone, CHF, exfoliative dermatitis, history of blood dyscrasias, severe liver or renal impairment, systemic lupus erythematosus

DRUG INTERACTIONS OF CONCERN TO DENTISTRY
None reported

SERIOUS REACTIONS

! Gold toxicity is the primary serious reaction. Signs and symptoms of gold toxicity include decreased hemoglobin, leukopenia (WBC count less than 4,000/mm³), reduced granulocyte counts (less than150,000/mm³), proteinuria, hematuria, stomatitis (sores, ulcers and white spots in the mouth and throat), blood dyscrasias (anemia, leukopenia, thrombocytopenia, and eosinophilia), glomerulonephritis, nephritic syndrome, and cholestatic jaundice.

DENTAL CONSIDERATIONS

General:
• Patients on chronic drug therapy may rarely have symptoms of blood dyscrasias, which can include infection, bleeding, and poor healing.
• Palliative medication may be required for management of oral side effects.
• Consider semisupine chair position for patient comfort because of arthritic disease.
Consultations:
• Medical consultation may be required to assess disease control and patient's ability to tolerate stress.
• In a patient with symptoms of blood dyscrasias, request a medical consultation for blood studies and postpone dental treatment until normal values are reestablished.
Teach Patient/Family to:
• Use effective oral hygiene to prevent soft tissue inflammation
• Be aware of the possibility of secondary oral infection and the need to see dentist immediately if infection occurs
• Report oral lesions, soreness, or bleeding to dentist

• Avoid mouth rinses with high alcohol content because of drying effects

azatadine maleate
ah-za´-ta-deen mal´-ee-ate
(Optimine)
Do not confuse with azelastine or azacitidine.

CATEGORY AND SCHEDULE
Pregnancy Risk Category: B

Drug Class: Antihistamine, H1-receptor antagonist

MECHANISM OF ACTION
A piperazine-derivative antihistamine that has both anticholinergic and antiserotonin activity. Inhibits mediator release from mast cells and prevents calcium entry into mast cells through voltage-dependent calcium channels. **Therapeutic Effect:** Relieves allergic conditions, including urticaria and pruritus. Anticholinergic effects cause drying of nasal mucosa.

USES
Allergy symptoms, rhinitis, chronic urticaria, pruritus

PHARMACOKINETICS
Rapidly and extensively absorbed from the GI tract. Protein binding: minimal. Metabolized in liver. Excreted in urine. **Half-life:** 8.7 hr.

INDICATIONS AND DOSAGES
▶ **Allergic Rhinitis**
PO
Adults, Elderly, Children 12 yr or older. 1–2 mg 2 times a day.

SIDE EFFECTS/ADVERSE REACTIONS
Frequent
Slight to moderate drowsiness, thickening of bronchial secretions
Rare
Headache, fatigue, nervousness, dizziness, appetite increase, weight gain, nausea, diarrhea, abdominal pain, dry mouth, arthralgia, pharyngitis

PRECAUTIONS AND CONTRAINDICATIONS
History of hypersensitivity to azatadine, antihistamines, or any other component of the formulation or to other related antihistamines including cyproheptadine, concomitant use of MAOIs

DRUG INTERACTIONS OF CONCERN TO DENTISTRY
• Increased CNS depression: all CNS depressants, alcohol
• Increased anticholinergic effect: anticholinergics

SERIOUS REACTIONS
! Hepatitis, bronchospasm, and epistaxis have been reported.

DENTAL CONSIDERATIONS
General:
• Assess salivary flow as a factor in caries, periodontal disease, and candidiasis.
• Patients on chronic drug therapy may rarely have symptoms of blood dyscrasias, which can include infection, bleeding, and poor healing.
• Consider semisupine chair position for patient comfort because of respiratory disease.

• Monitor vital signs at every appointment because of cardiovascular side effects.
Consultations:
• In a patient with symptoms of blood dyscrasia, request a medical consultation for blood studies and postpone dental treatment until normal values are reestablished.
Teach Patient/Family to:
• Use effective oral hygiene to prevent soft tissue inflammation
• Prevent injury when using oral hygiene aids
• When chronic dry mouth occurs, advise patient to:
  • Avoid mouth rinses with high alcohol content because of drying effects
  • Use daily home fluoride products for anticaries effect
  • Use sugarless gum, frequent sips of water, or saliva substitutes

azathioprine
ay-za-thye´-oh-preen
(Alti-Azathioprine[CAN], Azasan, Imuran, Thioprine[AUS])
Do not confuse azathioprine with Azulfidine or azatadine, or Imuran with Elmiron or Imferon.

CATEGORY AND SCHEDULE
Pregnancy Risk Category: D

Drug Class: Immunosuppressant

MECHANISM OF ACTION
An immunologic agent that antagonizes purine metabolism and inhibits DNA, protein, and RNA synthesis. *Therapeutic Effect:* Suppresses cell-mediated

hypersensitivities; alters antibody production and immune response in transplant recipients; reduces the severity of arthritis symptoms.

USES

Renal transplants to prevent graft rejection, refractory rheumatoid arthritis; unapproved use in refractory ITP, glomerulonephritis, nephrotic syndrome, bone marrow transplant; unapproved: pemphigoid and pemphigus, chronic ulcerative colitis, Behçet's syndrome, Crohn's disease

PHARMACOKINETICS

Metabolized in liver; excreted in urine (active metabolite); crosses placenta.

INDICATIONS AND DOSAGES

▶ **Adjunct in Prevention of Renal Allograft Rejection**
PO, IV
Adults, Elderly, Children. 2–5 mg/kg/day on day of transplant, then 1–3 mg/kg/day as maintenance dose.
▶ **Rheumatoid Arthritis**
PO
Adults. Initially, 1 mg/kg/day as a single dose or in 2 divided doses. May increase by 0.5 mg/kg/day after 6–8 wk at 4-wk intervals up to maximum of 2.5 mg/kg/day. Maintenance: Lowest effective dosage. May decrease dose by 0.5 mg/kg or 25 mg/day q4wk (while other therapies, such as rest, physiotherapy, and salicylates, are maintained).
Elderly. Initially, 1 mg/kg/day (50–100 mg); may increase by 25 mg/day until response or toxicity.
▶ **Dosage in Renal Impairment**
Dosage is modified on the basis of creatinine clearance.

Creatinine Clearance	Dose
10–50 ml/min	75% of usual dose
Less than 10 ml/min	50% of usual dose

SIDE EFFECTS/ADVERSE REACTIONS

Frequent
Nausea, vomiting, anorexia (particularly during early treatment and with large doses)
Occasional
Rash
Rare
Severe nausea and vomiting with diarrhea, abdominal pain, hypersensitivity reaction

PRECAUTIONS AND CONTRAINDICATIONS

Pregnant patients with rheumatoid arthritis

DRUG INTERACTIONS OF CONCERN TO DENTISTRY

• Increased blood dyscrasias: NSAIDs, especially phenylbutazone, dapsone, phenothiazines
• Increased immunosuppression, risk of infection: corticosteroids

SERIOUS REACTIONS

! Azathioprine use increases the risk of developing neoplasia (new abnormal-growth tumors).
! Significant leukopenia and thrombocytopenia may occur, particularly in those undergoing kidney transplant rejection.
! Hepatotoxicity occurs rarely.

DENTAL CONSIDERATIONS

General:
• Patients on chronic drug therapy may rarely have symptoms of blood dyscrasias, which can include infection, bleeding, and poor healing.

- To prevent infection if surgery or deep scaling is planned, prophylactic antibiotics may be indicated in patients who develop neutropenia.
- Determine why the patient is taking the drug.
- Alert the patient to the possibility of secondary oral infection; must see dentist immediately if infection occurs.

Consultations:
- In a patient with symptoms of blood dyscrasias, request a medical consultation for blood studies and postpone dental treatment until normal values are reestablished.
- Medical consultation may be required to assess disease control and patient's ability to tolerate stress.

Teach Patient/Family to:
- Use effective oral hygiene to prevent soft tissue inflammation
- Use caution to prevent injury when using oral hygiene aids
- Avoid mouth rinses with high alcohol content because of drying effects and irritation of mucous membranes

azelaic acid
aye-zeh-lay´-ick as´-id
(Azelex, Finacea, Finevin)

CATEGORY AND SCHEDULE
Pregnancy Risk Category: B

Drug Class: Topical antimicrobial, antiacne

MECHANISM OF ACTION
The exact mechanism of action of azelaic acid is not known. Possesses antimicrobial activity against Propionibacterium acnes and Staphylococcus epidermidis.

Therapeutic Effect: Inhibits microbial cellular protein synthesis.

USES
Topical therapy of mild-to-moderate inflammatory acne vulgaris; unapproved: melasma

PHARMACOKINETICS
Minimal absorption after topical administration. Metabolized in liver. Excreted in urine as unchanged drug. *Half-life:* 12 hr.

INDICATIONS AND DOSAGES
▸ Mild-to-Moderate Acne
Topical
Adults, Adolescents. Apply cream or gel to affected area twice daily (morning and evening).

SIDE EFFECTS/ADVERSE REACTIONS
Occasional
Pruritus, stinging, burning, tingling, erythema, dryness, rash, peeling, irritation, contact dermatitis
Rare
Worsening of asthma, vitiligo depigmentation, small depigmented spots, hypertrichosis, reddening (signs of keratosis pilaris), exacerbation of recurrent cold sore, fever blister, or oral herpes simplex

PRECAUTIONS AND CONTRAINDICATIONS
Hypersensitivity to azelaic acid or any component of the formulation

DRUG INTERACTIONS OF CONCERN TO DENTISTRY
None reported

SERIOUS REACTIONS
None reported

DENTAL CONSIDERATIONS
General:
• Topical use rarely causes exacerbation of recurrent herpes labialis.
• Keep away from mouth and other mucous membranes; wash eyes if cream comes in contact; irritation can occur.

azelastine
ah´-zel-ah-steen
(Astelin, Optivar)
Do not confuse Optivar with Optiray

CATEGORY AND SCHEDULE
Pregnancy Risk Category: C

Drug Class: Antihistamine

MECHANISM OF ACTION
An antihistamine that competes with histamine for histamine receptor sites on cells in the blood vessels, GI tract, and respiratory tract. *Therapeutic Effect:* Relieves symptoms associated with seasonal allergic rhinitis such as increased mucus production and sneezing and symptoms associated with allergic conjunctivitis, such as redness, itching, and excessive tearing.

USES
Temporary relief of signs and symptoms of allergic conjunctivitis. Control of symptoms associated with seasonal allergic rhinitis, nonallergic vasomotor rhinitis, nasal pruritus.

PHARMACOKINETICS

Route	Onset	Peak	Duration
Nasal spray	0.5–1 hr	2–3 hr	12 hr
Ophthalmic	N/A	3 min	8 hr

Well absorbed through nasal mucosa. Primarily excreted in feces. *Half-life:* 22 hr.

INDICATIONS AND DOSAGES
▶ **Allergic Rhinitis**
Nasal
Adults, Elderly, Children 12 yr and older. 2 sprays in each nostril twice a day.
Children 5–11 yr. 1 spray in each nostril twice a day.
▶ **Allergic Conjunctivitis**
Ophthalmic
Adults, Elderly, Children 3 yr or older. 1 drop into affected eye twice a day.

SIDE EFFECTS/ADVERSE REACTIONS
Frequent
Headache, bitter taste
Rare
Nasal burning, paroxysmal sneezing
Ophthalmic: Transient eye burning or stinging, bitter taste, headache

PRECAUTIONS AND CONTRAINDICATIONS
Breast-feeding women, history of hypersensitivity to antihistamines, neonates or premature infants, third trimester of pregnancy

DRUG INTERACTIONS OF CONCERN TO DENTISTRY
• Increased risk of anticholinergic effects: anticholinergics
• Possible additive sedation: alcohol, anxiolytics, opioid analgesics

SERIOUS REACTIONS
! Epistaxis occurs rarely.

DENTAL CONSIDERATIONS
General:
• Protect patient's eyes from accidental spatter during dental treatment.

• Assess salivary flow as factor in caries, periodontal disease, and candidiasis.

Teach Patient/Family:

• When chronic dry mouth occurs, advise patient to:
  • Avoid mouth rinses with high alcohol content because of drying effects
  • Use daily home fluoride products for anticaries effect
  • Use sugarless gum, frequent sips of water, or saliva substitutes

azithromycin
ay-zi-thro-mye´-sin
(Zithromax, Zithromax TRI-PAK, Zithromax Z-PAK)
Do not confuse azithromycin with erythromycin.

CATEGORY AND SCHEDULE
Pregnancy Risk Category: B

Drug Class: Macrolide antibiotic

MECHANISM OF ACTION
A macrolide antibiotic that binds to ribosomal receptor sites of susceptible organisms, inhibiting RNA-dependent protein synthesis. *Therapeutic Effect:* Bacteriostatic or bactericidal, depending on the drug dosage.

USES
Treatment of mild-to-moderate infections of the upper or lower respiratory tract; COPD exacerbations caused by *H. influenzae, M. catarrhalis,* or *S. pneumoniae;* gonorrhea, chancroid, uncomplicated skin and skin structure infections caused by *M. catarrhalis, S. pneumoniae, S. pyogenes, S. aureus, S. agalactiae,* *H. influenzae, Clostridium,* or *L. pneumophila;* nongonococcal urethritis; cervicitis caused by *C. trachomatis;* otitis media caused by *H. influenzae, S. pneumoniae,* or *M. catarrhalis;* chlamydia; *Mycobacterium avium* complex (MAC) in HIV infection

PHARMACOKINETICS
Rapidly absorbed from the GI tract. Protein binding: 7%–50%. Widely distributed. Eliminated primarily unchanged by biliary excretion. *Half-life:* 68 hr.

INDICATIONS AND DOSAGES
▶ **Respiratory Tract, Skin, and Skin-Structure Infections**
PO
Adults, Elderly. 500 mg once, then 250 mg/day for 4 days.
Children 6 mo and older. 10 mg/kg once (maximum 500 mg) then 5 mg/kg/day for 4 days (maximum 250 mg).
▶ **Acute Bacterial Exacerbations of COPD**
PO
Adults. 500 mg/day for 3 days.
▶ **Otitis Media**
PO
Children 6 mo and older. 10 mg/kg once (maximum 500 mg) then 5 mg/kg/day for 4 days (maximum 250 mg). Single dose: 30 mg/kg. Maximum: 1500 mg. Three day regimen: 10 mg/kg/day as single daily dose. Maximum: 500 mg/day.
▶ **Pharyngitis, Tonsillitis**
PO
Children older than 2 yr. 12 mg/kg/day (maximum 500 mg) for 5 days.
▶ **Chancroid**
PO
Adults, Elderly. 1 g as single dose.
Children. 20 mg/kg as single dose. Maximum: 1 g.

▸ **Treatment of MAC**
PO
Adults, Elderly. 500 mg/day in combination.
Children. 5 mg/kg/day (maximum 250 mg) in combination.
▸ **Prevention of MAC**
PO
Adults, Elderly. 1,200 mg/wk alone or with rifabutin.
Children. 5 mg/kg/day (maximum 250 mg) or 20 mg/kg/wk (maximum 1,200 mg) alone or with rifabutin.
▸ **Nongonococcal Urethritis and Cervicitis Due to Chlamydia Trachomatis**
PO
Adults. 1 g as a single dose.
▸ **Usual Pediatric Dosage**
PO
Children older than 6 mo. 10 mg/kg once (maximum: 500 mg) then 5 mg/kg/day for 4 days (maximum 250 mg).
▸ **Usual Parenteral Dosage (Community-Acquired Pneumonia, PID)**
IV
Adults. 500 mg/day, followed by oral therapy.

SIDE EFFECTS/ADVERSE REACTIONS
Occasional
Nausea, vomiting, diarrhea, abdominal pain
Rare
Headache, dizziness, allergic reaction

PRECAUTIONS AND CONTRAINDICATIONS
Hypersensitivity to azithromycin or other macrolide antibiotics

DRUG INTERACTIONS OF CONCERN TO DENTISTRY
• Increased serum levels: carbamazepine, cyclosporine, pimozide

• Risk of severe myopathy, rhabdomyolysis: hydroxymethylglutaryl coenzyme A (HMG-CoA) reductase inhibitors (statins)
• Decreased action of clindamycin, penicillin, lincomycin
• Oral contraceptives: advise patient of a low potential risk for decreased contraceptive action, to maintain compliance with oral contraceptive use while using antibiotics, and to consider the use of additional nonhormonal contraception
• Possible increase in anticoagulant effect: warfarin
• Increased serum levels of theophylline

SERIOUS REACTIONS
! Antibiotic-associated colitis and other superinfections may result from altered bacterial balance.
! Acute interstitial nephritis and hepatotoxicity occur rarely.

DENTAL CONSIDERATIONS
General:
• An alternative drug of choice for mild infection caused by susceptible organisms in patients allergic to penicillin.
• Determine why the patient is taking the drug.
• Consider semisupine chair position for patient comfort if GI side effects occur.
Teach Patient/Family:
• When used for dental infection, advise patient to:
    • Report sore throat, oral burning sensation, fever, and fatigue, any of which could indicate superinfection
    • Take at prescribed intervals and complete dosage regimen
    • Immediately notify the dentist if signs or symptoms of infection increase

aztreonam
az-tree´-oo-nam
(Azactam)

CATEGORY AND SCHEDULE
Pregnancy Risk Category: B

Drug Class: Antibacterial

MECHANISM OF ACTION
A monobactam antibiotic
that inhibits bacterial cell wall
synthesis. *Therapeutic Effect:*
Bactericidal.

USES
Treatment of infections caused by
bacteria

PHARMACOKINETICS
Completely absorbed after IM
administration. Protein binding:
56%–60%. Partially metabolized
by hydrolysis. Primarily excreted
unchanged in urine. Removed by
hemodialysis. *Half-life:* 1.4–2.2 hr
(increased in impaired renal or
hepatic function).

INDICATIONS AND DOSAGES
▸ **UTIs**
IV, IM
Adults, Elderly. 500 mg1 g q8–12h.
▸ **Moderate to Severe Systemic
Infections**
IV, IM
Adults, Elderly. 1–2 g q8–12h.
▸ **Severe or Life-Threatening
Infections**
IV
Adults, Elderly. 2 g q6–8h.
▸ **Cystic Fibrosis**
IV
Children. 50 mg/kg/dose
q6–8h up to 200 mg/kg/day.
Maximum: 8g/d.

▸ **Mild to Severe Infections in
Children**
IV
Children. 30 mg/kg q6–8h.
Maximum: 120 mg/kg/day.
Neonates. 60–120 mg/kg/day
q6–12h.
▸ **Dosage in Renal Impairment**
Dosage and frequency are modified
on the basis of creatinine clearance
and the severity of the infection:

Creatinine Clearance	Dosage
10–30 ml/min	1–2 g initially, then usual dose at usual intervals
Less than 10 ml/min	1–2 g initially; then usual dose at usual intervals

SIDE EFFECTS/ADVERSE REACTIONS
Occasional
Discomfort and swelling at IM
injection site, nausea, vomiting,
diarrhea, rash
Rare
Phlebitis or thrombophlebitis at IV
injection site, abdominal cramps,
headache, hypotension

PRECAUTIONS AND CONTRAINDICATIONS
None known

DRUG INTERACTIONS OF CONCERN TO DENTISTRY
None reported

SERIOUS REACTIONS
! Antibiotic-associated colitis and
other superinfections may result from
altered bacterial balance.
! Severe hypersensitivity reactions,
including anaphylaxis, occur
rarely.

DENTAL CONSIDERATIONS

General:
• For selected infections in the hospital setting.
• Provide palliative dental care for dental emergencies only.
• Caution regarding allergy to medication.
• Examine for oral manifestation of opportunistic infection.
• Determine why patient is taking the drug.

Consultations:
• Medical consultation may be required to assess disease control.

• Consult patient's physician if an acute dental infection occurs and another antiinfective is required.

Teach Patient/Family to:
• Use effective oral hygiene to prevent soft tissue inflammation
• Report oral lesions, soreness, or bleeding to dentist
• Prevent trauma when using oral hygiene aids

bacitracin

bass-ih-tray'-sin
(Baciguent, Baci-IM, Bacitracin)
Do not confuse bacitracin with
Bactrim or Bactroban.

CATEGORY AND SCHEDULE

Pregnancy Risk Category: C
OTC

Drug Class: Antiinfective;
antibiotic

MECHANISM OF ACTION

An antibiotic that interferes
with plasma membrane
permeability and inhibits bacterial
cell wall synthesis in susceptible
bacteria. *Therapeutic Effect:*
Bacteriostatic.

USES

Treatment of superficial ocular
infections (conjunctivitis, keratitis,
corneal ulcers, blepharitis). Minor
skin abrasions, superficial infections.
Treatment, prophylaxis of surgical
procedures.

INDICATIONS AND DOSAGES

▸ **Superficial Ocular Infections**
Ophthalmic
Adults. ½-inch ribbon in conjunctival
sac q3–4h.
▸ **Skin Abrasions, Superficial Skin
Infections**
Topical
Adults, Children. Apply to affected
area 1–5 times a day.
▸ **Surgical Treatment and
Prophylaxis**
Irrigation
Adults, Elderly. 50,000–150,000 units,
as needed.

SIDE EFFECTS/ADVERSE REACTIONS

Rare
Ophthalmic: Burning, itching,
redness, swelling, pain
Topical: Hypersensitivity reaction
(allergic contact dermatitis, burning,
inflammation, pruritus)

PRECAUTIONS AND CONTRAINDICATIONS

None known

DRUG INTERACTIONS OF CONCERN TO DENTISTRY

None reported

SERIOUS REACTIONS

! Severe hypersensitivity reactions,
including apnea and hypotension,
occur rarely.

DENTAL CONSIDERATIONS

General:
• Use protective glove or finger cot
to apply.
• Determine why patient is taking
the drug.
Teach Patient/Family to:
• Report burning, itching, or rash

baclofen

bak'-loe-fen
(Apo-Baclofen[CAN], Baclo[AUS],
Clofen[AUS], Lioresal, Liotec[CAN],
Novo-Baclofen[CAN], Nu-
Baclofen[CAN], Stelax[AUS])
Do not confuse baclofen with
Bactroban or Beclovent.

CATEGORY AND SCHEDULE

Pregnancy Risk Category: C

Drug Class: Skeletal muscle
relaxant, central acting

MECHANISM OF ACTION

A direct-acting skeletal muscle relaxant that inhibits transmission of reflexes at the spinal cord level.
Therapeutic Effect: Relieves muscle spasticity.

USES

Treatment of skeletal muscle spasticity in multiple sclerosis, spinal cord injury, children with cerebral palsy; intrathecal dose form for severe spasticity in spinal cord injury or those not responsive to oral dose form; unapproved: trigeminal neuralgia

PHARMACOKINETICS

Well absorbed from the GI tract. Protein binding: 30%. Partially metabolized in the liver. Primarily excreted in urine.
Half-life: 2.5–4 hr; intrathecal: 1.5 hr.

INDICATIONS AND DOSAGES
▶ **Spasticity**
PO
Adults. Initially, 5 mg 3 times a day. May increase by 15 mg/day at 3-day intervals. Range: 40–80 mg/day. Maximum: 80 mg/day.
Elderly. Initially, 5 mg 2–3 times a day. May gradually increase dosage.
Children. Initially, 10–15 mg/day in divided doses q8h. May increase by 5–15 mg/day at 3-day intervals. Maximum: 40 mg/day (children 2–7 yr); 60 mg/day (children 8 yr and older).
Usual Intrathecal Dosage
Adults, Elderly, Children older than 12 yr. 300–800 mcg/day.
Children 12 yr and younger. 100–300 mcg/day.

SIDE EFFECTS/ADVERSE REACTIONS

Frequent
Transient somnolence, asthenia, dizziness, light-headedness, nausea, vomiting
Occasional
Headache, paresthesia, constipation, anorexia, hypotension, confusion, nasal congestion
Rare
Paradoxical CNS excitement or restlessness, slurred speech, tremor, dry mouth, diarrhea, nocturia, impotence

PRECAUTIONS AND CONTRAINDICATIONS

Skeletal muscle spasm due to cerebral palsy, Parkinson's disease, rheumatic disorders, CVA, cough, intractable hiccups, neuropathic pain

DRUG INTERACTIONS OF CONCERN TO DENTISTRY

• Increased CNS depression: alcohol, all CNS depressants
• Muscle hypertonia: tricyclic antidepressants
  • Warn patient of sedative effects while taking medication

SERIOUS REACTIONS

! Abrupt discontinuation of baclofen may produce hallucinations and seizures.
! Overdose results in blurred vision, seizures, myosis, mydriasis, severe muscle weakness, strabismus, respiratory depression, and vomiting.

DENTAL CONSIDERATIONS

General:
• Monitor vital signs at every appointment because of cardiovascular side effects.

- Assess salivary flow as a factor in caries, periodontal disease, and candidiasis.
- After supine positioning, have patient sit upright for at least 2 min to avoid orthostatic hypotension.

Teach Patient/Family:
- When chronic dry mouth occurs, advise patient to:
  - Avoid mouth rinses with high alcohol content because of drying effects
  - Use daily home fluoride products for anticaries effect
  - Use sugarless gum, frequent sips of water, or saliva substitutes

balsalazide
ball-sal'-ah-zide
(Colazal)

CATEGORY AND SCHEDULE
Pregnancy Risk Category: B

Drug Class: Antiinflammatory

MECHANISM OF ACTION
A 5-aminosalicylic acid derivative that changes intestinal microflora, altering prostaglandin production and inhibiting function of natural killer cells, mast cells, neutrophils, and macrophages. *Therapeutic Effect:* Diminishes inflammatory effect in colon.

USES
Treatment of mild to moderately active ulcerative colitis

PHARMACOKINETICS
PO: Drug reaches colon intact; bacterial azoreductases release 5-aminobenzyl-B-analine and mesalamine (active metabolite); low, variable systemic absorption; peak concentration 1–2 hr, protein binding ≈99%; less than 1% renal excretion; most excreted in feces (65%)

INDICATIONS AND DOSAGES
▶ **Ulcerative Colitis**
PO
Adults, Elderly. Three 750-mg capsules 3 times a day for 8 wk.

SIDE EFFECTS/ADVERSE REACTIONS
Frequent
Headache, abdominal pain, nausea, diarrhea
Occasional
Vomiting, arthralgia, rhinitis, insomnia, fatigue, flatulence, coughing, dyspepsia

PRECAUTIONS AND CONTRAINDICATIONS
Hypersensitivity, including hypersensitivity to mesalamine or salicylates

DRUG INTERACTIONS OF CONCERN TO DENTISTRY
None reported

SERIOUS REACTIONS
! Liver toxicity occurs rarely.

DENTAL CONSIDERATIONS
General:
- Consider semisupine chair position for patient comfort because of GI side effects of disease.
Consultations:
- To reduce any potential risk of antibiotic-associated pseudomembranous colitis, a consultation is recommended before selecting an antibiotic for a dental infection.

becaplermin
beh-kap'-lear-min
(Regranex)

CATEGORY AND SCHEDULE
Pregnancy Risk Category: C

Drug Class: Topical wound repair

MECHANISM OF ACTION
A platelet-derived growth factor that heals open wounds. ***Therapeutic Effect:*** Stimulates body to grow new tissue.

USES
An adjunct to good ulcer care practices in lower extremity diabetic, neuropathic ulcers that extend into subcutaneous tissues or beyond and have adequate blood supply

PHARMACOKINETICS
None reported

INDICATIONS AND DOSAGES
▸ **Ulcers**
Topical
Adults, Elderly. Apply once daily (spread evenly; cover with saline-moistened gauze dressing). After 12 hr, rinse ulcer, re-cover with saline gauze.

SIDE EFFECTS/ADVERSE REACTIONS
Occasional
Local rash near ulcer

PRECAUTIONS AND CONTRAINDICATIONS
Hypersensitivity, neoplasms at the site of application, ulcers caused by vascular insufficiency

Caution
Nonsterile, low-bioburden product that is not for use in ulcers that heal by primary intention, lactation, children younger than 16 yr, external use only, do not apply with fingers

DRUG INTERACTIONS OF CONCERN TO DENTISTRY
Unknown

SERIOUS REACTIONS
None reported

DENTAL CONSIDERATIONS
General:
• Patients requiring use of this medication probably will be limited in activities or bedridden.
• Determine why patient is taking the drug.
• Diabetes: question patient about self-monitoring of blood glucose values or finger-stick records.
• Diabetics may be more susceptible to infection and have delayed wound healing.
• Examine for oral manifestation of opportunistic infection.
• Patients with advanced diabetes should be questioned about any limitations in activities or stress tolerance. Some will also be receiving dialysis treatment if renal function is compromised. Dental treatment usually can be performed the day after dialysis.
Consultations:
• Medical consultation may be required to assess disease control and patient's ability to tolerate stress.
• Medical consultation may include data from patient's blood glucose monitoring, including glycosylated hemoglobin or HbA1c testing
• Patients in dialysis may require antibiotic prophylaxis; determine need.

Teach Patient/Family to:
• Use effective oral hygiene to prevent soft tissue inflammation
• Prevent trauma when using oral hygiene aids
• Update health and drug history if physician makes any changes in evaluation or drug regimens

beclomethasone dipropionate/ beclomethasone dipropionate HFA
be-kloe-meth′-ah-sone di-pro′-pi-o-nate
Oral inhalation: Qvar
Nasal inhalation: Beconase, Beconase AQ Nasal, Vancenase AQ 84 mcg, Vancenase Pockethaler

CATEGORY AND SCHEDULE
Pregnancy Risk Category: C

Drug Class: Corticosteroid, synthetic

MECHANISM OF ACTION
Glucocorticoids have multiple actions that include antiinflammatory and immunosuppressant effects. They inhibit phospholipase A_2, interfering with or reducing the synthesis of prostaglandins and leukotrienes. They also bind to cytoplasmic glucocorticoid receptors (GRs) and enter the cell nucleus to bind with DNA. This results in the synthesis of various enzymes such as collagenase, elastase, and cytokines that play important roles in inflammation control and immunosuppression. They also suppress the production of lymphocytes, monocytes, and eosinophils.

USES
Treatment of chronic asthma, prevention of recurrent nasal polyps, allergic and nonallergic rhinitis

PHARMACOKINETICS
Inhalation: Onset 10 min, half-life 3–15 hr; crosses placenta; metabolized in lungs, liver, GI system; excreted in feces (metabolites).

INDICATIONS AND DOSAGES
Oral inhalation (QVAR only):
Adults, Adolescents. 40–160 mcg bid; limit to 320 mcg bid
Children 5–11 yr. 40 mcg bid; limit 80 mcg bid
Nasal inhalation:
Adults, Children older than 12 yr. 1–2 sprays in each nostril bid-qid; 84 mcg double strength: use once daily
Children 6–12 yr. 1 spray in each nostril once daily
Pockethaler:
Adults, Children older than 12 yr. 1 spray in each nostril bid-qid

SIDE EFFECTS/ADVERSE REACTIONS
ORAL: Dry mouth, candidiasis (rare)
RESP: Bronchospasm
EENT: Hoarseness, sore throat

PRECAUTIONS AND CONTRAINDICATIONS
Hypersensitivity; status asthmaticus (primary treatment); nonasthmatic bronchial disease; bacterial, fungal, or viral infections of mouth, throat, or lungs; children younger than 3 yr
Caution
Nasal disease/surgery

DRUG INTERACTIONS OF CONCERN TO DENTISTRY
None reported

B

SERIOUS REACTIONS
! Potential acute adrenal insufficiency if used to replace systemic corticosteriod use
! Signs an symptoms of hypercorticism

DENTAL CONSIDERATIONS
General:
• Evaluate respiration characteristics and rate.
• Assess salivary flow as a factor in caries, periodontal disease, and candidiasis.
• Place on frequent recall because of oral side effects.
• Be aware that aspirin or sulfite preservatives in vasoconstrictor-containing products can exacerbate asthma.
• Acute asthmatic episodes may be precipitated in the dental office. Sympathomimetic inhalants should be available for emergency use.
• Midday appointments and a stress-reduction protocol may be required for anxious patients.
Consultations:
• Medical consultation may be required to assess patient's ability to tolerate stress.
Teach Patient/Family:
• That gargling and rinsing with water after each dose helps prevent candidiasis
• When chronic dry mouth occurs, advise patient to:
  • Avoid mouth rinses with high alcohol content because of drying effects
  • Use daily home fluoride products for anticaries effect
  • Use sugarless gum, frequent sips of water, or saliva substitutes

benazepril
be-naze'-ah-pril
(Lotensin)
Do not confuse benazepril with Benadryl, or Lotensin with Loniten or lovastatin.

CATEGORY AND SCHEDULE
Pregnancy Risk Category: C (D if used in second or third trimester)

Drug Class: Angiotensin-converting enzyme (ACE) inhibitor

MECHANISM OF ACTION
An ACE inhibitor that decreases the rate of conversion of angiotensin I to angiotensin II, a potent vasoconstrictor. Reduces peripheral arterial resistance. *Therapeutic Effect:* Lowers B/P.

USES
Treatment of hypertension, alone or in combination with thiazide diuretics

PHARMACOKINETICS

Route	Onset	Peak	Duration
PO	1 hr	2–4 hr	24 hr

Partially absorbed from the GI tract. Protein binding: 97%. Metabolized in the liver to active metabolite. Primarily excreted in urine. Minimal removal by hemodialysis. *Half-life:* 35 min; metabolite 10–11 hr.

INDICATIONS AND DOSAGES
▶ **Hypertension (monotherapy)**
PO
Adults. Initially, 10 mg/day. Maintenance: 20–40 mg/day as

single or in 2 divided doses.
Maximum: 80 mg/day.
Elderly. Initially, 5–10 mg/day.
Range: 20–40 mg/day.

▶ **Hypertension (combination therapy)**

PO

Adults. Discontinue diuretic 2–3 days prior to initiating benazepril, then dose as noted above. If unable to discontinue diuretic, begin benazepril at 5 mg/day.

▶ **Dosage in Renal Impairment**

For adult patients with creatinine clearance less than 30 ml/min, initially, 5 mg/day titrated up to maximum of 40 mg/day.

SIDE EFFECTS/ADVERSE REACTIONS

Frequent

Cough, headache, dizziness

Occasional

Fatigue, somnolence or drowsiness, nausea

Rare

Rash, fever, myalgia, diarrhea, loss of taste

PRECAUTIONS AND CONTRAINDICATIONS

History of angioedema from previous treatment with ACE inhibitors

Caution

Impaired renal or liver function, dialysis patients, hypovolemia, blood dyscrasias, CHF, COPD, asthma, elderly

DRUG INTERACTIONS OF CONCERN TO DENTISTRY

• Increased hypotension: alcohol, phenothiazines
• Decreased hypotensive effects: indomethacin and possibly other NSAIDs, sympathomimetics

• Suspected reduction in the antihypertensive and vasodilator effects by salicylates; monitor blood pressure if used concurrently

SERIOUS REACTIONS

! Excessive hypotension ("first-dose syncope") may occur in patients with CHF and in those who are severely salt or volume depleted.

! Angioedema (swelling of the face and lips) and hyperkalemia occur rarely.

! Agranulocytosis and neutropenia may be noted in those with collagen vascular disease, including scleroderma and systemic lupus erythematosus, and impaired renal function.

! Nephrotic syndrome may be noted in patients with history of renal disease.

DENTAL CONSIDERATIONS

General:

• Monitor vital signs at every appointment because of cardiovascular and respiratory side effects.
• After supine positioning, have patient sit upright for at least 2 min to avoid orthostatic hypotension.
• Patients on chronic drug therapy may rarely have symptoms of blood dyscrasias, which can include infection, bleeding, and poor healing.
• Assess salivary flow as a factor in caries, periodontal disease, and candidiasis.
• Limit use of sodium-containing products, such as saline IV fluids, for those patients with a dietary salt restriction.
• Use vasoconstrictors with caution, in low doses, and with careful aspiration.

- Stress from dental procedures may compromise cardiovascular function; determine patient risk.
- Short appointments and a stress-reduction protocol may be required for anxious patients.

Consultations:
- Medical consultation may be required to assess disease control and patient's ability to tolerate stress.
- In a patient with symptoms of blood dyscrasias, request a medical consultation for blood studies and postpone dental treatment until normal values are reestablished.
- Take precautions if dental surgery is anticipated and sedation or general anesthesia is required; risk of hypotensive episode.

Teach Patient/Family to:
- Use effective oral hygiene to prevent soft tissue inflammation
- Use caution to prevent injury when using oral hygiene aids
- When chronic dry mouth occurs, advise patient to:
  - Avoid mouth rinses with high alcohol content because of drying effects
  - Use daily home fluoride products for anticaries effect
  - Use sugarless gum, frequent sips of water, or saliva substitutes

bendroflumethiazide
ben-droe-floo-meth-igh'-ah-zide
(Naturetin-5)

CATEGORY AND SCHEDULE
Pregnancy Risk Category: C

Drug Class: Antidiuretic, central and nephrogenic diabetes insipidus; Antihypertensive; Antiurolithic, calcium calculi; Diuretic

MECHANISM OF ACTION
A benzothiadiazine derivative that acts as a thiazide diuretic and antihypertensive. As a diuretic blocks reabsorption of water, sodium, and potassium at cortical diluting segment of distal tubule. As an antihypertensive reduces plasma, extracellular fluid volume, peripheral vascular resistance by direct effect on blood vessels. **Therapeutic Effect:** Promotes diuresis, reduces B/P.

USES
Commonly used to treat high B/P. May also be used to help reduce the amount of water in the body by increasing the flow of urine.

PHARMACOKINETICS

Route	Onset	Peak	Duration
PO	2 hr	4 hr	6–12 hr

Variably absorbed from the GI tract. Primarily excreted unchanged in urine. Not removed by hemodialysis. *Half-life:* 5.6–14.8 hr.

INDICATIONS AND DOSAGES
▸ **Edema**
PO
Adults. 5 mg/day, preferably given in the morning. To initiate therapy, doses up to 20 mg may be given once a day or divided into 2 doses.
▸ **Hypertension**
PO
Adults. 5–20 mg/day, preferably given in the morning. Maintenance: 2.5–15 mg/day.

SIDE EFFECTS/ADVERSE REACTIONS
Expected
Increase in urine frequency and volume

Frequent
Potassium depletion
Occasional
Postural hypotension, headache,
GI disturbances, photosensitivity
reaction

PRECAUTIONS AND CONTRAINDICATIONS
Anuria, history of hypersensitivity
to sulfonamides or thiazide
diuretics

DRUG INTERACTIONS OF CONCERN TO DENTISTRY
• Decreased hypotensive
response: NSAIDs, especially
indomethacin

SERIOUS REACTIONS
! Vigorous diuresis may lead to
profound water and electrolyte
depletion, resulting in
hypokalemia, hyponatremia,
and dehydration.
! Acute hypotensive episodes may
occur.
! Hyperglycemia may be noted
during prolonged therapy.
! Pancreatitis, blood dyscrasias,
pulmonary edema, allergic
pneumonitis, and dermatologic
reactions occur rarely.
! Overdose can lead to lethargy and
coma without changes in electrolytes
or hydration.

DENTAL CONSIDERATIONS
• Monitor vital signs at every
appointment due to cardiovascular
side effects.
• Patient on chronic drug
therapy may rarely present with
symptoms of blood dyscrasias,
which can include infection,
bleeding, and poor healing.

If dyscrasia is present, caution
patient to prevent oral tissue trauma
when using oral hygiene aids.
• After supine positioning, have
patient sit upright for at least 2 min
before standing to avoid orthostatic
hypotension.
• Limit use of sodium-containing
products, such as saline IV fluids, for
patients with a dietary salt
restriction.
• Stress from dental procedures may
compromise cardiovascular function,
determine patient risk.
• Short appointments and a stress-
reduction protocol may be required
for anxious patients.
• Advise patient if dental drugs
prescribed have a potential for
photosensitivity.
• Patients taking diuretics
should be monitored for serum
K levels.
Consultations:
• In a patient with symptoms
of blood dyscrasias, request a
medical consultation for blood
studies and postpone treatment
until normal values are
reestablished.
• Medical consultation may be
required to assess disease
control and patient's ability to
tolerate stress.
Teach Patient/Family to:
• Use effective oral
hygiene to prevent soft tissue
inflammation
• Prevent trauma when using oral
hygiene aids
• Update Health and medication
history if physician makes any
changes in evaluation or drug
regimens; include OTC, herbal,
and nonherbal remedies in the
update

benzocaine
ben´-zoe-kane
(Americaine Anesthetic Lubricant,
Americaine Otic, Anbesol, Anbesol
Baby Gel, Anbesol Maximum
Strength, Babee Teething,
Benzodent, Cepacol, Cetacaine,
Chiggerex, Chiggertox, Cylex,
Dermoplast, Detaine, Foille, Foille
Medicated First Aid, Foille Plus,
HDA Toothache, Hurricane,
Lanacane, Mycinettes, Omedia,
Orabase-B, Orajel, Orajel Baby,
Orajel Baby Nighttime, Orajel
Maximum Strength, Orasol,
Otricaine, Otocain, Retre-Gel,
Solarcaine, Topicaine[AUS],
Trocaine, Zilactin, Zilactin Baby)

CATEGORY AND SCHEDULE
Pregnancy Risk Category: C

Drug Class: Topical ester, local
anesthetic. Action: Inhibits
conduction of nerve impulses
from sensory nerves

MECHANISM OF ACTION
A local anesthetic that blocks
nerve conduction in the
autonomic, sensory, and motor
nerve fibers. Reduces permeability
of resting nerves to potassium
and sodium ions. *Therapeutic
Effect:* Produces local analgesic
effect.

USES
Treatment of oral irritation,
toothache, cold sore, canker sore,
pain, teething pain, pain caused by
dental prostheses or orthodontic
appliances

PHARMACOKINETICS
Poorly absorbed by topical
administration. Well absorbed from
mucous membranes and traumatized
skin. Metabolized in liver and by
hydrolysis with cholinesterase.
Minimal excretion in urine.

INDICATIONS AND DOSAGES
▸ **Canker Sores**
Topical
*Adults, Elderly, Children older
than 2 yr.* Apply gel, liquid, or
ointment to affected area.
Maximum: 4 times a day.
▸ **Denture Irritation**
Topical
Adults, Elderly. Apply thin layer of
gel to affected area up to 4 times a
day or until pain is relieved.
▸ **General Lubrication**
Topical
*Adults, Elderly, Children older than
2 yr.* Apply gel to exterior of tube or
instrument prior to use.
▸ **Otitis Externa, Otitis Media**
Otic
*Adults, Elderly, Children older than
1 yr.* Instill 4–5 drops into external
ear canal of affected ears.
Repeat q1–2h as needed.
▸ **Pain and Itching Associated with
Sunburn, Insect Bites, Minor Cuts,
Scrapes, Minor Burns, Minor Skin
Irritations**
Topical
*Adults, Elderly, Children older
than 2 yr.* Apply to affected area
3–4 times a day.
▸ **Pharyngitis**
PO
Adults, Elderly. 1 lozenge q2h.
Maximum 8 lozenges a day.
▸ **Toothache/Teething Pain**
Topical
*Adults, Elderly, Children older
than 2 yr.* Apply gel, liquid, or
ointment to affected areas.
Maximum: 4 times a day.

▶ **Anesthesia**
Topical
Adults, Elderly. Apply aerosol, gel, ointment, liquid q4–12h as needed.

SIDE EFFECTS/ADVERSE REACTIONS
Occasional
Burning, stinging, angioedema, contact dermatitis, taste disorders

PRECAUTIONS AND CONTRAINDICATIONS
Hypersensitivity to benzocaine or ester-type local anesthetics, perforated tympanic membrane or ear discharge (otic preparations)

DRUG INTERACTIONS OF CONCERN TO DENTISTRY
None reported

SERIOUS REACTIONS
❗ Methemoglobinermia occurs rarely in infants and young children

DENTAL CONSIDERATIONS
General:
• Do not use for topical anesthesia if medical history reveals allergy to procaine, PABA, parabens, or other ester-type local anesthetics.
• Use smallest effective amount in infants and children.
• Avoid applying to large denuded areas of mucosa to prevent excessive systemic absorption and potential toxicity.

benzonatate
ben-zoe′-na-tate
(Tessalon Perles)

CATEGORY AND SCHEDULE
Pregnancy Risk Category: C

Drug Class: Antitussive, non-narcotic

MECHANISM OF ACTION
A non-narcotic antitussive that anesthetizes stretch receptors in respiratory passages, lungs, and pleura. *Therapeutic Effect:* Reduces cough.

USES
Nonproductive cough relief

PHARMACOKINETICS
PO: Onset 15–20 min, duration 3–8 hr; metabolized by liver; excreted in urine.

INDICATIONS AND DOSAGES
▶ **Antitussive**
PO
Adults, Elderly, Children older than 10 yr. 100 mg 3 times a day or every 4 hr up to 600 mg/day.

SIDE EFFECTS/ADVERSE REACTIONS
Occasional
Mild somnolence, mild dizziness, constipation, GI upset, skin eruptions, nasal congestion

PRECAUTIONS AND CONTRAINDICATIONS
Hypersensitivity
Caution
Lactation

DRUG INTERACTIONS OF CONCERN TO DENTISTRY
• Increased CNS depression: slight risk of increased sedation with other CNS depressants

SERIOUS REACTIONS
❗ A paradoxical reaction, including restlessness, insomnia, euphoria, nervousness, and tremor, has been noted.

3

DENTAL CONSIDERATIONS

General:
• Elective dental treatment may not be possible with significant coughing episodes.

---

benzoyl peroxide

ben'-zoe-ill per-ox'-ide
(Acetoxyl[CAN], Benoxyl[CAN], Benzac, Benzac AC, Benzac AC Wash, Benzac W, Benzac W Wash, Benzagel, Benzagel Wash, Benzashave, Brevoxyl, Brevoxyl Cleansing, Brevoxyl Wash, Clearplex, Clinac BPO, Del Aqua, Desquam-E, Desquam-X, Exact Acne Medication, Fostex 10% BPO, Loroxide, Neutrogena Acne Mask, Neutrogena On the Spot Acne Treatment, Oxy[AUS], Oxy 10 Balanced Medicated Face Wash, Oxy 10 Balance Spot Treatment, Palmer's Skin Success Acne, Oxyderm[CAN], PanOxyl, PanOxyl-AQ, PanOxyl Aqua Gel, PanOxylBar, Seba-Gel, Solugel[CAN], Triaz, Triaz Cleanser, Zapzyt)

CATEGORY AND SCHEDULE

Pregnancy Risk Category: C
OTC

Drug Class: Antiacne agent, topical; keratolytic, topical

MECHANISM OF ACTION

A keratolytic agent that releases free-radical oxygen, which oxidizes bacterial proteins in the sebaceous follicles, decreasing the number of anaerobic bacteria and decreasing irritating-type free fatty acids.
Therapeutic Effect: Bactericidal action against Propionbacterium acnes and *Staphylococcus* epidermidis.

USES

Treatment of acne

PHARMACOKINETICS

Minimal absorption through skin. Gel is more penetrating than cream. Metabolized to benzoic acid in skin. Excreted in urine as benzoate.

INDICATIONS AND DOSAGES

▶ **Acne**
Topical
Adults. Apply 2.5%–10% concentration 1–2 times a day.

SIDE EFFECTS/ADVERSE REACTIONS

Occasional
Irritation, dryness, burning, peeling, stinging, contact dermatitis, bleaching of hair

PRECAUTIONS AND CONTRAINDICATIONS

Hypersensitivity to benzoyl peroxide or any component of the formulation

DRUG INTERACTIONS OF CONCERN TO DENTISTRY

None reported

SERIOUS REACTIONS

! Hypersensitivity reactions have been reported with benzoyl peroxide use.

DENTAL CONSIDERATIONS

General:
• Determine why patient is taking the drug.
• Advise patient if dental drugs prescribed have a potential for photosensitivity.
• Inquire about other drugs the patient may be using for acne.
Teach Patient/Family to:
• Avoid application to eyes, nose, mouth and mucous membranes.

• Update health and medication history if physician makes any changes in evaluation or drug regimens; include OTC, herbal, and nonherbal remedies in the update

benzthiazide
benz-thigh'-ah-zide
(Exna)

CATEGORY AND SCHEDULE
Pregnancy Risk Category: C

Drug Class: Diuretic, Thiazide

MECHANISM OF ACTION
Thiazide diuretic and antihypertensive. As a diuretic, blocks reabsorption of water, sodium, and potassium at cortical diluting segment of distal tubule. As an antihypertensive, reduces plasma and extracellular fluid volume and reduces peripheral vascular resistance by direct effect on blood vessels. *Therapeutic Effect:* Promotes diuresis, reduces B/P.

USES
Treatment of high B/P

PHARMACOKINETICS

Route	Onset	Peak	Duration
PO	2 hr	4 hr	6–12 hr

Variably absorbed from the GI tract. Primarily excreted unchanged in urine. Not removed by hemodialysis. *Half-life:* Unknown.

INDICATIONS AND DOSAGES
▶ **Edema**
PO
Adults. Initially, 50–200 mg/day. Maintenance: 50–150 mg/day.

▶ **Hypertension**
PO
Adults. Initially, 50–100 mg/day. Dosage should be adjusted according to the patient response, either upward to as much as 50 mg 4 times a day or downward to the minimal effective dosage level.

SIDE EFFECTS/ADVERSE REACTIONS
Expected
Increase in urine frequency and volume
Frequent
Potassium depletion
Occasional
Postural hypotension, headache, GI disturbances, photosensitivity reaction

PRECAUTIONS AND CONTRAINDICATIONS
Anuria, history of hypersensitivity to sulfonamide-derived drugs or thiazide diuretics

DRUG INTERACTIONS OF CONCERN TO DENTISTRY
• Decreased hypotensive response: NSAIDs.

SERIOUS REACTIONS
! Vigorous diuresis may lead to profound water and electrolyte depletion, resulting in hypokalemia, hyponatremia, and dehydration.
! Acute hypotensive episodes may occur.
! Hyperglycemia may be noted during prolonged therapy.
! Pancreatitis, blood dyscrasias, pulmonary edema, allergic pneumonitis, and dermatologic reactions occur rarely.
! Overdose can lead to lethargy and coma without changes in electrolytes or hydration.

DENTAL CONSIDERATIONS

General:
- Monitor vital signs at every appointment due to cardiovascular side effects.
- Patient on chronic drug therapy may rarely present with symptoms of blood dyscrasias, which can include infection, bleeding and poor healing. If dyscrasia is present, caution patient to prevent oral tissue trauma when using oral hygiene aids.
- Observe appropriate limitations of vasoconstrictor doses.
- After supine positioning, have patient sit upright for at least 2 min before standing to avoid orthostatic hypotension.
- Limit use of sodium-containing products, such as saline IV fluids, for patients with a dietary salt restriction.
- Stress from dental procedures may compromise cardiovascular function; determine patient risk.
- Short appointments and a stress-reduction protocol may be required for anxious patients.
- Advise patient if dental drugs prescribed have a potential for photosensitivity.
- Patients taking diuretics should be monitored for serum K levels.

Consultations:
- In a patient with symptoms of blood dyscrasias, request a medical consultation for blood studies and postpone treatment until normal values are reestablished.
- Medical consultation may be required to assess disease control and patient's ability to tolerate stress.

Teach Patient/Family to:
- Use effective oral hygiene to prevent soft tissue inflammation
- Prevent trauma when using oral hygiene aids
- Update health and medication history if physician makes any changes in evaluation or drug

regimens; include OTC, herbal, and nonherbal remedies in the update

benztropine mesylate

benz'-troe-peen mess-ah-late
(Apo-Benztropine[CAN],
Bentrop[AUS], Cogentin)
Do not confuse benztropine with bromocriptine.

CATEGORY AND SCHEDULE

Pregnancy Risk Category: C

Drug Class: Anticholinergic, antidyskinetic

MECHANISM OF ACTION

An antiparkinson agent that selectively blocks central cholinergic receptors, helping to balance cholinergic and dopaminergic activity. ***Therapeutic Effect:*** Reduces the incidence and severity of akinesia, rigidity, and tremor.

USES

Treatment of Parkinson symptoms, extrapyramidal symptoms associated with neuroleptic drugs

PHARMACOKINETICS

IM/IV: Onset 15 min, duration 6–10 hr.
PO: Onset 1 hr, duration 6–10 hr.

INDICATIONS AND DOSAGES

▶ **Parkinsonism**
PO
Adults. 0.5–6 mg/day as a single dose or in 2 divided doses. Titrate by 0.5 mg at 5–6 day intervals.
Elderly. Initially, 0.5 mg once or twice a day. Titrate by 0.5 mg at 5–6 day intervals. Maximum: 4 mg/day.

▸ **Drug-Induced Extrapyramidal Symptoms**
PO, IM
Adults. 1–4 mg once or twice a day.
Children older than 3 yr. 0.02–0.05 mg/kg/dose once or twice a day.
▸ **Acute Dystonic Reactions**
IV, IM
Adults. Initially, 1–2 mg; then 1–2 mg PO twice a day to prevent recurrence.

SIDE EFFECTS/ADVERSE REACTIONS
Frequent
Somnolence, dry mouth, blurred vision, constipation, decreased sweating or urination, GI upset, photosensitivity
Occasional
Headache, memory loss, muscle cramps, anxiety, peripheral paresthesia, orthostatic hypotension, abdominal cramps
Rare
Rash, confusion, eye pain

PRECAUTIONS AND CONTRAINDICATIONS
Angle-closure glaucoma, benign prostatic hyperplasia, children younger than 3 yr, GI obstruction, intestinal atony, megacolon, myasthenia gravis, paralytic ileus, severe ulcerative colitis
Caution:
Elderly, lactation, tachycardia, prostatic hypertrophy, liver or kidney disease, drug abuse history, dysrhythmias, hypotension, hypertension, psychiatric patients

DRUG INTERACTIONS OF CONCERN TO DENTISTRY
• Increased anticholinergic effect: antihistamines, anticholinergics, and meperidine
• Decreased effects of phenothiazines

SERIOUS REACTIONS
! Overdose may produce severe anticholinergic effects, such as unsteadiness, somnolence, tachycardia, dyspnea, skin flushing, and severe dryness of the mouth, nose, or throat.
! Severe paradoxical reactions, marked by hallucinations, tremor, seizures, and toxic psychosis, may occur.

DENTAL CONSIDERATIONS
General:
• Monitor vital signs at every appointment because of cardiovascular side effects.
• Assess salivary flow as a factor in caries, periodontal disease, and candidiasis.
• After supine positioning, have patient sit upright for at least 2 min to avoid orthostatic hypotension.
• Avoid dental light in patient's eyes; offer dark glasses for patient comfort.
• Do not use ingestible sodium bicarbonate products, such as the Prophy-Jet air polishing system, within 1 hr of taking benztropine.
• Place on frequent recall because of oral side effects.
Consultations:
• Medical consultation may be required to assess disease control and patient's ability to tolerate stress.
Teach Patient/Family to:
• Use effective oral hygiene to prevent soft tissue inflammation
• Use an electric tooth brush if patient has difficulty holding conventional devices
• When chronic dry mouth occurs, advise patient to:
   • Avoid mouth rinses with high alcohol content because of drying effects

- Use daily home fluoride products for anticaries effect
- Use sugarless gum, frequent sips of water, or saliva substitutes

bepridil
beh'-prih-dill
(Bepadin, Vascor)

CATEGORY AND SCHEDULE
Pregnancy Risk Category: C

Drug Class: Calcium channel blocker

MECHANISM OF ACTION
A calcium channel blocker that inhibits calcium ion entry across cell membranes of cardiac and vascular smooth muscle; decreases heart rate, myocardial contractility, slows SA and AV conduction. *Therapeutic Effect:* Dilates coronary arteries, peripheral arteries/arterioles.

USES
Treatment of stable angina, used alone or in combination with propranolol

PHARMACOKINETICS
Rapidly, completely absorbed from GI tract. Undergoes first-pass metabolism in liver to active metabolite. Primarily excreted in urine. Not removed by hemodialysis. *Half-life:* less than 24 hr.

INDICATIONS AND DOSAGES
▶ Chronic Stable Angina
PO
Adults, Elderly. Initially, 200 mg/day; after 10 days, dosage may be adjusted. Maintenance: 200–400 mg/day.

SIDE EFFECTS/ADVERSE REACTIONS
Frequent
Dizziness, lightheadedness, nervousness, headache, asthenia (loss of strength), hand tremor, nausea, diarrhea
Occasional
Drowsiness, insomnia, tinnitus, abdominal discomfort, palpitations, dry mouth, shortness of breath, wheezing, anorexia, constipation
Rare
Peripheral edema, anxiety, flatulence, nasal congestion, paresthesia

PRECAUTIONS AND CONTRAINDICATIONS
Sick sinus syndrome/second- or third-degree AV block (except in presence of pacemaker), severe hypotension (90 mm Hg, systolic), history of serious ventricular arrhythmias, uncompensated cardiac insufficiency, congenital QT interval prolongation, use with other drugs prolonging QT interval
Caution:
CHF, hypotension, hepatic injury, lactation, children, renal disease, may induce new arrhythmias, prolongs QT interval with risk of torsades de pointes

DRUG INTERACTIONS OF CONCERN TO DENTISTRY
- Decreased effect: NSAIDs, phenobarbital
- Increased effect: parenteral and inhalational general anesthetics or other drugs with hypotensive actions
- Increased effects of carbamazepine

SERIOUS REACTIONS
❗ CHF, second- and third-degree AV block occur rarely.
❗ Serious arrhythmias can be induced.
❗ Overdosage produces nausea, drowsiness, confusion, slurred speech, profound bradycardia.

DENTAL CONSIDERATIONS
General:
• Monitor cardiac status; take vital signs at every appointment because of cardiovascular side effects. Consider a stress-reduction protocol to prevent stress-induced angina during the dental appointment.
• Observe appropriate limitations of vasoconstrictor doses.
• After supine positioning, have patient sit upright for at least 2 min to avoid orthostatic hypotension.
• Limit use of sodium-containing products, such as saline IV fluids, for those patients with a dietary salt restriction.
• Assess salivary flow as a factor in caries, periodontal disease, and candidiasis.
Consultations:
• Medical consultation may be required to assess disease control and stress tolerance of patient.
Teach Patient/Family to:
• Schedule frequent oral prophylaxis if gingival overgrowth occurs
• When chronic dry mouth occurs, advise patient to:
  • Avoid mouth rinses with high alcohol content because of drying effects
  • Use daily home fluoride products for anticaries effect
  • Use sugarless gum, frequent sips of water, or saliva substitutes

betamethasone
bay-ta-meth′-ah-sone
(Alphatrex, Betaderm[CAN], Betatrex, Beta-Val, Betnesol[CAN], Celestone, Diprolene, Luxiq, Maxivate)

CATEGORY AND SCHEDULE
Pregnancy Risk Category: C
(D if used in first trimester)

Drug Class: Antiinflammatory

MECHANISM OF ACTION
An adrenocortical steroid that controls the rate of protein synthesis, depresses the migration of polymorphonuclear leukocytes and fibroblasts, reduces capillary permeability and prevents or controls inflammation. **Therapeutic Effect:** Decreases tissue response to inflammatory process.

USES
Treatment of psoriasis, eczema, contact dermatitis, pruritus, oral ulcerative inflammatory lesions, mild-to-moderate ulcerative colitis. Also used to relieve swelling, itching, and discomfort of some other rectal problems, including hemorrhoids and inflammation of the rectum caused by radiation therapy.

PHARMACOKINETICS:
PO: Onset 1–2 hr, peak 1 hr, duration 3 days.
IM/IV: Onset 10 min, peak 4–8 hr, duration 1–1.5 days.
Metabolized in liver, excreted in urine as steroids, crosses placenta.

INDICATIONS AND DOSAGES
▶ **Antiinflammation, Immunosuppression, Corticosteroid Replacement Therapy**

PO
Adults, Elderly. 0.6–7.2 mg/day.
Children. 0.063–0.25 mg/kg/day in
3–4 divided doses.
▶ **Relief of Inflamed and Pruritic**
Dermatoses
Topical
Adults, Elderly. 1–3 times a day.
Foam: Apply twice a day.

SIDE EFFECTS/ADVERSE
REACTIONS
Frequent
Systemic: Increased appetite,
abdominal distention, nervousness,
insomnia, false sense of
well-being
Topical: Burning, stinging,
pruritus
Occasional
Systemic: Dizziness, facial
flushing, diaphoresis,
decreased or blurred vision,
mood swings
Topical: Allergic contact dermatitis,
purpura or blood-containing blisters,
thinning of skin with easy bruising,
telangiectases, or raised dark red
spots on skin

PRECAUTIONS AND
CONTRAINDICATIONS
Hypersensitivity to betamethasone,
systemic fungal infections

DRUG INTERACTIONS OF
CONCERN TO DENTISTRY
• Decreased action: barbiturates
• Increased GI side effects:
alcohol, salicylates, and other
NSAIDs
• Increased action: ketoconazole,
macrolide antibiotics

SERIOUS REACTIONS
! Overdose may cause systemic
hypercorticism and adrenal
suppression.

DENTAL CONSIDERATIONS
General:
• Monitor vital signs at every
appointment because of
cardiovascular side effects.
• Patients on chronic drug therapy
may rarely have symptoms of blood
dyscrasias, which can include
infection, bleeding, and poor
healing.
• Symptoms of oral infections may
be masked.
• Determine dose and duration of
steroid therapy for each patient to
assess risk for stress tolerance and
immunosuppression.
• Avoid prescribing aspirin-
containing products.
• Place on frequent recall to evaluate
healing response.
• Prophylactic antibiotics may be
indicated to prevent infection if
surgery or deep scaling is
planned.
• Patients who have been or are
currently on chronic steroid therapy
(longer than 2 wk) may require
supplemental steroids for dental
treatment.
Consultations:
• In a patient with symptoms of
blood dyscrasias, request a medical
consultation for blood studies and
postpone dental treatment until
normal values are reestablished.
• Medical consultation may be
required to assess disease
control.
• Consultation may be required to
confirm steroid dose and duration of
use.
Teach Patient/Family to:
• Use effective oral
hygiene to prevent soft tissue
inflammation
• Use caution to prevent injury when
using oral hygiene aids

betaxolol
bay-tax′-oh-lol
(Betoptic[AUS], Betoptic-S,
Betoquin[AUS], Kerlone)
Do not confuse betaxolol with
bethanechol.

CATEGORY AND SCHEDULE
Pregnancy Risk Category: C (D if
used in second or third trimester)

Drug Class: Antihypertensive,
selective β₁-blocker

MECHANISM OF ACTION
An antihypertensive and
antiglaucoma agent that blocks
β₁-adrenergic receptors in cardiac
tissue. Reduces aqueous humor
production. *Therapeutic Effect:*
Slows sinus heart rate, decreases
B/P, and reduces intraocular
pressure (IOP).

USES
Treatment of hypertension, alone or
in combination with other
antihypertensive drugs, especially
thiazide diuretics

PHARMACOKINETICS
PO: Peak 3–4 hr. *Half-life:* 14–22 hr;
protein binding 50%; some hepatic
metabolism; excreted in urine mostly
unchanged.

INDICATIONS AND DOSAGES
▸ **Hypertension**
PO
Adults. Initially, 5–10 mg/day. May
increase to 20 mg/day after
7–14 days.
Elderly. Initially, 5 mg/day.
▸ **Chronic Open-Angle Glaucoma
and Ocular Hypertension**
Ophthalmic (Eye Drops)
Adults, Elderly. 1 drop twice a day.

▸ **Dosage in Renal Impairment**
For adult and elderly patients who
are on dialysis, initially give 5 mg/
day; increase by 5 mg/day q2wk.
Maximum: 20 mg/day.

SIDE EFFECTS/ADVERSE REACTIONS
Betaxolol is generally well tolerated,
with mild and transient side effects.
Frequent
Systemic: Hypotension manifested
as dizziness, nausea, diaphoresis,
headache, fatigue, constipation or
diarrhea, dyspnea
Ophthalmic: Eye irritation, visual
disturbances
Occasional
Systemic: Insomnia, flatulence,
urinary frequency, impotence or
decreased libido
Ophthalmic: Increased light
sensitivity, watering of eye
Rare
Systemic: Rash, arrhythmias,
arthralgia, myalgia, confusion,
altered taste, increased urination
Ophthalmic: Dry eye, conjunctivitis,
eye pain

PRECAUTIONS AND CONTRAINDICATIONS
Cardiogenic shock, overt cardiac
failure, second- or third-degree heart
block, sinus bradycardia
Caution
Major surgery, lactation, diabetes
mellitus, renal disease, thyroid
disease, COPD, asthma, well-
compensated heart failure, aortic or
mitral valve disease

DRUG INTERACTIONS OF CONCERN TO DENTISTRY
• Decreased antihypertensive effects:
NSAIDs, indomethacin
• May slow metabolism of lidocaine
• Decreased β-blocking effects
(or decreased β-adrenergic effects)

of epinephrine, levonordefrin, isoproterenol, and other sympathomimetics

SERIOUS REACTIONS

! Overdose may produce profound bradycardia, hypotension, and bronchospasm.

! Abrupt withdrawal may result in diaphoresis, palpitations, headache, and tremors.

! Betaxolol administration may precipitate CHF or MI in patients with cardiac disease; thyroid storm in those with thyrotoxicosis; and peripheral ischemia in those with existing peripheral vascular disease.

! Hypoglycemia may occur in patients with previously controlled diabetes.

! Ophthalmic overdose may produce bradycardia, hypotension, bronchospasm, and acute cardiac failure.

DENTAL CONSIDERATIONS

General:

• Monitor vital signs at every appointment because of cardiovascular and respiratory side effects.

• After supine positioning, have patient sit upright for at least 2 min to avoid orthostatic hypotension.

• Assess salivary flow as a factor in caries, periodontal disease, and candidiasis.

• Stress from dental procedures may compromise cardiovascular function; determine patient risk.

• Short appointments and a stress-reduction protocol may be required for anxious patients.

• Use vasoconstrictors with caution, in low doses, and with careful aspiration. Avoid use of gingival retraction cord with epinephrine.

Consultations:

• Medical consultation may be required to assess disease control and stress tolerance of patient.

• Use precautions if general anesthesia is required for dental surgery.

Teach Patient/Family to:

• Use effective oral hygiene to prevent soft tissue inflammation

• Use caution to prevent injury when using oral hygiene aids

• When chronic dry mouth occurs, advise patient to:

  • Avoid mouth rinses with high alcohol content because of drying effects

  • Use daily home fluoride products for anticaries effect

  • Use sugarless gum, frequent sips of water, or saliva substitutes

bethanechol chloride

beh-than′-eh-kole
(Duvoid[CAN], Myotonachol[CAN], Urecholine, Urocarb[AUS])
Do not confuse bethanechol with betaxolol.

CATEGORY AND SCHEDULE
Pregnancy Risk Category: C

Drug Class: Cholinergic stimulant

MECHANISM OF ACTION

A cholinergic that acts directly at cholinergic receptors in the smooth muscle of the urinary bladder and GI tract. Increases detrusor muscle tone. ***Therapeutic Effect:*** May initiate micturition and bladder emptying. Improves gastric and intestinal motility.

USES

Treatment of urinary retention (postoperative, postpartum), neurogenic atony of bladder with retention; unapproved: gastric atony

PHARMACOKINETICS:

PO: Onset 30–90 min, duration 6 hr. **SC:** Onset 5–15 min, duration 2 hr; excreted by kidneys.

INDICATIONS AND DOSAGES
▶ **Postoperative and Postpartum Urine Retention, Atony of Bladder**
PO
Adults, Elderly. 10–50 mg 3–4 times a day. Minimum effective dose determined by giving 5–10 mg initially, then repeating same amount at 1-hr intervals until desired response is achieved, or maximum of 50 mg is reached.
Children. 0.6 mg/kg/day in 3–4 divided doses.

SIDE EFFECTS/ADVERSE REACTIONS
Occasional
Belching, blurred or changed vision, diarrhea, urinary urgency

PRECAUTIONS AND CONTRAINDICATIONS
Active or latent bronchial asthma, acute inflammatory GI tract conditions, anastomosis, bladder wall instability, cardiac or coronary artery disease, epilepsy, hypertension, hyperthyroidism, hypotension, GI or urinary tract obstruction, parkinsonism, peptic ulcer, pronounced bradycardia, recent GI resection, vasomotor instability
Caution:
Hypertension, lactation, children younger than 8 yr, urinary retention

DRUG INTERACTIONS OF CONCERN TO DENTISTRY
• Decreased effects: anticholinergics

SERIOUS REACTIONS
! Overdosage produces CNS stimulation (including insomnia, anxiety, and orthostatic hypotension), and cholinergic stimulation (such as headache, increased salivation diaphoresis, nausea, vomiting, flushed skin, abdominal pain, and seizures).

DENTAL CONSIDERATIONS
General:
• Monitor vital signs at every appointment because of cardiovascular and respiratory side effects.
• After supine positioning, have patient sit upright for at least 2 min to avoid orthostatic hypotension.
Consultations:
• For excessive, troublesome salivation, reassure patient that treatment duration usually is limited to a few days; otherwise consult to lower bethanechol dose.

bevacizumab
beh-vah-siz'-you-mab
(Avastin)

CATEGORY AND SCHEDULE
Pregnancy Risk Category: C

Drug Class: Antineoplastic monoclonal antibody; vascular endothelial growth factor (VEGF) inhibitor

MECHANISM OF ACTION
An antineoplastic that binds to and inhibits vascular endothelial growth factor, a protein that plays a major

role in the formation of new blood vessels to tumors. *Therapeutic Effect:* Inhibits metastatic disease progression.

USES

Prevents the growth of certain types of blood vessels to cancer cells by starving the cells of nutrients needed to grow

PHARMACOKINETICS

Clearance varies by body weight, gender, and tumor burden. *Half-life:* 20 days (range, 11–50 days).

INDICATIONS AND DOSAGES

▸ **First-Line Treatment of Metastatic Carcinoma of the Colon or Rectum in Combination with 5-Fluorouracil (5-FU)**
IV
Adults, Elderly. 5 mg/kg once every 14 days.

SIDE EFFECTS/ADVERSE REACTIONS

Frequent
Asthenia, vomiting, anorexia, hypertension, epistaxis, stomatitis, constipation, headache, dyspnea
Occasional
Altered taste, dry skin, exfoliative dermatitis, dizziness, flatulence, excessive lacrimation, skin discoloration, weight loss, myalgia
Rare
Nail disorder, skin ulcer, alopecia, confusion, abnormal gait, dry mouth

PRECAUTIONS AND CONTRAINDICATIONS

GI perforation, hypertensive crisis, nephrotic syndrome, recent hemoptysis, serious bleeding, wound dehiscence requiring medical intervention

DRUG INTERACTIONS OF CONCERN TO DENTISTRY

None reported

SERIOUS REACTIONS

❗ UTIs, manifested as urinary frequency or urgency and proteinuria, occur frequently.
❗ CHF, deep vein thrombosis, GI perforation, hypertensive crisis, nephrotic syndrome, and severe hemorrhage are the most serious reactions that occur.
❗ Anemia, neutropenia, and thrombocytopenia occur occasionally.
❗ Hypersensitivity reactions occur rarely.

DENTAL CONSIDERATIONS

General:
• Assess salivary flow as a factor in caries, periodontal disease, and candidiasis.
• If additional analgesia is required for dental pain, consider alternative analgesics (NSAIDs) in patients taking narcotics for acute or chronic pain.
• Avoid products that affect platelet function, such as aspirin and NSAIDs.
• This drug may be used in the hospital or on an outpatient basis. Confirm the patient's disease and treatment status.
• Consider semisupine chair position for patient comfort if GI side effects occur.
• Chlorhexidine mouth rinse prior to and during chemotherapy may reduce severity of mucositis.
• Patient on chronic drug therapy may rarely present with symptoms of blood dyscrasias, which can include infection, bleeding, and poor healing. If dyscrasia is present, caution patient to prevent oral tissue trauma when using oral hygiene aids.

- Palliative medication may be required for management of oral side effects.
- Short appointments and a stress-reduction protocol may be required for anxious patients.
- Monitor vital signs at every appointment for cardiovascular side effects.
- Patients may have received other chemotherapy or radiation; confirm medical and drug history.
- Patients may be taking a prophylactic antiinfective.
- Patients may be at risk of bleeding, check for oral signs.
- Oral infections should be eliminated and/or treated aggressively.
- Place on frequent recall due to oral side effects.

Consultations:
- Medical consultation should include routine blood counts including platelet counts and bleeding time.
- Consult physician; prophylactic or therapeutic antiinfectives may be indicated if surgery or periodontal treatment is required.
- Medical consultation may be required to assess immunologic status during cancer chemotherapy and determine safety risk, if any, posed by the required dental treatment.
- Medical consultation may be required to assess disease control and patient's ability to tolerate stress.

Teach Patient/Family to:
- Inform dentist of unusual bleeding episodes following dental treatment
- Be aware of oral side effects
- Use effective oral hygiene to prevent soft tissue inflammation
- Report oral lesions, soreness, or bleeding to dentist

- Prevent trauma when using oral hygiene aids
- Update health and medication history if physician makes any changes in evaluation or drug regimens; include OTC, herbal, and nonherbal remedies in the update
- If abdominal pain associated with constipation and/or vomiting occur, advise patient to consult physician immediately
- When chronic dry mouth occurs advise patient to:
  - Avoid mouth rinses with high alcohol content due to drying effects
  - Use daily home fluoride products for anticaries effect
  - Use sugarless gum, frequent sips of water, or saliva substitutes

bexarotene
becks-aye'-row-teen
(Targretin)

CATEGORY AND SCHEDULE
Pregnancy Risk Category: X

Drug Class: Antineoplastic

MECHANISM OF ACTION
Retinoid antineoplastic agent that binds to and activates retinoid X receptor subtypes, which regulate the genes that control cellular differentiation and proliferation.
Therapeutic Effect: Inhibits growth of tumor cell lines of hematopoietic and squamous cell origin and induces tumor regression.

USES
Treatment of a form a cancer called cutaneous T-cell lymphoma (CTCL)

PHARMACOKINETICS

Moderately absorbed from the GI tract. Protein binding: greater than 99%. Metabolized in the liver. Primarily eliminated through the hepatobiliary system. *Half-life:* 7 hr.

INDICATIONS AND DOSAGES

▶ **Cutaneous T-cell Lymphoma Refractory to at Least One Prior Systemic Therapy**

PO

Adults. 300 mg/m²/day. If no response and initial dose is well tolerated, may be increased to 400 mg/m²/day. If not tolerated, may decrease to 200 mg/m²/day, then to 100 mg/m²/day.

Topical

Adults. Initially, apply once every other day. May increase at weekly intervals up to 4 times a day.

SIDE EFFECTS/ADVERSE REACTIONS

Frequent

Hyperlipidemia, headache, hypothyroidism, asthenia

Occasional

Rash, nausea, peripheral edema, dry skin, abdominal pain, chills, exfoliative dermatitis, diarrhea

PRECAUTIONS AND CONTRAINDICATIONS

Hypersensitivity to bexarotene or any component of the formulation

DRUG INTERACTIONS OF CONCERN TO DENTISTRY

Erythromycin, itraconazole

SERIOUS REACTIONS

! Pancreatitis, hepatic failure, and pneumonia occur rarely.

DENTAL CONSIDERATIONS

• Consult patient for ability to tolerate dental procedure and to determine why patient is taking drug

bicalutamide

by-kale-yew′-tah-myd
(Casodex, Cosudex[AUS])

CATEGORY AND SCHEDULE

Pregnancy Risk Category: X

Drug Class: Nonsteroidal antiandrogen, antineoplastic

MECHANISM OF ACTION

An antiandrogen antineoplastic agent that competitively inhibits androgen action by binding to androgen receptors in target tissue. *Therapeutic Effect:* Decreases growth of prostatic carcinoma.

USES

Combination therapy with a luteinizing hormone–releasing hormone (LHRH) analog for advanced prostate cancer

PHARMACOKINETICS

Well absorbed from the GI tract. Protein binding: 96%. Metabolized in the liver to inactive metabolite. Excreted in urine and feces. Not removed by hemodialysis. *Half-life:* 5.8 days.

INDICATIONS AND DOSAGES

▶ **Prostatic Carcinoma**

PO

Adults, Elderly. 50–100 mg once a day in morning or evening, given concurrently with a LHRH analog or after surgical castration.

SIDE EFFECTS/ADVERSE REACTIONS
Frequent
Hot flashes, breast pain, muscle pain, constipation, asthenia, nausea, diarrhea
Occasional
Nocturia, abdominal pain, peripheral edema
Rare
Vomiting, weight loss, dizziness, insomnia, rash, impotence, gynecomastia

PRECAUTIONS AND CONTRAINDICATIONS
Hypersensitivity, women who may become pregnant, pregnancy category X
Caution
Hepatic impairment, lactation, children

DRUG INTERACTIONS OF CONCERN TO DENTISTRY
• Avoid drugs that could exacerbate urinary retention, such as anticholinergics

SERIOUS REACTIONS
! Sepsis, CHF, hypertension, and iron deficiency anemia may occur.

DENTAL CONSIDERATIONS
General:
• Patients taking opioids for acute or chronic pain should be given alternative analgesics for dental pain.
• Palliative medication may be required for management of oral side effects.
• Assess salivary flow as a factor in caries, periodontal disease, and candidiasis.
• Monitor vital signs at every appointment because of cardiovascular and respiratory side effects.

• Short appointments may be required for patient comfort.
• Consider semisupine chair position for patient comfort because of disease and drug side effects.
• Place on frequent recall because of oral side effects.
Consultations:
• Medical consultation may be required to assess disease control and patient's ability to tolerate stress.
Teach Patient/Family to:
• Update medical/drug record if physician makes any changes in evaluation or drug regimens
• When chronic dry mouth occurs, advise patient to:
  • Avoid mouth rinses with high alcohol content because of drying effects
  • Use daily home fluoride products for anticaries effect
  • Use sugarless gum, frequent sips of water, or saliva substitutes

bimatoprost
bye-mat′-oh-prost
(Lumigan)

CATEGORY AND SCHEDULE

Drug Class: A prostamide (synthetic structural analog of prostaglandin)

MECHANISM OF ACTION
A synthetic analog of prostaglandin with ocular hypotensive activity.
Therapeutic Effect: Reduces intraocular pressure (IOP) by increasing the outflow of aqueous humor.

USES
Reduction of elevated IOP in patients with open-angle glaucoma or ocular hypertension who are intolerant of, or insufficiently responsive to, other IOP-lowering drugs

PHARMACOKINETICS
Absorbed through the cornea and hydrolyzed to the active free acid form. Protein binding: 88%. Moderately distributed into body tissues. Metabolized in liver. Primarily excreted in urine; some elimination in feces. *Half-life:* 45 min.

INDICATIONS AND DOSAGES
▸ **Glaucoma, Ocular Hypertension**
Ophthalmic
Adults, Elderly. 1 drop in affected eye(s) once daily, in the evening.

SIDE EFFECTS/ADVERSE REACTIONS
Frequent
Conjunctival hyperemia, growth of eyelashes, and ocular pruritus
Occasional
Ocular dryness, visual disturbance, ocular burning, foreign body sensation, eye pain, pigmentation of the periocular skin, blepharitis, cataract, superficial punctate keratitis, eyelid erythema, ocular irritation, and eyelash darkening
Rare
Intraocular inflammation (iritis)

PRECAUTIONS AND CONTRAINDICATIONS
Hypersensitivity to bimatoprost or any other component of the formulation
Caution
Increased pigmentation in iris and eyelid, change in eye color, changes in eyelashes (color, length, shape); uveitis, macular edema; renal or hepatic impairment, lactation, pediatric use, remove contact lenses to apply

DRUG INTERACTIONS OF CONCERN TO DENTISTRY
None reported

SERIOUS REACTIONS
❗ Systemic adverse events, including infections (colds and upper respiratory tract infections), headaches, asthenia, and hirsutism, have been reported

DENTAL CONSIDERATIONS
General:
• Avoid drugs with anticholinergic activity, such as antihistamines, opioids, benzodiazepines, propantheline, atropine, and scopolamine.
• Protect patient's eyes from accidental spatter during dental treatment.
• Avoid dental light in patient's eyes; offer dark glasses for patient comfort.
Consultations:
• Medical consultation may be required to assess disease control.
Teach Patient/Family to:
• Update health and drug history if physician makes any changes in evaluation or drug regimens

biperiden
bye-per′-ih-den
(Akineton HCl)

CATEGORY AND SCHEDULE
Pregnancy Risk Category: C

Drug Class: Anticholinergic

MECHANISM OF ACTION
A weak anticholinergic that exhibits competitive antagonism of acetylcholine at cholinergic receptors in the corpus striatum, which restores balance. *Therapeutic Effect:* Antiparkinson activity.

USES
Treatment of Parkinson symptoms, extrapyramidal symptoms secondary to neuroleptic drug therapy

PHARMACOKINETICS
Well absorbed from GI tract. Protein binding: 23%–33%. Widely distributed. *Half-life:* 18–24 hr.

INDICATIONS AND DOSAGES
▸ **Extrapyramidal Symptoms**
PO
Adults, Elderly. 2 mg 3–4 times a day. Dosage in renal impairment.
▸ **Parkinsonism**
PO
Adults, Elderly. 2 mg 1–3 times a day.

SIDE EFFECTS/ADVERSE REACTIONS
Frequent
Orthostatic hypotension, anorexia, headache, blurred vision, urinary retention, dry mouth or nose
Occasional
Insomnia, agitation, euphoria
Rare
Vomiting, depression, irritation or swelling of eyes, rash

PRECAUTIONS AND CONTRAINDICATIONS
Hypersensitivity, narrow-angle glaucoma, myasthenia gravis, GI/GU obstruction, megacolon, stenosing peptic ulcers
Caution
Elderly, lactation, tachycardia, prostatic hypertrophy, dysrhythmias, liver or kidney disease, drug abuse, hypotension, hypertension, psychiatric patients, children

DRUG INTERACTIONS OF CONCERN TO DENTISTRY
• Increased anticholinergic effect: antihistamines, anticholinergic-acting drugs, meperidine
• Increased CNS depression: alcohol, CNS depressants
• Decreased effects of phenothiazines

SERIOUS REACTIONS
! Overdosage may vary from severe anticholinergic effects, such as unsteadiness, severe drowsiness, dryness of mouth, nose, or throat, tachycardia, shortness of breath, and skin flushing.
! Also produces severe paradoxical reaction, marked by hallucinations, tremor, seizures, and toxic psychosis.

DENTAL CONSIDERATIONS
General:
• Monitor vital signs at every appointment because of cardiovascular side effects.
• After supine positioning, have patient sit upright for at least 2 min to avoid orthostatic hypotension.
• Assess salivary flow as a factor in caries, periodontal disease, and candidiasis.
• Avoid dental light in patient's eyes; offer dark glasses for patient comfort.
Consultations:
• Medical consultation may be required to assess disease control and patient's ability to tolerate stress.
Teach Patient/Family to:
• Use electric tooth brush if patient has difficulty holding conventional devices

- Use effective hygiene to prevent soft tissue inflammation
- When chronic dry mouth occurs, advise patient to:
  - Avoid mouth rinses with high alcohol content because of drying effects
  - Use daily home fluoride products for anticaries effect
  - Use sugarless gum, frequent sips of water, or saliva substitutes

bisacodyl

bis-ah-koe′-dill
(Alophen, Apo-Bisacodyl[CAN], Bisalax[AUS], Dulcolax, Femilax, Gentlax, Modane, Veracolate)
Do not confuse Veracolate with Accolate or Modane with Mudrane.

CATEGORY AND SCHEDULE
Pregnancy Risk Category: C
OTC

Drug Class: Laxative, carbon dioxide-releasing; hyperosmotic; laxative, hypersosmotic, saline; laxative lubricant; laxative, stimulant (contact); laxative, stool softener (emollient)

MECHANISM OF ACTION
A GI stimulant that has a direct effect on colonic smooth musculature by stimulating the intramural nerve plexi. **Therapeutic Effect:** Promotes fluid and ion accumulation in the colon, increasing peristalsis and producing a laxative effect.

USES
As enemas or suppositories to produce bowel movements in a short time

PHARMACOKINETICS

Route	Onset	Peak	Duration
PO	6–12 hr	N/A	N/A
Rectal	15–60 min	N/A	N/A

Minimal absorption following oral and rectal administration. Absorbed drug is excreted in urine; remainder is eliminated in feces.

INDICATIONS AND DOSAGES
▶ **Treatment of Constipation**
PO
Adults, Children older than 12 yr. 5–15 mg as needed.
Maximum: 30 mg.
Children 3–12 yr. 5–10 mg or 0.3 mg/kg at bedtime or after breakfast.
Elderly. Initially, 5 mg/day.
Rectal
Adults, Children 12 yr and older. 10 mg to induce bowel movement.
Children 2–11 yr. 5–10 mg as a single dose.
Children younger than 2 yr. 5 mg.
Elderly. 5–10 mg/day.

SIDE EFFECTS/ADVERSE REACTIONS
Frequent
Some degree of abdominal discomfort, nausea, mild cramps, faintness
Occasional
Rectal administration: burning of rectal mucosa, mild proctitis

PRECAUTIONS AND CONTRAINDICATIONS
Abdominal pain, appendicitis, intestinal obstruction, nausea, undiagnosed rectal bleeding, vomiting

DRUG INTERACTIONS OF CONCERN TO DENTISTRY
• None reported; however, a decreased transit time may be expected for orally administered drugs

SERIOUS REACTIONS
! Long-term use may result in laxative dependence, chronic constipation, and loss of normal bowel function.
! Prolonged use or overdose may result in electrolyte or metabolic disturbances (such as hypokalemia, hypocalcemia, and metabolic acidosis or alkalosis), as well as persistent diarrhea, vomiting, muscle weakness, malabsorption, and weight loss.

DENTAL CONSIDERATIONS
General:
• Determine why patient is taking the drug.
• Consider semisupine chair position for patient comfort if GI side effects occur.
• Avoid the use of drugs that may exacerbate constipation.

bismuth subsalicylate
bis′-muth sub-sal-ih′-sah-late
(Bismed[CAN], Colo-Fresh, Devrom, Kaopectate, Pepto-Bismol)

CATEGORY AND SCHEDULE
Pregnancy Risk Category: C
OTC

Drug Class: Antidiarrheal

MECHANISM OF ACTION
An antinauseant and antiulcer agent that absorbs water and toxins in the large intestine and forms a protective coating in the intestinal mucosa. Also possesses antisecretory and antimicrobial effects. ***Therapeutic Effect:*** Prevents diarrhea. Helps treat Helicobacter-pylori-associated peptic ulcer disease.

USES
Treatment of diarrhea (cause undetermined), prevention of diarrhea when traveling

PHARMACOKINETICS
PO: Onset 1 hr, peak 2 hr, duration 4 hr.

INDICATIONS AND DOSAGES
▶ **Diarrhea, Gastric Distress**
PO
Adults, Elderly. 2 tablets (30 ml) q30–60min. Maximum: 8 doses in 24 hr.
Children 9–12 yr. 1 tablet or 15 ml q30–60min. Maximum: 8 doses in 24 hr.
Children 6–8 yr. Two-thirds of a tablet or 10 ml q30–60 min. Maximum: 8 doses in 24 hr.
Children 3–5 yr. One-third of a tablet or 5 ml q30–60 min. Maximum: 8 doses in 24 hr.
▶ **H. Pylori–Associated Duodenal Ulcer, Gastritis**
PO
Adults, Elderly. 525 mg 4 times a day, with 500 mg amoxicillin and 500 mg metronidazole, 3 times a day after meals, for 7–14 days.
▶ **Chronic Infant Diarrhea**
PO
Children 2–24 mo. 2.5 ml q4h.

SIDE EFFECTS/ADVERSE REACTIONS
Frequent
Grayish black stools
Rare
Constipation

PRECAUTIONS AND CONTRAINDICATIONS
Bleeding ulcers, gout, hemophilia, hemorrhagic states, renal impairment
Caution
Anticoagulant therapy

DRUG INTERACTIONS OF CONCERN TO DENTISTRY
• Salicylate toxicity: other salicylates
• Decreased absorption of tetracyclines
• Suspected reduction in antihypertensives and vasodilator effects of ACE inhibitors; monitor blood pressure if used concurrently

SERIOUS REACTIONS
! Debilitated patients and infants may develop impaction.

DENTAL CONSIDERATIONS
General:
• Avoid prescribing aspirin-containing products for analgesia.

bisoprolol fumarate
bis-ope′-pro-lal
(Bicor[AUS], Zebeta)
Do not confuse Zebeta with DiaBeta.

CATEGORY AND SCHEDULE
Pregnancy Risk Category: C (D if used in second or third trimester)

Drug Class: Antihypertensive, selective β_1-blocker

MECHANISM OF ACTION
An antihypertensive that blocks β_1-adrenergic receptors in cardiac tissue. *Therapeutic Effect:* Slows sinus heart rate and decreases B/P.

USES
Treatment of hypertension as a single agent or in combination with other antihypertensives

PHARMACOKINETICS
Well absorbed from the GI tract. Protein binding: 26%–33%. Metabolized in the liver. Primarily excreted in urine. Not removed by hemodialysis. *Half-life:* 9–12 hr (increased in impaired renal function).

INDICATIONS AND DOSAGES
▸ **Hypertension**
PO
Adults. Initially, 5 mg/day. May increase up to 20 mg/day.
Elderly. Initially, 2.5–5 mg/day. May increase by 2.5–5 mg/day. Maximum: 20 mg/day.
▸ **Dosage in Hepatic Impairment**
For adults and elderly patients with cirrhosis or hepatitis whose creatinine clearance is less than 40 ml/minute, initially give 2.5 mg.

SIDE EFFECTS/ADVERSE REACTIONS
Frequent
Hypotension manifested as dizziness, nausea, diaphoresis, headache, cold extremities, fatigue, constipation or diarrhea
Occasional
Insomnia, flatulence, urinary frequency, impotence or decreased libido
Rare
Rash, arthralgia, myalgia, confusion (especially in the elderly), altered taste

PRECAUTIONS AND CONTRAINDICATIONS

Cardiogenic shock, overt cardiac failure, second- or third-degree heart block

Caution

Major surgery, lactation, diabetes mellitus, renal disease, thyroid disease, COPD, heart failure, CAD, nonallergic bronchospasm, hepatic disease

DRUG INTERACTIONS OF CONCERN TO DENTISTRY

• Decreased antihypertensive effects: NSAIDs, indomethacin, sympathomimetics
• May slow metabolism of lidocaine
• Decreased β-blocking effects (or decreased β-adrenergic effects) of epinephrine, levonordefrin, isoproterenol, and other sympathomimetics

SERIOUS REACTIONS

! Overdose may produce profound bradycardia and hypotension.
! Abrupt withdrawal may result in diaphoresis, palpitations, headache, and tremulousness.
! Bisoprolol administration may precipitate CHF and MI in patients with heart disease, thyroid storm in those with thyrotoxicosis, and peripheral ischemia in those with existing peripheral vascular disease.
! Hypoglycemia may occur in patients with previously controlled diabetes.
! Thrombocytopenia, including unusual bruising and bleeding, occurs rarely.

DENTAL CONSIDERATIONS

General:
• Monitor vital signs at every appointment because of cardiovascular side effects.

• After supine positioning, have patient sit upright for at least 2 min to avoid orthostatic hypotension.
• Patients on chronic drug therapy may rarely have symptoms of blood dyscrasias, which can include infection, bleeding, and poor healing.
• Assess salivary flow as a factor in caries, periodontal disease, and candidiasis.
• Stress from dental procedures may compromise cardiovascular function; determine patient risk.
• Short appointments and a stress-reduction protocol may be required for anxious patients.
• Use vasoconstrictors with caution, in low doses, and with careful aspiration. Avoid use of gingival retraction cord with epinephrine.

Consultations:
• In a patient with symptoms of blood dyscrasias, request a medical consultation for blood studies and postpone dental treatment until normal values are reestablished.
• Medical consultation may be required to assess disease control and patient's ability to tolerate stress.
• Take precautions if general anesthesia is required for dental surgery.

Teach Patient/Family:
• When chronic dry mouth occurs, advise patient to:
  • Avoid mouth rinses with high alcohol content because of drying effects
  • Use daily home fluoride products for anticaries effect
  • Use sugarless gum, frequent sips of water, or saliva substitutes

bitolterol
bye-tole′-ter-ol
(Tornalate)

CATEGORY AND SCHEDULE
Pregnancy Risk Category: C

Drug Class: Bronchodilator;
Croup therapy agent

MECHANISM OF ACTION
An antiadrenergic, sympatholytic
agent that stimulates β_2-adrenergic
receptors in lungs. *Therapeutic
Effect:* Relaxes bronchial smooth
muscle, relieves bronchospasm,
reduces airway resistance.

USES
Inhaled through the mouth to open
up the bronchial tubes (air passages)
of the lungs. Some of these
medicines are used to treat the
symptoms of asthma, chronic
bronchitis, emphysema, and other
lung diseases, while others are used
to prevent the symptoms.

PHARMACOKINETICS
Onset of action is rapid with duration
of 4–8 hr. Rapidly absorbed
following aerosol administration.
Primarily distributed to lungs.
Metabolized in liver. Excreted in
urine and feces. *Half-life:* 3 hr.

INDICATIONS AND DOSAGES
▸ **Brochospasm**
Inhalation
*Adults, Elderly, Children 12 yr and
older.* Use 2 inhalations, separated by
1–3 min interval. A third inhalation
may be required.
▸ **Prevention of Bronchospasm**
Inhalation
*Adults, Elderly, Children 12 yr and
older.* Use 2 inhalations q8h. Do not
exceed 3 inhalations q6h, or
2 inhalations q4h.

SIDE EFFECTS/ADVERSE REACTIONS
Frequent
Tremor
Occasional
Cough, dry or irritated mouth/throat,
headache, nausea, vomiting
Rare
Dizziness, vertigo, palpitations,
insomnia

PRECAUTIONS AND CONTRAINDICATIONS
History of hypersensitivity to
sympathomimetics, bitolterol, or any
of its components

DRUG INTERACTIONS OF CONCERN TO DENTISTRY
• Significant reduction of effects:
β-adrenergic blockers
• Potentiation of CV effects: MAOIs,
tricyclic antidepressants,
methylxanthine

SERIOUS REACTIONS
❗ Although tolerance to the
bronchodilating effect has not been
observed, prolonged or too frequent
use may lead to tolerance.
❗ Severe paradoxical
bronchoconstriction may occur with
excessive use.

DENTAL CONSIDERATIONS
General:
• Assess salivary flow as a factor in
caries, periodontal disease, and
candidiasis.
• Consider semisupine chair position
for patients with respiratory disease.
• Acute asthmatic episodes may be
precipitated in the dental office.
A rapid-acting sympathomimetic
inhalant (rescue inhaler) should be

available for emergency use. Many patients may already have a prescribed rescue inhaler they normally use for acute asthmatic events.

Consultations:
• Medical consultation may be required to assess disease control and patient's ability to tolerate stress.

Teach Patient/Family to:
• Gargle, rinse mouth with water, and expectorate after each aerosol dose
• When chronic dry mouth occurs advise patient to:
  • Avoid mouth rinses with high alcohol content due to drying effects
  • Use daily home fluoride products for anticaries effect
  • Use sugarless gum, frequent sips of water, or saliva substitutes

---

bivalirudin
bye-va-leer'-uh-din
(Angiomax)

CATEGORY AND SCHEDULE
Pregnancy Risk Category: B

Drug Class: Anticoagulants, thrombin inhibitors

MECHANISM OF ACTION
An anticoagulant that specifically and reversibly inhibits thrombin by binding to its receptor sites.
Therapeutic Effect: Decreases acute ischemic complications in patients with unstable angina pectoris.

USES
Treatment of unstable angina in patients undergoing percutaneous transluminal coronary angioplasty

PHARMACOKINETICS

Route	Onset	Peak	Duration
IV	Immediate	N/A	1 hr

Primarily eliminated by kidneys. Twenty-five percent removed by hemodialysis. *Half-life:* 25 min (increased in moderate to severe renal impairment).

INDICATIONS AND DOSAGES
▸ **Anticoagulant in Patients with Unstable Angina who are Undergoing Percutaneous Transluminal Coronary Angioplasty (PTCA) in Conjunction with Aspirin**
IV
Adults, Elderly. 1 mg/kg as IV bolus followed by 4-hr IV infusion at rate of 2.5 mg/ kg/hr. After initial 4-hr infusion is completed, give additional IV infusion at rate of 0.2 mg/ kg/hr for 20 hr or less, if necessary.
▸ **Dosage in Renal Impairment**

GFR	Dosage Reduced by
30–59 ml/min	20%
10–29 ml/min	60%
Dialysis	90%

SIDE EFFECTS/ADVERSE REACTIONS
Frequent
Back pain
Occasional
Nausea, headache, hypotension, generalized pain
Rare
Injection site pain, insomnia, hypertension, anxiety, vomiting, pelvic or abdominal pain, bradycardia, nervousness, dyspepsia, fever, urine retention

CAUTIONS AND CONTRAINDICATIONS
Active major bleeding

DRUG INTERACTIONS OF CONCERN TO DENTISTRY
• Increased risk of bleeding: anticoagulants, antiplatelet agents, thrombolytics, ginkgo biloba (herb)

SERIOUS REACTIONS
! A hemorrhagic event occurs rarely and is characterized by a fall in B/P or Hct.

DENTAL CONSIDERATIONS
General:
• Intended for use in hospitals or emergency rooms.
• Patients are at risk of bleeding, check for oral signs.
• Provide palliative dental care for dental emergencies only.
Consultations:
• Medical consultation should include routine blood counts including platelet counts and bleeding time.
• In a patient with symptoms of blood dyscrasias, request a medical consultation for blood studies and postpone treatment until normal values are reestablished.
Teach Patient/Family to:
• Use soft tooth brush to reduce risk of bleeding
• Use effective oral hygiene to prevent soft tissue inflammation
• Report oral lesions, soreness, or bleeding to dentist
• Prevent trauma when using oral hygiene aids
• Update health and medication history if physician makes any changes in evaluation or drug regimens; include OTC, herbal, and nonherbal remedies in the update

bleomycin sulfate
blee-oh-my′-sin sull′-fate
(Blenamax[AUS], Blenoxane)

CATEGORY AND SCHEDULE
Pregnancy Risk Category: D

Drug Class: Antineoplastic

MECHANISM OF ACTION
A glycopeptide antibiotic whose mechanism of action is unknown. Is most effective in the G2 phase of cell division. *Therapeutic Effect:* Appears to inhibit DNA synthesis and, to a lesser extent, RNA and protein synthesis.

USES
Treatment of cancer of head, neck, penis, cervix, vulva of squamous cell origin, Hodgkin's and non-Hodgkin's disease, lymphosarcoma, reticulum cell sarcoma, testicular carcinoma, as a sclerosing agent for malignant pleural effusion

PHARMACOKINETICS
Half-life: 2 hr; when creatinine clearance is greater than 35 ml/min, half-life is increased in lower clearance; metabolized in liver, 50% excreted in urine (unchanged).

INDICATIONS AND DOSAGES
▶ **As Monotherapy to Treat Testicular Carcinoma; Lymphomas (including Hodgkin's disease, choriocarcinoma, reticulum cell sarcoma, and lymphosarcoma); and Squamous Cell Carcinomas of the Head and Neck (including mouth, tongue, tonsil, nasopharynx, oropharynx, sinus, palate, lip, buccal mucosa, gingiva, epiglottis, and larynx)**
IV, IM, Subcutaneous

Adults, Elderly. 10–20 units/m^2 (0.25–0.5 units/kg) 1–2 times/wk.
IV (continuous)
Adults, Elderly. 15 units/m^2 over 24 hr for 4 days.

▶ **In Combination Therapy to Treat Testicular Carcinoma; Lymphomas (including Hodgkin's disease, choriocarcinoma, reticulum cell sarcoma, and lymphosarcoma); and Squamous Cell Carcinomas of the Head and Neck (including mouth, tongue, tonsil, nasopharynx, oropharynx, sinus, palate, lip, buccal mucosa, gingiva, epiglottis, and larynx)**
IV, IM
Adults, Elderly. 3–4 units/m^2.

▶ **As a sclerosing agent to treat malignant pleural effusions and prevent recurrent pleural effusions.**
Intrapleural
Adults, Elderly. 60–240 units as a single injection.

SIDE EFFECTS/ADVERSE REACTIONS
Frequent
Anorexia, weight loss, erythematous skin swelling, urticaria, rash, striae, vesiculation, hyperpigmentation (particularly at areas of pressure, skin folds, cuticles, IM injection sites, and scars), stomatitis (usually evident 1–3 wk after initial therapy); may also be accompanied by decreased skin sensitivity followed by skin hypersensitivity, nausea, vomiting, alopecia, and—with parenteral form—fever or chills (typically occurring a few hr after large single dose and lasting 4–12 hr)

PRECAUTIONS AND CONTRAINDICATIONS
Previous allergic reaction

DRUG INTERACTIONS OF CONCERN TO DENTISTRY
None reported

SERIOUS REACTIONS
❗ Interstitial pneumonitis occurs in 10% of patients and occasionally progresses to pulmonary fibrosis. This condition appears to be dose or age related, occurring more often in patients receiving a total dose greater than 400 units and those older than 70 yr.
❗ Nephrotoxicity and hepatotoxicity occur infrequently.

DENTAL CONSIDERATIONS
General:
• Monitor vital signs at every appointment due to cardiovascular side effects.
• Examine for oral manifestation of opportunistic infection.
• This drug may be used in the hospital or on an outpatient basis. Confirm the patient's disease and treatment status.
• Chlorhexidine mouth rinse prior to and during chemotherapy may reduce severity of mucositis.
• Patient on chronic drug therapy may rarely present with symptoms of blood dyscrasias, which can include infection, bleeding, and poor healing. If dyscrasia is present, caution patient to prevent oral tissue trauma when using oral hygiene aids.
• Palliative medication may be required for management of oral side effects.
• Patients may have received other chemotherapy or radiation; confirm medical and drug history.
• Patients may be taking a prophylactic antiinfective.
• Place on frequent recall due to oral side effects.

Consultations:
• Consult physician; prophylactic or therapeutic antiinfectives may be indicated if surgery or periodontal treatment is required.
• Medical consultation may be required to assess immunologic status during cancer chemotherapy and determine safety risk, if any, posed by the required dental treatment.
• Medical consultation may be required to assess disease control and patient's ability to tolerate stress.
Teach Patient/Family to:
• Be aware of oral side effects
• Use effective oral hygiene to prevent soft tissue inflammation
• Report oral lesions, soreness, or bleeding to dentist
• Prevent trauma when using oral hygiene aids
• Update health and medication history if physician makes any changes in evaluation or drug regimens; include OTC, herbal, and nonherbal remedies in the update

bosentan
bo´-sen-tan
(Tracleer)
Do not confuse with Tricor.

CATEGORY AND SCHEDULE
Pregnancy Risk Category: X

Drug Class: Antihypertensive

MECHANISM OF ACTION
An endothelin receptor antagonist that blocks endothelin-1, the neurohormone that constricts pulmonary arteries. *Therapeutic Effect:* Improves exercise ability and slows clinical worsening of pulmonary arterial hypertension (PAH).

USES
Treatment of pulmonary arterial hypertension in patients with World Health Organization (WHO) class III and IV symptoms

PHARMACOKINETICS
Highly bound to plasma proteins, mainly albumin. Metabolized in the liver. Eliminated by biliary excretion. *Half-life:* Approximately 5 hr.

INDICATIONS AND DOSAGES
▸ **PAH in those with WHO Class III or IV Symptoms**
PO
Adults, Elderly. 62.5 mg twice a day for 4 wk; then increase to maintenance dosage of 125 mg twice a day.
Children weighing less than 40 kg. 62.5 mg twice a day.

SIDE EFFECTS/ADVERSE REACTIONS
Occasional
Headache, nasopharyngitis, flushing
Rare
Dyspepsia (heartburn, epigastric distress), fatigue, pruritus, hypotension

PRECAUTIONS AND CONTRAINDICATIONS
Administration with cyclosporine or glyburide, pregnancy
Caution
Hepatic impairment, pregnancy category X, use during lactation or in children has not been determined, necessitates monthly tests for pregnancy during use

DRUG INTERACTIONS OF CONCERN TO DENTISTRY
• Increased plasma concentrations: ketoconazole and possibly other

drugs that inhibit or induce CYP450 enzymes involved with metabolism
• See contraindications for other drugs

SERIOUS REACTIONS
! Abnormal hepatic function, lower extremity edema, and palpitations occur rarely.

DENTAL CONSIDERATIONS
General:
• Acute pulmonary arterial hypertension rarely occurs and is a major medical problem. Patients are at high risk.
• Chronic pulmonary arterial hypertension also occurs. Patients may be taking a variety of antihypertensive medications. It is advisable to consult with the physician of record to determine quality of disease control, patient's ability to tolerate stress, and, with this particular drug, liver function.
Teach Patient/Family to:
• Use effective oral hygiene to prevent tissue inflammation and dental caries
• Update health and drug history if physician makes any changes in evaluation or drug regimens; include OTC, herbal, and nonherbal drugs in the update

brimonidine
bry-mo′-nih-deen
(Alphagan P)
Do not confuse with bromocriptine.

CATEGORY AND SCHEDULE
Pregnancy Risk Category: B

Drug Class: α-adrenergic receptor agonist

MECHANISM OF ACTION
An ophthalmic agent that is a selective α_2-adrenergic agonist. **Therapeutic Effect:** Reduces intraocular pressure (IOP).

USES
Lowering of intraocular pressure in open-angle glaucoma or ocular hypertension; prevention of postoperative intraocular pressure elevation after argon laser trabeculoplasty

PHARMACOKINETICS
Plasma concentrations peak within 0.5–2.5 hr after ocular administration. Distributed into aqueous humor. Metabolized in liver. Primarily excreted in urine. **Half-life:** 3 hr.

INDICATIONS AND DOSAGES
▶ **Glaucoma, Ocular Hypertension**
Ophthalmic
Adults, Elderly, Children 2 yr and older. 1 drop in affected eye(s) 3 times a day.

SIDE EFFECTS/ADVERSE REACTIONS
Occasional
Allergic conjunctivitis, conjunctival hyperemia, eye pruritus, burning sensation, conjunctival folliculosis, oral dryness, visual disturbances

PRECAUTIONS AND CONTRAINDICATIONS
Concurrent use of MAOI therapy, hypersensitivity to brimonidine tartrate or any other component of the formulation
Caution
Wait 15 min after using before inserting contact lens; tricyclic antidepressants, β-blockers, CNS depressants; severe CV disease,

hepatic or renal impairment, depression, cerebral or coronary insufficiency, Raynaud's phenomenon, orthostatic hypotension, thromboangiitis obliterans, lactation, children younger than 2 yr

DRUG INTERACTIONS OF CONCERN TO DENTISTRY

- Drug interactions have not been studied; however, the following possibilities exist:
- Increased CNS depression: opioids, sedatives, alcohol, and general anesthetics
- Possible risk of interference with lowering intraocular pressure: anticholinergic drugs or drugs with anticholinergic actions; tricyclic antidepressants benzodiazepines

SERIOUS REACTIONS

! Bradycardia, hypotension, iritis, miosis, skin reactions, including erythema, eyelid, pruritus, rash, vasodilation, and tachycardia have been reported.

DENTAL CONSIDERATIONS

General:
- Assess salivary flow as factor in caries, periodontal disease, and candidiasis.
- Avoid dental light in patient's eyes; offer dark glasses for patient comfort.
- Question patient about compliance with prescribed drug regimen for glaucoma.
- Avoid drugs with anticholinergic activity, such as antihistamines, opioids, benzodiazepines, propantheline, atropine, and scopolamine.
- Monitor vital signs at every appointment because of cardiovascular side effects.

Consultations:
- Consultation with physician may be necessary if sedation or general anesthesia is required.

Teach Patient/Family to:
- Update health and drug history if physician makes any changes in evaluation or drug regimens
- When chronic dry mouth occurs, advise patient to:
  - Avoid mouth rinses with high alcohol content because of drying effects
  - Use daily home fluoride products for anticaries effect
  - Use sugarless gum, frequent sips of water, or saliva substitutes

brinzolamide
brin-zol´-ah-mide
(Azopt)

CATEGORY AND SCHEDULE
Pregnancy Risk Category: C

Drug Class: Carbonic anhydrase inhibitor

MECHANISM OF ACTION
An ophthalmic agent that inhibits carbonic anhydrase. Decreases aqueous humor secretion.
Therapeutic Effect: Reduces intraocular pressure (IOP).

USES
Treatment of ocular hypertension, open-angle glaucoma

PHARMACOKINETICS
Systemically absorbed to some degree. Protein binding: 60%. Distributed extensively in red

blood cells. Site of metabolism has not been established. Metabolized to active and inactive metabolites. Primarily excreted unchanged in urine.

INDICATIONS AND DOSAGES
▸ **Glaucoma, Ocular Hypertension**
Ophthalmic
Adults, Elderly. Instill 1 drop in affected eye(s) 3 times a day.

SIDE EFFECTS/ADVERSE REACTIONS
Occasional
Blurred vision, bitter taste, dry eye, ocular discharge, ocular discomfort and pain, ocular pruritus, headache, rhinitis
Rare
Allergic reactions, alopecia, chest pain, conjunctivitis, diarrhea, diplopia, dizziness, dry mouth, dyspnea, dyspepsia, eye fatigue, hypertonia, keratoconjunctivitis, keratopathy, kidney pain, lid margin crusting or sticky sensation, nausea, pharyngitis, tearing, urticaria

PRECAUTIONS AND CONTRAINDICATIONS
Hypersensitivity to brinzolamide or any other component of the formulation
Caution
Lactation, no data for pediatric use

DRUG INTERACTIONS OF CONCERN TO DENTISTRY
• Avoid drugs that can exacerbate glaucoma (e.g., anticholinergics)

SERIOUS REACTIONS
! Electrolyte imbalance, development of an acidotic state, and possible CNS effects may occur.

DENTAL CONSIDERATIONS
General:
• Avoid dental light in patient's eyes; offer dark glasses for patient comfort.
• Question patient about compliance with prescribed drug regimen for glaucoma.
Consultations:
• Medical consult may be required to assess disease control.

bromocriptine mesylate
broe-moe-krip′-teen mess-ah-late
(Apo-Bromocriptine[CAN], Bromohexal[AUS], Kripton[AUS], Parlodel)
Do not confuse bromocriptine with benztropine, or Parlodel with pindolol.

CATEGORY AND SCHEDULE
Pregnancy Risk Category: C

Drug Class: Dopamine receptor agonist, ovulation stimulant

MECHANISM OF ACTION
A dopamine agonist that directly stimulates dopamine receptors in the corpus striatum and inhibits prolactin secretion. Also suppresses secretion of growth hormone. ***Therapeutic Effect:*** Improves symptoms of parkinsonism, suppresses galactorrhea, and reduces serum growth hormone concentrations in acromegaly.

USES
Treatment of female infertility, Parkinson's disease, prevention of postpartum lactation, amenorrhea caused by hyperprolactinemia, acromegaly

PHARMACOKINETICS

Indication	Onset	Peak	Duration
Prolactin lowering	2 hr	8 hr	24 hr
Antiparkinson	0.5–1.5 hr	2 hr	N/A
Growth hormone suppressant	1–2 hr	4–8 wk	4–8 hr

Minimally absorbed from the GI tract. Protein binding: 90%–96%. Metabolized in the liver. Excreted in feces by biliary secretion. *Half-life:* 15 hr.

INDICATIONS AND DOSAGES
▶ **Hyperprolactinemia**
PO
Adults, Elderly. Initially, 1.25–2.5 mg/day. May increase by 2.5 mg/day at 3- to 7-day intervals. Range: 2.5 mg 2–3 times a day.
▶ **Parkinson's Disease**
PO
Adults, Elderly. Initially, 1.25 mg twice a day. May increase by 2.5 mg/day every 14–28 days. Range: 30–90 mg/day.
▶ **Acromegaly**
PO
Adults, Elderly. Initially, 1.25–2.5 mg. May increase at 3- to7-day intervals. Usual dose 20–30 mg/day.

SIDE EFFECTS/ADVERSE REACTIONS
Frequent
Nausea (49%), headache (19%), dizziness (17%)
Occasional (7%–3%)
Fatigue, lightheadedness, vomiting, abdominal cramps, diarrhea, constipation, nasal congestion, somnolence, dry mouth
Rare
Muscle cramps, urinary hesitancy

PRECAUTIONS AND CONTRAINDICATIONS
Hypersensitivity to ergot alkaloids, peripheral vascular disease, pregnancy, severe ischemic heart disease, uncontrolled hypertension
Caution
Lactation, hepatic disease, renal disease, children

DRUG INTERACTIONS OF CONCERN TO DENTISTRY
None reported

SERIOUS REACTIONS
! Visual or auditory hallucinations have been noted in patients with Parkinson's disease.
! Long-term, high-dose therapy may produce continuing rhinorrhea, syncope, GI hemorrhage, peptic ulcer, and severe abdominal pain.

DENTAL CONSIDERATIONS
General:
• Monitor vital signs at every appointment because of cardiovascular side effects.
• After supine positioning, have patient sit upright for at least 2 min to avoid orthostatic hypotension.
• Assess salivary flow as a factor in caries, periodontal disease, and candidiasis.
• Short appointments may be required because of disease effects on musculature.
Consultations:
• Medical consultation may be required to assess disease control.
Teach Patient/Family to:
• Avoid mouth rinses with high alcohol content because of drying effects

brompheniramine
brome-fen-ir′-ah-meen
(BroveX, BroveX CT, Codimal A,
Colhist, Dimetane, Dimetane
Extentabs, Dimetapp, Lodrane
12 Hour, Nasahist B, ND Stat)

CATEGORY AND SCHEDULE
Pregnancy Risk Category: B
OTC (tablets, elixir)

Drug Class: Antihistamine,
H1- receptor antagonist

MECHANISM OF ACTION
An alkylamine that competes with
histamine at histaminic receptor (H_1)
sites. Inhibits central acetylcholine.
Therapeutic Effect: Results in
anticholinergic, antipruritic,
antitussive, antiemetic effects.
Produces antidyskinetic, sedative
effect.

USES
Allergy symptoms, rhinitis, hay fever

PHARMACOKINETICS
Rapidly absorbed after PO
administration. Widely distributed.
Metabolized in liver. Primarily
excreted in urine. *Half-life:* 25 hr.

INDICATIONS AND DOSAGES
▶ **Allergic Rhinitis, Anaphylaxis,
Urticarial Transfusion Reactions,
Urticaria**
PO
*Adults, Elderly, Children 12 yr and
older.* 4 mg q4–6h or 8–12 mg
extended/timed-release q12h.
Children younger than 12 yr.
1–2 mg q4–6h.
▶ **Amelioration of Allergic Reactions
to Blood or Plasma, Anaphylaxis as
an Adjunct to Epinephrine and other
Standard Measures after the Acute
Symptoms Have Been Controlled,
Other Uncomplicated Allergic
Conditions of the Immediate Type
When Oral Therapy Is Impossible or
Contraindicated**
IM/IV/SC
*Adults, Elderly, Children 12 yr and
older.* 5–20 mg/day in 2 divided
doses. Maximum: 40 mg/day.
Children younger than 12 yr.
0.125 mg/kg/day or 3.75 mg/m² in
3–4 divided doses.

SIDE EFFECTS/ADVERSE REACTIONS
Frequent
Drowsiness; dizziness; dry
mouth, nose, or throat; urinary
retention; thickening of bronchial
secretions
Elderly: Sedation, dizziness,
hypotension
Occasional
Epigastric distress, flushing, blurred
vision, tinnitus, paresthesia,
sweating, chills

PRECAUTIONS AND CONTRAINDICATIONS
Concurrent MAOI therapy, focal
CNS lesions, newborn or premature
infants, hypersensitivity to
brompheniramine or related
drugs
Caution
Increased intraocular pressure, renal
disease, cardiac disease,
hypertension, bronchial asthma,
seizure disorder, stenosed peptic
ulcers, hyperthyroidism, prostatic
hypertrophy, bladder neck
obstruction

DRUG INTERACTIONS OF CONCERN TO DENTISTRY
• Increased CNS depression: alcohol,
all CNS depressants
• Additive photosensitization:
tetracyclines

- Increased drying effect: anticholinergics
- Hypotension: general anesthetics

SERIOUS REACTIONS

! Children may experience dominant paradoxical reactions, including restlessness, insomnia, euphoria, nervousness, and tremors.
! Overdosage in children may result in hallucinations, seizures, and death.
! Hypersensitivity reaction, such as eczema, pruritus, rash, cardiac disturbances, and photosensitivity, may occur.

DENTAL CONSIDERATIONS

General:
- Assess salivary flow as a factor in caries, periodontal disease, and candidiasis.
- Consider semisupine chair position for patients with respiratory disease.
- Determine why the patient is taking the drug.

Teach Patient/Family to:
- Use effective oral hygiene to prevent soft tissue inflammation
- Avoid mouth rinses with high alcohol content because of drying effects

buclizine hydrochloride
bew′-klih-zeen hi-droh-klor′-ide
(Bucladin-S)

CATEGORY AND SCHEDULE
Pregnancy Risk Category: C

Drug Class: Antiemetic

MECHANISM OF ACTION
A centrally acting agent that suppresses nausea and vomiting. Buclizine is an anticholinergic that reduces labyrinth excitability and diminishes vestibular stimulation of labyrinth, affecting chemoreceptor trigger zone (CTZ). Possesses anticholinergic activity. **Therapeutic Effect:** Reduces nausea, vomiting, vertigo.

USES
Prophylaxis of nausea, vomiting, and dizziness associated with motion sickness

PHARMACOKINETICS
None reported

INDICATIONS AND DOSAGES
▸ **Motion Sickness**
PO
Adults, Elderly, Children 12 yr and older. 50 mg 30 min before travel. Dose may be repeated every 4–6 hr as needed. Maximum: 150 mg/day.

SIDE EFFECTS/ADVERSE REACTIONS
Frequent
Drowsiness
Occasional
Dryness of mouth, headache, jitteriness

PRECAUTIONS AND CONTRAINDICATIONS
Early pregnancy, hypersensitivity to buclizine or other components of the formulation including tartrazine

DRUG INTERACTIONS OF CONCERN TO DENTISTRY
None reported

SERIOUS REACTIONS
! Children may experience dominant paradoxical reaction, including restlessness, insomnia, euphoria, nervousness, and tremors.
! Overdosage in children may result in hallucinations, convulsions, and death.

! Hypersensitivity reaction, marked by eczema, pruritus, rash, cardiac disturbances, and photosensitivity, may occur.

! Overdosage may vary from CNS depression, such as sedation, apnea, cardiovascular collapse, or death, to severe paradoxical reaction, including hallucinations, tremors, or seizures.

DENTAL CONSIDERATIONS

General:

• Symptoms may preclude elective dental treatment.

• Assess salivary flow as a factor in caries, periodontal disease, and candidiasis.

• Consider semisupine chair position for patient comfort because of GI effects of disease.

Teach Patient/Family to:

• Use effective oral hygiene to prevent soft tissue inflammation.

• When chronic dry mouth occurs, advise patient to:

  • Avoid mouth rinses with high alcohol content due to drying effects

  • Use daily home fluoride products for anticaries effect

  • Use sugarless gum, frequent sips of water, or saliva substitutes

budesonide

bu-dess′-ah-nide

(Burinex[AUS], Entocort EC, Pulmicort Respules, Pulmicort Turbuhaler, Rhinocort Aqua, Rhinocort Aqueous[AUS], Rhinocort Hayfever[AUS])

CATEGORY AND SCHEDULE

Pregnancy Risk Category: B

Drug Class: Glucocorticoid, long-acting

MECHANISM OF ACTION

A glucocorticoid that inhibits the accumulation of inflammatory cells and decreases and prevents tissues from responding to the inflammatory process. ***Therapeutic Effect:*** Relieves symptoms of allergic rhinitis or Crohn's disease.

USES

Treatment of mild-to-moderate active Crohn's disease of the ileum or ascending colon

PHARMACOKINETICS

Minimally absorbed from nasal tissue; moderately absorbed from inhalation. Protein binding: 88%. Primarily metabolized in the liver. ***Half-life:*** 2–3 hr.

INDICATIONS AND DOSAGES

▸ **Rhinitis**

Intranasal (Rhinocort Aqua)

Adults, Elderly, Children 6 yr and older. 1 spray in each nostril once a day. Maximum: 8 sprays a day for adults and children 12 yr and older; 4 sprays a day for children younger than 12 yr.

▸ **Bronchial Asthma**

Nebulization

Children 6 mo–8 yr. 0.25–1 mg/day titrated to lowest effective dosage.

Inhalation

Adults, Elderly, Children 6 yr and older. Initially, 200–400 mcg twice a day. Maximum: Adults: 800 mcg twice a day. Children: 400 mcg twice a day.

▸ **Crohn's Disease**

PO

Adults, Elderly. 9 mg once a day for up to 8 wk.

SIDE EFFECTS/ADVERSE REACTIONS
Frequent
Nasal: Mild nasopharyngeal irritation, burning, stinging, or dryness; headache; cough
Inhalation: Flu-like symptoms, headache, pharyngitis
Occasional
Nasal: Dry mouth, dyspepsia, rebound congestion, rhinorrhea, loss of taste
Inhalation: Back pain, vomiting, altered taste, voice changes, abdominal pain, nausea, dyspepsia

PRECAUTIONS AND CONTRAINDICATIONS
Hypersensitivity to any corticosteroid or its components, persistently positive sputum cultures for *Candida albicans,* primary treatment of status asthmaticus, systemic fungal infections, untreated localized infection involving nasal mucosa
Caution
Tuberculosis, hypertension, diabetes mellitus, osteoporosis, peptic ulcer, glaucoma, cataracts, suppression of the hypothalamic-pituitary-adrenal (HPA) axis, discontinue use during nursing or discontinue drug, safety in children has not been established, geriatric patients

SERIOUS REACTIONS
! An acute hypersensitivity reaction marked by urticaria, angioedema, and severe bronchospasm, occurs rarely.

DENTAL CONSIDERATIONS
General:
• Evaluate respiration characteristics and rate.
• Assess salivary flow as a factor in caries, periodontal disease, and candidiasis.

• Midday appointments are suggested with stress reduction protocol for anxious patients.
• Place on frequent recall because of oral side effects.
• Acute asthmatic episodes may be precipitated in the dental office. Rapid-acting sympathomimetic inhalants should be available for emergency use. Budesonide is not a rapid-acting drug and is not intended for use in acute asthmatic attacks.
Consultations:
• Medical consultation may be required to assess disease control.
Teach Patient/Family to:
• Use effective oral hygiene to prevent soft tissue inflammation
• Gargle and rinse with water after each dose
• When chronic dry mouth occurs, advise patient to:
  • Avoid mouth rinses with high alcohol content because of drying effects
  • Use daily home fluoride products for anticaries effect
  • Use sugarless gum, frequent sips of water, or artificial saliva substitutes

bumetanide
byoo-met′-ah-nide
(Bumex, Burinex[CAN])

CATEGORY AND SCHEDULE
Pregnancy Risk Category: C (D if used in pregnancy-induced hypertension)

Drug Class: Loop diuretic

MECHANISM OF ACTION
A loop diuretic that enhances excretion of sodium, chloride, and to

lesser degree, potassium, by direct action at the ascending limb of the loop of Henle and in the proximal tubule. ***Therapeutic Effect:*** Produces diuresis.

USES

Treatment of edema in CHF, liver disease, renal disease (nephrotic syndrome), pulmonary edema, ascites (nephrotic syndrome), hypertension

PHARMACOKINETICS

Route	Onset	Peak	Duration
PO	30–60 min	60–120 min	4–6 hr
IV	Rapid	15–30 min	2–3 hr
IM	40 min	60–120 min	4–6 hr

Completely absorbed from the GI tract (absorption decreased in CHF and nephrotic syndrome). Protein binding: 94%–96%. Partially metabolized in the liver. Primarily excreted in urine. Not removed by hemodialysis. *Half-life:* 1–1.5 hr.

INDICATIONS AND DOSAGES
▸ **Edema**
PO
Adults, Children older than 18 yr. 0.5–2 mg as a single dose in the morning. May repeat at q4–5 hr.
Elderly. 0.5 mg/day, increased as needed.
IV, IM
Adults, Elderly. 0.5–2 mg/dose; may repeat in 2–3 hr. Or 0.5–1 mg/hr by continuous IV infusion.
▸ **Hypertension**
PO
Adults, Elderly. Initially, 0.5 mg/day. Range: 1–4 mg/day. Maximum: 5 mg/day. Larger doses may be given 2–3 doses a day.

▸ **Usual Pediatric Dosage**
PO, IV, IM
Children. 0.015–0.1 mg/kg/dose q6–24h.

SIDE EFFECTS/ADVERSE REACTIONS
Expected
Increased urinary frequency and urine volume
Frequent
Orthostatic hypotension, dizziness
Occasional
Blurred vision, diarrhea, headache, anorexia, premature ejaculation, impotence, dyspepsia
Rare
Rash, urticaria, pruritus, asthenia, muscle cramps, nipple tenderness

PRECAUTIONS AND CONTRAINDICATIONS
Anuria, hepatic coma, severe electrolyte depletion
Caution
Dehydration, ascites, severe renal disease

DRUG INTERACTIONS OF CONCERN TO DENTISTRY
• Decreased diuretic effect: NSAIDs, indomethacin
• Masked ototoxicity: phenothiazines
• Increased electrolyte imbalance: nondepolarizing skeletal muscle relaxants, corticosteroids

SERIOUS REACTIONS
! Vigorous diuresis may lead to profound water and electrolyte depletion, resulting in hypokalemia, hyponatremia, dehydration, coma, and circulatory collapse.
! Ototoxicity—manifested as deafness, vertigo, or tinnitus—may occur, especially in patients with severe renal impairment and those taking other ototoxic drugs.

3

! Blood dyscrasias and acute
hypotensive episodes have been
reported.

DENTAL CONSIDERATIONS
General:
• Monitor vital signs at every
appointment because of
cardiovascular side effects.
• Patients on chronic drug therapy
may rarely have symptoms of blood
dyscrasias, which can include
infection, bleeding, and poor healing.
• After supine positioning, have
patient sit upright for at least 2 min
to avoid orthostatic hypotension.
• Assess salivary flow as a factor in
caries, periodontal disease, and
candidiasis.
• Observe appropriate limitation of
vasoconstriction.
• Limit use of sodium-containing
products, such as saline IV fluids, for
patients with a dietary salt restriction.
• Patients on high-potency diuretics
should be monitored for serum K levels.
Consultations:
• In a patient with symptoms of
blood dyscrasias, request a medical
consultation for blood studies and
postpone dental treatment until
normal values are reestablished.
• Medical consultation may be
required to assess disease control.
Teach Patient/Family to:
• Use effective oral hygiene to
prevent soft tissue inflammation
• Use caution to prevent injury when
using oral hygiene aids
• When chronic dry mouth occurs,
advise patient to:
• Avoid mouth rinses with high
alcohol content because of drying
effects
• Use daily home fluoride products
for anticaries effect
• Use sugarless gum, frequent sips
of water, or saliva substitutes

bupivacaine
byoo-piv′-ah-caine
(Marcaine, Marcaine Spinal,
Sensorcaine, Sensorcaine-MPF)

CATEGORY AND SCHEDULE
Pregnancy Risk Category: C

Drug Class: Amide local
anesthetic

MECHANISM OF ACTION
An amide-type anesthetic that
stabilizes neuronal membranes and
prevents initiation and transmission
of nerve impulses, thereby effecting
local anesthetic actions. ***Therapeutic
Effect:*** Produces local analgesia.

USES
Local dental anesthesia, epidural
anesthesia, peripheral nerve block,
caudal anesthesia

PHARMACOKINETICS
Onset of action occurs within
4–10 min depending on route of
administration. Duration is
1.5–8.5 hr, depending on site of
administration. Well absorbed.
Protein binding: 95%. Metabolized
in liver. Excreted in urine. ***Half-life:***
1.5–5.5 hr (Adults), 8.1 hr (Neonates).

INDICATIONS AND DOSAGES
Dose varies with procedure, depth of
anesthesia, vascularity of tissues,
duration of anesthesia and condition
of patient.
▸ **Analgesic, Epidural (partial to
moderate motor blockade)**
IV
Adults, Elderly. 10–20 ml (25–50
mg) of a 0.25% solution. Repeat
once q3h as needed.
Children weighing more than 10 kg.
1–2.5 mg/kg single dose as a 0.125%

or 0.25% solution or 0.2–0.4 mg/kg/hr continuous infusion as a 0.1%, 0.125%, or 0.25% solution. Maximum: 0.4 mg/kg/hr.
Children weighing less than 10 kg. 1–1.25 mg/kg single dose as a 0.125% or 0.25% solution or 0.1–0.2 mg/kg/hr continuous infusion as a 0.1%, 0.125%, or 0.25% solution. Maximum: 0.2 mg/kg/hr.

▸ **Analgesic, Epidural (moderate to complete motor blockade)**
IV
Adults, Elderly. 10–20 ml (50–100 mg) as a 0.5% solution. Repeat once q3h as needed.
Children weighing more than 10 kg. 1–2.5 mg/kg single dose as a 0.125% or 0.25% solution or 0.2–0.4 mg/kg/hr continuous infusion as a 0.1%, 0.125%, or 0.25% solution. Maximum: 0.4 mg/kg/hr.
Children weighing less than 10 kg. 1–1.25 mg/kg single dose as a 0.125% or 0.25% solution or 0.1–0.2 mg/kg/hr continuous infusion as a 0.1%, 0.125%, or 0.25% solution. Maximum: 0.2 mg/kg/hr.

▸ **Analgesic, Epidural (complete motor blockade)**
IV
Adults. 10–20 ml (75–150 mg) as a 0.75% solution. Repeat once q3h as needed.
Children weighing more than 10 kg. 1–2.5 mg/kg single dose as a 0.125% or 0.25% solution or 0.2–0.4 mg/kg/hr continuous infusion as a 0.1%, 0.125%, or 0.25% solution. Maximum: 0.4 mg/kg/hr.
Children weighing less than 10 kg. 1–1.25 mg/kg single dose as a 0.125% or 0.25% solution or 0.1–0.2 mg/kg/hr continuous infusion as a 0.1%, 0.125%, or 0.25% solution. Maximum: 0.2 mg/kg/hr.

▸ **Analgesic, Intrapleural**
IV
Adults, Elderly. 10–30 ml bolus of 0.25%, 0.375%, or 0.5% q4–8h or 0.375% solution with epinephrine continuous infusion at 6 ml/hr after 20 ml loading dose.

▸ **Analgesic, Caudal (moderate to complete blockade)**
IV
Adults, Elderly. 15–30 ml of 0.5% solution (75–150 mg) OR 0.25% solution (37.5–75 mg), repeated once every 3 hr as needed.
Children weighing more than 10 kg. 1–2.5 mg/kg single dose as a 0.125% or 0.25% solution or 0.2–0.4 mg/kg/hr continuous infusion as a 0.1%, 0.125%, or 0.25% solution. Maximum: 0.4 mg/kg/hr.
Children weighing less than 10 kg. 1–1.25 mg/kg single dose as a 0.125% or 0.25% solution or 0.1–0.2 mg/kg/hr continuous infusion as a 0.1%, 0.125%, or 0.25% solution. Maximum: 0.2 mg/kg/hr.

▸ **Analgesic, Dental**
IV
Adults, Elderly. 1.8–3.6 ml of 0.5% solution (9–18 mg) with epinephrine. A second dose of 9 mg may be administered. Maximum: 90 mg total dose.

▸ **Analgesic, Peripheral Nerve Block (moderate to complete motor blockade)**
IV
Adults, Elderly. 5–37.5 ml (25–175 mg) of 0.5% solution or 5–70 ml (12.5–175 mg) of 0.25% solution. Repeat q3h as needed. Maximum: up to 400 mg/day.
Children 12 yr and older. 0.3–2.5 mg/kg as a 0.25% or 0.5% solution. Maximum: 1 ml/kg of 0.25% solution or 0.5 ml/kg of 0.5% solution.

▸ **Analgesic, Retrobulbar (complete motor blockade)**
IV
Adults, Elderly. 2–4 ml (15–30 mg) of 0.75% solution.

▸ **Analgesic, Sympathetic blockade**
IV
Adults, Elderly. 20–50 ml (50–125 mg) of 0.25% (no epinephrine) solution. Repeat once q3h as needed.

▸ **Analgesic, Hyperbaric Spinal (obstetrical, normal vaginal delivery)**
IV
Adults, Elderly. 0.8 ml (6 mg) bupivacaine in dextrose as 0.75% solution.

▸ **Analgesic, Hyperbaric Spinal (obstetrical, cesarean section)**
IV
Adults, Elderly. 1–1.4 ml (7.5–10.5 mg) bupivacaine in dextrose as 0.75% solution.

▸ **Anesthesia, Hyperbaric Spinal (surgical, lower extremity and perineal procedures)**
IV
Adults, Elderly. 1 ml (7.5 mg) bupivacaine in dextrose as 0.75% solution.
Children 12 yr and older. 0.3–0.6 mg/kg bupivacaine in dextrose as a 0.75% solution.

▸ **Anesthesia, Spinal (surgical, lower abdominal procedures)**
IV
Adults, Elderly 1.6 ml (12 mg) bupivacaine in dextrose as 0.75% solution.
Children 12 yr and older. 0.3–0.6 mg/kg bupivacaine in dextrose as a 0.75% solution.

▸ **Anesthesia, Spinal (surgical, hyperbaric, upper abdominal procedures)**
IV
Adults, Elderly. 2 ml (15 mg) bupivacaine in dextrose administered in horizontal position.
Children 12 yr and older.

0.3–0.6 mg/kg bupivacaine in dextrose as a 0.75% solution.

▸ **Analgesic, Local Infiltration**
IV
Adults, Elderly.
0.25% solution. Maximum: 225 mg with epinephrine or 175 mg without epinephrine.
Children 12 yr and older.
0.5–2.5 mg/kg as a 0.25% or 0.5% solution. Maximum: 1 ml/kg of 0.25% solution or 0.5 ml/kg of 0.5% solution.

SIDE EFFECTS/ADVERSE REACTIONS
Occasional
Hypotension, bradycardia, palpitations, respiratory depression, dizziness, headache, vomiting, nausea, restlessness, weakness, blurred vision, tinnitus, apnea

PRECAUTIONS AND CONTRAINDICATIONS
Local infection at the site of proposed lumbar puncture (spinal anesthesia), obstetrical paracervical block anesthesia, septicemia (spinal anesthesia), severe hemorrhage, severe hypotension or shock, arrhythmias such as complete heart block, which severely restricts cardiac output (spinal anesthesia), sulfite allergy (epinephrine containing solutions only), hypersensitivity to bupivacaine products or to other amide-type anesthetics
Caution
Elderly, severe drug allergies, use in children (risk of local injury because of long duration of anesthesia)

DRUG INTERACTIONS OF CONCERN TO DENTISTRY
• CNS depressants: may see increased risk of CNS depression with all CNS depressants, especially in children and when larger doses are used

• Avoid placing dental cartridges in disinfectant solutions with heavy metals or surface-active agents; may see release of metal ions into local anesthetic solutions, with tissue irritation following injection
• Avoid excessive exposure of dental cartridges to light or heat; it hastens deterioration of vasoconstrictors; color change in local anesthetic solution indicates breakdown of vasoconstrictor
• Risk of cardiovascular side effects: rapid intravascular administration of local anesthetic containing vasoconstrictors, either alone or in patients taking tricyclic antidepressants, MAOIs, digitalis drugs, cocaine, phenothiazines, β-blockers, and in the presence of halogenated hydrocarbon general anesthetics; always use the smallest effective vasoconstrictor dose and careful aspiration technique
• Avoid use of vasoconstrictors in patients with uncontrolled hyperthyroidism, diabetes, angina, or hypertension; refer these patients for medical treatment before elective dental procedures

SERIOUS REACTIONS

! Arterial hypotension, bradycardia, ventricular arrhythmias, central nervous system (CNS) depression and excitation, convulsions, respiratory arrest, tinnitus have been reported.
! Solutions with epinephrine contain metabisulfite, a sulfite that may cause allergic-type reactions, including anaphylaxis.

DENTAL CONSIDERATIONS

General:
• Monitor vital signs at every appointment because of cardiovascular and respiratory side effects.

• Lubricate dry lips before injection or dental treatment as required.
Teach Patient/Family to:
• Use care to prevent injury while numbness exists; do not chew gum or eat following dental anesthesia
• Remember that numbness with this drug is expected to last for a considerable period
• Report any signs of infection, muscle pain, or fever to dentist when oral sensations return
• Report any unusual soft tissue reactions

buprenorphine hydrochloride
byoo-pre-nor′-feen hi-droh-klor′-ide
Schedule V
(Buprenex, Subutex, Temgesic[CAN])

CATEGORY AND SCHEDULE
Pregnancy Risk Category: C
Controlled Substance: Schedule V (opioid agonist), III (tablet)

Drug Class: Opioid agonist-antagonist

MECHANISM OF ACTION
An opioid agonist-antagonist that binds with opioid receptors in the CNS. *Therapeutic Effect:* Alters the perception of and emotional response to pain; blocks the effects of heroin and produces minimal opioid withdrawal symptoms.

USES
Relief of moderate to severe pain (injection) and for treatment of opioid dependence (tablets)

PHARMACOKINETICS:

IM: Onset 15–30 min, duration 4–6 hr; absorption 90%–100%; hepatic metabolism; excreted in feces (68%–71%); also renal excretion.

INDICATIONS AND DOSAGES

▸ **Analgesia**

IV, IM

Adults, Children older than 12 yr. 0.3 mg q6–8h as needed. May repeat once in 30–60 min. Range: 0.15–0.6 mg q4–8h as needed.
Children 2–12 yr. 2–6 mcg/kg q4–6h as needed.
Elderly. 0.15 mg q6h as needed.

▸ **Opioid Dependence**

Sublingual

Adults, Elderly, Children older than 16 yr. Initially, 12–16 mg/day, beginning at least 4 hr after last use of heroin or short-acting opioid. Maintenance: 16 mg/day. Range: 4–24 mg/day. Patients should be switched to buprenorphine and naloxone combination, preferred for maintenance treatment.

SIDE EFFECTS/ADVERSE REACTIONS

Frequent

Tablet: Headache, pain, insomnia, anxiety, depression, nausea, abdominal pain, constipation, back pain, weakness, rhinitis, withdrawal syndrome, infection, diaphoresis Injection (more than 10%): Sedation

Occasional

Injection: Hypotension, respiratory depression, dizziness, headache, vomiting, nausea, vertigo

PRECAUTIONS AND CONTRAINDICATIONS

Hypersensitivity to buprenorphine; hypersensitivity to naloxone for those receiving the fixed combination product containing naloxone (Suboxone)

Caution

Hepatic impairment, hepatitis, risk of allergic reaction, bile tract disease, impaired respiration (COPD, corpulmonale, decreased respiratory reserve, hypoxia, hypercapnia, preexisting respiratory depression); naloxone may not be effective as a narcotic reversal agent, head injury, impairment of reaction time, low abuse potential, opioid-dependent patients, debilitated patients, elderly, children younger than 2 yr, use not advised during lactation

DRUG INTERACTIONS OF CONCERN TO DENTISTRY

• Increased risk of respiratory and cardiovascular collapse: benzodiazepines
• Increased CNS depression: all CNS depressants, concomitant use of other opioids

SERIOUS REACTIONS

! Overdose results in cold and clammy skin, weakness, confusion, severe respiratory depression, cyanosis, pinpoint pupils, and extreme somnolence progressing to seizures, stupor, and coma.

DENTAL CONSIDERATIONS

General:

• Patients taking this drug for opioid dependence; avoid the use of any drug with abuse potential.
• Consider aspirin, acetaminophen, or NSAIDs for the management of dental-related pain.
• Monitor vital signs at every appointment because of cardiovascular side effects.
• After supine positioning, have patient sit upright for at least 2 minutes to avoid orthostatic hypotension.

• Assess salivary flow as a factor in caries, periodontal disease, and candidiasis.
• Consider semisupine chair position for patient comfort if GI or respiratory side effects occur.
• Take precautions if dental surgery is anticipated and general anesthesia is required.
• If opioid or sedative drugs are required for patient management and comfort, advise current drug abuse care facility or aftercare program as appropriate.
Consultations:
• Consultations may be difficult to obtain where treatment confidentiality of drug dependence is followed.
• Medical consultation may be required to assess disease control.
Teach Patient/Family to:
• Use effective oral hygiene to prevent soft tissue inflammation.
• When chronic dry mouth occurs, advise patient to:
  • Avoid mouth rinses with high alcohol content because of drying effects
  • Use daily home fluoride products for anticaries effect
  • Use sugarless gum, frequent sips of water, or saliva substitutes

bupropion
byoo-proe′-pee-on
(Wellbutrin, Wellbutrin SR, Wellbutrin XL, Zyban, Zyban sustained release[AUS])
Do not confuse bupropion with buspirone, Wellbutrin with Wellcovorin or Wellferon, or Zyban with Zagam.

CATEGORY AND SCHEDULE
Pregnancy Risk Category: B

Drug Class: Antidepressant

MECHANISM OF ACTION
An aminoketone that blocks the reuptake of neurotransmitters, including serotonin and norepinephrine at CNS presynaptic membranes, increasing their availability at postsynaptic receptor sites. Also reduces the firing rate of noradrenergic neurons. ***Therapeutic Effect:*** Relieves depression and nicotine withdrawal symptoms.

USES
Treatment of depression; smoking cessation treatment (Zyban)

PHARMACOKINETICS
Rapidly absorbed from the GI tract. Protein binding: 84%. Crosses the blood-brain barrier. Undergoes extensive first-pass metabolism in the liver to active metabolite. Primarily excreted in urine. ***Half-life:*** 14 hr.

INDICATIONS AND DOSAGES
▶ **Depression**
PO (Immediate-Release)
Adults. Initially, 100 mg twice a day. May increase to 100 mg 3 times a day no sooner than 3 days after beginning therapy. Maximum: 450 mg/day.
Elderly. 37.5 mg twice a day. May increase by 37.5 mg q3–4 days. Maintenance: Lowest effective dosage.
PO (Sustained-Release)
Adults. Initially, 150 mg/day as a single dose in the morning. May increase to 150 mg twice a day as early as day 4 after beginning therapy. Maximum: 400 mg/day.
Elderly. 50–100 mg/day. May increase by 50–100 mg/day q3–4 days. Maintenance: Lowest effective dosage.
PO (Extended-Release)

Adults. 150 mg once a day. May increase to 300 mg once a day. Maximum: 450 mg a day.

▶ **Smoking Cessation**
PO
Adults. Initially, 150 mg a day for 3 days; then 150 mg twice a day for 7–12 wk.

SIDE EFFECTS/ADVERSE REACTIONS
Frequent
Constipation, weight gain or loss, nausea, vomiting, anorexia, dry mouth, headache, diaphoresis, tremors, sedation, insomnia, dizziness, agitation
Occasional
Diarrhea, akinesia, blurred vision, tachycardia, confusion, hostility, fatigue

PRECAUTIONS AND CONTRAINDICATIONS
Current or prior diagnosis of anorexia nervosa or bulimia, seizure disorder, use within 14 days of MAOIs
Caution
Renal and hepatic disease, recent MI, cranial trauma, lactation, children, low abuse potential; increased CNS or psychiatric symptoms may occur with use

DRUG INTERACTIONS OF CONCERN TO DENTISTRY
• Increased adverse reactions (seizures): tricyclic antidepressants, phenothiazines, benzodiazepines, alcohol, haloperidol, and trazodone
• Decreased serum levels with carbamazepine
• Inhibits CYP2D6 isoenzymes; use with caution; other drugs metabolized by this enzyme

SERIOUS REACTIONS
❗ The risk of seizures increases in patients taking more than 150 mg/dose of bupropion, in patients with a history of bulimia or seizure disorders, and in patients discontinuing drugs that may lower the seizure threshold.

DENTAL CONSIDERATIONS
General:
• Assess salivary flow as a factor in caries, periodontal disease, and candidiasis.
• Short appointments and a stress-reduction protocol may be required for anxious patients.
• See nicotine dose forms for additional smoking cessation considerations.
Consultations:
• Medical consultation may be required to assess disease control and patient's ability to tolerate stress.
• Physician should be informed if significant xerostomic side effects occur (e.g., increased caries, sore tongue, problems eating or swallowing, difficulty wearing prosthesis) so that a medication change can be considered.
Teach Patient/Family:
• When chronic dry mouth occurs, advise patient to:
    • Avoid mouth rinses with high alcohol content because of drying effects
    • Use daily home fluoride products for anticaries effect
    • Use sugarless gum, frequent sips of water, or saliva substitutes

buspirone hydrochloride
byoo-spir'-own hi-droh-klor'-ide
(BuSpar, Buspirex[CAN],
Bustab[CAN])
Do not confuse buspirone with
bupropion.

CATEGORY AND SCHEDULE
Pregnancy Risk Category: B

Drug Class: Antianxiety agent

MECHANISM OF ACTION
Although its exact mechanism of
action is unknown, this
nonbarbiturate is thought to bind to
serotonin and dopamine receptors in
the CNS. The drug may also increase
norepinephrine metabolism in the
locus ceruleus. *Therapeutic Effect:*
Produces anxiolytic effect.

USES
Management and short-term relief of
anxiety disorders; unapproved: PMS

PHARMACOKINETICS
Rapidly and completely absorbed
from the GI tract. Protein binding:
95%. Undergoes extensive first-pass
metabolism. Metabolized in the liver
to active metabolite. Primarily
excreted in urine. Not removed by
hemodialysis. *Half-life:* 2–3 hr.

INDICATIONS AND DOSAGES
▶ **Short-Term Management (up to 4
wk) of Anxiety Disorders**
PO
Adults. 5 mg 2–3 times a day or
7.5 mg twice a day. May increase by
5 mg/day every 2–4 days.
Maintenance: 15–30 mg/day in
2–3 divided doses. Maximum:
60 mg/day.

Elderly. Initially, 5 mg twice a day.
May increase by 5 mg/day every
2–3 days. Maximum: 60 mg/day.
Children. Initially, 5 mg/day. May
increase by 5 mg/day at weekly
intervals. Maximum: 60 mg/day.

SIDE EFFECTS/ADVERSE REACTIONS
Frequent
Dizziness, somnolence, nausea,
headache
Occasional
Nervousness, fatigue, insomnia,
dry mouth, lightheadedness,
mood swings, blurred vision,
poor concentration, diarrhea,
paraesthesia
Rare
Muscle pain and stiffness, nightmares,
chest pain, involuntary movements

PRECAUTIONS AND CONTRAINDICATIONS
Concurrent use of MAOIs, severe
hepatic or renal impairment
Caution
Lactation, elderly, impaired hepatic/
renal function

DRUG INTERACTIONS OF CONCERN TO DENTISTRY
• Increased sedation: alcohol, all
CNS depressants
• Increased plasma levels:
fluconazole, ketoconazole,
itraconazole, miconazole,
erythromycin, clarithromycin,
troleandomycin

SERIOUS REACTIONS
! Buspirone does not appear to cause
drug tolerance, psychological or
physical dependence, or withdrawal
syndrome.
! Overdose may produce severe
nausea, vomiting, dizziness,
drowsiness, abdominal distention,
and excessive pupil contraction.

3

DENTAL CONSIDERATIONS

General:
- Monitor vital signs at every appointment because of cardiovascular side effects.
- Assess salivary flow as a factor in caries, periodontal disease, and candidiasis.
- Short appointments and a stress-reduction protocol may be required for anxious patients.
- Determine why the patient is taking the drug.

Consultations:
- Medical consultation may be required to assess disease control.

Teach Patient/Family:
- When chronic dry mouth occurs, advise patient to:
  - Avoid mouth rinses with high alcohol content because of drying effects
  - Use daily home fluoride products for anticaries effect
  - Use sugarless gum, frequent sips of water, or saliva substitutes

busulfan

byoo-sull'-fan
(Busulfex, Myleran)
Do not confuse Myleran with Alkeran, Leukeran, or Mylicon.

CATEGORY AND SCHEDULE

Pregnancy Risk Category: D

Drug Class: Antineoplastic

MECHANISM OF ACTION

An alkylating agent that interferes with DNA replication and RNA synthesis. Cell cycle-phase nonspecific. **_Therapeutic Effect:_** Disrupts nucleic acid function and causes myelosuppression.

USES

Treatment of chronic myelogenous leukemia, orphan drug in preparative therapy for malignancies treated with bone marrow transplant

PHARMACOKINETICS

Completely absorbed from the GI tract. Protein binding: 33%. Metabolized in the liver. Primarily excreted in urine. Minimally removed by hemodialysis. **_Half-life:_** 2.5 hr.

INDICATIONS AND DOSAGES

▸ **Remission Induction in Chronic Myelogenous Leukemia (CML)**
PO
Adults, Elderly. 4–8 mg/day up to 12 mg/day. Maintenance: 1–4 mg/day to 2 mg/wk. Continue until WBC count is 10,000–20,000/mm^3, resume when WBC count reaches 50,000/mm^3.
Children. 0.06–0.12 mg/kg/day. Maintenance: Titrate to maintain leukocyte count above 40,000/mm^3, reduce dose by 50% if count is 30,000–40,000/mm^3, and discontinue if the count is 20,000/mm^3 or less
▸ **Marrow Ablative Conditioning for Bone Marrow Transplantation**
IV
Adults, Elderly, Children weighing more than 12 kg. 0.8 mg/kg/dose q6h for total of 16 doses. (Use IBW or ABW, whichever is lower.)
Children weighing 12 kg or less. 1.1 mg/kg/dose (IBW) q6h for 16 doses.
PO
Adults, Elderly, Children. 1 mg/kg/dose (IBW) q6h for 16 doses.

SIDE EFFECTS/ADVERSE REACTIONS

Expected
Nausea, stomatitis, vomiting, anorexia, insomnia, diarrhea, fever, abdominal pain, anxiety

Frequent
Headache, rash, asthenia, infection, chills, tachycardia, dyspepsia
Occasional
Constipation, dizziness, edema, pruritus, cough, dry mouth, depression, abdominal enlargement, pharyngitis, hiccups, back pain, alopecia, myalgia
Rare
Injection site pain, arthralgia, confusion, hypotension, lethargy

PRECAUTIONS AND CONTRAINDICATIONS
Disease resistance to previous therapy with this drug
Caution
Childbearing-age men and women, leukopenia, thrombocytopenia, anemia, hepatotoxicity, renal toxicity

DRUG INTERACTIONS OF CONCERN TO DENTISTRY
• Acetaminophen may reduce clearance if given within 72 hr before busulfan administration

SERIOUS REACTIONS
❗ Busulfan's major adverse effect is myelosuppression, resulting in hematologic toxicity, as evidenced by anemia, severe leukopenia, and severe thrombocytopenia.
❗ Very high busulfan dosages may produce blurred vision, muscle twitching, and tonic-clonic seizures.
❗ Long-term therapy (more than 4 yr) may produce pulmonary syndrome ("busulfan lung"), characterized by persistent cough, congestion, crackles, and dyspnea.
❗ Hyperuricemia may produce uric acid nephropathy, renal calculi, and acute renal failure.

DENTAL CONSIDERATIONS
General:
• Patients taking opioids for acute or chronic pain should be given alternative analgesics for dental pain.
• Consider semisupine chair position for patient comfort if GI side effects occur.
• Chlorhexidine mouth rinse (nonalcoholic) before and during chemotherapy may reduce severity of mucositis.
• Patients on chronic drug therapy may rarely have symptoms of blood dyscrasias, which can include infection, bleeding, and poor healing.
• Palliative medication may be required for management of oral side effects.
• Apply lubricant to dry lips for patient comfort before dental procedures.
• Assess salivary flow as factor in caries, periodontal disease, and candidiasis.
• Patients in active chemotherapy treatment should have adequate WBC count before completing dental procedures that may produce a wound. Consultation with the oncologist may be required to determine WBC counts before treatment.
Consultations:
• Medical consultation may be required to assess disease control and patient's ability to tolerate stress.
• In a patient with symptoms of blood dyscrasias, request a medical consultation for blood studies and postpone dental treatment until normal values are reestablished.
• Consult oncologist; prophylactic or therapeutic antibiotics may be indicated to prevent or treat infection if surgery or deep scaling is planned.

Teach Patient/Family to:
• Use effective oral hygiene to prevent soft tissue inflammation
• Prevent trauma when using oral hygiene aids
• Report oral lesions, soreness, or bleeding to dentist
• See dentist immediately if secondary oral infection occurs
• Update medical/drug record if physician makes any changes in evaluation or drug regimen
• When chronic dry mouth occurs, advise patient to:
  • Avoid mouth rinses with high alcohol content because of drying effects
  • Use daily home fluoride products for anticaries effect
  • Use sugarless gum, frequent sips of water, or artificial saliva substitutes

butabarbital sodium
byoo-tah-bar'-bi-tal
(Butisol)

CATEGORY AND SCHEDULE
Pregnancy Risk Category: D
Controlled Substance: Schedule III

Drug Class: Anticonvulsant; antihyperbilirubinemic; sedative-hypnotic

MECHANISM OF ACTION
A barbiturate and nonselective CNS depressant that binds at GABA receptor complex, enhancing GABA activity. *Therapeutic Effect:* Produces hypnotic effect due to CNS depression.

USES
May be used before surgery to relieve anxiety or tension. In addition, some are used as anticonvulsants to help control seizures in certain disorders or diseases, such as epilepsy.

PHARMACOKINETICS
Widely distributed. Metabolized in liver. Minimally excreted unchanged in urine. *Half-life:* 34–100 hr.

INDICATIONS AND DOSAGES
▸ **Insomnia, Short-Term**
PO
Adults. 50–100 mg at bedtime.
▸ **Preoperative Sedation**
PO
Adults. 50–100 mg, 60–90 min before surgery.
Children. 2–6 mg/kg. Maximum: 100 mg.
▸ **Sedation, Daytime**
PO
Adults. 15–30 mg 3–4 times a day.

SIDE EFFECTS/ADVERSE REACTIONS
Occasional
Somnolence
Rare
Confusion, dizziness, agitation, nausea, vomiting, constipation, headache, hypotension, acnes

PRECAUTIONS AND CONTRAINDICATIONS
Porphyria, barbiturate sensitivity

DRUG INTERACTIONS OF CONCERN TO DENTISTRY
• Nephrotoxicity and/or hepatotoxicity: halogenated hydrocarbon anesthetics
• Increased CNS depression: alcohol and all other CNS depressants

- Increased metabolism of: oral anticoagulants, glucocorticoids, carbamazepine, tricyclic antidepressants

SERIOUS REACTIONS
! Skin eruptions appear as hypersensitivity reaction.
! Blood dyscrasias, liver disease, and hypocalcemia occur rarely.

DENTAL CONSIDERATIONS
General:
- Determine why patient is taking the drug.
- Monitor vital signs at every appointment due to cardiovascular side effects.
- Patient on chronic drug therapy may rarely present with symptoms of blood dyscrasias, which can include infection, bleeding and poor healing. If dyscrasia is present, caution patient to prevent oral tissue trauma when using oral hygiene aids.
- When used for sedation in dentistry:
  - Have responsible person drive patient to and from dental office when drug used for conscious sedation.
  - After supine positioning, have patient sit upright for at least 2 min before standing to avoid orthostatic hypotension.
  - Geriatric patients are more susceptible to drug effects, use lower dose.
  - Barbiturates induce certain liver enzymes that can alter the metabolism of other drugs (see drug interactions).
Consultations:
- In a patient with symptoms of blood dyscrasias, request a medical consultation for blood studies and postpone treatment until normal values are reestablished.

Teach Patient/Family to:
- Avoid driving or other activities requiring mental alertness
- Avoid alcohol ingestion or CNS depressants; serious CNS depression may result
- Avoid OTC preparations that contain CNS depressants (antihistamine, cold remedies)
- Update health and medication history if physician makes any changes in evaluation or drug regimens; include OTC, herbal, and nonherbal remedies in the update

butenafine
byoo-ten'-ah-feen
(Mentax)

CATEGORY AND SCHEDULE
Pregnancy Risk Category: B

Drug Class: Antifungal

MECHANISM OF ACTION
An antifungal agent that locks biosynthesis of ergosterol, essential for fungal cell membrane. Fungicidal. *Therapeutic Effect:* Relieves athlete's foot.

USES
Treatment of tinea pedis caused by *E. floccosum, T. mentagrophytes,* or *T. rubrum;* and tinea versicolor caused by *Malassezia furfur*

PHARMACOKINETICS
Total amount absorbed into systemic circulation has not been determined. Metabolized in liver. Excreted in urine. *Half-life:* 35 hr.

INDICATIONS AND DOSAGES
▸ **Tinea Pedis, Tinea Corporis, Tinea Cruris, Tinea Versicolor**

Topical
Adults, Elderly, Children 12 yr and older. Apply to affected area and immediate surrounding skin daily for 4 wk.

SIDE EFFECTS/ADVERSE REACTIONS
Occasional
Contact dermatitis, burning/ stinging, worsening of the condition
Rare
Erythema, irritation, pruritus

PRECAUTIONS AND CONTRAINDICATIONS
Hypersensitivity to butenafine or any component of the formulation
Caution
External use only, lactation, children younger than 12 yr, not for oral use

DRUG INTERACTIONS OF CONCERN TO DENTISTRY
None reported

SERIOUS REACTIONS
None known

---

butoconazole
byoo-toe-ko′-na-zole
(Gynazole-1, Femstat One[CAN])Mycelex-32%

CATEGORY AND SCHEDULE
Pregnancy Risk Category: C

Drug Class: Antifungal

MECHANISM OF ACTION
An antifungal similar to imidazole derivatives that inhibits the steroid synthesis, a vital component of fungal cell formation, thereby damaging the fungal cell membrane. *Therapeutic Effect:* Fungistatic.

USES
Treatment of vulvovaginal infections caused by **Candida** spp.

PHARMACOKINETICS
Not known

INDICATIONS AND DOSAGES
▶ **Treatment of Candidiasis**
Topical
Adults, Elderly. Insert 1 full applicator intravaginally at bedtime for up to 6 days.

SIDE EFFECTS/ADVERSE REACTIONS
Occasional
Vaginal itching, burning, irritation

PRECAUTIONS AND CONTRAINDICATIONS
Hypersensitivity to butoconazole or any of its components
Caution
Lactation

SERIOUS REACTIONS
! Soreness, swelling, pelvic pain, or cramping rarely occurs.

DENTAL CONSIDERATIONS
General:
• Examine oral mucous membranes for signs of yeast infection.
• Broad-spectrum antibiotics for dental infections may cause vaginal yeast infection.

butorphanol tartrate

byoo-tor'-fa-nole
Schedule IV
(Stadol, Stadol NS)
Do not confuse butorphanol with
butabarbital or Stadol with Haldol.

CATEGORY AND SCHEDULE

Pregnancy Risk Category: C, D if
used for prolonged time, high dose
at term
Controlled Substance: Schedule IV

Drug Class: Analgesic;
anesthesia adjunct; anesthesia
adjunct, opioid analgesic;
antidiarrheal; antitussive;
pulmonary edema therapy
adjunct; suppressant, narcotic
abstinence syndrome

MECHANISM OF ACTION

An opioid that binds to opiate
receptor sites in the CNS. Reduces
intensity of pain stimuli incoming
from sensory nerve endings.
Therapeutic Effect: Alters pain
perception and emotional response
to pain.

USES

Pain relief

PHARMACOKINETICS

Route	Onset	Peak	Duration
IM	10–30 min	30–60 min	3–4 hr
IV	Less than 1 min	30 min	2–4 hr
Nasal	15 min	1–2 hr	4–5 hr

Rapidly absorbed after IM injection.
Protein binding: 80%. Extensively
metabolized in the liver. Primarily
excreted in urine. *Half-life:*
2.5–4 hr.

INDICATIONS AND DOSAGES

▸ **Analgesia**
IV
Adults. 0.5–2 mg q3–4h as
needed.
Elderly. 1 mg q4–6h as needed.
IM
Adults. 1–4 mg q3–4h as needed.
Elderly. 1 mg q4–6h as needed.
▸ **Migraine**
Nasal
Adults. 1 mg or 1 spray in one
nostril. May repeat in 60–90 min.
May repeat 2-dose sequence q3–4h
as needed. Alternatively, 2 mg or
1 spray each nostril if patient
remains recumbent, may repeat
in 3–4 hr.

SIDE EFFECTS/ADVERSE REACTIONS

Frequent
Parenteral: Somnolence, dizziness
Nasal: Nasal congestion, insomnia
Occasional
Parenteral: Confusion, diaphoresis,
clammy skin, lethargy, headache,
nausea, vomiting, dry
mouth
Nasal: Vasodilation, constipation,
unpleasant taste, dyspnea, epistaxis,
nasal irritation, upper respiratory
tract infection, tinnitus
Rare
Parenteral: Hypotension, pruritus,
blurred vision, sensation of heat,
CNS stimulation, insomnia
Nasal: Hypertension, tremor, ear
pain, paresthesia, depression,
sinusitis

PRECAUTIONS AND CONTRAINDICATIONS

CNS disease that affects
respirations, physical dependence on
other opioid analgesics, preexisting
respiratory depression, pulmonary
disease

DRUG INTERACTIONS OF CONCERN TO DENTISTRY

- Increased CNS depression: alcohol and all CNS depressants
- Decreased effects of: buprenorphine
- Use caution or avoid use in patients taking MAOIs
- Avoid use in narcotic-dependent persons
- Possible decrease in effects: drugs that induce CYP3A4 isoenzymes (phenobarbital, carbamazepine)
- Possible increase in effects: drugs that inhibit CYP3A4 isoenzymes (ketoconazole, itraconazole, erythromycin, protease inhibitors)

SERIOUS REACTIONS

! Abrupt withdrawal after prolonged use may produce symptoms of narcotic withdrawal, such as abdominal cramping, rhinorrhea, lacrimation, anxiety, increased temperature, and piloerection or goose bumps.

! Overdose results in severe respiratory depression, skeletal muscle flaccidity, cyanosis, and extreme somnolence progressing to seizures, stupor, and coma.

! Tolerance to analgesic effect and physical dependence may occur with chronic use.

- This is an acute-use drug; it is doubtful that patients will undergo dental treatment during severe migraine attacks.
- After supine positioning, have patient sit upright for at least 2 min before standing to avoid orthostatic hypotension.
- Psychologic and physical dependence may occur with chronic administration.
- Determine why patient is taking the drug.
- If additional analgesia is required for dental pain, consider alternative analgesics (NSAIDs) in patients taking narcotics for acute or chronic pain.

Teach Patient/Family to:
- Avoid driving or other activities requiring mental alertness
- Avoid alcohol ingestion or CNS depressants; serious CNS depression may result
- Avoid OTC preparations that contain CNS depressants (antihistamine, cold remedies)
- Update health and medication history if physician makes any changes in evaluation or drug regimens; include OTC, herbal, and nonherbal remedies in the update

DENTAL CONSIDERATIONS

General:
- Monitor vital signs at every appointment due to cardiovascular side effects.

cabergoline
kab-err-go´-leen
(Dostinex)

CATEGORY AND SCHEDULE
Pregnancy Risk Category: B

Drug Class: Dopamine agonist;
antihyperprolactinemic

MECHANISM OF ACTION
Agonist at dopamine D2 receptors,
suppressing prolactin secretion.
Therapeutic Effects: Shrinks
prolactinomas, restores gonadal
function.

USES
Treatment of different types of
medical problems that occur when
too much of the hormone prolactin
is produced. It can be used to treat
certain menstrual problems, fertility
problems in men and women, and
pituitary prolactinomas (tumors of
the pituitary gland).

PHARMACOKINETICS
Cabergoline is administered orally
and undergoes significant first-pass
metabolism following systemic
absorption. Extensively metabolized
in the liver. Elimination is primarily
in the feces. *Half-life:* 80 hr.

INDICATIONS AND DOSAGES
▸ **Hyperprolactinemia (idiopathic
or primary pituitary
adenomas)**
PO
Adults, Elderly. 0.25 mg 2 times
a wk, titrate by 0.25 mg/dose no
more than every 4 wk up to 1 mg
2 times a wk.
PV
Adults. 0.5 mg 2 to 5 times
a wk.

▸ **Parkinson's Disease**
PO
Adults. 0.5 mg/day and titrate to
response. Mean effective dose is 3 mg/
day and ranges from 0.5–6 mg/day.
▸ **Restless Legs Syndrome (RLS)**
PO
Adults. 0.5 mg once daily at bedtime,
slowly titrate until symptoms resolve
or drug-intolerance limits further
adjustment. Mean effective dose is
2 mg/day and ranges from
1–4 mg/day.

SIDE EFFECTS/ADVERSE
REACTIONS
Frequent
Nausea, orthostatic hypotension,
confusion, dyskinesia, hallucinations,
peripheral edema
Occasional
Headache, vertigo, dizziness,
dyspepsia, postural hypotension,
constipation, asthenia, fatigue,
abdominal pain, drowsiness
Rare
Vomiting, dry mouth, diarrhea,
flatulence, anxiety, depression,
dysmenorrhea, dyspepsia,
mastalgia, paresthesias, vertigo,
visual impairment, pleuropulmonary
changes, pleural effusion, pulmonary
fibrosis, heart failure, peptic ulcer

PRECAUTIONS AND
CONTRAINDICATIONS
Hypersensitivity to cabergoline,
ergot alkaloids or any one of its
components. Uncontrolled
hypertension.

DRUG INTERACTIONS OF
CONCERN TO DENTISTRY
None reported

SERIOUS REACTIONS
❗ Overdosage may produce nasal
congestion, syncope, or
hallucinations.

DENTAL CONSIDERATIONS

General:
- Determine why patient is taking the drug.
- Monitor vital signs at every appointment for cardiovascular side effects.
- After supine positioning, have patient sit upright for at least 2 min before standing to avoid orthostatic hypotension.
- Use precaution if sedation or general anesthesia is required; risk of hypotensive episode.
- Assess salivary flow as a factor in caries, periodontal disease, and candidiasis.
- Consider semisupine chair position for patient comfort if GI side effects occur.

Consultations:
- Medical consultation may be required to assess disease control.

Teach Patient/Family:
- When chronic dry mouth occurs, advise patient to:
  - Avoid mouth rinses with high alcohol content due to drying effects
  - Use daily home fluoride products for anticaries effect
  - Use sugarless gum, frequent sips of water, or saliva substitutes
- Update health and medication history if physician makes any changes in evaluation or drug regimens; include OTC, herbal, and nonherbal remedies in the update

calcitonin

kal-si-toe′-nin
(Calcimar, Caltine[CAN], Cibacalcin, Miacalcin)
Do not confuse calcitonin with calcitriol.

CATEGORY AND SCHEDULE
Pregnancy Risk Category: C

Drug Class: Synthetic polypeptide calcitonins

MECHANISM OF ACTION
A synthetic hormone that decreases osteoclast activity in bones, decreases tubular reabsorption of sodium and calcium in the kidneys, and increases absorption of calcium in the GI tract. **Therapeutic Effect:** Regulates serum calcium concentrations.

USES
Treatment of Paget's disease, postmenopausal osteoporosis, hypercalcemia

PHARMACOKINETICS
Injection form rapidly metabolized (primarily in kidneys); primarily excreted in urine. Nasal form rapidly absorbed. **Half-life:** 70–90 min (injection); 43 min (nasal).

INDICATIONS AND DOSAGES
▶ **Skin Testing Before Treatment in Patients with Suspected Sensitivity to Calcitonin-Salmon**
Intracutaneous
Adults, Elderly. Prepare a 10-international units/ml dilution; withdraw 0.05 ml from a 200-international units/ml vial in a tuberculin syringe; fill up to 1 ml with 0.9% NaCl. Take 0.1 ml and inject intracutaneously on inner

aspect of forearm. Observe after 15 min; a positive response is the appearance of more than mild erythema or wheal.

▶ **Paget's Disease**
IM, Subcutaneous
Adults, Elderly. Initially, 100 international units/day. Maintenance: 50 international units/day or 50–100 international units every 1–3 days.
Intranasal
Adults, Elderly. 200–400 international units/day.

▶ **Osteoporosis Imperfecta**
IM, Subcutaneous
Adults. 2 international units/kg 3 times a wk.

▶ **Postmenopausal Osteoporosis**
IM, Subcutaneous
Adults, Elderly. 100 international units/day with adequate calcium and vitamin D intake.
Intranasal
Adults, Elderly. 200 international units/day as a single spray, alternating nostrils daily.

▶ **Hypercalcemia**
IM, Subcutaneous
Adults, Elderly. Initially, 4 international units/kg q12h; may increase to 8 international units/kg q12h if no response in 2 days; may further increase to 8 international units/kg q6h if no response in another 2 days.

SIDE EFFECTS/ADVERSE REACTIONS
Frequent
IM, Subcutaneous: Nausea (may occur 30 min after injection, usually diminishes with continued therapy), inflammation at injection site
Nasal: Rhinitis, nasal irritation, redness, sores
Occasional
IM, Subcutaneous: Flushing of face or hands

Nasal: Back pain, arthralgia, epistaxis, headache
Rare
IM, Subcutaneous: Epigastric discomfort, dry mouth, diarrhea, flatulence
Nasal: Itching of earlobes, edema of feet, rash, diaphoresis

PRECAUTIONS AND CONTRAINDICATIONS
Hypersensitivity to gelatin desserts or salmon protein
Caution
Allergy, hypocalcemic tetany, routine monitoring of urine sediment, osteogenic sarcoma in Paget's disease, lactation, children

DRUG INTERACTIONS OF CONCERN TO DENTISTRY
• Supplemental calcium and vitamin D may already be used; do not use additional amounts

SERIOUS REACTIONS
! Patients with a protein allergy may develop a hypersensitivity reaction.

DENTAL CONSIDERATIONS
General:
• Consider semisupine chair position for patient comfort because of effects of disease or if GI side effects occur.
• Assess salivary flow as factor in caries, periodontal disease, and candidiasis.
Teach Patient/Family to:
• Use effective oral hygiene to prevent soft tissue inflammation
• When chronic dry mouth occurs, advise patient to:
  • Avoid mouth rinses with high alcohol content because of drying effects
  • Use daily home fluoride products for anticaries effect
  • Use sugarless gum, frequent sips of water, or saliva substitutes

candesartan cilexetil
kan-de-sar´-tan sill-ex´-eh-till
(Atacand)

CATEGORY AND SCHEDULE
Pregnancy Risk Category: C (D if used in second or third trimester)

Drug Class: Angiotensin II (AT1) receptor antagonist, antihypertensive

MECHANISM OF ACTION
An angiotensin II receptor, type AT1, antagonist that blocks the vasoconstrictor and aldosterone-secreting effects of angiotensin II, inhibiting the binding of angiotensin II to the AT1 receptors. *Therapeutic Effect:* Causes vasodilation, decreases peripheral resistance, and decreases B/P.

USES
Treatment of hypertension, as a single drug or in combination with other antihypertensives

PHARMACOKINETICS
Rapidly, completely absorbed. Protein binding: greater than 99%. Undergoes minor hepatic metabolism to inactive metabolite. Excreted unchanged in urine and in the feces through the biliary system. Not removed by hemodialysis. *Half-life:* 9 hr.

INDICATIONS AND DOSAGES
▸ **Hypertension Alone or in Combination with Other Antihypertensives**
PO
Adults, Elderly, Patients with mildly impaired liver or renal function.
Initially, 16 mg once a day in those who are not volume depleted. Can be given once or twice a day with total daily doses of 8–32 mg. Give lower dosage in those treated with diuretics or with severely impaired renal function.

SIDE EFFECTS/ADVERSE REACTIONS
Occasional
Upper respiratory tract infection, dizziness, back and leg pain
Rare
Pharyngitis, rhinitis, headache, fatigue, diarrhea, nausea, dry cough, peripheral edema

PRECAUTIONS AND CONTRAINDICATIONS
Hypersensitivity to candesartan
Caution
Discontinue drug if pregnancy occurs, risk of fetal and neonatal injury, correct volume depletion if present, renal impairment, pregnancy category C (first trimester) and D (second and third trimesters), lactation

DRUG INTERACTIONS OF CONCERN TO DENTISTRY
● Potential for increased hypotensive effects with other hypotensive and sedative drugs

SERIOUS REACTIONS
❗ Overdosage may manifest as hypotension and tachycardia. Bradycardia occurs less often. Institute supportive measures.

DENTAL CONSIDERATIONS
General:
● Monitor vital signs at every appointment in patients with history of hypertension.
● Evaluate respiration characteristics and rate.
● Consider semisupine chair position for patient comfort if GI side effects occur.

- Observe appropriate limitations of vasoconstrictor doses.
- Limit use of sodium-containing products, such as saline IV fluids, for those patients with a dietary salt restriction.
- Stress from dental procedures may compromise cardiovascular function; determine patient risk.
- Short appointments and a stress-reduction protocol may be required for anxious patients.
- Use precaution if sedation or general anesthesia is required; risk of hypotensive episode.

Consultations:
- Medical consultation may be required to assess disease control and patient's ability to tolerate stress.

Teach Patient/Family to:
- Update health and drug history if physician makes any changes in evaluation or drug regimens

capecitabine
cap-eh-site´-ah-bean
(Xeloda)
Do not confuse Xeloda with Xenical.

CATEGORY AND SCHEDULE
Pregnancy Risk Category: D

Drug Class: Antineoplastic

MECHANISM OF ACTION
An antimetabolite that is enzymatically converted to 5-fluorouracil. Inhibits enzymes necessary for synthesis of essential cellular components. *Therapeutic Effect:* Interferes with DNA synthesis, RNA processing, and protein synthesis.

USES
First-line treatment of patients with metastatic colorectal cancer and metastatic breast cancer resistant to both paclitaxel and anthracycline-containing chemotherapy regimens; colorectal cancer when treatment with a fluoropyrimidine alone is preferred

PHARMACOKINETICS
Readily absorbed from the GI tract. Protein binding: less than 60%. Metabolized in the liver. Primarily excreted in urine. *Half-life:* 45 min.

INDICATIONS AND DOSAGES
▸ **Metastatic Breast Cancer, Colon Cancer**
PO
Adults, Elderly. Initially, 2,500 mg/m^2/day in 2 equally divided doses approximately q12h for 2 wk. Follow with a 1-wk rest period; given in 3-wk cycles.

SIDE EFFECTS/ADVERSE REACTIONS
Frequent
Diarrhea (sometimes severe), nausea, vomiting, stomatitis, hand-and-foot syndrome (painful palmar-plantar swelling with paresthesia, erythema, and blistering), fatigue, anorexia, dermatitis
Occasional
Constipation, dyspepsia, nail disorder, headache, dizziness, insomnia, edema, myalgia

PRECAUTIONS AND CONTRAINDICATIONS
Severe renal impairment
Caution
Food reduces absorption, renal insufficiency, altered coagulation when taken with Coumadin, patients older than 80 yr, pregnancy category D, hepatic dysfunction because of liver metastases, lactation, children younger than 18 yr, avoid use of folic acid

DRUG INTERACTIONS OF CONCERN TO DENTISTRY
• Dental drug interactions not reported; however, patients taking this drug with coumarin oral anticoagulants have altered coagulation parameters, bleeding, or both; INR or PT should be physician-monitored

SERIOUS REACTIONS
! Serious reactions may include myelosuppression (evidenced by neutropenia, thrombocytopenia, and anemia), cardiovascular toxicity (marked by angina, cardiomyopathy, and deep vein thrombosis), respiratory toxicity (marked by dyspnea, epistaxis, and pneumonia), and lymphedema.

DENTAL CONSIDERATIONS
General:
• Monitor vital signs at every appointment because of cardiovascular side effects.
• Patients on chronic drug therapy may have symptoms of blood dyscrasias, which can include infection, bleeding, and poor healing.
• Patients taking opioids for acute or chronic pain should be given alternative analgesics for dental pain.
• Short appointments and a stress reduction protocol may be required for anxious patients.
• Consider semisupine chair position for patient comfort if GI side effects occur.
• Question patient about tolerance of NSAIDs or aspirin related to GI side effects of drug.
• Consider local hemostasis measures to control and prevent excessive bleeding.
• Examine for oral manifestation of opportunistic infection.
• Be aware of oral side effects and potential sequelae.

• Palliative medication may be required for management of oral side effects.
• Avoid dental light in patient's eyes; offer dark glasses for patient comfort.
• Prophylactic or therapeutic antibiotics may be indicated to prevent or treat infection if surgery or periodontal debridement is required.
Consultations:
• In a patient with symptoms of blood dyscrasias, request a medical consultation for blood studies and postpone treatment until normal values are reestablished.
• Medical consultation may be required to assess disease control and patient's ability to receive dental treatment.
• Consultation with physician may be necessary if sedation or general anesthesia is required.
Teach Patient/Family to:
• Prevent trauma when using oral hygiene aids
• See dentist immediately if secondary oral infection occurs
• Use effective oral hygiene to prevent soft tissue inflammation
• Report oral lesions, soreness, or bleeding to dentist
• Update health and drug history if physician makes any changes in evaluation or drug regimens

capsaicin
kap-say´-sin
(Zostrix)
Do not confuse with Zovirax.

CATEGORY AND SCHEDULE
Pregnancy Risk Category: C
OTC

Drug Class: Topical analgesic

MECHANISM OF ACTION

A topical analgesic that depletes and prevents reaccumulation of the chemomediator of pain impulses (substance P) from peripheral sensory neurons to CNS. *Therapeutic Effect:* Relieves pain.

USES

Treatment of neuralgia associated with herpes zoster or diabetic neuropathy; pain of osteoarthritis and rheumatoid arthritis

PHARMACOKINETICS

None reported

INDICATIONS AND DOSAGES
▶ **Treatment of Neuralgia, Osteoarthritis, Rheumatoid Arthritis**
Topical
Adults, Elderly, Children older than 2 yr. Apply directly to affected area 3–4 times a day. Continue for 14–28 days for optimal clinical response.

SIDE EFFECTS/ADVERSE REACTIONS
Frequent
Burning, stinging, erythema at site of application

PRECAUTIONS AND CONTRAINDICATIONS

Hypersensitivity to capsaicin or any component of the formulation
Caution
Lactation, avoid use on broken skin

DRUG INTERACTIONS OF CONCERN TO DENTISTRY

None reported

SERIOUS REACTIONS

None known

DENTAL CONSIDERATIONS
General:
• Determine why the patient is taking the drug.
• Consider location of lesions and alter dental procedures accordingly.
Teach Patient/Family to:
• Wash hands thoroughly after use and avoid contact with mouth or eyes

---

captopril
kap´-toe-pril
(Acenorm[AUS], Capoten, Captohexal[AUS], Novo-Captoril[CAN], Topace[AUS])
Do not confuse captopril with Capitrol.

CATEGORY AND SCHEDULE

Pregnancy Risk Category: C (D if used in second or third trimester)

Drug Class: Angiotensin-converting enzyme (ACE) inhibitor

MECHANISM OF ACTION

An ACE inhibitor that suppresses the renin-angiotensin-aldosterone system and prevents conversion of angiotensin I to angiotensin II, a potent vasoconstrictor; may also inhibit angiotensin II at local vascular and renal sites. Decreases plasma angiotensin II, increases plasma renin activity, and decreases aldosterone secretion. *Therapeutic Effect:* Reduces peripheral arterial resistance, pulmonary capillary wedge pressure; improves cardiac output and exercise tolerance.

USES

Treatment of hypertension, heart failure not responsive to conventional therapy, left ventricular dysfunction (LVD) after MI, diabetic nephropathy

PHARMACOKINETICS

Rapidly, well absorbed from the GI tract (absorption is decreased in the presence of food). Protein binding: 25%–30%. Metabolized in the liver. Primarily excreted in urine. Removed by hemodialysis. *Half-life:* less than 3 hr (increased in those with impaired renal function).

INDICATIONS AND DOSAGES
▸ **Hypertension**
PO
Adults, Elderly. Initially, 12.5–25 mg 2–3 times a day. After 1–2 wk, may increase to 50 mg 2–3 times a day. Diuretic may be added if no response in additional 1–2 wk. If taken in combination with diuretic, may increase to 100–150 mg 2–3 times a day after 1–2 wk. Maintenance: 25–150 mg 2–3 times a day. Maximum: 450 mg/day.
▸ **CHF**
PO
Adults, Elderly. Initially, 6.25–25 mg 3 times a day. Increase to 50 mg 3 times a day. After at least 2 wk, may increase to 50–100 mg 3 times a day. Maximum: 450 mg/day.
▸ **Post-Myocardial Infarction, Impaired Liver Function**
PO
Adults, Elderly. 6.25 mg a day, then 12.5 mg 3 times a day. Increase to 25 mg 3 times a day over several days up to 50 mg 3 times a day over several wk.
▸ **Diabetic Nephropathy Prevention of Kidney Failure**
PO
Adults, Elderly. 25 mg 3 times a day.
Children. Initially 0.3–0.5 mg/kg/ dose titrated up to a maximum of 6 mg/kg/day in 2–4 divided doses.
Neonates. Initially, 0.05–0.1 mg/kg/ dose q8–24h titrated up to 0.5 mg/ kg/dose given q6–24h.

▸ **Dosage in Renal Impairment**
Creatinine clearance 10–50 ml/min. 75% of normal dosage.
Creatinine clearance less than 10 ml/min. 50% of normal dosage.

SIDE EFFECTS/ADVERSE REACTIONS
Frequent
Rash
Occasional
Pruritus, dysgeusia (altered taste)
Rare
Headache, cough, insomnia, dizziness, fatigue, paraesthesia, malaise, nausea, diarrhea or constipation, dry mouth, tachycardia

PRECAUTIONS AND CONTRAINDICATIONS
History of angioedema from previous treatment with ACE inhibitors
Caution
Dialysis patients, hypovolemia, leukemia, scleroderma, lupus erythematosus, blood dyscrasias, CHF, diabetes mellitus, renal disease, thyroid disease, COPD, asthma, discontinue drug if pregnancy is detected

DRUG INTERACTIONS OF CONCERN TO DENTISTRY
• Increased hypotension: alcohol, phenothiazines
• Decreased hypotensive effects: indomethacin and possibly other NSAIDs, sympathomimetics
• Suspected reduction in the antihypertensive and vasodilator effects by salicylates; monitor blood pressure if used concurrently

SERIOUS REACTIONS
❗ Excessive hypotension ("first-dose syncope") may occur in patients with CHF and in those who are severely salt and volume depleted.

! Angioedema (swelling of face and lips) and hyperkalemia occur rarely.

! Agranulocytosis and neutropenia may be noted in those with collagen vascular disease, including scleroderma and systemic lupus erythematosus, and impaired renal function.

! Nephrotic syndrome may be noted in those with history of renal disease.

DENTAL CONSIDERATIONS

General:

• Monitor vital signs at every appointment because of cardiovascular side effects.

• Observe appropriate limitations of vasoconstrictor doses.

• After supine positioning, have patient sit upright for at least 2 min before standing to avoid orthostatic hypotension.

• Patients on chronic drug therapy may rarely have symptoms of blood dyscrasias, which can include infection, bleeding, and poor healing.

• Assess salivary flow as a factor in caries, periodontal disease, and candidiasis.

• Limit use of sodium-containing products, such as saline IV fluids, for patients with a dietary salt restriction.

• Stress from dental procedures may compromise cardiovascular function; determine patient risk.

• Short appointments and a stress-reduction protocol may be required for anxious patients.

Consultations:

• Medical consultation may be required to assess patient's ability to tolerate stress.

• In a patient with symptoms of blood dyscrasias, request a medical consultation for blood studies and postpone dental treatment until normal values are reestablished.

• Take precautions if dental surgery is anticipated and sedation or general anesthesia is required; risk of hypotensive episode.

Teach Patient/Family to:

• Use effective oral hygiene to prevent soft tissue inflammation

• Use caution to prevent injury when using oral hygiene aids

• When chronic dry mouth occurs, advise patient to:

  • Avoid mouth rinses with high alcohol content because of drying effects

  • Use daily home fluoride products for anticaries effect

  • Use sugarless gum, frequent sips of water, or saliva substitutes

carbachol
kar´-ba-kole
(Caroptic, Isopto Carbachol, Miostat)

CATEGORY AND SCHEDULE
Pregnancy Risk Category: C

Drug Class: Antiglaucoma agent, ophthalmic; Antihypertensive agent, ocular, postsurgical; Miotic

MECHANISM OF ACTION
A direct-acting parasympathomimetic agent that stimulates cholinergic receptors resulting in muscarinic and nicotinic effects. Indirectly promotes release of acetylcholine. *Therapeutic Effect:* Produces contraction of the iris sphincter muscle, resulting in miosis, and reduction in intraocular pressure associated with decreased resistance to aqueous humor outflow.

USES
Used in the eye to treat glaucoma

PHARMACOKINETICS
None reported

INDICATIONS AND DOSAGES

▶ **Glaucoma**
Ophthalmic
Adults, Elderly. Instill 1–2 drops of 0.75%–3% solution in affected eye(s) up to 3 times a day.

▶ **Miosis, Ophthalmic Surgery**
Ophthalmic
Adults, Elderly. Instill 0.5 ml of 0.01% solution into anterior chamber before or after securing sutures.

SIDE EFFECTS/ADVERSE REACTIONS
Occasional
Blurred vision, burning/irritation of eye, decreased night vision, headache

PRECAUTIONS AND CONTRAINDICATIONS
Acute iritis, hypersensitivity to carbachol or any component of the formulation

DRUG INTERACTIONS OF CONCERN TO DENTISTRY
None reported

SERIOUS REACTIONS
None reported

DENTAL CONSIDERATIONS
General:
• Determine why patient is taking the drug.
• Avoid drugs with anticholinergic activity, such as antihistamines, opioids, benzodiazepines, propantheline, atropine, and scopolamine.
• Avoid dental light in patient's eyes; offer dark glasses for patient comfort.
• Protect patient's eyes from accidental spatter during dental treatment.
• Question glaucoma patient about compliance with prescribed drug regimen.

Consultations:
• Medical consultation may be required to assess disease control.
Teach Patient/Family to:
• Update health and medication history if physician makes any changes in evaluation or drug regimens; include OTC, herbal, and nonherbal remedies in the update

carbamazepine
kar-ba-maz´-eh-peen
(Apo-Carbamazepine[CAN], Carbatrol, Epitol, Equetro, Tegretol, Tegretol CR[AUS], Tegretol XR, Teril[AUS])
Do not confuse Tegretol with Cartrol, Toradol, or Trental.

CATEGORY AND SCHEDULE
Pregnancy Risk Category: D

Drug Class: Anticonvulsant

MECHANISM OF ACTION
An iminostilbene derivative that decreases sodium and calcium ion influx into neuronal membranes, reducing post-tetanic potentiation at synapses. *Therapeutic Effect:* Reduces seizure activity.

USES
Treatment of tonic-clonic, complex-partial, and mixed seizures; trigeminal neuralgia; unapproved: neurogenic pain, some psychotic disorders, diabetes insipidus, alcohol withdrawal

PHARMACOKINETICS
Slowly and completely absorbed from the GI tract. Protein binding: 75%. Metabolized in the liver to active metabolite. Primarily excreted in urine. Not removed by hemodialysis. *Half-life:* 25–65 hr (decreased with chronic use).

INDICATIONS AND DOSAGES
▶ **Seizure Control**
PO
Adults, Children older than 12 yr.
Initially, 200 mg twice a day. May
increase dosage by 200 mg/day at
weekly intervals. Range:
400–1200 mg/day in 2–4 divided
doses. Maximum: 1.6–2.4 g/day.
Children 6–12 yr. Initially, 100 mg
twice a day. May increase by
100 mg/day at weekly intervals.
Range: 20–30 mg/kg/day.
Maximum: 1000 mg/day.
Children younger than 6 yr. Initially
5 mg/kg/day. May increase at weekly
intervals to 10 mg/kg/day up to
20 mg/kg/day.
Elderly. Initially 100 mg 1–2 times
a day. May increase by 100 mg/day at
weekly intervals. Usual dose
400–1000 mg/day.
▶ **Trigeminal Neuralgia, Diabetic
Neuropathy**
PO
Adults. Initially, 100 mg twice a day.
May increase by 100 mg twice a day
up to 400–800 mg/day. Maximum:
1200 mg/day.
Elderly. Initially 100 mg 1–2 times
a day. May increase by 100 mg/day at
weekly intervals. Usual dose
400–1000 mg/day.

SIDE EFFECTS/ADVERSE REACTIONS
Frequent
Drowsiness, dizziness, nausea,
vomiting
Occasional
Visual abnormalities (spots before
eyes, difficulty focusing, blurred
vision), dry mouth or pharynx,
tongue irritation, headache, fluid
retention, diaphoresis, constipation
or diarrhea, behavioral changes in
children

PRECAUTIONS AND CONTRAINDICATIONS
Concomitant use of MAOIs, history
of myelosuppression,
hypersensitivity to tricyclic
antidepressants.
Caution
Glaucoma, hepatic disease, renal
disease, cardiac disease, psychosis,
lactation, children younger
than 6 yr

DRUG INTERACTIONS OF CONCERN TO DENTISTRY
• Decreased metabolism:
erythromycin, clarithromycin,
propoxyphene, troleandomycin,
metronidazole, ketoconazole,
fluconazole, itraconazole, or any
drug that inhibits CYP450 3A4
enzymes
• Increased serum levels: tricyclic
antidepressants, fluoxetine,
fluvoxamine, nefazodone,
ketoconazole, itraconazole
• Increased CNS depression:
haloperidol, phenothiazines
• Decreased half-life: doxycycline
• Potential hepatotoxicity: chronic
high doses of carbamazepine with
acetaminophen
• Decreased effects of phenobarbital,
corticosteroids, benzodiazepines,
doxycycline, sertraline

SERIOUS REACTIONS
! Toxic reactions may include blood
dyscrasias (such as aplastic anemia,
agranulocytosis, thrombocytopenia,
leukopenia, leukocytosis, and
eosinophilia), cardiovascular
disturbances (such as CHF,
hypotension or hypertension,
thrombophlebitis, and arrhythmias),
and dermatologic effects (such as
rash, urticaria, pruritus, and
photosensitivity).
! Abrupt withdrawal may precipitate
status epilepticus.

DENTAL CONSIDERATIONS
General:
- Monitor vital signs at every appointment because of cardiovascular side effects.
- Patients on chronic drug therapy may rarely have symptoms of blood dyscrasias, which can include infection, bleeding, and poor healing.
- Assess salivary flow as a factor in caries, periodontal disease, and candidiasis.
- Short appointments and a stress-reduction protocol may be required for anxious patients.
- Talk with patient about type of epilepsy, seizure frequency, and quality of seizure control.

Consultations:
- In a patient with symptoms of blood dyscrasias, request a medical consultation for blood studies and postpone dental treatment until normal values are reestablished.
- Medical consultation may be required to assess disease control and patient's ability to tolerate stress.

Teach Patient/Family to:
- Use effective oral hygiene to prevent soft tissue inflammation
- Use caution to prevent injury when using oral hygiene aids
- Use caution when driving or performing other tasks requiring alertness.
- When chronic dry mouth occurs, advise patient to:
  - Avoid mouth rinses with high alcohol content because of drying effects
  - Use daily home fluoride products for anticaries effect
  - Use sugarless gum, frequent sips of water, or saliva substitutes

carbamide peroxide
kahr´-buh-mahyd
(Auro Ear Drops, Debrox, E•R•O Ear, GlyOxide, Mollifene Ear Wax Removing, Murine Ear Drops, Orajel Perioseptic, Proxigel)
(gel, solution)

CATEGORY AND SCHEDULE
Pregnancy Risk Category: C

Drug Class: Cerumenolytic; topical oral antiinflammatory

MECHANISM OF ACTION
A cerumenolytic that releases oxygen on contact with moist mouth tissues to provide cleansing effects, reduce inflammation, relieve pain, and inhibit odor-forming bacteria. In the ear, oxygen is released and hydrogen peroxide is reduced to water, which enables the chemical reaction.
Therapeutic Effect: Relieves inflammation of gums and lips. Emulsifies and disperses ear wax.

USES
Dental whitener

PHARMACOKINETICS
Not known

INDICATIONS AND DOSAGES
▶ **Earwax Removal**
Topical, solution
Adults, Elderly, Children 12 yr or older. Tilt head and administer 5–10 drops twice a day for up to 4 days.
Children 12 yr or younger. Tilt head and administer 1–5 drops twice a day for up to 4 days.
▶ **Oral Lesions**
Topical, gel
Adults, Elderly, Children. Apply to affected area 4 times a day.

Topical, solution
Adults, Elderly, Children. Apply
several drops undiluted on affected
area 4 times a day after meals and
at bedtime.

SIDE EFFECTS/ADVERSE REACTIONS
Occasional
Oral: Gingival sensitivity

PRECAUTIONS AND CONTRAINDICATIONS
Dizziness, ear discharge or drainage,
ear injury, ear pain, irritation, or rash,
hypersensitivity to carbamide
peroxide or any one of its
components

DRUG INTERACTIONS OF CONCERN TO DENTISTRY
None reported

SERIOUS REACTIONS
! Opportunistic infections caused
by organisms like Candida
albicans is possible with
prolonged use.

DENTAL CONSIDERATIONS
General:
• For oral ulcers, perform an oral
exam to rule out possible local
contributing factors such as
broken tooth or filling or ill-fitting
dentures.
• Question patient about symptom
history; onset, duration, and
frequency.
• This drug is the principal
ingredient in tooth bleaching or
whiting agents; avoid excessive
use.
Teach Patient/Family:
• To see the dentist if symptoms
worsen or do not abate within
7 days

Carbinoxamine Maleate 237

carbinoxamine maleate
kar-bi-nox´-ah-meen mal-ee-ate
(Carboxine, Histex CT, Histex I/E,
Histex PD, Histex Pd 12, Palgic,
Pediatex, Pediox)

CATEGORY AND SCHEDULE
Pregnancy Risk Category: C

Drug Class: Antihistaminic
(H 1-receptor)-decongestant

MECHANISM OF ACTION
An antihistamine that exhibits H1
receptor blocking action.
Therapeutic Effect: Prevents allergic
responses mediated by histamine,
such as rhinitis.

USES
Treatment of the nasal congestion
(stuffy nose), sneezing, and runny
nose caused by colds and hay
fever

PHARMACOKINETICS
Virtually no intact drug is excreted
in urine. ***Half-life:*** 1–20 hr.

INDICATIONS AND DOSAGES
▶ Allergic Rhinitis
PO
Adults, Children 6 yr and Older.
1 tsp 4 times a day.
Children 18 mo–6 yr. $^1/_2$ tsp 4 times
a day.
Children 9–18 mo. $^1/_4$–$^1/_2$ tsp 4 times
a day.

SIDE EFFECTS/ADVERSE REACTIONS
Frequent
Somnolence, dizziness, muscle
weakness, hypotension, urine
retention, thickening of bronchial
secretions, dry mouth, nose, throat,

or lips; in elderly, sedation, dizziness, hypotension
Occasional
Epigastric distress, vomiting, headache
Rare
Excitability in children

PRECAUTIONS AND CONTRAINDICATIONS
Hypersensitivity or idiosyncrasy to any ingredients, patients taking MAOIs

DRUG INTERACTIONS OF CONCERN TO DENTISTRY
• Increased sedation: alcohol and all CNS depressants
• Prolonged sedative and anticholinergic effects: MAOIs

SERIOUS REACTIONS
! Overdose symptoms may vary from CNS depression, including sedation, apnea, hypotension, cardiovascular collapse, and death, to severe paradoxical reactions, such as hallucinations, tremor, and seizures.

DENTAL CONSIDERATIONS
General:
• Assess salivary flow as a factor in caries, periodontal disease, and candidiasis.
• Determine why patient is taking the drug.
Teach Patient/Family to:
• Use effective oral hygiene to prevent soft tissue inflammation
• Prevent trauma when using oral hygiene aids
• When chronic dry mouth occurs, advise patient to:
  • Avoid mouth rinses with high alcohol content due to drying effects
  • Use daily home fluoride products for anticaries effect
  • Use sugarless gum, frequent sips of water, or saliva substitutes

carboplatin
kar-bow-play´-tin
(Paraplatin)
Do not confuse carboplatin with Cisplatin or Platinol.

CATEGORY AND SCHEDULE
Pregnancy risk category: D

Drug Class: Antineoplastic

MECHANISM OF ACTION
A platinum coordination complex that inhibits DNA synthesis by cross-linking with DNA strands, preventing cell division. Cell cycle–phase nonspecific. *Therapeutic Effect:* Interferes with DNA function.

USES
Treatment of cancer of the ovaries

PHARMACOKINETICS
Protein binding: Low. Hydrolyzed in solution to active form. Primarily excreted in urine. *Half-life:* 2.6–5.9 hr.

INDICATIONS AND DOSAGES
▶ **Ovarian Carcinoma (Monotherapy)**
IV
Adults. 360 mg/m^2 on day 1, every 4 wk. Do not repeat dose until neutrophil and platelet counts are within acceptable levels. Adjust drug dosage in previously treated patients based on lowest post-treatment platelet or neutrophil count. Increase dosage only once to no more than 125% of starting dose.
▶ **Ovarian Carcinoma (Combination Therapy)**
IV
Adults. 300 mg/m^2 (with cyclophosphamide) on day 1, every 4 wk. Don't repeat dose until neutrophil and platelet counts are within acceptable levels.

Children. 300–600 mg/m² every
4 wk for solid tumor, or 175 mg/m²
every 4 wk for brain tumor.
▸ **Dosage in Renal Impairment**
Initial dosage is based on creatinine
clearance; subsequent dosages are
based on the patient's tolerance and
degree of myelosuppression.

Creatinine Clearance	Dosage Day 1
60 ml/min or greater	360 mg/m²
41–59 ml/min	250 mg/m²
16–40 ml/min	200 mg/m²

SIDE EFFECTS/ADVERSE REACTIONS
Frequent
Nausea, vomiting
Occasional
Generalized pain, diarrhea or
constipation, peripheral neuropathy
Rare
Alopecia, asthenia, hypersensitivity
reaction (erythema, pruritus, rash,
urticaria)

PRECAUTIONS AND CONTRAINDICATIONS
History of severe allergic reaction
to cisplatin, platinum compounds,
or mannitol; severe bleeding, severe
myelosuppression

DRUG INTERACTIONS OF CONCERN TO DENTISTRY
None reported

SERIOUS REACTIONS
! Myelosuppression may be
severe, resulting in anemia,
infection, (sepsis, pneumonia),
and bleeding.
! Prolonged treatment may result in
peripheral neurotoxicity.

General:
• Determine why patient is taking
the drug.
• If additional analgesia is required
for dental pain, consider alternative
analgesics (NSAIDs) in patients
taking narcotics for acute or chronic
pain.
• Examine for oral manifestation
of opportunistic infection.
• Avoid prescribing aspirin-
containing products.
• This drug may be used in the
hospital or on an outpatient basis.
Confirm the patient's disease and
treatment status.
• Patient on chronic drug therapy
may rarely present with symptoms of
blood dyscrasias, which can include
infection, bleeding, and poor healing.
If dyscrasia is present, caution
patient to prevent oral tissue trauma
when using oral hygiene aids.
• Short appointments and a stress
reduction protocol may be required
for anxious patients.
• Patients may have received other
chemotherapy or radiation; confirm
medical and drug history.
• Patients may be at risk of bleeding;
check for oral signs.
• Patients may be at risk of
infection.
• Patients may be taking prophylactic
antiinfectives.
• Oral infections should be
eliminated and/or treated
aggressively.
Consultations:
• Medical consultation should
include routine blood counts
including platelet counts and
bleeding time.
• Consult physician; prophylactic or
therapeutic antiinfectives may be
indicated if surgery or periodontal
treatment is required.

• Medical consultation may be required to assess immunologic status during cancer chemotherapy and determine safety risk, if any, posed by the required dental treatment.
• Medical consultation may be required to assess disease control and patient's ability to tolerate stress.
Teach Patient/Family to:
• See dentist immediately if secondary oral infection occurs
• Use effective oral hygiene to prevent soft tissue inflammation
• Report oral lesions, soreness, or bleeding to dentist
• Prevent trauma when using oral hygiene aids
• Updating health and medication history if physician makes any changes in evaluation or drug regimens; include OTC, herbal, and nonherbal remedies in the update

carisoprodol
kar-ih-so-pro´-dol
(Soma)

CATEGORY AND SCHEDULE
Pregnancy Risk Category: C

Drug Class: Skeletal muscle relaxant, central acting

MECHANISM OF ACTION
A centrally acting skeletal muscle relaxant whose exact mechanism is unknown. Effects may be due to its CNS depressant actions.
Therapeutic Effect: Relieves muscle spasms and pain.

USES
Adjunct for relief of acute, painful musculoskeletal conditions

PHARMACOKINETICS
Onset 2 hr, duration 4–6hr.
Half-life: 2.5 hr. Metabolized in liver to meprobamate by the CYP 2C19 isoenzyme; excreted by kidneys.

INDICATIONS AND DOSAGES
▶ **Adjunct to Rest, Physical Therapy, Analgesics, and Other Measures for Relief of Discomfort from Acute, Painful Musculoskeletal Conditions**
PO
Adults, Elderly. 350 mg 4 times a day.

SIDE EFFECTS/ADVERSE REACTIONS
Frequent
Somnolence
Occasional
Tachycardia, facial flushing, dizziness, headache, lightheadedness, dermatitis, nausea, vomiting, abdominal cramps, dyspnea

PRECAUTIONS AND CONTRAINDICATIONS
Acute intermittent porphyria, sensitivity to meprobamate
Caution
Renal disease, hepatic disease, addictive personalities, elderly, children younger than 12 yr

DRUG INTERACTIONS OF CONCERN TO DENTISTRY
• Increased CNS depression: alcohol, all CNS depressants

SERIOUS REACTIONS
❗ Overdose may cause CNS and respiratory depression, shock, and coma.

DENTAL CONSIDERATIONS
General:
• When used in dentistry, may be more effective when used in combination with aspirin or NSAIDs.

Teach Patient/Family to:
• Use electric tooth brush if patient has difficulty holding conventional devices

carmustine
kar-muss´-teen
(BiCNU, Gliadel)

CATEGORY AND SCHEDULE
Pregnancy Risk Category: D

Drug Class: Antineoplastic

MECHANISM OF ACTION
An alkylating agent and nitrosourea that inhibits DNA and RNA synthesis by cross-linking with DNA and RNA strands, preventing cell division. Cell cycle–phase nonspecific. *Therapeutic Effect:* Interferes with DNA and RNA function.

USES
Treatment of certain types of brain cancer

PHARMACOKINETICS
Degraded within 15 min; crosses blood-brain barrier; 70% excreted in urine within 96 hr; 10% excreted as CO_2; fate of 20% is unknown.

INDICATIONS AND DOSAGES
▶ **Disseminated Hodgkin's Disease, Non-Hodgkin's Lymphoma, Multiple Myeloma, and Primary and Metastatic Brain Tumors in Previously Untreated Patients (Monotherapy)**
IV (BiCNu)
Adults, Elderly. 150–200 mg/m² as a single dose or 75–100 mg/m² on 2 successive days.
Children. 200–250 mg/m² every 4–6 wk as a single dose.

▶ Implantation (Gliadel)
Adults, Elderly, Children. Up to 8 wafers may be placed in resection cavity.

SIDE EFFECTS/ADVERSE REACTIONS
Frequent
Nausea and vomiting within min to 2 hr after administration (may last up to 6 hr)
Occasional
Diarrhea, esophagitis, anorexia, dysphagia
Rare
Thrombophlebitis

PRECAUTIONS AND CONTRAINDICATIONS
None known

DRUG INTERACTIONS OF CONCERN TO DENTISTRY
None reported

SERIOUS REACTIONS
❗ Hematologic toxicity due to myelosuppression occurs frequently. Thrombocytopenia occurs about 4 wk after carmustine treatment begins and lasts 1–2 wk.
❗ Leukopenia is evident 5–6 wk after treatment begins and lasts 1–2 wk. Anemia occurs less frequently and is less severe.
❗ Mild, reversible hepatotoxicity also occurs frequently.
❗ Prolonged high-dose carmustine therapy may produce impaired renal function and pulmonary toxicity (pulmonary infiltrate or fibrosis).

DENTAL CONSIDERATIONS
General:
• Determine why patient is taking the drug.

C

- If additional analgesia is required for dental pain, consider alternative analgesics in patients taking narcotics for acute or chronic pain.
- Avoid products that affect platelet function, such as aspirin and NSAIDs.
- This drug may be used in the hospital or on an outpatient basis. Confirm the patient's disease and treatment status.
- Consider semisupine chair position for patient comfort if GI side effects occur.
- Patient on chronic drug therapy may rarely present with symptoms of blood dyscrasias, which can include infection, bleeding and poor healing. If dyscrasia is present, caution patient to prevent oral tissue trauma when using oral hygiene aids.
- Examine for oral manifestation of opportunistic infection.
- Consider local hemostasis measures to prevent excessive bleeding.
- Monitor vital signs at every appointment due to cardiovascular side effects.
- Use caution with use of potentially hepatotoxic drugs.

Consultations:
- Medical consultation should include routine blood counts including platelet counts and bleeding time.
- Consult physician; prophylactic or therapeutic antiinfectives may be indicated if surgery or periodontal treatment is required.
- In a patient with symptoms of blood dyscrasias, request a medical consultation for blood studies and postpone treatment until normal values are reestablished.
- Medical consultation may be required to assess disease control and patient's ability to tolerate stress.

Teach Patient/Family to:
- Use effective oral hygiene to prevent soft tissue inflammation

- Prevent trauma when using oral hygiene aids
- Update health and medication history if physician makes any changes in evaluation or drug regimens; include OTC, herbal, and nonherbal remedies in the update
- Report oral lesions, soreness, or bleeding to dentist

carteolol
kar-tee´-oh-lole
(Cartrol, Ocupress)
Do not confuse carteolol with carvedilol.

CATEGORY AND SCHEDULE
Pregnancy Risk Category: C (D if after first trimester)

Drug Class: β-adrenergic blocker

MECHANISM OF ACTION
An antihypertensive that blocks β_1-adrenergic receptor at normal doses and β_2-adrenergic receptors at large doses. Predominantly blocks β_1-adrenergic receptors in cardiac tissue. Reduces aqueous humor production. *Therapeutic Effect:* Slows sinus heart rate, decreases cardiac output, decreases B/P, increases airway resistance, decreases intraocular pressure.

USES
Treatment of chronic open-angle glaucoma, ocular hypertension

PHARMACOKINETICS
Well absorbed from the GI tract. Protein binding: unknown. Minimally metabolized in liver. Primarily excreted unchanged in urine. Not removed by hemodialysis. *Half-life:* 6 hr (increased in decreased renal function).

INDICATIONS AND DOSAGES
▸ **Hypertension**
PO
Adults, Elderly. Initially, 2.5 mg/day as single dose either alone or in combination with diuretic. May increase gradually to 5–10 mg/day as a single dose. Maintenance: 2.5–5 mg/day.

DOSAGE IN RENAL IMPAIRMENT

Creatinine Clearance	Dosage Interval
Greater than 60 ml/min	24 hr
20–60 ml/min	48 hr
Less than 20 ml/min	72 hr

▸ **Open-Angle Glaucoma, Ocular Hypertension**
Ophthalmic
Adults, Elderly. 1 drop 2 times a day.

SIDE EFFECTS/ADVERSE REACTIONS
Frequent
Oral: Hypotension manifested as dizziness, nausea, diaphoresis, headache, cold extremities, fatigue, constipation/diarrhea
Ophthalmic: Redness of eye or inside of eyelids, decreased night vision
Occasional
Oral: Insomnia, flatulence, urinary frequency, impotence or decreased libido
Ophthalmic: Blepharoconjunctivitis, edema, droopy eyelid, staining of cornea, blurred vision, brow ache, increased light sensitivity, burning, stinging
Rare
Rash, arthralgia, myalgia, confusion (especially elderly), taste disturbances

PRECAUTIONS AND CONTRAINDICATIONS
Bronchial asthma, COPD, bronchospasm, overt cardiac failure, cardiogenic shock, heart block greater than first degree, persistently severe bradycardia.
Caution
Major surgery, lactation, diabetes mellitus, renal disease, thyroid disease, COPD, well-compensated heart failure, coronary artery disease (CAD), nonallergic bronchospasm

DRUG INTERACTIONS OF CONCERN TO DENTISTRY
• Decreased hypotensive effect: indomethacin, NSAIDs
• Increased hypotension, myocardial depression: hydrocarbon inhalation anesthetics
• Hypertension, bradycardia: sympathomimetics (epinephrine, ephedrine)
• Bradycardia: fluoxetine, paroxetine

SERIOUS REACTIONS
❗ Abrupt withdrawal (particularly in those with CAD) may produce angina or precipitate MI.
❗ May precipitate thyroid crisis in those with thyrotoxicosis.
❗ β-blockers may mask signs and symptoms of acute hypoglycemia (tachycardia, B/P changes) in diabetic patients.

DENTAL CONSIDERATIONS
General:
• Monitor vital signs at every appointment because of cardiovascular side effects.
• After supine positioning, have patient sit upright for at least 2 min before standing to avoid orthostatic hypotension.
• Assess salivary flow as a factor in caries, periodontal disease, and candidiasis.

• Patients on chronic drug therapy may rarely have symptoms of blood dyscrasias, which can include infection, bleeding, and poor healing.
• Limit use of sodium-containing products, such as saline IV fluids, for those patients with a dietary salt restriction.
• Stress from dental procedures may compromise cardiovascular function; determine patient risk.
• Short appointments and a stress-reduction protocol may be required for anxious patients.
Consultations:
• In a patient with symptoms of blood dyscrasias, request a medical consultation for blood studies and postpone dental treatment until normal values are reestablished.
• Medical consultation may be required to assess disease control and patient's ability to tolerate stress.
Teach Patient/Family to:
• Report oral lesions, soreness, or bleeding to dentist
• When chronic dry mouth occurs, advise patient to:
  • Avoid mouth rinses with high alcohol content because of drying effects
  • Use daily home fluoride products for anticaries effect
  • Use sugarless gum, frequent sips of water, or saliva substitutes

---

caspofungin acetate
kas-poe-fun´-gin ass´-eh-tayte
(Cancidas)

CATEGORY AND SCHEDULE
Pregnancy Risk Category: C

Drug Class: Antifungal, systemic

MECHANISM OF ACTION
An antifungal that inhibits the synthesis of glucan, a vital component of fungal cell formation, thereby damaging the fungal cell membrane. ***Therapeutic Effect:*** Fungistatic.

USES
Help the body overcome serious fungus infections

PHARMACOKINETICS
Distributed in tissue. Extensively bound to albumin. Protein binding: 97%. Slowly metabolized in liver to active metabolite. Excreted primarily in urine and to a lesser extent in feces. Not removed by hemodialysis. ***Half-life:*** 40–50 hr.

INDICATIONS AND DOSAGES
▸ **Aspergillosis**
IV
Adults, Elderly, Children older than 12 yr. Give single 70-mg loading dose on day 1, followed by 50 mg/day thereafter. For patients with moderate hepatic insufficiency, daily dose reduced to 35 mg.
▸ **Invasive Candidiasis**
IV
Adults, Elderly. Initially, 70 mg followed by 50 mg daily.
▸ **Esophageal Candidiasis**
IV
Adult, Elderly. 50 mg a day.

SIDE EFFECTS/ADVERSE REACTIONS
Frequent
Fever
Occasional
Headache, nausea, phlebitis
Rare
Paresthesia, vomiting, diarrhea, abdominal pain, myalgia, chills, tremor, insomnia

PRECAUTIONS AND CONTRAINDICATIONS
None known

DRUG INTERACTIONS OF CONCERN TO DENTISTRY
• Reduction in concentration: dexamethasone, carbamazepine

SERIOUS REACTIONS
! Hypersensitivity reactions (characterized by rash, facial swelling, pruritus, and a sensation of warmth) may occur.

DENTAL CONSIDERATIONS
General:
• For selected infections in the hospital setting.
• Provide palliative dental care for dental emergencies only.
• Patient on chronic drug therapy may rarely present with symptoms of blood dyscrasias, which can include infection, bleeding, and poor healing. If dyscrasia is present, caution patient to prevent oral tissue trauma when using oral hygiene aids.
Consultations:
• In a patient with symptoms of blood dyscrasias, request a medical consultation for blood studies and postpone treatment until normal values are reestablished.
• Medical consultation may be required to assess disease control and patient's ability to tolerate stress.
• Medical consultation should include PPT, PT, or INR.
Teach Patient/Family to:
• Use effective oral hygiene to prevent soft tissue inflammation
• Report oral lesions, soreness, or bleeding to dentist
• Prevent trauma when using oral hygiene aids

cefaclor
sef´-ah-klor
(Apo-Cefaclor[CAN], Ceclor, Ceclor CD, Cefkor[AUS], Cefkor CD[AUS], Keflor[AUS])

CATEGORY AND SCHEDULE
Pregnancy Risk Category: B

Drug Class: Antibiotic, cephalosporin (second generation)

MECHANISM OF ACTION
A second-generation cephalosporin that binds to bacterial cell membranes and inhibits cell wall synthesis. *Therapeutic Effect:* Bactericidal.

USES
For use in the treatment of the following infections when caused by susceptible strains of named microorganisms: otitis media caused by *S. pneumoniae, H. influenzae,* staphylococci, and *S. pyogenes;* lower respiratory tract infections caused by *S. pneumoniae, H. influenzae,* and *S. pyogenes;* pharyngitis and tonsillitis caused by *S. pyogenes;* UTIs caused by *E. coli, P. mirabilis, Klebsiella* species, and coagulase-negative staphylococci; skin and skin structure infections caused by *S. aureus* and *S. pyogenes;* and in vitro activity against *Peptococcus, Peptostreptococcus,* and *Propionibacterium* (clinical significance unknown)

PHARMACOKINETICS
Well absorbed from the GI tract. Protein binding: 25%. Widely distributed. Primarily excreted unchanged in urine. Moderately removed by hemodialysis. *Half-life:* 0.6–0.9 hr (increased in impaired renal function).

INDICATIONS AND DOSAGES

▶ **Bronchitis**
PO (Extended-Release)
Adults, Elderly. 500 mg q12h for
7 days.
▶ **Lower Respiratory Tract Infections**
PO
Adults, Elderly. 250–500 mg q8h.
▶ **Otitis Media**
PO
Children. 20–40 mg/kg/day in 2–3
divided doses. Maximum: 1 g/day.
▶ **Pharyngitis, Skin/Skin Structure Infections, Tonsillitis**
PO (Extended-Release)
Adults, Elderly. 375 mg q12h.
PO (Regular-Release)
Adults, Elderly. 250–500 mg q8h.
Children. 20–40 mg/kg/day in
2–3 divided doses. Maximum: 1 g/day.
▶ **UTIs**
PO
Adults, Elderly. 250–500 mg q8h.
Children. 20–40 mg/kg/day in
2–3 divided doses q8h. Maximum:
1 g/day.
PO (Extended-Release)
Adults, Children older than 16 yr.
375–500 mg q12h.
▶ **Otitis Media**
PO
Children older than 1 mo. 40 mg/kg/
day in divided doses q8h. Maximum:
1 g/day.
▶ **Dosage in Renal Impairment**
Decreased dosage may be necessary
in patients with creatinine clearance
less than 40 ml/min.

SIDE EFFECTS/ADVERSE REACTIONS

Frequent
Oral candidiasis, mild diarrhea, mild
abdominal cramping, vaginal
candidiasis
Occasional
Nausea, serum sickness–like reaction
(marked by fever and joint pain;
usually occurs after the second
course of therapy and resolves after
the drug is discontinued)
Rare
Allergic reaction (pruritus, rash,
and urticaria)

PRECAUTIONS AND CONTRAINDICATIONS

History of anaphylactic reaction to
penicillins or hypersensitivity to
cephalosporins
Caution
Hypersensitivity to penicillins,
lactation, renal disease

DRUG INTERACTIONS OF CONCERN TO DENTISTRY

• Decreased bactericidal effects:
tetracyclines, erythromycins
• Increased and prolonged serum
levels: probenecid
• Oral contraceptives: advise patient
of a potential low risk for decreased
contraceptive action, to maintain
compliance with oral contraceptive
use while using antibiotics, and to
consider the use of additional
nonhormonal contraception

SERIOUS REACTIONS

❗ Antibiotic-associated colitis and
other superinfections may result from
altered bacterial balance.
❗ Nephrotoxicity may occur,
especially in patients with
preexisting renal disease.
❗ Patients with a history of allergies,
especially to penicillin, are at
increased risk for developing a
severe hypersensitivity reaction,
marked by severe pruritus,
angioedema, bronchospasm, and
anaphylaxis.

DENTAL CONSIDERATIONS

General:
• Take precautions regarding allergy
to medication.

- Determine why the patient is taking the drug.

Consultations:
- Medical consultation may be required to assess disease control.

Teach Patient/Family to:
- Use effective oral hygiene to prevent soft tissue inflammation
- Avoid mouth rinses with high alcohol content because of drying effects and possible drug–drug reaction
- When used for dental infection, advise patient to:
  - Report sore throat, oral burning sensation, fever, and fatigue, any of which could indicate superinfection
  - Take at prescribed intervals and complete dosage regimen
  - Immediately notify the dentist if signs or symptoms of infection increase

cefadroxil
sef-ah-drox´-ill
(Duricef)

CATEGORY AND SCHEDULE
Pregnancy Risk Category: B

Drug Class: Cephalosporin (first generation)

MECHANISM OF ACTION
A first-generation cephalosporin that binds to bacterial cell membranes and inhibits cell wall synthesis. **Therapeutic Effect:** Bactericidal.

USES
Treatment of gram-negative bacilli: *E. coli, P. mirabilis, Klebsiella* (UTI only); gram-positive organisms: *S. pneumoniae, S. pyogenes, S. aureus;* upper/lower respiratory tract, urinary tract, skin infections; otitis media; tonsillitis; particularly for UTI

PHARMACOKINETICS
Well absorbed from the GI tract. Protein binding: 15%–20%. Widely distributed. Primarily excreted unchanged in urine. Removed by hemodialysis. **Half-life:** 1.2–1.5 hr (increased in impaired renal function).

INDICATIONS AND DOSAGES
▸ **UTIs**
PO
Adults, Elderly. 1–2 g/day as a single dose or in 2 divided doses.
Children. 30 mg/kg/day in 2 divided doses. Maximum: 2 g/day.

▸ **Skin and Skin-Structure Infections, Group A β-Hemolytic Streptococcal Pharyngitis, Tonsillitis**
PO
Adults, Elderly. 1–2 g in 2 divided doses.
Children. 30 mg/kg/day in 2 divided doses. Maximum: 2 g/day.

▸ **Impetigo**
PO
Children. 30 mg/kg/day as a single or in 2 divided doses. Maximum: 2 g/day.

▸ **Dosage in Renal Impairment**
After an initial 1-g dose, dosage and frequency are modified on the basis of creatinine clearance and the severity of the infection.

Creatinine Clearance	Dosage Interval
25–50 ml/min	500 mg q12h
10–25 ml/min	500 mg q24h
0–10 ml/min	500 mg q36h

SIDE EFFECTS/ADVERSE REACTIONS
Frequent
Oral candidiasis, mild diarrhea, mild abdominal cramping, vaginal candidiasis

Occasional
Nausea, unusual bruising or
bleeding, serum sickness–like
reaction (marked by fever and joint
pain; usually occurs after the second
course of therapy and resolves after
the drug is discontinued)
Rare
Allergic reaction (rash, pruritus,
urticaria), thrombophlebitis
(pain, redness, swelling at
injection site)

PRECAUTIONS AND CONTRAINDICATIONS

History of anaphylactic reaction to
penicillins or hypersensitivity to
cephalosporins
Caution
Hypersensitivity to penicillins,
lactation, renal disease

DRUG INTERACTIONS OF CONCERN TO DENTISTRY

• Decreased bactericidal effects:
tetracyclines, erythromycins
• Increased and prolonged serum
levels: probenecid
• Oral contraceptives: advise
patient of a potential low risk for
decreased contraceptive action,
to maintain compliance with oral
contraceptive use while using
antibiotics, and to consider the
use of additional, nonhormonal
contraception

SERIOUS REACTIONS

❗ Antibiotic-associated colitis and
other superinfections may result
from altered bacterial balance.
❗ Nephrotoxicity may occur,
especially in patients with
preexisting renal disease.
❗ Patients with a history of allergies,
especially to penicillin, are at
increased risk for developing
a severe hypersensitivity reaction,
marked by severe pruritus,
angioedema, bronchospasm, and
anaphylaxis.

DENTAL CONSIDERATIONS
General:
• Take precautions regarding allergy
to medication.
• Determine why the patient is taking
the drug.
Consultations:
• Medical consultation may be
required to assess disease control.
Teach Patient/Family to:
• Use effective oral hygiene
to prevent soft tissue inflammation
• Avoid mouth rinses with high
alcohol content because of drying
effects and possible drug–drug
reaction
• When used for dental infection,
advise patient to:
  • Report sore throat, oral burning
  sensation, fever, and fatigue, any
  of which could indicate
  superinfection
  • Take at prescribed intervals and
  complete dosage regimen
  • Immediately notify the dentist if
  signs or symptoms of infection
  increase

cefazolin sodium
sef-a´-zoe-lin so´-dee-um
(Ancef, Kefzol)
Do not confuse cefazolin with
cefprozil or Cefzil.

CATEGORY AND SCHEDULE
Pregnancy Risk Category: B

Drug Class: Cephalosporin
(first generation)

MECHANISM OF ACTION
A first-generation cephalosporin that
binds to bacterial cell membranes

and inhibits cell wall synthesis.
Therapeutic Effect: Bactericidal.

USES

Indicated for use when infection is caused by susceptible microorganisms: respiratory tract infections caused by *S. pneumoniae, Klebsiella* species, *H. influenzae, S. aureus*, and group A β-hemolytic streptococci; UTI infections caused by *E. coli, P. mirabilis, Klebsiella* species, and some enterobacter and enterococci; skin and skin structure infections caused by *S. aureus*, group A β-hemolytic streptococci; biliary tract infections caused by *E. coli, P. mirabilis, S. aureus, Klebsiella* species, and various strains of streptococci; bone and joint infections caused by *S. aureus*; genital infections caused by *E. coli, P. mirabilis, Klebsiella* species, and some enterococci; septicemia caused by *S. aureus, S. viridans, P. mirabilis, E. coli,* and *Klebsiella* species, group A β-hemolytic streptococci

PHARMACOKINETICS

Widely distributed. Protein binding: 85%. Primarily excreted unchanged in urine. Moderately removed by hemodialysis. ***Half-life:*** 1.4–1.8 hr (increased in impaired renal function).

INDICATIONS AND DOSAGES
▶ **Uncomplicated UTIs**
IV, IM
Adults, Elderly. 1 g q12h.
▶ **Mild to Moderate Infections**
IV, IM
Adults, Elderly. 250–500 mg q8–12h.
▶ **Severe infections**
IV, IM
Adults, Elderly. 0.5–1 g q6–8h.
▶ **Life-Threatening Infections**
IV, IM
Adults, Elderly. 1–1.5 g q6h.
Maximum: 12 g/day.

▶ **Perioperative Prophylaxis**
IV, IM
Adults, Elderly. 1 g 30–60 min before surgery, 0.5–1 g during surgery, and q6–8h for up to 24 hr postoperatively.
▶ **Usual Pediatric Dosage**
Children. 50–100 mg/kg/day in divided doses q8h. Maximum: 6 g/day.
Neonates older than 7 days. 40–60 mg/kg/day in divided doses q8–12h.
Neonates 7 days and younger. 40 mg/kg/day in divided doses q12h.
▶ **Dosage in Renal Impairment**
Dosing frequency is modified on the basis of creatinine clearance.

Creatinine Clearance	Dosage Interval
10–30 ml/min	Usual dose q12h
Less than 10 ml/min	Usual dose q24h

SIDE EFFECTS/ADVERSE REACTIONS
Frequent

Discomfort with IM administration, oral candidiasis, mild diarrhea, mild abdominal cramping, vaginal candidiasis
Occasional

Nausea, serum sickness–like reaction (marked by fever and joint pain; usually occurs after the second course of therapy and resolves after the drug is discontinued)
Rare

Allergic reaction (rash, pruritus, urticaria), thrombophlebitis (pain, redness, swelling at injection site)

PRECAUTIONS AND CONTRAINDICATIONS

History of anaphylactic reaction to penicillins or hypersensitivity to cephalosporins.
Caution

Hypersensitivity to penicillins, lactation, renal disease

DRUG INTERACTIONS OF CONCERN TO DENTISTRY
• Decreased bactericidal effects: tetracyclines, erythromycins
• Increased and prolonged serum levels: probenecid
• Oral contraceptives: advise patient of a potential low risk for decreased contraceptive action, to maintain compliance with oral contraceptive use while using antibiotics, and to consider the use of additional nonhormonal contraception

SERIOUS REACTIONS
❗ Antibiotic-associated colitis and other superinfections may result from altered bacterial balance.
❗ Nephrotoxicity may occur, especially in patients with preexisting renal disease.
❗ Patients with a history of allergies, especially to penicillin, are at increased risk for developing a severe hypersensitivity reaction, marked by severe pruritus, angioedema, bronchospasm, and anaphylaxis.

DENTAL CONSIDERATIONS
General:
• Take precautions regarding allergy to medication.
• Determine why the patient is taking the drug.
Consultations:
• Medical consultation may be required to assess disease control.
Teach Patient/Family to:
• Use effective oral hygiene to prevent soft tissue inflammation
• Avoid mouth rinses with high alcohol content because of drying effects and possible drug–drug reaction
• When used for dental infection, advise patient to:
  • Report sore throat, oral burning sensation, fever, and fatigue, any

of which could indicate superinfection
• Take at prescribed intervals and complete dosage regimen
• Immediately notify the dentist if signs or symptoms of infection increase

cefdinir
sef´-di-neer
(Omnicef)

CATEGORY AND SCHEDULE
Pregnancy Risk Category: B

Drug Class: Cephalosporin (third generation)

MECHANISM OF ACTION
A third-generation cephalosporin that binds to bacterial cell membranes and inhibits cell wall synthesis. **Therapeutic Effect:** Bactericidal.

USES
Community-acquired pneumonia, acute exacerbations of chronic bronchitis, acute maxillary sinusitis, pharyngitis/tonsillitus.

PHARMACOKINETICS
Moderately absorbed from the GI tract. Protein binding: 60%–70%. Widely distributed. Not appreciably metabolized. Primarily excreted unchanged in urine. Minimally removed by hemodialysis. **Half-life:** 1–2 hr (increased in impaired renal function).

INDICATIONS AND DOSAGES
▶ **Community-Acquired Pneumonia**
PO
Adults, Elderly, Children 13 yr and older. 300 mg q12h for 10 days.

2000

▶ **Acute Exacerbation of Chronic bronchitis**
PO
Adults, Elderly. 300 mg q12h for 5–10 days.

▶ **Acute Maxillary Sinusitis**
PO
Adults, Elderly, Children 13 yr and older. 300 mg q12h or 600 mg q24h for 10 days.
Children 6 mo–12 yr. 7 mg/kg q12h or 14 mg/kg q24h for 10 days.

▶ **Pharyngitis or Tonsillitis**
PO
Adults, Elderly, Children 13 yr and older. 300 mg q12h for 5–10 days or 600 mg q24h for 10 days.
Children 6 mo–12 yr. 7 mg/kg q12h for 5–10 days or 14 mg/kg q24h for 10 days.

▶ **Uncomplicated Skin or Skin-Structure Infections**
PO
Adults, Elderly, Children 13 yr and older. 300 mg q12h for 10 days.
Children 6 mo–12 yr. 7 mg/kg q12h for 10 days.

▶ **Acute Bacterial Otitis Media**
PO (Capsules)
Children 6 mo–12 yr. 7 mg/kg q12h or 14 mg/kg q24h for 10 days.

▶ **Usual Pediatric Dosage for Oral Suspension**
Children weighing 81–95 lb (37–43 kg). 12.5 ml (2.5 tsp) q12h or 25 ml (5 tsp) q24h.
Children weighing 61–80 lb (28–36 kg). 10 ml (2 tsp) q12h or 20 ml (4 tsp) q24h.
Children weighing 41–60 lb (19–27 kg). 7.5 ml (1 tsp) q12h or 15 ml (3 tsp) q24h.
Children weighing 20–40 lb (9–18 kg). 5 ml (1 tsp) q12h or 10 ml (2 tsp) q24h.
Infants weighing less than 20 lb (9 kg). 2.5 ml (1/2 tsp) q12h or 5 ml (1 tsp) q24h.

▶ **Dosage in Renal Impairment**
For patients with creatinine clearance less than 30 ml/min, dosage is 300 mg/day as single daily dose. For hemodialysis patients, dosage is 300 mg or 7 mg/kg/dose every other day.

SIDE EFFECTS/ADVERSE REACTIONS
Frequent
Oral candidiasis, mild diarrhea, mild abdominal cramping, vaginal candidiasis
Occasional
Nausea, serum sickness–like reaction (marked by fever and joint pain; usually occurs after the second course of therapy and resolves after the drug is discontinued)
Rare
Allergic reaction (rash, pruritus, urticaria)

PRECAUTIONS AND CONTRAINDICATIONS
History of anaphylactic reaction to penicillins or hypersensitivity to cephalosporins
Caution
Hypersensitivity to other cephalosporins, penicillins, or penicillamine; renal impairment (need dose reduction); ulcerative colitis, pseudomembranous colitis, bleeding disorders, renal impairment, hemodialysis, β-lactamase–resistant organisms, not detected in breast milk, children younger than 6 mo

DRUG INTERACTIONS OF CONCERN TO DENTISTRY
• Absorption retarded by iron salts, magnesium, or aluminum antacids: take antiinfective dose at least 2 hr before antacids or iron preparations
• Increased plasma levels: probenecid

• Oral contraceptives: advise patient of a potential low risk for decreased contraceptive action, to maintain compliance with oral contraceptive use while using antibiotics, and to consider the use of additional nonhormonal contraception

SERIOUS REACTIONS
! Antibiotic-associated colitis and other superinfections may result from altered bacterial balance.
! Nephrotoxicity may occur, especially in patients with preexisting renal disease.
! Patients with a history of allergies, especially to penicillin, are at increased risk for developing a severe hypersensitivity reaction, marked by severe pruritus, angioedema, bronchospasm, and anaphylaxis.

DENTAL CONSIDERATIONS
General:
• Use precaution regarding allergy to medication.
• Determine why patient is taking the drug.
• Examine for oral manifestation of opportunistic infection.
Consultations:
• Medical consultation may be required to assess disease control.
Teach Patient/Family to:
• Use effective oral hygiene to prevent soft tissue inflammation

cefditoren pivoxil
seff-di-tore´-en
(Spectracef)

CATEGORY AND SCHEDULE
Pregnancy Risk Category: B

Drug Class: Cephalosporin, third generation

MECHANISM OF ACTION
A third-generation cephalosporin that binds to bacterial cell membranes and inhibits cell wall synthesis. ***Therapeutic Effect:*** Bactericidal.

USES
Treatment of mild-to-moderate infections in adults and children older than 12 yr; for susceptible microorganisms causing (1) acute bacterial exacerbation of chronic bronchitis (H. influenzae, *H. parainfluenzae, S. pneumoniae* (penicillin susceptible only), or *M. catarrhalis;* (2) pharyngitis/ tonsillitis (*S. pyogenes*); (3) uncomplicated skin and skin-structure infections (*S. aureus* and *S. pyogenes*)

PHARMACOKINETICS
Moderately absorbed from the GI tract. Protein binding: 88%. Not metabolized. Excreted in the urine. Minimally removed by hemodialysis. ***Half-life:*** 1.6 hr (half-life increased with impaired renal function).

INDICATIONS AND DOSAGES
▸ **Pharyngitis, Tonsillitis, Skin Infections**
PO
Adults, Elderly, Children older than 12 yr. 200 mg twice a day for 10 days.
▸ **Acute Exacerbation of Chronic Bronchitis**
PO
Adults, Elderly, Children older than 12 yr. 400 mg twice a day for 10 days.
▸ **Community-Acquired Pneumonia**
PO
Adults, Elderly, Children older than 12 yr. 400 mg 2 twice a day for 14 days.
▸ **Dosage in Renal Impairment**
Dosage and frequency are modified on the basis of creatinine clearance.

Creatinine Clearance	Dosage
50-80 ml/min	No adjustment necessary
30-49 ml/min	200 mg twice a day
Less than 30 ml/min	200 mg once a day

SIDE EFFECTS/ADVERSE REACTIONS

Occasional
Diarrhea
Rare
Nausea, headache, abdominal pain, vaginal candidiasis, dyspepsia, vomiting

PRECAUTIONS AND CONTRAINDICATIONS

Carnitive deficiency, inborn errors of metabolism, known allergy to cephalosporins, hypersensitivity to milk protein
Caution
Penicillin-allergic patients, diarrhea, not for prolonged treatment, risk of resistance emergence, alteration of normal GI flora, decrease in prothrombin activity (long-term use, renal or hepatic impairment, taking anticoagulants), take with meals, lactation, safety and efficiency has not been established in children younger than 12 yr, elderly patients with impaired renal function, reduce dose in severe renal impairment

DRUG INTERACTIONS OF CONCERN TO DENTISTRY

• Reduced absorption: concurrent use with antacids, H2-receptor antagonist
• Increased and prolonged serum levels: probenecid
• Does not alter pharmacokinetics of ethinyl estradiol

SERIOUS REACTIONS

! Antibiotic-associated colitis and other superinfections may occur.
! Patients with a history of allergies, especially to penicillin, are at increased risk for developing a severe hypersensitivity reaction, marked by severe pruritus, angioedema, bronchospasm, and anaphylaxis.

DENTAL CONSIDERATIONS

General:
• Caution regarding allergy to medication.
• Assess salivary flow as a factor in caries, periodontal disease, and candidiasis.
• Determine why patient is taking the drug.
• Consider semisupine chair position for patient comfort if GI side effects occur.
• Consult with patient's physician if an acute dental infection occurs and another antiinfective is required.
• Examine for oral manifestation of opportunistic infection.
• Patients on chronic drug therapy may rarely have symptoms of blood dyscrasias, which can include infection, bleeding, and poor healing.
Consultations:
• Medical consultation may be required to assess disease control
• In a patient with symptoms of blood dyscrasias, request a medical consultation for blood studies and postpone treatment until normal values are reestablished.
Teach Patient/Family to:
• Use effective oral hygiene to prevent soft tissue inflammation and infection
• When chronic dry mouth occurs, advise patient to:

- Avoid mouth rinses with high alcohol content because of drying effects
- Use daily home fluoride products for anticaries effect
- Use sugarless gum, frequent sips of water, or saliva substitutes

cefepime
sef´-eh-peem
(Maxipime)
Do not confuse cefepime with ceftidine.

CATEGORY AND SCHEDULE
Pregnancy Risk Category: B

Drug Class: Cephalosporin (fourth generation)

MECHANISM OF ACTION
A fourth-generation cephalosporin that binds to bacterial cell membranes and inhibits cell wall synthesis. *Therapeutic Effect:* Bactericidal.

USES
Treatment of UTIs (uncomplicated and complicated), uncomplicated skin and soft tissue infections, complicated intraabdominal infections (in combination with metronidazole), and pneumonia caused by susceptible strains of microorganisms, including *S. pneumoniae;* febrile neutropenia

PHARMACOKINETICS
Well absorbed after IM administration. Protein binding: 20%. Widely distributed. Primarily excreted unchanged in urine. Removed by hemodialysis. *Half-life:* 2–2.3 hr (increased in impaired renal function, and in the elderly).

INDICATIONS AND DOSAGES
▶ **Pneumonia**
IV
Adults, Elderly. 1–2 g q12h for 7–10 days.
Children 2 mo and older. 50 mg/kg q12h. Maximum: 2 g/dose.
▶ **Intraabdominal Infections**
IV
Adults, Elderly. 2 g q12h for 10 days.
▶ **Skin and Skin-Structure Infections**
IV
Adults, Elderly. 2 g q12h for 10 days.
Children 2 mo and older. 50 mg/kg q12h. Maximum: 2 g/dose.
▶ **UTIs**
IV
Adults, Elderly. 0.5–2 g q12h for 7–10 days.
Children 2 mo and older. 50 mg/kg q12h. Maximum: 2 g/dose.
▶ **Febrile Neutropenia**
IV
Adults, Elderly. 2 g q8h.
Children 2 mo and older. 50 mg/kg q8h. Maximum: 2 g/dose.
▶ **Dosage in Renal Impairment**
Dosage and frequency are modified on the basis of creatinine clearance and the severity of the infection.

Creatinine Clearance	Dosage
30–60 ml/min	0.5–2 g q24h
11–29 ml/min	0.5–1 g q24h
10 ml/min or less	0.25–0.5 g q24h

SIDE EFFECTS/ADVERSE REACTIONS
Frequent
Discomfort with IM administration, oral candidiasis, mild diarrhea, mild abdominal cramping, vaginal candidiasis

Occasional
Nausea, serum sickness–like
reaction (marked by fever and
joint pain; usually occurs after
the second course of therapy
and resolves after the drug is
discontinued)
Rare
Allergic reaction (rash, pruritus,
urticaria), thrombophlebitis
(pain, redness, swelling at
injection site)

PRECAUTIONS AND CONTRAINDICATIONS
History of anaphylactic reaction to
penicillins or hypersensitivity to
cephalosporins
Caution
Renal impairment, overgrowth
of resistant organisms, colitis,
monitor prothrombin, lactation,
children younger than 12 yr; renal
insufficiency patient at risk for
encephalopathy, myoclonus,
seizures, renal failure

DRUG INTERACTIONS OF CONCERN TO DENTISTRY
• Increased risk of nephrotoxicity,
ototoxicity: aminoglycosides in
high doses, furosemide

SERIOUS REACTIONS
! Antibiotic-associated colitis
manifested and other superinfections
may result from altered bacterial
balance.
! Nephrotoxicity may occur,
especially in patients with
preexisting renal disease.
! Patients with a history of allergies,
especially to penicillin, are at
increased risk for developing a
severe hypersensitivity reaction,
marked by severe pruritus,
angioedema, bronchospasm, and
anaphylaxis.

DENTAL CONSIDERATIONS
General:
• Precaution regarding allergy to
medication.
• Determine why patient is taking
the drug.
• Oral contraceptives: advise
patient of a potential risk for
decreased contraceptive action,
to maintain compliance with oral
contraceptive use while using
antibiotics, and to consider the
use of additional nonhormonal
contraception
Consultation:
• Medical consultation may
be required to assess disease
control.
Teach Patient/Family to:
• Use effective oral hygiene to
prevent soft tissue inflammation
• Report sore throat, oral burning
sensation, fever, and fatigue, any
of which could indicate presence
of a superinfection

cefixime
sef-ix´-zeem
(Suprax)
Do not confuse Suprax with
Sporanox, Surbex, or Surfak.

CATEGORY AND SCHEDULE
Pregnancy Risk Category: B

Drug Class: Cephalosporin
(third generation)

MECHANISM OF ACTION
A third-generation cephalosporin
that binds to bacterial cell
membranes and inhibits cell wall
synthesis. *Therapeutic Effect:*
Bactericidal.

USES

Treatment of uncomplicated UTI
(*E. coli, P. mirabilis*), pharyngitis and
tonsillitis (*S. pyogenes*), otitis media
(*H. influenzae, M. catarrhalis*), acute
bronchitis, and acute exacerbations
of chronic bronchitis (*S. pneumoniae,
H. influenzae*)

PHARMACOKINETICS

Moderately absorbed from the GI tract.
Protein binding: 65%–70%. Widely
distributed. Primarily excreted
unchanged in urine. Minimally
removed by hemodialysis. ***Half-life:***
3–4 hr (increased in renal impairment).

INDICATIONS AND DOSAGES

▶ **Otitis Media, Acute Bronchitis,
Acute Exacerbations of Chronic
Bronchitis, Pharyngitis, Tonsillitis,
and Uncomplicated UTIs**
PO
*Adults, Elderly, Children weighing
more than 50 kg.* 400 mg/day as a
single dose or in 2 divided doses.
*Children 6 mo–12 yr weighing less
than 50 kg.* 8 mg/kg/day as a single
dose or in 2 divided doses.
Maximum: 400 mg.
▶ **Uncomplicated Gonorrhea**
PO
Adults. 400 mg as a single dose.
▶ **Dosage in Renal Impairment**
Dosage is modified on the basis
of creatinine clearance.

| Creatinine
Clearance | % of Usual
Dose |
|---|---|
| 21–60 ml/min | 75% |
| 20 ml/min or less | 50% |

SIDE EFFECTS/ADVERSE REACTIONS

Frequent
Oral candidiasis, mild diarrhea, mild
abdominal cramping, vaginal
candidiasis

Occasional
Nausea, serum sickness–like reaction
(marked by arthralgia and fever; usually
occurs after second course of therapy
and resolves after drug is discontinued)
Rare
Allergic reaction (rash, pruritus, urticaria)

PRECAUTIONS AND CONTRAINDICATIONS

History of anaphylactic reaction to
penicillins, hypersensitivity to
cephalosporins.
Caution
Hypersensitivity to penicillins,
lactation, renal disease

DRUG INTERACTIONS OF CONCERN TO DENTISTRY

• Decreased bactericidal effects:
tetracyclines, erythromycins
• Increased and prolonged serum
levels: probenecid
• Oral contraceptives: advise patient
of a potential low risk for decreased
contraceptive action, to maintain
compliance with oral contraceptive
use while using antibiotics, and to
consider the use of additional
nonhormonal contraception

SERIOUS REACTIONS

! Antibiotic-associated colitis and
other superinfections may result from
altered bacterial balance.
! Nephrotoxicity may occur,
especially in patients with
preexisting renal disease.
! Patients with a history of allergies,
especially to penicillin, are at increased
risk for developing a severe
hypersensitivity reaction, marked by
severe pruritus, angioedema,
bronchospasm, and anaphylaxis.

DENTAL CONSIDERATIONS

General:
• Take precautions regarding allergy
to medication.

• Determine why the patient is taking the drug.
Consultations:
• Medical consultation may be required to assess disease control.
Teach Patient/Family to:
• Use effective oral hygiene to prevent soft tissue inflammation
• Avoid mouth rinses with high alcohol content because of drying effects and possible drug–drug reaction
• When used for dental infection, advise patient to:
  • Report sore throat, oral burning sensation, fever, and fatigue, any of which could indicate superinfection
  • Take at prescribed intervals and complete dosage regimen
  • Immediately notify the dentist if signs or symptoms of infection increase

cefonicid sodium
sef-on-ih´-sid
(Monocid)
Do not confuse with cefoxitin.

CATEGORY AND SCHEDULE
Pregnancy Risk Category: B

Drug Class: Antibacterial, systemic

MECHANISM OF ACTION
A second-generation cephalosporin that binds to bacterial cell membranes and inhibits cell wall synthesis. **Therapeutic Effect:** Bactericidal.

USES
Treatment of infections caused by bacteria

PHARMACOKINETICS
Protein binding: greater than 90%. Widely distributed. Not metabolized. Primarily excreted unchanged in urine. Not removed by hemodialysis. **Half-life:** 4.5 hr.

INDICATIONS AND DOSAGES
▸ **UTIs**
IV, IM
Adults, Elderly. 0.5 g q24h.
▸ **Mild to Moderate Infections**
IV, IM
Adults, Elderly. 1 g q24h.
▸ **Severe or Life-Threatening Infections**
IV, IM
Adults, Elderly. 2 g q24h.
▸ **Surgical Prophylaxis**
IV
Adults, Elderly. 1 g 60 min before surgery.
▸ **Dosage in Renal Impairment**
Dosage and frequency are modified on the basis of creatinine clearance and the severity of infection.

Creatinine Clearance	Dosage (mild to moderate infections)
60–79 ml/min	10 mg/kg q24h
59–40 ml/min	8 mg/kg q24h
39–20 ml/min	4 mg/kg q24h
19–10 ml/min	4 mg/kg q48h
9–5 ml/min	4 mg/kg q3-5days
Less than 5 ml/min	3 mg/kg q3-5days

SIDE EFFECTS/ADVERSE REACTIONS
Frequent
Discomfort with IM administration, oral candidiasis, mild diarrhea, mild abdominal cramping, vaginal candidiasis
Occasional
Nausea, unusual bleeding or bruising, serum sickness–like reaction (marked by fever and joint pain)

Rare
Allergic reaction (rash, pruritus, urticaria), thrombophlebitis (pain, redness, swelling at injection site)

PRECAUTIONS AND CONTRAINDICATIONS
History of anaphylactic reaction to penicillins or hypersensitivity to cephalosporins

DRUG INTERACTIONS OF CONCERN TO DENTISTRY
• Increased or prolonged plasma levels: probenecid

SERIOUS REACTIONS
! Antibiotic-associated colitis and other superinfections may result from altered bacterial balance.
! Nephrotoxicity may occur, especially in patients with preexisting renal disease.
! Patients with a history of allergies, especially to penicillin, are at an increased risk for developing a severe hypersensitivity reaction, marked by severe pruritus, angioedema, bronchospasm, and anaphylaxis.

DENTAL CONSIDERATIONS
General:
• For selected infections in the hospital setting; provide palliative emergency dental care only.
• Use with caution in patients with a history of antibiotic-associated colitis.
• Determine why patient is taking the drug.
• Examine for oral manifestation of opportunistic infection.
• Caution regarding allergy to medication.
Consultations:
• CONIF
• Medical consultation may be required to assess disease control and patient's ability to tolerate stress.

Teach Patient/Family to:
• Use effective oral hygiene to prevent soft tissue inflammation
• Report sore throat, oral burning sensation, fever, or fatigue, any of which could indicate presence of a superinfection

cefoperazone
sef-oh-per´-ah-zone
(Cefobid)
Do not confuse with ceftin, cefotetan, and cefamandole.

CATEGORY AND SCHEDULE
Pregnancy Risk Category: B

Drug Class: Antibacterial, systemic

MECHANISM OF ACTION
A third-generation cephalosporin that binds to bacterial cell membranes. *Therapeutic Effect:* Inhibits synthesis of bacterial cell wall. Bactericidal.

USES
Treatment of infections caused by bacteria

PHARMACOKINETICS
Widely distributed, including CSF. Protein binding: 82%–93%. Metabolized and excreted in kidney and urine. Removed by hemodialysis. *Half-life:* 1.6–2.4 hrs (half-life is increased with impaired renal function).

INDICATIONS AND DOSAGES
▶ **Mild to Moderate Infections**
IM/IV
Adults, Elderly. 2–4 g/day in 2 divided doses q12h.

▶ **Severe or Life-Threatening Infections**
IM/IV
Adults, Elderly. Total daily dose and/or frequency may be increased to 6–12 g/day divided into 2, 3, or 4 equal doses of 1.5–4 g per dose.
▶ **Dosage in renal and/or hepatic impairment**
Do not exceed 4 g/day in those with liver disease and/or biliary obstruction. Modification of dose usually not necessary in those with renal impairment. Dose should not exceed 1–2 g/day in those with both hepatic and substantial renal impairment.

SIDE EFFECTS/ADVERSE REACTIONS
Frequent
Discomfort with IM administration, oral candidiasis, mild diarrhea, mild abdominal cramping, vaginal candidiasis
Occasional
Nausea, unusual bruising/bleeding, serum sickness reaction
Rare
Allergic reaction, rash, pruritus, urticaria, thrombophlebitis (pain, redness, swelling at injection site)

PRECAUTIONS AND CONTRAINDICATIONS
Anaphylactic reaction to penicillins, history of hypersensitivity to cephalosporins or any one of its components

DRUG INTERACTIONS OF CONCERN TO DENTISTRY
• Avoid alcohol, risk of disulfiram-like reaction
• Increased risk of bleeding: drugs that interfere with platelet action

SERIOUS REACTIONS
! Antibiotic-associated colitis manifested as severe abdominal pain and tenderness, fever, and watery and severe diarrhea, and other superinfections may result from altered bacterial balance.
! Nephrotoxicity may occur, especially in patients with preexisting renal disease. Severe hypersensitivity reaction including severe pruritus, angioedema, bronchospasm, and anaphylaxis, particularly in patients with a history of allergies, especially to penicillins, may occur.

DENTAL CONSIDERATIONS
General:
• For selected infections in the hospital setting; provide palliative emergency dental treatment only.
• Use with caution in patients with a history of antibiotic-associated colitis.
• Caution: may interfere with prothrombin levels.
• Examine for oral manifestation of opportunistic infection.
• Determine why patient is taking the drug.
• Caution regarding allergy to medication.
Consultations:
• CONIF
• Medical consultation may be required to assess disease control and patient's ability to tolerate stress.
• Medical consultation should include partial prothrombin time, prothrombin time, or INR.
Teach Patient/Family to:
• Use effective oral hygiene to prevent soft tissue inflammation
• Report sore throat, oral burning sensation, fever, or fatigue, any of which could indicate presence of a superinfection

cefotaxime sodium
sef-oh-taks′-eem so′-dee-um
(Claforan)
Do not confuse cefotaxime with
cefoxitin, ceftizoxime, or
cefuroxime, or Claforan with
Claritin.

CATEGORY AND SCHEDULE
Pregnancy Risk Category: B

Drug Class: Antibacterial,
systemic

MECHANISM OF ACTION
A third-generation cephalosporin
that binds to bacterial cell
membranes and inhibits cell wall
synthesis. *Therapeutic Effect:*
Bactericidal.

USES
Treatment of infections caused by
bacteria

PHARMACOKINETICS
Widely distributed, including to CSF.
Protein binding: 30%–50%. Partially
metabolized in the liver to active
metabolite. Primarily excreted in
urine. Moderately removed by
hemodialysis. *Half-life:* 1 hr
(increased in impaired renal
function).

INDICATIONS AND DOSAGES
▸ **Uncomplicated Infections**
IV, IM
Adults, Elderly. 1 g q12h.
▸ **Mild to Moderate Infections**
IV, IM
Adults, Elderly. 1–2 g q8h.
▸ **Severe Infections**
IV, IM
Adults, Elderly. 2 g q6–8h.
▸ **Life-Threatening Infections**
IV, IM

Adults, Elderly. 2 g q4h.
Children. 2 g q4h. Maximum:
12 g/day.
▸ **Gonorrhea**
IM
Adults. (Male): 1 g as a single dose.
(Female): 0.5 g as a single dose.
▸ **Perioperative Prophylaxis**
IV, IM
Adults, Elderly. 1 g 30–90 min before
surgery.
▸ **Cesarean Section**
IV
Adults. 1 g as soon as umbilical cord
is clamped, then 1 g 6 and 12 hr after
first dose.
▸ **Usual Pediatric Dosage**
Children weighing 50 kg or more.
1–2 g q6–8h.
*Children 1 mo–12 yr weighing less
than 50 kg.* 100–200 mg/kg/day in
divided doses q6–8h.
▸ **Dosage in Renal Impairment**
For patients with creatinine clearance
less than 20 ml/min give half of dose
at usual dosing intervals.

SIDE EFFECTS/ADVERSE REACTIONS
Frequent
Discomfort with IM administration,
oral candidiasis, mild diarrhea, mild
abdominal cramping, vaginal
candidiasis
Occasional
Nausea, serum sickness–like reaction
(marked by fever and joint pain;
usually occurs after the second
course of therapy and resolves after
the drug is discontinued)
Rare
Allergic reaction (rash, pruritus,
urticaria), thrombophlebitis (pain,
redness, swelling at injection site)

PRECAUTIONS AND CONTRAINDICATIONS
History of anaphylactic reaction to
penicillins or hypersensitivity to
cephalosporins

DRUG INTERACTIONS OF CONCERN TO DENTISTRY
- Increased or prolonged plasma levels: probenecid

SERIOUS REACTIONS
! Antibiotic-associated colitis and other superinfections may result from altered bacterial balance.
! Nephrotoxicity may occur, especially in patients with preexisting renal disease.
! Patients with a history of allergies, especially to penicillin, are at increased risk for developing a severe hypersensitivity reaction, marked by severe pruritus, angioedema, bronchospasm, and anaphylaxis.

DENTAL CONSIDERATIONS
General:
- For selected infections in the hospital setting; provide palliative emergency dental treatment only.
- Use caution in patients with a history of antibiotic-associated colitis.
- Examine for oral manifestation of opportunistic infection.
- Determine why patient is taking the drug.
- Caution regarding allergy to medication.

Consultations:
- CONIF
- Medical consultation may be required to assess disease control and patient's ability to tolerate stress.

Teach Patient/Family to:
- Use effective oral hygiene to prevent soft tissue inflammation
- Report sore throat, oral burning sensation, fever, or fatigue, any of which could indicate presence of a superinfection

cefotetan disodium
sef´-oh-tee-tan die-so´-dee-um
(Apatef[AUS], Cefotan)
Do not confuse cefotetan with cefoxitin or Ceftin.

CATEGORY AND SCHEDULE
Pregnancy Risk Category: B

Drug Class: Antibacterial, systemic

MECHANISM OF ACTION
A second-generation cephalosporin that binds to bacterial cell membranes and inhibits cell wall synthesis. *Therapeutic Effect:* Bactericidal.

USES
Treatment of infections caused by bacteria

PHARMACOKINETICS
Protein binding: 78%–91%. Primarily excreted unchanged in urine. Minimally removed by hemodialysis. *Half-life:* 3–4.6 hr (increased in impaired renal function).

INDICATIONS AND DOSAGES
▸ **UTIs**
IV, IM
Adults, Elderly. 1–2 g in divided doses q12–24h.
▸ **Mild to Moderate Infections**
IV, IM
Adults, Elderly. 1–2 g q12h.
▸ **Severe Infections**
IV, IM
Adults, Elderly. 2 g q12h.
▸ **Life-Threatening Infections**
IV, IM
Adults, Elderly. 3 g q12h.
▸ **Perioperative Prophylaxis**
IV
Adults, Elderly. 1–2 g 30–60 min before surgery.

▶ **Cesarean Section**

IV

Adults. 1–2 g as soon as umbilical cord is clamped.

▶ **Usual Pediatric Dosage**

Children. 40–80 mg/kg/day in divided doses q12h.
Maximum: 6 g/day.

▶ **Dosage in Renal Impairment**

Dosing frequency is modified on the basis of creatinine clearance and the severity of the infection.

Creatinine Clearance	Dosage Interval
10–30 ml/min	Usual dose q24h
Less than 10 ml/min	Usual dose q48h

SIDE EFFECTS/ADVERSE REACTIONS

Frequent

Discomfort with IM administration, oral candidiasis, mild diarrhea, mild abdominal cramping, vaginal candidiasis

Occasional

Nausea, unusual bleeding or bruising, serum sickness–like reaction (marked by fever and joint pain; usually occurs after the second course of therapy and resolves after the drug is discontinued)

Rare

Allergic reaction (rash, pruritus, urticaria), thrombophlebitis (pain, redness, swelling at injection site)

PRECAUTIONS AND CONTRAINDICATIONS

History of anaphylactic reaction to penicillins or hypersensitivity to cephalosporins

DRUG INTERACTIONS OF CONCERN TO DENTISTRY

• Avoid alcohol, risk of disulfiram-like reaction

• Increased or prolonged plasma levels: probenecid
• Increased risk of bleeding: drugs that interfere with platelet action

SERIOUS REACTIONS

❗ Antibiotic-associated colitis and other superinfections may result from altered bacterial balance.
❗ Nephrotoxicity may occur, especially in patients with preexisting renal disease.
❗ Patients with a history of allergies, especially to penicillin, are at increased risk for developing a severe hypersensitivity reaction, marked by severe pruritus, angioedema, bronchospasm, and anaphylaxis.

DENTAL CONSIDERATIONS

General:
• For selected infections in the hospital setting; provide palliative emergency dental treatment only
• Use with caution in patients with a history of antibiotic-associated colitis
• Caution: may interfere with prothrombin levels
• Examine for oral manifestation of opportunistic infection
• Determine why patient is taking the drug
• Caution regarding allergy to medication
Consultations:
• CONIF
• Medical consultation may be required to assess disease control and patient's ability to tolerate stress
• Medical consultation should include partial prothrombin time, prothrombin time, or INR
Teach Patient/Family to:
• Use effective oral hygiene to prevent soft tissue inflammation
• Report sore throat, oral burning sensation, fever, or fatigue, any of which could indicate presence of a superinfection

cefoxitin sodium

se-fox´-ih-tin so´-dee-um
(Mefoxin)
Do not confuse cefoxitin with
cefotaxime, cefotetan, or Cytoxan.

CATEGORY AND SCHEDULE
Pregnancy Risk Category: B

Drug Class: Antibacterial,
systemic

MECHANISM OF ACTION
A second-generation cephalosporin
that binds to bacterial cell membranes
and inhibits cell wall synthesis.
Therapeutic Effect: Bactericidal.

USES
Treatment of infections caused by
bacteria

PHARMACOKINETICS
Peak levels reached within 5 min
following IV infusion. *Half-life:*
45 m–1 hr; 85% excreted unchanged
in urine.

INDICATIONS AND DOSAGES
▶ **Mild to Moderate Infections**
IV, IM
Adults, Elderly. 1–2 g q6–8h.
▶ **Severe Infections**
IV, IM
Adults, Elderly. 1 g q4h or 2 g q6–8h
up to 2 g q4h.
▶ **Uncomplicated Gonorrhea**
IM
Adults. 2 g one time with 1 g
probenecid.
▶ **Perioperative Prophylaxis**
IV, IM
Adults, Elderly. 2 g 30–60 min before
surgery, then q6h for up to 24 hr after
surgery.
Children older than 3 mo. 30–40 mg/
kg 30–60 min before surgery, then
q6h for up to 24 hr after surgery.

▶ **Cesarean Section**
IV
Adults. 2 g as soon as umbilical cord
is clamped, then 2 g 4 and 8 hr after
first dose, then q6h for up to 24 hr.
▶ **Usual Pediatric Dosage**
Children older than 3 mo.
80–160 mg/kg/day in 4–6 divided
doses. Maximum: 12 g/day.
Neonates. 90–100 mg/kg/day in
divided doses q6–8h.
▶ **Dosage in Renal Impairment**
After a loading dose of 1–2 g, dosage
and frequency are modified on the
basis of creatinine clearance and the
severity of the infection.

Creatine Clearance	Dosage
30–50 ml/min	1–2 g q8–12h
10–29 ml/min	1–2 g q12–24h
5–9 ml/min	500 mg–1 g q12–24h
Less than 5 ml/min	500 mg–1 g q24–48h

SIDE EFFECTS/ADVERSE REACTIONS
Frequent
Discomfort with IM administration,
oral candidiasis, mild diarrhea,
mild abdominal cramping, vaginal
candidiasis
Occasional
Nausea, serum sickness–like reaction
(marked by fever and joint pain;
usually occurs after the second
course of therapy and resolves after
the drug is discontinued)
Rare
Allergic reaction (pruritus, rash,
urticaria), thrombophlebitis (pain,
redness, swelling at injection site)

PRECAUTIONS AND CONTRAINDICATIONS
History of anaphylactic reaction to
penicillins or hypersensitivity to
cephalosporins

DRUG INTERACTIONS OF CONCERN TO DENTISTRY
• Increased or prolonged plasma levels: probenecid

SERIOUS REACTIONS
❗ Antibiotic-associated colitis and other superinfections may result from altered bacterial balance.
❗ Nephrotoxicity may occur, especially in patients with preexisting renal disease.
❗ Patients with a history of allergies, especially to penicillin, are at increased risk for developing a severe hypersensitivity reaction, marked by severe pruritus, angioedema, bronchospasm, and anaphylaxis.

DENTAL CONSIDERATIONS
General:
• For selected infections in the hospital setting; provide palliative emergency dental treatment only.
• Use with caution in patients with a history of antibiotic-associated colitis.
• Examine for oral manifestation of opportunistic infection.
• Determine why patient is taking the drug.
• Caution regarding allergy to medication.
Consultations:
• Consult patient's physician if an acute dental infection occurs and another antiinfective is required.
• Medical consultation may be required to assess disease control and patient's ability to tolerate stress.
Teach Patient/Family to:
• Use effective oral hygiene to prevent soft tissue inflammation
• Report sore throat, oral burning sensation, fever, or fatigue, any of which could indicate presence of a superinfection

cefpodoxime proxetil
sef-poe-dox´-ime prox´-eh-til
(Vantin)
Do not confuse Vantin with Ventolin.

CATEGORY AND SCHEDULE
Pregnancy Risk Category: B

Drug Class: Cephalosporin (third generation)

MECHANISM OF ACTION
A third-generation cephalosporin that binds to bacterial cell membranes and inhibits cell wall synthesis. **Therapeutic Effect:** Bactericidal.

USES
Treatment of upper and lower respiratory tract infections, pharyngitis (tonsillitis), gonorrhea, UTI, uncomplicated skin and skin structure infections caused by susceptible organisms, acute otitis media, community-acquired pneumonia, acute bacterial exacerbation of chronic bronchitis, anorectal infections in women

PHARMACOKINETICS
Well absorbed from the GI tract (food increases absorption). Protein binding: 21%–40%. Widely distributed. Primarily excreted unchanged in urine. Partially removed by hemodialysis. **Half-life:** 2.3 hr (increased in impaired renal function and elderly patients).

INDICATIONS AND DOSAGES
▶ **Chronic Bronchitis, Pneumonia**
PO
Adults, Elderly, Children older than 13 yr. 200 mg q12h for 10–14 days.

▶ **Gonorrhea, Rectal Gonococcal Infection (Female Patients Only)**
PO
Adults, Children older than 13 yr.
200 mg as a single dose.

▶ **Skin and Skin-Structure Infections**
PO
Adults, Elderly, Children older than 13 yr. 400 mg q12h for 7–14 days.

▶ **Pharyngitis, Tonsillitis**
PO
Adults, Elderly, Children older than 13 yr. 100 mg q12h for 5–10 days.
Children 6 mo–13 yr. 5 mg/kg q12h for 5–10 days. Maximum: 100 mg/dose.

▶ **Acute Maxillary Sinusitis**
PO
Adults, Children older than 13 yr. 200 mg twice a day for 10 days.
Children 2 mos–13 yr. 5 mg/kg q12h for 10 days. Maximum: 400 mg/day.

▶ **UTIs**
PO
Adults, Elderly, Children older than 13 yr. 100 mg q12h for 7 days.

▶ **Acute Otitis Media**
PO
Children 6 mos–13 yr. 5 mg/kg q12h for 5 days. Maximum: 400 mg/dose.

▶ **Dosage in Renal Impairment**
For patients with creatinine clearance less than 30 ml/min, usual dose is given q24h. For patients on hemodialysis, usual dose is given 3 times a wk after dialysis.

SIDE EFFECTS/ADVERSE REACTIONS

Frequent
Oral candidiasis, mild diarrhea, mild abdominal cramping, vaginal candidiasis
Occasional
Nausea, serum sickness-like reaction (marked by fever and joint pain; usually occurs after the second course of therapy and resolves after the drug is discontinued)

Rare
Allergic reaction (pruritus, rash, urticaria)

PRECAUTIONS AND CONTRAINDICATIONS
History of anaphylactic reaction to penicillins or hypersensitivity to cephalosporins
Caution
Hypersensitivity to penicillins, lactation, renal disease, safety and efficacy in infants younger than 5 mo not established

DRUG INTERACTIONS OF CONCERN TO DENTISTRY
• Decreased bactericidal effects: tetracyclines, erythromycins
• Increased and prolonged serum levels: probenecid
• Oral contraceptives: advise patient of a potential risk for decreased contraceptive action, to maintain compliance with oral contraceptive use while using antibiotics, and to consider the use of additional nonhormonal contraception

SERIOUS REACTIONS
❗ Antibiotic-associated colitis and other superinfections may result from altered bacterial balance.
❗ Nephrotoxicity may occur, especially in patients with pre-existing renal disease.
❗ Patients with a history of allergies, especially to penicillin, are at increased risk for developing a severe hypersensitivity reaction, marked by severe pruritus, angioedema, bronchospasm, and anaphylaxis.

DENTAL CONSIDERATIONS
General:
• Take precautions regarding allergy to medication.
• Determine why the patient is taking the drug.

Consultations:
• Medical consultation may be required to assess disease control.
Teach Patient/Family to:
• Use effective oral hygiene to prevent soft tissue inflammation
• Avoid mouth rinses with high alcohol content because of drying effects and possible drug–drug reaction
• When used for dental infection, advise patient to:
  • Report sore throat, oral burning sensation, fever, and fatigue, any of which could indicate superinfection
  • Take at prescribed intervals and complete dosage regimen
  • Immediately notify the dentist if signs or symptoms of infection increase

cefprozil

sef-pro´-zil
(Cefzil)
Do not confuse cefprozil with Cefazolin or Cefzil with Cefol, Ceftin, or Kefzol.

CATEGORY AND SCHEDULE

Pregnancy Risk Category: B

Drug Class: Cephalosporin (second generation)

MECHANISM OF ACTION

A second-generation cephalosporin that binds to bacterial cell membranes and inhibits cell wall synthesis. ***Therapeutic Effect:*** Bactericidal.

USES

Treatment of pharyngitis/tonsillitis, otitis media, secondary bacterial infection of acute bronchitis, sinusitis; acute bacterial sinusitis; acute bacterial exacerbation of chronic bronchitis and uncomplicated skin and skin structure infections

PHARMACOKINETICS

Well absorbed from the GI tract. Protein binding: 36%–45%. Widely distributed. Primarily excreted unchanged in urine. Moderately removed by hemodialysis. ***Half-life:*** 1.3 hr (increased in impaired renal function).

INDICATIONS AND DOSAGES

▶ **Pharyngitis, Tonsillitis**
PO
Adults, Elderly. 500 mg q24h for 10 days.
Children 2–12 yr. 7.5 mg/kg q12h for 10 days.
▶ **Acute Bacterial Exacerbation of Chronic Bronchitis, Secondary Bacterial Infection of Acute Bronchitis**
PO
Adults, Elderly. 500 mg q12h for 10 days.
▶ **Skin and Skin-Structure Infections**
PO
Adults, Elderly. 250–500 mg q12h for 10 days.
Children. 20 mg/kg q24h for 10 days.
▶ **Acute Sinusitis**
PO
Adults, Elderly. 250–500 mg q12h for 10 days.
Children 6 mo–12 yr. 7.5–15 mg/kg q12h for 10 days.
▶ **Otitis Media**
PO
Children 6 mo–12 yr. 15 mg/kg q12h for 10 days. Maximum: 1 g/day.
▶ **Dosage in Renal Impairment**
Patients with creatinine clearance less than 30 ml/min receive 50% of usual dose at usual interval.

SIDE EFFECTS/ADVERSE REACTIONS
Frequent
Oral candidiasis, mild diarrhea, mild abdominal cramping, vaginal candidiasis
Occasional
Nausea, serum sickness reaction (marked by fever and joint pain; usually occurs after the second course of therapy and resolves after the drug is discontinued)
Rare
Allergic reaction (pruritus, rash, urticaria)

PRECAUTIONS AND CONTRAINDICATIONS
History of anaphylactic reaction to penicillins or hypersensitivity to cephalosporins
Caution
Lactation, elderly, hypersensitivity to penicillins, renal disease

DRUG INTERACTIONS OF CONCERN TO DENTISTRY
• Decreased bactericidal effects: tetracyclines, erythromycins
• Increased and prolonged serum levels: probenecid
• Oral contraceptives: advise patient of a potential low risk for decreased contraceptive action, to maintain compliance with oral contraceptive use while using antibiotics, and to consider the use of additional nonhormonal contraception

SERIOUS REACTIONS
! Antibiotic-associated colitis and other superinfections may result from altered bacterial balance.
! Nephrotoxicity may occur, especially in patients with preexisting renal disease.
! Patients with a history of allergies, especially to penicillin, are at increased risk for developing a severe

hypersensitivity reaction, marked by severe pruritus, angioedema, bronchospasm, and anaphylaxis.

DENTAL CONSIDERATIONS
General:
• Take precautions regarding allergy to medication.
• Determine why the patient is taking the drug.
• Examine for evidence of oral manifestations of blood dyscrasia (infection, bleeding, poor healing) and superinfection.
Consultations:
• Medical consultation may be required to assess disease control.
Teach Patient/Family to:
• Use effective oral hygiene to prevent soft tissue inflammation
• Avoid mouth rinses with high alcohol content because of drying effects and possible drug–drug reaction
• When used for dental infection, advise patient to:
    • Report sore throat, oral burning sensation, fever, and fatigue, any of which could indicate superinfection
    • Take at prescribed intervals and complete dosage regimen
    • Immediately notify the dentist if signs or symptoms of infection increase

ceftazidime
sef-taz´-ih-deem
(Ceptaz, Fortaz, Fortum[AUS], Tazicef, Tazidime)
Do not confuse ceftazidime with ceftizoxime.

CATEGORY AND SCHEDULE
Pregnancy Risk Category: B

Drug Class: Third-generation cephalosporin; antibiotic

MECHANISM OF ACTION

A third-generation cephalosporin that binds to bacterial cell membranes and inhibits cell wall synthesis. *Therapeutic Effect:* Bactericidal.

USES

Treatment of intraabdominal, biliary tract, respiratory tract, GU tract, skin, bone infections; meningitis; septicemia

PHARMACOKINETICS

Widely distributed (including to CSF). Protein binding: 5%–17%. Primarily excreted unchanged in urine. Removed by hemodialysis. *Half-life:* 2 hr (increased in impaired renal function).

INDICATIONS AND DOSAGES

▶ **UTIs**
IV, IM
Adults. 250–500 mg q8–12h.
▶ **Mild-to-Moderate Infections**
IV, IM
Adults. 1 g q8–12h.
▶ **Uncomplicated Pneumonia, Skin and Skin-Structure Infections**
IV, IM
Adults. 0.5–1 g q8h.
▶ **Bone and Joint Infections**
IV, IM
Adults. 2 g q12h.
▶ **Meningitis, Serious Gynecologic and Intraabdominal Infections**
IV, IM
Adults. 2 g q8h.
▶ **Pseudomonal Pulmonary Infections in Patients with Cystic Fibrosis**
IV
Adults. 30–50 mg/kg q8h.
Maximum: 6 g/day.
▶ **Usual Elderly Dosage**
Elderly (normal renal function).
500 mg–1 g q12h.
▶ **Usual Pediatric Dosage**
Children 1 mo–12 yr. 100–150 mg/kg/day in divided doses q8h.
Maximum: 6 g/day.

Neonates 0–4 wk. 100–150 mg/kg/day in divided doses q8–12h.
▶ **Dosage in Renal Impairment**
After an initial 1-g dose, dosage and frequency are modified on the basis of creatinine clearance and the severity of the infection.

Creatinine Clearance	Dosage
31–50 ml/min	1 g q12h
16–30 ml/min	1 g q24h
6–15 ml/min	500 mg q24h
Less than 5 ml/min	500 mg q48h

SIDE EFFECTS/ADVERSE REACTIONS

Frequent
Discomfort with IM administration, oral candidiasis, mild diarrhea, mild abdominal cramping, vaginal candidiasis
Occasional
Nausea, serum sickness–like reaction (marked by fever and joint pain; usually occurs after the second course of therapy and resolves after the drug is discontinued)
Rare
Allergic reaction (pruritus, rash, urticaria), thrombophlebitis (pain, redness, swelling at injection site)

PRECAUTIONS AND CONTRAINDICATIONS

History of anaphylactic reaction to penicillins or hypersensitivity to cephalosporins

DRUG INTERACTIONS OF CONCERN TO DENTISTRY

None reported

SERIOUS REACTIONS

❗ Antibiotic-associated colitis and other superinfections may result from altered bacterial balance.

! Nephrotoxicity may occur, especially in patients with preexisting renal disease.
! Patients with a history of allergies, especially to penicillin, are at increased risk for developing a severe hypersensitivity reaction, marked by severe pruritus, angioedema, bronchospasm, and anaphylaxis.

DENTAL CONSIDERATIONS
General:
• For selected infections in the hospital setting; provide palliative emergency dental treatment only.
• Use with caution in patients with a history of antibiotic-associated colitis.
• Examine for oral manifestation of opportunistic infection.
• Determine why patient is taking the drug.
• Caution regarding allergy to medication.
Consultations:
• CONIF
• Medical consultation may be required to assess disease control and patient's ability to tolerate stress.
Teach Patient/Family to:
• Use effective oral hygiene to prevent soft tissue inflammation
• Report sore throat, oral burning sensation, fever, or fatigue, any of which could indicate presence of a superinfection

ceftibuten
cef´-te-bute-in
(Cedax)

CATEGORY AND SCHEDULE
Pregnancy Risk Category: B

Drug Class: Cephalosporin (third-generation)

MECHANISM OF ACTION
A third-generation cephalosporin that binds to bacterial cell membranes and inhibits cell wall synthesis. *Therapeutic Effect:* Bactericidal.

USES
Treatment of acute exacerbations of chronic bronchitis caused by susceptible strains of *H. influenzae, M. catarrhalis,* or *S. pneumoniae;* acute otitis media caused by susceptible strains of *H. influenzae, M. catarrhalis,* or *S. pyogenes;* pharyngitis and tonsillitis caused by *S. pyogenes*

PHARMACOKINETICS
Rapidly absorbed from the GI tract. Excreted primarily in urine. *Half-life:* 2–3 hr.

INDICATIONS AND DOSAGES
▸ **Chronic Bronchitis**
PO
Adults, Elderly. 400 mg/day once a day for 10 days.
▸ **Pharyngitis, Tonsillitis**
PO
Adults, Elderly. 400 mg once a day for 10 days.
Children older than 6 mo. 9 mg/kg once a day for 10 days. Maximum: 400 mg/day.
▸ **Otitis Media**
PO
Children older than 6 mo. 9 mg/kg once a day for 10 days. Maximum: 400 mg/day.
▸ **Dosage in Renal Impairment**
Dosage is modified on the basis of creatinine clearance.

Creatine Clearance	Dosage
50 mg/kg and higher	400 mg or 9 mg/kg q24h
30–49 ml/min	200 mg or 4.5 mg/kg q24h
Less than 30 ml/min	100 mg or 2.25 mg/kg q24h

SIDE EFFECTS/ADVERSE REACTIONS

Frequent
Oral candidiasis, mild diarrhea (discharge, itching)
Occasional
Nausea, serum sickness–like reaction (marked by fever and joint pain; usually occurs after the second course of therapy and resolves after the drug is discontinued)
Rare
Allergic reaction (rash, pruritus, urticaria)

PRECAUTIONS AND CONTRAINDICATIONS

History of anaphylactic reaction to penicillins or hypersensitivity to cephalosporins
Caution
Hypersensitivity to penicillins, renal impairment, lactation, infants younger than 6 mo, pseudomembranous colitis, oral suspension contains 1 g sucrose/5 ml

DRUG INTERACTIONS OF CONCERN TO DENTISTRY

• Decreased bactericidal effects: tetracyclines, erythromycins
• Increased and prolonged serum levels: probenecid
• Aminoglycosides increase nephrotoxic potential
• Oral contraceptives: advise patient of a potential low risk for decreased contraceptive action, to maintain compliance with oral contraceptive use while using antibiotics, and to consider the use of additional nonhormonal contraception

SERIOUS REACTIONS

! Antibiotic-associated colitis and other superinfections may result from altered bacterial balance.
! Nephrotoxicity may occur, especially in patients with preexisting renal disease.

! Patients with a history of allergies, especially to penicillin, are at increased risk for developing a severe hypersensitivity reaction, marked by severe pruritus, angioedema, bronchospasm, and anaphylaxis.

DENTAL CONSIDERATIONS

General:
• Take precautions regarding allergy to medication.
• Assess salivary flow as factor in caries, periodontal disease, and candidiasis.
• Oral suspension contains sucrose; patient should rinse mouth after use.
• Determine why the patient is taking the drug.
Consultations:
• Medical consultation may be required to assess disease control.
Teach Patient/Family to:
• Use effective oral hygiene to prevent soft tissue inflammation
• When used for dental infection, advise patient to:
  • Report sore throat, oral burning sensation, fever, and fatigue, any of which could indicate superinfection
  • Take at prescribed intervals and complete dosage regimen
  • Immediately notify the dentist if signs or symptoms of infection increase

ceftizoxime sodium

sef-ti-zox´-eem so´-dee-um
(Cefizox)
Do not confuse ceftizoxime with cefotaxime or ceftazidime.

CATEGORY AND SCHEDULE

Pregnancy Risk Category: B

Drug Class: Third-generation cephalosporin; antibiotic

MECHANISM OF ACTION

A third-generation cephalosporin that binds to bacterial cell membranes and inhibits cell wall synthesis. *Therapeutic Effect:* Bactericidal.

USES

Treatment of intraabdominal, biliary tract, respiratory tract, GU tract, skin, bone infections; gonorrhea; meningitis; septicemia; pelvic inflammatory disease (PID)

PHARMACOKINETICS

Widely distributed (including to CSF). Protein binding: 30%. Primarily excreted unchanged in urine. Moderately removed by hemodialysis. *Half-life:* 1.7 hr (increased in impaired renal function).

INDICATIONS AND DOSAGES
▸ **Uncomplicated UTIs**
IV, IM
Adults, Elderly. 500 mg q12h.
▸ **Mild, Moderate, or Severe Infections of the Biliary, Respiratory, and GU Tracts; Skin, Bone, and Intraabdominal Infections; Meningitis; and Septicemia**
IV, IM
Adults, Elderly. 1–2 g q8–12h.
▸ **Life-Threatening Infections of the Biliary, Respiratory, and GU Tracts; Skin, Bone and Intraabdominal Infections; Meningitis; and Septicemia**
IV
Adults, Elderly. 3–4 g q8h, up to 2 g q4h.
▸ **PID**
IV
Adults. 2 g q4–8h.
▸ **Uncomplicated Gonorrhea**
IM
Adults. 1 g 1 time.
▸ **Usual Pediatric Dosage**
Children older than 6 mo: 50 mg/kg q6–8h. Maximum: 12 g/day.

▸ **Dosage in Renal Impairment**
After a loading dose of 0.5–1 g, dosage and frequency are modified on the basis of creatinine clearance and the severity of the infection.

Creatinine Clearance	Dosage
50–79 ml/min	0.5 g–1.5 g q8h
5–49 ml/min	0.25 g–1 g q12h
Less than 5 ml/min	0.25–0.5 g q24h or 0.5 g–1 g q48h

SIDE EFFECTS/ADVERSE REACTIONS
Frequent
Discomfort with IM administration, oral candidiasis, mild diarrhea, mild abdominal cramping, vaginal candidiasis
Occasional
Nausea, serum sickness–like reaction (fever, joint pain; usually occurs after the second course of therapy and resolves after the drug is discontinued)
Rare
Allergic reaction (rash, pruritus, urticaria), thrombophlebitis (pain, redness, swelling at injection site)

PRECAUTIONS AND CONTRAINDICATIONS
History of anaphylactic reaction to penicillins or hypersensitivity to cephalosporins

DRUG INTERACTIONS OF CONCERN TO DENTISTRY
• Increased or prolonged plasma levels: probenecid

SERIOUS REACTIONS
! Antibiotic-associated colitis manifested and other superinfections may result from altered bacterial balance.

! Nephrotoxicity may occur, especially in patients with preexisting renal disease.
! Patients with a history of allergies, especially to penicillin, are at increased risk for developing a severe hypersensitivity reaction, marked by severe pruritus, angioedema, bronchospasm, and anaphylaxis.

DENTAL CONSIDERATIONS

General:
• For selected infections in the hospital setting; provide palliative emergency dental treatment only.
• Use with caution in patients with a history of antibiotic-associated colitis.
• Examine for oral manifestation of opportunistic infection.
• Determine why patient is taking the drug.
• Caution regarding allergy to medication.
Consultations:
• CONIF
• Medical consultation may be required to assess disease control and patient's ability to tolerate stress.
Teach Patient/Family to:
• Use effective oral hygiene to prevent soft tissue inflammation
• Report sore throat, oral burning sensation, fever, or fatigue, any of which could indicate presence of a superinfection

ceftriaxone sodium
sef-try-ax´-one so´-dee-um
(Rocephin)

CATEGORY AND SCHEDULE
Pregnancy Risk Category: B

Drug Class: Third-generation cephalosporin; antibiotic

MECHANISM OF ACTION
A third-generation cephalosporin that binds to bacterial cell membranes and inhibits cell wall synthesis.
Therapeutic Effect: Bactericidal.

USES
Treatment of respiratory tract, GU tract, skin, bone, intraabdominal, biliary tract infections; septicemia; meningitis; gonorrhea; Lyme disease; acute bacterial otitis media

PHARMACOKINETICS
Widely distributed (including to CSF). Protein binding: 83%–96%. Primarily excreted unchanged in urine. Not removed by hemodialysis. **Half-life:** 4.3–4.6 hr IV; 5.8–8.7 hr IM (increased in impaired renal function).

INDICATIONS AND DOSAGES
▸ **Mild to Moderate Infections**
IV, IM
Adults, Elderly. 1–2 g as a single dose or in 2 divided doses.
▸ **Serious Infections**
IV, IM
Adults, Elderly. Up to 4 g/day in 2 divided doses.
Children. 50–75 mg/kg/day in divided doses q12h. Maximum: 2 g/day.
▸ **Skin and Skin-Structure Infections**
IV, IM
Children. 50–75 mg/kg/day as a single dose or in 2 divided doses. Maximum: 2 g/day.
▸ **Meningitis**
IV
Children. Initially, 75 mg/kg, then 100 mg/kg/day as a single dose or in divided doses q12h. Maximum: 4 g/day.
▸ **Lyme Disease**
IV

Adults, Elderly. 2–4 g a day for
10–14 days.
▸ **Acute Bacterial Otitis Media**
IM
Children. 50 mg/kg once a day for
3 days. Maximum: 1 g/day.
▸ **Perioperative Prophylaxis**
IV, IM
Adults, Elderly. 1 g 0.5–2 hr before
surgery.
▸ **Uncomplicated Gonorrhea**
IM
Adults. 250 mg plus doxycycline
one time.
▸ **Dosage in Renal Impairment**
Dosage modification is usually
unnecessary, but liver and renal
function test results should be
monitored in those with both renal
and liver impairment or severe renal
impairment.

SIDE EFFECTS/ADVERSE REACTIONS
Frequent
Discomfort with IM administration,
oral candidiasis, mild diarrhea, mild
abdominal cramping, vaginal
candidiasis
Occasional
Nausea, serum sickness–like reaction
(marked by fever and joint pain;
usually occurs after the second
course of therapy and resolves
after the drug is discontinued)
Rare
Allergic reaction (rash, pruritus,
urticaria), thrombophlebitis (pain,
redness, swelling at injection site)

PRECAUTIONS AND CONTRAINDICATIONS
History of anaphylactic reaction
to penicillins or hypersensitivity to
cephalosporins
Caution
Hypersensitivity to penicillins,
lactation, renal disease

DRUG INTERACTIONS OF CONCERN TO DENTISTRY
None reported

SERIOUS REACTIONS
❗ Antibiotic-associated colitis and
other superinfections may result
from altered bacterial balance.
❗ Nephrotoxicity may occur,
especially in patients with
preexisting renal disease.
❗ Patients with a history of allergies,
especially to penicillin, are at
increased risk for developing a severe
hypersensitivity reaction, marked
by severe pruritus, angioedema,
bronchospasm, and anaphylaxis.

DENTAL CONSIDERATIONS
General:
• For selected infections in the
hospital setting; provide palliative
emergency dental treatment only.
• Use with caution in patients with a
history of antibiotic-associated colitis.
• Caution: may interfere with
prothrombin levels.
• Examine for oral manifestation
of opportunistic infection.
• Determine why patient is taking
the drug.
• Caution regarding allergy to
medication.
Consultations:
• CONIF
• Medical consultation may be
required to assess disease control
and patient's ability to tolerate stress.
• Medical consultation should
include partial prothrombin time,
prothrombin time, or INR.
Teach Patient/Family to:
• Use effective oral hygiene to
prevent soft tissue inflammation
• Report sore throat, oral burning
sensation, fever, or fatigue, any of
which could indicate presence of a
superinfection

cefuroxime axetil/ cefuroxime sodium

sef-yur-ox´-ime
(cefuroxime axetil) Ceftin,
Zinnat[AUS] (cefuroxime sodium),
Kefurox, Zinacef
Do not confuse cefuroxime with
cefotaxime or deferoxamine or
Ceftin with Cefzil.

CATEGORY AND SCHEDULE

Pregnancy Risk Category: B

Drug Class: Cephalosporin
(second-generation)

MECHANISM OF ACTION

A second-generation cephalosporin
that binds to bacterial cell
membranes and inhibits cell wall
synthesis. ***Therapeutic Effect:***
Bactericidal.

USES

Gram-negative bacilli (*H.
influenzae, E. coli, Neisseria,
P. mirabilis, Klebsiella*); gram-
positive organisms (*S. pneumoniae,
S. pyogenes, S. aureus*); serious
lower respiratory tract, urinary tract,
skin, gonococcal infections;
septicemia; meningitis; early Lyme
disease; acute bronchitis, acute
bacterial maxillary sinusitis,
pharyngitis, tonsillitis, impetigo,
bone and joint infections.

PHARMACOKINETICS

Rapidly absorbed from the GI tract.
Protein binding: 33%–50%.
Widely distributed (including to
CSF). Primarily excreted unchanged
in urine. Moderately removed
by hemodialysis. ***Half-life:***
1.3 hr (increased in impaired
renal function).

INDICATIONS AND DOSAGES

▸ **Ampicillin-Resistant Influenza;
Bacterial Meningitis; Early Lyme
Disease; GU Tract, Gynecologic,
Skin, and Bone Infections;
Septicemia; Gonorrhea, and Other
Gonococcal Infections**
IV, IM
Adults, Elderly. 750 mg–1.5 g
q8h.
Children. 75–100 mg/kg/day divided
q8h. Maximum: 8 g/day.
Neonates. 50–100 mg/kg/day divided
q12h.
PO
Adults, Elderly. 125–500 mg twice
a day, depending on the infection.
▸ **Pharyngitis, Tonsillitis**
PO
Children 3 mo–12 yr. 125 mg
(tablets) q12h or 20 mg/kg/day
(suspension) in 2 divided doses.
▸ **Acute Otitis Media, Acute
Bacterial Maxillary Sinusitis,
Impetigo**
PO
Children 3 mo–12 yr. 250 mg
(tablets) q12h or 30 mg/kg/day
(suspension) in 2 divided doses.
▸ **Bacterial Meningitis**
IV
Children 3 mo–12 yr. 200–240 mg/
kg/day in divided doses q6–8h.
▸ **Perioperative Prophylaxis**
IV
Adults, Elderly. 1.5 g 30–60 min
before surgery and 750 mg q8h after
surgery.
▸ **Usual Neonatal Dosage**
IV, IM
Neonates. 20–100 mg/kg/day in
divided doses q12h.
▸ **Dosage in Renal Impairment**
Adult dosage and frequency are
modified based on creatinine
clearance and the severity of the
infection.

C

SIDE EFFECTS/ADVERSE REACTIONS

Frequent

Discomfort with IM administration, oral candidiasis, mild diarrhea, mild abdominal cramping, vaginal candidiasis

Occasional

Nausea, serum sickness–like reaction (marked by fever and joint pain; usually occurs after the second course of therapy and resolves after the drug is discontinued)

Rare

Allergic reaction (rash, pruritus, urticaria), thrombophlebitis (pain, redness, swelling at injection site)

PRECAUTIONS AND CONTRAINDICATIONS

History of anaphylactic reaction to penicillins or hypersensitivity to cephalosporins

DRUG INTERACTIONS OF CONCERN TO DENTISTRY

- Decreased bactericidal effects: tetracyclines, erythromycins
- Increased and prolonged serum levels: probenecid
- Oral contraceptives: advise patient of a potential risk for decreased contraceptive action, to maintain compliance with oral contraceptive use while using antibiotics, and to consider the use of additional nonhormonal contraception

SERIOUS REACTIONS

! Antibiotic-associated colitis and other superinfections may result from altered bacterial balance.
! Nephrotoxicity may occur, especially in patients with preexisting renal disease.
! Patients with a history of allergies, especially to penicillin, are at increased risk for developing a severe hypersensitivity reaction, marked by severe pruritus,

angioedema, bronchospasm, and anaphylaxis.

DENTAL CONSIDERATIONS

General:
- Take precautions regarding allergy to medication.
- Determine why the patient is taking the drug.

Consultations:
- Medical consultation may be required to assess disease control.

Teach Patient/Family to:
- Use effective oral hygiene to prevent soft tissue inflammation
- Avoid mouth rinses with high alcohol content because of drying effects and possible drug-drug reaction
- When used for dental infection, advise patient to:
  - Report sore throat, oral burning sensation, fever, and fatigue, any of which could indicate superinfection
  - Take at prescribed intervals and complete dosage regimen
  - Immediately notify the dentist if signs or symptoms of infection increase

celecoxib

sel-eh-kox´-ib
(Celebrex, DisperDose, Panixine)
Do not confuse Celebrex with Cerebyx or Celexa.

CATEGORY AND SCHEDULE

Pregnancy Risk Category: *C*
(D if used in third trimester or near delivery)

Drug Class: Nonsteroidal antiinflammatory, analgesic

MECHANISM OF ACTION

An NSAID that inhibits cyclo-oxygenase-2, the enzyme responsible for prostaglandin synthesis. Mechanism of action in treating familial adenomatous polyposis is unknown. *Therapeutic Effect:* Reduces inflammation and relieves pain.

USES
Relief of signs and symptoms of osteoarthritis and relief of signs and symptoms of rheumatoid arthritis in adults; also approved for reducing the number of intestinal polyps in patients with familial adenomatous polyposis; acute pain and primary dysmenorrhea

PHARMACOKINETICS
Widely distributed. Protein binding: 97%. Metabolized in the liver. Primarily eliminated in feces. *Half-life:* 11.2 hr.

INDICATIONS AND DOSAGES
▸ **Osteoarthritis**
PO
Adults, Elderly. 200 mg/day as a single dose or 100 mg twice a day.
▸ **Rheumatoid Arthritis**
PO
Adults, Elderly. 100–200 mg twice a day.
▸ **Acute Pain**
PO
Adults, Elderly. Initially, 400 mg with additional 200 mg on day 1, if needed. Maintenance: 200 mg twice a day as needed.
▸ **Familial Adenomatous Polyposis**
PO
Adults, Elderly. 400 mg twice daily (with food).

SIDE EFFECTS/ADVERSE REACTIONS
Frequent
Diarrhea, dyspepsia, headache, upper respiratory tract infection
Occasional
Abdominal pain, flatulence, nausea, back pain, peripheral edema, dizziness, rash

PRECAUTIONS AND CONTRAINDICATIONS
NSAIDs may cause an increased risk of serious cardiovascular thrombotic events, including myocardial infarction and stroke, which may be fatal. Patients with cardiovascular disease may be at greater risk. Hypersensitivity to aspirin, NSAIDs, or sulfonamides
Caution
Geriatric patients weighing less than 50 kg use lowest dose, children younger than 18 yr, severe hepatic or renal impairment, upper active GI disease, GI bleeding, avoid in late pregnancy (category D after 34 wk), lactation, dehydrated patients, heart failure, hypertension, asthma, patients suspected or known to be poor CYP2C9 isoenzyme metabolizers

DRUG INTERACTIONS OF CONCERN TO DENTISTRY
• Increased plasma levels: fluconazole
• Increased risk of thromboembolism
• Increased risk of GI bleeding: long-duration NSAIDs, aspirin (except low doses), oral glucocorticoids, alcoholism, smoking, older age, generally poor health
• Increased plasma levels of lithium
• Possible risk of increased INR in elderly patients taking warfarin
• Possible reduction in blood pressure control: ACE inhibitors
• First-time users of SSRIs also taking NSAIDs may have a higher risk of GI side effects; until more data are available, it may be advisable to avoid use of NSAIDs in these patients (Br J Clin Pharmacol 55:591–595, 2003)

SERIOUS REACTIONS
None known

DENTAL CONSIDERATIONS
General:
• Patients on chronic drug therapy may rarely have symptoms of blood dyscrasias, which can include infection, bleeding, and poor healing.
• Assess salivary flow as a factor in caries, periodontal disease, and candidiasis.
• Consider semisupine chair position for patient comfort because of effects of disease and GI side effects of drug.
Teach Patient/Family to:
• Use effective oral hygiene to prevent soft tissue inflammation
• Update health and drug history if physician makes any changes in evaluation or drug regimens
• Use electric tooth brush if patient has difficulty holding conventional devices
• When chronic dry mouth occurs, advise patient to:
  • Avoid mouth rinses with high alcohol content because of drying effects
  • Use daily home fluoride products for anticaries effect
  • Use sugarless gum, frequent sips of water, or saliva substitutes

cephalexin
sef-ah-lex´-in
(Apo-Cephalex[CAN], Biocef, Ceporex[AUS], Ibilex[AUS], Keflex, Keftab, Novolexin[CAN])

CATEGORY AND SCHEDULE
Pregnancy Risk Category: B

Drug Class: Cephalosporin (first-generation)

MECHANISM OF ACTION
A first-generation cephalosporin that binds to bacterial cell membranes and inhibits cell wall synthesis. *Therapeutic Effect:* Bactericidal.

USES
Treatment of the following infections when caused by susceptible microorganisms: respiratory tract infections caused by *S. pneumoniae* and group A β-hemolytic streptococci; otitis media caused by *S. pneumoniae, H. influenzae, M. catarrhalis*, staphylococci, and streptococci; skin and skin structure infections caused by staphylococci and streptococci; bone infections caused by staphylococci and *P. mirabilis;* and GU tract infections caused by *E. coli, P. mirabilis*, and *K. pneumoniae*

PHARMACOKINETICS
Rapidly absorbed from the GI tract. Protein binding: 10%–15%. Widely distributed. Primarily excreted unchanged in urine. Moderately removed by hemodialysis. *Half-life:* 0.9–1.2 hr (increased in impaired renal function).

INDICATIONS AND DOSAGES
▶ **Bone Infections, Prophylaxis of Rheumatic Fever, Follow-up to Parenteral Therapy**
PO
Adults, Elderly. 250–500 mg q6h up to 4 g/day.
▶ **Streptococcal Pharyngitis, Skin and Skin-Structure Infections, Uncomplicated Cystitis**
PO
Adults, Elderly. 500 mg q12h.
▶ **Usual Pediatric Dosage**
Children. 25–100 mg/kg/day in 2–4 divided doses.
▶ **Otitis Media**
PO

Children. 75–100 mg/kg/day in 4 divided doses.

▶ **Dosage in Renal Impairment**
After usual initial dose, dosing frequency is modified on the basis of creatinine clearance and the severity of the infection.

Creatine Clearance	Dosage Interval
10–50 ml/min	250 mg q6h
0–10 ml/min	125 mg q6h

SIDE EFFECTS/ADVERSE REACTIONS
Frequent
Oral candidiasis, mild diarrhea, mild abdominal cramping, vaginal candidiasis
Occasional
Nausea, serum sickness–like reaction (marked by fever and joint pain; ususally occurs after the second course of therapy and resolves after the drug is discontinued)
Rare
Allergic reaction (rash, pruritus, urticaria)

PRECAUTIONS AND CONTRAINDICATIONS
History of anaphylactic reaction to penicillins or hypersensitivity to cephalosporins
Caution
Hypersensitivity to penicillins, lactation, renal disease

DRUG INTERACTIONS OF CONCERN TO DENTISTRY
• Decreased bactericidal effects: tetracyclines, erythromycins
• Increased and prolonged serum levels: probenecid
• Oral contraceptives: advise patient of a low potential risk for decreased contraceptive action, to maintain compliance with oral contraceptive use while using antibiotics, and to consider the use of additional nonhormonal contraception

SERIOUS REACTIONS
! Antibiotic-associated colitis and other superinfections may result from altered bacterial balance.
! Nephrotoxicity may occur, especially in patients with preexisting renal disease.
! Patients with a history of allergies, especially to penicillin, are at increased risk for developing a severe hypersensitivity reaction, marked by severe pruritus, angioedema, bronchospasm, and anaphylaxis.

DENTAL CONSIDERATIONS
General:
• Take precautions regarding allergy to medication.
• Determine why the patient is taking the drug.
Consultations:
• Medical consultation may be required to assess disease control.
Teach Patient/Family to:
• Use effective oral hygiene to prevent soft tissue inflammation
• Avoid mouth rinses with high alcohol content because of drying effects and possible drug–drug reaction
• When used for dental infection, advise patient to:
  • Report sore throat, oral burning sensation, fever, and fatigue, any of which could indicate superinfection
  • Take at prescribed intervals and complete dosage regimen
  • Immediately notify the dentist if signs or symptoms of infection increase

cephradine
sef´-ra-deen
(Velosef)

CATEGORY AND SCHEDULE
Pregnancy Risk Category: B

Drug Class: Cephalosporin
(first-generation)

MECHANISM OF ACTION
A first-generation cephalosporin that
binds to bacterial cell membranes.
Inhibits synthesis of bacterial cell
wall. *Therapeutic Effect:* Bactericidal.

USES
Treatment of gram-negative bacilli:
*H. influenzae, E. coli, P. mirabilis,
Klebsiella;* gram-positive organisms:
*S. pneumoniae, S. pyogenes,
S. aureus;* serious respiratory tract,
urinary tract, skin, and skin structure
infections; otitis media

PHARMACOKINETICS
Well absorbed from the GI tract.
Protein binding: 18%–20%. Widely
distributed. Primarily excreted
unchanged in urine. Removed by
hemodialysis. *Half-life:* 1–2 hr
(half-life is increased with impaired
renal function).

INDICATIONS AND DOSAGES
▸ **Mild, Moderate, or Severe
Infections of the Respiratory,
and GU Tracts; Bone, Joint, and Skin
Infections; Prostatitis; Otitis Media**
PO
Adults, Elderly. 250–500 mg q6h.
Maximum: 8 g/day.
Children older than 9 mo. 25–50 mg/
kg/day in divided doses q6–12h.
Maximum: 4 g/day.
▸ **Dosage in renal impairment**
Dosage and frequency are based on
the degree of renal impairment and

the severity of infection. In patients
with renal impairment, starting doses
of 250 mg are recommended, with
longer dosing intervals of up to 12 hr.
Consult physician for use in patients
on dialysis.

SIDE EFFECTS/ADVERSE REACTIONS
Frequent
Diarrhea, mild abdominal cramping,
vaginal candidiasis (discharge,
itching)
Occasional
Nausea, headache, unusual bruising
or bleeding, serum sickness-like
reaction (fever, joint pain)
Rare
Allergic reaction (rash, pruritus,
urticaria)

PRECAUTIONS AND CONTRAINDICATIONS
History of hypersensitivity to
penicillins and cephalosporins
Caution
Hypersensitivity to penicillins,
lactation, renal disease

DRUG INTERACTIONS OF CONCERN TO DENTISTRY
• Decreased bactericidal effects:
tetracyclines, erythromycins
• Increased and prolonged serum
levels: probenecid
• Oral contraceptives: advise patient
of a low potential risk for decreased
contraceptive action, to maintain
compliance with oral contraceptive
use while using antibiotics, and
to consider the use of additional
nonhormonal contraception

SERIOUS REACTIONS
! Antibiotic-associated colitis as
evidenced by severe abdominal pain
and tenderness, fever, and watery
and severe diarrhea, and other
superinfections may result from
altered bacterial balance.

! Nephrotoxicity may occur, especially in patients with preexisting renal disease.
! Severe hypersensitivity reaction including severe pruritus, angioedema, bronchospasm, and anaphylaxis, particularly in patients with history of allergies, especially penicillin, may occur.

DENTAL CONSIDERATIONS
General:
• Take precautions regarding allergy to medication.
• Determine why the patient is taking the drug.
Consultations:
• Medical consultation may be required to assess disease control.
Teach Patient/Family to:
• Use effective oral hygiene to prevent soft tissue inflammation
• Avoid mouth rinses with high alcohol content because of drying effects and possible drug–drug reaction
• When used for dental infection, advise patient to:
  • Report sore throat, oral burning sensation, fever, and fatigue, any of which could indicate superinfection
  • Take at prescribed intervals and complete dosage regimen
  • Immediately notify the dentist if signs or symptoms of infection increase

cetirizine
si-tear´-ah-zeen
(Reactine[CAN], Zyrtec)
Do not confuse Zyrtec with Zantac or Zyprexa.

CATEGORY AND SCHEDULE
Pregnancy Risk Category: B

Drug Class: Antihistamine

MECHANISM OF ACTION
A second-generation piperazine that competes with histamine for H_1-receptor sites on effector cells in the GI tract, blood vessels, and respiratory tract. **Therapeutic Effect:** Prevents allergic response, produces mild bronchodilation, blocks histamine-induced bronchitis.

USES
Treatment of symptoms of seasonal allergic rhinitis, perennial allergic rhinitis, chronic urticaria

PHARMACOKINETICS
Rapidly and almost completely absorbed from the GI tract (absorption not affected by food). Protein binding: 93%. Undergoes low first-pass metabolism; not extensively metabolized. Primarily excreted in urine (more than 80% as unchanged drug). **Half-life:** 6.5–10 hr.

INDICATIONS AND DOSAGES
▶ **Allergic Rhinitis, Urticaria**
PO
Adults, Elderly, Children older than 5 yr. Initially, 5–10 mg/day as a single or in 2 divided doses.
Children 2–5 yr. 2.5 mg/day. May increase up to 5 mg/day as a single or in 2 divided doses.
Children 12–23 mo. Initially, 2.5 mg/day. May increase up to 5 mg/day in 2 divided doses.
Children 6–11 mo. 2.5 mg once a day.
▶ **Dosage in Renal or Hepatic impairment**
For adult and elderly patients with renal impairment (creatinine clearance of 11–31 ml/min), those receiving hemodialysis (creatinine clearance of 7 ml/min), and those with hepatic impairment, dosage is decreased to 5 mg once a day.

SIDE EFFECTS/ADVERSE REACTIONS
Occasional
Pharyngitis; dry mucous membranes, nose, or throat; nausea and vomiting; abdominal pain; headache; dizziness; fatigue; thickening of mucus; somnolence; photosensitivity; urine retention

PRECAUTIONS AND CONTRAINDICATIONS
Hypersensitivity to cetirizine or hydroxyzine
Caution
Renal impairment (requires dose reduction), elderly, glaucoma, urinary obstruction, lactation

DRUG INTERACTIONS OF CONCERN TO DENTISTRY
• No drug interactions reported, but should be similar to other antihistamines; anticipate increased sedation with other CNS depressants and increased anticholinergic effects with anticholinergic drugs

SERIOUS REACTIONS
! Children may experience paradoxical reactions, including restlessness, insomnia, euphoria, nervousness, and tremor.
! Dizziness, sedation, and confusion are more likely to occur in elderly patients.

DENTAL CONSIDERATIONS
General:
• Assess salivary flow as factor in caries, periodontal disease, and candidiasis.
Teach Patient/Family:
• When chronic dry mouth occurs, advise patient to:
    • Avoid mouth rinses with high alcohol content because of drying effects

• Use daily home fluoride products for anticaries effect
• Use sugarless gum, frequent sips of water, or saliva substitutes

cetuximab
ceh-tux´-ih-mab
(Erbitux)

CATEGORY AND SCHEDULE
Pregnancy Risk Category: C

Drug Class: Monoclonal antibody; antineoplastic

MECHANISM OF ACTION
A monoclonal antibody that binds to the epidermal growth factor receptor (EGFR), a glycoprotein on normal and tumor cells, thus inhibiting cell growth and inducing apoptosis. *Therapeutic Effect:* Inhibits the growth and survival of tumor cells that overexpress EGFR.

USES
As a single agent or in combination with irinotecan for treatment of EGFR-expressing, metastatic colorectal carcinoma in patients who are refractory or intolerant to irinotecan-based chemotherapy

PHARMACOKINETICS
Reaches steady state levels by the third weekly infusion. Clearance decreases as dose increases. *Half-life:* 114 hr (range, 75–188 hr).

INDICATIONS AND DOSAGES
▶ **Metastatic Colorectal Carcinoma**
IV
Adults, Elderly. Initially, 400 mg/m^2 as a loading dose. Maintenance: 250 mg/m^2 infused over 60 min weekly.

C

SIDE EFFECTS/ADVERSE REACTIONS

Frequent

Acneiform rash, malaise, fever, nausea, diarrhea, constipation, headache, abdominal pain, anorexia, vomiting

Occasional

Nail disorder, back pain, stomatitis, peripheral edema, pruritus, cough, insomnia

Rare

Weight loss, depression, dyspepsia, conjunctivitis, alopecia

PRECAUTIONS AND CONTRAINDICATIONS

None known

DRUG INTERACTIONS OF CONCERN TO DENTISTRY

• Dental drug interactions have not been studied

SERIOUS REACTIONS

! Anemia occurs in 10% of patients.
! A severe infusion reaction, characterized by rapid onset of airway obstruction, a precipitous drop in B/P, and severe urticaria, occurs rarely.
! Dermatologic toxicity, pulmonary embolus, leukopenia, and renal failure occur rarely.

DENTAL CONSIDERATIONS

General:

• Monitor vital signs at every appointment due to cardiovascular side effects.
• If additional analgesia is required for dental pain, consider alternative analgesics (NSAIDs) in patients taking narcotics for acute or chronic pain.
• Examine for oral manifestation of opportunistic infection.
• Consider semisupine chair position for patient comfort because of GI effects of disease.

• Patient on chronic drug therapy may rarely present with symptoms of blood dyscrasias, which can include infection, bleeding, and poor healing. If dyscrasia is present, caution patient to prevent oral tissue trauma when using oral hygiene aids.
• Advise patient if dental drugs prescribed have a potential for photosensitivity.
• Patients may be taking a prophylactic antiinfective.
• Use caution in the use of drugs that may cause diarrhea or constipation.
• Patients may have received other chemotherapy or radiation; confirm medical and drug history.

Consultations:

• Consult physician; prophylactic or therapeutic antiinfectives may be indicated if surgery or periodontal treatment is required.
• Medical consultation may be required to assess immunologic status during cancer chemotherapy and determine safety risk, if any, posed by the required dental treatment.
• Medical consultation may be required to assess disease control and patient's ability to tolerate stress.
• Medical consultation should include routine blood counts including platelet counts and bleeding time.

Teach Patient/Family to:

• Use effective oral hygiene to prevent soft tissue inflammation
• Report oral lesions, soreness, or bleeding to dentist
• Prevent trauma when using oral hygiene aids
• Update health and medication history if physician makes any changes in evaluation or drug regimens; include OTC, herbal, and nonherbal remedies in the update

cevimeline

sev-im´-el-ine
(Evoxac)
Do not confuse Evoxac with Eurax.

CATEGORY AND SCHEDULE
Pregnancy Risk Category: C

Drug Class: Cholinergic
(muscarinic) agonist

MECHANISM OF ACTION
A cholinergic agonist that binds to
muscarinic receptors of effector
cells, thereby increasing secretion of
exocrine glands, such as salivary
glands. *Therapeutic Effect:* Relieves
dry mouth.

USES
Treatment of symptoms of dry mouth
associated with Sjögren's syndrome

PHARMACOKINETICS
Rapid absorption after oral
administration, peak levels 1.5–2 hr.
Protein binding: 20%. Metabolized
in liver by CYP 2D6 and CYP 3A4
isoenzymes. *Half-life:* 5 hr. 84%
excreted in urine within 24 hr.

INDICATIONS AND DOSAGES
▶ **Dry Mouth**
PO
Adults. 30 mg 3 times a day.

SIDE EFFECTS/ADVERSE REACTIONS
Frequent
Diaphoresis, headache, nausea,
sinusitis, rhinitis, upper respiratory
tract infection, diarrhea
Occasional
Dyspepsia, abdominal pain, cough,
UTI, vomiting, back pain, rash,
dizziness, fatigue
Rare
Skeletal pain, insomnia, hot flashes,
excessive salivation, rigors, anxiety

PRECAUTIONS AND CONTRAINDICATIONS
Acute iritis, angle-closure glaucoma,
uncontrolled asthma
Caution
Has the potential to alter heart rate
or cardiac conduction; use with care
in cardiovascular disease, asthma,
bronchitis, COPD, seizure disorders,
Parkinson's disease, urinary tract/
bladder obstruction, cholecystitis,
cholangitis, biliary obstruction, GI
ulcers, lactation, children (no data),
history of adverse effects to other
cholinergic agonists

DRUG INTERACTIONS OF CONCERN TO DENTISTRY
• Use with caution in patients taking
β-adrenergic blockers: possible
conduction disturbances
• There are no specific data on
dental drug interactions; however,
use caution with other cholinergic
agonists
• There is always the possibility
that a cholinergic antagonist could
interfere with this drug's action
• Although there are no supporting
data, use with caution in patients
taking drugs that inhibit cytochrome
P-450 (CYP3A3/4 and CYP2D6
isoenzymes)

SERIOUS REACTIONS
❗ Cevimeline use may result in
decreased visual acuity, especially at
night, and impaired depth perception.

DENTAL CONSIDERATIONS
General:
• Assess salivary flow as a factor in
caries, periodontal disease, and
candidiasis.
• Place on frequent recall to assess
effectiveness.
• Consider semisupine chair position
for patient comfort if GI side effects
occur.

Consultations:
• Medical consultation may be required to assess disease control.
• Medical consultation may be necessary before prescribing for those patients with cardiovascular or respiratory disease.

Teach Patient/Family to:
• Be aware that this drug may cause visual disturbances, especially with night driving, which may impair driving safety
• Drink extra fluids (water) to compensate for excessive sweating
• When chronic dry mouth occurs, advise patient to:
  • Avoid mouth rinses with high alcohol content because of drying effects
  • Use daily home fluoride to prevent caries
  • Use sugarless gum, frequent sips of water, or saliva substitutes

chloral hydrate
klor´-al hye´-drate
(Aquachloral Supprettes, PMS-Chloral Hydrate[CAN], Somnote)

CATEGORY AND SCHEDULE
Pregnancy Risk Category: C
Controlled Substance Schedule IV

Drug Class: Sedative hypnotic, chloral derivative

MECHANISM OF ACTION
A nonbarbiturate chloral derivative that produces CNS depression. *Therapeutic Effect:* Induces quiet, deep sleep, with only a slight decrease in respiratory rate and B/P.

USES
Sedation, insomnia

PHARMACOKINETICS
Rapid absorption after oral administration, peak levels 30–45 min. Duration: 2–5 hr. Metabolized to trichloroethanol in liver and other tissues and, to a lesser extent, trichloracetic acid, in liver. *Half-life:* 7–9.5 hr. Glucuronide conjugate excerted in urine.

INDICATIONS AND DOSAGES
▸ **Premedication for Dental or Medical Procedures**
PO, Rectal
Adults. 0.5–1 g.
Children. 75 mg/kg up to 1 g total. (Dosage reduced when combined with other sedatives.)
▸ **Premedication for EEG**
PO, Rectal
Adults. 0.5–1.5 g.
Children. 25–50 mg/kg/dose 30–60 min prior to EEG. May repeat in 30 min. Maximum: 1 g for infants, 2 g for children.

SIDE EFFECTS/ADVERSE REACTIONS
Occasional
Gastric irritation (nausea, vomiting, flatulence, diarrhea), rash, sleepwalking
Rare
Headache, paradoxical CNS hyperactivity or nervousness in children, excitement or restlessness in the elderly (particularly in patients with pain)

PRECAUTIONS AND CONTRAINDICATIONS
Gastritis, marked hepatic or renal impairment, severe cardiac disease
Caution
Severe cardiac disease, depression, suicidal individuals, asthma, intermittent porphyria, lactation, elderly; no specific reversal agent available, use extreme caution in dose calculation when used in pediatric patients for sedation

DRUG INTERACTIONS OF CONCERN TO DENTISTRY
• Increased action of both drugs: alcohol, all CNS depressants, including nitrous oxide

SERIOUS REACTIONS
! Overdose may produce somnolence, confusion, slurred speech, severe incoordination, respiratory depression, and coma.

DENTAL CONSIDERATIONS
General:
• Consider semisupine chair position for patient comfort because of GI side effects of drug.
• Administer syrup in juice or beverage to mask taste and reduce GI upset.
• Contraindicated for use in patients with GI ulcerative disease.
• Have someone drive patient to and from dental office when drug used for conscious sedation.
• Geriatric patients are more susceptible to drug effects; use lower dose.
• Psychologic and physical dependence may occur with chronic administration.

chlordiazepoxide
klor-dye-az-eh-pox´-ide
(Apo-Chlordiazepoxide[CAN], Librium, Novopoxide[CAN])
Do not confuse Librium with Librax.

CATEGORY AND SCHEDULE
Pregnancy Risk Category: D
Controlled Substance Schedule IV

Drug Class: Benzodiazepine antianxiety

MECHANISM OF ACTION
A benzodiazepine that enhances the action of the inhibitory neurotransmitter gamma-aminobutyric acid in the CNS. *Therapeutic Effect:* Produces anxiolytic effect.

USES
Short-term management of anxiety, acute alcohol withdrawal, preoperatively for relaxation

PHARMACOKINETICS
Slow onset after oral administration, peak levels 2 hr. Metabolized in liver (active metabolites). *Half-life:* 24–48 hr. Metabolites excreted in urine.

INDICATIONS AND DOSAGES
▸ **Alcohol Withdrawal Symptoms**
PO
Adults, Elderly. 50–100 mg. May repeat q2–4h. Maximum: 300 mg/ 24 hr.
▸ **Anxiety**
PO
Adults. 15–100 mg/day in 3–4 divided doses.
Elderly. 5 mg 2–4 times a day.
IV, IM
Adults. Initially, 50–100 mg, then 25–50 mg 3–4 times a day as needed.

SIDE EFFECTS/ADVERSE REACTIONS
Frequent
Pain at IM injection site; somnolence, ataxia, dizziness, confusion with oral dose (particularly in elderly or debilitated patients)
Occasional
Rash, peripheral edema, GI disturbances
Rare
Paradoxical CNS reactions, such as hyperactivity or nervousness in children and excitement or

restlessness in the elderly (generally noted during first 2 wk of therapy, particularly in presence of uncontrolled pain)

PRECAUTIONS AND CONTRAINDICATIONS

Acute alcohol intoxication, acute angle-closure glaucoma
Caution
Elderly, debilitated, hepatic disease, renal disease

DRUG INTERACTIONS OF CONCERN TO DENTISTRY

- Delayed elimination: erythromycin
- Increased CNS depression: CNS depressants, alcohol, disulfiram, nefazodone
- Increased serum levels and prolonged effects of benzodiazepines: ketoconazole, itraconazole, fluconazole, miconazole (systemic), cimetidine, fluvoxamine, omeprazole, rifabutin, rifampin
- Contraindicated with ritonavir, indinavir, saquinavir
- Possible increase in CNS side effects: kava kava (herb)
- Decreased plasma levels: St. John's wort (herb)

SERIOUS REACTIONS

! IV administration may produce pain, swelling, thrombophlebitis, and carpal tunnel syndrome.
! Abrupt or too-rapid withdrawal may result in pronounced restlessness, irritability, insomnia, hand tremors, abdominal or muscle cramps, diaphoresis, vomiting, and seizures.
! Overdose results in somnolence, confusion, diminished reflexes, and coma.

DENTAL CONSIDERATIONS

General:
- After supine positioning, have patient sit upright for at least 2 min to avoid orthostatic hypotension.

- Assess salivary flow as a factor in caries, periodontal disease, and candidiasis.
- Psychologic and physical dependence may occur with chronic administration.
- Geriatric patients are more susceptible to drug effects; use lower dose.
- Have someone drive patient to and from dental office if used for conscious sedation.
Consultations:
- Medical consultation may be required to assess disease control.
Teach Patient/Family to:
- Use effective oral hygiene to prevent soft tissue inflammation
- Avoid mouth rinses with high alcohol content because of drying effects

chlorhexidine gluconate

klor-hex´-ih-deen gloo´-ko-nate
(Chlorhexidine Mouthwash[AUS], Chlorhexidine Obstetric Lotion[AUS], Chlorohex Gel[AUS], Chlorohex Gel Forte[AUS], Chlorohex Mouth Rinse[AUS], Peridex, PerioChip, PerioGard, Perisol)

CATEGORY AND SCHEDULE

Pregnancy Risk Category: C

Drug Class: Antiinfective–oral rinse

MECHANISM OF ACTION

An antiseptic and antimicrobial agent that is active against a broad spectrum of microbes. The chlorhexidine molecule, due to its positive charge, reacts with the microbial cell surface, destroys the integrity of the cell membrane, penetrates into the cell, precipitates the cytoplasm, and the cell dies. *Therapeutic Effect:* Causes cell death.

USES
Treatment of gingivitis; unlabeled use: acute aphthous ulcers and denture stomatitis

PHARMACOKINETICS
Initially, the chlorhexidine gluconate dental chip releases approximately 40% of the drug within the first 24 hr, then releases the remainder in an almost linear fashion for 7–10 days. Approximately 30% of the active ingredient, chlorhexidine gluconate, is retained in the oral cavity following oral rinsing. This retained drug is slowly released into the oral fluids. Poorly absorbed from the GI track. Primarily excreted in feces. *Half-life:* Unknown.

INDICATIONS AND DOSAGES
▸ **Gingivitis**
Oral rinse
Adults, Elderly. Swish and spit for 30 sec twice daily.
▸ **Periodontitis**
Oral insert
Adults, Elderly. One chip is inserted into a periodontal pocket; insert a new chip q3mo; maximum of 8 chips per dental visit.

SIDE EFFECTS/ADVERSE REACTIONS
Occasional
Altered taste, staining of tooth, toothache

PRECAUTIONS AND CONTRAINDICATIONS
Hypersensitivity to chlorhexidine gluconate or any component of the formulation.
Caution
Lactation, efficacy not established for children younger than 18 yr, not intended for periodontitis

DRUG INTERACTIONS OF CONCERN TO DENTISTRY
None reported

SERIOUS REACTIONS
! Anaphylaxis has been reported.

DRUG INTERACTIONS OF CONCERN TO DENTISTRY
• Disulfiram-like effects resulting from alcohol content: Antabuse, metronidazole

DENTAL CONSIDERATIONS
General:
• Perform dental examination and prophylaxis/scaling/root planing before starting rinse.
• Place on frequent recall because of oral side effects.
• Use discretion when prescribing to patients with anterior facial restorations with rough surfaces or margins.
Teach Patient/Family to:
• Eat, brush, and floss before using rinse
• Not rinse with water after using chlorhexidine
• Not dilute solution; not swallow solution
• Beware of oral side effects
• Not brush or use dental floss at site of chip placement.
• Notify dentist immediately if chip is dislodged or if pain, swelling, or other symptoms occur

chlorhexidine gluconate chip
klor-hex′-ih-deen gloo′-ko-nate
(Perio Chip)

CATEGORY AND SCHEDULE
Pregnancy Risk Category: C

Drug Class: Antiinfective

MECHANISM OF ACTION
Interferes with the integrity of the bacterial cell membrane, causing leakage of the intracellular components; penetrates into the cell, precipitates the cytoplasm, and the cell dies; effective against numerous supragingival and subgingival bacteria

USES
Adjunct to scaling and root planing for reduction of the subgingival bacterial flora

PHARMACOKINETICS
40% of chlorhexidine released in first 24 hr, remainder released over 7–10 days; no detectable plasma levels.

INDICATIONS AND DOSAGES
Adults: Insert chip into a periodontal pocket with probing depth 5 mm or greater; up to 8 chips may be inserted per single visit; treatment 5 mm in depth; if chip dislodges within 48 hr of placement, replace with new chip; do not replace chips lost after 48 hr, but reevaluate in 3 mo and insert a new chip if pocket depth has not been reduced to less than 5mm; if chip is dislodged 7 days or more after placement, consider this a full course of treatment.

SIDE EFFECTS/ADVERSE REACTIONS
Oral: Localized pain, tenderness, aching, throbbing, toothache
Note: All other side effects reported did not differ from placebo chip

PRECAUTIONS AND CONTRAINDICATIONS
Hypersensitivity
Caution
Not recommended for acutely abscessed periodontal pocket, use in children not established

DRUG INTERACTIONS OF CONCERN TO DENTISTRY
None reported

DENTAL CONSIDERATIONS
General:
• Do not brush or use dental floss at site of chip placement.
Teach patient/family to:
• Notify dentist immediately if chip is dislodged or if pain, swelling, or other symptoms occur

chloroquine/ chloroquine phosphate
klor´-oh-kwin/klor´-oh-kwin foss´-fate
(Aralen hydrochloride, Aralen[CAN])
(Aralen phosphate)

CATEGORY AND SCHEDULE
Pregnancy Risk Category: C

Drug Class: Antimalarial

MECHANISM OF ACTION
An amebecide that concentrates in parasite acid vesicles and may interfere with parasite protein synthesis. *Therapeutic Effect:* Increases pH and inhibits parasite growth.

USES
Treatment of malaria caused by *P. vivax, P. malariae, P. ovale, P. falciparum* (some strains); rheumatoid arthritis; amebiasis

PHARMACOKINETICS
Rate of absorption is variable. Chloroquine is almost completely absorbed from the GI tract. Protein binding: 50%–65%. Widely distributed into body tissues such as

eyes, heart, kidneys, liver, and lungs. Partially metabolized to active de-ethylated metabolites (principle metabolite is desethylchloroquine). Excreted in urine. Removed by hemodialysis. *Half-life:* 1–2 mo.

INDICATIONS AND DOSAGES
Chloroquine Phosphate
▸ **Treatment of malaria (acute attack): Dose (mg base)**

Dose	Time	Adults	Children
Initial	Day 1	600 mg	10 mg/kg
Second	6 hr later	300 mg	5 mg/kg
Third	Day 2	300 mg	5 mg/kg
Fourth	Day 3	300 mg	5 mg/kg

▸ **Suppression of Malaria**
PO
Adults. 300 mg (base)/wk on same day each week beginning 2 wk before exposure; continue for 6–8 wk after leaving endemic area.
Children. 5 mg (base)/kg/wk.
▸ **Malaria Prophylaxis**
PO
Adults. 600 mg base initially given in 2 divided doses 6 hr apart.
Children. 10 mg base/kg.
▸ **Amebiasis**
PO
Adults. 1 g (600 mg base) daily for 2 days; then, 500 mg (300 mg base)/day for at least 2–3 wk.

Chloroquine HCL
▸ **Treatment of malaria**
IM
Adults. Initially, 160–200 mg base (4–5 ml), repeat in 6 hr. Maximum: 800 mg base in first 24 hr. Begin oral therapy as soon as possible and continue for 3 days until approximately 1.5 g base given.
Children. Initially, 5 mg base/kg, repeat in 6 hr. Do not exceed 10 mg base/kg/24 hr.

▸ **Amebiasis**
IM
Adults. 160–200 mg base (4–5 ml) daily for 10–12 days. Change to oral therapy as soon as possible.

SIDE EFFECTS/ADVERSE REACTIONS
Frequent
Discomfort with IM administration, mild transient headache, anorexia, nausea, vomiting
Occasional
Visual disturbances (blurring, difficulty focusing); nervousness, fatigue, pruritus especially of palms, soles, scalp; bleaching of hair, irritability, personality changes, diarrhea, skin eruptions
Rare
Phlebitis or thrombophlebitis at IV injection site, abdominal cramps, headache, hypotension

PRECAUTIONS AND CONTRAINDICATIONS
Hypersensitivity to 4-aminoquinoline compounds, retinal or visual field changes

DRUG INTERACTIONS OF CONCERN TO DENTISTRY
• Hepatotoxicity: alcohol, hepatotoxic drugs

SERIOUS REACTIONS
! Ocular toxicity and ototoxicity have been reported.
! Prolonged therapy: peripheral neuritis and neuromyopathy, hypotension, ECG changes, agranulocytosis, aplastic anemia, thrombocytopenia, convulsions, psychosis.
! Overdosage includes symptoms of headache, vomiting, visual disturbance, drowsiness, convulsions, hypokalemìa followed by cardiovascular collapse, and death.

DENTAL CONSIDERATIONS

General:
- Patients on chronic drug therapy may rarely have symptoms of blood dyscrasias, which can include infection, bleeding, and poor healing.
- Avoid dental light in patient's eyes; offer dark glasses for patient comfort.
- Determine why the patient is taking the drug.

Consultations:
- In a patient with symptoms of blood dyscrasias, request a medical consultation for blood studies and postpone dental treatment until normal values are reestablished.

Teach Patient/Family to:
- Use effective oral hygiene to prevent soft tissue inflammation
- Avoid mouth rinses with high alcohol content because of drying effects

---

chlorothiazide
klor-oh-thye´-ah-zide
(Diuril, Diuril Sodium)

CATEGORY AND SCHEDULE
Pregnancy Risk Category: C

Drug Class: Thiazide diuretic

MECHANISM OF ACTION
A sulfonamide derivative that acts as a thiazide diuretic and antihypertensive. As a diuretic blocks reabsorption of water, the electrolytes sodium and potassium at cortical diluting segment of distal tubule. As an antihypertensive reduces plasma, extracellular fluid volume, decreases peripheral vascular resistance (PVR) by direct effect on blood vessels. ***Therapeutic Effect:*** Promotes diuresis, reduces B/P.

USES
Treatment of edema, hypertension, diuresis

PHARMACOKINETICS
Poorly absorbed from the GI tract. Not metabolized. Primarily excreted unchanged in urine. Not removed by hemodialysis. ***Half-life:*** 45–120 min.

INDICATIONS AND DOSAGES
▶ **Edema, Hypertension**
PO
Adults. 0.5–1 g 1–2 times a day. May give every other day or 3–5 days a wk.
Children 12 yr and older. 10–20 mg/kg/dose in divided doses q8–12h. Maximum: 2g/day.
Children 2–12 yr. 1 g/day.
Children 6 mo–2 yr. 10–20 mg/kg/day in divided doses q12–24h. Maximum: 375 mg/day.
Children younger than 6 mo. 20–30 mg/kg/day in divided doses q12h. Maximum: 375 mg/day.
▶ **Hypertension**
IV
Adults. 0.5–1 g in divided doses q12–24h.

SIDE EFFECTS/ADVERSE REACTIONS
Expected
Increase in urine frequency and volume
Frequent
Potassium depletion
Occasional
Postural hypotension, headache, GI disturbances, photosensitivity reaction, muscle spasms, alopecia, rash, urticaria

PRECAUTIONS AND CONTRAINDICATIONS
Anuria, history of hypersensitivity to sulfonamides or thiazide diuretics, renal decompensation

Caution
Hypokalemia, renal disease, hepatic disease, gout, COPD, lupus erythematosus, diabetes mellitus, elderly

DRUG INTERACTIONS OF CONCERN TO DENTISTRY
• Increased photosensitization: tetracyclines
• Decreased hypotensive response, nephrotoxicity: indomethacin and other NSAIDs

SERIOUS REACTIONS
! Vigorous diuresis may lead to profound water loss and electrolyte depletion, resulting in hypokalemia, hyponatremia, and dehydration.
! Acute hypotensive episodes may occur.
! Hyperglycemia may be noted during prolonged therapy.
! GI upset, pancreatitis, dizziness, paresthesias, headache, blood dyscrasias, pulmonary edema, allergic pneumonitis, and dermatologic reactions occur rarely.
! Overdosage can lead to lethargy and coma without changes in electrolytes or hydration.

DENTAL CONSIDERATIONS
General:
• Monitor vital signs at every appointment because of cardiovascular side effects.
• After supine positioning, have patient sit upright for at least 2 min before standing to avoid orthostatic hypotension.
• Patients on chronic drug therapy may rarely have symptoms of blood dyscrasias, which can include infection, bleeding, and poor healing.
• Observe appropriate limitations of vasoconstrictor doses.

• Assess salivary flow as a factor in caries, periodontal disease, and candidiasis.
• Limit use of sodium-containing products, such as saline IV fluids, for patients with a dietary salt restriction.
• Stress from dental procedures may compromise cardiovascular function; determine patient risk.
• Short appointments and a stress-reduction protocol may be required for anxious patients.
• Patients taking diuretics should be monitored for serum K levels.
Consultations:
• In a patient with symptoms of blood dyscrasias, request a medical consultation for blood studies and postpone dental treatment until normal values are reestablished.
• Medical consultation may be required to assess disease control and patient's ability to tolerate stress.
• Physician should be informed if significant xerostomic side effects occur (increased caries, sore tongue, problems eating or swallowing, difficulty wearing prosthesis) so that a medication change can be considered.
Teach Patient/Family to:
• Use effective oral hygiene to prevent soft tissue inflammation
• Use caution to prevent injury when using oral hygiene aids
• When chronic dry mouth occurs, advise patient to:
    • Avoid mouth rinses with high alcohol content because of drying effects
    • Use daily home fluoride products for anticaries effect
    • Use sugarless gum, frequent sips of water, or saliva substitutes

chlorpheniramine

klor-fen-ir´-ah-meen
(Aller-Chlor, Chlor-Trimeton, Chlor-Trimeton Allergy, Chlor-Trimeton Allergy 12 Hour, Chlor-Trimeton Allergy 8 Hour, Chlor-Tripolon[CAN], Chlorate, Chlorphen, Diabetic Tussin Allergy Relief)
Do not confuse with chlorpromazine or chlorpropamide.

CATEGORY AND SCHEDULE

Pregnancy Risk Category: C
OTC (tablets, syrup)

Drug Class: Antihistamine, H_1-receptor antagonist

MECHANISM OF ACTION

A propylamine derivative antihistamine that competes with histamine for H_1 histamine receptor sites on cells in the blood vessels, GI tract, and respiratory tract.
Therapeutic Effect: Inhibits symptoms associated with seasonal allergic rhinitis such as increased mucus production and sneezing.

USES

Allergy symptoms, rhinitis

PHARMACOKINETICS

Well absorbed after PO and parenteral administration. Food delays absorption. Widely distributed. Metabolized in liver. Primarily excreted in urine. Not removed by dialysis. ***Half-life:*** 20 hr.

INDICATIONS AND DOSAGES

▸ **Allergic Rhinitis, Common cold**
PO
Adults, Elderly. 4 mg q6–8h or 8–12 mg (sustained-release) q8–12h. Maximum: 24 mg/day.

Children 12 yr and older. 4 mg q6–8h or 8 mg (sustained-release) q12h. Maximum: 24 mg/day.
Children 6–11 yr. 2 mg q4–6h. Maximum: 12 mg/day.
IM/IV/SC
Adults, Elderly. 5–40 mg as a single dose. Maximum: 40 mg/day.
SC
Children 6 yr and older. 87.5 mcg/kg or 2.5 mg/m^2 4 times a day.

SIDE EFFECTS/ADVERSE REACTIONS

Frequent
Drowsiness, dizziness, muscular weakness, hypotension, dry mouth, nose, throat, and lips, urinary retention, thickening of bronchial secretions
Elderly: Sedation, dizziness, hypotension
Occasional
Epigastric distress, flushing, visual or hearing disturbances, paresthesia, diaphoresis, chills

PRECAUTIONS AND CONTRAINDICATIONS

Hypersensitivity to chlorpheniramine or its components

DRUG INTERACTIONS OF CONCERN TO DENTISTRY

• Increased CNS depression: alcohol, all CNS depressants
• Increased anticholinergic effect: other anticholinergics, phenothiazines, tricyclic antidepressants

SERIOUS REACTIONS

! Children may experience dominant paradoxical reactions, including restlessness, insomnia, euphoria, nervousness, and tremors.
! Overdosage in children may result in hallucinations, seizures, and death.
! Hypersensitivity reaction, such as eczema, pruritus, rash, cardiac disturbances, and photosensitivity, may occur.

! Overdosage may vary from CNS depression, including sedation, apnea, hypotension, cardiovascular collapse, or death to severe paradoxical reaction, such as hallucinations, tremors, and seizures.

DENTAL CONSIDERATIONS
General:
• Assess salivary flow as a factor in caries, periodontal disease, and candidiasis.
• Consider semisupine chair position for patients with respiratory disease.
• Determine why the patient is taking the drug.
Teach Patient/Family to:
• Use effective oral hygiene to prevent soft tissue inflammation
• Use caution to prevent injury when using oral hygiene aids
• When chronic dry mouth occurs, advise patient to:
  • Avoid mouth rinses with high alcohol content because of drying effects
  • Use daily home fluoride products for anticaries effect
  • Use sugarless gum, frequent sips of water, or saliva substitutes

chlorpromazine
klor-proe´-ma-zeen
(Chlorpromanyl[CAN], Largactil[CAN], Thorazine)
Do not confuse chlorpromazine with chlorpropamide, clomipramine, or prochlorperazine, or Thorazine with thiamide or thioridazine.

CATEGORY AND SCHEDULE
Pregnancy Risk Category: C

Drug Class: Phenothiazine antipsychotic

MECHANISM OF ACTION
A phenothiazine that blocks dopamine neurotransmission at postsynaptic dopamine receptor sites. Possesses strong anticholinergic, sedative, and antiemetic effects; moderate extrapyramidal effects; and slight antihistamine action.
Therapeutic Effect: Relieves nausea and vomiting; improves psychotic conditions; controls intractable hiccups and porphyria.

USES
Psychotic disorders, mania, schizophrenia, anxiety, intractable hiccups, nausea, vomiting, preoperatively for relaxation, acute intermittent porphyria, behavioral problems in children

PHARMACOKINETICS
Rapidly absorbed after oral or IM administration. Protein binding: 92%–97%. Metabolized in the liver. Excreted in urine. **Half-life:** 6 hr.

INDICATIONS AND DOSAGES
▶ **Severe Nausea or Vomiting**
PO
Adults, Elderly. 10–25 mg q4–6h.
Children. 0.5–1 mg/kg q4–6h.
IV, IM
Adults, Elderly. 25–50 mg q4–6h.
Children. 0.5–1 mg/kg q6–8h.
Rectal
Adults, Elderly. 50–100 mg q6–8h.
Children. 1 mg/kg q6–8h.
▶ **Psychotic Disorders**
PO
Adults, Elderly. 30–800 mg/day in 1–4 divided doses.
Children older than 6 mo. 0.5–1 mg/kg q4–6h.
IV, IM
Adults, Elderly. Initially, 25 mg; may repeat in 1–4 hr. May gradually increase to 400 mg q4–6h.
Maximum: 300–800 mg/day.

Children older than 6 mo. 0.5–1 mg/
kg q6–8h. Maximum: 75 mg/day for
children 5–12 yr; 40 mg/day for
children younger than 5 yr.
▸ **Intractable Hiccups**
PO, IV, IM
Adults. 25–50 mg 3 times a day.
▸ **Porphyria**
PO
Adults. 25–50 mg 3–4 times a day.
IM
Adults, Elderly. 25 mg 3–4 times a day.

SIDE EFFECTS/ADVERSE REACTIONS
Frequent
Somnolence, blurred vision,
hypotension, color vision or night
vision disturbances, dizziness,
decreased sweating, constipation,
dry mouth, nasal congestion
Occasional
Urinary retention, photosensitivity,
rash, decreased sexual function,
swelling or pain in breasts, weight
gain, nausea, vomiting, abdominal
pain, tremors

PRECAUTIONS AND CONTRAINDICATIONS
Comatose states, myelosuppression,
severe cardiovascular disease, severe
CNS depression, subcortical brain
damage
Caution
Lactation, seizure disorders,
hypertension, hepatic disease,
cardiac disease, elderly

DRUG INTERACTIONS OF CONCERN TO DENTISTRY
• Increased sedation: other CNS
depressants, alcohol, barbiturate
anesthetics, opioid analgesics
• Hypotension, tachycardia:
epinephrine (systemic)
• Increased extrapyramidal effects:
related drugs, such as haloperidol,
droperidol, and metoclopramide

• Additive photosensitization:
tetracyclines
• Increased anticholinergic effects:
anticholinergics

SERIOUS REACTIONS
! Extrapyramidal symptoms appear
to be dose related and are divided
into three categories: akathisia
(including inability to sit still, tapping
of feet), parkinsonian symptoms
(such as masklike face, tremors,
shuffling gait, hypersalivation), and
acute dystonias (including torticollis,
opisthotonos, and oculogyric crisis).
A dystonic reaction may also
produce diaphoresis and pallor.
! Tardive dyskinesia, including
tongue protrusion, puffing of the
cheeks, and puckering of the mouth
is a rare reaction that may be
irreversible.
! Abrupt discontinuation after long-
term therapy may precipitate nausea,
vomiting, gastritis, dizziness, and
tremors.
! Blood dyscrasias, particularly
agranulocytosis and mild leukopenia,
may occur.
! Chlorpromazine may lower the
seizure threshold.

DENTAL CONSIDERATIONS
General:
• Monitor vital signs at every
appointment because of
cardiovascular side effects.
• Patients on chronic drug therapy
may rarely have symptoms of blood
dyscrasias, which can include
infection, bleeding, and poor healing.
• After supine positioning, have
patient sit upright for at least 2 min
before standing to avoid orthostatic
hypotension.
• Assess salivary flow as a factor
in caries, periodontal disease, and
candidiasis.

- Avoid dental light in patient's eyes; offer dark glasses for patient comfort.
- Assess for presence of extrapyramidal motor symptoms, such as tardive dyskinesia and akathisia. Extrapyramidal motor activity may complicate dental treatment.
- Geriatric patients are more susceptible to drug effects; use a lower dose.

Consultations:
- In a patient with symptoms of blood dyscrasias, request a medical consultation for blood studies and postpone dental treatment until normal values are reestablished.
- Take precautions if dental surgery is anticipated and anesthesia is required.
- If signs of tardive dyskinesia or akathisia are present, refer to physician.
- Physician should be informed if significant xerostomic side effects occur (increased caries, sore tongue, problems eating or swallowing, difficulty wearing prosthesis) so that a medication change can be considered.

Teach Patient/Family to:
- Use effective oral hygiene to prevent soft tissue inflammation
- Use caution to prevent injury when using oral hygiene aids
- Use electric tooth brush if patient has difficulty holding conventional devices
- When chronic dry mouth occurs, advise patient to:
  - Avoid mouth rinses with high alcohol content because of drying effects
  - Use daily home fluoride products for anticaries effect
  - Use sugarless gum, frequent sips of water, or saliva substitutes

chlorpropamide
klor-pro´-pa-mide
(Apo-Chlorpropamide[CAN], Diabinese)
Do not confuse with chlorpromazine.

CATEGORY AND SCHEDULE
Pregnancy Risk Category: C

Drug Class: Antidiabetic, sulfonylurea (first-generation)

MECHANISM OF ACTION
A first-generation sulfonylurea that promotes release of insulin from beta cells of pancreas. *Therapeutic Effect:* Lowers blood glucose concentration.

USES
Treatment of stable adult-onset diabetes mellitus (type 2)

PHARMACOKINETICS
Rapidly absorbed from the GI tract. Protein binding: 60%–90%. Extensively metabolized in liver. Excreted primarily in urine. Removed by hemodialysis. *Half-life:* 30–42 hr.

INDICATIONS AND DOSAGES
▶ **Diabetes Mellitus, Combination Therapy**
PO
Adults. Initially, 250 mg once a day. Maintenance: 250–500 mg once a day. Maximum: 750 mg/day.
Elderly. Initially, 100–125 mg once a day. Maintenance: 100–250 mg once a day. Increase or decrease by 50–125 mg a day for 3–5 day intervals.
▶ **Renal Function Impairment**
Not recommended.

SIDE EFFECTS/ADVERSE REACTIONS

Frequent
Headache, upper respiratory tract infection

Occasional
Sinusitis, myalgia (muscle aches), pharyngitis, aggravated diabetes mellitus

PRECAUTIONS AND CONTRAINDICATIONS

Diabetic complications, such as ketosis, acidosis, and diabetic coma, severe liver or renal impairment, sole therapy for type 1 diabetes mellitus, or hypersensitivity to sulfonylureas

Caution
Elderly, cardiac disease, thyroid disease, renal disease, hepatic disease, severe hypoglycemic reactions, avoid use in lactation, use in children not established

DRUG INTERACTIONS OF CONCERN TO DENTISTRY

• Increased hypoglycemic effects: salicylates, NSAIDs, ketoconazole, miconazole
• Decreased action: corticosteroids, sympathomimetics
• Disulfiram-like reaction: alcohol

SERIOUS REACTIONS

! Possible increased risk of cardiovascular mortality with this class of drugs.
! Overdosage can cause severe hypoglycemia prolonged by extended half-life.

DENTAL CONSIDERATIONS

General:
• Patients on chronic drug therapy may rarely have symptoms of blood dyscrasias, which can include infection, bleeding, and poor healing.
• Short appointments and a stress-reduction protocol may be required for anxious patients.

• Question patient about self-monitoring of drug's antidiabetic effect, including blood glucose values or finger-stick records.
• Ensure that patient is following prescribed diet and regularly takes medication.
• Determine if medication controls disease. Patients with diabetes may be more susceptible to infection and have delayed wound healing.
• Avoid prescribing aspirin-containing products.

Consultations:
• In a patient with symptoms of blood dyscrasias, request a medical consultation for blood studies and postpone dental treatment until normal values are reestablished.
• Medical consultation may be required to assess disease control.
• Medical consultation may include data from patient's blood glucose monitoring, including glycosylated hemoglobin or HbA1c testing.

Teach Patient/Family to:
• Use effective oral hygiene to prevent soft tissue inflammation
• Use caution to prevent injury when using oral hygiene aids
• Avoid mouth rinses with high alcohol content because of drying effects

chlorthalidone

klor-thal´-ih-doan
(Apo-Chlorthalidone[CAN], Hygroton[AUS], Thalitone)

CATEGORY AND SCHEDULE

Pregnancy Risk Category: B
(D if used in pregnancy-induced hypertension)

Drug Class: Diuretic with thiazide-like effects

MECHANISM OF ACTION
A thiazide diuretic that blocks reabsorption of sodium, potassium, and water at the distal convoluted tubule; also decreases plasma and extracellular fluid volume and peripheral vascular resistance. *Therapeutic Effect:* Produces diuresis; lowers B/P.

USES
Treatment of edema, hypertension, diuresis, CHF

PHARMACOKINETICS
Rapidly absorbed from the GI tract. Excreted unchanged in urine. *Half-life:* 35–50 hr. Onset of antihypertensive effect: 3–4 days; optimal therapeutic effect: 3–4 wk.

INDICATIONS AND DOSAGES
▶ **Hypertension, Edema**
PO
Adults. 25–100 mg/day or 100 mg 3 times a week.
Elderly. Initially, 12.5–25 mg/day or every other day.

SIDE EFFECTS/ADVERSE REACTIONS
Expected
Increase in urinary frequency and urine volume
Frequent
Potassium depletion (rarely produces symptoms)
Occasional
Anorexia, impotence, diarrhea, orthostatic hypotension, GI disturbances, photosensitivity
Rare
Rash

PRECAUTIONS AND CONTRAINDICATIONS
Anuria, history of hypersensitivity to sulfonamides or thiazide diuretics, renal decompensation

Caution
Hypokalemia, renal disease, hepatic disease, gout, diabetes mellitus, elderly, lactation

DRUG INTERACTIONS OF CONCERN TO DENTISTRY
• Increased photosensitization: tetracyclines
• Decreased hypotensive response, nephrotoxicity: NSAIDs, indomethacin

SERIOUS REACTIONS
❗ Vigorous diuresis may lead to profound water and electrolyte depletion, resulting in hypokalemia, hyponatremia, and dehydration.
❗ Acute hypotensive episodes may occur.
❗ Hyperglycemia may occur during prolonged therapy.
❗ Overdose can lead to lethargy and coma without changes in electrolytes or hydration.

DENTAL CONSIDERATIONS
General:
• Monitor vital signs at every appointment because of cardiovascular side effects.
• After supine positioning, have patient sit upright for at least 2 min before standing to avoid orthostatic hypotension.
• Patients on chronic drug therapy may rarely have symptoms of blood dyscrasias, which can include infection, bleeding, and poor healing.
• Assess salivary flow as a factor in caries, periodontal disease, and candidiasis.
• Limit use of sodium-containing products, such as saline IV fluids, for those patients with a dietary salt restriction.
• Short appointments and a stress reduction protocol may be required for anxious patients.

- Observe appropriate limitations of vasoconstrictor doses.
- Stress from dental procedures may compromise cardiovascular function; determine patient risk.

Consultations:
- In a patient with symptoms of blood dyscrasias, request a medical consultation for blood studies and postpone dental treatment until normal values are reestablished.
- Medical consultation may be required to assess disease control and patient's ability to tolerate stress.

Teach Patient/Family to:
- Use effective oral hygiene to prevent soft tissue inflammation
- Use caution to prevent injury when using oral hygiene aids
- When chronic dry mouth occurs, advise patient to:
  - Avoid mouth rinses with high alcohol content because of drying effects
  - Use daily home fluoride products for anticaries effect
  - Use sugarless gum, frequent sips of water, or saliva substitutes

chlorzoxazone

klor-zox´-ah-zone
(Parafon Forte DSC, Remular, Remular-S)
Do not confuse with chlorthalidone.

CATEGORY AND SCHEDULE
Pregnancy Risk Category: C

Drug Class: Skeletal muscle relaxant, centrally acting

MECHANISM OF ACTION
A skeletal muscle relaxant that inhibits transmission of reflexes at the spinal cord level. *Therapeutic Effect:* Relieves muscle spasticity.

USES
Adjunct for relief of muscle spasm in musculoskeletal conditions

PHARMACOKINETICS
Readily absorbed from the GI tract. Metabolized in liver. Primarily excreted in urine. *Half-life:* 1.1 hr.

INDICATIONS AND DOSAGES
▶ **Musculoskeletal Pain**
PO
Adults, Elderly. 250–500 mg 3–4 times a day. Maximum: 750 mg 3–4 day.
Children. 20 mg/kg/day in 3–4 divided doses.

SIDE EFFECTS/ADVERSE REACTIONS
Frequent
Drowsiness, fever, headache
Occasional
Nausea, vomiting, stomach cramps, rash

PRECAUTIONS AND CONTRAINDICATIONS
Hypersensitivity to chlorzoxazone or any one of its components
Caution
Lactation, hepatic disease, elderly

DRUG INTERACTIONS OF CONCERN TO DENTISTRY
- Increased CNS depression: alcohol, narcotics, barbiturates, sedatives, hypnotics

SERIOUS REACTIONS
! Overdosage results in nausea, vomiting, diarrhea, and hypotension.

DENTAL CONSIDERATIONS
General:
- Determine why the patient is taking the drug.
- Consider semisupine chair position if back is involved.

• When used for dental-related problems, consider aspirin or NSAIDs to improve response.

cholestyramine resin
koe-less-tir´-ah-meen
(Novo-Cholamine[CAN], Prevalite, Questran[CAN], Questran Lite[AUS])
Do not confuse Questran with Quarzan.

CATEGORY AND SCHEDULE
Pregnancy Risk Category: B

Drug Class: Antihyperlipidemic

MECHANISM OF ACTION
An antihyperlipoproteinemic that binds with bile acids in the intestine, forming an insoluble complex. Binding results in partial removal of bile acid from enterohepatic circulation. *Therapeutic Effect:* Removes LDL cholesterol from plasma.

USES
Treatment of primary hypercholesterolemia, pruritus associated with biliary obstruction, diarrhea caused by excess bile acid, digitalis toxicity, xanthomas

PHARMACOKINETICS
Not absorbed from the GI tract. Decreases in serum LDL apparent in 5–7 days and in serum cholesterol in 1 mo. Serum cholesterol returns to baseline levels about 1 mo after drug is discontinued.

INDICATIONS AND DOSAGES
▶ **Primary Hypercholesterolemia**
PO
Adults, Elderly. 3–4 g 3–4 times a day. Maximum: 16–32 g/day in 2–4 divided doses.

Children older than 10 yr. 2 g/day. Maximum: 8 g/day in 2 or more divided doses.
Children 10 yr and younger. Initially, 2 g/day. Range: 1–4 g/day.
▶ **Pruritis**
PO
Adults, Elderly. 4 g 1–2 times a day. Maintenance: Up to 24 g/day in divided doses.

SIDE EFFECTS/ADVERSE REACTIONS
Frequent
Constipation (may lead to fecal impaction), nausea, vomiting, abdominal pain, indigestion
Occasional
Diarrhea, belching, bloating, headache, dizziness
Rare
Gallstones, peptic ulcer disease, malabsorption syndrome

PRECAUTIONS AND CONTRAINDICATIONS
Complete biliary obstruction, hypersensitivity to cholestyramine or tartrazine (frequently seen in aspirin hypersensitivity)
Caution
Lactation, children

DRUG INTERACTIONS OF CONCERN TO DENTISTRY
• Decreased absorption of tetracyclines, cephalexin, phenobarbital, corticosteroids, clindamycin, penicillins; administer doses several hr apart

SERIOUS REACTIONS
! GI tract obstruction, hyperchloremic acidosis, and osteoporosis secondary to calcium excretion may occur.
! High dosage may interfere with fat absorption, resulting in steatorrhea.

DENTAL CONSIDERATIONS

General:

• Consider semisupine chair position for patient comfort because of GI side effects of disease.

ciclopirox

sye-kloe-peer'-ox

(Loprox, Penlac)

Do not confuse with ciprofloxacin.

CATEGORY AND SCHEDULE

Pregnancy Risk Category: B

Drug Class: Topical antifungal

MECHANISM OF ACTION

An antifungal that inhibits the transport of essential elements in the fungal cell, thereby interfering with biosynthesis in fungi. *Therapeutic Effect:* Results in fungal cell death.

USES

Treatment of tinea cruris, tinea corporis, tinea pedis, tinea versicolor, cutaneous candidiasis, nail solution for immunocompetent patients with mild to moderate onychomycosis of nails without lunula involvement; caused by *T. rubrum*

PHARMACOKINETICS

Absorbed through intact skin. Distributed to epidermis, dermis, including hair, hair follicles, and sebaceous glands. Protein binding: 98%. Primarily excreted in urine and to a lesser extent in feces. *Half-life:* 1.7 hr.

INDICATIONS AND DOSAGES

▸ **Tinea Pedis**

Topical

Adults, Elderly, Children 10 yr and older. Apply 2 times a day until signs and symptoms significantly improve.

▸ **Tinea Cruris, Tinea Corporis**

Topical

Adults, Elderly, Children 10 yr and older. Apply 2 times a day until signs and symptoms significantly improve.

▸ **Onychomycosis**

Topical (solution)

Adults, Elderly, Children 10 yr and older. Apply to the affected area (nails) daily. Remove with alcohol every 7 days.

▸ **Seborrheic Dermatitis**

Shampoo

Adults, Elderly, Children 10 yr and older. Apply to affected scalp areas 2 times a day, in the morning and evening for 4 wk.

SIDE EFFECTS/ADVERSE REACTIONS

Rare

Topical: Irritation, burning, redness, pain at the site of application

PRECAUTIONS AND CONTRAINDICATIONS

Hypersensitivity to ciclopirox or any one of its components

Caution

Lactation, children younger than 10 yr

DRUG INTERACTIONS OF CONCERN TO DENTISTRY

None reported

SERIOUS REACTIONS

None known

DENTAL CONSIDERATIONS

General:

• There are neither dental drug interactions nor relevant considerations to dentistry for this drug.

cimetidine

sye-met´-ih-deen
(Apo-Cimetidine[CAN],
Cimehexal[AUS], Magicul[AUS],
Novocimetine[CAN], Peptol[CAN],
Sigmetadine[AUS], Tagamet,
Tagamet HB)
Do not confuse cimetidine with
simethicone.

CATEGORY AND SCHEDULE
Pregnancy Risk Category: B

Drug Class: H_2 histamine
receptor antagonist
OTC (100 mg tablets)

MECHANISM OF ACTION
An antiulcer agent and gastric acid
secretion inhibitor that inhibits
histamine action at H_2 receptor sites
of parietal cells. ***Therapeutic Effect:***
Inhibits gastric acid secretion during
fasting, at night, or when stimulated
by food, caffeine, or insulin.

USES
Short-term treatment of duodenal
and benign gastric ulcers and
maintenance; gastroesophageal reflux
disease (GERD), upper GI bleeding,
pathologic hypersecretory diseases
and heartburn with acid indigestion

PHARMACOKINETICS
Well absorbed from the GI tract.
Protein binding: 15%–20%. Widely
distributed. Metabolized in the liver.
Primarily excreted in urine. Not
removed by hemodialysis. ***Half-life:***
2 hr; increased with impaired renal
function.

INDICATIONS AND DOSAGES
▶ **Active Ulcer**
PO

Adults, Elderly. 300 mg 4 times a day
or 400 mg twice a day or 800 mg at
bedtime.
IV, IM
Adults, Elderly. 300 mg q6h or
150 mg as single dose followed by
37.5 mg/hr continuous infusion.
▶ **Prevention of Duodenal Ulcer**
PO
Adults, Elderly. 400–800 mg at
bedtime.
▶ **Gastric Hypersecretory Secretions**
PO, IV, IM
Adults, Elderly. 300–600 mg q6h.
Maximum: 2,400 mg/day.
Children. 20–40 mg/kg/day in
divided doses q6h.
Infants. 10–20 mg/kg/day in divided
doses q6–12h.
Neonates. 5–10 mg/kg/day in divided
doses q8–12h.
▶ **GERD**
PO
Adults, Elderly. 800 mg twice a day
or 400 mg 4 times a day for 12 wk.
▶ **OTC use**
PO
Adults, Elderly. 100 mg up to 30 min
before meals. Maximum: 2 doses a
day.
▶ **Prevention of Upper GI Bleeding**
IV Infusion
Adults, Elderly. 50 mg/hr.
▶ **Dosage in Renal Impairment**
Dosage is based on a 300-mg dose in
adults. Dosage interval is modified
on the basis of creatinine clearance.

Creatinine Clearance	Dosage Interval
Greater than 40 ml/min	q6h
20–40 ml/min	q8h or decrease dose by 25%
Less than 20 ml/min	q12h or decrease dose by 50%

Give after hemodialysis and q12h between dialysis sessions.

SIDE EFFECTS/ADVERSE REACTIONS
Occasional
Headache
Elderly and severely ill patients, patients with impaired renal function: Confusion, agitation, psychosis, depression, anxiety, disorientation, hallucinations. Effects reverse 3–4 days after discontinuance.
Rare
Diarrhea, dizziness, somnolence, nausea, vomiting, gynecomastia, rash, impotence

PRECAUTIONS AND CONTRAINDICATIONS
Hypersensitivity to other H_2-antagonists.
Caution
Lactation, children younger than 12 yr, organic brain syndrome, hepatic disease, renal disease, smoking

DRUG INTERACTIONS OF CONCERN TO DENTISTRY
• GI ulceration, bleeding: aspirin, NSAIDs
• Decreased absorption: sodium bicarbonate, anticholinergics
• Decreased absorption of fluconazole, ketoconazole, tetracycline (take doses 2 hr apart), ferrous salts
• Increased blood levels of metronidazole, alcohol, lidocaine, narcotic analgesics, benzodiazepines, carbamazepine

SERIOUS REACTIONS
❗ Rapid IV administration may produce cardiac arrhythmias and hypotension.

DENTAL CONSIDERATIONS
General:
• Monitor vital signs at every appointment because of cardiovascular side effects.
• Consider semisupine chair position for patient comfort because of GI side effects of disease.
• Avoid prescribing aspirin- or NSAID-containing products in patients with active upper GI disease; risk of irritation and ulceration exists.
• Sodium bicarbonate products can be used 1 hr before or 1 hr after cimetidine dose.
Teach Patient/Family to:
• Use effective oral hygiene to prevent soft tissue inflammation
• Use caution to prevent injury when using oral hygiene aids

ciprofloxacin hydrochloride
sip-ro-floks´-ah-sin
hi-droe-klor´-ide
(C-Flox[AUS], Ciloquin[AUS], Ciloxan, Cipro, Ciproxin[AUS])
Do not confuse ciprofloxacin or Ciproxin with Ciloxan, cinoxacin, or Cytoxan.

CATEGORY AND SCHEDULE
Pregnancy Risk Category: C

Drug Class: Topical fluoroquinolone antiinfective

MECHANISM OF ACTION
A fluoroquinolone that inhibits the enzyme DNA gyrase in susceptible bacteria, interfering with bacterial cell replication. *Therapeutic Effect:* Bactericidal.

USES

Infections caused by susceptible strains of microorganisms in conjunctivitis or corneal ulcers

PHARMACOKINETICS

Well absorbed from the GI tract (food delays absorption). Protein binding: 20%–40%. Widely distributed (including to CSF). Metabolized in the liver to active metabolite. Primarily excreted in urine. Minimal removal by hemodialysis. *Half-life:* 4–6 hr (increased in impaired renal function and the elderly).

INDICATIONS AND DOSAGES
▸ **Mild to Moderate UTIs**
PO
Adults, Elderly. 250 mg q12h.
IV
Adults, Elderly. 200 mg q12h.
▸ **Complicated UTIs; Mild to Moderate Respiratory Tract, Bone, Joint, Skin, and Skin-Structure Infections; Infectious Diarrhea**
PO
Adults, Elderly. 500 mg q12h.
IV
Adults, Elderly. 400 mg q12h.
▸ **Severe, Complicated Infections**
PO
Adults, Elderly. 750 mg q12h.
IV
Adults, Elderly. 400 mg q12h.
▸ **Prostatitis**
PO
Adults, Elderly. 500 mg q12h for 28 days.
▸ **Uncomplicated Bladder Infection**
PO
Adults. 100 mg twice a day for 3 days.
▸ **Acute Sinusitis**
PO
Adults. 500 mg q12h.
▸ **Uncomplicated Gonorrhea**
PO

Adults. 250 mg as a single dose.
▸ **Cystic Fibrosis**
IV
Children. 30 mg/kg/day in 2–3 divided doses. Maximum: 1.2 g/day.
PO
Children. 40 mg/kg/day. Maximum: 2 g/day.
▸ **Corneal Ulcer**
Ophthalmic
Adults, Elderly. 2 drops q15min for 6 hr, then 2 drops q30min for the remainder of first day, 2 drops q1h on second day, and 2 drops q4h on days 3–14.
▸ **Conjunctivitis**
Ophthalmic
Adults, Elderly. 1–2 drops q2h for 2 days, then 2 drops q4h for next 5 days.
▸ **Dosage in Renal Impairment**
Dosage and frequency are modified on the basis of creatinine clearance and the severity of the infection.

Creatine Clearance	Dosage Interval
Less than 30 ml/min	Usual dose q18–24h

▸ **Hemodialysis**
Adults, Elderly. 250–500 mg q24h (after dialysis).
▸ **Peritoneal Dialysis**
Adults, Elderly. 250–500 mg q24h (after dialysis).

SIDE EFFECTS/ADVERSE REACTIONS
Frequent
Nausea, diarrhea, dyspepsia, vomiting, constipation, flatulence, confusion, crystalluria
Ophthalmic: Burning, crusting in corner of eye
Occasional
Abdominal pain or discomfort, headache, rash

C

Ophthalmic: Bad taste, sensation of something in eye, eyelid redness or itching

Rare

Dizziness, confusion, tremors, hallucinations, hypersensitivity reaction, insomnia, dry mouth, paresthesia

PRECAUTIONS AND CONTRAINDICATIONS

Hypersensitivity to ciprofloxacin or other quinolones; for ophthalmic administration: vaccinia, varicella, epithelial herpes simplex, keratitis, mycobacterial infection, fungal disease of ocular structure, use after uncomplicated removal of a foreign body

Caution

Lactation, children, renal disease, tendon ruptures of shoulder, hand, and Achilles tendons, epilepsy, severe cerebral arteriosclerosis; monitor blood glucose levels, extended release tablets can be taken with meals, defects in glucose-6-phosphate dehydrogenase activity, myasthenia gravis

DRUG INTERACTIONS OF CONCERN TO DENTISTRY

• Decreased absorption: divalent, trivalent antacids, iron and zinc salts, calcium fortified juices
• Increased serum levels: probenecid
• Increased risk of bleeding with warfarin (monitor)
• Serious adverse effects with theophylline, caffeine
• Specific studies have not been conducted with topical ciprofloxacin. See systemic drug for interactions.

SERIOUS REACTIONS

! Superinfection (especially enterococcal or fungal), nephropathy,

cardiopulmonary arrest, chest pain, and cerebral thrombosis may occur.
! Hypersensitivity reactions, including photosensitivity (as evidenced by rash, pruritus, blisters, edema, and burning skin), have occurred in patients receiving fluoroquinolones.
! Arthropathy may occur if the drug is given to children younger than 18 yr.
! Sensitization to the ophthalmic form of the drug may contraindicate later systemic use of ciprofloxacin.

DENTAL CONSIDERATIONS

General:
• Determine why the patient is taking the drug.
• Avoid dental light in patient's eyes; offer dark glasses for patient comfort.
• Minimize exposure to sunlight and wear sunscreen if sun exposure is planned.
• Ruptures of the shoulder, hand, and Achilles tendon requiring surgical repair or resulting in prolonged disability have been reported with this drug.
• Protect patient's eyes from accidental spatter during dental treatment.
• Avoid dental light in patient's eyes; offer dark glasses for patient comfort.

Consultations:
• Consult with patient's physician if an acute dental infection occurs and another antiinfective is required.

Teach Patient/Family to:
• Discontinue treatment and inform dentist immediately if patient experiences pain or inflammation of a tendon, and to rest and refrain from exercise

cisplatin

sis-plah´-tin
(Platinol-AQ)
Do not confuse cisplatin with
carboplatin, or Platinol with
Paraplatin or Patanol.

CATEGORY AND SCHEDULE

Pregnancy Risk Category: D

Drug Class: Platinum
coordination complex;
antineoplastic

MECHANISM OF ACTION

A platinum coordination complex
that inhibits DNA and to a lesser
extent, RNA, protein synthesis by
cross-linking with DNA strands,
preventing cell division. Cell cycle–
phase nonspecific. *Therapeutic
Effect:* Interferes with DNA function.

USES

Treatment of metastatic testicular
tumors, metastatic ovarian tumors,
advanced bladder carcinoma

PHARMACOKINETICS

Widely distributed. Protein binding:
greater than 90%. Undergoes rapid
nonenzymatic conversion to inactive
metabolite. Excreted in urine.
Removed by hemodialysis. *Half-life:*
58–73 hr (increased with impaired
renal function).

INDICATIONS AND DOSAGES

▶ **Advanced Bladder Carcinoma,
Metastatic Ovarian Tumors,
Metastatic Testicular Tumors**
IV
Adults, Elderly, Children. For
intermittent dosage schedule,
37–75 mg/m² once every 2–3 wk or
50–100 mg/m² over 4–8 hr once
every 21–28 days. For daily dosage
schedule, 15–20 mg/m²/day for
5 days every 3–4 wk.

DOSAGE IN RENAL IMPAIRMENT

Dosage is modified on the basis of
creatinine clearance.

Creatine Clearance	% of Dose
10–50 ml/min	75%
Less than 10 ml/min	50%

SIDE EFFECTS/ADVERSE REACTIONS

Frequent
Nausea, vomiting (generally
beginning 1–4 hr after administration
and lasting up to 24 hr);
myelosuppression (affecting
25%–30% of patients with recovery
generally occurring in 18–23 days)
Occasional
Peripheral neuropathy (with
prolonged therapy [4–7 mo]).
Pain or redness at injection site,
loss of taste or appetite
Rare
Hemolytic anemia, blurred vision,
stomatitis

PRECAUTIONS AND CONTRAINDICATIONS

Hearing impairment,
myelosuppression, pregnancy

DRUG INTERACTIONS OF CONCERN TO DENTISTRY

• Risk of masking ototoxicity:
antihistamines

SERIOUS REACTIONS

❗ An anaphylactic reaction
manifested as angioedema, wheezing,
tachycardia, and hypotension, may
occur in the first few min of IV
administration in patients previously
exposed to cisplatin.

! Nephrotoxicity occurs in
28%–36% of patients treated with
a single dose of cisplatin, usually
during the second wk of therapy.
! Ototoxicity, including tinnitus and
hearing loss, occurs in 31% of
patients treated with a single dose
of cisplatin. It may be more severe
in children and may become more
frequent or severe with repeated
doses.

DENTAL CONSIDERATIONS
General:
• Determine why patient is taking
the drug.
• If additional analgesia is required
for dental pain, consider alternative
analgesics (NSAIDs) in patients
taking narcotics for acute or chronic
pain.
• Examine for oral manifestation
of opportunistic infection.
• Avoid prescribing aspirin-
containing products.
• This drug may be used in the
hospital or on an outpatient basis.
Confirm the patient's disease and
treatment status.
• Chlorhexidine mouth rinse prior
to and during chemotherapy may
reduce severity of mucositis.
• Patient on chronic drug therapy
may rarely present with symptoms
of blood dyscrasias, which can
include infection, bleeding and poor
healing. If dyscrasia is present,
caution patient to prevent oral tissue
trauma when using oral hygiene aids.
• Palliative medication may be
required for management of oral
side effects.
• Short appointments and a stress
reduction protocol may be required
for anxious patients.
• Patients may have received other
chemotherapy or radiation; confirm
medical and drug history.

• Patients may be at risk of bleeding,
check for oral signs.
• Oral infections should be eliminated
and/or treated aggressively.
• Patients may be at risk of infection.
Consultations:
• Medical consultation should
include routine blood counts
including platelet counts and
bleeding time.
• Consult physician; prophylactic
or therapeutic antiinfectives may be
indicated if surgery or periodontal
treatment is required.
• Medical consultation may be
required to assess immunologic status
during cancer chemotherapy and
determine safety risk, if any, posed
by the required dental treatment.
• Medical consultation may be
required to assess disease control and
patient's ability to tolerate stress.
Teach Patient/Family to:
• See dentist immediately if
secondary oral infection occurs
• Be aware of oral side effects
• Use effective oral hygiene to
prevent soft tissue inflammation
• Report oral lesions, soreness,
or bleeding to dentist
• Prevent trauma when using oral
hygiene aids
• Update health and medication
history if physician makes any
changes in evaluation or drug
regimens; include OTC, herbal, and
nonherbal remedies in the update

clarithromycin
clare-ih-thro-mye´-sin
(Biaxin, Biaxin XL, Klacid[AUS])

CATEGORY AND SCHEDULE
Pregnancy Risk Category: C

Drug Class: Macrolide antibiotic

MECHANISM OF ACTION
A macrolide that binds to ribosomal receptor sites of susceptible organisms, inhibiting protein synthesis of the bacterial cell wall. *Therapeutic Effect:* Bacteriostatic; may be bactericidal with high dosages or very susceptible microorganisms.

USES
Treatment of mild-to-moderate infections of the upper and lower respiratory tract; community-acquired pneumonia caused by *H. influenzae;* uncomplicated skin and skin structure infections caused by *S. pneumoniae, M. pneumoniae, C. diphtheriae, B. pertussis, L. monocytogenes, H. influenzae, S. pyogenes,* and *S. aureus;* otitis media; maxillary sinusitis, bronchitis (XL dose form); middle ear infection; disseminated Mycobacterium avium complex (MAC); in combination with other drugs for *H. pylori* duodenal ulcer

PHARMACOKINETICS
Well absorbed from the GI tract. Protein binding: 65%–75%. Widely distributed. Metabolized in the liver to active metabolite. Primarily excreted in urine. Not removed by hemodialysis. *Half-life:* 3–7 hr; metabolite 5–7 hr (increased in impaired renal function).

INDICATIONS AND DOSAGES
▸ **Bronchitis**
PO
Adults, Elderly. 500 mg q12h for 7–14 days.
▸ **Skin, Soft Tissue Infections**
PO
Adults, Elderly. 250 mg q12h for 7–14 days.
Children. 7.5 mg/kg q12h for 10 days.

▸ **MAC Prophylaxis**
PO
Adults, Elderly. 500 mg 2 times a day.
Children. 7.5 mg/kg q12h.
Maximum: 500 mg 2 times a day.
▸ **MAC Treatment**
PO
Adults, Elderly. 500 mg 2 times a day in combination.
Children. 7.5 mg/kg q12h in combination. Maximum: 500 mg 2 times a day.
▸ **Pharyngitis, Tonsillitis**
PO
Adults, Elderly. 250 mg q12h for *10 days.*
Children. 7.5 mg/kg q12h for 10 days.
▸ **Pneumonia**
PO
Adults, Elderly. 250 mg q12h for 7–14 days.
Children. 7.5 mg/kg q12h.
▸ **Maxillary Sinusitis**
PO
Adults, Elderly. 500 mg q12h for 14 days.
Children.
7.5 mg/kg q12h. Maximum: 500 mg 2 times a day.
▸ ***H. pylori***
PO
Adults, Elderly.
500 mg q12h for 10–14 days in combination.
▸ **Acute Otitis Media**
PO
Children. 7.5 mg/kg q12h for 10 days.
▸ **Dosage in Renal Impairment**
For patients with creatinine clearance less than 30 ml/min, reduce dose by 50% and administer once or twice a day.

SIDE EFFECTS/ADVERSE REACTIONS
Occasional
Diarrhea, nausea, altered taste, abdominal pain

Rare
Headache, dyspepsia

PRECAUTIONS AND CONTRAINDICATIONS
Hypersensitivity to clarithromycin or other macrolide antibiotics
Caution
Lactation, hepatic and renal disease

DRUG INTERACTIONS OF CONCERN TO DENTISTRY
• Decreased effect: anticholinergic drugs
• Use with caution, possible reduced metabolism: drugs metabolized by CXP450 3A4 isoenzymes
• Increased effects of cyclosporine, warfarin, cilostazol, tacrolimus, pimozide, methylprednisolone, fluconazole, buspirone
• Decreased action of clindamycin, penicillins, lincomycin, rifabutin, rifampin, zidovudine
• Increased serum levels of carbamazepine, theophylline, digoxin
• Contraindicated with indinavir
• Increased CNS depression with alprazolam, diazepam, midazolam, triazolam
• Oral contraceptives: advise patient of a low potential risk for decreased contraceptive action, to maintain compliance with oral contraceptive use while using antibiotics, and to consider the use of additional nonhormonal contraception
• Suspected increase in plasma levels of repaglinide
• Risk of severe myopathy or rhabdomyolysis: atorvastatin, fluvastatin, lovastatin, pravastatin

SERIOUS REACTIONS
! Antibiotic-associated colitis and other superinfections may result from altered bacterial balance.
! Hepatotoxicity and thrombocytopenia occur rarely.

DENTAL CONSIDERATIONS
General:
• Determine why the patient is taking the drug.
• May prove to be an alternative drug of choice for mild infections caused by a susceptible organism in patients who are allergic to penicillin.
Teach Patient/Family to:
• Use effective oral hygiene to prevent soft tissue inflammation
• When used for dental infection, advise patient to:
  • Report sore throat, oral burning sensation, fever, and fatigue, any of which could indicate superinfection
  • Take at prescribed intervals and complete dosage regimen
  • Immediately notify the dentist if signs or symptoms of infection increase

clemastine fumarate
klem´-as-teen fyoo´-mer-ate
(Dayhistol Allergy, Tavist Allergy)

CATEGORY AND SCHEDULE
Pregnancy Risk Category: B

Drug Class: Antihistamine, H_1-receptor antagonist

MECHANISM OF ACTION
An ethanolamine that competes with histamine on effector cells in the GI tract, blood vessels, and respiratory tract. **Therapeutic Effect:** Relieves allergy symptoms, including urticaria, rhinitis, and pruritus.

USES
Treatment of allergy symptoms, rhinitis, angioedema, urticaria, common cold

PHARMACOKINETICS

Route	Onset	Peak	Duration
PO	15–60 min	5–7 hr	10–12 hr

Well absorbed from the GI tract. Metabolized in the liver. Excreted primarily in urine.

INDICATIONS AND DOSAGES
▸ **Allergic Rhinitis, Urticaria**
PO
Adults, Children older than 11 yr. 1.34 mg twice a day up to 2.68 mg 3 times a day. Maximum: 8.04 mg/day.
Children 6–11 yr. 0.67–1.34 mg twice a day. Maximum: 4.02 mg/day.
Children younger than 6 yr. 0.05 mg/kg/day divided into 2–3 doses per day. Maximum: 1.34 mg/day.
Elderly. 1.34 mg 1–2 times a day.

SIDE EFFECTS/ADVERSE REACTIONS
Frequent
Somnolence, dizziness, urine retention, thickening of bronchial secretions, dry mouth, nose, or throat; in elderly, sedation, dizziness, hypotension
Occasional
Epigastric distress, flushing, blurred vision, tinnitus, paresthesia, diaphoresis, chills

PRECAUTIONS AND CONTRAINDICATIONS
Angle-closure glaucoma, hypersensitivity to clemastine, use within 14 days of MAOIs
Caution
Increased intraocular pressure, renal disease, cardiac disease, hypertension, bronchial asthma, seizure disorder, stenosed peptic ulcers, hyperthyroidism, prostatic hypertrophy, bladder neck obstruction, elderly

DRUG INTERACTIONS OF CONCERN TO DENTISTRY
• Increased CNS depression: all CNS depressants, alcohol
• Increased anticholinergic effect of anticholinergics, phenothiazines, tricyclic antidepressants

SERIOUS REACTIONS
! A hypersensitivity reaction, marked by eczema, pruritus, rash, cardiac disturbances, angioedema, and photosensitivity, may occur.
! Overdose symptoms may vary from CNS depression, including sedation, apnea, cardiovascular collapse, and death to severe paradoxical reaction, such as hallucinations, tremors, and seizures.
! Children may experience paradoxical reactions, such as restlessness, insomnia, euphoria, nervousness, and tremors.
! Overdose in children may result in hallucinations, seizures, and death.

DENTAL CONSIDERATIONS
General:
• Assess salivary flow as a factor in caries, periodontal disease, and candidiasis.
• Determine why the patient is taking the drug.
Teach Patient/Family to:
• Use effective oral hygiene to prevent soft tissue inflammation
• Use caution to prevent injury when using oral hygiene aids
• When chronic dry mouth occurs, advise patient to:
  • Avoid mouth rinses with high alcohol content because of drying effects
  • Use daily home fluoride products for anticaries effect

C

• Use sugarless gum, frequent sips of water, or saliva substitutes

clindamycin
klin-da-mye´-sin
(Cleocin, Cleocin HCl[AUS], Clindesse, Dalacin[CAN], Dalacin C[AUS])

CATEGORY AND SCHEDULE
Pregnancy Risk Category: B

Drug Class: Lincomycin derivative antiinfective

MECHANISM OF ACTION
A lincosamide antibiotic that inhibits protein synthesis of the bacterial cell wall by binding to bacterial ribosomal receptor sites. Topically, it decreases fatty acid concentration on the skin. **Therapeutic Effect:** Bacteriostatic. Prevents outbreaks of acne vulgaris.

USES
Indications for use include serious infections caused by susceptible anaerobic bacteria and the treatment of serious infections caused by susceptible strains of pneumococci and streptococci; includes infections of the respiratory tract, serious skin and soft tissue infections, intraabdominal abscess, and infections of the female GU tract

PHARMACOKINETICS
Rapidly absorbed from the GI tract. Protein binding: 92%–94%. Widely distributed. Metabolized in the liver to some active metabolites. Primarily excreted in urine. Not removed by hemodialysis. **Half-life:** 2.4–3 hr (increased in impaired renal function and premature infants).

INDICATIONS AND DOSAGES
▶ **Chronic Bone and Joint, Respiratory Tract, Skin and Soft Tissue, Intraabdominal, and Female GU Infections; Endocarditis; Septicemia**
PO
Adults, Elderly. 150–450 mg/dose q6–8h.
Children. 10–30 mg/kg/day in 3–4 divided doses. Maximum: 1.8 g/day.
IV, IM
Adults, Elderly. 1.2–1.8 g/day in 2–4 divided doses.
Children. 25–40 mg/kg/day in 3–4 divided doses. Maximum: 4.8 g/day.
▶ **Bacterial Vaginosis**
PO
Adults, Elderly. 300 mg twice a day for 7 days.
▶ **Intravaginal**
Adults. One applicatorful at bedtime for 3–7 days or 1 suppository at bedtime for 3 days.
▶ **Acne Vulgaris**
Topical
Adults. Apply thin layer to affected area twice a day.

SIDE EFFECTS/ADVERSE REACTIONS
Frequent
Systemic: Abdominal pain, nausea, vomiting, diarrhea
Topical: Dry scaly skin
Vaginal: Vaginitis, pruritus
Occasional
Systemic: Phlebitis or thrombophlebitis with IV administration, pain and induration at IM injection site, allergic reaction, urticaria, pruritus
Topical: Contact dermatitis, abdominal pain, mild diarrhea, burning, or stinging
Vaginal: Headache, dizziness, nausea, vomiting, abdominal pain

Rare
Vaginal: Hypersensitivity reaction

PRECAUTIONS AND CONTRAINDICATIONS
History of antibiotic-associated colitis, regional enteritis, or ulcerative colitis; hypersensitivity to clindamycin or lincomycin
Caution
Renal disease, liver disease, GI disease, elderly, lactation, tartrazine sensitivity

DRUG INTERACTIONS OF CONCERN TO DENTISTRY
• Decreased action: erythromycin, absorbent antidiarrheals
• Increased effects of nondepolarizing muscle relaxants, hydrocarbon inhalation anesthetics
• Avoid antiperistaltic drugs if diarrhea occurs
• Possible reduced blood levels of cyclosporine
• Oral contraceptives: advise patient of a potential low risk for decreased contraceptive action, to maintain compliance with oral contraceptive use while using antibiotics, and to consider the use of additional nonhormonal contraception

SERIOUS REACTIONS
! Antibiotic-associated colitis and other superinfections may occur during and several wk after clindamycin therapy (including the topical form).
! Blood dyscrasias (leukopenia, thrombocytopenia) and nephrotoxicity (proteinuria, azotemia, oliguria) occur rarely.

DENTAL CONSIDERATIONS
General:
• Determine why the patient is taking the drug.
Consultations:
• Medical consultation may be required to assess disease control.

Teach Patient/Family to:
• Use effective oral hygiene to prevent soft tissue inflammation
• Use caution to prevent injury when using oral hygiene aids
• When used for dental infection, advise patient to:
  • Report sore throat, oral burning sensation, fever, and fatigue, any of which could indicate superinfection
  • Take at prescribed intervals and complete dosage regimen
  • Immediately notify the dentist if signs or symptoms of infection increase

clobetasol
klo-bet´-ah-sol
(Alti-Clobetasol[CAN], Cormax, Dermovate[CAN], Gen-Clobetasol[CAN], Olux, Novo-Clobetasol[CAN], Temovate)

CATEGORY AND SCHEDULE
Pregnancy Risk Category: C

Drug Class: Topical corticosteroid, very high potency

MECHANISM OF ACTION
A corticosteroid that inhibits accumulation of inflammatory cells at inflammation sites, phagocytosis, lysosomal enzyme release and synthesis or release of mediators of inflammation. *Therapeutic Effect:* Decreases or prevents tissue response to inflammatory process.

USES
Treatment of inflammatory and pruritic manifestations of moderate to severe corticosteroid-responsive dermatitis of the scalp; other uses include psoriasis

PHARMACOKINETICS
May be absorbed from intact skin. Metabolized in liver. Excreted in the urine.

INDICATIONS AND DOSAGES
▸ **Antiinflammatory, Corticosteroid Replacement Therapy**
Topical
Adults, Elderly, Children 12 yr and older. Apply 2 times a day for 2 wk.
Foam
Adults, Elderly, Children 12 yr and older. Apply 2 times a day for 2 wk.

SIDE EFFECTS/ADVERSE REACTIONS
Frequent
Local irritation, dry skin, itching, redness
Occasional
Allergic contact dermatitis
Rare
Cushing's syndrome, numbness of fingers, skin atrophy

PRECAUTIONS AND CONTRAINDICATIONS
Hypersensitivity to clobetasol or other corticosteroids
Caution
Lactation, bacterial infections

DRUG INTERACTIONS OF CONCERN TO DENTISTRY
None reported

SERIOUS REACTIONS
! Overdosage can occur from topically applied clobetasol propionate absorbed in sufficient amounts to produce systemic effects producing reversible adrenal suppression, manifestations of Cushing's syndrome, hyperglycemia, and glucosuria in some patients.

DENTAL CONSIDERATIONS
Clobetasol Propionate (topical foam)
General:
• Determine why patient is taking the drug.
• Avoid use of systemic corticosteroids unless a consultation is made.
Clobetasol Propionate
General:
• Place on frequent recall to evaluate healing response.
• Topical adrenocorticosteroids are not indicated for treating plaque-related gingivitis, which should be treated by removal of local irritants and improved oral hygiene.
Teach Patient/Family to:
• Use effective oral hygiene to prevent soft tissue inflammation
• Use on oral herpetic ulcerations is contraindicated
• Apply at bedtime or after meals for maximum effect
• Apply with cotton-tipped applicator by pressing, not rubbing, paste on lesion
• Return for oral evaluation if response of oral tissues has not occurred in 7–14 days

clocortolone
klo-kort´-oh-lone
(Cloderm, Cloderm[CAN])

CATEGORY AND SCHEDULE
Pregnancy Risk Category: C

Drug Class: Topical corticosteroid, group III medium potency

MECHANISM OF ACTION

A topical corticosteroid that inhibits accumulation of inflammatory cells at inflammation sites, suppresses mitotic activity, and causes vasoconstriction. ***Therapeutic Effect:*** Decreases or prevents tissue response to inflammatory process.

USES

Psoriasis, eczema, contact dermatitis, pruritus

PHARMACOKINETICS

Absorption is variable and dependent upon many factors including integrity of skin, dose, vehicle used, and use of occlusive dressings. Small amounts may be absorbed from the skin. Metabolized in liver. Excreted in the urine and feces.

INDICATIONS AND DOSAGES
▸ **Dermatoses**
Topical
Adults, Elderly, Children 12 yr and older. Apply 1–4 times a day.

SIDE EFFECTS/ADVERSE REACTIONS
Occasional
Local irritation, burning, itching, redness
Allergic contact dermatitis
Rare
Hypertrichosis, hypopigmentation, maceration of skin, miliaria, perioral dermatitis, skin atrophy, striae

PRECAUTIONS AND CONTRAINDICATIONS

Hypersensitivity to clocortolone pivalate or other corticosteroids; viral, fungal, or tubercular skin lesions.
Caution
Lactation, viral infections, bacterial infections

DRUG INTERACTIONS OF CONCERN TO DENTISTRY
None reported

SERIOUS REACTIONS

! Overdosage can occur from topically applied clocortolone pivalate absorbed in sufficient amounts to produce systemic effects in some patients.

DENTAL CONSIDERATIONS
General:
• Determine why the patient is taking the drug.
• Place on frequent recall to evaluate healing response if used on a chronic basis.
• Apply lubricant to dry lips for patient comfort before dental procedures.

clofarabine
kloe-far′-ah-been
(Clolar)

CATEGORY AND SCHEDULE
Pregnancy Risk Category: D

Drug Class: Antineoplastic

MECHANISM OF ACTION
An antineoplastic agent that inhibits DNA synthesis by decreasing deoxynucleotide triphosphate pools. It inhibits ribonucleoside reductase, terminates elongation of the DNA chain, and inhibits repair through incorporation into the DNA chain by competitive inhibition of DNA polymerases. ***Therapeutic Effect:*** Inhibits synthesis of DNA.

USES
Treatment of acute lymphoid leukemia (ALL) in patients who have failed prior regimens

PHARMACOKENETICS
Protein binding: 47%. Negligible liver metabolism. Primarily excreted in urine. *Half-life:* 5.2 hr.

INDICATIONS AND DOSAGES
▶ ALL
IV
Adults. 52 mg/m^2 over 2 hr daily for 5 consecutive days. Repeat every 2–6 wk following recovery or return to baseline organ function. *Children (1–21 yr).* 52 mg/m^2 over 2 hr daily for 5 consecutive days. Repeat every 2–6 wk following recovery or return to baseline organ function.

SIDE EFFECTS/ADVERSE REACTIONS:
Frequent
Infection, vomiting, nausea, febrile neutropenia, diarrhea, pruritus, headache, ALT increased, dermatitis, pyrexia, AST increased, rigors, abdominal pain, fatigue, pericardial effusion, tachycardia, epistaxis, anorexia, petechiae, hypotension, pain in limb, left ventricular systolic dysfunction, anxiety, constipation, edema, pain, cough, erythema, flushing, mucosal inflammation, hematuria, dizziness, bilirubin increased, jaundice, gingival bleeding, hepatomegaly, injection site pain, myalgia, respiratory distress, palmar-plantar sore throat, back pain, dyspnea, erythrodysesthesia syndrome, staphylococcal infection, oral candidiasis, appetite decreased, cellulitis, depression, irritability, arthralgia, herpes simplex, hypertension, lethargy
Occasional
Somnolence, weight gain, tremor, pleural effusion, pneumonia, systemic inflammatory response syndrome (SIRS)/capillary leak syndrome, transfusion reaction, bacteremia, creatinine increased

PRECAUTIONS AND CONTRAINDICATIONS
Hypersensitivity to clofarabine or its components
Caution
Do not breast-feed, renal or hepatic impairment

DRUG INTERACTIONS OF CONCERN TO DENTISTRY
• CNS depressants, alcohol: may increase CNS depression and dizziness

SERIOUS REACTIONS
! Tumor lysis syndrome may occur.
! Severe bone marrow suppression, including neutropenia, anemia, and thrombocytopenia, have been observed.

DENTAL CONSIDERATIONS
General:
• Monitor vital signs at every appointment due to cardiovascular side effects
• Avoid NSAIDs for pain control
• Examine for oral manifestation of opportunistic infection
• This drug may be used in the hospital or on an outpatient basis. Confirm the patient's disease and treatment status
• Chlorhexidine mouth rinse prior to and during chemotherapy may reduce severity of mucositis
• Determine presence, type, and severity of blood dyscrasis prior to undertaking any dental treatment and modify therapy accordingly

- Consider effects of drug on healing and susceptibility to infection
- Palliative measures may be required for management of oral side effects

Consultations:

- Consult physician to determine disease control and ability of patient to tolerate dental procedures
- Consult physician to determine need for prophylactic antiinfectives if invasive dental procedures are needed
- Consult physician about patient's immunologic status during cancer chemotherapy and determine safety risk, if any, posed by required dental treatment

Teach Family/Patient to:

- Be aware of oral side effects of medication
- Practice effective oral hygiene to prevent soft-tissue inflammation and prevent trauma when using oral hygiene aids
- Report oral lesions, soreness, or bleeding to dentist
- Update health and medication history if physician makes any changes in evaluation or drug regimens, including the use of OTC drugs, herbal products, and dietary supplements

clofazimine
kloe-faz´-ih-meen
(Lamprene)

CATEGORY AND SCHEDULE
Pregnancy Risk Category: C

Drug Class: Leprostatic

MECHANISM OF ACTION
An antibiotic that binds to mycobacterial DNA. *Therapeutic Effect:* Inhibits mycobacterial growth and produces antiinflammatory action.

USES
Treatment of lepromatous leprosy, dapsone-resistant leprosy, lepromatous leprosy complicated by erythema nodosum leprosum

PHARMACOKINETICS
Deposited in fatty tissue, reticuloendothelial system; small amount excreted in feces, sputum, sweat. *Half-life:* 70 days.

INDICATIONS AND DOSAGES
▶ **Leprosy**
PO
Adults, Elderly. 100 mg/day in combination with dapsone and rifampin for 3 yr then 100 mg/day as monotherapy.
Children. 1 mg/kg/day in combination with dapsone and rifampin.
▶ **Erythema Nodosum**
PO
Adults, Elderly. 100–200 mg/day for up to 3 mo, then 100 mg/day.

SIDE EFFECTS/ADVERSE REACTIONS
Frequent
Dry skin, abdominal pain, nausea, vomiting, diarrhea, skin discoloration (pink to brownish-black)
Occasional
Rash; pruritus; eye irritation; discoloration of sputum; sweat and urine

PRECAUTIONS AND CONTRAINDICATIONS
Caution
Lactation, children, abdominal pain, diarrhea, depression

DRUG INTERACTIONS OF CONCERN TO DENTISTRY
None reported

SERIOUS REACTIONS
None significant

DENTAL CONSIDERATIONS

General:
• Develop awareness of the patient's disease.

Teach Patient/Family to:
• Use effective oral hygiene to prevent soft tissue inflammation
• Avoid mouth rinses with high alcohol content because of drying effects

clofibrate
kloe-fye´-brate
(Abitrate, Atromid-S, Claripex[CAN], Novofibrate[CAN])

CATEGORY AND SCHEDULE
Pregnancy Risk Category: C

Drug Class: Antihyperlipidemic

MECHANISM OF ACTION
An antihyperlipidemic that enhances synthesis of lipoprotein lipase and reduces triglyceride-rich lipoproteins and VLDLs. ***Therapeutic Effect:*** Increases VLDL catabolism and reduces total plasma triglyceride levels.

USES
Treatment of hyperlipidemia (types III, IV, V)

PHARMACOKINETICS
Well absorbed from the GI tract. Protein binding: 95%–97%. Metabolized in liver. Excreted primarily in urine, lesser amount in feces. ***Half-life:*** 14–35 hr.

INDICATIONS AND DOSAGES
▸ **Hypercholesterolemia**
PO
Adults, Elderly. 2 g/day in divided doses. Some patients may respond to a lower dosage.

SIDE EFFECTS/ADVERSE REACTIONS
Frequent
Nausea, vomiting, loose stools, dyspepsia, flatulence, abdominal distress
Occasional
Headache, dizziness, fatigue
Rare
Muscle cramping, aching, weakness; skin rash, urticaria, pruritus; dry brittle hair, alopecia

PRECAUTIONS AND CONTRAINDICATIONS
Hypersensitivity to clofibrate, severe renal or hepatic dysfunction, pregnancy, nursing women, rhabdomyolysis, severe hyperkalemia, primary biliary cirrhosis
Caution
Peptic ulcer

DRUG INTERACTIONS OF CONCERN TO DENTISTRY
None reported

SERIOUS REACTIONS
❗ May increase excretion of cholesterol into bile, leading to cholelithiasis.
❗ Various cardiac arrhythmias have been reported.
❗ Anemia and, more frequently, leukopenia have been reported.

DENTAL CONSIDERATIONS
General:
• Consider semisupine chair position for patient comfort if GI side effects occur.
• Patients on chronic drug therapy may rarely have symptoms of blood dyscrasias, which can include infection, bleeding, and poor healing.

Consultations:
• In a patient with symptoms of blood dyscrasias, request a medical consultation for blood studies and postpone treatment until normal values are reestablished.
Teach Patient/Family to:
• Use effective oral hygiene to prevent soft tissue inflammation

clomiphene
kloe´-mi-feen
(Clomhexal[AUS], Clomid, Clomid[CAN], Milophene, Milophene[CAN], Serophene, Serophene[CAN])
Do not confuse with chlomipramine.

CATEGORY AND SCHEDULE
Pregnancy Risk Category: X

Drug Class: Nonsteroidal ovulatory stimulant, antiestrogen

MECHANISM OF ACTION
An ovulation stimulator that promotes release of pituitary gonadotropins. *Therapeutic Effect:* Stimulates ovulation.

USES
Treatment of female infertility

PHARMACOKINETICS
Readily absorbed. Time to peak occurs within 6.5 hr. Undergoes enterohepatic recirculation. Primarily excreted in feces. *Half-life:* 5–7 days.

INDICATIONS AND DOSAGES
▶ Ovulatory Failure, Females
PO
Adults. 50 mg/day for 5 days (first course); start the regimen on the fifth day of cycle. Increase dose only if

unresponsive to cyclic 50 mg. Maximum: 100 mg/day for 5 days.

SIDE EFFECTS/ADVERSE REACTIONS
Frequent
Hot flashes, ovarian enlargement
Occasional
Abdominal/pelvic discomfort, bloating, nausea, vomiting, breast discomfort (females)
Rare
Vision disturbances, abnormal menstrual flow, breast enlargement (males), headache, mental depression, ovarian cyst formation, thromboembolism, uterine fibroid enlargement

PRECAUTIONS AND CONTRAINDICATIONS
Liver dysfunction, abnormal uterine bleeding, enlargement or development of ovarian cyst, uncontrolled thyroid or adrenal dysfunction in the presence of an organic intracranial lesion such as pituitary tumor, pregnancy, hypersensitivity to clomiphene
Caution
Hypertension, depression, convulsions, diabetes mellitus

DRUG INTERACTIONS OF CONCERN TO DENTISTRY
None reported

SERIOUS REACTIONS
! Thrombophlebitis, alopecia, and polyuria occurs rarely.

DENTAL CONSIDERATIONS
General:
• Consider semisupine chair position for patient comfort if GI side effects occur.
• Avoid dental light in patient's eyes; offer dark glasses for patient comfort.

• Be aware that patient may be in early stage of pregnancy.

clomipramine hydrochloride

klom-ip´-ra-meen hi-droh-klor´-ide
(Anafranil, Apo-Clomipramine[CAN], Clopram[AUS], Novo-Clopamine[CAN], Placil[AUS])
Do not confuse clomipramine with chlorpromazine, clomiphene, or imipramine, or Anafranil with alfentanil, enalapril, or nafarelin.

CATEGORY AND SCHEDULE
Pregnancy Risk Category: C

Drug Class: Tricyclic antidepressant

MECHANISM OF ACTION
A tricyclic antidepressant that blocks the reuptake of neurotransmitters, such as norepinephrine and serotonin, at CNS presynaptic membranes, increasing their availability at postsynaptic receptor sites.
Therapeutic Effect: Reduces obsessive-compulsive behavior.

USES
Treatment of obsessive-compulsive disorder; unapproved: depression, panic disorder, narcolepsy, and neurogenic pain

PHARMACOKINETICS
Well absorbed from GI tract. Protein binding: 97%. Principally bound to albumin. Distributed into cerebrospinal fluid. Metabolized in the liver. Undergoes extensive first-pass effect. Excreted in urine and feces.
Half-life: 19–37 hr.

INDICATIONS AND DOSAGES
▸ **Obsessive-Compulsive Disorder**
PO
Adults, Elderly. Initially, 25 mg/day. May gradually increase to 100 mg/day in the first 2 wk. Maximum: 250 mg/day.
Children 10 yr and older. Initially, 25 mg/day. May gradually increase up to maximum of 200 mg/day.

SIDE EFFECTS/ADVERSE REACTIONS
Frequent
Somnolence, fatigue, dry mouth, blurred vision, constipation, sexual dysfunction, ejaculatory failure, impotence, weight gain, delayed micturition, orthostatic hypotension, diaphoresis, impaired concentration, increased appetite, urine retention
Occasional
GI disturbances (such as nausea, GI distress, and metallic taste), asthenia, aggressiveness, muscle weakness
Rare
Paradoxical reactions (agitation, restlessness, nightmares, insomnia), extrapyramidal symptoms, (particularly fine hand tremor), laryngitis, seizures

PRECAUTIONS AND CONTRAINDICATIONS
Acute recovery period after MI, use within 14 days of MAOIs
Caution
Seizures, suicidal patients, elderly, MAOIs, not for use in children younger than 10 yr, renal or hepatic dysfunction

DRUG INTERACTIONS OF CONCERN TO DENTISTRY
• Increased anticholinergic effects: muscarinic blockers, antihistamines, phenothiazines

- Increased effects of direct-acting sympathomimetics (epinephrine, levonordefrin)
- Potential risk of CNS depression: alcohol, barbiturates, benzodiazepines, and other CNS depressants
- Decreased antihypertensive effects: clonidine, guanadrel, guanethidine
- Use with caution, possible reduced metabolism: drugs metabolized by CYP450 2D6 isoenzymes
- Avoid concurrent use with St. John's wort (herb)

SERIOUS REACTIONS

! Overdose may produce seizures; cardiovascular effects, such as severe orthostatic hypotension, dizziness, tachycardia, palpitations, and arrhythmias; and altered temperature regulation, including hyperpyrexia or hypothermia.

! Abrupt discontinuation after prolonged therapy may produce headache, malaise, nausea, vomiting, and vivid dreams.

! Anemia and agranulocytosis have been noted.

DENTAL CONSIDERATIONS

General:
- Take vital signs at every appointment because of cardiovascular side effects.
- Assess salivary flow as a factor in caries, periodontal disease, and candidiasis.
- Patients on chronic drug therapy may rarely have symptoms of blood dyscrasias, which can include infection, bleeding, and poor healing.
- After supine positioning, have patient sit upright for at least 2 min before standing to avoid orthostatic hypotension.
- Use vasoconstrictor with caution, in low doses, and with careful aspiration. Avoid use of gingival retraction cord with epinephrine.

- Place on frequent recall because of oral side effects.
- A stress reduction protocol may be required.

Consultations:
- In a patient with symptoms of blood dyscrasias, request a medical consultation for blood studies and postpone dental treatment until normal values are reestablished.
- Physician should be informed if significant xerostomic side effects occur (e.g., increased caries, sore tongue, problems eating or swallowing, difficulty wearing prosthesis) so that a medication change can be considered.
- Medical consultation may be required to assess disease control.

Teach Patient/Family to:
- Use effective oral hygiene to prevent soft tissue inflammation
- Prevent injury when using oral hygiene aids
- When chronic dry mouth occurs, advise patient to:
  - Avoid mouth rinses with high alcohol content because of drying effects
  - Use daily home fluoride products for anticaries effect
  - Use sugarless gum, frequent sips of water, or saliva substitutes

clonazepam
kloe-na´-zi-pam
(Apo-Clonazepam[CAN], Clonapam[CAN], Klonopin, Paxam[AUS], Rivotril[CAN])
Do not confuse clonazepam with clonidine or lorazepam.

CATEGORY AND SCHEDULE
Pregnancy Risk Category: D
Controlled Substance Schedule IV

Drug Class: Anticonvulsant, benzodiazepine

MECHANISM OF ACTION

A benzodiazepine that depresses all levels of the CNS; inhibits nerve impulse transmission in the motor cortex and suppresses abnormal discharge in petit mal seizures. *Therapeutic Effect:* Produces anxiolytic and anticonvulsant effects.

USES

Absence, atypical absence, akinetic, myoclonic seizures; unlabeled uses: Parkinson's dysarthria, adjunct in schizophrenia, neuralgias

PHARMACOKINETICS

Well absorbed from the GI tract. Protein binding: 85%. Metabolized in the liver. Excreted in urine. Not removed by hemodialysis. *Half-life:* 18–50 hr.

INDICATIONS AND DOSAGES

▶ **Adjunctive Treatment of Lennox-Gastaut Syndrome (petit mal variant) and Akinetic, Myoclonic, and Absence (petit mal) Seizures**

PO

Adults, Elderly, Children 10 yr and older. 1.5 mg/day; may be increased in 0.5- to 1-mg increments every 3 days until seizures are controlled. Don't exceed maintenance dosage of 20 mg/day.

Infants, Children younger than 10 yr or weighing less than 30 kg. 0.01–0.03 mg/kg/day in 2–3 divided doses; may be increased by up to 0.5 mg every 3 days until seizures are controlled. Don't exceed maintenance dosage of 0.2 mg/kg/day.

▶ **Panic Disorder**

PO

Adults, Elderly. Initially, 0.25 mg twice a day; increased in increments of 0.125–0.25 mg twice a day every 3 days. Maximum: 4 mg/day.

SIDE EFFECTS/ADVERSE REACTIONS

Frequent

Mild, transient drowsiness; ataxia; behavioral disturbances (aggression, irritability, agitation), especially in children

Occasional

Rash, ankle or facial edema, nocturia, dysuria, change in appetite or weight, dry mouth, sore gums, nausea, blurred vision

Rare

Paradoxical CNS reactions, including hyperactivity or nervousness in children and excitement or restlessness in the elderly (particularly in the presence of uncontrolled pain)

PRECAUTIONS AND CONTRAINDICATIONS

Narrow-angle glaucoma, significant hepatic disease

Caution

Open-angle glaucoma, chronic respiratory disease, renal, hepatic disease, elderly, interferes with cognitive and motor performance, withdrawal symptoms

DRUG INTERACTIONS OF CONCERN TO DENTISTRY

• Increased sedation: alcohol, all CNS depressants, indinavir, kava (herb)
• Risk of increased serum levels: drugs that inhibit CYP3A4 isoenzymes, ketoconazole, itraconazole, fluconazole, protease inhibitor, nefazodone
• Risk of decreased effect: St. John's wort (herb)

SERIOUS REACTIONS

! Abrupt withdrawal may result in pronounced restlessness, irritability, insomnia, hand tremors, abdominal or muscle cramps, diaphoresis, vomiting, and status epilepticus.

! Overdose results in somnolence, confusion, diminished reflexes, and coma.

DENTAL CONSIDERATIONS
General:
• Patients on chronic drug therapy may rarely have symptoms of blood dyscrasias, which can include infection, bleeding, and poor healing.
• Assess salivary flow as a factor in caries, periodontal disease, and candidiasis.
• Psychologic and physical dependence may occur with chronic administration.
• Geriatric patients are more susceptible to drug effects; use lower dose.
• Ask about type of epilepsy, seizure frequency, and quality of seizure control.
Consultations:
• Medical consultation may be required to assess disease control.
• In a patient with symptoms of blood dyscrasias, request a medical consultation for blood studies and postpone dental treatment until normal values are reestablished.
Teach Patient/Family to:
• Use effective oral hygiene to prevent soft tissue inflammation
• Use caution to prevent injury when using oral hygiene aids
• When chronic dry mouth occurs, advise patient to:
  • Avoid mouth rinses with high alcohol content because of drying effects
  • Use daily home fluoride products for anticaries effect
  • Use sugarless gum, frequent sips of water, or saliva substitutes

clonidine
klon´-ih-deen
(Catapres, Catapres TTS, Dixarit[CAN], Duraclon)
Do not confuse clonidine with clomiphene, Klonopin, or quinidine, or Catapres with Cetapred.

CATEGORY AND SCHEDULE
Pregnancy Risk Category: C

Drug Class: Antihypertensive, central α-adrenergic agonist

MECHANISM OF ACTION
An antiadrenergic, sympatholytic agent that prevents pain signal transmission to the brain and produces analgesia at pre- and post-alpha-adrenergic receptors in the spinal cord. *Therapeutic Effect:* Reduces peripheral resistance; decreases B/P and heart rate.

USES
Hypertension, severe pain in combination with opioids for cancer patients; unapproved: opioid abstinence syndrome, nicotine withdrawal, vascular headache, alcohol withdrawal, ADHD, postherpetic neuralgia

PHARMACOKINETICS

Route	Onset	Peak	Duration
PO	0.5–1 hr	2–4 hr	Up to 8 hr

Well absorbed from the GI tract. Transdermal best absorbed from the chest and upper arm; least absorbed from the thigh. Protein binding: 20%–40%. Metabolized in the liver. Primarily excreted in urine. Minimally removed by hemodialysis.

Half-life: 12–16 hr (increased with impaired renal function).

INDICATIONS AND DOSAGES
▶ **Hypertension**
PO
Adults. Initially, 0.1 mg twice a day. Increase by 0.1–0.2 mg q2–4 days. Maintenance: 0.2–1.2 mg/day in 2–4 divided doses up to maximum of 2.4 mg/day.
Elderly. Initially, 0.1 mg at bedtime. May increase gradually.
Children. 5–25 mcg/kg/day in divided doses q6h. Increase at 5- to 7-day intervals. Maximum: 0.9 mg/day.
▶ **Transdermal**
Adults, Elderly. System delivering 0.1 mg/24 hr up to 0.6 mg/24 hr q7 days.
▶ **Attention Deficit Hyperactivity Disorder (ADHD)**
PO
Children. Initially 0.05 mg/day. May increase by 0.05 mg/day q3–7 days. Maximum: 0.3–0.4 mg/day.
▶ **Severe Pain**
Epidural
Adults, Elderly. 30–40 mcg/hr.
Children. Initially, 0.5 mcg/kg/hr, not to exceed adult dose.

SIDE EFFECTS/ADVERSE REACTIONS
Frequent
Dry mouth, somnolence, dizziness, sedation, constipation
Occasional
Tablets, injection: Depression, swelling of feet, loss of appetite, decreased sexual ability, itching eyes, dizziness, nausea, vomiting, nervousness
Transdermal: Itching, reddening or darkening of skin
Rare
Nightmares, vivid dreams, cold feeling in fingers and toes

PRECAUTIONS AND CONTRAINDICATIONS
Epidural contraindicated in those patients with bleeding diathesis or infection at the injection site, and in those receiving anticoagulation therapy
Caution
MI (recent), cerebrovascular disease, chronic renal failure, Raynaud's disease, thyroid disease, depression, COPD, children younger than 12 yr (patches), asthma, lactation, elderly

DRUG INTERACTIONS OF CONCERN TO DENTISTRY
• Increased CNS depression: alcohol, all CNS depressants
• Decreased hypotensive effects: NSAIDs, especially indomethacin, sympathomimetics, tricyclic antidepressants

SERIOUS REACTIONS
! Overdose produces profound hypotension, irritability, bradycardia, respiratory depression, hypothermia, miosis (pupillary constriction), arrhythmias, and apnea.
! Abrupt withdrawal may result in rebound hypertension associated with nervousness, agitation, anxiety, insomnia, hand tingling, tremor, flushing, and diaphoresis.

DENTAL CONSIDERATIONS
General:
• Monitor vital signs at every appointment because of cardiovascular side effects.
• After supine positioning, have patient sit upright for at least 2 min before standing to avoid orthostatic hypotension.
• Limit use of sodium-containing products, such as saline IV fluids, for patients with a dietary salt restriction.

- Observe appropriate limitations of vasoconstrictor doses.
- Assess salivary flow as a factor in caries, periodontal disease, and candidiasis.
- Stress from dental procedures may compromise cardiovascular function; determine patient risk.
- Short appointments and a stress-reduction protocol may be required for anxious patients.
- Consider drug in diagnosis of taste alterations.

Consultations:
- Medical consultation may be required to assess disease control.

Teach Patient/Family:
- When chronic dry mouth occurs, advise patient to:
  - Avoid mouth rinses with high alcohol content because of drying effects
  - Use daily home fluoride products for anticaries effect
  - Use sugarless gum, frequent sips of water, or saliva substitutes

clopidogrel

clo-pid´-oh-grill
(Iscover[AUS], Plavix)
Do not confuse Plavix with Paxil.

CATEGORY AND SCHEDULE
Pregnancy Risk Category: B

Drug Class: Platelet aggregation inhibitor

MECHANISM OF ACTION
A thienopyridine derivative that inhibits binding of the enzyme adenosine phosphate (ADP) to its platelet receptor and subsequent ADP-mediated activation of a glycoprotein complex. **Therapeutic Effect:** Inhibits platelet aggregation.

USES
Adjunctive treatment in recent MI, ischemic stroke, and peripheral vascular disease in patients with atherosclerosis; treatment of acute coronary syndrome (unstable angina with non–Q wave MI)

PHARMACOKINETICS

Route	Onset	Peak	Duration
PO	1hr	2hr	N/A

Rapidly absorbed. Protein binding: 98%. Extensively metabolized by the liver. Eliminated equally in the urine and feces. **Half-life:** 8 hr.

INDICATIONS AND DOSAGES
▶ **MI, Stroke Reduction**
PO
Adults, Elderly. 75 mg once a day.
▶ **Acute Coronary Syndrome**
PO
Adults, Elderly. Initially, 300 mg loading dose, then 75 mg once a day (in combination with aspirin).

SIDE EFFECTS/ADVERSE REACTIONS
Frequent
Skin disorders
Occasional
Upper respiratory tract infection, chest pain, flu-like symptoms, headache, dizziness, arthralgia
Rare
Fatigue, edema, hypertension, abdominal pain, dyspepsia, diarrhea, nausea, epistaxis, dyspnea, rhinitis

PRECAUTIONS AND CONTRAINDICATIONS
Active bleeding, coagulation disorders, severe hepatic disease
Caution
Hepatic impairment, renal impairment, hypertension, history of bleeding disorders, major surgery, safety and efficacy during lactation or use in children not established

DRUG INTERACTIONS OF CONCERN TO DENTISTRY
• Caution in use with NSAIDs

SERIOUS REACTIONS
None known

DENTAL CONSIDERATIONS
General:
• Avoid discontinuation for dental procedures due to increased risk of thromboembolism.
• Effects on platelet aggregation return to normal in 5–7 days.
• Patients on chronic drug therapy may rarely have symptoms of blood dyscrasias, which can include infection, bleeding, and poor healing.
• Consider local hemostasis measures to prevent excessive bleeding.
• Question patient about concurrent aspirin use.
• Monitor vital signs at every appointment because of cardiovascular disease.
• Consider semisupine chair position for patient comfort if GI side effects occur.
Consultations:
• Medical consultation may be required to assess disease control and patient's ability to tolerate stress.
• Consultation should include data on bleeding time.
• In a patient with symptoms of blood dyscrasias, request a medical consultation for blood studies and postpone treatment until normal values are reestablished.
Teach Patient/Family to:
• Update health and drug history if physician makes any changes in evaluation or drug regimens
• Use caution to prevent trauma when using oral hygiene aids
• Report any unusual or prolonged bleeding episodes after dental treatment

clorazepate dipotassium
klor-az´e-pate di-poe-tass´-ee-um
(Novoclopate[CAN], Tranxene, Tranxene SD, Tranxene SD Half-Strength, T-Tab)
Do not confuse clorazepate with clofibrate.

CATEGORY AND SCHEDULE
Pregnancy Risk Category: D
Controlled Substance Schedule IV

Drug Class: Benzodiazepine

MECHANISM OF ACTION
A benzodiazepine that depresses all levels of the CNS, including limbic and reticular formation, by binding to benzodiazepine receptor sites on the gamma-aminobutyric acid (GABA) receptor complex. Modulates GABA, a major inhibitory neurotransmitter in the brain. *Therapeutic Effect:* Produces anxiolytic effect, suppresses seizure activity.

USES
Anxiety, acute alcohol withdrawal, adjunctive treatment of partial seizures

PHARMACOKINETICS
Well absorbed after oral administration rapidly metabolized by liver to nordiazepam, which is slowly eliminated. *Half-life:* 40–50 hr. Protein binding of nordiazepam: 97–98%. Metabolites (nordiazepam, oxazepam, and glucuronide conjugates) excreted in urine.

INDICATIONS AND DOSAGES
▶ **Anxiety**
PO (Regular-Release)
Adults, Elderly. 7.5–15 mg 2–4 times a day.

PO (Sustained-Release)
Adults, Elderly. 11.25 mg or 22.5 mg
once a day at bedtime.
▸ **Anticonvulsant**
PO
*Adults, Elderly, Children older than
12 yr.* Initially, 7.5 mg 2–3 times
a day. May increase by 7.5 mg at
weekly intervals. Maximum:
90 mg/day.
Children 9–12 yr. Initially, 3.75–7.5
mg twice a day. May increase by
2.75 mg at weekly intervals.
Maximum: 60 mg/day.
▸ **Alcohol Withdrawal**
PO
Adults, Elderly. Initially, 30 mg, then
15 mg 2–4 times a day on first day.
Gradually decrease dosage over
subsequent days.
Maximum: 90 mg/day.

SIDE EFFECTS/ADVERSE REACTIONS
Frequent
Somnolence
Occasional
Dizziness, GI disturbances,
nervousness, blurred vision, dry
mouth, headache, confusion, ataxia,
rash, irritability, slurred speech
Rare
Paradoxical CNS reactions, such
as hyperactivity or nervousness
in children and excitement or
restlessness in the elderly or
debilitated (generally noted during
first 2 wk of therapy, particularly
in presence of uncontrolled pain)

PRECAUTIONS AND CONTRAINDICATIONS
Acute narrow-angle glaucoma
Caution
Elderly, debilitated, hepatic disease,
renal disease

DRUG INTERACTIONS OF CONCERN TO DENTISTRY
• Increased effects: CNS depressants,
alcohol, opioid analgesics, general
anesthetics, indinavir
• Increased serum levels and
prolonged effect of benzodiazepines:
fluconazole, ketoconazole,
itraconazole, miconazole (systemic)
• Possible increase in CNS side
effects: kava kava (herb)
• Contraindicated with saquinavir

SERIOUS REACTIONS
❗ Abrupt or too-rapid withdrawal
may result in pronounced
restlessness, irritability, insomnia,
hand tremors, abdominal or muscle
cramps, diaphoresis, vomiting,
and seizures.
❗ Overdose results in somnolence,
confusion, diminished reflexes,
and coma.

DENTAL CONSIDERATIONS
General:
• Monitor vital signs at every
appointment because of
cardiovascular side effects.
• Assess salivary flow as a factor
in caries, periodontal disease, and
candidiasis.
• After supine positioning, have
patient sit upright for at least 2 min
to avoid orthostatic hypotension.
• Psychologic and physical
dependence may occur with
chronic administration.
• Geriatric patients are more
susceptible to drug effects; use
a lower dose.
• Short appointments and a stress
reduction protocol may be required
for anxious patients.
• Seizure: ask about type of epilepsy,
seizure frequency, and quality of
seizure control.

Consultations:
• Medical consultation may be required to assess disease control and the patient's ability to tolerate stress.
Teach Patient/Family:
• When chronic dry mouth occurs, advise patient to:
  • Avoid mouth rinses with high alcohol content because of drying effects
  • Use daily home fluoride products for anticaries effect
  • Use sugarless gum, frequent sips of water, or saliva substitutes

clotrimazole
kloe-try´-mah-zole
(Canesten[CAN], Clotrimaderm[CAN], Mycelex, Mycelex OTC, Lotrimin, Gyne-Lotrimin, Trivagizole 3)

CATEGORY AND SCHEDULE
Pregnancy Risk Category: B (topical), C (troches)

Drug Class: Imidazole antifungal

MECHANISM OF ACTION
An antifungal that binds with phospholipids in fungal cell membrane. The altered cell membrane permeability. ***Therapeutic Effect:*** Inhibits yeast growth.

USES
Treatment of tinea pedis; tinea cruris; tinea corporis; tinea versicolor; C. albicans infection of the vagina, vulva, throat, mouth

PHARMACOKINETICS
Poorly, erratically absorbed from GI tract. Bound to oral mucosa. Absorbed portion metabolized in liver. Eliminated in feces. Topical: Minimal systemic absorption (highest concentration in stratum corneum). Intravaginal: Small amount systemically absorbed. ***Half-life:*** 3.5–5 hr.

INDICATIONS AND DOSAGES
▶ **Oropharyngeal Candidiasis Treatment**
PO
Adults, Elderly. 10 mg 5 times a day for 14 days.
▶ **Oropharyngeal Candidiasis Prophylaxis**
PO
Adults, Elderly. 10 mg 3 times a day.
▶ **Dermatophytosis, Cutaneous Candidiasis**
Topical
Adults, Elderly. 2 times a day. Therapeutic effect may take up to 8 wk.
▶ **Vulvovaginal Candidiasis**
Vaginal (Tablets)
Adults, Elderly. 1 tablet (100 mg) at bedtime for 7 days; 2 tablets (200 mg) at bedtime for 3 days; or 500 mg tablet one time.
Vaginal (Cream)
Adults, Elderly. 1 applicatorful at bedtime for 7–14 days.

SIDE EFFECTS/ADVERSE REACTIONS
Frequent
Oral: Nausea, vomiting, diarrhea, abdominal pain
Occasional
Topical: Itching, burning, stinging, erythema, urticaria
Vaginal: Mild burning (tablets/cream); irritation, cystitis (cream)
Rare
Vaginal: Itching, rash, lower abdominal cramping, headache

PRECAUTIONS AND CONTRAINDICATIONS
Hypersensitivity to clotrimazole or any component of the formulation, children younger than 3 yr

DRUG INTERACTIONS OF CONCERN TO DENTISTRY
None reported

SERIOUS REACTIONS
None reported

General:
• Determine why the patient is taking the drug.
• Examine oral mucous membranes for signs of fungal infection.
Teach Patient/Family to:
• Soak full or partial dentures in an antifungal solution overnight until lesions are absent; prolonged infections may require fabrication of new prosthesis
• Dispose of tooth brush used during oral infection after oral lesions are absent to prevent reinoculation
• Complete entire course of medication; long-term therapy may be necessary to clear infection

clozapine
klo´-za-peen
(Clopine[AUS], Clozaril, FazaClo)
Do not confuse clozapine with Cloxapen or clofazimine, or Clozaril with Clinoril or Colazal.

CATEGORY AND SCHEDULE
Pregnancy Risk Category: B

Drug Class: Antipsychotic, atypical

MECHANISM OF ACTION
A dibenzodiazepine derivative that interferes with the binding of dopamine at dopamine receptor sites; binds primarily at nondopamine receptor sites.
Therapeutic Effect: Diminishes schizophrenic behavior.

USES
Management of psychotic symptoms in schizophrenic patients for whom other antipsychotics have failed (available only through the Clozaril Patient Management System)

PHARMACOKINETICS
Absorbed rapidly and almost completely. Distributed rapidly and extensively. Crosses the blood-brain barrier. Protein binding: 95%. Metabolized in the liver. Excreted in urine and feces. **Half-life:** 8 hr.

INDICATIONS AND DOSAGES
▶ **Schizophrenic Disorders, Reduce Suicidal Behavior**
PO
Adults. Initially, 25 mg once or twice a day. May increase by 25–50 mg/day over 2 wk until dosage of 300–450 mg/day is achieved. May further increase by 50–100 mg/day no more than once or twice a wk. Range: 200–600 mg/day. Maximum: 900 mg/day.
Elderly. Initially, 25 mg/day. May increase by 25 mg/day. Maximum: 450 mg/day.

SIDE EFFECTS/ADVERSE REACTIONS
Frequent
Somnolence, salivation, tachycardia, dizziness, constipation
Occasional
Hypotension, headache, tremors, syncope, diaphoresis, dry mouth, nausea, visual disturbances, nightmares, restlessness, akinesia, agitation, hypertension, abdominal discomfort or heartburn, weight gain
Rare
Rigidity, confusion, fatigue, insomnia, diarrhea, rash

PRECAUTIONS AND CONTRAINDICATIONS

Coma, concurrent use of other drugs that may suppress bone marrow function, history of clozapine-induced agranulocytosis or severe granulocytopenia, myeloproliferative disorders, severe CNS depression

Caution

Lactation; children younger than 16 yr; hepatic, renal, cardiac disease; seizures; prostatic enlargement; elderly; increased incidence of cardiomyopathy

DRUG INTERACTIONS OF CONCERN TO DENTISTRY

- Increased anticholinergic effects: anticholinergics
- Increased CNS depression: alcohol, all CNS depressant drugs
- Increased serum concentration, leukocytosis: erythromycin base
- Possible decreased effects: carbamazepine
- Increased plasma levels: ciprofloxacin

SERIOUS REACTIONS

! Blood dyscrasias, particularly agranulocytosis and mild leukopenia, may occur.
! Seizures occur in about 3% of patients.
! Overdose produces CNS depression (including sedation, coma, and delirium), respiratory depression, and hypersalivation.

DENTAL CONSIDERATIONS

General:

- Monitor vital signs at every appointment because of cardiovascular and respiratory side effects.
- Patients on chronic drug therapy may rarely have symptoms of blood dyscrasias, which can include infection, bleeding, and poor healing.
- After supine positioning, have patient sit upright for at least 2 min before standing to avoid orthostatic hypotension.
- Assess salivary flow as a factor in caries, periodontal disease, and candidiasis.
- Determine why the patient is taking the drug.
- Place on frequent recall because of oral side effects.

Consultations:

- In a patient with symptoms of blood dyscrasias, request a medical consultation for blood studies and postpone dental treatment until normal values are reestablished.
- Medical consultation may be required to assess disease control and stress tolerance of patient.
- Physician should be informed if significant xerostomic side effects occur (e.g., increased caries, sore tongue, problems eating or swallowing, difficulty wearing prosthesis) so that a medication change can be considered.

Teach Patient/Family to:

- Use effective oral hygiene to prevent soft tissue inflammation
- Use caution to prevent injury when using oral hygiene aids
- Use electric tooth brush if patient has difficulty holding conventional devices
- When chronic dry mouth occurs, advise patient to:
  - Avoid mouth rinses with high alcohol content because of drying effects
  - Use daily home fluoride products for anticaries effect
  - Use sugarless gum, frequent sips of water, or saliva substitutes

cocaine hydrochloride

koe-kane´ hi-droh-klor´-ide
(Cocaine[CAN], Cocaine HCl)

CATEGORY AND SCHEDULE

Pregnancy Risk Category: C
Controlled Substance: Schedule II

Drug Class: Amide; topical
anesthetic

MECHANISM OF ACTION

A topical anesthetic that decreases
membrane permeability, increases
norepinephrine at postsynaptic
receptor sites, producing intense
vasoconstriction. ***Therapeutic
Effect:*** Blocks conduction of
nerve impulses.

USES

Topical anesthesia for mucous
membranes of orolaryngeal, nasal
areas; minor, uncomplicated facial
lacerations

PHARMACOKINETICS

Readily absorbed from all mucous
membranes. Cocaine penetrates the
CNS but is rapidly metabolized.
Rapidly hydrolyzed in blood by
serum cholinesterases. Metabolized
in liver. Excreted in urine. ***Half-life:***
1–1.5 hr.

INDICATIONS AND DOSAGES

▶ **Anesthesia**
Topical
Adults, Elderly, Children. 1%–4% to
mucous membranes. Maximum:
1–3 mg/kg. Dosage varies depending
upon the area to be anesthetized,
vascularity of the tissues, individual
tolerance, and anesthetic technique.
Administer lowest effective dose.

SIDE EFFECTS/ADVERSE REACTIONS

Frequent
Loss of sense of smell and taste
Occasional
Anxiety, CNS stimulation or
depression

PRECAUTIONS AND CONTRAINDICATIONS

Hypersensitivity to cocaine or any
component of the formulation

DRUG INTERACTIONS OF CONCERN TO DENTISTRY

• Sensitization to catecholamines,
such as epinephrine; risk of serious
adverse cardiovascular events
• Avoid ester-type local anesthetics
in patients with allergic reactions to
cocaine

SERIOUS REACTIONS

! Repeated nasal application may
produce stuffy nose and chronic
rhinitis.
! Early signs of overdosage are
increased B/P, increased pulse,
irregular heartbeat, chills or fever,
agitation, nervousness, confusion,
inability to remain still, nausea,
vomiting, abdominal pain, increased
sweating, rapid breathing, and large
pupils.
! Advanced signs of overdosage are
arrhythmias, CNS hemorrhage, CHF,
convulsions, delirium, hyperreflexia,
loss of bladder or bowel control, and
respiratory weakness.
! Late signs of overdosage are loss
of reflexes, muscle paralysis, dilated
pupils, LOC, cyanosis, pulmonary
edema, cardiac and respiratory failure.

DENTAL CONSIDERATIONS

General:
• Acute-use drug for medical topical
anesthesia (not for injection).

- Abusers of cocaine may present with oral or nasal mucosal lesions and dry mucous membranes, nervousness, and anxiety.
- Caution: drug interactions in chronic abusers of cocaine.
- Determine why patient is taking the drug.
- Monitor vital signs at every appointment due to cardiovascular side effects.
- Assess salivary flow as a factor in caries, periodontal disease, and candidiasis.
- If additional analgesia is required for dental pain, consider alternative analgesics (NSAIDs) in patients taking narcotics for acute or chronic pain.
- Use vasoconstrictor with caution, in low doses, and with careful aspiration. Avoid using gingival retraction cord containing epinephrine.
- Examine for oral manifestation of opportunistic infection.
- Psychologic and physical dependence may occur with chronic administration.
- Dental local anesthetics will not interfere with urine test for cocaine abuse.

Consultations:

- Notify recovery program director if controlled substances may be required for a patient in recovery from cocaine use.

Teach Patient/Family:

- When chronic dry mouth occurs, advise patient to:
  - Avoid mouth rinses with high alcohol content due to drying effects
  - Use daily home fluoride products for anticaries effect
  - Use sugarless gum, frequent sips of water, or saliva substitutes.
- Report oral lesions, soreness, or bleeding to dentist

codeine phosphate/ codeine sulfate

koe´-deen foss´-fate/koe´-deen sull´-fate
(codeine phosphate) Actacode[AUS], Codeine Phosphate Injection, Codeine Linctus[AUS](codeine sulfate) Contin[CAN]
Do not confuse codeine with Cardene or Lodine.

CATEGORY AND SCHEDULE

Pregnancy Risk Category: C
(D if used for prolonged periods or at high dosages at term)
Controlled Substance: Schedule II (analgesic), III (fixed-combination form)

Drug Class: Narcotic analgesic

MECHANISM OF ACTION

An opioid agonist that binds to opioid receptors at many sites in the CNS, particularly in the medulla. This action inhibits the ascending pain pathways. *Therapeutic Effect:* Alters the perception of and emotional response to pain, suppresses cough reflex.

USES

Treatment of mild-to-moderate pain, non-productive cough

PHARMACOKINETICS

Well absorbed after oral administration; rapidly metabolized by liver; 10% methylated to the active analgesic morphine. *Half-life:* 2.5–3 hr. Metabolites excreted in urine.

INDICATIONS AND DOSAGES
▸ **Analgesia**
PO, IM, Subcutaneous
Adults, Elderly. 30 mg q4–6h.
Range: 15–60 mg.

Children. 0.5–1 mg/kg q4–6h.
Maximum: 60 mg/dose.
▸ **Cough**
PO
Adults, Elderly, Children 12 yr and older. 10–20 mg q4–6h.
Children 6–11 yr. 5–10 mg q4–6h.
Children 2–5 yr. 2.5–5 mg q4–6h.
▸ **Dosage in Renal Impairment**
Dosage is modified on the basis of creatinine clearance.

Creatinine Clearance	Dosage
10–50 ml/min	75% of usual dose
Less than 10 ml/min	50% of usual dose

SIDE EFFECTS/ADVERSE REACTIONS
Frequent
Constipation, somnolence, nausea, vomiting
Occasional
Paradoxical excitement, confusion, palpitations, facial flushing, decreased urination, blurred vision, dizziness, dry mouth, headache, hypotension (including orthostatic hypotension), decreased appetite, injection site redness, burning, or pain
Rare
Hallucinations, depression, abdominal pain, insomnia

PRECAUTIONS AND CONTRAINDICATIONS
Caution
Elderly, cardiac dysrhythmias

DRUG INTERACTIONS OF CONCERN TO DENTISTRY
• Increased sedation with other CNS depressants and alcohol
• Increased effects of anticholinergics

SERIOUS REACTIONS
! Too-frequent use may result in paralytic ileus.
! Overdose may produce cold and clammy skin, confusion, seizures, decreased B/P, restlessness, pinpoint pupils, bradycardia, respiratory depression, decreased LOC, and severe weakness.
! The patient who uses codeine repeatedly may develop a tolerance to the drug's analgesic effect, as well as physical dependence.

DENTAL CONSIDERATIONS
General:
• Monitor vital signs at every appointment because of cardiovascular and respiratory side effects.
• After supine positioning, have patient sit upright for at least 2 min to avoid orthostatic hypotension.
• Assess salivary flow as a factor in caries, periodontal disease, and candidiasis.
• Psychologic and physical dependence may occur with chronic administration.
Teach Patient/Family:
• When chronic dry mouth occurs, advise patient to:
  • Avoid mouth rinses with high alcohol content because of drying effects
  • Use daily home fluoride products for anticaries effect
  • Use sugarless gum, frequent sips of water, or saliva substitutes

colchicine
kol´-chi-seen
(Colchicine, Colgout[AUS])

CATEGORY AND SCHEDULE
Pregnancy Risk Category: D

Drug Class: Antigout agent

MECHANISM OF ACTION

An alkaloid that decreases leukocyte motility, phagocytosis, and lactic acid production. *Therapeutic Effect:* Decreases urate crystal deposits and reduces inflammatory process.

USES

Gout, gouty arthritis (prevention, treatment); unlabeled uses: hepatic cirrhosis, Behçet's disease, scleroderma, Sweet's syndrome

PHARMACOKINETICS

Rapidly absorbed from the GI tract. Highest concentration is in the liver, spleen, and kidney. Protein binding: 30%–50%. Reenters the intestinal tract by biliary secretion and is reabsorbed from the intestines. Partially metabolized in the liver. Eliminated primarily in feces.

INDICATIONS AND DOSAGES
▸ **Acute Gouty Arthritis**
PO
Adults, Elderly. 0.6–1.2 mg; then 0.6 mg q1–2h or 1–1.2 mg q2h, until pain is relieved or nausea, vomiting, or diarrhea occurs. Total dose: 4–8 mg.
IV
Adults, Elderly. Initially, 2 mg; then 0.5 mg q6h until satisfactory response. Maximum: 4 mg/wk or 4 mg/one course of treatment. If pain recurs, may give 1–2 mg/day for several days but no sooner than 7 days after a full course of IV therapy (total of 4 mg).
▸ **Chronic Gouty Arthritis**
PO
Adults, Elderly. 0.5–0.6 mg once a wk up to once a day, depending on number of attacks per year.

SIDE EFFECTS/ADVERSE REACTIONS
Frequent
PO: Nausea, vomiting, abdominal discomfort

Occasional
PO: Anorexia
Rare
Hypersensitivity reaction, including angioedema
Parenteral: Nausea, vomiting, diarrhea, abdominal discomfort, pain or redness at injection site, neuritis in injected arm

PRECAUTIONS AND CONTRAINDICATIONS

Blood dyscrasias; severe cardiac, GI, hepatic, or renal disorders
Caution
Severe renal disease, blood dyscrasias, hepatic disease, elderly, lactation, children, retards B_{12} absorption

DRUG INTERACTIONS OF CONCERN TO DENTISTRY

- Increased risk of GI side effects: NSAIDs, alcohol
- Possible increased serum levels: erythromycin

SERIOUS REACTIONS

❗ Bone marrow depression, including aplastic anemia, agranulocytosis, and thrombocytopenia, may occur with long-term therapy.
❗ Overdose initially causes a burning feeling in the skin or throat, severe diarrhea, and abdominal pain. The patient then experiences fever, seizures, delirium, and renal impairment, marked by hematuria and oliguria. The third stage of overdose causes hair loss, leukocytosis, and stomatitis.

DENTAL CONSIDERATIONS
General:
- Consider drug in diagnosis of taste alteration.
- Patients on chronic drug therapy may rarely have symptoms of blood

dyscrasias, which can include infection, bleeding, and poor healing.
• Avoid prescribing aspirin-containing products.

Consultations:
• Medical consultation may be required to assess disease control.
• In a patient with symptoms of blood dyscrasias, request a medical consultation for blood studies and postpone dental treatment until normal values are reestablished.

Teach Patient/Family to:
• Use effective oral hygiene to prevent soft tissue inflammation
• Use caution to prevent injury when using oral hygiene aids
• Avoid mouth rinses with high alcohol content because of drying effects

colesevelam
koh-le-sev´-eh-lam
(Welchol)

CATEGORY AND SCHEDULE
Pregnancy Risk Category: B

Drug Class: Antihyperlipidemic

MECHANISM OF ACTION
A bile acid sequestrant and nonsystemic polymer that binds with bile acids in the intestines, preventing their reabsorption and removing them from the body.
Therapeutic Effect: Decreases LDL cholesterol.

USES
Adjunctive therapy to diet and exercise, alone or in combination with an HMG-Co. A reductase inhibitor (statin) in patients with primary hypercholesterolemia (type IIa) to reduce elevated LDL cholesterol

PHARMACOKINETICS:
PO: Not absorbed; excreted in feces

INDICATIONS AND DOSAGES
▸ **To decrease LDL Cholesterol Level in Primary Hypercholesterolemia (Fredrickson type IIa)**
PO
Adults, Elderly. 3 tablets with meals twice a day or 6 tablets once a day with a meal. May increase daily dose to 7 tablets a day.

SIDE EFFECTS/ADVERSE REACTIONS
Frequent
Flatulence, constipation, infection, dyspepsia (heartburn, epigastric distress)

PRECAUTIONS AND CONTRAINDICATIONS
Complete biliary obstruction, hypersensitivity to colesevelam
Caution
Preexisting GI diseases, primary biliary cirrhosis, biliary obstruction, hypertriglyceridemia, use in children not established

DRUG INTERACTIONS OF CONCERN TO DENTISTRY
• None reported, but monitor if drugs with narrow therapeutic index are prescribed for dental conditions

SERIOUS REACTIONS
! GI tract obstruction may occur.

DENTAL CONSIDERATIONS
General:
• Consider semisupine chair position for patient comfort if GI side effects occur.
• Monitor vital signs at every appointment because of possibility of cardiovascular disease.

colestipol
koe-les´-ti-pole
(Colestid, Colestid[CAN])

CATEGORY AND SCHEDULE
Pregnancy Risk Category: C

Drug Class: Antihyperlipidemic

MECHANISM OF ACTION
An antihyperlipoproteinemic that
binds with bile acids in the intestine,
forming an insoluble complex.
Binding results in partial removal
of bile acid from enterohepatic
circulation. *Therapeutic Effect:*
Removes LDL and cholesterol from
plasma.

USES
Adjunctive therapy to diet and
exercise for the reduction of elevated
serum total and LDL cholesterol
in patients with primary
hypercholesterolemia

PHARMACOKINETICS
Not absorbed from the GI tract.
Excreted in the feces.

INDICATIONS AND DOSAGES
▶ **Primary Hypercholesterolemia**
PO, granules
Adults, Elderly. Initially, 5 g
1–2 times a day. Range: 5–30 g/day
once or in divided doses.
PO, tablets
Adults, Elderly. Initially, 2 g
1–2 times a day. Range: 2–16 g/day.

SIDE EFFECTS/ADVERSE REACTIONS
Frequent
Constipation (may lead to fecal
impaction), nausea, vomiting,
stomach pain, indigestion

Occasional
Diarrhea, belching, bloating,
headache, dizziness
Rare
Gallstones, peptic ulcer,
malabsorption syndrome

PRECAUTIONS AND CONTRAINDICATIONS
Complete biliary obstruction,
hypersensitivity to bile acid
sequestering resins
Caution
Lactation, children, bleeding disorders

DRUG INTERACTIONS OF CONCERN TO DENTISTRY
• Decreased absorption of
tetracyclines, cephalexin,
phenobarbital, corticosteroids,
clindamycin, penicillins;
administer doses several hr apart

SERIOUS REACTIONS
! GI tract obstruction, hyperchloremic
acidosis, and osteoporosis secondary
to calcium excretion may occur.
! High dosage may interfere with
fat absorption, resulting in
steatorrhea.

DENTAL CONSIDERATIONS
General:
• Consider semisupine chair position
for patient comfort because of GI
side effects of disease.

conivaptan
con-ih-vap´-tan
(Vaprisol)

CATEGORY AND SCHEDULE
Pregnancy Risk Category: C

Drug Class: Vasopressin
antagonist

MECHANISM OF ACTION
An arginine vaspressin (AVP) V1A and V2 selective antagonist that inhibits vasopressin binding V1A in the liver and V1 and V2 sites in renal collecting ducts. Results in excretion of free water. *Therapeutic Effect:* Restores normal fluid and electrolyte status.

USES
Treatment of euvolemic hyponatremia in hospitalized patients

PHARMACOKENETICS
Protein binding: 99%. Metabolized in liver; CYP450 3A4 is responsible for primary metabolism. Primarily eliminated in feces (approximately 83%); minimal excretion in urine (about 12%). *Half-life:* 3.6–8.6 hr.

INDICATIONS AND DOSAGES
▸ Hyponatremia
IV
Adults. Initially, a loading dose of 20 mg given over 30 min. Maintenance: 20 mg/day as continuous infusion over 24 hr for an additional 1–3 days. May titrate to maximum dose of 40 mg/day; total duration should not exceed 4 days after loading dose.
Safety and efficacy have not been established in children.

SIDE EFFECTS/ADVERSE REACTIONS:
Frequent
Injection site reaction, headache
Occasional
Hypokalemia, thirst, vomiting, diarrhea, hypertension, orthostatic hypotension, polyuria, phlebitis, constipation, dry mouth, anemia, fever, nausea, confusion, erythema, insomnia, atrial fibrillation, hyper- or hypoglycemia, hyponatremia, pneumonia, UTI, hypomagnesemia, pain, dehydration, oral candidiasis, hematuria

PRECAUTIONS AND CONTRAINDICATIONS
Hypersensitivity to conivaptan or its components
Use with ketoconazole, itraconazole, clarithromycin, ritonavir, and indinavir is contraindicated
Caution
Hyponatremia with underlying CHF, renal, or hepatic impairment

DRUG INTERACTIONS OF CONCERN TO DENTISTRY
• CYP3A4 inducers: may decrease the levels and effects of conivaptan
• CYP3A4 inhibitors (e.g., erythromycin): may increase the levels and effects of conivaptan
• CYP3A4 substrates: conivaptan may increase the levels and effects of CYP3A4 substrates
• Digoxin: may increase the levels of digoxin

SERIOUS REACTIONS
! Atrial fibrillation has been reported.

DENTAL CONSIDERATIONS
• Monitor vital signs at every appointment because of cardiovascular side effects.
• Avoid NSAIDs because of renal side effects.
• After supine positioning, have patient sit upright for at least 2 min before standing to avoid orthostatic hypotension.
• Patients taking this medication are treated on an inpatient basis.
Consultations:
• Consult physician to determine disease control and ability of patient to tolerate dental procedures, if needed while receiving drug.

Teach Patient/Family to:
• Report signs and symptoms of dry mouth and candidiasis

cortisone acetate
kor´-ti-sone ass´-eh-tayte
(Cortate[AUS], Cortone[CAN])
Do not confuse cortisone with Cort-Dome.

CATEGORY AND SCHEDULE
Pregnancy Risk Category: C (D if used in the first trimester)

Drug Class: Glucocorticoid, short-acting

MECHANISM OF ACTION
An adrenocortical steroid that inhibits the accumulation of inflammatory cells at inflammation sites, phagocytosis, lysosomal enzyme release and synthesis, and release of mediators of inflammation. *Therapeutic Effect:* Prevents or suppresses cell-mediated immune reactions. Decreases or prevents tissue response to inflammatory process.

USES
Treatment of inflammation, severe allergy, adrenal insufficiency, collagen disorders, respiratory, dermatologic disorders

PHARMACOKINETICS
Well absorbed after oral administration. *Half-life:* 60–90 min. Metabolized in liver and kidneys, approximately one-third excreted in urine as metabolites.

INDICATIONS AND DOSAGES
Dosage is dependent on the condition being treated and patient response.

▸ **Antiinflammation, Immunosuppression**
PO
Adults, Elderly. 25–300 mg/day in divided doses q12–24h.
Children. 2.5–10 mg/kg/day in divided doses q6–8h.
▸ **Physiologic Replacement**
PO
Adults, Elderly. 25–35 mg/day.
Children. 0.5–0.75 mg/kg/day in divided doses q8h.

SIDE EFFECTS/ADVERSE REACTIONS
Frequent
Insomnia, heartburn, anxiety, abdominal distention, increased diaphoresis, acne, mood swings, increased appetite, facial flushing, delayed wound healing, increased susceptibility to infection, diarrhea or constipation
Occasional
Headache, edema, change in skin color, frequent urination
Rare
Tachycardia, allergic reaction (such as rash and hives), psychological changes, hallucinations, depression

PRECAUTIONS AND CONTRAINDICATIONS
Hypersensitivity to corticosteroids, administration of live virus vaccine, peptic ulcers (except in life-threatening situations), systemic fungal infection
Caution
Diabetes mellitus, glaucoma, osteoporosis, seizure disorders, ulcerative colitis, CHF, myasthenia gravis, renal disease, esophagitis, peptic ulcer, rifampin

DRUG INTERACTIONS OF CONCERN TO DENTISTRY
• Decreased action: barbiturates, rifabutin, rifampin

• Increased GI side effects: alcohol, salicylates, NSAIDs
• Increased action: ketoconazole, macrolide antibiotics
• Hepatotoxicity: acetaminophen (chronic, high doses)

SERIOUS REACTIONS

! Long-term therapy may cause hypocalcemia, hypokalemia, muscle wasting in arms and legs, osteoporosis, spontaneous fractures, amenorrhrea, cataracts, glaucoma, peptic ulcer disease, and CHF.
! Abrupt withdrawal following long-term therapy may cause anorexia, nausea, fever, headache, joint pain, rebound inflammation, fatigue, weakness, lethargy, dizziness, and orthostatic hypotension.

DENTAL CONSIDERATIONS

General:
• Monitor vital signs at every appointment because of cardiovascular side effects.
• Patients on chronic drug therapy may rarely have symptoms of blood dyscrasias, which can include infection, bleeding, and poor healing.
• Assess salivary flow as a factor in caries, periodontal disease, and candidiasis.
• Avoid prescribing aspirin-containing products.
• Symptoms of oral infections may be masked.
• Place on frequent recall to evaluate healing response.
• Prophylactic antibiotics may be indicated to prevent infection if surgery or deep scaling is planned.
• Determine dose and duration of steroid therapy for each patient to assess risk for stress tolerance and immunosuppression.
• Patients who have been or are currently on chronic steroid therapy (>2 wk) may require supplemental steroids for dental treatment.

• Determine why the patient is taking the drug.
Consultations:
• In a patient with symptoms of blood dyscrasias, request a medical consultation for blood studies and postpone dental treatment until normal values are reestablished.
• Medical consultation may be required to assess disease control and stress tolerance of patient.
• Consultation may be required to confirm steroid dose and duration of use.
Teach Patient/Family to:
• Use effective oral hygiene to prevent soft tissue inflammation
• Prevent injury when using oral hygiene aids
• When chronic dry mouth occurs, advise patient to:
  • Avoid mouth rinses with high alcohol content because of drying effects
  • Use daily home fluoride products for anticaries effect
  • Use sugarless gum, frequent sips of water, or saliva substitutes

cromolyn sodium
kroe´-moe-lin so´-dee-um
(Apo-Cromolyn[CAN], Crolom, Gastrocom, Intal, Nasalcrom, Opticrom, Rynacrom[AUS])

CATEGORY AND SCHEDULE
Pregnancy Risk Category: B

Drug Class: Antiasthmatic, mast cell stabilizer

MECHANISM OF ACTION
An antiasthmatic and antiallergic agent that prevents mast cell release of histamine and formation of other mediators (leukotrienes) of anaphylaxis by inhibiting degranulation after

contact with antigens. ***Therapeutic Effect:*** Helps prevent symptoms of asthma, allergic rhinitis, mastocytosis, and exercise-induced bronchospasm.

USES
Treatment of allergic rhinitis, severe perennial bronchial asthma, exercise-induced bronchospasm (prevention), prevention of acute bronchospasm induced by environmental pollutants, mastocytosis

PHARMACOKINETICS
Minimal absorption after PO, inhalation, or nasal administration. Absorbed portion excreted in urine or by biliary system. ***Half-life:*** 80–90 min.

INDICATIONS AND DOSAGES
▸ **Asthma**
Inhalation (nebulization)
Adults, Elderly, Children older than 2 yr. 20 mg 3–4 times a day.
Aerosol Spray
Adults, Elderly, Children 12 yr and older. Initially, 2 sprays 4 times a day. Maintenance: 2–4 sprays 3–4 times a day.
Children 5–11 yr. Initially, 2 sprays 4 times a day, then 1–2 sprays 3–4 times a day.
▸ **Prevention of Bronchospasm**
Inhalation (nebulization)
Adults, Elderly, Children older than 2 yr. 20 mg 1 hr before exercise or exposure to allergens.
Aerosol Spray
Adults, Elderly, Children older than 5 yr. 2 sprays 1 hr before exercise or exposure to allergens.
▸ **Food Allergy, Inflammatory Bowel Disease**
PO
Adults, Elderly, Children older than 12 yr. 200–400 mg 4 times a day.

Children 2–12 yr. 100–200 mg 4 times a day. Maximum: 40 mg/kg/day.
▸ **Allergic Rhinitis**
Intranasal
Adults, Elderly, Children older than 6 yr. 1 spray each nostril 3–4 times a day. May increase up to 6 times a day.
▸ **Systemic Mastocytosis**
PO
Adults, Elderly, Children older than 12 yr. 200 mg 4 times a day.
Children 2–12 yr. 100 mg 4 times a day. Maximum: 40 mg/kg/day.
Children younger than 2 yr. 20 mg/kg/day in 4 divided doses. Maximum: 30 mg/kg/day (children 6 mo–2 yr).
▸ **Conjunctivitis**
Ophthalmic
Adults, Elderly, Children older than 4 yr. 1–2 drops in both eyes 4–6 times a day.

SIDE EFFECTS/ADVERSE REACTIONS
Frequent
PO: Headache, diarrhea
Inhalation: Cough, dry mouth and throat, stuffy nose, throat irritation, unpleasant taste
Nasal: Nasal burning, stinging, or irritation; increased sneezing
Ophthalmic: Eye burning or stinging
Occasional
PO: Rash, abdominal pain, arthralgia, nausea, insomnia
Inhalation: Bronchospasm, hoarseness, lacrimation
Nasal: Cough, headache, unpleasant taste, postnasal drip
Ophthalmic: Lacrimation and itching of eye
Rare
Inhalation: Dizziness, painful urination, arthralgia, myalgia, rash
Nasal: Epistaxis, rash

Ophthalmic: Chemosis or edema of conjunctiva, eye irritation

PRECAUTIONS AND CONTRAINDICATIONS

Status asthmaticus.
Caution
Lactation, renal disease, hepatic disease, children younger than 5 yr

DRUG INTERACTIONS OF CONCERN TO DENTISTRY

None reported

SERIOUS REACTIONS

! Anaphylaxis occurs rarely when cromolyn is given by the inhalation, nasal, or oral route.

DENTAL CONSIDERATIONS

General:
• Determine why patient is taking the drug.
• Protect patient's eyes from accidental spatter during dental treatment.
• Avoid dental light in patient's eyes; offer dark glasses for patient comfort.
General:
• Assess salivary flow as a factor in caries, periodontal disease, and candidiasis.
• Consider semisupine chair position for patients with respiratory disease.
• A stress reduction protocol may be required.
• Midday appointments and a stress reduction protocol may be required for anxious patients.
• Be aware that aspirin or sulfite preservatives in vasoconstrictor-containing products can exacerbate asthma.
Consultations:
• Consider drug in diagnosis of taste alteration and burning mouth syndrome.

• Medical consultation may be required to assess disease control and stress tolerance of patient.
Teach Patient/Family to:
• Rinse mouth with water after each inhaled dose to prevent dryness
• When chronic dry mouth occurs, advise patient to:
  • Avoid mouth rinses with high alcohol content because of drying effects
  • Use daily home fluoride products for anticaries effect
  • Use sugarless gum, frequent sips of water, or saliva substitutes

cyanocobalamin (vitamin B$_{12}$)

sye-an-oh-koe-bal′-ah-min
(Bedoz[CAN], Cytamen[AUS], Nascobal)

CATEGORY AND SCHEDULE

Pregnancy Risk Category: A (C if used in doses above recommended daily allowance)

Drug Class: Vitamin B$_{12}$, water-soluble vitamin

MECHANISM OF ACTION

Acts as a coenzyme for various metabolic functions, including fat and carbohydrate metabolism and protein synthesis. Therapeutic Effect: Necessary for cell growth and replication, hematopoiesis, and myelin synthesis.

USES

Vitamin B$_{12}$ deficiency, pernicious anemia, vitamin B$_{12}$ malabsorption syndrome, Schilling test, increased requirements with pregnancy thyrotoxicosis, hemolytic anemia, hemorrhage, renal and hepatic disease; intranasal gel: maintaining vitamin B$_{12}$ levels in patients with HIV, multiple sclerosis, or Crohn's disease

PHARMACOKINETICS

In the presence of calcium, absorbed systemically in lower half of ileum. Initially, bound to intrinsic factor; this complex passes down intestine, binding to receptor sites on ileal mucosa. Protein binding: High. Metabolized in the liver. Primarily eliminated unchanged in urine. *Half-life:* 6 days.

INDICATIONS AND DOSAGES

▶ **Pernicious Anemia**
IM, Subcutaneous
Adults, Elderly. 100 mcg/day for 7 days, then every other day for 7 days, then every 3–4 days for 2–3 wk. Maintenance: 100 mcg/mo (oral 1000–2000 mcg/day).
Children. 30–50 mcg/day for 2 or more wk.
Maintenance: 100 mcg/mo.
Neonates. 1000 mcg/day for 2 or more wk.
Maintenance: 50 mcg/mo.
Intranasal
Adults, Elderly. 500 mcg once a wk.
▶ **Uncomplicated Vitamin B$_{12}$ Deficiency**
PO
Adults, Elderly. 1000–2000 mcg/day
IM, Subcutaneous
Adults, Elderly. 100 mcg/day for 5–10 days, followed by 100–200 mcg/mo.
▶ **Complicated Vitamin B$_{12}$ Deficiency**
IM, Subcutaneous
Adults, Elderly. 1000 mcg (with IM or IV folic acid 15 mg) as a single dose, then 1000 mcg/day plus oral folic acid 5 mg/day for 7 days.

SIDE EFFECTS/ADVERSE REACTIONS

Occasional
Diarrhea, pruritus

PRECAUTIONS AND CONTRAINDICATIONS

Folic acid deficiency anemia, hereditary optic nerve atrophy, history of allergy to cobalamins
Caution
Lactation, children

DRUG INTERACTIONS OF CONCERN TO DENTISTRY

• Increased absorption: prednisone

SERIOUS REACTIONS

! Impurities in preparation may cause a rare allergic reaction.
! Peripheral vascular thrombosis, pulmonary edema, hypokalemia, and CHF may occur.

DENTAL CONSIDERATIONS

General:
• Deficiency in vitamin B$_{12}$ and other B-complex vitamins may cause oral symptomatology.

cyclobenzaprine hydrochloride

sye-kloe-ben´-za-preen
hi-droh-klor´-ide
(Flexeril, Flexitec[CAN], Novo-Cycloprine[CAN])
Do not confuse cyclobenzaprine with cycloserine or cyproheptadine, or Flexeril with Floxin.

CATEGORY AND SCHEDULE

Pregnancy Risk Category: B

Drug Class: Skeletal muscle relaxant, centrally acting tricyclic

MECHANISM OF ACTION

A centrally acting skeletal muscle relaxant that reduces tonic somatic muscle activity at the level of the brainstem. *Therapeutic Effect:* Relieves local skeletal muscle spasm.

USES

Adjunct for relief of muscle spasm and pain in musculoskeletal conditions

PHARMACOKINETICS

Route	Onset	Peak	Duration
PO	1 hr	3–4 hr	12–24hr

Well but slowly absorbed from the GI tract. Protein binding: 93%. Metabolized in the GI tract and the liver. Primarily excreted in urine. *Half-life:* 1–3 days.

INDICATIONS AND DOSAGES

▶ **Acute, Painful Musculoskeletal Conditions**
PO
Adults. Initially, 5 mg 3 times a day. May increase to 10 mg 3 times a day.
Elderly. 5 mg 3 times a day.
▶ **Dosage in Hepatic Impairment**
Mild. 5 mg 3 times a day.
Moderate and severe. Not recommended.

PRECAUTIONS AND CONTRAINDICATIONS

Acute recovery phase of MI, arrhythmias, CHF, heart block, conduction disturbances, hyperthyroidism, use within 14 days of MAOIs
Caution
Renal disease, hepatic disease, addictive personality, elderly

SIDE EFFECTS/ADVERSE REACTIONS

Frequent
Somnolence, dry mouth, dizziness
Rare
Fatigue, asthenia, blurred vision, headache, nervousness, confusion, nausea, constipation, dyspepsia, unpleasant taste

PRECAUTIONS AND CONTRAINDICATIONS

Acute recovery phase of MI, dysrhythmias, heart block, CHF, hypersensitivity, children younger than 12 yr, intermittent porphyria, thyroid disease, concomitant use with or within 14 days of discontinuing MAOIs, renal disease, hepatic disease, addictive personality, elderly

DRUG INTERACTIONS OF CONCERN TO DENTISTRY

• Increased CNS depression: alcohol, narcotics, barbiturates, sedatives, hypnotics
• Increased effects of anticholinergic drugs
• Increased effects of direct-acting sympathomimetics (epinephrine, levonordefrin)

SERIOUS REACTIONS

! Overdose may result in visual hallucinations, hyperactive reflexes, muscle rigidity, vomiting, and hyperpyrexia.

DENTAL CONSIDERATIONS
General:
• Monitor vital signs at every appointment because of cardiovascular side effects.
• Assess salivary flow as a factor in caries, periodontal disease, and candidiasis.

• After supine positioning, have patient sit upright for at least 2 min to avoid orthostatic hypotension.
• Use vasoconstrictors with caution, in low doses, and with careful aspiration. Avoid use of gingival retraction cord with epinephrine.
• Place on frequent recall because of oral side effects.
• Consider drug in diagnosis of taste alterations.

Consultations:
• Medical consultation may be required to assess disease control.

Teach Patient/Family:
• When chronic dry mouth occurs, advise patient to:
    • Avoid mouth rinses with high alcohol content because of drying effects
    • Use daily home fluoride products for anticaries effect
    • Use sugarless gum, frequent sips of water, or saliva substitutes

cyclopentolate hydrochloride

sye-kloe-pen´-toe-late
hi-droh-klor´-ide
(AK-Pentolate, Cyclogyl, Cylate, Diopentolate[CAN], Ocu-Pentolate, Pentolair)

CATEGORY AND SCHEDULE
Pregnancy Risk Category: C

Drug Class: Cycloplegic; mydriatic

MECHANISM OF ACTION
An antimuscarinic similar to atropine that competes with acetylcholine. Blocks the responses of the sphincter muscle of the iris and the accommodative muscle of the ciliary body to cholinergic stimulation. *Therapeutic Effect:* Results in mydriasis and cycloplegia.

USES
Used to dilate (enlarge) the pupil for eye examination

PHARMACOKINETICS
Rapid systemic absorption following ophthalmic administration. Shorter duration of action than atropine. Complete recovery takes 6–24 hr.

INDICATIONS AND DOSAGES
▸ **Cycloplegia Induction, Mydriasis Induction**
Ophthalmic
Adults, Elderly, Children. Instill 1–2 drops of 0.5%–2% solution in eye(s). May repeat with 0.5% or 1% solution in 5–10 min as needed.
Neonates, infants. Instill 1 drop of 0.5%–2% solution in eye(s) followed by 1 drop of 0.5% or 1% in 5 min as needed.

SIDE EFFECTS/ADVERSE REACTIONS
Occasional
Blurred vision, burning of eye, photophobia
Rare
Conjunctivitis, increased intraocular pressure

PRECAUTIONS AND CONTRAINDICATIONS
Narrow-angle glaucoma, anatomical narrow angles, hypersensitivity to cyclopentolate or any component of the formulation

DRUG INTERACTIONS OF CONCERN TO DENTISTRY
None reported

SERIOUS REACTIONS

! Systemic absorption, which includes signs and symptoms of confusion, psychosis, and ataxia; tachycardia and vasodilation occur rarely.

DENTAL CONSIDERATIONS

General:
• Not likely to be encountered in the dental office; used for diagnostic procedures.
• Question patient about eye health, including the presence of glaucoma.

cyclophosphamide

sye-kloe-foss´-fa-mide
(Cycloblastin[AUS], Cytoxan, Endoxan Asta[AUS], Endoxon Asta[AUS], Neosar, Procytox[CAN])
Do not confuse Cytoxan with cefoxitin, Ciloxan, cyclosporine, or Cytotec.

CATEGORY AND SCHEDULE

Pregnancy Risk Category: D

Drug Class: Antineoplastic alkylating agent

MECHANISM OF ACTION

An alkylating agent that inhibits DNA and RNA protein synthesis by cross-linking with DNA and RNA strands, preventing cell growth. Cell cycle–phase nonspecific.
Therapeutic Effect: Potent immunosuppressant.

USES

Treatment of Hodgkin's disease; lymphomas; leukemia; cancer of female reproductive tract, lung, prostate; multiple myeloma; neuroblastoma, retinoblastoma; Ewing's sarcoma; Burkett's lymphoma; advanced mycosis fungoides; nephrotic syndrome (children)

PHARMACOKINETICS

Well absorbed from the GI tract. Protein binding: Low. Crosses the blood-brain barrier. Metabolized in the liver to active metabolites. Primarily excreted in urine. Removed by hemodialysis.
Half-life: 3–12 hr.

INDICATIONS AND DOSAGES

▸ **Ovarian Adenocarcinoma, Breast Carcinoma, Hodgkin's Disease, Non-Hodgkin's Lymphoma, Multiple Myeloma, Leukemia (acute lymphoblastic, acute myelogenous, acute monocytic, chronic granulocytic, chronic lymphocytic), Mycosis Fungoides, Disseminated Neuroblastoma, Retinoblastoma**
PO
Adults. 1–5 mg/kg/day.
Children. Initially, 2–8 mg/kg/day. Maintenance: 2–5 mg/kg twice a wk.
IV
Adults. 40–50 mg/kg in divided doses over 2–5 days; or 10–15 mg/kg every 7–10 days or 3–5 mg/kg twice a wk.
Children. 2–8 mg/kg/day for 6 days or total dose for 7 days once a wk.
▸ **Biopsy-Proven Minimal-Change Nephrotic Syndrome**
PO
Adults, Children. 2.5–3 mg/kg/day for 60–90 days.

SIDE EFFECTS/ADVERSE REACTIONS

Expected
Marked leukopenia 8–15 days after initial therapy

Frequent
Nausea, vomiting (beginning about 6 hr after administration and lasting about 4 hr), alopecia
Occasional
Diarrhea, darkening of skin and fingernails, stomatitis, headache, diaphoresis
Rare
Pain or redness at injection site

PRECAUTIONS AND CONTRAINDICATIONS
Lactation
Caution
Radiation therapy

DRUG INTERACTIONS OF CONCERN TO DENTISTRY
• Increased blood dyscrasia: NSAIDs, dapsone, phenothiazines, corticosteroids
• Increased metabolism: phenobarbital

SERIOUS REACTIONS
❗ Cyclophosphamide's major toxic effect is myelosuppression resulting in blood dyscrasias, such as leukopenia, anemia, thrombocytopenia, and hypoprothrombinemia.
❗ Expect leukopenia to resolve in 17–28 days. Anemia generally occurs after large doses or prolonged therapy. Thrombocytopenia may occur 10–15 days after drug initiation.
❗ Hemorrhagic cystitis occurs commonly in long-term therapy, especially in pediatric patients.
❗ Pulmonary fibrosis and cardiotoxicity have been noted with high doses.
❗ Amenorrhea, azoospermia, and hyperkalemia may also occur.

DENTAL CONSIDERATIONS
General:
• Monitor vital signs at every appointment because of cardiovascular and respiratory side effects.
• Patients on chronic drug therapy may rarely have symptoms of blood dyscrasias, which can include infection, bleeding, and poor healing.
• Avoid prescribing aspirin-containing products.
• Prophylactic antibiotics may be indicated to prevent infection if surgery or deep scaling is planned because of leukopenic drug side effects.
• Patients receiving chemotherapy may require palliative treatment for stomatitis.
Consultations:
• In a patient with symptoms of blood dyscrasias, request a medical consultation for blood studies and postpone dental treatment until normal values are reestablished.
• Take precautions if dental surgery is anticipated and anesthesia is required.
Teach Patient/Family to:
• Use effective oral hygiene to prevent soft tissue inflammation
• Prevent injury when using oral hygiene aids

cycloserine
sye-kloe-ser´-een
(Closina[AUS], Seromycin)

CATEGORY AND SCHEDULE
Pregnancy Risk Category: C

Drug Class: Antitubercular

MECHANISM OF ACTION

An antitubercular that inhibits cell wall synthesis by competing with the amino acid, D-alanine, for incorporation into the bacterial cell wall. *Therapeutic Effect:* Causes disruption of bacterial cell wall. Bactericidal or bacteriostatic.

USES

Treatment of pulmonary TB, extrapulmonary as adjunctive

PHARMACOKINETICS

Readily absorbed from the GI tract. No protein binding. Widely distributed (including CSF). Metabolized in liver. Primarily excreted in urine. Removed by hemodialysis. *Half-life:* 10 hr.

INDICATIONS AND DOSAGES
▸ TB

Adults, Elderly. 250 mg q12h for 14 days, then 500 mg to 1g/day in 2 divided doses for 18–24 mo. Maximum: 1 g as a single daily dose. *Children.* 10–20 mg/kg/day in 2 divided doses. Maximum: 1000 mg/day for 18–24 mo.
▸ **Dosage in renal impairment**

Creatinine Clearance	Dosage Interval
10–50 ml/min	q24h
Less than 10 ml/min	q36–48h

SIDE EFFECTS/ADVERSE REACTIONS
Occasional

Drowsiness, headache, dizziness, vertigo, seizures, confusion, psychosis, paresis, tremor, vitamin B_{12} deficiency, folate deficiency, cardiac arrhythmias, increased liver enzymes

PRECAUTIONS AND CONTRAINDICATIONS

Epilepsy, depression, severe anxiety, psychosis, severe renal insufficiency, excessive concurrent use of alcohol, history of hypersensitivity reactions with previous cycloserine therapy

DRUG INTERACTIONS OF CONCERN TO DENTISTRY

• Seizures: alcohol
• Drowsiness is a common side effect; although no drug interactions with sedatives are reported, increased drowsiness is possible

SERIOUS REACTIONS/ADVERSE REACTIONS

! Neurotoxicity, as evidenced by confusion, agitation, CNS depression, psychosis, coma, and seizures, occur rarely.
! Neurotoxic effects of cycloserine may be treated and prevented with the administration of 200–300 mg of pyridoxine daily.

DENTAL CONSIDERATIONS

General:
• Patients on chronic drug therapy may rarely have symptoms of blood dyscrasias, which can include infection, bleeding, and poor healing.
• Examine for evidence of oral signs of disease.
• Determine why the patient is taking the drug (i.e., for preventive or therapeutic therapy).
Consultation:
• Medical consultation may be required to assess patient's ability to tolerate stress.
• In a patient with symptoms of blood dyscrasias, request a medical consultation for blood studies and postpone dental treatment until normal values are reestablished.

• Determine that noninfectious status exists by ensuring that:
  • Anti-TB drugs have been taken for more than 3 wk
  • Culture confirms antibiotic susceptibility to TB microorganism
  • Patient has had 3 consecutive negative sputum smears
  • Patient is not in the coughing stage

Teach Patient/Family to:
• Avoid mouth rinses with high alcohol content
• Use caution to prevent injury when using oral hygiene aids
• Use effective oral hygiene to prevent soft tissue inflammation
• Take medication for full length of prescribed therapy to ensure effectiveness of treatment and prevent the emergence of resistant forms of microbe

cyclosporine
sye-kloe-spor´-in
(Cysporin[AUS], Gengraf, Neoral, Restasis, Sandimmune, Sandimmune Neoral[AUS])
Do not confuse cyclosporine with cycloserine, cyclophosphamide, or Cyklokapron.

CATEGORY AND SCHEDULE
Pregnancy Risk Category: C

Drug Class: Immunosuppressant

MECHANISM OF ACTION
A cyclic polypeptide that inhibits both cellular and humoral immune responses by inhibiting interleukin-2, a proliferative factor needed for T-cell activity. *Therapeutic Effect:* Prevents organ rejection and relieves symptoms of psoriasis and arthritis.

USES
Prevent rejection of tissues/allogeneic organ transplants; severe recalcitrant psoriasis; rheumatoid arthritis (Neoral only); Note: Sandimmune and Neoral are not bioequivalent

PHARMACOKINETICS
Variably absorbed from the GI tract. Protein binding: 90%. Widely distributed. Metabolized in the liver. Eliminated primarily by biliary or fecal excretion. Not removed by hemodialysis. *Half-life:* Adults, 10–27 hr; children, 7–19 hr.

INDICATIONS AND DOSAGES
▸ **Transplantation, Prevention of Organ Rejection**
PO
Adults, Elderly, Children. 10–18 mg/kg/dose given 4–12 hr prior to organ transplantation. Maintenance: 5–15 mg/kg/day in divided doses then tapered to 3–10 mg/kg/day.
IV
Adults, Elderly, Children. Initially, 5–6 mg/kg/dose given 4–12 hr prior to organ transplantation. Maintenance: 2–10 mg/kg/day in divided doses.
▸ **Rheumatoid Arthritis**
PO
Adults, Elderly. Initially, 2.5 mg/kg a day in 2 divided doses. May increase by 0.5–0.75 mg/kg/day. Maximum: 4 mg/kg/day.
▸ **Psoriasis**
PO
Adults, Elderly. Initially, 2.5 mg/kg/day in 2 divided doses. May increase by 0.5 mg/kg/day. Maximum: 4 mg/kg/day.
▸ **Dry Eye**
Ophthalmic
Adults, Elderly. Instill 1 drip in each affected eye q12h.

SIDE EFFECTS/ADVERSE REACTIONS
Frequent
Mild-to-moderate hypertension, hirsutism, tremors
Occasional
Acne, leg cramps, gingival hyperplasia (marked by red, bleeding, and tender gums), paresthesia, diarrhea, nausea, vomiting, headache
Rare
Hypersensitivity reaction, abdominal discomfort, gynecomastia, sinusitis

PRECAUTIONS AND CONTRAINDICATIONS
History of hypersensitivity to cyclosporine or polyoxyethylated castor oil
Caution
Severe renal disease, severe hepatic disease

DRUG INTERACTIONS OF CONCERN TO DENTISTRY
Systemic Form
• Hepatotoxicity/nephrotoxicity: erythromycin, azithromycin, clarithromycin
• Decreased action: barbiturates, carbamazepine
• Possibly reduced blood levels: clindamycin
• Increased infection and immunosuppression: corticosteroids
• Increased blood levels and risk of toxicity: fluconazole, ketoconazole, and itraconazole
Ophthalmic-Dose Form
None reported

SERIOUS REACTIONS
! Mild nephrotoxicity occurs in 25% of renal transplant patients, 38% of cardiac transplant patients, and 37% of liver transplant patients, generally 2 to 3 months after transplantation (more severe toxicity generally occurs soon after transplantation). Hepatotoxicity occurs in 4% of renal transplant patients, 7% of cardiac transplant patients, and 4% of liver transplant patients, generally within the first month after transplantation. Both toxicities usually respond to dosage reduction.
! Severe hyperkalemia and hyperuricemia occur occasionally.

DENTAL CONSIDERATIONS
Systemic Form
General:
• Monitor vital signs at every appointment because of cardiovascular side effects.
• Patients on chronic drug therapy may rarely have symptoms of blood dyscrasias, which can include infection, bleeding, and poor healing.
• Place on frequent recall to evaluate gingival condition and healing response.
• Monitor time since organ/tissue transplant.
Consultations:
• Antibiotic prophylaxis usually is recommended in patients with organ transplants and immunosuppression.
• In a patient with symptoms of blood dyscrasias, request a medical consultation for blood studies and postpone dental treatment until normal values are reestablished.
• Request baseline B/P in renal transplant patients for patient evaluation before dental treatment.
Teach Patient/Family to:
• Use effective oral hygiene to prevent soft tissue inflammation
• Use caution to prevent injury when using oral hygiene aids
Ophthalmic-Dose Form
General:
• Determine why the patient is taking the drug.

- Protect the patient's eyes from accidental spatter during dental treatment.
- Avoid dental light in the patient's eyes; offer dark glasses for patient comfort.

Teach Patient/Family:
- When chronic dry mouth occurs, advise patient to:
  - Avoid mouth rinses with high alcohol content because of drying effects
  - Use daily home fluoride products for anticaries effect
  - Use sugarless gum, frequent sips of water, or saliva substitutes

cyproheptadine
si-proe-hep´-ta-deen
(Periactin)

CATEGORY AND SCHEDULE
Pregnancy Risk Category: B

Drug Class: Antihistamine, H_1-receptor antagonist

MECHANISM OF ACTION
An antihistamine that competes with histamine at histaminic receptor sites. Anticholinergic effects cause drying of nasal mucosa. ***Therapeutic Effect:*** Relieves allergic conditions (urticaria, pruritus).

USES
Allergy symptoms, rhinitis, pruritus, cold urticaria

PHARMACOKINETICS
Well absorbed from GI tract. Metabolized in liver. Primarily eliminated in feces. ***Half-life:*** 16 hr.

INDICATIONS AND DOSAGES
▶ **Allergic Condition**
PO

Adults, Children older than 15 yr.
4 mg 3 times a day. May increase dose but do not exceed 0.5 mg/kg/day.
Children 7–14 yr. 4 mg 2–3 times a day, or 0.25 mg/kg daily in divided doses.
Children 2–6 yr. 2 mg 2–3 times a day, or 0.25 mg/kg daily in divided doses.

▶ **Usual elderly dosage**
PO
Initially, 4 mg 2 times a day.

SIDE EFFECTS/ADVERSE REACTIONS
Frequent
Drowsiness, dizziness, muscular weakness, dry mouth/nose/throat/lips, urinary retention, thickening of bronchial secretions

Elderly
Frequent
Sedation, dizziness, hypotension
Occasional
Epigastric distress, flushing, visual disturbances, hearing disturbances, paresthesia, sweating, chills

PRECAUTIONS AND CONTRAINDICATIONS
Acute asthmatic attack, patients receiving MAOIs, history of hypersensitivity to antihistamines
Caution
Increased intraocular pressure, renal disease, cardiac disease, hypertension, bronchial asthma, seizure disorder, stenosed peptic ulcers, hyperthyroidism, prostatic hypertrophy, bladder neck obstruction, elderly

DRUG INTERACTIONS OF CONCERN TO DENTISTRY
- Increased CNS depression: alcohol, CNS depressants

• Increased effect of anticholinergic drugs

SERIOUS REACTIONS

! Children may experience dominant paradoxical reaction (restlessness, insomnia, euphoria, nervousness, tremors).
! Overdose in children may result in hallucinations, convulsions, death.
! Hypersensitivity reaction (eczema, pruritus, rash, cardiac disturbances, angioedema, photosensitivity) may occur.
! Overdose may vary from CNS depression (sedation, apnea, cardiovascular collapse, death) to severe paradoxical reaction (hallucinations, tremor, seizures).

DENTAL CONSIDERATIONS

General:
• Assess salivary flow as a factor in caries, periodontal disease, and candidiasis.
• Determine why the patient is taking the drug.

cysteamine bitartrate

sis-tee´-ah-meen bye-tar´-trate
(Cystagon)

CATEGORY AND SCHEDULE

Pregnancy Risk Category: C

Drug Class: Nephropathic cystinosis therapy

MECHANISM OF ACTION

An aminothiol that participates within lysosomes in a thiol-disulfide interchange reaction converting cystine into cysteine and cysteine-cysteamine mixed disulfide, both of which can exit cystinotic lysosomes.

Therapeutic Effect: Lowers the cystine content in cells.

USES

Used to prevent damage that may be caused by the buildup of cystine crystals in organs such as the kidneys

PHARMACOKINETICS

Poorly bound to plasma proteins.
Half-life: Unknown.

INDICATIONS AND DOSAGES
▶ **Cystinosis**
PO
Adults. Initially, $1/4$–$1/6$ of maintenance dose. Gradually, increase dose over 4–6 wk.
Maintenance. 2 g/day in 4 divided doses.
Children older than 12 yr and weighing more than 110 lb. 2 g/day in 4 divided doses.
Children 6–12 yr. 1.30 g/m²/day of the free base, given in 4 divided doses.

SIDE EFFECTS/ADVERSE REACTIONS

Frequent
Rash, loss of appetite, fever, vomiting, diarrhea, lethargy
Occasional
Dehydration, hypertension, nausea, abdominal pain, somnolence, nervousness, nightmares, urticaria

PRECAUTIONS AND CONTRAINDICATIONS

Hypersensitivity to cysteamine or penicillamine

DRUG INTERACTIONS OF CONCERN TO DENTISTRY

• Dental drug interactions have not been studied

SERIOUS REACTIONS
! Leukopenia, abnormal liver function, and anemia occur rarely.
! Sudden deaths have been reported.

DENTAL CONSIDERATIONS
General:
• Patients taking this medication may have significant renal disease; thoroughly review medical and drug history.
Consultations:
• Specific consultation depends on type of renal disease.
Teach Patient/Family to:
• Use effective oral hygiene to prevent soft tissue inflammation
• Prevent trauma when using oral hygiene aids
• Update health and medication history if physician makes any changes in evaluation or drug regimens; include OTC, herbal, and nonherbal remedies in the update

cytarabine
sigh-tar´-ah-bean
(Ara-C, Cytosar[CAN], Cytosar-U)
Do not confuse cytarabine with Cytadren, Cytovene, or vidarabine.

CATEGORY AND SCHEDULE
Pregnancy Risk Category: D

Drug Class: Antimetabolite; antineoplastic

MECHANISM OF ACTION
An antimetabolite that is converted intracellularly to a nucleotide. Cell cycle-specific for S phase of cell division. *Therapeutic Effect:* May inhibit DNA synthesis. Potent immunosuppressive activity.

USES
Treatment of acute and chronic myelocytic leukemia, acute lymphocytic leukemia, meningeal leukemia, non-Hodgkin's lymphoma in children. Off label: Treatment of Hodgkin's lymphoma, myelodysplastic syndrome

PHARMACOKINETICS
Widely distributed; moderate amount crosses the blood-brain barrier. Protein binding: 15%. Primarily excreted in urine.
Half-life: 1–3 hr.

INDICATIONS AND DOSAGES
▶ **To Induce Remission in Acute Lymphocytic Leukemia, Acute and Chronic Myelocytic Leukemia, Meningeal Leukemia, or Non-Hodgkin's Lymphoma in Children**
IV
Adults, Elderly, Children. 200 mg/m^2/day for 5 days q2wk as monotherapy or 100–200 mg/m^2/day for 5- to 10-day course of therapy every q2–4wk in combination therapy.
Intrathecal
Adults, Elderly, Children. 5–7.5 mg/m^2 every 2–7 days.
▶ **To Maintain Remission in Acute Lymphocytic Leukemia, Acute and Chronic Myelocytic Leukemia, Meningeal Leukemia, or Non-Hodgkin's Lymphoma in Children**
IV
Adults, Elderly, Children. 70–200 mg/m^2/day for 2–5 days every month.
IM, Subcutaneous
Adults, Elderly, Children. 1–1.5 mg/m^2 as single dose q1–4wk.
Intrathecal
Adults, Elderly, Children. 5–7.5 mg/m^2 every 2–7 days.

SIDE EFFECTS/ADVERSE REACTIONS
Frequent
IV, Subcutaneous: Asthenia, fever, pain, altered taste and smell, nausea, vomiting (risk greater with IV push than with continuous IV infusion)
Intrathecal: Headache, asthenia, altered taste and smell, confusion, somnolence, nausea, vomiting
Occasional
IV, Subcutaneous: Abnormal gait, somnolence, constipation, back pain, urinary incontinence, peripheral edema, headache, confusion
Intrathecal: Peripheral edema, back pain, constipation, abnormal gait, urinary incontinence

PRECAUTIONS AND CONTRAINDICATIONS
None known

DRUG INTERACTIONS OF CONCERN TO DENTISTRY
• Increased risk of bleeding: drugs that interfere with coagulation or platelet function, such as NSAIDs and aspirin
• Increased risk of infection; glucocorticoids

SERIOUS REACTIONS
! Myelosuppression may result in blood dyscrasias, such as leukopenia, anemia, thrombocytopenia, megaloblastosis, and reticulocytopenia, after a single IV dose.
! Leukopenia, anemia, and thrombocytopenia should be expected with daily or continuous IV therapy.
! Cytarabine syndrome, (as evidenced by fever, myalgia, rash, conjunctivitis, malaise, and chest pain) and hyperuricemia may occur.

! High-dose cytarabine therapy may produce severe CNS, GI, and pulmonary toxicity.

DENTAL CONSIDERATIONS
General:
• Determine why patient is taking the drug.
• If additional analgesia is required for dental pain, consider alternative analgesics (acetaminophen) in patients taking narcotics for acute or chronic pain.
• Avoid prescribing aspirin-containing products.
• This drug may be used in the hospital or on an outpatient basis. Confirm the patient's disease and treatment status.
• Patient on chronic drug therapy may rarely present with symptoms of blood dyscrasias, which can include infection, bleeding, and poor healing. If dyscrasia is present, caution patient to prevent oral tissue trauma when using oral hygiene aids.
• Short appointments and a stress-reduction protocol may be required for anxious patients.
• Patients may have received other chemotherapy or radiation; confirm medical and drug history.
• Patients may be at risk of infection.
• Patients may be taking a prophylactic antiinfective.
• Patients are at risk of bleeding, so check for oral signs.
• Oral infections should be eliminated and/or treated aggressively.
Consultations:
• Medical consultation should include routine blood counts including platelet counts and bleeding time.
• Consult physician; prophylactic or therapeutic antiinfectives may be indicated if surgery or periodontal treatment is required.

- Medical consultation may be required to assess immunologic status during cancer chemotherapy and determine safety risk, if any, posed by the required dental treatment.
- Medical consultation may be required to assess disease control and patient's ability to tolerate stress.

Teach Patient/Family to:
- Use effective oral hygiene to prevent soft tissue inflammation
- Report oral lesions, soreness, or bleeding to dentist
- Prevent trauma when using oral hygiene aids
- Update health and medication history if physician makes any changes in evaluation or drug regimens; include OTC, herbal, and nonherbal remedies in the update

daclizumab
day-cly´-zu-mab
(Zenapax)

CATEGORY AND SCHEDULE
Pregnancy Risk Category: C

Drug Class:
Immunosuppressive, IgG1
monoclonal antibody

MECHANISM OF ACTION
A monoclonal antibody that binds to
the interleukin-2 (IL-2) receptor
complex, inhibiting the IL-
2–mediated activation of
T lymphocytes, a critical pathway in
the cellular immune response
involved in allograft rejection.
Therapeutic Effect: Prevents organ
rejection.

USES
Prophylaxis of acute organ rejection
in patients with renal transplants;
used in combination with
cyclosporine and glucocorticoids

PHARMACOKINETICS
Half-life: Adults, 20 days.

INDICATIONS AND DOSAGES
▶ **Prevention of Acute Renal
Transplant Rejection (in combination
with an immunosuppressive)**
IV
Adults, Children. 1 mg/kg over
15 min q14 days for 5 doses,
beginning no more than 24 hr before
transplantation. Maximum: 100 mg.

SIDE EFFECTS/ADVERSE REACTIONS
Occasional
Constipation, nausea, diarrhea,
vomiting, abdominal pain, edema,
headache, dizziness, fever, pain,
fatigue, insomnia, weakness,
arthralgia, myalgia, diaphoresis

PRECAUTIONS AND CONTRAINDICATIONS
Caution
Risk of lymphoproliferative disease
and opportunistic infections,
anaphylaxis risk unknown, long-term
effects unknown, lactation, children,
geriatric patients

DRUG INTERACTIONS OF CONCERN TO DENTISTRY
None reported

SERIOUS REACTIONS
! Hypersensitivity reaction,
which occurs rarely, is characterized
by dyspnea, tachycardia, dysphagia,
peripheral edema, rash, and
pruritus.

DENTAL CONSIDERATIONS
General:
• This is a hospital-type drug,
but because some dosing is
continued, patients may appear
in the dental office while receiving
this drug.
• Transplant patients may also be
taking cyclosporine and
glucocorticoids; review each
transplant patient's medications.
• Short appointments and a stress
reduction protocol may be required
for anxious patients.
Consultations:
• Antibiotic prophylaxis usually
is recommended in patients with
organ transplants and
immunosuppression.
• Medical consultation may be
required to assess disease control and
patient's ability to tolerate stress.
Teach Patient/Family to:
• Use effective oral hygiene to
prevent soft tissue inflammation

- Prevent trauma when using oral hygiene aids
- Update health and drug history if physician makes any changes in evaluation or drug regimens

dalteparin sodium
doll´-teh-pare-in so´-dee-um
(Fragmin)

CATEGORY AND SCHEDULE
Pregnancy Risk Category: B

Drug Class: Heparin-type anticoagulant

MECHANISM OF ACTION
An antithrombin that inhibits factor Xa and thrombin in the presence of low-molecular-weight heparin. Only slightly influences platelet aggregation, PT, and aPTT. *Therapeutic Effect:* Produces anticoagulation.

USES
Prevention of deep vein thrombosis (DVT) following abdominal surgery, treatment of life-threatening conditions such as unstable angina, non–q-wave MI; prevention of ischemia complications caused by blood clot formation in patients on aspirin therapy; in combination with warfarin in deep vein thrombosis with or without pulmonary embolism (PE)

PHARMACOKINETICS

Route	Onset	Peak	Duration
Subcutaneous	N/A	4 hr	N/A

Protein binding: less than 10%. *Half-life:* 3–5 hr.

INDICATIONS AND DOSAGES
▶ **Low- to Moderate-Risk Abdominal Surgery**
Subcutaneous
Adults, Elderly. 2,500 international units 1–2 hr before surgery, then daily for 5–10 days.
▶ **High-Risk Abdominal Surgery**
Subcutaneous
Adults, Elderly. 5,000 international units 1–2 hr before surgery, then daily for 5–10 days.
▶ **Total Hip Surgery**
Subcutaneous
Adults, Elderly. 2,500 international units 1–2 hr before surgery, then 2,500 units 6 hr after surgery, then 5,000 units/day for 7–10 days.
▶ **Unstable Angina, Non–Q-Wave MI**
Subcutaneous
Adults, Elderly. 120 international units/kg q12h (maximum: 10,000 international units/dose) given with aspirin until clinically stable.
▶ **Prevention of DVT or PE in the Acutely Ill Patient**
Subcutaneous
Adults, Elderly. 5,000 international units once a day.

SIDE EFFECTS/ADVERSE REACTIONS
Occasional
Hematoma at injection site
Rare
Hypersensitivity reaction (chills, fever, pruritus, urticaria, asthma, rhinitis, lacrimation, headache); mild, local skin irritation

PRECAUTIONS AND CONTRAINDICATIONS
Active major bleeding; concurrent heparin therapy; hypersensitivity to dalteparin, heparin, or pork products; thrombocytopenia associated with

positive in vitro test for antiplatelet antibody
Caution
Hemorrhage, cannot be used interchangeably with other forms of heparin, lactation, children, requires monitoring, GI bleeding

DRUG INTERACTIONS OF CONCERN TO DENTISTRY
• Avoid concurrent use of aspirin (except as noted), NSAIDs, dipyridamole, and sulfinpyrazone

SERIOUS REACTIONS
! Overdose may lead to bleeding complications ranging from local ecchymoses to major hemorrhage.
! Thrombocytopenia occurs rarely.

DENTAL CONSIDERATIONS
General:
• Product may be used in outpatient therapy. Delay elective dental treatment until patient completes anticoagulant therapy.
• Determine why patient is taking the drug.
• Consider local hemostasis measures to prevent excessive bleeding.
• Avoid prescribing aspirin-containing products.
Consultations:
• Medical consultation should include routine blood counts, including platelet counts and bleeding time.
Teach Patient/Family to:
• Use effective oral hygiene to prevent soft tissue inflammation
• Prevent trauma when using oral hygiene aids
• Report oral lesions, soreness, or bleeding to dentist

danaparoid
da-nah´-pah-roid
(Orgaran k)

CATEGORY AND SCHEDULE
Pregnancy Risk Category: B

Drug Class: Heparinoid-type anticoagulant

MECHANISM OF ACTION
An antithrombotic agent that inhibits thrombin formation through factor anti-Xa and anti-IIa effects. Does not significantly influence bleeding time, PT, aPTT, or platelet function. Possesses greater antithrombotic activity than anticoagulant activity.

USES
Prevention of deep vein thrombosis (DVT) following hip or knee replacement surgery; unapproved: thromboembolism, hemodialysis, and cardiovascular surgery

PHARMACOKINETICS
Well absorbed following subcutaneous administration. Eliminated primarily in the urine.
Half-life: 24 hr (half-life prolonged with severe renal impairment).

INDICATIONS AND DOSAGES
Note: Give initial dose as soon as possible after surgery but not more than 24 hr after surgery.
▶ **Prevention of DVT**
Subcutaneous
Adults, Elderly. 750 anti-Xa units twice daily beginning 1–4 hr preoperatively and then not sooner than 2 hr after surgery. Continue treatment throughout postoperative care until risk of DVT has diminished (average duration 7–14 days).

SIDE EFFECTS/ADVERSE REACTIONS

Frequent
Injection site pain
Occasional
Fever, pain, nausea, UTI, constipation
Rare
Rash, pruritus, infection

PRECAUTIONS AND CONTRAINDICATIONS

Severe hemorrhagic diathesis (hemophilia, idiopathic thrombocytopenic purpura), active major bleeding state, including hemorrhagic stroke in the acute phase, type II phase thrombocytopenia associated with positive in vitro test for antiplatelet antibody in presence of danaparoid, hypersensitivity to pork products, danaparoid, or any component of the formulation
Caution
Cannot interchange with heparin, hemorrhage, thrombocytopenia, renal or hepatic impairment, lactation, children, antidotes not available, GI bleeding

DRUG INTERACTIONS OF CONCERN TO DENTISTRY

• Avoid concurrent use of platelet aggregation antagonist, such as aspirin; NSAIDs; dipyridamole

SERIOUS REACTIONS

❗ Accidental overdosage may lead to bleeding complications ranging from minor ecchymosis to major hemorrhage. An unexplained fall in Hct or fall in B/P should lead to consideration of a hemorrhagic event. The antidote protamine sulfate only partially neutralizes danaparoid activity and is incapable of reducing severe nonsurgical bleeding during treatment.

If serious bleeding occurs, discontinue danaparoid; give blood or blood product transfusions.

DENTAL CONSIDERATIONS

General:
• Determine why patient is taking the drug.
• Consider local hemostasis measures to prevent excessive bleeding if dental treatment must be performed.
• Antibiotic prophylaxis before dental treatment may be required for joint prosthesis (see section on "Medically Compromised Patients").
• Delay elective dental treatment until patient completes danaparoid therapy.
Consultations:
• Medical consultation should include routine blood counts, including platelet counts and bleeding time.
Teach Patient/Family to:
• Use effective oral hygiene to prevent soft tissue inflammation
• Use caution to prevent trauma when using oral hygiene aids
• Report oral lesions, soreness, or bleeding to dentist

danazol
da´-na-zole
(Cyclomen[CAN], Danocrine)

CATEGORY AND SCHEDULE
Pregnancy Risk Category: X

Drug Class: Androgen, a-ethinyl testosterone derivative

MECHANISM OF ACTION
A testosterone derivative that suppresses the pituitary-ovarian axis by inhibiting the output of pituitary

gonadotropins. Causes atrophy of both normal and ectopic endometrial tissue in endometriosis. Follicle-stimulating hormone (FSH) and luteinizing hormone (LH) are depressed in fibrocystic breast disease. Inhibits steroid synthesis and binding of steroids to their receptors in breast tissues. Increases serum levels of esterase inhibitor. ***Therapeutic Effect:*** Produces anovulation and amenorrhea, reduces the production of estrogen, corrects biochemical deficiency as seen in hereditary angioedema.

USES
Treatment of endometriosis, prevention of hereditary angioedema, fibrocystic breast disease

PHARMACOKINETICS
Well absorbed from GI tract. Metabolized in liver, primarily to 2-hydroxymethylethisterone. Excreted in urine. ***Half-life:*** 4.5 hr.

INDICATIONS AND DOSAGES
▸ **Endometriosis**
PO
Adults. 200–800 mg/day in 2 divided doses for 3–9 mo.
▸ **Fibrocystic Breast Disease**
PO
Adults. 100–400 mg/day in 2 divided doses.
▸ **Hereditary Angioedema**
PO
Adults. Initially, 200 mg 2–3 times a day. Decrease dose by 50% or less at 1–3 mo intervals. If attack occurs, increase dose by up to 200 mg/day.

SIDE EFFECTS/ADVERSE REACTIONS
Frequent
Females: Amenorrhea, breakthrough bleeding/spotting, decreased breast size, increased weight, irregular menstrual period.
Occasional
Males/females: Edema, rhabdomyolysis (muscle cramps, unusual fatigue), virilism (acne, oily skin), flushed skin, altered moods
Rare
Males/females: Hematuria, gingivitis, carpal tunnel syndrome, cataracts, severe headache, vomiting, rash, photosensitivity
Females: Enlarged clitoris, hoarseness, deepening voice, hair growth, monilial vaginitis
Males: Decreased testicle size

PRECAUTIONS AND CONTRAINDICATIONS
Cardiac impairment, hypercalcemia, pregnancy, prostatic or breast cancer in males, severe liver or renal disease
Caution
Migraine headaches, seizure disorders

DRUG INTERACTIONS OF CONCERN TO DENTISTRY
• Increased serum concentration of carbamazepine; consider avoiding concurrent administration

SERIOUS REACTIONS
❗ Jaundice may occur in those receiving 400 mg/day or more. Liver dysfunction, eosinophilia, thrombocytopenia, pancreatitis occur rarely.

DENTAL CONSIDERATIONS
General:
• Patients on chronic drug therapy may rarely have symptoms of blood dyscrasias, which can include infection, bleeding, and poor healing.

Consultations:
• In a patient with symptoms of blood dyscrasias, request a medical consultation for blood studies and postpone dental treatment until normal values are reestablished.

Teach Patient/Family to:
• Use effective oral hygiene to prevent soft tissue inflammation
• Avoid mouth rinses with high alcohol content because of drying and irritating effects

dantrolene sodium
dan´-troe-leen so´-dee-um
(Dantrium)
Do not confuse Dantrium with Daraprim.

CATEGORY AND SCHEDULE
Pregnancy Risk Category: C

Drug Class: Skeletal muscle relaxant, direct acting

MECHANISM OF ACTION
A skeletal muscle relaxant that reduces muscle contraction by interfering with release of calcium ion. Reduces calcium ion concentration. *Therapeutic Effect:* Dissociates excitation-contraction coupling. Interferes with catabolic process associated with malignant hyperthermic crisis.

USES
Treatment of spasticity in multiple sclerosis, stroke, spinal cord injury, cerebral palsy, malignant hyperthermia

PHARMACOKINETICS
Poorly absorbed from the GI tract. Protein binding: High. Metabolized in the liver.

Primarily excreted in urine.
Half-life: IV: 4–8 hr; PO: 8.7 hr.

INDICATIONS AND DOSAGES
▸ **Spasticity**
PO
Adults, Elderly. Initially, 25 mg/day. Increase to 25 mg 2–4 times a day, then by 25-mg increments up to 100 mg 2–4 times a day.
Children. Initially, 0.5 mg/kg twice a day. Increase to 0.5 mg/kg 3–4 times a day, then in increments of 0.5 mg/kg/day up to 3 mg/kg 2–4 times a day. Maximum: 400 mg/day.

▸ **Prevention of Malignant Hyperthermic Crisis**
PO
Adults, Elderly, Children. 4–8 mg/kg/day in 3–4 divided doses 1–2 days before surgery; give last dose 3–4 hr before surgery.
IV
Adults, Elderly, Children. 2.5 mg/kg about 1.25 hr before surgery.

▸ **Management of Malignant Hyperthermic Crisis**
IV
Adults, Elderly, Children. Initially a minimum of 1 mg/kg rapid IV; may repeat up to total cumulative dose of 10 mg/kg. May follow with 4–8 mg/kg/day PO in 4 divided doses up to 3 days after crisis.

SIDE EFFECTS/ADVERSE REACTIONS
Frequent
Drowsiness, dizziness, weakness, general malaise, diarrhea (mild)
Occasional
Confusion, diarrhea (may be severe), headache, insomnia, constipation, urinary frequency
Rare
Paradoxical CNS excitement or restlessness, paresthesia, tinnitus, slurred speech, tremors, blurred

vision, dry mouth, nocturia, impotence, rash, pruritus

PRECAUTIONS AND CONTRAINDICATIONS
Active hepatic disease
Caution
Peptic ulcer disease, renal disease, hepatic disease, stroke, seizure disorder, diabetes mellitus, elderly; monitor liver enzymes

DRUG INTERACTIONS OF CONCERN TO DENTISTRY
None reported

SERIOUS REACTIONS
! There is a risk of liver toxicity, most notably in females, those 35 yr of age and older, and those taking other medications concurrently.
! Overt hepatitis noted most frequently between 3rd and 12th mo of therapy.
! Overdosage results in vomiting, muscular hypotonia, muscle twitching, respiratory depression, and seizures.

DENTAL CONSIDERATIONS
General:
• Monitor vital signs at every appointment because of cardiovascular and respiratory side effects.
• Patients on chronic drug therapy may rarely have symptoms of blood dyscrasias, which can include infection, bleeding, and poor healing.
• Requires proficiency in IV administration technique when used for emergency treatment of malignant hyperthermia.
Consultations:
• In a patient with symptoms of blood dyscrasias, request a medical consultation for blood studies and

postpone dental treatment until normal values are reestablished.
Teach Patient/Family to:
• Use effective oral hygiene to prevent soft tissue inflammation
• Avoid mouth rinses with high alcohol content because of drying effects

dapiprazole hydrochloride
da´-pi-prah-zohl hi-droh-klor´-ide
(Rev-Eyes)

CATEGORY AND SCHEDULE
Pregnancy Risk Category: B

Drug Class: Antimydriatic

MECHANISM OF ACTION
An α-adrenergic blocker that primarily affects α-1 adrenoceptors. Does not significantly affect intraocular pressure. *Therapeutic Effect:* Induces miosis via relaxation of the smooth dilator (radial) muscle of the iris, which causes papillary constriction.

USES
Reduction of pupil size after certain kinds of eye examinations

PHARMACOKINETICS
Well absorbed. Mydriasis reversal begins in 1 hr and occurs in about 6 hr.

INDICATIONS AND DOSAGES
▸ **Drug-Induced Mydriasis**
Ophthalmic
Adults, Elderly, Children. 2 drops applied topically to the conjunctiva

of each eye. Repeat after 5 min. Do not use more than once a wk.

SIDE EFFECTS/ADVERSE REACTIONS
Occasional
Burning, eyelid edema, photophobia

PRECAUTIONS AND CONTRAINDICATIONS
Acute iritis, hypersensitivity to dapiprazole or any component of the formulation

DRUG INTERACTIONS OF CONCERN TO DENTISTRY
None reported

SERIOUS REACTIONS
None reported

DENTAL CONSIDERATIONS
General:
• Used in ophthalmic examinations.
• Protect patient's eyes from accidental spatter during dental treatment.
• Avoid dental light in patient's eyes; offer dark glasses for patient comfort.

dapsone
dap´-sone
(Dapsone)

CATEGORY AND SCHEDULE
Pregnancy Risk Category: C

Drug Class: Leprostatic, antibacterial

MECHANISM OF ACTION
An antibiotic that is a competitive antagonist of para-aminobenzoic acid (PABA); it prevents normal bacterial utilization of PABA for synthesis of folic acid. *Therapeutic Effect:* Inhibits bacterial growth.

USES
Treatment of leprosy (Hansen's disease); dermatitis herpetiformis; unapproved: cicatricial pemphigoid, LE, pemphigoid, malaria, Pneumocystis carinii pneumonia (PCP)

PHARMACOKINETICS
Rapid complete absorption; highly bound to plasma protein; metabolized in liver; excreted in urine. *Half-life:* 10–50 hr

INDICATIONS AND DOSAGES
▸ **Leprosy**
PO
Adults, Elderly. 50–100 mg/day for 3–10 yr.
Children. 1–2 mg/kg/24 hr.
Maximum: 100 mg/day.
▸ **Dermatitis Herpetiformis**
PO
Adults, Elderly. Initially, 50 mg/day. May increase up to 300 mg/day.
▸ **PCP**
PO
Adults, Elderly. 100 mg/day in combination with trimethoprim for 21 days.
▸ **Prevention of PCP**
PO
Adults, Elderly. 100 mg/day.
Children older than 1 mo. 2 mg/kg/day. Maximum: 100 mg/day.

SIDE EFFECTS/ADVERSE REACTIONS
Frequent
Hemolytic anemia, methemoglobinemia, rash
Occasional
Hemolysis, photosensitivity reaction

PRECAUTIONS AND CONTRAINDICATIONS
Hypersensitivity to sulfones, severe anemia

Caution
Renal disease, hepatic disease, G6PD deficiency, lactation

DRUG INTERACTIONS OF CONCERN TO DENTISTRY
None reported

SERIOUS REACTIONS
! Agranulocytosis and blood dyscrasias may occur.

DENTAL CONSIDERATIONS
General:
• Patients on chronic drug therapy may rarely have symptoms of blood dyscrasias, which can include infection, bleeding, and poor healing.
• Avoid dental light in patient's eyes; offer dark glasses for patient comfort.
• Advise patient if dental drugs prescribed have a potential for photosensitivity.
Consultations:
• In a patient with symptoms of blood dyscrasias, request a medical consultation for blood studies and postpone dental treatment until normal values are reestablished.
Teach Patient/Family to:
• Use effective oral hygiene to prevent soft tissue inflammation
• Use caution to prevent injury when using oral hygiene aids

daptomycin
dap´-toe-my-sin
(Cubicin)

CATEGORY AND SCHEDULE
Pregnancy Risk Category: B

Drug Class: Antiinfective (polypeptide)

MECHANISM OF ACTION
A lipopeptide antibacterial agent that binds to bacterial membranes and causes a rapid depolarization of the membrane potential. The loss of membrane potential leads to inhibition of protein, DNA, and RNA synthesis. **Therapeutic Effect:** Bactericidal.

USES
Treatment of complicated skin and skin-structure infections caused by susceptible strains of S. aureus (including methicillin-resistant S. aureus), S. pyogenes, S. agalactiae, S. dysgalactiae, E. coli, and E. faecalis (vancomycin-susceptible strains only)

PHARMACOKINETICS
Widely distributed. Protein binding: 90%. Primarily excreted unchanged in urine. Moderately removed by hemodialysis. **Half-life:** 7–8 hr (increased in impaired renal function).

INDICATIONS AND DOSAGES
▸ **Complicated Skin and Skin-Structure Infections**
IV
Adults, Elderly. 4 mg/kg every 24 hr for 7–14 days.
▸ **Dosage in Renal Impairment**
For patients with creatinine clearance of less than 30 ml/min, dosage is 4 mg/kg q48h for 7–14 days.

SIDE EFFECTS/ADVERSE REACTIONS
Frequent
Constipation, nausea, peripheral injection site reactions, headache, diarrhea
Occasional
Insomnia, rash, vomiting
Rare
Pruritus, dizziness, hypotension

PRECAUTIONS AND CONTRAINDICATIONS

Hypersensitivity
Caution
Reduce dose in renal impairment, risk of superinfection, monitor for muscle weakness, pain and CPK levels, lactation, elderly, safety and efficacy in children younger than 18 yr not established

DRUG INTERACTIONS OF CONCERN TO DENTISTRY

None reported

SERIOUS REACTIONS

! Skeletal muscle myopathy, characterized by muscle pain and weakness, particularly of the distal extremities, occurs rarely.
! Antibiotic-associated colitis and other superinfections may result from altered bacterial balance.

DENTAL CONSIDERATIONS

General:
• Used in the hospital environment for serious infections.
• Determine why patient is taking the drug.
• Monitor vital signs, including temperature, B/P, and respiration characteristics and rate, at every appointment.
Consultations:
• Consult with patient's physician if an acute dental infection occurs and another antiinfective is required.

darbepoetin alfa

dar-beh-poe´-ee-tin al´-fah
(Aranesp)
Do not confuse Aranesp with Aricept.

CATEGORY AND SCHEDULE

Pregnancy Risk Category: C

Drug Class: Hematopoietic agent

MECHANISM OF ACTION

A glycoprotein that stimulates formation of RBCs in bone marrow; increases serum half-life of epoetin. *Therapeutic Effect:* Induces erythropoiesis and release of reticulocytes from bone marrow.

USES

An erythropoiesis-stimulating protein; stimulates the division and differentiation of erythroid progenitors in bone marrow

PHARMACOKINETICS

Well absorbed after subcutaneous administration. *Half-life:* 48.5 hr.

INDICATIONS AND DOSAGES

▸ **Anemia in Chronic Renal Failure**
IV Bolus, Subcutaneous
Adults, Elderly. Initially, 0.45 mcg/kg once a wk. Adjust dosage to achieve and maintain a target Hgb not to exceed 12 g/dl. Do not increase dosage more frequently than once a mo. Limit increases in Hgb by less than 1 g/dl over any 2-wk period.
▸ **Anemia Associated with Chemotherapy**
IV, Subcutaneous
Adults, Elderly. 2.25 mcg/kg/dose once a wk.

SIDE EFFECTS/ADVERSE REACTIONS

Frequent
Myalgia, hypertension or hypotension, headache, diarrhea
Occasional
Fatigue, edema, vomiting, reaction at administration site, asthenia, dizziness

PRECAUTIONS AND CONTRAINDICATIONS

History of sensitivity to mammalian cell-derived products or human albumin, uncontrolled hypertension

Caution
Increased risk of serious
cardiovascular events,
seizures in CRF, albumin
formula has risk of viral
diseases, safety in lactation
or pediatric patients has not been
established

DRUG INTERACTIONS OF CONCERN TO DENTISTRY
No studies reported

SERIOUS REACTIONS
! Vascular access thrombosis,
CHF, sepsis, arrhythmias,
and anaphylactic reaction
occur rarely.

DENTAL CONSIDERATIONS
General:
• Monitor vital signs at every
appointment because of
cardiovascular side effects.
• Consider semisupine chair position
for patient comfort if GI side effects
occur.
• Monitor disease control and date of
last dialysis.
• Prophylactic antibiotics may
be indicated to prevent
infection if invasive procedure
is planned.
Consultations:
• Medical consultation may be
required to assess disease
control and patient's ability to
tolerate stress.
Teach Patient/Family to:
• Use effective oral hygiene to
prevent soft tissue inflammation,
infection
• Update health and drug history if
physician makes any changes in
evaluation or drug regimens

darunavir
dar-oo´-na-veer
(Prezista)

CATEGORY AND SCHEDULE
Pregnancy Risk Category: B

Drug Class: Antiretroviral agent,
protease inhibitor

MECHANISM OF ACTION
A antiretroviral agent that inhibits
HIV-1 protease. Prevents the
cleavage of HIV encoded Gag-Pol
polyproteins in infected cells.
Therapeutic Effect: Impedes HIV
replication, slowing the progression
of HIV infection.

USES
Treatment of HIV infection

PHARMACOKENETICS
Absorption increased 30% with
food. Protein binding: 95%.
Extensively metabolized in liver,
primarily by CYP450 3A4.
Primarily eliminated in feces
(about 80%, 41% unchanged);
partial excretion in urine
(approximately 14%, 8% unchaged).
Half-life: 15 hr.

INDICATIONS AND DOSAGES
▸ **HIV Infection (in combination with ritonavir)**
PO
Adults. 600 mg twice a day taken
with ritonavir 100 mg twice a day
with food.
Safety and efficacy have not been
established in children.

SIDE EFFECTS/ADVERSE REACTIONS:
Frequent
Hypertriglyceridemia, diarrhea, nausea, increased amylase level, headache, nasopharyngitis
Occasional
hypercholesterolemia, rash, hypoglycemia, hypocalcemia, thrombocytopenia, hyponatremia, vomiting, abdominal pain
Rare
Constipation, anxiety, acute renal failure, fat redistribution, confusional state, disorientation, irritability, altered mood, nightmares, dyspnea, cough, hiccups, night sweats, diabetes mellitus, Stevens-Johnson syndrome

PRECAUTIONS AND CONTRAINDICATIONS
Hypersensitivity to darunavir or its components
Sulfa allergy, diabetes mellitus
Multiple drug interactions

DRUG INTERACTIONS OF CONCERN TO DENTISTRY
• Anticonvulsants: may decrease concentrations of darunavir
• Antihistamines: increased risk of arrhythmias
• Benzodiazepines: may cause increased sedation or respiratory depression
• Clarithyromycin: may increase concentrations of clarithromycin
• Corticosteroids: may increase levels and effects of these drugs

• CYP3A4 inducers: may decrease levels and effects of darunavir
• CYP3A4 substrates: may increase levels and effects of CYP3A4 substrates
• Estrogens, oral contraceptives: may decrease concentrations of these drugs; may reduce contraceptive effectiveness
• Immunosuppressants: may increase concentrations of these drugs
• Ketoconazole: may increase levels and effects of darunavir and ketoconazole
• Methadone: may decrease concentrations of methadone
• Neuroleptic agents: increased risk of arrhythmias
• Rifampin: may decrease concentrations of darunavir
• Sedatives/hypnotics: increased sedation and risk of respiratory depression
• SSRIs: may decrease the levels and effects of SSRIs
• St. John's wort: may decrease the levels of darunavir
• Trazodone: may increase concentrations of trazodone

SERIOUS REACTIONS
! Protease inhibitors have been associated with severe dermatologic reactions including Stevens-Johnson Syndrome.

dasatinib
da-sa´-ti-nib
(Sprycel)

CATEGORY AND SCHEDULE
Pregnancy Risk Category: D

Drug Class: Antineoplastic

MECHANISM OF ACTION
Inhibits BCR-ABL tyrosine kinase, an enzyme created by the Philadelphia chromosome abnormality found in patients with chronic myeloid leukemia (CML). Also inhibits SRC family kinases. *Therapeutic Effect:* Suppresses tumor growth during the three stages of CML: blast crisis, accelerated phase, and chronic phase.

USES
Treatment in CML—blast crisis, accelerated phase, and chronic phase—resistant or intolerant to prior therapy. Also used in treatment of Philadelphia chromosome-positive acute lymphoblastic leukemia (ALL) with resistance or intolerance to prior therapy.

PHARMACOKENETICS
Protein binding: 96%. Metabolized in liver, primarily by CYP450 3A4. Primarily eliminated in feces (85%, 19% as unchanged); minimal excretion in urine (4%, 0.1% unchanged). *Half-life:* 3-5 hr.

INDICATIONS AND DOSAGES
▸ ALL, Philadelphia Chromosome-Positive, Resistant or Intolerant to Prior Therapy
PO
Adults. 70 mg twice a day (morning and evening), with or without food.
▸ CML, blast crisis
Adults. 70 mg twice a day (morning and evening), with or without food.
▸ CML, accelerated phase
Adults. 70 mg twice a day (morning and evening), with or without food.
▸ CML, chronic phase
Adults. 70 mg twice a day (morning and evening), with or without food. Safety and efficacy have not been established in children.

SIDE EFFECTS/ADVERSE REACTIONS:

Adult
Frequent
Neutropenia, thrombocytopenia, diarrhea, headache, musculoskeletal pain, fatigue, fever, superficial edema, rash, nausea, dyspnea, upper respiratory infection, abdominal pain, pleural effusion, vomiting, arthralgia, asthenia, loss of appetite, inflammatory disease of mucous membrane, GI hemorrhage, constipation, weight loss, dizziness, chest pain, neuropathy, myalgia, weight increased, cardiac dysrhythmia, pruritus, pneumonia, swollen abdomen, pneumonia, shivering
Occasional
Febrile neutropenia, febrile neutropenia, CHF, pericardial effusion, pulmonary edema, prolonged QT interval, anemia

Rare
Pulmonary hypertension, CNS hemorrhage, ascites

PRECAUTIONS AND CONTRAINDICATIONS

Hypersensitivity to dasatinib or its components, hypokalemia, hypomagnesemia, use with anti-arrhythmic medication, patients at risk for fluid retention

DRUG INTERACTIONS OF CONCERN TO DENTISTRY

- NSAIDs: increased risk of bleeding
- CYP3A4 inhibitors (e.g., clarithromycin, erythromycin, azole antifungals): may increase the levels and adverse effects of dasatinib
- CYP3A4 substrates (midazolam, triazolam): increased plasma concentrations of these drugs with increased CNS depression
- Vasoconstrictors: may increase the risk of potentially fatal arrhythmias

SERIOUS REACTIONS

! Severe CNS hemorrhage, including fatalities, have been reported.
! Dasatinib may cause severe bone marrow suppression (thrombo-cytopenia, neutropenia, anemia).
! Fluid retention, including pleural and pericardial effusion, severe ascites, and generalized edema, has been reported.

DENTAL CONSIDERATIONS

General:
- Monitor vital signs at every appointment because of cardiovascular adverse effects.
- Determine why patient is taking drug.
- Avoid aspirin and NSAIDs.
- Consider semi-supine chair position for patients with GI or respiratory adverse effects.
- Consider blood dyscrasias as factors in infection, bleeding and poor healing.

- If blood dyscrasia present, caution patient to prevent oral tissue trauma when using oral hygiene aids.
- Examine for oral manifestations of opportunistic infection.
- Consider local hemostatic measures to prevent excessive bleeding.
- Use caution with potentially hepatotoxic drugs (e.g., telithromycin).
Consultations:
- Consult physician to determine disease control and ability of patient to tolerate dental procedures.
- Medical consultation should include routine blood counts, including platelets and bleeding time and postpone dental therapy until values are in acceptable range.
- Consult physician to determine possible need for prophylactic antibiotics.
Teach Patient/Family to:
- Use effective, atramatic oral hygiene to prevent soft-tissue inflammation
- Update health and medication history if physician makes any changes in evaluation or drug regimen; include over-the-counter, herbal products, and dietary supplements
- Report oral lesions, soreness or bleeding to dentist

daunorubicin citrate liposome
dawn-oh-rue´-bih-sin
(DaunoXome)
Do not confuse with dactinomycin or doxorubicin.

CATEGORY AND SCHEDULE
Pregnancy Risk Category: D

Drug Class: Anthracycline antibiotic; antineoplastic

MECHANISM OF ACTION

An anthracycline antibiotic that is cell cycle-phase nonspecific. Most active in S phase of cell division. Appears to bind to DNA. *Therapeutic Effect:* Inhibits DNA, DNA-dependent RNA synthesis.

USES

Treatment of advanced AIDS–associated Kaposi's sarcoma (KS), a kind of skin cancer

PHARMACOKINETICS

Widely distributed. Does not cross blood-brain barrier. Protein binding: High. Metabolized in liver to active metabolite. Excreted in urine, eliminated by biliary excretion. *Half-life:* 18.5 hr; metabolite: 26.7 hr.

INDICATIONS AND DOSAGES
▸ **KS**
IV
Adults. 20–40 mg/m2 over 1 hr. Repeat q2wk or 100 mg/m2 q3wk.

SIDE EFFECTS/ADVERSE REACTIONS

Frequent
Mild to moderate nausea, fatigue, fever
Occasional
Diarrhea, abdominal pain, esophagitis, stomatitis (redness or burning of oral mucous membranes, inflammation of gums or tongue), transverse pigmentation of fingernails and toenails
Rare
Transient fever, chills

PRECAUTIONS AND CONTRAINDICATIONS

Arrhythmias, CHF, left ventricular ejection fraction less than 40%, preexisting bone marrow suppression

DRUG INTERACTIONS OF CONCERN TO DENTISTRY

Dental drug interactions have not been studied

SERIOUS REACTIONS

! Bone marrow depression manifested as hematologic toxicity (severe leukopenia, anemia, and thrombocytopenia) may occur.
! Decreases in platelet and white blood cell (WBC) counts occur in 10–14 days and return to normal levels by the third wk of daunorubicin treatment.
! Cardiotoxicity noted as either acute with transient abnormal ECG findings or as chronic with cardiomyopathy manifested as CHF. The risk of cardiotoxicity increases when the cumulative dose exceeds 550 mg/m2 in adults and 300 mg/m2 in children older than 2 yr or when the total dosage is greater than 10 mg/kg in children younger than 2 yr.

DENTAL CONSIDERATIONS

General:
• Determine why patient is taking the drug.
• Assess salivary flow as a factor in caries, periodontal disease, and candidiasis.
• Administered in the hospital; AIDS patients will be taking many other medications; confirm medical and drug history.
Consultations:
• In a patient with symptoms of blood dyscrasias, request a medical consultation for blood studies and postpone treatment until normal values are reestablished.
• Medical consultation may be required to assess disease control and patient's ability to tolerate stress.
Teach Patient/Family to:
• Use effective oral hygiene to prevent soft tissue inflammation

• Prevent trauma when using oral hygiene aids
• Report oral lesions, soreness, or bleeding to dentist
• When chronic dry mouth occurs, advise patient to:
  • Avoid mouth rinses with high alcohol content due to drying effects
  • Use daily home fluoride products for anticaries effect
  • Use sugarless gum, frequent sips of water, or saliva substitutes
• Update health and medication history if physician makes any changes in evaluation or drug regimens; include OTC, herbal, and nonherbal remedies in the update

decitabine
de-sye′-ta-been
(Dacogen)

CATEGORY AND SCHEDULE
Pregnancy Risk Category: D

Drug Class: Antineoplastic

MECHANISM OF ACTION
A pyrimidine antimetabolite that is incorporated into DNA and inhibits DNA methyltransferase causing hypomethylation and subsequent cell death. *Therapeutic Effect:* Restores normal function to tumor-suppressor genes regulating cellular differentiation and proliferation.

USES
Treatment of myelodysplastic syndrome (MDS)

PHARMACOKINETICS
No information is available regarding the pharmacokinetics of decitabine.

INDICATIONS AND DOSAGES
▸ **MDS**
IV
Adults. 15 mg/m^2 over 3 hr, repeat every 8 hr for 3 days; repeat cycle every 6 wk for a minimum of 4 cycles.

SIDE EFFECTS/ADVERSE REACTIONS:
Frequent
Neutropenia, thrombocytopenia, anemia, fever, nausea, cough, petechiae, constipation, diarrhea, hyperglycemia, headache, febrile neutropenia, leukopenia, insomnia, peripheral edema, hypomagnesemia, hypoalbuminemia, vomiting, pallor, bruising, hypokalemia, rigors, pneumonia, arthralgia, rash, limb pain, edema, dizziness, back pain, cardiac murmur, anorexia, pharyngitis, appetite decreased, abdominal pain, lung crackles, hyperbilirubinemia, erythema, pain, hyperkalemia, hyponatremia, oral mucosal lymphadenopathy, confusion, lethargy, cellulitis, stomatitis, dyspepsia, anxiety, hypoesthesia, lesions, pruritus, alkaline phosphatase increased, tenderness
Occasional
Candidal infection, ascites, AST increased, breath sounds diminished, hyperuricemia, hypoxia, rales, LDH increased, hemorrhoids, alopecia, catheter infection, gingival bleeding, chest discomfort, UTI, chest wall pain, loose stools, staphylococcal infection, transfusion reaction, tongue ulceration, dysphagia, oral candidiasis, dysuria, facial swelling, hypotension, musculoskeletal discomfort, blurred vision, bicarbonate increased, dehydration, hypochloremia, pulmonary edema,

urticaria, malaise, hematoma, thrombocythemia, bacteremia, polyuria, hypobilirubinemia, site erythema, catheter site pain, injection site swelling, lip ulceration, abdominal distension, bicarbonate decreased, hypoproteinemia, crepitation, myalgia, gastroesophageal reflux, glossodynia, postnasal drip, sinusitis

Rare

Anaphylactic reaction, atrial fibrillation, cardiomyopathy, CHF, cholecystitis, dyspnea, fungal infection, hemorrhage, gingival pain, mental status change, mucosal inflammation, mycobacterium avium complex infection, peridiverticular abscess, pseudomonal lung infection, pulmonary embolism, renal failure, respiratory arrest, respiratory tract infection, sepsis, splenomegaly, supraventricular tachycardia, weakness

PRECAUTIONS AND CONTRAINDICATIONS

Hypersensitivity to decitabine or its components; do not breastfeed, bone marrow depression, renal or hepatic impairment

DRUG INTERACTIONS OF CONCERN TO DENTISTRY

None reported

SERIOUS REACTIONS

! Neutropenia and thrombocytopenia are expected to occur.

DENTAL CONSIDERATIONS

General:
• Monitor vital signs at every appointment because of cardiovascular side effects.
• Avoid aspirin and NSAIDs.
• Consider immunosuppression as a factor in oral opportunistic infections.
• Consider semisupine chair position if GI or respiratory adverse effects occur.
• Chlorhexidine mouth rinse before and during chemotherapy may reduce severity of mucositis.
• Consider blood dyscrasias as a factor in infection, bleeding, and delayed healing.
• Palliative medication may be required of oral adverse effects.
• Assess salivary flow as a factor in caries, periodontal disease, and candidiasis.
• Obtain CBCs, including platelets and bleeding time, prior to initiating invasive dental procedures and postpone dental treatment as needed.

Consultations:
• Consult physician to determine why patient is taking drug.
• Consult physician to determine disease control and ability of patient to tolerate dental procedures.
• Consult physician(s) to determine if prophylactic antibiotics are required prior to dental procedures.

Teach Patient/Family to:
• Use effective atraumatic oral hygiene measures to prevent soft tissue inflammation
• Report oral lesions, soreness, or bleeding to dentist
• Update health history when physician changes drug regimen

and/or report use of over-the-counter medications, herbal products, and dietary supplements
• When chronic dry mouth occurs, advise patient to:
  • Avoid mouth rinses with high alcohol content due to drying effect
  • Use daily home fluoride products for anticaries effects
  • Use sugarless gum, frequent sips of water, or artificial saliva substitutes

delavirdine mesylate
deh-la´-ver-deen mess-ah-late
(Rescriptor)
Do not confuse Rescriptor with Retrovin or Ritonavir.

CATEGORY AND SCHEDULE
Pregnancy Risk Category: C

Drug Class: Antiviral, nonnucleoside

MECHANISM OF ACTION
A nonnucleoside reverse transcriptase inhibitor that binds directly to HIV-1 reverse transcriptase and blocks RNA- and DNA-dependent DNA polymerase activities. *Therapeutic Effect:* Interrupts HIV replication, slowing the progression of HIV infection.

USES
Treatment of HIV infection in combination with appropriate antiretroviral agents when therapy is warranted

PHARMACOKINETICS
Rapidly absorbed after PO administration. Protein binding: 98%.

Primarily distributed in plasma. Metabolized in the liver. Eliminated in feces and urine. *Half-life:* 2–11 hr.

INDICATIONS AND DOSAGES
▶ **HIV Infection (in combination with other antiretrovirals)**
PO
Adults. 400 mg 3 times a day.

SIDE EFFECTS/ADVERSE REACTIONS
Frequent
Rash, pruritus
Occasional
Headache, nausea, diarrhea, fatigue, anorexia

PRECAUTIONS AND CONTRAINDICATIONS
Hypersensitivity
Caution
Modify dose in liver disease; children younger than 16 yr, lactation; rapid development of viral resistance if used as a single drug

DRUG INTERACTIONS OF CONCERN TO DENTISTRY
• Reduced absorption: antacids, cimetidine, other H2-receptor antagonists
• Increased plasma levels of both delavirdine and clarithromycin
• Increased plasma levels of alprazolam, triazolam, midazolam
• Avoid coadministration with carbamazepine, phenobarbital, ketoconazole, fluoxetine

SERIOUS REACTIONS
None known

DENTAL CONSIDERATIONS
General:
• Examine for oral manifestation of opportunistic infection.

• Patients on chronic drug therapy may rarely have symptoms of blood dyscrasias, which can include infection, bleeding, and poor healing.

• Assess salivary flow as a factor in caries, periodontal disease, and candidiasis.

• After supine positioning, have patient sit upright for at least 2 min before standing to avoid orthostatic hypotension.

• Do not use ingestible sodium bicarbonate products, such as the Prophy-Jet air polishing system, within 2 hr of drug use.

Consultations:

• In a patient with symptoms of blood dyscrasias, request a medical consultation for blood studies and postpone treatment until normal values are reestablished.

• Medical consultation may be required to assess disease control and patient's ability to tolerate stress.

Teach Patient/Family to:

• Use effective oral hygiene to prevent soft tissue inflammation

• Use caution to prevent trauma when using oral hygiene aids

• See dentist immediately if secondary oral infection occurs

• When chronic dry mouth occurs, advise patient to:

  • Avoid mouth rinses with high alcohol content because of drying effects

  • Use daily home fluoride products for anticaries effect

  • Use sugarless gum, frequent sips of water, or saliva substitutes

demecarium bromide

de-mi-kare´-ee-um bro´-mide
(Humorsol Ocumeter)

CATEGORY AND SCHEDULE
Pregnancy Risk Category: X

Drug Class: Antiglaucoma agent, ophthalmic; cyclostimulant, accommodative esotropia

MECHANISM OF ACTION
A cholinesterase inhibitor that increases the concentration of acetylcholine at cholinergic receptor sites and produces effects equivalent to excessive stimulation of cholinergic receptors. *Therapeutic Effect:* Reduces intraocular pressure (IOP) due to facilitation of outflow of aqueous humor.

USES
Treatment of certain types of glaucoma and other eye conditions, such as accommodative esotropia. Also used in the diagnosis of certain eye conditions, such as accommodative esotropia.

PHARMACOKINETICS
Decreases intraocular pressure within a few hr. The duration is variable among individuals.

INDICATIONS AND DOSAGES
▸ **Glaucoma**
Ophthalmic, topical
Adults, Elderly. 1–2 drops of the 0.125% or 0.25% solution in affected eye(s) twice a day to twice a wk.
▸ **Cyclostimulant**
Ophthalmic, topical
Adults, Elderly. 1 drop of 0.125% or 0.25% solution in each eye daily for

2–3 wk, followed by 1 drop every 2 days for 4 wk.

▶ **Diagnostic Aid (accommodative esotropia)**

Ophthalmic, topical

Adults, Elderly. 1 drop of 0.125% or 0.25% solution once a day for 2 wk, then 1 drop every 2 days for 2–3 wk.

SIDE EFFECTS/ADVERSE REACTIONS

Occasional

Brow ache, nausea, vomiting, abdominal cramps, diarrhea, hypersalivation, urinary incontinence, lid muscle twitching, redness, myopia blurred vision, increase in IOP, iris cysts, breathing difficulties, increased sweating

PRECAUTIONS AND CONTRAINDICATIONS

Pregnancy, active uveal inflammation and/or glaucoma associated with iridocyclitis, hypersensitivity to demecarium or any component of the formulation.

DRUG INTERACTIONS OF CONCERN TO DENTISTRY

• Avoid use of succinylcholine in general anesthesia
• Possible inhibition of the metabolism of: ester-type local and topical anesthetics
• Avoid use of anticholinergics, such as systemic atropine or related drugs

SERIOUS REACTIONS

! Systemic absorption has been associated with demecarium resulting in anticholinesterase toxicity.
! Overdosage can produce cholinergic crisis characterized by cardiac arrhythmias, diarrhea, muscle weakness, profuse sweating, respiratory difficulties, urinary incontinence, and shock.

DENTAL CONSIDERATIONS

General:
• Determine why patient is taking the drug.
• Avoid drugs with anticholinergic activity, such as antihistamines, opioids, benzodiazepines, propantheline, atropine, and scopolamine.
• Avoid dental light in patient's eyes; offer dark glasses for patient comfort.
• Question glaucoma patient about compliance with prescribed drug regimen.

Consultations:
• Medical consultation may be required to assess disease control.

Teach Patient/Family to:
• Update health and medication history if physician makes any changes in evaluation or drug regimens; include OTC, herbal, and nonherbal remedies in the update

demeclocycline hydrochloride

dem-eh-kloe-sye´-kleen hi-droh-klor´-ide
(Declomycin, Ledermycin [AUS])

CATEGORY AND SCHEDULE

Pregnancy Risk Category: D

Drug Class: Tetracycline

MECHANISM OF ACTION

A tetracycline antibiotic that inhibits bacterial protein synthesis by binding to ribosomal receptor sites; also inhibits ADH-induced water reabsorption. ***Therapeutic Effect:*** Bacteriostatic; also produces water diuresis.

USES
Treatment of a wide variety of gram-positive and gram-negative bacteria, protozoa, *Rickettsia, Mycoplasma,* agents of psittacosis and ornithosis, actinomyces species

PHARMACOKINETICS
PO: Peak 3–6 hr, duration 48–72 hr, ***Half-life:*** 10–17 hr; 36%–91% bound to serum protein; crosses placenta; excreted in urine, breast milk

INDICATIONS AND DOSAGES
▸ **Mild-to-Moderate Infections, Including Acne, Pertussis, Chronic Bronchitis, and UTIs**
PO
Adults, Elderly. 150 mg 4 times a day or 300 mg 2 times a day.
Children older than 8 yr. 8–12 mg/kg/day in 2–4 divided doses.
▸ **Uncomplicated Gonorrhea**
PO
Adults. Initially, 600 mg, then 300 mg q12h for 4 days for total of 3 g.
▸ **Syndrome of Inappropriate ADH Secretion (SIADH)**
PO
Adults, Elderly. Initially, 900–1200 mg/day in 3–4 divided doses, then decrease dose to 600–900 mg/day in divided doses.

SIDE EFFECTS/ADVERSE REACTIONS
Frequent
Anorexia, nausea, vomiting, diarrhea, dysphagia, possibly severe photosensitivity (with moderate to high demeclocycline dosage)

Occasional
Urticaria, rash; diabetes insipidus syndrome, marked by polydipsia, polyuria, and weakness (with long-term therapy)

PRECAUTIONS AND CONTRAINDICATIONS
Children 8 yr and younger, last half of pregnancy.
Caution
Renal disease, hepatic disease, lactation, nephrogenic diabetes insipidus.

DRUG INTERACTIONS OF CONCERN TO DENTISTRY
• Decreased effect of penicillins, cephalosporins, oral contraceptives
• Oral contraceptives: advise patient of a potential risk for decreased contraceptive action, to maintain compliance with oral contraceptive use while using antibiotics, and to consider the use of additional nonhormonal contraception
• Contraindicated with isotretinoin (Accutane)

SERIOUS REACTIONS
❗ Superinfection (especially fungal), anaphylaxis, and benign intracranial hypertension occur rarely.
❗ Bulging fontanelles occur rarely in infants.

DENTAL CONSIDERATIONS
General:
• Examine oral cavity for side effects if on long-term drug therapy.
• Determine why the patient is taking the drug.
• Do not prescribe during pregnancy or before age 8 yr because of tooth discoloration.
• Absorption is reduced by dairy products, metals, and antacids.

Consultations:
- Medical consultation may be required to assess disease control.

Teach Patient/Family to:
- Use effective oral hygiene to prevent soft tissue inflammation
- Use caution to prevent injury when using oral hygiene aids
- When used for dental infection, advise patient to:
  - Report sore throat, oral burning sensation, fever, and fatigue, any of which could indicate superinfection
  - Take at prescribed intervals and complete dosage regimen
  - Immediately notify the dentist if signs or symptoms of infection increase

desipramine hydrochloride

dess-ip´-ra-meen hi-droh-klor´-ide
(Apo-Desipramine [CAN], Norpramin, Novo-Desipramine [CAN], Pertofran [AUS])
Do not confuse desipramine with clomipramine, disopyramide, imipramine, or nortriptyline.

CATEGORY AND SCHEDULE
Pregnancy Risk Category: C

Drug Class: Antidepressant, tricyclic

MECHANISM OF ACTION
A tricyclic antidepressant that blocks the reuptake of neurotransmitters, such as norepinephrine and serotonin, at presynaptic membranes, increasing their availability at postsynaptic receptor sites. Also has strong anticholinergic activity.
Therapeutic Effect: Relieves depression.

USES
Treatment of depression; unapproved: neurogenic pain

PHARMACOKINETICS
Rapidly and well absorbed from the GI tract. Protein binding: 90%. Metabolized in the liver. Primarily excreted in urine. Minimally removed by hemodialysis. **Half-life:** 12–27 hr.

INDICATIONS AND DOSAGES
▸ **Depression**
PO
Adults. 75 mg/day. May gradually increase to 150–200 mg/day. Maximum: 300 mg/day.
Elderly. Initially, 10–25 mg/day. May gradually increase to 75–100 mg/day. Maximum: 300 mg/day.
Children older than 12 yr. Initially, 25–50 mg/day. May gradually increase to 100 mg/day. Maximum: 150 mg/day.
Children 6–12 yr. 1–3 mg/kg/day. Maximum: 5 mg/kg/day.

SIDE EFFECTS/ADVERSE REACTIONS
Frequent
Somnolence, fatigue, dry mouth, blurred vision, constipation, delayed micturition, orthostatic hypotension, diaphoresis, impaired concentration, increased appetite, urine retention
Occasional
GI disturbances (such as nausea, GI distress, metallic taste)
Rare
Paradoxical reactions (agitation, restlessness, nightmares, insomnia), extrapyramidal symptoms (particularly fine hand tremor)

PRECAUTIONS AND CONTRAINDICATIONS
Angle-closure glaucoma, use within 14 days of MAOIs.

Caution
Suicidal patients, severe depression, increased intraocular pressure, narrow-angle glaucoma, elderly, MAOIs

DRUG INTERACTIONS OF CONCERN TO DENTISTRY
• Increased anticholinergic effects: muscarinic blockers, antihistamines, phenothiazines
• Increased effects of direct-acting sympathomimetics: epinephrine, levonordefrin
• Potential risk for increased CNS depression: alcohol, barbiturates, benzodiazepines, and other CNS depressants
• Decreased antihypertensive effects: clonidine, guanadrel, guanethidine
• At higher tricyclic doses, serum levels of fluconazole and ketoconazole may be elevated
• Avoid concurrent use with St. John's wort (herb)

SERIOUS REACTIONS
! Overdose may produce confusion, seizures, somnolence, arrhythmias, fever, hallucinations, dyspnea, vomiting, and unusual fatigue or weakness.
! Abrupt discontinuation after prolonged therapy may produce severe headache, malaise, nausea, vomiting, and vivid dreams.

DENTAL CONSIDERATIONS
General:
• Take vital signs at every appointment because of cardiovascular side effects.
• Assess salivary flow as a factor in caries, periodontal disease, and candidiasis.
• Patients on chronic drug therapy may rarely have symptoms of blood dyscrasias, which can include infection, bleeding, and poor healing.
• After supine positioning, have patient sit upright for at least 2 min to avoid orthostatic hypotension.
• Use vasoconstrictors with caution, in low doses, and with careful aspiration. Avoid use of gingival retraction cord with epinephrine.
• Place on frequent recall because of oral side effects.
Consultations:
• In a patient with symptoms of blood dyscrasias, request a medical consultation for blood studies and postpone dental treatment until normal values are reestablished.
• Medical consultation may be required to assess disease control.
• Physician should be informed if significant xerostomic side effects occur (e.g., increased caries, sore tongue, problems eating or swallowing, difficulty wearing prosthesis) so that a medication change can be considered.
Teach Patient/Family to:
• Use effective oral hygiene to prevent soft tissue inflammation
• Use caution to prevent injury when using oral hygiene aids
• When chronic dry mouth occurs, advise patient to:
  • Avoid mouth rinses with high alcohol content because of drying effects
  • Use daily home fluoride products for anticaries effect
  • Use sugarless gum, frequent sips of water, or saliva substitutes

desirudin

deh-sear´-ew-din
(Iprivask)

CATEGORY AND SCHEDULE
Pregnancy Risk Category: C

Drug Class: Anticoagulant;
thrombin inhibitor

MECHANISM OF ACTION
An anticoagulant that binds specifically
and directly to thrombin, inhibiting
free-circulating and clot-bound
thrombin. *Therapeutic Effect:* Prolongs
the clotting time of human plasma.

USES
Prophylaxis for deep vein thrombosis
(DVT) in those undergoing hip
replacement

PHARMACOKINETICS
Completely absorbed. Distributed in
extracellular space. Metabolized and
eliminated by the kidney.
Half-life: 2–3 hr.

INDICATIONS AND DOSAGES
▶ **Prevention of DVT in Patients**
Undergoing Hip Replacement
Surgery
Subcutaneous
Adults, Elderly. Initially, 15 mg q12h
given 5–15 min before surgery but
following induction of regional block
anesthesia, if used. May administer
up to 12 days after surgery.
▶ **Moderate Renal Impairment**
(creatinine clearance 31–60 ml/min
or higher)
Subcutaneous
Adults, Elderly. 5 mg q12h.
▶ **Severe Renal Impairment (creatinine**
clearance less than 31 ml/min)
Subcutaneous
Adults, Elderly. 1.7 mg q12h.

SIDE EFFECTS/ADVERSE REACTIONS
Frequent
Hematoma
Occasional
Injection site mass, wound
secretion, nausea, hypersensitivity
reaction

PRECAUTIONS AND CONTRAINDICATIONS
Hypersensitivity to natural or
recombinant hirudins
(anticoagulation factors), active
bleeding, irreversible coagulation
disorders

DRUG INTERACTIONS OF CONCERN TO DENTISTRY
• Increased risk of bleeding:
salicylates, NSAIDs, or any drug that
affects coagulation

SERIOUS REACTIONS
! Serious or major hemorrhage
and anaphylactic reaction occur
rarely.

DENTAL CONSIDERATIONS
General:
• Patients are at risk of bleeding, so
check for oral signs.
• Product may be used in outpatient
therapy. Delay elective dental
treatment until patient completes
anticoagulant therapy.
• Determine why patient is taking
the drug.
• Avoid products that affect platelet
function, such as aspirin and
NSAIDs.
• Consider local hemostasis
measures to prevent excessive
bleeding.
Consultations:
• Medical consultation should
include PPT, PT, or INR.

- Medical consultation may be required to assess disease control and patient's ability to tolerate stress.
Teach Patient/Family to:
- Use soft tooth brush to reduce risk of bleeding
- Use effective oral hygiene to prevent soft tissue inflammation
- Report oral lesions, soreness, or bleeding to dentist
- Prevent trauma when using oral hygiene aids
- Update health and medication history if physician makes any changes in evaluation or drug regimens; include OTC, herbal, and nonherbal remedies in the update

desloratadine
des-loer-at´-ah-deen
(Aerius [CAN], Clarinex, Clarinex Redi-Tabs)

CATEGORY AND SCHEDULE
Pregnancy Risk Category: C
Do not confuse Clarinex with Claritin.

Drug Class: Antihistamine, histamine H1-receptor antagonist

MECHANISM OF ACTION
A nonsedating antihistamine that exhibits selective peripheral histamine H_1 receptor blocking action. Competes with histamine at receptor sites.
Therapeutic Effect: Prevents allergic responses mediated by histamine, such as rhinitis and urticaria.

USES
Treatment of seasonal allergic rhinitis; chronic idiopathic urticaria

PHARMACOKINETICS
Rapidly and almost completely absorbed from the GI tract.

Distributed mainly in liver, lungs, GI tract, and bile. Metabolized in the liver to active metabolite and undergoes extensive first-pass metabolism. Eliminated in urine and feces. **Half-life:** 27 hr (increased in the elderly and in renal or hepatic impairment).

INDICATIONS AND DOSAGES
▸ **Allergic Rhinitis, Urticaria**
PO
Adults, Elderly, Children older than 12 yr. 5 mg once a day.
▸ **Dosage in Hepatic or Renal Impairment**
Dosage is decreased to 5 mg every other day.

SIDE EFFECTS/ADVERSE REACTIONS
Frequent
Headache
Occasional
Dry mouth, somnolence
Rare
Fatigue, dizziness, diarrhea, nausea

PRECAUTIONS AND CONTRAINDICATIONS
Hypersensitivity to this drug or loratadine
Caution
Distributed to breast milk (caution in nursing), incomplete dosing studies in the elderly, safety has not been established in children younger than 12 yr, dosage adjustment required in hepatic impairment

DRUG INTERACTIONS OF CONCERN TO DENTISTRY
- Limited studies with concurrent doses of erythromycin; ketoconazole and azithromycin show slight elevations of plasma levels, but no clinically relevant changes in electrocardiographic parameters

• One report indicated a potential for increased anticholinergic effects with other anticholinergic drugs and increased somnolence with CNS depressants; however, data are lacking

SERIOUS REACTIONS
None known.

DENTAL CONSIDERATIONS
General:
• Assess salivary flow as a factor in caries, periodontal disease, and candidiasis.
Teach Patient/Family to:
• Use effective oral hygiene to prevent soft tissue inflammation
• When chronic dry mouth occurs, advise patient to:
   • Avoid mouth rinses with high alcohol content because of drying effects
   • Use sugarless gum, frequent sips of water, or saliva substitutes
   • Use daily home fluoride products for anticaries effect

desmopressin
des-moe-press´-in
(DDAVP, Minirin[AUS], Octostim[CAN], Stimate)

CATEGORY AND SCHEDULE
Pregnancy Risk Category: B

Drug Class: Antidiuretic, central diabetes insipidus; antidiuretic, primary nocturnal enuresis; antihemorrhagic

MECHANISM OF ACTION
A synthetic pituitary hormone that increases reabsorption of water by increasing permeability of collecting ducts of the kidneys. Also serves as a plasminogen activator. **Therapeutic Effect:** Increases plasma factor VIII (antihemophilic factor). Decreases urinary output.

USES
Prevents or controls the frequent urination, increased thirst, and loss of water associated with diabetes insipidus (water diabetes). It is used also to control bed-wetting and frequent urination and increased thirst associated with certain types of brain injuries or brain surgery

PHARMACOKINETICS

Route	Onset	Peak	Duration
PO	1 hr	2–7 hr	6–8 hr
IV	15–30 min	1.5–3 hr	N/A
Intranasal	15 min–1 hr	1–5 hr	5–21 hr

Poorly absorbed after oral or nasal administration. Metabolism: Unknown. **Half-life:** Oral: 1.5–2.5 hr. Intranasal: 3.3–3.5 hr. IV: 0.4–4 hr.

INDICATIONS AND DOSAGES
▸ **Primary Nocturnal Enuresis**
PO
Children 12 yr and older. 0.2–0.6 mg once before bedtime.
Intranasal
Children 6 yr and older. Initially, 20 mcg (0.2 ml) at bedtime; use one-half dose in each nostril. Adjust to maximum of 40 mcg/day.
▸ **Central Cranial Diabetes Insipidus**
PO
Adults, Elderly, Children 12 yr and older. Initially, 0.05 mg twice a day. Range: 0.1–1.2 mg/day in 2–3 divided doses.
Children younger than 12 yr. Initially, 0.05 mg; then twice a day. Range: 0.1–0.8 mg daily.

IV, Subcutaneous
Adults, Elderly, Children 12 yr and older. 2–4 mcg/day in 2 divided doses or $^{1}/_{10}$ of maintenance intranasal dose.
Intranasal
Adults, Elderly, Children older than 12 yr. 5–40 mcg (0.05–0.4 ml) in 1–3 doses/day.
Children 3 mo–12 yr. Initially, 5 mcg (0.05 ml)/day. Range: 5–30 mcg (0.05–0.3 ml)/day.
▶ **Hemophilia A, Von Willebrand's Disease (Type I)**
IV Infusion
Adults, Elderly, Children weighing more than 10 kg. 0.3 mcg/kg diluted in 50 ml 0.9% NaCl.
Children weighing 10 kg and less. 0.3 mcg/kg diluted in 10 ml 0.9% NaCl.
Intranasal
Adults, Elderly, Children 12 yr and older weighing more than 50 kg. 300 mcg; use 1 spray in each nostril.
Adults, Elderly, Children 12 yr and older weighing 50 kg or less. 150 mcg as a single spray.

SIDE EFFECTS/ADVERSE REACTIONS
Occasional
IV: Pain, redness, or swelling at injection site; headache; abdominal cramps; vulval pain; flushed skin; mild B/P elevation; nausea with high dosages
Nasal: Rhinorrhea, nasal congestion, slight B/P elevation

PRECAUTIONS AND CONTRAINDICATIONS
Hemophilia A with factor VIII levels less than 5%; hemophilia B; severe type I, type IIB, or platelet-type von Willebrand's disease
Caution
Lactation, hypertension

DRUG INTERACTIONS OF CONCERN TO DENTISTRY
• Decreased antidiuretic effects: demeclocycline
• Increased antidiuretic effects: carbamazepine

SERIOUS REACTIONS
! Water intoxication or hyponatremia, marked by headache, somnolence, confusion, decreased urination, rapid weight gain, seizures, and coma, may occur in overhydration. Children, elderly patients, and infants are especially at risk.

DENTAL CONSIDERATIONS
General:
• Monitor vital signs at every appointment because of cardiovascular side effects.
• Avoid prescribing aspirin-containing products if treatment is for bleeding disorder.
• Consider local hemostatic measures to prevent excessive bleeding.
• Determine why the patient is taking the drug.
• Consider semisupine chair position for patient comfort because of GI effects of disease.
Consultations:
• Medical consultation may be required to assess disease control; definite consultation for patients with chronic bleeding disorders.
• Medical consultation should include PTT or PT.
Teach Patient/Family to:
• Advise dentist if excessive bleeding occurs or continues after dental treatment

desonide
dess´-oh-nide
(Delonide, Desocrot[CAN],
DesOwen, Scheinpharm
Desonide[CAN], Tridesilon)

CATEGORY AND SCHEDULE
Pregnancy Risk Category: C

Drug Class: Topical corticosteroid,
group IV low potency

MECHANISM OF ACTION
A topical corticosteroid that has
antiinflammatory, antipruritic, and
vasoconstrictive properties. The exact
mechanism of the antiinflammatory
process is unclear. *Therapeutic
Effect:* Reduces or prevents tissue
response to the inflammatory process.

USES
Treatment of psoriasis, eczema,
contact dermatitis, pruritus

PHARMACOKINETICS
Large variation in absorption determined
by many factors. Metabolized in the
liver. Primarily excreted by the kidneys
and small amounts in the bile.

INDICATIONS AND DOSAGES
▶ **Dermatoses**
Topical
Adults, Elderly. Apply sparingly
2–3 times a day.
▶ **Otitis Externa**
Aural
Adults, Elderly, Children. Instill
3–4 drops into the ear 3–4 times a day.

SIDE EFFECTS/ADVERSE
REACTIONS
Occasional
Burning and stinging at site of
application, dryness, skin peeling,
contact dermatitis

PRECAUTIONS AND
CONTRAINDICATIONS
Perforated eardrum, history of
hypersensitivity to desonide or other
corticosteroids
Caution
Lactation, viral infections, bacterial
infections

DRUG INTERACTIONS OF
CONCERN TO DENTISTRY
None listed

SERIOUS REACTIONS
❗ The serious reactions of long-term
therapy and the addition of occlusive
dressings are reversible
hypothalamic-pituitary-adrenal
(HPA) axis suppression,
manifestations of Cushing's
syndrome, hyperglycemia and
glucosuria.

DENTAL CONSIDERATIONS
General:
• Determine why the patient is taking
the drug.
• Place on frequent recall to evaluate
healing response if used on chronic
basis.
• Apply lubricant to dry lips for
patient comfort before dental
procedures.

desoximetasone
des-ox-ih-met´-ah-sone
(Taro-Desoximetason[CAN],
Topicort, Topicort-LP)
Do not confuse with
dexamethasone.

CATEGORY AND SCHEDULE
Pregnancy Risk Category: C

Drug Class: Topical
corticosteroid, group II potency
(0.25%), group III potency (0.05%)

MECHANISM OF ACTION

A high-potency, fluorinated topical corticosteroid that has anti-inflammatory, antipruritic, and vasoconstrictive properties. The exact mechanism of the anti-inflammatory process is unclear. *Therapeutic Effect:* Reduces tissue response to the inflammatory process.

USES

Treatment of psoriasis, eczema, contact dermatitis, pruritus

PHARMACOKINETICS

Large variation in absorption among sites. Protein binding in varying degrees. Metabolized in liver. Primarily excreted in urine.

INDICATIONS AND DOSAGES

▸ **Dermatoses**
Topical
Adults, Elderly. Apply sparingly 2 times a day.
Children. Apply sparingly 1–2 times a day.

SIDE EFFECTS/ADVERSE REACTIONS

Frequent
Itching, redness, irritation, burning at site of application
Occasional
Dryness, folliculitis, hypertrichosis, acneiform eruptions, hypopigmentation, perioral dermatitis
Rare
Allergic contact dermatitis, adrenal suppression, atrophy, striae, miliaria, photosensitivity

PRECAUTIONS AND CONTRAINDICATIONS

History of hypersensitivity to desoximetasone or other corticosteroids.

Caution
Lactation, viral infections, bacterial infections

SERIOUS REACTIONS

! Serious reactions of long-term therapy and addition of occlusive dressings are reversible hypothalamic-pituitary-adrenal (HPA) axis suppression, manifestations of Cushing's syndrome, hyperglycemia, and glucosuria.
! Abruptly withdrawing the drug after long-term therapy may require supplemental systemic corticosteroids.

DENTAL CONSIDERATIONS

General:
• Gel formulations are used in the treatment of oral lichen planus lesions when the diagnosis has been confirmed by immunofluorescent biopsy testing.
• Place on frequent recall to evaluate healing response.
Teach Patient/Family to:
• Return for oral evaluation if response of oral tissues has not occurred in 7–14 days
• Use effective oral hygiene to prevent soft tissue inflammation
• Not use on oral herpetic ulcerations
• Apply at bedtime or after meals for maximum effect
• Apply with cotton-tipped applicator, dabbing gently, not rubbing medication on lesion

dexamethasone

dex-ah-meth´-ah-sone
(Decadron, Desamethasone
Intensol, Dexasone, Dexasone LA,
Dexmethsone[AUS], Diodex[CAN],
Hexadrol[CAN], Maxidex, Solurex,
Solurex LA)
Do not confuse dexamethasone
with desoximetasone or
dextramethophan, or Maxidex with
Maxzide.

CATEGORY AND SCHEDULE
Pregnancy Risk Category: C
(D if used in the first trimester)

Drug Class: Synthetic topical
corticosteroid

MECHANISM OF ACTION
A long-acting glucocorticoid that
inhibits accumulation of
inflammatory cells at inflammation
sites, phagocytosis, lysosomal
enzyme release and synthesis, and
release of mediators of inflammation.
Therapeutic Effect: Prevents and
suppresses cell and tissue immune
reactions and inflammatory process.

USES
Treatment of corticosteroid-
responsive dermatoses, oral
ulcerative inflammatory lesions

PHARMACOKINETICS
Rapidly, completely absorbed from
the GI tract after oral administration.
Widely distributed. Protein binding:
High. Metabolized in the liver.
Primarily excreted in urine.
Minimally removed by hemodialysis.
Half-life: 3–4.5 hr.

INDICATIONS AND DOSAGES
▸ **Anti-inflammatory**
PO, IV, IM
Adults, Elderly. 0.75–9 mg/day in
divided doses q6–12h.
Children. 0.08–0.3 mg/kg/day in
divided doses q6–12h.
▸ **Cerebral Edema**
IV
Adults, Elderly. Initially, 10 mg, then
4 mg (IV or IM) q6h.
PO, IV, IM
Children. Loading dose of 1–2 mg/kg,
then 1–1.5 mg/kg/day in divided
doses q4–6h.
▸ **Nausea and Vomiting in
Chemotherapy Patients**
IV
Adults, Elderly. 8–20 mg once, then
4 mg (PO) q4–6h or 8 mg q8h.
Children. 10 mg/m²/dose
(Maximum: 20 mg), then 5 mg/m²/
dose q6h.
▸ **Physiologic Replacement**
PO, IV, IM
Children. 0.03–0.15 mg/kg/day in
divided doses q6–12h.
▸ **Usual Ophthalmic Dosage, Ocular
Inflammatory Conditions**
Ointment
Adults, Elderly, Children. Thin
coating 3–4 times a day.
Suspension
Adults, Elderly, Children. Initially,
2 drops q1h while awake and q2h at
night for 1 day, then reduce to
3–4 times a day.

SIDE EFFECTS/ADVERSE
REACTIONS
Frequent
Inhalation: Cough, dry mouth,
hoarseness, throat irritation
Intranasal: Burning, mucosal
dryness
Ophthalmic: Blurred vision
Systemic: Insomnia, facial swelling
or cushingoid appearance, moderate
abdominal distention, indigestion,
increased appetite, nervousness,
facial flushing, diaphoresis

Occasional

Inhalation: Localized fungal infection, such as thrush

Intranasal: Crusting inside nose, nosebleed, sore throat, ulceration of nasal mucosa

Ophthalmic: Decreased vision, watering of eyes, eye pain, burning, stinging, redness of eyes, nausea, vomiting

Systemic: Dizziness, decreased or blurred vision

Topical: Allergic contact dermatitis, purpura or blood-containing blisters, thinning of skin with easy bruising, telangiectasis or raised dark red spots on skin

Rare

Inhalation: Increased bronchospasm, esophageal candidiasis

Intranasal: Nasal and pharyngeal candidiasis, eye pain

Systemic: General allergic reaction (such as rash and hives); pain, redness, or swelling at injection site; psychological changes; false sense of well-being; hallucinations; depression

PRECAUTIONS AND CONTRAINDICATIONS

Active untreated infections, fungal, tuberculosis, or viral diseases of the eye

Caution

Lactation, viral infections, bacterial infections

SERIOUS REACTIONS

❗ Long-term therapy may cause muscle wasting (especially in the arms and legs), osteoporosis, spontaneous fractures, amenorrhea, cataracts, glaucoma, peptic ulcer disease, and CHF.

❗ The ophthalmic form may cause glaucoma, ocular hypertension, and cataracts.

❗ Abrupt withdrawal following long-term therapy may cause severe joint pain, severe headache, anorexia, nausea, fever, rebound inflammation, fatigue, weakness, lethargy, dizziness, and orthostatic hypotension.

DENTAL CONSIDERATIONS

General:

• Monitor vital signs at every appointment because of cardiovascular side effects.

• Patients on chronic drug therapy may rarely have symptoms of blood dyscrasias, which can include infection, bleeding, and poor healing.

• Symptoms of oral infections may be masked.

• Patients who have been or are currently on chronic steroid therapy (longer than 2 wk) may require supplemental steroids for dental treatment.

• Avoid prescribing aspirin-containing products.

• Place on frequent recall to evaluate healing response.

• Prophylactic antibiotics may be indicated to prevent infection if surgery or deep scaling is planned.

Consultations:

• In a patient with symptoms of blood dyscrasias, request a medical consultation for blood studies and postpone dental treatment until normal values are reestablished.

• Medical consultation may be required to assess disease control.

• Consultation may be required to confirm steroid dose and duration of use.

Teach Patient/Family to:

• Use effective oral hygiene to prevent soft tissue inflammation

- Use caution to prevent injury when using oral hygiene aids
- Avoid mouth rinses with high alcohol content because of drug interaction

dexamethasone sodium phosphate

dex-ah-meth´-ah-sone soe´-dee-um foss´-fate
(AK-Dex, Decadron Phosphate Ophthalmic, Dexamthasone Ophthalmic, Maxidex, Ocu-Dex, Diodex[CAN])
Do not confuse dexamehtasone with desoximetasone, dextramethophan, or Maxzide.

CATEGORY AND SCHEDULE
Pregnancy Risk Category: C (D if used in the first trimester)

Drug Class: Synthetic topical corticosteroid

MECHANISM OF ACTION
A corticosteroid that inhibits accumulation of inflammatory cells at inflammation sites, phagocytosis, lysosomal enzyme release, and synthesis and release of mediators of inflammation. ***Therapeutic Effect:*** Prevents and suppresses cell and tissue immune reactions, inflammatory process.

USES
Treatment of corticosteroid-responsive dermatoses, oral ulcerative inflammatory lesions

PHARMACOKINETICS
Absorbed into aqueous humor, cornea, iris, choroids, ciliary body, and retina. Systemic absorption may occur and is more likely at higher doses or in pediatric therapy.

INDICATIONS AND DOSAGES
▶ **Ocular Inflammatory Conditions**
Ophthalmic, Ointment
Adults, Elderly. Apply thin strip 3–4 times a day.
Ophthalmic, Solution and Suspension
Adults, Elderly. Instill 1 or 2 drops up to 6 times a day.

SIDE EFFECTS/ADVERSE REACTIONS
Frequent
Blurred vision, increased intraocular pressure
Occasional
Decreased vision, watering of eyes, eye pain, burning, stinging, redness of eyes, nausea, vomiting
Rare
Optic nerve damage, posterior subcapsular cataract formation, delayed wound healing

PRECAUTIONS AND CONTRAINDICATIONS
Epithelial herpes simplex keratitis (dendritic keratitis), vaccinia, varicella or other viral diseases of the cornea and conjunctiva, mycobacterial infection of the eye, fungal diseases of ocular structures, hypersensitivity to any component of the medication.
Caution
Diabetes mellitus, glaucoma, osteoporosis, seizure disorders, ulcerative colitis, CHF, myasthenia gravis, renal disease, peptic ulcer, esophagitis

DRUG INTERACTIONS OF CONCERN TO DENTISTRY
- Decreased action: barbiturates
- Increased side effects: alcohol, salicylates, other NSAIDs

• Increased action: ketoconazole, macrolide antibiotics

SERIOUS REACTIONS
! The serious reactions of the ophthalmic form of dexamethasone sodium phosphate are glaucoma, ocular hypertension, and cataracts.
! May promote development and spread of secondary infection (usually fungal).

DENTAL CONSIDERATIONS
General:
• Place on frequent recall to evaluate healing response.
Teach Patient/Family to:
• Return for oral evaluation if response of oral tissues has not occurred in 7–14 days
• Use effective oral hygiene to prevent soft tissue inflammation
• Apply approximately 0.25 inch; measure and apply with cotton-tipped applicator by gently dabbing, not rubbing, medication on lesion
• Apply at bedtime or after meals for maximum effect
• Avoid use on oral herpetic ulcerations is contraindicated

dexchlorpheniramine
dex-klor-fen-eer´-ah-meen
(Polaramine, Polaramine Repetabs)

CATEGORY AND SCHEDULE
Pregnancy Risk Category: B

Drug Class: Antihistamine

MECHANISM OF ACTION
A propylamine derivative that competes with histamine for H_1-receptor sites on effector cells in the GI tract, blood vessels, and respiratory tract.
Dexchlorpheniramine is the dextro-isomer of chlorpheniramine and is approximately 2 times more active.
Therapeutic Effect: Prevents allergic response, produces mild bronchodilation, blocks histamine-induced bronchitis.

USES
Treatment of allergy symptoms, rhinitis, pruritus, contact dermatitis

PHARMACOKINETICS

Route	Onset	Peak	Duration
PO	0.5 hr	1–2 hr	3–6 hr

Well absorbed from the GI tract. Protein binding: 70%. Widely distributed. Metabolized in liver to active metabolite, undergoes extensive first-pass metabolism. Excreted primarily in urine. Not removed by hemodialysis.
Half-life: 20 hr.

INDICATIONS AND DOSAGES
▸ **Allergic Rhinitis, Common Cold**
PO
Adults, Elderly, Children 12 yr or older. 2 mg q4–6h or 4–6 mg timed release at bedtime or q8–10h.
Children 6–11 yr. 4 mg timed release at bedtime or 1 mg q4–6h.
Children 2–5 yr. 0.5 mg q4–6h. Do not use timed release.

SIDE EFFECTS/ADVERSE REACTIONS
Frequent
Drowsiness, dizziness, headache, dry mouth, nose, or throat, urinary retention, thickening of bronchial secretions, sedation, hypotension

Occasional

Epigastric distress, flushing, blurred vision, tinnitus, paresthesia, sweating, chills

PRECAUTIONS AND CONTRAINDICATIONS

History of hypersensitivity to antihistamines, newborn or premature infants, nursing mothers, third trimester of pregnancy

Caution

Increased intraocular pressure, renal disease, cardiac disease, hypertension, bronchial asthma, seizure disorder, stenosed peptic ulcers, hyperthyroidism, prostatic hypertrophy, bladder neck obstruction, elderly

DRUG INTERACTIONS OF CONCERN TO DENTISTRY

• Increased CNS depression: barbiturates, narcotics, hypnotics, tricyclic antidepressants, alcohol
• Increased anticholinergic effect: anticholinergic drugs

SERIOUS REACTIONS

! Children may experience dominant paradoxical reactions, including restlessness, insomnia, euphoria, nervousness, and tremors.
! Hypersensitivity reaction, such as eczema, pruritus, rash, cardiac disturbances, and photosensitivity, may occur.
! Overdosage may vary from CNS depression, including sedation, apnea, hypotension, cardiovascular collapse, or death to severe paradoxical reaction, such as hallucinations, tremors, and seizures.

DENTAL CONSIDERATIONS

General:

• Assess salivary flow as a factor in caries, periodontal disease, and candidiasis.

• Consider semisupine chair position for patient comfort because of respiratory effects of disease.

Teach Patient/Family:

• When chronic dry mouth occurs, advise patient to:
  • Avoid mouth rinses with high alcohol content because of drying effects
  • Use sugarless gum, frequent sips of water, or saliva substitutes
  • Use daily home fluoride products for anticaries effect

dexmethylphenidate hydrochloride

dex-meth-ill-fen´-ih-date
hi-droh-klor´-ide
(Focalin)

CATEGORY AND SCHEDULE

Pregnancy Risk Category: C
Controlled Substance: Schedule II

Drug Class: CNS stimulant; related to the amphetamines

MECHANISM OF ACTION

A CNS stimulant that blocks the reuptake of norepinephrine and dopamine into presynaptic neurons, increasing the release of these neurotransmitters into the synaptic cleft.

Therapeutic Effect: Decreases motor restlessness and fatigue; increases motor activity, mental alertness, and attention span; elevates mood.

USES

Treatment of attention deficit hyperactivity disorder (ADHD)

PHARMACOKINETICS

Route	Onset	Peak	Duration
PO	N/A	N/A	4–5 hr

Readily absorbed from the GI tract. Plasma concentrations increase rapidly. Metabolized in the liver. Excreted unchanged in urine. *Half-life:* 2.2 hr.

INDICATIONS AND DOSAGES
▸ **ADHD**
PO
Patients new to dexmethylphenidate or methylphenidate. 2.5 mg twice a day (5 mg/day). May adjust dosage in 2.5- to 5-mg increments. Maximum: 20 mg/day.
Patients currently taking methylphenidate. Half the methylphenidate dosage. Maximum: 20 mg/day.

SIDE EFFECTS/ADVERSE REACTIONS
Frequent
Abdominal pain, nausea, anorexia, fever
Occasional
Tachycardia, arrhythmias, palpitations, insomnia, twitching
Rare
Blurred vision, rash, arthralgia

PRECAUTIONS AND CONTRAINDICATIONS
Diagnosis or family history of Tourette syndrome; glaucoma; history of marked agitation, anxiety, or tension; motor tics; use within 14 days of MAOIs.
Caution
Long-term effect on growth in children unknown, exacerbation of psychotic behavior, history of seizures, hypertension, heart failure, recent MI, hyperthyroidism, use in children younger than 6 yr not established, drug dependence, lactation

DRUG INTERACTIONS OF CONCERN TO DENTISTRY
• May inhibit metabolism of phenobarbital, tricyclic antidepressants, and SSRIs
• Increased effects of anticholinergics, CNS stimulants, tricyclic antidepressants, and sympathomimetics

SERIOUS REACTIONS
! Withdrawal after prolonged therapy may unmask symptoms of the underlying disorder.
! Dexmethylphenidate may lower the seizure threshold in those with a history of seizures.
! Overdose produces excessive sympathomimetic effects, including vomiting, tremor, hyperreflexia, seizures, confusion, hallucinations, and diaphoresis.
! Prolonged administration to children may delay growth.

DENTAL CONSIDERATIONS
General:
• Monitor vital signs at every appointment because of cardiovascular side effects.
• Assess salivary flow as a factor in caries, periodontal disease, and candidiasis.
• Patients on chronic drug therapy may rarely have symptoms of blood dyscrasias, which can include infection, bleeding, and poor healing.
• Use vasoconstrictor with caution, in low doses, and with careful aspiration.
• Determine why the patient is taking the drug.
Consultations:
• In a patient with symptoms of blood dyscrasias, request a medical consultation for blood studies and postpone treatment until normal values are reestablished.

• Medical consultation may be required to assess disease control.

Teach Patient/Family to:
• Use effective oral hygiene to prevent soft tissue inflammation, infection
• Use caution to prevent injury when using oral hygiene aids
• Update health and drug history if physician makes any changes in evaluation or drug regimens
• When chronic dry mouth occurs, advise patient to:
  • Avoid mouth rinses with high alcohol content because of drying effects
  • Use daily home fluoride products for anticaries effect
  • Use sugarless gum, frequent sips of water, or saliva substitutes

dextroamphetamine sulfate
dex-troe-am-fet´-ah-meen sull´-fate
(Dexamphetamine[AUS], Dexedrine, Dexedrine Spansule, Dextrostat)
Do not confuse dextroamphetamine with dextromethorphan, or Dexedrine with Dextran or Excedrin.

CATEGORY AND SCHEDULE
Pregnancy Risk Category: C
Controlled Substance: Schedule II

Drug Class: Amphetamine

MECHANISM OF ACTION
An amphetamine that enhances the action of dopamine and norepinephrine by blocking their reuptake from synapses; also inhibits monoamine oxidase and facilitates the release of catecholamines.
Therapeutic Effect: Increases motor activity and mental alertness; decreases motor restlessness, drowsiness, and fatigue; suppresses appetite.

USES
Treatment of narcolepsy, attention deficit hyperactivity disorder (ADHD)

PHARMACOKINETICS
PO: Onset 30 min, peak 1–3 hr, duration 4–20 hr, *Half-life:* 10–30 hr; metabolized by liver; urine excretion pH dependent; crosses placenta, excreted in breast milk

INDICATIONS AND DOSAGES
▶ **Narcolepsy**
PO
Adults, Children older than 12 yr.
Initially, 10 mg/day. Increase by 10 mg/day at weekly intervals until therapeutic response is achieved.
Children 6–12 yr. Initially, 5 mg/day. Increase by 5 mg/day at weekly intervals until therapeutic response is achieved. Maximum: 60 mg/day.
▶ **ADHD**
PO
Children 6 yr and older. Initially, 5 mg once or twice a day. Increase by 5 mg/day at weekly intervals until therapeutic response is achieved.
Children 3–5 yr. Initially, 2.5 mg/day. Increase by 2.5 mg/day at weekly intervals until therapeutic response is achieved. Maximum: 40 mg/day.
▶ **Appetite Suppressant**
PO
Adults. 5–30 mg daily in divided doses of 5–10 mg each, given 30–60 min before meals; or 1 extended-release capsule in the morning.

SIDE EFFECTS/ADVERSE REACTIONS
Frequent
Irregular pulse, increased motor activity, talkativeness, nervousness, mild euphoria, insomnia

Occasional
Headache, chills, dry mouth, GI
distress, worsening depression in
patients who are clinically depressed,
tachycardia, palpitations, chest pain,
dizziness, decreased appetite

PRECAUTIONS AND CONTRAINDICATIONS
Advanced arteriosclerosis, agitated
states, glaucoma, history of drug
abuse, hypersensitivity to
sympathomimetic amines,
hyperthyroidism, moderate to severe
hypertension, symptomatic
cardiovascular disease, use within
14 days of MAOIs
Caution
Gilles de la Tourette's syndrome,
lactation, children younger than 3 yr

DRUG INTERACTIONS OF CONCERN TO DENTISTRY
• Increased risk of serious side
effects: meperidine, propoxyphene,
tricyclic antidepressants

SERIOUS REACTIONS
! Overdose may produce skin pallor
or flushing, arrhythmias, and
psychosis.
! Abrupt withdrawal after prolonged
use of high doses may produce
lethargy lasting for weeks.
! Prolonged administration to
children with ADHD may inhibit
growth.

DENTAL CONSIDERATIONS

General:
• Monitor vital signs at every
appointment because of
cardiovascular side effects.
• Assess salivary flow as a factor in
caries, periodontal disease, and
candidiasis.
• Psychologic and physical
dependence may occur with chronic
administration.

Consultations:
• Medical consultation may be
required to assess disease control.
Teach Patient/Family:
• When chronic dry mouth occurs,
advise patient to:
• Avoid mouth rinses with high
alcohol content because of drying
effects
• Use daily home fluoride products
for anticaries effect
• Use sugarless gum, frequent sips
of water, or saliva substitutes

dextromethorphan
dex-troe-meth-or´-fan
(Babee Cof Syrup, Benylin Adult,
Benylin Pediatric, Creomulsion
Cough, Creomulsion for Children,
Creo-Terpin, Delsym, Dexalone,
ElixSure Cough, Hold DM,
PediaCare Infants' Long-Acting
Cough, Robitussin[AUS],
Robitussin CoughGels, Robitussin
Honey Cough, Robitussin
Maximum Strength Cough,
Robitussin Pediatric Cough,
Scot-Tussin DM Cough Chasers,
Silphen DM, Simply Cough, Vicks
44 Cough Relief)

CATEGORY AND SCHEDULE
Pregnancy Risk Category: C
OTC

Drug Class: Antitussive,
nonnarcotic

MECHANISM OF ACTION
A chemical relative of morphine
without the narcotic properties that
acts on the cough center in the
medulla oblongata by elevating the
threshold for coughing. *Therapeutic
Effect:* Suppresses cough.

USES
Treatment of nonproductive cough

PHARMACOKINETICS
Rapidly absorbed from the GI tract. Distributed into CSF. Extensively and poorly metabolized in liver to dextrorphan (active metabolite). Excreted unchanged in urine. *Half-life:* 1.4–3.9 hr (parent compound), 3.4–5.6 hr. (dextrorphan).

INDICATIONS AND DOSAGES
▶ **Cough**
PO
Adults, Elderly, Children 12 yr and older. 10–20 mg q4h. Maximum: 120 mg/day.
Children 6–12 yr. 5–10 mg q4h. Maximum: 60 mg/day.
Children 2–5 yr. 2.5–5 mg q4h. Maximum: 30 mg/day.

SIDE EFFECTS/ADVERSE REACTIONS
Rare
Abdominal discomfort, constipation, dizziness, drowsiness, GI upset, nausea

PRECAUTIONS AND CONTRAINDICATIONS
Coadministration with MAOIs, hypersensitivity to dextromethorphan or its components
Caution
Nausea, vomiting, increased temperature, persistent headache, drug abuse

DRUG INTERACTIONS OF CONCERN TO DENTISTRY
• Inhibition of metabolism: terbinafine

SERIOUS REACTIONS
! Overdosage may result in muscle spasticity, increase or decrease in B/P, blurred vision, blue fingernails and lips, nausea, vomiting, hallucinations, and respiratory depression.

DENTAL CONSIDERATIONS
General:
• Consider semisupine chair position for patients with respiratory disease.

diazepam
dye-az´-eh-pam
(Antenex[AUS], Apo-Diazepam[CAN], Diastat, Diazemuls[CAN], Dizac, Ducene[AUS],Valium, Valpam[AUS], Vivol[CAN])
Do not confuse diazepam with diazoxide or Ditropan, or Valium with Valcyte.

CATEGORY AND SCHEDULE
Pregnancy Risk Category: D
Controlled Substance: Schedule IV

Drug Class: Benzodiazepine, anxiolytic

MECHANISM OF ACTION
A benzodiazepine that depresses all levels of the CNS by enhancing the action of gamma-aminobutyric acid, a major inhibitory neurotransmitter in the brain. *Therapeutic Effect:* Produces anxiolytic effect, elevates the seizure threshold, produces skeletal muscle relaxation.

USES
Anxiety, acute alcohol withdrawal, adjunct in seizure disorders, skeletal muscle spasm; conscious sedation in dentistry

PHARMACOKINETICS

Route	Onset	Peak	Duration
PO	30 min	1–2 hr	2–3 hr
IV	1–5 min	15 min	15–60 min
IM	15 min	30–90 min	30–90 min

Well absorbed from the GI tract. Widely distributed. Protein binding: 98%. Metabolized in the liver to active metabolite. Excreted in urine. Minimally removed by hemodialysis. *Half-life:* 20–70 hr (increased in hepatic dysfunction and the elderly).

INDICATIONS AND DOSAGES
▶ **Anxiety, Skeletal Muscle Relaxation**
PO
Adults. 2–10 mg 2–4 times a day.
Elderly. 2.5 mg twice a day.
Children. 0.12–0.8 mg/kg/day in divided doses q6–8h.
IV, IM
Adults. 2–10 mg repeated in 3–4 hr.
Children. 0.04–0.3 mg/kg/dose q2–4h. Maximum: 0.5 mg/kg in an 8-hr period.
▶ **Preanesthesia**
IV
Adults, Elderly. 5–15 mg 5–10 min before procedure.
Children. 0.2–0.3 mg/kg. Maximum: 10 mg.
▶ **Alcohol Withdrawal**
PO
Adults, Elderly. 10 mg 3–4 times during first 24 hr, then reduced to 5–10 mg 3–4 times a day as needed.
IV, IM
Adults, Elderly. Initially, 10 mg, followed by 5–10 mg q3–4h.
▶ **Status Epilepticus**
IV
Adults, Elderly. 5–10 mg q10–15min up to 30 mg/8 hr.

Children 5 yr and older.
0.05–0.3 mg/kg/dose q15–30min. Maximum: 10 mg/dose.
Children 1 mo to younger than 5 yr.
0.05–0.3 mg/kg/dose q15–30min. Maximum: 5 mg/dose.
▶ **Control of Increased Seizure Activity in Patients with Refractory Epilepsy Who Are on Stable Regimens of Anticonvulsants**
Rectal Gel
Adults, Children 12 yr and older.
0.2 mg/kg; may be repeated in 4–12 hr.
Children 6–11 yr. 0.3 mg/kg; may be repeated in 4–12 hr.
Children 2–5 yr. 0.5 mg/kg; may be repeated in 4–12 hr.

SIDE EFFECTS/ADVERSE REACTIONS
Frequent

Pain with IM injection, somnolence, fatigue, ataxia
Occasional

Slurred speech, orthostatic hypotension, headache, hypoactivity, constipation, nausea, blurred vision
Rare

Paradoxical CNS reactions, such as hyperactivity or nervousness in children and excitement or restlessness in the elderly or debilitated (generally noted during first 2 wk of therapy, particularly in presence of uncontrolled pain)

PRECAUTIONS AND CONTRAINDICATIONS
Angle-closure glaucoma, coma, preexisting CNS depression, respiratory depression, severe, uncontrolled pain
Caution

Elderly, debilitated, hepatic disease, renal disease

DRUG INTERACTIONS OF CONCERN TO DENTISTRY
• Increased CNS depression of diazepam: alcohol, all CNS depressants, kava kava (herb)
• Increased serum levels and prolonged effect of benzodiazepines: erythromycin, clarithromycin, ketoconazole, itraconazole, fluconazole, miconazole (systemic), cimetidine, rifamycin
• Contraindicated with saquinavir
• Possible increase in CNS side effects: kava kava (herb)

SERIOUS REACTIONS
❗ IV administration may produce pain, swelling, thrombophlebitis, and carpal tunnel syndrome.
❗ Abrupt or too-rapid withdrawal may result in pronounced restlessness, irritability, insomnia, hand tremor, abdominal or muscle cramps, diaphoresis, vomiting, and seizures.
❗ Abrupt withdrawal in patients with epilepsy may produce an increase in the frequency or severity of seizures.
❗ Overdose results in somnolence, confusion, diminished reflexes, and coma.

DENTAL CONSIDERATIONS
General:
• Assess salivary flow as a factor in caries, periodontal disease, and candidiasis.
• After supine positioning, have patient sit upright for at least 2 min before standing to avoid orthostatic hypotension.
• Psychologic and physical dependence may occur with chronic administration.
• Geriatric patients are more susceptible to drug effects; use lower dose.

• Have someone drive patient to and from dental appointment when drug used for conscious sedation.
• Provide assistance when escorting patient to and from dental chair when dizziness occurs.
• Avoid use of this drug in a patient with a history of drug abuse or alcoholism.

Teach Patient/Family to:
• Use effective oral hygiene to prevent soft tissue inflammation
• When chronic dry mouth occurs, advise patient to:
  • Avoid mouth rinses with high alcohol content because of drying effects
  • Use daily home fluoride products for anticaries effect
  • Use sugarless gum, frequent sips of water, or saliva substitutes

diclofenac
dye-kloe´-fen-ak
(Cataflam, Diclohexal[AUS], Diclotek[CAN], Fenac[AUS], Novo-Difenac[CAN], Solaraze, Voltaren, Voltaren Emulgel[AUS], Voltaren Ophthalmic, Voltaren Rapid[AUS], Voltaren XR)
Do not confuse diclofenac with Diflucan or Duphalac, or Voltaren with Verelan.

CATEGORY AND SCHEDULE
Pregnancy Risk Category: X

Drug Class: Nonsteroidal anti-inflammatory

MECHANISM OF ACTION
An NSAID that inhibits prostaglandin synthesis, reducing the intensity of pain. Also constricts the

iris sphincter. May inhibit angiogenesis (the formation of blood vessels) by inhibiting substance P or blocking the angiogenic effects of prostaglandin E. *Therapeutic Effect:* Produces analgesic and anti-inflammatory effects. Prevents miosis during cataract surgery. May reduce angiogenesis in inflamed tissue.

USES
Treatment of acute, chronic rheumatoid arthritis, osteoarthritis, ankylosing spondylitis, analgesia

PHARMACOKINETICS

Route	Onset	Peak	Duration
PO	30 min	2–3 hr	Up to 8 hr

Completely absorbed from the GI tract; penetrates cornea after ophthalmic administration (may be systemically absorbed). Protein binding: greater than 99%. Widely distributed. Metabolized in the liver. Primarily excreted in urine. Minimally removed by hemodialysis. *Half-life:* 1.2–2 hr.

INDICATIONS AND DOSAGES
▶ **Osteoarthritis**
PO (Cataflam, Voltaren)
Adults, Elderly. 50 mg 2–3 times a day.
PO (Voltaren XR)
Adults, Elderly. 100 mg/day as a single dose.
▶ **Rheumatoid Arthritis**
PO (Cataflam, Voltaren)
Adults, Elderly. 50 mg 2–4 times a day. Maximum: 225 mg/day.
PO (Voltaren XR)
Adults, Elderly. 100 mg once a day. Maximum: 100 mg twice a day.
▶ **Ankylosing Spondylitis**
PO (Voltaren)

Adults, Elderly. 100–125 mg/day in 4–5 divided doses.
▶ **Analgesia, Primary Dysmenorrhea**
PO (Cataflam)
Adults, Elderly. 30 mg 3 times a day.
▶ **Usual Pediatric Dosage**
Children. 2–3 mg/kg/day in 2–4 divided doses.
▶ **Actinic Keratoses**
Topical
Adults, Adolescents. Apply twice a day to lesion for 60–90 days.
▶ **Cataract Surgery**
Ophthalmic
Adults, Elderly. Apply 1 drop to eye 4 times a day commencing 24 hr after cataract surgery. Continue for 2 wk afterward.
▶ **Pain, Relief of Photophobia in Patients Undergoing Corneal Refractive Surgery**
Ophthalmic
Adults, Elderly. Apply 1 drop to affected eye 1 hr before surgery, within 15 min after surgery, then 4 times a day for 3 days.

SIDE EFFECTS/ADVERSE REACTIONS
Frequent
PO: Headache, abdominal cramps, constipation, diarrhea, nausea, dyspepsia
Ophthalmic: Burning or stinging on instillation, ocular discomfort
Occasional
PO: Flatulence, dizziness, epigastric pain
Ophthalmic: Ocular itching or tearing
Rare
PO: Rash, peripheral edema or fluid retention, visual disturbances, vomiting, drowsiness

PRECAUTIONS AND CONTRAINDICATIONS
Hypersensitivity to aspirin, diclofenac, and other NSAIDs; porphyria

Caution

Lactation, children, bleeding disorders, GI disorders, cardiac disorders, hypersensitivity to other anti-inflammatory agents

DRUG INTERACTIONS OF CONCERN TO DENTISTRY

• Use with caution in patients with cardiovascular disease at risk of thromboembolism
• GI ulceration, bleeding: aspirin, alcohol, corticosteroids, potassium supplements
• Nephrotoxicity: acetaminophen (prolonged use)
• Possible risk of decreased renal function: cyclosporine
• When prescribed for dental pain:
  • Risk of increased effects: oral anticoagulants, oral antidiabetics, lithium, methotrexate
  • Decreased antihypertensive effects of diuretics, β-adrenergic blockers, and ACE inhibitors
  • First-time users of SSRIs also taking NSAIDs may have a higher risk of GI side effects; until more data are available, it may be advisable to avoid use of NSAIDs in these patients (Br J Clin Pharmacol 55:591–595, 2003)

Diclofenac Sodium (Voltaren)

None reported

SERIOUS REACTIONS

! Overdose may result in acute renal failure.
! Rare reactions with long-term use include peptic ulcer disease, GI bleeding, gastritis, a severe hepatic reaction (jaundice), nephrotoxicity (hematuria, dysuria, proteinuria), and a severe hypersensitivity reaction (bronchospasm or angioedema).

DENTAL CONSIDERATIONS

General:

• Patients on chronic drug therapy may rarely have symptoms of blood dyscrasias, which can include infection, bleeding, and poor healing.
• Assess salivary flow as a factor in caries, periodontal disease, and candidiasis.
• Avoid prescribing for dental use in pregnancy.
• Avoid prescribing aspirin-containing products.
• Consider semisupine chair position for patients with rheumatic disease.
• Advise patient if dental drugs prescribed have a potential for photosensitivity.

Consultations:

• In a patient with symptoms of blood dyscrasias, request a medical consultation for blood studies and postpone dental treatment until normal values are reestablished.
• Medical consultation may be required to assess disease control.

Teach Patient/Family to:

• Use effective oral hygiene to prevent soft tissue inflammation
• Use caution to prevent injury when using oral hygiene aids
• When chronic dry mouth occurs, advise patient to:
  • Avoid mouth rinses with high alcohol content because of drying effects
  • Use daily home fluoride products for anticaries effect
  • Use sugarless gum, frequent sips of water, or saliva substitutes

Diclofenac Sodium (Voltaren)

General:

• Determine why patient is taking the drug.
• Protect patient's eyes from accidental spatter during dental treatment.
• Avoid dental light in patient's eyes; offer dark glasses for patient comfort.

dicloxacillin sodium
dye-klox´-ah-sill-in soe´-dee-um
(Dycil, Pathocil)

CATEGORY AND SCHEDULE
Pregnancy Risk Category: B

Drug Class: Penicillinase-
resistant penicillin

MECHANISM OF ACTION
A penicillin that acts as a bactericidal
in susceptible microorganisms.
Therapeutic Effect: Inhibits bacterial
cell wall synthesis.

USES
Treatment of infections caused by
penicillinase-producing Staphylococcus

PHARMACOKINETICS
Well absorbed from GI tract. Rate
and extent reduced by food.
Distributed throughout body
including CSF. Protein binding: 96%.
Partially metabolized in liver.
Primarily excreted in feces and urine.
Not removed by hemodialysis.
Half-life: 0.7 hr.

INDICATIONS AND DOSAGES
▶ **Respiratory Tract Infection,
Staphylococcal and Streptococcal
Infections**
PO
*Adults, Elderly, Children weighing
more than 40 kg.* 125–250 mg q6h.
Children weighing less than 40 kg.
12.5–25 mg/kg/day q6h.

SIDE EFFECTS/ADVERSE
REACTIONS
Frequent
GI disturbances (mild diarrhea,
nausea, or vomiting), headache
Occasional
Generalized rash, urticaria

PRECAUTIONS AND
CONTRAINDICATIONS
Hypersensitivity to any penicillin
Caution
Hypersensitivity to cephalosporins

DRUG INTERACTIONS OF
CONCERN TO DENTISTRY
• Tetracyclines: reduced
effectiveness of dicloxacillin

SERIOUS REACTIONS
! Altered bacterial balance may
result in potentially fatal
superinfections and antibiotic-
associated colitis as evidenced by
abdominal cramps, watery or severe
diarrhea, and fever.
! Severe hypersensitivity reactions,
including anaphylaxis and acute
interstitial nephritis occur rarely.

DENTAL CONSIDERATIONS
General:
• Take precautions regarding allergy
to medication.
• Determine why the patient is
taking the drug.
Consultations:
• Concern for drug of choice if
dental infection is also present.
Teach Patient/Family to:
• Use effective oral hygiene to
prevent soft tissue inflammation
• Use caution to prevent trauma
when using oral hygiene aids
• When used for dental infection,
advise patient to:
   • Use additional method of
   contraception for duration of cycle
   (females)
   • Report sore throat, oral burning
   sensation, fever, and fatigue, any of
   which could indicate
   superinfection
   • Take at prescribed intervals and
   complete dosage regimen
   • Immediately notify the dentist if
   signs or symptoms of infection
   increase

dicyclomine hydrochloride

dye-sye´-kloe-meen
hye-droe-klor´-ide
(Bentyl, Bentylol[CAN],
Formulex[CAN], Lomine[CAN],
Merbentyl[AUS])
Do not confuse dicyclomine
with doxycycline or dyclonime,
or Bentyl with Aventyl or
Benadryl.

CATEGORY AND SCHEDULE

Pregnancy Risk Category: B

Drug Class: GI anticholinergic

MECHANISM OF ACTION

A GI antispasmodic and
anticholinergic agent that directly
acts as a relaxant on smooth muscle.
Therapeutic Effect: Reduces tone
and motility of GI tract.

USES

Treatment of irritable bowel
syndrome

PHARMACOKINETICS

Route	Onset	Peak	Duration
PO	1–2 hr	N/A	4 hr

Readily absorbed from the GI tract.
Widely distributed. Metabolized in
the liver. Half-life: 9–10 hr.

INDICATIONS AND DOSAGES
▸ **Functional Disturbances of GI Motility**
PO
Adults. 10–20 mg 3–4 times a day up
to 40 mg 4 times a day.
Children older than 2 yr. 10 mg
3–4 times a day.
Children 6 mos–2 yr. 5 mg 3–4 times
a day.

Elderly. 10–20 mg 4 times a day.
May increase up to 160 mg/day.
IM
Adults. 20 mg q4–6h.

SIDE EFFECTS/ADVERSE REACTIONS

Frequent
Dry mouth (sometimes severe),
constipation, diminished sweating
ability
Occasional
Blurred vision; photophobia; urinary
hesitancy; somnolence (with high
dosage); agitation, excitement,
confusion, or somnolence noted in
elderly (even with low dosages);
transient light-headedness (with IM
route), irritation at injection site
(with IM route)
Rare
Confusion, hypersensitivity reaction,
increased intraocular pressure,
nausea, vomiting, unusual fatigue

PRECAUTIONS AND CONTRAINDICATIONS

Bladder neck obstruction due to
prostatic hyperplasia, coronary
vasospasm, intestinal atony,
myasthenia gravis in patients not
treated with neostigmine, narrow-
angle glaucoma, obstructive disease
of the GI tract, paralytic ileus, severe
ulcerative colitis, tachycardia
secondary to cardiac insufficiency or
thyrotoxicosis, toxic megacolon,
unstable cardiovascular status in
acute hemorrhage
Caution
Hyperthyroidism, CAD,
dysrhythmias, CHF, ulcerative colitis,
hypertension, hiatal hernia, hepatic
disease, renal disease, urinary
retention, prostatic hypertrophy

DRUG INTERACTIONS OF CONCERN TO DENTISTRY
• Increased anticholinergic effect: atropine, scopolamine, other anticholinergics, meperidine
• Decreased effect of ketoconazole

SERIOUS REACTIONS
! Overdose may produce temporary paralysis of ciliary muscle; pupillary dilation; tachycardia; palpitations; hot, dry, or flushed skin; absence of bowel sounds; hyperthermia; increased respiratory rate; ECG abnormalities; nausea; vomiting; rash over face or upper trunk; CNS stimulation (marked by agitation, restlessness, rambling speech, visual hallucinations, paranoid behavior, and delusions, followed by depression).

DENTAL CONSIDERATIONS
General:
• Assess salivary flow as a factor in caries, periodontal disease, and candidiasis.
• Avoid dental light in patient's eyes; offer dark glasses for patient comfort.
Consultation:
• Physician should be informed if significant xerostomic side effects occur (e.g., increased caries, sore tongue, problems eating or swallowing, difficulty wearing prosthesis) so that a medication change can be considered.
Teach Patient/Family to:
• Use effective oral hygiene to prevent soft tissue inflammation
• When chronic dry mouth occurs, advise patient to:
  • Avoid mouth rinses with high alcohol content because of drying effects
  • Use daily home fluoride products for anticaries effect
  • Use sugarless gum, frequent sips of water, or saliva substitutes

didanosine
dye-dan´-oh-seen
(Videx, Videx-EC)

CATEGORY AND SCHEDULE
Pregnancy Risk Category: B

Drug Class: Synthetic antiviral, nucleoside analog

MECHANISM OF ACTION
A purine nucleoside analog that is intracellularly converted into a triphosphate, which interferes with RNA-directed DNA polymerase (reverse transcriptase). ***Therapeutic Effect:*** Inhibits replication of retroviruses, including HIV.

USES
Treatment of advanced HIV infections in adults and children who have been unable to use zidovudine or who have not responded to treatment; used in combination with other antiretroviral drugs

PHARMACOKINETICS
Variably absorbed from the GI tract. Protein binding: less than 5%. Rapidly metabolized intracellularly to active form. Primarily excreted in urine. Partially (20%) removed by hemodialysis. ***Half-life:*** 1.5 hr; metabolite: 8–24 hr.

INDICATIONS AND DOSAGES
▸ **HIV Infection (in combination with other antiretrovirals)**
PO (Chewable Tablets)
Adults, Children 13 yr and older weighing 60 kg or more. 200 mg q12h or 400 mg once a day.

Adults, Children 13 yr and older weighing 60 kg or less. 125 mg q12h or 250 mg once a day.
Children 3 mo to less than 13 yr. 180–300 mg/m2/day in divided doses q12h.
Children younger than 3 mo. 50 mg/m^2/day in divided doses q12h.
PO (Delayed-Release Capsules)
Adults, Children 13 yr and older, weighing 60 kg or more. 400 mg once a day.
Adults, Children 13 yr and older, weighing 60 kg or less. 250 mg once a day.
PO (Oral Solution)
Adults, Children 13 yr and older weighing 60 kg or more. 250 mg q12h.
Adults, Children 13 yr and older weighing 60 kg or less.
167 mg q12h.
PO (Pediatric Powder for Oral Solution)
Children 3 mo to younger than 13 yr. 180–300 mg/m2/day in divided doses q12h.
Children younger than 3 mo. 50 mg/m^2/day in divided doses q12h.

▸ **Dosage in Renal Impairment**

CrCl	Tablets	Oral Solution	Delayed-Release Capsules
30–59 ml/min	75 mg twice a day	100 mg twice a day	125 mg once a day
10–29 ml/min	100 mg once a day	100 mg once a day	125 mg once a day
Less than 10ml/min	75 mg once a day	100 mg once a day	N/A

CrCl = creatinine clearance

Patients weighing 60 kg or more:

CrCl	Tablets	Oral Solution	Delayed-Release Capsules
30–59 ml/min	100 mg twice a day	10 mg twice a day	200 mg once a day
10–29 ml/min	150 mg once a day	167 mg once a day	125 mg once a day
Less than 10 ml/min	100 mg once a day	100 mg once a day	125 mg once a day

CrCl = creatinine clearance

SIDE EFFECTS/ADVERSE REACTIONS
Frequent
Adults Diarrhea, neuropathy, chills and fever
Children Chills, fever, decreased appetite, pain, malaise, nausea, vomiting, diarrhea, abdominal pain, headache, nervousness, cough, rhinitis, dyspnea, asthenia, rash, pruritus
Occasional
Adults Rash, pruritus, headache, abdominal pain, nausea, vomiting, pneumonia, myopathy, decreased appetite, dry mouth, dyspnea
Children Failure to thrive, weight loss, stomatitis, oral thrush, ecchymosis, arthritis, myalgia, insomnia, epistaxis, pharyngitis

PRECAUTIONS AND CONTRAINDICATIONS
Hypersensitivity to didanosine or any of its components
Caution
Renal disease, hepatic disease, lactation, children, sodium-restricted diets; pancreatitis

(in combination with stavudine); lactic acidosis, severe hepatomegaly

DRUG INTERACTIONS OF CONCERN TO DENTISTRY
• Decreased absorption of the following drugs: ketoconazole, dapsone, itraconazole, tetracyclines, fluoroquinolone antibiotics
• Increased risk of pancreatitis: metronidazole, sulfonamides, sulindac, tetracyclines
• Increased risk of peripheral neuropathy: metronidazole, nitrous oxide

SERIOUS REACTIONS
! Pneumonia and opportunistic infections occur occasionally.
! Peripheral neuropathy, potentially fatal pancreatitis, retinal changes, and optic neuritis are the major toxic effects.

DENTAL CONSIDERATIONS
General:
• Monitor vital signs at every appointment because of cardiovascular side effects.
• Avoid dental light in patient's eyes; offer dark glasses for patient comfort.
• Patients on chronic drug therapy may rarely have symptoms of blood dyscrasias, which can include infection, bleeding, and poor healing.
Consultations:
• Medical consultation may be required to assess patient's ability to tolerate stress.
• In a patient with symptoms of blood dyscrasias, request a medical consultation for blood studies and postpone dental treatment until normal values are reestablished.
Teach Patient/Family to:
• Use effective oral hygiene to prevent soft tissue inflammation

• Use caution to prevent injury when using oral hygiene aids
• When chronic dry mouth occurs, advise patient to:
  • Avoid mouth rinses with high alcohol content because of drying effects
  • Use daily home fluoride products for anticaries effect
  • Use sugarless gum, frequent sips of water, or saliva substitutes

diethylpropion
die-ethyl-prop´-ion
(Tenuate, Teuante Dospan)

CATEGORY AND SCHEDULE
Pregnancy Risk Category: B
Controlled Substance: Schedule IV

Drug Class: Anorexiant, amphetamine-like

MECHANISM OF ACTION
A sympathomimetic amine that stimulates the release of norepinephrine and dopamine. *Therapeutic Effect:* Decreases appetite.

USES
Treatment of exogenous obesity

PHARMACOKINETICS
Rapidly absorbed from the GI tract. Widely distributed. Metabolized in liver to active metabolite and undergoes extensive first-pass metabolism. Excreted in urine. Unknown if removed by hemodialysis. *Half-life:* 4–6 hr.

INDICATIONS AND DOSAGES
▶ **Obesity**
PO
Adults. 25 mg 3 times a day before meals. Extended-release: 75 mg at midmorning.

SIDE EFFECTS/ADVERSE REACTIONS
Frequent
Elevated B/P, nervousness, insomnia
Occasional
Dizziness, drowsiness, tremors, headache, nausea, stomach pain, fever, rash
Rare
Agranulocytosis, leukopenia, blurred vision, psychosis, CVA, seizure

PRECAUTIONS AND CONTRAINDICATIONS
Agitated states, use of MAOIs within 14 days, glaucoma, history of drug abuse, hyperthyroidism, advanced arteriosclerosis or severe cardiovascular disease, severe hypertension, and hypersensitivity to sympathomimetic amines
Caution
Convulsive disorders, lactation

DRUG INTERACTIONS OF CONCERN TO DENTISTRY
• Dysrhythmia: hydrocarbon inhalation anesthetics
• Decreased effects: barbiturates, tricyclic antidepressants, phenothiazines

SERIOUS REACTIONS
! Overdose may produce agitation, tachycardia, palpitations, cardiac irregularities, chest pain, psychotic episode, seizures, and coma.
! Hypersensitivity reactions and blood dyscrasias occur rarely.

DENTAL CONSIDERATIONS
General:
• Monitor vital signs at every appointment because of cardiovascular and respiratory side effects.

• Examine for evidence of oral manifestations of blood dyscrasias (infection, bleeding, poor healing).
• Assess salivary flow as a factor in caries, periodontal disease, and candidiasis.
• Psychologic and physical dependence may occur with chronic administration.
• Consider semisupine chair position for patient comfort because of GI effects of disease.
Consultations:
• Medical consultation for blood studies (e.g., CBC); leukopenic or thrombocytopenic side effects may result in infection, delayed healing, and excessive bleeding. Postpone dental treatment until normal values are maintained.
Teach Patient/Family to:
• Use effective oral hygiene to prevent soft tissue inflammation
• Use caution in use of oral hygiene aids to prevent injury
• When chronic dry mouth occurs, advise patient to:
  • Avoid mouth rinses with high alcohol content because of drying effects
  • Use daily home fluoride products for anticaries effect
  • Use sugarless gum, frequent sips of water, or saliva substitutes

diflorasone
die-floor´-ah-sone
(Florone[CAN], Maxiflor, Psorcon, Psorcon-e)

CATEGORY AND SCHEDULE
Pregnancy Risk Category: C

Drug Class: Topical corticosteroid, group II high potency

MECHANISM OF ACTION
A high-potency, fluorinated corticosteroid that decreases inflammation by suppression of migration of polymorphonuclear leukocytes and reversal of increased capillary permeability. The exact mechanism of the antiinflammatory process is unclear. *Therapeutic Effect:* Decreases or prevents tissue response to the inflammatory process.

USES
Treatment of psoriasis, eczema, contact dermatitis, pruritus

PHARMACOKINETICS
Poor absorption; occlusive dressings increase absorption. Metabolized in liver. Primarily excreted in urine.

INDICATIONS AND DOSAGES
▶ **Dermatoses**
Topical
Adults, Elderly. (Cream) Apply sparingly 2–4 times a day. (Ointment) Apply sparingly 1–3 times a day.

SIDE EFFECTS/ADVERSE REACTIONS
Rare
Itching, redness, dryness, irritation, burning at site of application, arthralgia, folliculitis, maceration, muscle atrophy, secondary infection

PRECAUTIONS AND CONTRAINDICATIONS
History of hypersensitivity to diflorasone or other corticosteroids
Caution
Lactation, viral infections, bacterial infections

SERIOUS REACTIONS
! Overdosage symptoms include moon face, central obesity, hypertension, diabetes, hyperlipidemia, peptic ulcer, increased susceptibility to infection, electrolyte and fluid imbalance, psychosis, and hallucinations.
! The serious reactions of long-term therapy and the addition of occlusive dressings are reversible hypothalamic-pituitary-adrenal (HPA) axis suppression, manifestations of Cushing's syndrome, hyperglycemia, and glucosuria.

DENTAL CONSIDERATIONS
General:
• Determine why the patient is taking the drug.
• Apply lubricant to dry lips for patient comfort before dental procedures.
• Place on frequent recall to evaluate healing response if used on chronic basis.

diflunisal
die-floo´-ni-sal
(Apo-Diflunisal[CAN], Dolobid, Novo-Diflunisal[CAN])
Do not confuse diflunisal with Dicarbosil or Dolobid with Slo-bid.

CATEGORY AND SCHEDULE
Pregnancy Risk Category: C

Drug Class: Salicylate derivative, nonsteroidal antiinflammatory

MECHANISM OF ACTION
A nonsteroidal antiinflammatory drug that inhibits prostaglandin synthesis, reducing inflammatory response and intensity of pain stimulus reaching sensory nerve endings.

D

Therapeutic Effect: Produces analgesic and antiinflammatory effect.

USES
Treatment of mild-to-moderate pain, symptoms of rheumatoid arthritis and osteoarthritis

PHARMACOKINETICS

Route	Onset	Peak	Duration
PO	1 hr	2–3 hr	8–12 hr

Completely absorbed from the GI tract. Widely distributed. Protein binding: greater than 99%. Metabolized in liver. Primarily excreted in urine. Not removed by hemodialysis. *Half-life:* 8–12 hr.

INDICATIONS AND DOSAGES
▶ **Mild-to-Moderate Pain**
PO
Adults, Elderly. Initially, 0.5–1 g, then 250–500 mg q8–12h. Maximum: 1.5 g/day.
▶ **Rheumatoid Arthritis, Osteoarthritis**
PO
Adults, Elderly. 0.5–1 g/day in 2 divided doses. Maximum: 1.5 g/day.

SIDE EFFECTS/ADVERSE REACTIONS
Side effects are less common with short-term treatment.
Occasional
Nausea, dyspepsia (heartburn, indigestion, epigastric pain), diarrhea, headache, rash
Rare
Vomiting, constipation, flatulence, dizziness, somnolence, insomnia, fatigue, tinnitus

PRECAUTIONS AND CONTRAINDICATIONS
Active GI bleeding, factor VII or factor IX deficiencies, hypersensitivity to aspirin or NSAIDs
Caution
Anemia, hepatic disease, renal disease, Hodgkin's disease, lactation

DRUG INTERACTIONS OF CONCERN TO DENTISTRY
• Increased risk of GI ulceration and bleeding: aspirin, steroids, alcohol, indomethacin, other NSAIDs
• Hepatotoxicity, nephrotoxicity: acetaminophen (prolonged use)
• Suspected increase in potential toxic effects: probenecid

SERIOUS REACTIONS
! Overdosage may produce drowsiness, vomiting, nausea, diarrhea, hyperventilation, tachycardia, diaphoresis, stupor, and coma.
! Peptic ulcer, GI bleeding, gastritis, and severe hepatic reaction, including cholestasis, jaundice occur rarely.
! Nephrotoxicity, including dysuria, hematuria, proteinuria, and nephrotic syndrome, and severe hypersensitivity reaction, marked by bronchospasm and angioedema, occur rarely.

DENTAL CONSIDERATIONS
General:
• Patients on chronic drug therapy may rarely have symptoms of blood dyscrasias, which can include infection, bleeding, and poor healing.
• Assess salivary flow as a factor in caries, periodontal disease, and candidiasis.
• Avoid prescribing for dental use in first and last trimester of pregnancy.
• Use with caution in patients with cardiovascular disease at risk for thromboembolism.

Consultations:
• Medical consultation may be required to assess disease control.
• In a patient with symptoms of blood dyscrasias, request a medical consultation for blood studies and postpone dental treatment until normal values are reestablished.
Teach Patient/Family to:
• Use effective oral hygiene to prevent soft tissue inflammation
• Prevent injury when using oral hygiene aids
• When chronic dry mouth occurs, advise patient to:
  • Avoid mouth rinses with high alcohol content because of drying effects
  • Use daily home fluoride products for anticaries effect
  • Use sugarless gum, frequent sips of water, or saliva substitutes

digoxin
di-jox´-in
(Digitek, Lanoxicaps, Lanoxin, Sigmaxin[AUS])
Do not confuse digoxin with Desoxyn or doxepin, or Lanoxin with Levsinex or Lonox.

CATEGORY AND SCHEDULE
Pregnancy Risk Category: C

Drug Class: Cardiac glycoside

MECHANISM OF ACTION
A cardiac glycoside that increases the influx of calcium from extracellular to intracellular cytoplasm.
Therapeutic Effect: Potentiates the activity of the contractile cardiac muscle fibers and increases the force of myocardial contraction. Slows the heart rate by decreasing conduction through the SA and AV nodes.

USES
Treatment of CHF, atrial fibrillation, atrial flutter, paroxysmal atrial tachycardia, rapid digitalization in these disorders

PHARMACOKINETICS

Route	Onset	Peak	Duration
PO	0.5–2 hr	28 hr	3–4 days
IV	5–30 hr	1–4 hr	3–4 days

Readily absorbed from the GI tract. Widely distributed. Protein binding: 30%. Partially metabolized in the liver. Primarily excreted in urine. Minimally removed by hemodialysis. **Half-life:** 36–48 hr (increased with impaired renal function and in the elderly).

INDICATIONS AND DOSAGES
▶ **Rapid Loading Dose for the Management and Treatment of CHF; Control of Ventricular Rate in Patients with Atrial Fibrillation; Treatment and Prevention of Recurrent Paroxysmal Atrial Tachycardia**
PO
Adults, Elderly. Initially, 0.5–0.75 mg, additional doses of 0.125–0.375 mg at 6- to 8-hr intervals. Range: 0.75–1.25 mg.
Children 10 yr and older. 10–15 mcg/kg.
Children 5–9 yr. 20–35 mcg/kg.
Children 2–4 yr. 30–40 mcg/kg.
Children 1–23 mo. 35–60 mcg/kg.
Neonate, full-term. 25–35 mcg/kg.
Neonate, premature. 20–30 mcg/kg.
IV
Adults, Elderly. 0.6–1 mg.
Children 10 yr and older. 8–12 mcg/kg.
Children 5–9 yr. 15–30 mcg/kg.
Children 2–4 yr. 25–35 mcg/kg.
Children 1–23 mo. 30–50 mcg/kg.
Neonates, full-term. 20–30 mcg/kg.
Neonates, premature. 15–25 mcg/kg.

D

▶ **Maintenance Dosage for CHF; Control of Ventricular Rate in Patients with Atrial Fibrillation; Treatment and Prevention of Recurrent Paroxysmal Atrial Tachycardia**

PO, IV

Adults, Elderly. 0.125–0.375 mg/day.
Children. 25%–35% loading dose (20%–30% for premature neonates).

▶ **Dosage in Renal Impairment**

Dosage adjustment is based on creatinine clearance. Total digitalizing dose: decrease by 50% in end-stage renal disease.

Creatinine Clearance	Dosage
10–50 ml/min	25%–75% usual
Less than 10 ml/min	10%–25% usual

SIDE EFFECTS/ADVERSE REACTIONS

None known. However, there is a very narrow margin of safety between a therapeutic and toxic result. Long-term therapy may produce mammary gland enlargement in women but is reversible when drug is withdrawn

PRECAUTIONS AND CONTRAINDICATIONS

Ventricular fibrillation, ventricular tachycardia unrelated to CHF
Caution
Renal disease, acute MI, AV block, severe respiratory disease, hypothyroidism, elderly, sinus nodal disease, lactation, hypokalemia

DRUG INTERACTIONS OF CONCERN TO DENTISTRY

• Hypokalemia: corticosteroids
• Increased digoxin blood levels: erythromycin, clarithromycin, tetracyclines, itraconazole, propantheline
• Cardiac dysrhythmias: adrenergic agonists, succinylcholine

SERIOUS REACTIONS

! The most common early manifestations of digoxin toxicity are GI disturbances (anorexia, nausea, vomiting) and neurologic abnormalities (fatigue, headache, depression, weakness, drowsiness, confusion, nightmares).
! Facial pain, personality change, and ocular disturbances (photophobia, light flashes, halos around bright objects, yellow or green color perception) may be noted.

DENTAL CONSIDERATIONS

General:
• Monitor vital signs at every appointment because of cardiovascular side effects.
• After supine positioning, have patient sit upright for at least 2 min to avoid orthostatic hypotension.
• Avoid dental light in patient's eyes; offer dark glasses for patient comfort.
• An increased gag reflex may make dental procedures, such as taking radiographs or impressions, difficult.
• Use vasoconstrictors with caution, in low doses, and with careful aspiration. Avoid use of gingival retraction cord with epinephrine.
Consultations:
• Stress from dental procedures may compromise cardiovascular function; determine patient risk.
• Use stress-reduction protocol
• Medical consultation may be required to assess disease control and patient's ability to tolerate stress.

dihydrotachysterol
dye-hye-droe-tak-ee-ster′-ole
(DHT, DHT Intensol, Hytakerol)

CATEGORY AND SCHEDULE
Pregnancy Risk Category: A
(D if used in doses above RDA)

Drug Class: Vitamin D analog

MECHANISM OF ACTION
A fat-soluble vitamin that is essential for absorption, utilization of calcium phosphate, and normal calcification of bone. *Therapeutic Effect:* Stimulates calcium and phosphate absorption from small intestine, promotes secretion of calcium from bone to blood, promotes renal tubule phosphate resorption, acts on bone cells to stimulate skeletal growth and on parathyroid gland to suppress hormone synthesis and secretion.

USES
Nutritional supplement, treatment of rickets, hypoparathyroidism, pseudo-hypoparathyroidism, postoperative tetany

PHARMACOKINETICS
Well absorbed from small intestine. Metabolized in liver. Eliminated via biliary system; excreted in urine. *Half-life:* Unknown.

INDICATIONS AND DOSAGES
▶ **Hypoparathyroidism**
PO
Adults, Elderly, Older Children. Initially, 0.8–2.4 mg/day for several days. Maintenance: 0.2–1 mg/day.
Infants, Young Children. Initially, 1–5 mg/day for 4 days, then 0.1–0.5 mg/day.

▶ **Nutritional Rickets**
PO
Adults, Elderly, Children. 0.5 mg as a single dose or 13–50 mcg/day until healing occurs.
▶ **Renal Osteodystrophy**
PO
Adults, Elderly. 0.25–0.6 mg/24 hr adjusted as needed to achieve normal serum calcium levels and promote bone healing.

SIDE EFFECTS/ADVERSE REACTIONS
Occasional
Nausea, vomiting

PRECAUTIONS AND CONTRAINDICATIONS
Hypercalcemia, malabsorption syndrome, vitamin D toxicity, hypersensitivity to vitamin D products or analogs
Caution
Renal calculi, lactation, cardiovascular disease

DRUG INTERACTIONS OF CONCERN TO DENTISTRY
• Decreased effect of dihydrotachysterol: prolonged use of corticosteroids, barbiturates

SERIOUS REACTIONS
! Early signs of overdosage are manifested as weakness, headache, somnolence, nausea, vomiting, dry mouth, constipation, muscle and bone pain, and metallic taste sensation.
! Later signs of overdosage are evidenced by polyuria, polydipsia, anorexia, weight loss, nocturia, photophobia, rhinorrhea, pruritus, disorientation, hallucinations, hyperthermia, hypertension, and cardiac arrhythmias.

General:
• Consider semisupine chair position for patient comfort because of GI effects of drug.
• Assess salivary flow as a factor in caries, periodontal disease, and candidiasis.

Teach Patient/Family:
• When chronic dry mouth occurs, advise patient to:
  • Avoid mouth rinses with high alcohol content because of drying effects
  • Use daily home fluoride products for anticaries effect
  • Use sugarless gum, frequent sips of water, or saliva substitutes

diltiazem hydrochloride

dil-tye´-ah-zem hi-droh-klor´-ide
(Apo-Diltiaz[CAN], Auscard[AUS], Cardcal[AUS], Cardizem, Cardizem CD, Cardizem LA, Cardizem SR, Cartia, Coras[AUS], Dilacor XR, Diltahexal[AUS], Diltia XT, Diltiamax[AUS], Dilzem[AUS], Novo-Diltiazem[CAN], Taztia XT, Tiazac, Vasocardal CD[AUS])
Do not confuse Cardizem with Cardene or Cardene SR, or Tiazac with Ziac.

CATEGORY AND SCHEDULE
Pregnancy Risk Category: C

Drug Class: Calcium channel blocker

MECHANISM OF ACTION
An antianginal, antihypertensive, and antiarrhythmic agent that inhibits calcium movement across cardiac and vascular smooth-muscle cell membranes. This action causes the dilation of coronary arteries, peripheral arteries, and arterioles. *Therapeutic Effect:* Decreases heart rate and myocardial contractility, slows SA and AV conduction, and decreases total peripheral vascular resistance by vasodilation.

USES
Treatment of chronic stable angina pectoris, vasospastic angina, coronary artery spasm, hypertension, supraventricular tachydysrhythmias

PHARMACOKINETICS

Route	Onset	Peak	Duration
PO	0.5–1 hr	N/A	
PO (extended release)	2–3 hr	N/A	
IV	3 min	N/A	

Well absorbed from the GI tract.
Protein binding: 70%–80%.
Undergoes first-pass metabolism in the liver to active metabolite.
Primarily excreted in urine.
Not removed by hemodialysis.
Half-life: 3–8 hr.

INDICATIONS AND DOSAGES
▶ **Angina Related to Coronary Artery Spasm (Prinzmetal's Variant), Chronic Stable Angina (Effort-Associated)**
PO
Adults, Elderly. Initially, 30 mg 4 times a day. Increase up to 180–360 mg/day in 3–4 divided doses at 1- to 2-day intervals.
PO (Cardizem LA)
Adults, Elderly. Initially, 180 mg/day. May increase at intervals of 7–14 days up to 360 mg/day.
PO (Cardizem CD)

Adults, Elderly. Initially, 120–180 mg/day; titrate over 7–14 days. Range: Up to 480 mg/day.

▶ **Essential Hypertension**

PO (Cardizem CD, Cartia XT)
Adults, Elderly. Initially, 180–240 mg once a day. May increase at 2-wk intervals. Maintenance 240–360 mg/day. Maximum: 480 mg once a day.
PO (Cardizem SR)
Adults, Elderly. Initially, 60–120 mg twice a day. May increase at 2-wk intervals.
Maintenance: 240–360 mg/day.
PO (Cardizem LA)
Adults, Elderly. Initially, 180–240 mg once a day. May increase at 2-wk intervals. Maintenance: 120–540 mg/day.
PO (Dilacor XR)
Adults, Elderly. 180–240 mg once a day.
PO (Dilacor XT)
Adults, Elderly. Initially, 180–240 mg a day. May increase at 2-wk intervals. Maximum: 540 mg once a day.
PO (Taztia XT)
Adults, Elderly. Initially, 120–240 mg once a day. May increase at 2-wk intervals. Maximum: 540 mg once a day.

▶ **Temporary Control of Rapid Ventricular Rate in Atrial Fibrillation or Flutter, Rapid Conversion of Paroxysmal Supraventricular Tachycardia to Normal Sinus Rhythm.**

IV push
Adults, Elderly. Initially, 0.25 mg/kg actual body weight over 2 min. May repeat in 15 min at dose of 0.35 mg/kg actual body weight. Subsequent doses individualized.
IV Infusion
Adults, Elderly.
After initial bolus injection, may begin infusion at 5–10 mg/hr; may increase by 5 mg/hr up to a maximum of 15 mg/hr. Infusion duration should not exceed 24 hr.

SIDE EFFECTS/ADVERSE REACTIONS

Frequent
Peripheral edema, dizziness, light-headedness, headache, bradycardia, asthenia (loss of strength, weakness)
Occasional
Nausea, constipation, flushing, ECG changes
Rare
Rash, micturition disorder (polyuria, nocturia, dysuria, frequency of urination), abdominal discomfort, somnolence

PRECAUTIONS AND CONTRAINDICATIONS

Acute MI, pulmonary congestion, severe hypotension (less than 90 mm Hg, systolic), sick sinus syndrome, second- or third-degree AV block (except in the presence of a pacemaker)
Caution
CHF, hypotension, hepatic injury, lactation, children, renal disease

DRUG INTERACTIONS OF CONCERN TO DENTISTRY

• Decreased effect: indomethacin, possibly other NSAIDs, phenobarbital
• Increased effect: parenteral and inhalational general anesthetics, other drugs with hypotensive actions
• Increased effects of carbamazepine, midazolam, triazolam, buspirone

SERIOUS REACTIONS

❗ Abrupt withdrawal may increase frequency or duration of angina.
❗ CHF and second- and third-degree AV block occur rarely.

! Overdose produces nausea, somnolence, confusion, slurred speech, and profound bradycardia.

DENTAL CONSIDERATIONS

General:
• Monitor cardiac status; take vital signs at each appointment because of cardiovascular side effects. Consider a stress reduction protocol to prevent stress-induced angina during the dental appointment.
• After supine positioning, have patient sit upright for at least 2 min to avoid orthostatic hypotension.
• Place on frequent recall to monitor possible gingival enlargement.
• Limit use of sodium-containing products, such as saline IV fluids, for patients with a dietary salt restriction.
• Assess salivary flow as a factor in caries, periodontal disease, and candidiasis.
• Consider drug in diagnosis of taste alterations.
Consultations:
• Medical consultation may be required to assess disease control.
Teach Patient/Family to:
• Use effective oral hygiene to prevent soft tissue inflammation and minimize gingival overgrowth
• Schedule frequent oral prophylaxis if gingival overgrowth occurs
• When chronic dry mouth occurs, advise patient to:
  • Avoid mouth rinses with high alcohol content because of drying effects
  • Use daily home fluoride products for anticaries effect
  • Use sugarless gum, frequent sips of water, or saliva substitutes

dimenhydrinate
dye-men-hye´-dri-nate
(Dramamine)

CATEGORY AND SCHEDULE
Pregnancy Risk Category: B

Drug Class: H_1-receptor antagonist (equal parts diphenhydramine and chlorotheophylline)

MECHANISM OF ACTION
An antihistamine and anticholinergic that competes for H_1 receptor sites on effector cells of the GI tract, blood vessels, and respiratory tract. The anticholinergic action diminishes vestibular stimulation and depresses labyrinthine function. **Therapeutic Effect:** Prevents symptoms of motion sickness.

USES
Treatment of motion sickness, nausea, vomiting, vertigo

PHARMACOKINETICS
IM/PO: Duration 4–6 hr.

INDICATIONS AND DOSAGES
▸ **Motion Sickness**
PO
Adults, Elderly, Children older than 12 yr. 50–100 mg q4–6h. Maximum: 400 mg/day.
Children 6–12 yr. 25–50 mg q6–8h. Maximum: 150 mg/day.
Children 2–5 yr. 12.5–25 mg q6–8h. Maximum: 75 mg/day.

SIDE EFFECTS/ADVERSE REACTIONS
Frequent
Dry mouth

Occasional

Hypotension, palpitations, tachycardia, headache, somnolence, dizziness, paradoxical stimulation (especially in children), anorexia, constipation, dysuria, blurred vision, tinnitus, wheezing, chest tightness
Rare

Photosensitivity, rash, urticaria

PRECAUTIONS AND CONTRAINDICATIONS

Hypersensitivity to narcotics, shock
Caution

Children, cardiac dysrhythmias, elderly, asthma, prostatic hypertrophy, bladder neck obstruction, narrow-angle glaucoma, stenosing peptic ulcer, pyloroduodenal obstruction, may mask ototoxicity of ototoxic antibiotics.

DRUG INTERACTIONS OF CONCERN TO DENTISTRY

• Increased photosensitization: tetracycline
• Increased effects of alcohol, other CNS depressants, anticholinergics

SERIOUS REACTIONS

None significant

DENTAL CONSIDERATIONS

General:
• Assess salivary flow as a factor in caries, periodontal disease, and candidiasis.
Teach Patient/Family to:
• When chronic dry mouth occurs, advise patient to:
  • Avoid mouth rinses with high alcohol content because of drying effects
  • Use daily home fluoride products for anticaries effect
  • Use sugarless gum, frequent sips of water, or saliva substitutes

diphenhydramine

dye-fen-hye´-dra-meen
(Allerdryl[CAN], Banophen, Benadryl, Diphen, Diphenhist, Genahist, Nytol[CAN], Unisom Sleepgels[AUS])
Do not confuse diphenhydramine with dimenhydrinate, or Benadryl with benazepril, Bentyl, or Benylin, or Banophen with baclofen.

CATEGORY AND SCHEDULE

Pregnancy Risk Category: B
OTC (capsules, tablets, chewable tablets, syrup, elixir, cream, spray)

Drug Class: Antihistamine, H_1-receptor antagonist

MECHANISM OF ACTION

An ethanolamine that competitively blocks the effects of histamine at peripheral H_1 receptor sites.
Therapeutic Effect: Produces anticholinergic, antipruritic, antitussive, antiemetic, antidyskinetic, and sedative effects.

USES

Allergy symptoms, rhinitis, motion sickness, antiparkinsonism, nighttime sedation, infant colic, nonproductive cough; unlabeled use for dental local anesthesia

PHARMACOKINETICS

Route	Onset	Peak	Duration
PO	15–30 min	1–4 hr	4–6 hr
IV, IM	Less than 15 min	1–4 hr	4–6 hr

Well absorbed after PO or parenteral administration. Protein binding: 98%–99%. Widely distributed.

Metabolized in the liver. Primarily excreted in urine. *Half-life:* 1–4 hr.

INDICATIONS AND DOSAGES
▸ **Moderate to Severe Allergic Reaction, Dystonic Reaction**
PO, IV, IM
Adults, Elderly. 25–50 mg q4h.
Maximum: 400 mg/day.
Children. 5 mg/kg/day in divided doses
q6–8h. Maximum: 300 mg/day.
▸ **Motion Sickness, Minor Allergic Rhinitis**
PO, IV, IM
Adults, Elderly, Children 12 yr and older. 25–50 mg q4–6h. Maximum: 300 mg/day.
Children 6–11 yr. 12.5–25 mg q4–6h. Maximum: 150 mg/day.
Children 2–5 yr. 6.25 mg q4–6h. Maximum: 37.5 mg/day.
▸ **Antitussive**
PO
Adults, Elderly, Children 12 yr and older. 25 mg q4h. Maximum: 150 mg/day.
Children 6–11 yr. 12.5 mg q4h. Maximum: 75 mg/day.
Children 2–5 yr. 6.25 mg q4h. Maximum: 37.5 mg/day.
▸ **Nighttime Sleep Aid**
PO
Adults, Elderly, Children 12 yr and older. 50 mg at bedtime.
Children 2–11 yr. 1 mg/kg/dose. Maximum: 50 mg.
▸ **Pruritus**
Topical
Adults, Elderly, Children 12 yr and older. Apply 1% or 2% cream or spray 3–4 times a day.
Children 2–11 yr. Apply 1% cream or spray 3–4 times a day.

SIDE EFFECTS/ADVERSE REACTIONS
Frequent
Somnolence, dizziness, muscle weakness, hypotension, urine retention, thickening of bronchial secretions, dry mouth, nose, throat, or lips; in elderly, sedation, dizziness, hypotension
Occasional
Epigastric distress, flushing, visual or hearing disturbances, paresthesia, diaphoresis, chills

PRECAUTIONS AND CONTRAINDICATIONS
Acute exacerbation of asthma, use within 14 days of MAOIs
Caution
Increased intraocular pressure, renal disease, cardiac disease, hypertension, bronchial asthma, seizure disorder, stenosed peptic ulcers, hyperthyroidism, prostatic hypertrophy, bladder neck obstruction

DRUG INTERACTIONS OF CONCERN TO DENTISTRY
● Increased CNS depression: all CNS depressants, alcohol
● Increased anticholinergic effect: anticholinergics
● Increased plasma levels of labetalol

SERIOUS REACTIONS
❗ Hypersensitivity reactions, such as eczema, pruritus, rash, cardiac disturbances, and photosensitivity, may occur.
❗ Overdose symptoms may vary from CNS depression, including sedation, apnea, hypotension, cardiovascular collapse, and death, to severe paradoxical reactions, such as hallucinations, tremors, and seizures.
❗ Children and neonates may experience paradoxical reactions,

including restlessness, insomnia, euphoria, nervousness, and tremors.
! Overdosage in children may result in hallucinations, seizures, and death.

DENTAL CONSIDERATIONS
General:
• Patients on chronic drug therapy may rarely have symptoms of blood dyscrasias, which can include infection, bleeding, and poor healing.
• Assess salivary flow as a factor in caries, periodontal disease, and candidiasis.
• Consider semisupine chair position for patients with respiratory disease.
Consultations:
• In a patient with symptoms of blood dyscrasias, request a medical consultation for blood studies and postpone dental treatment until normal values are reestablished.
Teach Patient/Family to:
• Use effective oral hygiene to prevent soft tissue inflammation
• Use caution to prevent injury when using oral hygiene aids
• When chronic dry mouth occurs, advise patient to:
  • Avoid mouth rinses with high alcohol content because of drying effects
  • Use daily home fluoride products for anticaries effect
  • Use sugarless gum, frequent sips of water, or saliva substitutes

dipivefrin hydrochloride
die-pih´-ve-frin hi-droh-klor´-ide
(Propine)

CATEGORY AND SCHEDULE
Pregnancy Risk Category: B

Drug Class: Adrenergic agonist

MECHANISM OF ACTION
A prodrug of epinephrine that penetrates into anterior chamber of the eye through its lipophilic character. **Therapeutic Effect:** Reduces intraocular pressure.

USES
Treatment of open-angle glaucoma

PHARMACOKINETICS
Onset of action occurs within 30 min and peak effect in 1 hr. Dipivefrin is more lipophilic than epinephrine. Distributed to cornea. Dipivefrin is converted to epinephrine inside the eye by enzyme hydrolysis.

INDICATIONS AND DOSAGES
▸ **Glaucoma, Open-Angle**
Ophthalmic, Topical
Adults, Elderly. Instill 1 drop of 0.1% solution in affected eye(s) q12h.

SIDE EFFECTS/ADVERSE REACTIONS
Occasional
Blurred vision, burning or stinging of eye, mydriasis, headache
Rare
Foliicular conjunctivitis

PRECAUTIONS AND CONTRAINDICATIONS

Narrow-angle glaucoma, hypersensitivity to dipivefrin or any component of the formulation
Caution
Lactation, children, aphakia

DRUG INTERACTIONS OF CONCERN TO DENTISTRY

- Avoid use of anticholinergics such as atropine, scopolamine, and propantheline; use benzodiazepines with caution

SERIOUS REACTIONS

! Signs of systemic absorption include hypertension, arrhythmias, and tachycardia.
! Follicular conjunctivitis has been reported.

DENTAL CONSIDERATIONS

General:
- Avoid dental light in patient's eyes; offer dark glasses for patient comfort.

dipyridamole

die-peer-id´-ah-mole
(Apo-Dipyridamole[CAN],
Novodipiradol[CAN], Persantin[AUS],
Persantin 100[AUS], Persantin
SR[AUS], Persantine)
Do not confuse Aggrenox with
Aggrastat, or dipyridamole
with disopyramide, or Persantin
with Periactin.

CATEGORY AND SCHEDULE

Pregnancy Risk Category: C

Drug Class: Platelet aggregation inhibitor

MECHANISM OF ACTION

A blood modifier and platelet aggregation inhibitor that inhibits the activity of adenosine deaminase and phosphodiesterase, enzymes causing accumulation of adenosine and cyclic adenosine monophosphate. **Therapeutic Effect:** Inhibits platelet aggregation; may cause coronary vasodilation.

USES

Adjunctive therapy with warfarin in prosthetic heart valve replacement

PHARMACOKINETICS

Slowly, variably absorbed from the GI tract. Widely distributed. Protein binding: 91%–99%. Metabolized in the liver. Primarily eliminated via biliary excretion. **Half-life:** 10–15 hr.

INDICATIONS AND DOSAGES

▶ **Prevention of Thromboembolic Disorders**
PO
Adults, Elderly.
75–400 mg/day in combination with other medications.
Children. 3–6 mg/kg/day in 3 divided doses.
▶ **Diagnostic Aid**
IV
Adults, Elderly (based on weight).
0.142 mg/kg/min infused over 4 min; although a maximum hasn't been determined, doses greater than 60 mg have been determined to be unnecessary for any patient.

SIDE EFFECTS/ADVERSE REACTIONS

Frequent
Dizziness
Occasional
Abdominal distress, headache, rash

Rare
Diarrhea, vomiting, flushing, pruritus

PRECAUTIONS AND CONTRAINDICATIONS
Hypersensitivity, hypotension
Caution
Children younger than 12 yr

DRUG INTERACTIONS OF CONCERN TO DENTISTRY
• Additive antiplatelet effects: aspirin, other NSAIDs

SERIOUS REACTIONS
! Overdose produces peripheral vasodilation, resulting in hypotension.

DENTAL CONSIDERATIONS
General:
• Monitor vital signs at every appointment because of cardiovascular side effects.
• After supine positioning, have patient sit upright for at least 2 min to avoid orthostatic hypotension.
• Avoid prescribing NSAIDs and aspirin-containing products, even though ASA/dipyridamole combination drugs are used in some patients.
• Patients with prosthetic valves require antibiotic prophylaxis
• Evaluate for clotting ability during gingival instrumentation because inhibition of platelet aggregation may occur.
• Consider local hemostatic measures to prevent excessive bleeding during instrumentation.
Consultations:
• Medical consultation should include PTT or PT.
• Medical consultation may be required to assess disease control.
Teach Patient/Family to:
• Use effective oral hygiene to prevent gingival inflammation

dirithromycin
die-rith-ro-my´-sin
(Dynabac)
Do not confuse Dynabac with Dynacin or DynaCirc.

CATEGORY AND SCHEDULE
Pregnancy Risk Category: C

Drug Class: Macrolide antibiotic

MECHANISM OF ACTION
A macrolide that binds to ribosomal receptor sites of susceptible organisms, inhibiting bacterial protein synthesis. *Therapeutic Effect:* Bactericidal or bacteriostatic, depending on drug dosage.

USES
Treatment of acute and secondary bacterial infection of acute bronchitis, community-acquired pneumonia, streptococcal pharyngitis, and uncomplicated skin and skin-structure infections

PHARMACOKINETICS
Rapidly absorbed from the GI tract. Protein binding: 15%–30%. Widely distributed into tissues and within cells. Eliminated primarily unchanged by biliary excretion. Not removed by hemodialysis.
Half-life: 30–44 hr.

INDICATIONS AND DOSAGES
▶ **Pharyngitis, Tonsillitis**
PO
Adults, Elderly, Children 12 yr and older. 500 mg once a day for 10 days.
▶ **Acute or Chronic Bronchitis, Skin and Skin-Structure Infections**
PO
Adults, Elderly, Children 12 yr

and older. 500 mg once a day for
7 days.
▶ **Community-Acquired Pneumonia**
PO
*Adults, Elderly, Children 12 yr and
older.* 500 mg once a day for 14 days.

SIDE EFFECTS/ADVERSE REACTIONS
Frequent
Abdominal pain, headache, nausea,
diarrhea
Occasional
Vomiting, dyspepsia, dizziness,
nonspecific pain, asthenia
Rare
Increased cough, flatulence, rash,
dyspnea, pruritus and urticaria,
insomnia

PRECAUTIONS AND CONTRAINDICATIONS
Hypersensitivity to dirithromycin or
other macrolide antibiotics
Caution
Not for *H. influenzae* or *S. pyogenes*
infections, lactation, children
younger than 12 yr

DRUG INTERACTIONS OF CONCERN TO DENTISTRY
• Other drug interactions: data are
limited; antacids and histamine
H2 antagonists tend to enhance
absorption; refer to erythromycin for
potential interacting drugs

SERIOUS REACTIONS
❗ Antibiotic-associated colitis and
other superinfections may result from
altered bacterial balance.

<hr>

DENTAL CONSIDERATIONS

General:
• Do not use in patients at risk for
bacteremias caused by inadequate
serum levels.

• Potential value in dental infections
is unknown.
• Determine why the patient is taking
the drug.
• Examine for oral manifestations of
opportunistic infections.
Consultations:
• Medical consultation may be
required to assess disease control.
Teach Patient/Family to:
• Be aware of the possibility of
secondary oral infection and the need
to see dentist immediately if
infection occurs

<hr>

disopyramide phosphate
die-soe-peer´-ah-mide
(Norpace, Norpace CR,
Rythmodan[CAN])
Do not confuse disopyramide with
desipramine, dipyridamole, or Rythmol.

CATEGORY AND SCHEDULE
Pregnancy Risk Category: C

Drug Class: Antidysrhythmic
(class Ia)

MECHANISM OF ACTION
An antiarrhythmic that prolongs the
refractory period of the cardiac cell by
direct effect, decreasing myocardial
excitability and conduction velocity.
Therapeutic Effect: Depresses
myocardial contractility. Has
anticholinergic and negative
inotropic effects.

USES
Treatment of premature ventricular
contractions (PVCs), ventricular
tachycardia

D

PHARMACOKINETICS

PO: Peak 30 min–3 hr, duration 6–12 hr, half-life 4–10 hr; metabolized in liver; excreted in feces, urine, breast milk; crosses placenta

INDICATIONS AND DOSAGES

▶ **Suppression and Prevention of Ventricular Ectopy, Unifocal or Multifocal Premature Ventricular Contractions, Paired Ventricular Contractions (Couplets), and Episodes of Ventricular Tachycardia**
PO
Adults, Elderly weighing 50 kg and more. 150 mg q6h (300 mg ql2h with extended-release).
Adults, Elderly weighing less than 50 kg. 100 mg q6h (200 mg q12h with extended-release).

▶ **Rapid Control of Arrhythmias**
PO
Adults, Elderly weighing 50 kg and more. Initially, 300 mg, then 150 mg q6h or 300 mg (controlled release) q12h.
Adults, Elderly weighing less than 50 kg. Initially, 200 mg, then 100 mg q6h or 200 mg (controlled release) q12h.

▶ **Severe Refractory Arrhythmias**
PO
Adults, Elderly. Up to 400 mg q6h.
Children 12–18 yr. 6–15 mg/kg/day in divided doses q6h.
Children 5–11 yr. 10–15 mg/kg/day in divided doses q6h.
Children 1–4 yr. 10–20 mg/kg/day in divided doses q6h.
Children younger than 1 yr. 10–30 mg/kg/day in divided doses q6h.

▶ **Dosage in Renal Impairment**
With or without loading dose of 150 mg:

Creatinine Clearance	Dosage
40 ml/min and higher	100 mg q6h (extended-release 200 mg q12h)
30–39 ml/min	100 mg q8h
15–29 ml/min	100 mg q12h
Less than 15 ml/min	100 mg q24h

▶ **Dosage in Liver Impairment**
Adults, Elderly weighing 50 kg and more. 100 mg q6h (200 mg q12h with extended-release).
▶ **Dosage in Cardiomyopathy, Cardiac Decompensation**
Adults, Elderly weighing 50 kg and more. No loading dose; 100 mg q6–8h with gradual dosage adjustments.

SIDE EFFECTS/ADVERSE REACTIONS
Frequent
Dry mouth (32%), urinary hesitancy, constipation
Occasional
Blurred vision, dry eyes, nose, or throat, urinary retention, headache, dizziness, fatigue, nausea
Rare
Impotence, hypotension, edema, weight gain, shortness of breath, syncope, chest pain, nervousness, diarrhea, vomiting, decreased appetite, rash, itching

PRECAUTIONS AND CONTRAINDICATIONS
Cardiogenic shock, narrow-angle glaucoma (unless patient is undergoing cholinergic therapy), preexisting second- or third-degree

AV block, preexisting urinary retention.
Caution
Lactation, diabetes mellitus, renal disease, children, hepatic disease, myasthenia gravis, narrow-angle glaucoma, cardiomyopathy, conduction abnormalities

DRUG INTERACTIONS OF CONCERN TO DENTISTRY
• Possible increased risk of prolonged QT interval: clarithromycin, erythromycin
• Increased side effects: anticholinergics, alcohol
• Decreased effects: barbiturates, corticosteroids

SERIOUS REACTIONS
! May produce or aggravate CHF.
! May produce severe hypotension, shortness of breath, chest pain, syncope (especially in patients with primary cardiomyopathy or CHF).
! Hepatotoxicity occurs rarely.

DENTAL CONSIDERATIONS
General:
• Monitor vital signs at every appointment because of cardiovascular side effects.
• After supine positioning, have patient sit upright for at least 2 min before standing to avoid orthostatic hypotension.
• Patients on chronic drug therapy may rarely have symptoms of blood dyscrasias, which can include infection, bleeding, and poor healing.
• Assess salivary flow as a factor in caries, periodontal disease, and candidiasis.
Consultations:
• In a patient with symptoms of blood dyscrasias, request a medical consultation for blood studies and

postpone dental treatment until normal values are reestablished.
• Medical consultation may be required to assess disease control and patient's ability to tolerate stress.
Teach Patient/Family to:
• Use effective oral hygiene to prevent soft tissue inflammation
• When chronic dry mouth occurs, advise patient to:
  • Avoid mouth rinses with high alcohol content because of drying effects
  • Use daily home fluoride products for anticaries effect
  • Use sugarless gum, frequent sips of water, or saliva substitutes

disulfiram
die-sul´-fi-ram
(Antabuse)

CATEGORY AND SCHEDULE
Pregnancy Risk Category: C

Drug Class: Aldehyde dehydrogenase inhibitor

MECHANISM OF ACTION
A thiuram derivative and an irreversible aldehyde dehydrogenase inhibitor. When taken with alcohol, there is an increase in serum acetaldehyde levels.
Therapeutic Effect: Produces an acute sensitivity to alcohol.

USES
Treatment of chronic alcoholism (as adjunct)

PHARMACOKINETICS
Slowly absorbed from GI tract. Metabolized in liver. Primarily excreted in urine. Up to 20% of dose remains in body for at least 1 wk.
Half-life: Unknown.

INDICATIONS AND DOSAGES

▶ **Adjunct in Management of Selected Chronic Alcoholic Patients Who Want to Remain in State of Enforced Sobriety**

PO

Adults, Elderly. Initially, administer maximum of 500 mg daily given as a single dose for 1–2 wk. Maintenance: 250 mg daily (normal range: 125–500 mg). Do not exceed maximum daily dose of 500 mg.

SIDE EFFECTS/ADVERSE REACTIONS

Frequent
Drowsiness
Occasional
Headache, restlessness, optic neuritis (impaired color perception, altered vision), peripheral neuropathy, metallic or garlic taste, rash

PRECAUTIONS AND CONTRAINDICATIONS

Severe heart disease, psychosis, hypersensitivity to disulfiram or any component of the formulation
Caution
Hypothyroidism, hepatic disease, diabetes mellitus, seizure disorders, nephritis, cerebral damage

DRUG INTERACTIONS OF CONCERN TO DENTISTRY

• Increased CNS depression: long-acting benzodiazepines
• Increased disulfiram reaction: alcohol
• Risk of psychosis: metronidazole (do not use), tricyclic antidepressants

SERIOUS REACTIONS

! Disulfiram-alcohol reactions to ingestion of alcohol in any form include flushing/throbbing in head and neck, throbbing headache, nausea, copious vomiting, diaphoresis, dyspnea, hyperventilation, tachycardia, hypotension, marked uneasiness, vertigo, blurred vision, confusion, and death.

DENTAL CONSIDERATIONS

General:
• Be aware of the needs of patients who are in recovery from substance abuse.
• Avoid other addictive drugs, including opioids and benzodiazepines.
Consultations:
• Medical consultation may be required to assess disease control.
Teach Patient/Family to:
• Avoid mouth rinses with high alcohol content because of drying effects and drug–drug interaction

dobutamine hydrochloride

doe-bute´-a-meen
hi-droh-klor´-ide
(Dobutrex)
Do not confuse dobutamine with dopamine.

CATEGORY AND SCHEDULE

Pregnancy Risk Category: B

Drug Class: Adrenergic direct-acting β_1-agonist, cardiac stimulant; Catecholamine

MECHANISM OF ACTION

A direct-acting inotropic agent acting primarily on β_1-adrenergic receptors. *Therapeutic Effect:* Decreases preload and afterload, and enhances myocardial contractility, stroke volume, and cardiac output.

Improves renal blood flow and urine output.

USES
Treatment of cardiac decompensation caused by organic heart disease or cardiac surgery

PHARMACOKINETICS
Metabolized in the liver.
Primarily excreted in urine.
Not removed by hemodialysis.
Half-life: 2 min.

INDICATIONS AND DOSAGES
▶ **Short-Term Management of Cardiac Decompensation**
IV Infusion
Adults, Elderly, Children.
2.5–15 mcg/kg/min. Rarely, drug can be infused at a rate of up to 40 mcg/kg/min to increase cardiac output.
Neonates. 2–15 mcg/kg/min.

SIDE EFFECTS/ADVERSE REACTIONS
Frequent
Increased heart rate, increased B/P
Occasional
Pain at injection site
Rare
Nausea, headache, anginal pain, shortness of breath, fever

PRECAUTIONS AND CONTRAINDICATIONS
Hypovolemia patients, idiopathic hypertrophic subaortic stenosis, sulfite sensitivity

DRUG INTERACTIONS OF CONCERN TO DENTISTRY
None reported.

SERIOUS REACTIONS
! Overdose may produce a marked increase in heart rate (by 30 beats/min or higher), marked increase in

B/P (by 50 mm Hg or higher), anginal pain, and premature ventricular contractions (PVCs).

DENTAL CONSIDERATIONS
General:
• Acute-use drug for use in hospitals, cardiac labs, or emergency rooms.

docetaxel
doe-ceh-tax´-el
(Taxotere)
Do not confuse docetaxel with Taxol.

CATEGORY AND SCHEDULE
Pregnancy Risk Category: D

Drug Class: Miscellaneous antineoplastic

MECHANISM OF ACTION
An antimitotic agent belonging to the taxoid family that disrupts the microtubular cell network, which is essential for cellular function.
Therapeutic Effect: Inhibits cellular mitosis.

USES
Locally advanced or metastatic breast cancer, non–small-cell lung cancer, androgen independent metastatic prostate cancer, post-surgery operable node-positive breast cancer.

PHARMACOKINETICS
Distributed into peripheral compartments. Protein binding: 94%.
Extensively metabolized.
Excreted primarily in feces, with lesser amount in urine.
Half-life: 11.1 hr.

INDICATIONS AND DOSAGES
▶ Breast Carcinoma
IV
Adults. 60–100 mg/m² given over
1 hr q3wk. If patient develops febrile
neutropenia, a neutrophil count less
than 500 cells/mm³ for longer than
1 wk, severe or cumulative cutaneous
reactions, or severe peripheral
neuropathy with initial dose of
100 mg/m², dosage should be
decreased to 75 mg/m². If reaction
continues, dosage should be further
reduced to 55 mg/m² or therapy
should be discontinued. Patients who
don't experience the above symptoms
at a dose of 60 mg/m² may tolerate
an increased docetaxel dose.
▶ Non–Small-cell Lung Carcinoma
IV
Adults. 75 mg/m² q3wk. Adjust
dosage if toxicity occurs.

SIDE EFFECTS/ADVERSE REACTIONS
Frequent
Alopecia, asthenia, hypersensitivity
reaction such as dermatitis (59%,
decreases to 16% in those pretreated
with oral corticosteroids), fluid
retention, stomatitis, nausea and
diarrhea, fever, nail changes,
vomiting, myalgia
Occasional
Hypotension, edema, anorexia,
headache, weight gain, infection
(urinary tract, injection site,
indwelling catheter tip), dizziness
Rare
Dry skin, sensory disorders (vision,
speech, taste), arthralgia, weight
loss, conjunctivitis, hematuria,
proteinuria

PRECAUTIONS AND CONTRAINDICATIONS
History of severe hypersensitivity to
docetaxel or other drugs formulated
with polysorbate 80, neutrophil count
less than 1,500 cells/mm³

DRUG INTERACTIONS OF CONCERN TO DENTISTRY
• Significant risk of increased
effects: drugs that inhibit CYP3A4
isoenzymes (including ketoconazole,
itraconazole, erythromycin)
• Caution in use of any drugs that
induce CYP3A4 isoenzymes

SERIOUS REACTIONS
! In patients with normal liver
function tests, neutropenia
(neutrophil count 2,000 cells/mm³)
and leukopenia (WBC count less
than 4,000 cells/mm³) occur in 96%
of patients; anemia (hemoglobin
level less than 11 g/dl) occurs in 90%
of patients; thrombocytopenia
(platelet count less than 100,000
cells/mm³) occur in 8% of patients;
and infection occurs in 28% of
patients.
! Neurosensory and neuromotor
effects, such as distal paresthesias
and weakness, occur in 54% and
13% of patients, respectively.

DENTAL CONSIDERATIONS
General:
• If additional analgesia is required
for dental pain, consider alternative
analgesics (NSAIDs) in patients
taking narcotics for acute or chronic
pain.
• Examine for oral manifestation of
opportunistic infection.
• Avoid products that affect platelet
function, such as aspirin and
NSAIDs.
• This drug may be used in the
hospital or on an outpatient basis.

Confirm the patient's disease and treatment status.

• Chlorhexidine mouth rinse prior to and during chemotherapy may reduce severity of mucositis.

• Patient on chronic drug therapy may rarely present with symptoms of blood dyscrasias, which can include infection, bleeding and poor healing. If dyscrasia is present, caution patient to prevent oral tissue trauma when using oral hygiene aids.

• Palliative medication may be required for management of oral side effects.

• Short appointments and a stress reduction protocol may be required for anxious patients.

• Patients may be at risk of bleeding, check for oral signs.

• Oral infections should be eliminated and/or treated aggressively.

Consultations:

• Medical consultation should include routine blood counts including platelet counts and bleeding time.

• Consult physician; prophylactic or therapeutic antiinfectives may be indicated if surgery or periodontal treatment is required.

• Medical consultation may be required to assess immunologic status during cancer chemotherapy and determine safety risk, if any, posed by the required dental treatment.

• Medical consultation may be required to assess disease control and patient's ability to tolerate stress.

Teach Patient/Family to:

• Be aware of oral side effects

• Use effective oral hygiene to prevent soft tissue inflammation

• Report oral lesions, soreness, or bleeding to dentist

• Use caution to prevent trauma when using oral hygiene aids

• Update health and medication history if physician makes any changes in evaluation or drug regimens; include OTC, herbal, and nonherbal remedies in the update

docosanol
do-cos'-ah-nole
(Abreva)

CATEGORY AND SCHEDULE
Pregnancy Risk Category: B

Drug Class: Synthetic lipophilic alcohol

MECHANISM OF ACTION
A highly lipophilic, fatty alcohol that prevents fusion of lipid-enveloped viruses with cell membranes, thereby blocking viral replication

USES
Treatment of recurrent herpes labialis (cold sores, fever blisters) on the face or lips; appears to shorten healing time by at least 1 day

PHARMACOKINETICS
Topical: Negligible absorption.

INDICATIONS AND DOSAGES
▸ **Recurrent Herpes Labialis**
Topical
Adult, Children older than 12 yr.
Apply small amount to affected area on face or lips or at the first sign of lesion 5 times a day until healed.

SIDE EFFECTS/ADVERSE REACTIONS
CNS: Headache
INTEG: Site reaction, rash, pruritus, dry skin, acne

PRECAUTIONS AND CONTRAINDICATIONS
Hypersensitivity
Caution
Avoid application to eyes, external use only (not for intraoral use), children younger than 12 yr

DRUG INTERACTIONS OF CONCERN TO DENTISTRY
None reported

DENTAL CONSIDERATIONS
Teach Patient/Family to:
• Apply with finger cot; wash hands before and after use
• Not share this medication to prevent potential cross contamination of virus
• Replace tooth brush after resolution of lesion to prevent reinfection of virus

docusate
dok´-yoo-sate
(Apo-Docusate[CAN], Colace, Colax-C[CAN], Coloxyl[AUS], Diocto, Docusoft-S, Novo-Ducosate[CAN], PMS-Docusate[CAN], Pro-Cal-Sof, Regulex[CAN], Selax[CAN], Soflax[CAN], Surfak)

CATEGORY AND SCHEDULE
Pregnancy Risk Category: C
OTC

Drug Class: Bulk-producing laxative; stool softener

MECHANISM OF ACTION
A bulk-producing laxative that decreases surface film tension by mixing liquid and bowel contents.

Therapeutic Effect: Increases infiltration of liquid to form a softer stool.

USES
Stool softener for those who need to avoid straining during defecation; treatment of constipation associated with hard, dry stools

PHARMACOKINETICS
Minimal absorption from the GI tract. Acts in small and large intestines. Results usually occur 1–2 days after first dose, but may take 3–5 days.

INDICATIONS AND DOSAGES
▸ Stool Softener
PO
Adults, Elderly, Children 12 yr and older: 50–500 mg/day in 1–4 divided doses.
Children 6–11 yr: 40–150 mg/day in 1–4 divided doses.
Children 3–5 yr: 20–60 mg/day in 1–4 divided doses.
Children younger than 3 yr: 10–40 mg in 1–4 divided doses.

SIDE EFFECTS/ADVERSE REACTIONS
Occasional
Mild GI cramping, throat irritation (with liquid preparation)
Rare
Rash

PRECAUTIONS AND CONTRAINDICATIONS
Acute abdominal pain, concomitant use of mineral oil, intestinal obstruction, nausea, vomiting

DRUG INTERACTIONS OF CONCERN TO DENTISTRY
None reported

SERIOUS REACTIONS
None known

DENTAL CONSIDERATIONS
General:
- Determine why patient is taking the drug.
- Use caution when prescribing medications that may aggravate constipation.

dofetilide
doe-fet´-ill-ide
(Tikosyn)

CATEGORY AND SCHEDULE
Pregnancy Risk Category: C

Drug Class: Antidysrhythmic (class III)

MECHANISM OF ACTION
A selective potassium channel blocker that prolongs repolarization without affecting conduction velocity by blocking one or more time-dependent potassium currents. Dofetilide has no effect on sodium channels or adrenergic alpha or beta receptors. *Therapeutic Effect:* Terminates reentrant tachyarrhythmias, preventing reinduction.

USES
Maintenance of normal sinus rhythm in patients with atrial fibrillation or atrial flutter longer than 1 wk duration, who have been converted to normal sinus rhythm; conversion of atrial fibrillation or atrial flutter to normal sinus rhythm

PHARMACOKINETICS
PO: Bioavailability greater than 90%, peak plasma levels 2–3 hr, steady-state levels 2–3 days, plasma protein binding 60%–70%, excreted (80%) in urine unchanged, excretion involves both glomerular filtration and active tubular secretion, limited metabolism by CYP450 3A4 isoenzymes

INDICATIONS AND DOSAGES
▶ **Maintain Normal Sinus Rhythm after Conversion from Atrial Fibrillation or Flutter**
PO
Adults, Elderly. Individualized using a 7-step dosing algorithm dependent upon calculated creatinine clearance and QT interval measurements.

SIDE EFFECTS/ADVERSE REACTIONS
Occasional
Headache, chest pain, dizziness, dyspnea, nausea, insomnia, back and abdominal pain, diarrhea, rash

PRECAUTIONS AND CONTRAINDICATIONS
Concurrent use of drugs that prolong the QT interval; concurrent use of amiodarone, megestrol, prochlorperazine, or verapamil; congenital or acquired prolonged QT syndrome; paroxysmal atrial fibrillation; severe renal impairment
Caution
Requires dose adjustment in renal impairment, can cause life-threatening ventricular arrhythmias, caution in use with CYP450 3A4 isoenzyme inhibitors, hepatic impairment, abnormal serum potassium or magnesium levels, lactation, children younger than 18 yr

DRUG INTERACTIONS OF CONCERN TO DENTISTRY
• Use NSAIDs with caution in patients at risk for thromboembolism
• Decreased renal excretion: ketoconazole (contraindicated use)
• Not recommended with concurrent use of phenothiazines, tricyclic antidepressants, SSRIs, macrolide antiinfectives (erythromycin, clarithromycin), azole antifungals, or other drugs that inhibit CYP3A4 isoenzymes
• Contraindicated with cimetidine, trimethoprim, ketoconazole, prochlorperazine, megestrol, or verapamil

SERIOUS REACTIONS
! Angioedema, bradycardia, cerebral ischemia, facial paralysis, and serious ventricular arrhythmias or various forms of heart block may be noted.

DENTAL CONSIDERATIONS
General:
• Monitor vital signs at every appointment because of cardiovascular side effects.
• Delay or avoid dental treatment if patient shows signs of cardiac symptoms or respiratory distress.
• Ensure that the patient is compliant with drug therapy.
Consultations:
• Patient's physician should be informed about use of any dental drugs.
• Medical consultation may be required to assess disease control and patient's ability to tolerate stress.
Teach Patient/Family to:
• Update health and drug history if physician makes any changes in evaluation or drug regimens

dolasetron
doe-lass´-eh-tron
(Anzemet)
Do not confuse Anzemet with Aldomet.

CATEGORY AND SCHEDULE
Pregnancy Risk Category: B

Drug Class: Antinauseant and antiemetic

MECHANISM OF ACTION
A 5-HT3 receptor antagonist that acts centrally in the chemoreceptor trigger zone and peripherally at the vagal nerve terminals. *Therapeutic Effect:* Prevents nausea and vomiting.

USES
Control of nausea and vomiting associated with cancer chemotherapy and prevention of postoperative nausea and vomiting

PHARMACOKINETICS
Readily absorbed from the GI tract after PO administration. Protein binding: 69%–77%. Metabolized in the liver. Primarily excreted in urine. Unknown if removed by hemodialysis. *Half-life:* 5–10 hr.

INDICATIONS AND DOSAGES
▸ **Prevention of Chemotherapy-Induced Nausea and Vomiting**
PO
Adults. 100 mg within 1 hr of chemotherapy.
Children 2–16 yr. 1.8 mg/kg within 1 hr of chemotherapy. Maximum: 100 mg.
IV
Adults, Children 1–16 yr. 1.8 mg/kg as a single dose 30 min before chemotherapy. Maximum: 100 mg.

▶ **Treatment or Prevention of Postoperative Nausea or Vomiting**
PO
Adults. 100 mg within 2 hr of surgery.
Children 2–16 yr. 1.2 mg/kg within 2 hr of surgery. Maximum: 100 mg.
IV
Adults. 12.5 mg 15 min before cessation of anesthesia or as soon as nausea occurs.
Children 2–16 yr. 0.35 mg/kg 15 min before cessation of anesthesia or as soon as nausea occurs. Maximum: 12.5 mg.

SIDE EFFECTS/ADVERSE REACTIONS
Frequent
Headache, diarrhea, fatigue
Occasional
Fever, dizziness, tachycardia, dyspepsia

PRECAUTIONS AND CONTRAINDICATIONS
Hypersensitivity
Caution
Previous hypersensitivity to other antagonists,5-HT3cardiovascular disease, seizure disorders, ECG changes, hypokalemia, hypomagnesemia, diuretics, antiarrhythmics, lactation

DRUG INTERACTIONS OF CONCERN TO DENTISTRY
• Does not influence anesthesia recovery time

SERIOUS REACTIONS
! Overdose may produce a combination of CNS stimulant and depressant effects.

DENTAL CONSIDERATIONS
General:
• Monitor patients in recovery to avoid untoward events.

• Patients taking opioids for acute or chronic pain should be given alternative analgesics for dental pain.
• Chlorhexidine mouth rinse before and during chemotherapy may reduce severity of mucositis.
• Palliative medication may be required for management of oral side effects from chemotherapy.
Teach Patient/Family to:
• Be aware of possible oral side effects from concurrent cancer chemotherapy
• Report to dentist excessive nausea and vomiting in patients recovering from anesthesia after dental treatment

donepezil hydrochloride
dah-nep´-eh-zil hi-droh-klor´-ide (Aricept)
Do not confuse Aricept with Aciphex or Ascriptin.

CATEGORY AND SCHEDULE
Pregnancy Risk Category: C

Drug Class: Cholinesterase inhibitor

MECHANISM OF ACTION
A cholinesterase inhibitor that inhibits the enzyme acetyl-cholinesterase, thus increasing the concentration of acetylcholine at cholinergic synapses and enhancing cholinergic function in the CNS. *Therapeutic Effect:* Slows the progression of Alzheimer's disease.

USES
Treatment of mild-to-moderate dementia associated with Alzheimer's disease

PHARMACOKINETICS
Well absorbed after PO administration. Protein binding: 96%. Extensively metabolized. Eliminated in urine and feces. *Half-life:* 70 hr. Tablets (Orally Disintegrating): 5 mg, 10 mg.

INDICATIONS AND DOSAGES
▸ **Alzheimer's Disease**
PO
Adults, Elderly. 5–10 mg/day as a single dose. If initial dose is 5 mg, do not increase to 10 mg for 4–6 wk.

SIDE EFFECTS/ADVERSE REACTIONS
Frequent
Nausea, diarrhea, headache, insomnia, nonspecific pain, dizziness
Occasional
Mild muscle cramps, fatigue, vomiting, anorexia, ecchymosis
Rare
Depression, abnormal dreams, weight loss, arthritis, somnolence, syncope, frequent urination

PRECAUTIONS AND CONTRAINDICATIONS
History of hypersensitivity to donepezil or piperidine derivatives
Caution
Bradycardia, sick sinus syndrome, GI ulcer disease, bladder obstruction, seizures, asthma, obstructive pulmonary disease, lactation, children, hepatic impairment

DRUG INTERACTIONS OF CONCERN TO DENTISTRY
• Enhanced succinylcholine muscle relaxation during anesthesia
• Risk of GI side effects: NSAIDs
• Action may be inhibited by anticholinergic drugs or enhanced by cholinergic agonists

• Increased blood levels: ketoconazole, paroxetine
• Use with caution drugs that inhibit CYP3A4 or CYP2D6 isoenzymes

SERIOUS REACTIONS
❗ Overdose may result in cholinergic crisis, characterized by severe nausea, increased salivation, diaphoresis, bradycardia, hypotension, flushed skin, abdominal pain, respiratory depression, seizures, and cardiorespiratory collapse. Increasing muscle weakness may result in death if respiratory muscles are involved. The antidote is 1–2 mg IV atropine sulfate with subsequent doses based on therapeutic response.

DENTAL CONSIDERATIONS
General:
• Determine why patient is taking the drug.
• Monitor vital signs at every appointment because of cardiovascular side effects.
• After supine positioning, have patient sit upright for at least 2 min before standing to avoid orthostatic hypotension.
• Use caution if sedation or general anesthesia is required.
• Patients on chronic drug therapy may rarely have symptoms of blood dyscrasias, which can include infection, bleeding, and poor healing.
• Drug is used early in the disease; ensure that patient or caregiver understands informed consent.
• Place on frequent recall because early attention to dental health is important for Alzheimer's patients.
• Assess salivary flow as factor in caries, periodontal disease, and candidiasis.

- Consider semisupine chair position for patient comfort if GI side effects occur.

Consultations:
- Consultation with physician may be necessary if sedation or general anesthesia is required.
- Medical consultation may be required to assess disease control and patient's ability to tolerate stress.
- In a patient with symptoms of blood dyscrasias, request a medical consultation for blood studies and postpone treatment until normal values are reestablished.

Teach Patient/Family to:
- Use effective oral hygiene to prevent soft tissue inflammation
- Prevent trauma when using oral hygiene aids
- Use electric toothbrush if patient has difficulty holding conventional devices
- When chronic dry mouth occurs, advise patient to:
  - Avoid mouth rinses with high alcohol content because of drying effects
  - Use daily home fluoride products for anticaries effect
  - Use sugarless gum, frequent sips of water, or saliva substitutes

dopamine hydrochloride

doe´-pa-meen hye-droe-klor´-ide
(Dopamine Injection[AUS], Intropin)
Do not confuse dopamine with dobutamine or Dopram, or Inotropin with Isoptin.

CATEGORY AND SCHEDULE
Pregnancy Risk Category: C

Drug Class: Sympathomimetic (adrenergic agonist); cardiac stimulant, vasopressor

MECHANISM OF ACTION

A sympathomimetic (adrenergic agonist) that stimulates adrenergic receptors. Effects are dose dependent. Low dosages (less than 5 mcg/kg/min) stimulate dopaminergic receptors, causing renal vasodilation. Low to moderate dosages (less than 10 mcg/kg/min) have a positive inotropic effect by direct action and release of norepinephrine. High dosages (more than 10 mcg/kg/min) stimulate alpha-receptors.
Therapeutic Effect: With low dosages, increases renal blood flow, urine flow, and sodium excretion. With low to moderate dosages, increases myocardial contractility, stroke volume, and cardiac output. With high dosages, increases peripheral resistance, renal vasoconstriction, and systolic and diastolic B/P.

USES

Prophylaxis and treatment of acute hypotension, shock (associated with MI, trauma, renal failure, cardiac decompensation, open heart surgery), treatment of low cardiac output, CHF

PHARMACOKINETICS

Route	Onset	Peak	Duration
IV	1–2 min	N/A	Less than 10 min

Widely distributed. Does not cross blood-brain barrier. Metabolized in the liver, kidney, and plasma. Primarily excreted in urine. Not removed by hemodialysis.
Half-life: 2 min.

INDICATIONS AND DOSAGES
▶ **Treatment and Prevention of Acute Hypotension; Shock (Associated with Cardiac Decompensation, MI, Open Heart Surgery, Renal Failure, or Trauma), Treatment of Low Cardiac Output, Treatment of CHF**
IV
Adults, Elderly. 1 mcg/kg/min up to 50 mcg/kg/min titrated to desired response.
Children. 1–20 mcg/kg/min.
Maximum: 50 mcg/kg/min.
Neonates. 1–20 mcg/kg/min.

SIDE EFFECTS/ADVERSE REACTIONS
Frequent
Headache, ectopic beats, tachycardia, anginal pain, palpitations, vasoconstriction, hypotension, nausea, vomiting, dyspnea
Occasional
Piloerection or goose bumps, bradycardia, widening of QRS complex

PRECAUTIONS AND CONTRAINDICATIONS
Pheochromocytoma, sulfite sensitivity, uncorrected tachyarrhythmias, ventricular fibrillation

SERIOUS REACTIONS
❗ High doses may produce ventricular arrhythmias.
❗ Patients with occlusive vascular disease are at high risk for further compromise of circulation to the extremities, which may result in gangrene.
❗ Tissue necrosis with sloughing may occur with extravasation of IV solution.

General:
• Acute-use drug for use in hospitals, cardiac labs, or emergency rooms.
• Inquire about cardiovascular disease and medications used.

dornase alfa
door´-nace al´-fa
(Pulmozyme)

CATEGORY AND SCHEDULE
Pregnancy Risk Category: B

Drug Class: Recombinant human deoxyribonuclease (rh DNase)

MECHANISM OF ACTION
An enzyme that selectively splits and hydrolyzes DNA in sputum.
Therapeutic Effect: Reduces sputum viscosity and elasticity.

USES
Treatment of cystic fibrosis; reduces incidence of pulmonary infections; improves pulmonary function

PHARMACOKINETICS
Inhalation: Peak sputum levels 15 min

INDICATIONS AND DOSAGES
▶ **To Improve Management of Pulmonary Function in Patients with Cystic Fibrosis**
Nebulization
Adults, Children older than 5 yr. 2.5 mg (1 ampule) once daily by recommended nebulizer.
May increase to 2.5 mg twice daily.

SIDE EFFECTS/ADVERSE REACTIONS

Frequent
Pharyngitis, chest pain or discomfort, voice changes
Occasional
Conjunctivitis, hoarseness, rash

PRECAUTIONS AND CONTRAINDICATIONS

Sensitivity to dornase alfa or epoetin alfa
Caution
Lactation, children younger than 5 yr

DRUG INTERACTIONS OF CONCERN TO DENTISTRY

None documented

SERIOUS REACTIONS

None significant

DENTAL CONSIDERATIONS

General:
• Consider semisupine chair position for patients with respiratory disease.
• Monitor vital signs at every appointment because of respiratory and cardiovascular side effects.
• Stress reduction protocol may be required.
Consultations:
• Medical consultation may be required to assess disease control.
Teach Patient/Family to:
• Use effective oral hygiene to prevent soft tissue inflammation

---

dorzolamide hydrochloride
door-zol´-ah-mide hi-droh-klor´-ide
(Trusopt)

CATEGORY AND SCHEDULE

Pregnancy Risk Category: C

Drug Class: Carbonic anhydrase inhibitor

MECHANISM OF ACTION

An ophthalmic agent that inhibits carbonic anhydrase. *Therapeutic Effect:* Reduces intraocular pressure (IOP).

USES

Treatment of ocular hypertension, open-angle glaucoma

PHARMACOKINETICS

Peak response occurs in 2 hr and the duration of action is 8–12 hr. Systemically absorbed to some degree. Protein binding: 33%. Distributed in red blood cells. Sites of metabolism have not been established. Metabolized to active metabolite, N-desethyldorzolamide. Excreted in urine. *Half-life:* Unknown; 147 days (terminal red blood cell).

INDICATIONS AND DOSAGES

▸ **Glaucoma, Ocular Hypertension**
Ophthalmic
Adults, Elderly. 1 drop in affected eye(s) 3 times a day.

SIDE EFFECTS/ADVERSE REACTIONS

Frequent
Ocular burning, bitter taste
Occasional
Superficial punctuate keratitis, ocular allergic reaction

PRECAUTIONS AND CONTRAINDICATIONS

Hypersensitivity to dorzolamide or any other component of the formulation
Caution
Allergy to sulfonamides, renal or hepatic impairment, lactation, children, oral carbonic anhydrase inhibitors, contact lenses

DRUG INTERACTIONS OF CONCERN TO DENTISTRY
• Avoid drugs that may exacerbate glaucoma (anticholinergic drugs)
• High-dose salicylates to avoid systemic toxicity

SERIOUS REACTIONS
! Iridocyclitis, skin rash, and urolithiasis occur rarely.
! Electrolyte imbalance, development of an acidotic state, and possible CNS effects may occur.

DENTAL CONSIDERATIONS
General:
• Avoid dental light in patient's eyes; offer dark glasses for patient comfort.
• Protect patient's eyes from accidental spatter during dental treatment.
• Check patient's compliance with prescribed drug regimen for glaucoma.
Consultations:
• Medical consultation may be required to assess disease control.

doxazosin mesylate
dox-ay´-zoe-sin mess-ah-late
(Apo-Doxazosin[CAN], Cardura)
Do not confuse doxazosin with doxapram, doxepin, or doxorubicin, or Cardura with Cardene, Cordarone, Coumadin, K-Dur, or Ridaura.

CATEGORY AND SCHEDULE
Pregnancy Risk Category: C

MECHANISM OF ACTION
An antihypertensive that selectively blocks alpha$_1$-adrenergic receptors, decreasing peripheral vascular resistance. ***Therapeutic Effect:*** Causes peripheral vasodilation and lowers of B/P. Also relaxes smooth muscle of bladder and prostate.

USES
Treatment of benign prostatic hyperplasia (BPH)

PHARMACOKINETICS
54–59% absorbed; peak blood levels 8–9 hr. 99% protein binding. Primarily metabolized in the liver by the CYP 3A4 isoenzyme. 63% excreted in feces, 9% in urine.

Route	Onset	Peak	Duration
PO	N/A	2–6 hr	24 hr

Well absorbed from the GI tract. Protein binding: 98%–99%. Metabolized in the liver. Primarily eliminated in feces. Not removed by hemodialysis. ***Half-life:*** 19–22 hr.

INDICATIONS AND DOSAGES
▸ **Mild-to-Moderate Hypertension**
PO
Adults. Initially, 1 mg once a day. May increase to a maximum of 16 mg/day.
Elderly. Initially, 0.5 mg once a day.
▸ **Benign Prostatic Hyperplasia, Alone or in Combination with Finasteride (Proscar)**
PO
Adults, Elderly. Initially, 1 mg/day. May increase q1–2 wk. Maximum: 8 mg/day.

SIDE EFFECTS/ADVERSE REACTIONS
Frequent
Dizziness, asthenia, headache, edema
Occasional
Nausea, pharyngitis, rhinitis, pain in extremities, somnolence

Rare

Palpitations, diarrhea, constipation, dyspnea, myalgia, altered vision, dizziness, nervousness

PRECAUTIONS AND CONTRAINDICATIONS

Hypersensitivity to other quinazolines
Caution
Children, lactation, hepatic disease

DRUG INTERACTIONS OF CONCERN TO DENTISTRY

- Increased hypotensive effects: all CNS depressants
- Reduced effects with indomethacin, NSAIDs, sympathomimetics
- Caution in use of drugs that may cause urinary retention: anticholinergics, opioids

SERIOUS REACTIONS

! First-dose syncope (hypotension with sudden loss of consciousness) may occur 30–90 min following initial dose of 2 mg or greater, a too-rapid increase in dosage, or addition of another antihypertensive agent to therapy. First-dose syncope may be preceded by tachycardia (pulse rate of 120–160 beats/min).

DENTAL CONSIDERATIONS

General:
- Monitor vital signs at every appointment because of cardiovascular side effects.
- After supine positioning, have patient sit upright for at least 2 min before standing to avoid orthostatic hypotension
- Assess salivary flow as a factor in caries, periodontal disease, and candidiasis.

Consultations:
- Medical consultation may be required to assess disease control and patient's ability to tolerate stress.
Teach Patient/Family to:
- When chronic dry mouth occurs, advise patient to:
  - Avoid mouth rinses with high alcohol content because of drying effects
  - Use daily home fluoride products for anticaries effect
  - Use sugarless gum, frequent sips of water, or saliva substitutes

doxepin hydrochloride

dox´-eh-pin hye-droe-klor´-ide
(Apo-Doxepin[CAN], Deptran[AUS], Novo-Doxepin[CAN], Prudoxin, Sinequan, Zonalon)
Do not confuse doxepin with doxapram, doxazosin, or Doxidan, or Sinequan with saquinavir.

CATEGORY AND SCHEDULE

Pregnancy Risk Category: C
(B for topical form)

Drug Class: Antidepressant, tricyclic

MECHANISM OF ACTION

A tricyclic antidepressant, antianxiety agent, antineuralgic agent, antipruritic, and antiulcer agent that increases synaptic concentrations of norepinephrine and serotonin.
Therapeutic Effect: Produces antidepressant and anxiolytic effects.

USES

Treatment of major depression, anxiety; unapproved: panic disorders

PHARMACOKINETICS

Rapidly and well absorbed from the GI tract. Protein binding: 80%–85%. Metabolized in the liver to active metabolite. Primarily excreted in urine. Not removed by hemodialysis. *Half-life:* 6–8 hr. Topical: Absorbed through the skin. Distributed to body tissues. Metabolized to active metabolite. Excreted in urine.

INDICATIONS AND DOSAGES
▸ **Depression, Anxiety**
PO
Adults. 30–150 mg/day at bedtime or in 2–3 divided doses. May increase to 300 mg/day.
Elderly. Initially, 10–25 mg at bedtime. May increase by 10–25 mg/day every 3–7 days. Maximum: 75 mg/day.
Adolescents. Initially, 25–50 mg/day as a single dose or in divided doses. May increase to 100 mg/day.
Children 12 yr and younger. 1–3 mg/kg/day.
▸ **Pruritus Associated with Eczema**
Topical
Adults, Elderly. Apply thin film 4 times a day.

SIDE EFFECTS/ADVERSE REACTIONS
Frequent
Oral: Orthostatic hypotension, somnolence, dry mouth, headache, increased appetite, weight gain, nausea, unusual fatigue, unpleasant taste
Topical: Edema; increased pruritus and eczema; burning, tingling, or stinging at application site; altered taste; dizziness; drowsiness; dry skin; dry mouth; fatigue; headache; thirst
Occasional
Oral: Blurred vision, confusion, constipation, hallucinations, difficult urination, eye pain, irregular heartbeat, fine muscle tremors, nervousness, impaired sexual function, diarrhea, diaphoresis, heartburn, insomnia
Topical: Anxiety, skin irritation or cracking, nausea
Rare
Oral: Allergic reaction, alopecia, tinnitus, breast enlargement
Topical: Fever, photosensitivity

PRECAUTIONS AND CONTRAINDICATIONS
Angle-closure glaucoma, hypersensitivity to other tricyclic antidepressants, urine retention
Caution
Suicidal patients, elderly, MAOIs

DRUG INTERACTIONS OF CONCERN TO DENTISTRY FOR TOPICAL FORM:
• Potential for interactions depends on how much drug is absorbed and duration of use (longer than 8 days)
• Increased anticholinergic effects: anticholinergics, antihistamines, phenothiazines, other tricyclic antidepressants
• Potential risk for increased CNS depression: all CNS depressants
• Increased effects of direct-acting sympathomimetics: epinephrine, levonordefrin
• Avoid concurrent use with St. John's wort (herb)

DRUG INTERACTIONS OF CONCERN TO DENTISTRY FOR SYSTEMIC-DOSE FORM:
• Increased anticholinergic effects: anticholinergic blockers, antihistamines, phenothiazines
• Increased effects of direct-acting sympathomimetics (epinephrine, levonordefrin)

- Potential risk of increased CNS depression: alcohol, barbiturates, benzodiazepines, other CNS depressants
- Decreased antihypertensive effects: clonidine, guanadrel, guanethidine

SERIOUS REACTIONS
! Abrupt or too-rapid withdrawal may result in headache, malaise, nausea, vomiting, and vivid dreams.
! Overdose may produce seizures, dizziness, and cardiovascular effects, such as severe orthostatic hypotension, tachycardia, palpitations, and arrhythmias.

DENTAL CONSIDERATIONS

Topical Form
General:
- Doxepin may be absorbed and produce typical systemic side effects of tricyclic drugs.
- Monitor vital signs at every appointment because of cardiovascular side effects.
- Use vasoconstrictors with caution, in low doses, and with careful aspiration.
- Place on frequent recall because of oral side effects.
- Apply lubricant to dry lips for patient comfort before dental procedures.
- Assess salivary flow as a factor in caries, periodontal disease, and candidiasis.
Consultations:
- Medical consultation may be required to assess disease control.
Teach Patient/Family to:
- Avoid mouth rinses with high alcohol content because of interaction with alcohol (see precautions) and drying effects

- When chronic dry mouth occurs, advise patient to:
  - Use daily home fluoride products for anticaries effect
  - Use sugarless gum, frequent sips of water, or saliva substitutes

Systemic-Dose Form
General:
- Monitor vital signs at every appointment because of cardiovascular side effects.
- Assess salivary flow as a factor in caries, periodontal disease, and candidiasis.
- Patients on chronic drug therapy may rarely have symptoms of blood dyscrasias, which can include infection, bleeding, and poor healing.
- After supine positioning, have patient sit upright for at least 2 min before standing to avoid orthostatic hypotension.
- Use vasoconstrictors with caution, in low doses, and with careful aspiration. Avoid use of gingival retraction cord with epinephrine.
- Place on frequent recall because of oral side effects.
Consultations:
- In a patient with symptoms of blood dyscrasias, request a medical consultation for blood studies and postpone dental treatment until normal values are reestablished.
- Medical consultation may be required to assess disease control.
- Physician should be informed if significant xerostomic side effects occur (e.g., increased caries, sore tongue, problems eating or swallowing, difficulty wearing prosthesis) so that a medication change can be considered.
Teach Patient/Family to:
- Use effective oral hygiene to prevent soft tissue inflammation

• When chronic dry mouth occurs, advise patient to:
  • Avoid mouth rinses with high alcohol content because of drying effects
  • Use daily home fluoride products for anticaries effect
  • Use sugarless gum, frequent sips of water, or saliva substitutes

doxorubicin
dox-oh-roo´-bi-sin
(Doxil)
Do not confuse doxorubicin with Daunorubicin, Idamycin, or Idarubicin.

CATEGORY AND SCHEDULE
Pregnancy Risk Category: D

Drug Class: Anthracycline antibiotic; antineoplastic

MECHANISM OF ACTION
An anthracycline antibiotic that inhibits DNA and DNA-dependent RNA synthesis by binding with DNA strands. Liposomal encapsulation increases uptake by tumors, prolongs action, and may decrease toxicity.
Therapeutic Effect: Prevents cellular division.

USES
Treatment of some kinds of cancer

PHARMACOKINETICS
Widely distributed. Protein binding: Unknown. Metabolized in liver. Minimal excretion in urine.
Half-life: 45–55 hr.

INDICATIONS AND DOSAGES
▶ **AIDS-Related Kaposi's Sarcoma**
IV infusion
Adults. 20 mg/m² over 30 min q3wk.

▶ **Ovarian Cancer**
IV infusion
Adults. 50 mg/m² q4wk.
▶ **Dosage in Liver Impairment**

Serum Bilirubin Concentration	Dosage
1.2–3 mg/dl	50% usual dose
More than 3 mg/dl	25% usual dose

SIDE EFFECTS/ADVERSE REACTIONS
Frequent
Nausea
Occasional
Anorexia, diarrhea, hyperpigmentation of nailbeds, phalangeal and dermal creases
Rare
Fever, chills, conjunctivitis, lacrimation

PRECAUTIONS AND CONTRAINDICATIONS
Nursing mothers, hypersensitivity to doxorubicin compounds or daunorubicin

DRUG INTERACTIONS OF CONCERN TO DENTISTRY
None reported

SERIOUS REACTIONS
! Bone marrow depression manifested as hematologic toxicity (principally leukopenia and, to lesser extent, anemia, thrombocytopenia) may occur.
! Cardiotoxicity noted as either acute, transient abnormal ECG findings or cardiomyopathy manifested as CHF may occur.

DENTAL CONSIDERATIONS
General:
• If additional analgesia is required for dental pain, consider alternative

analgesics (NSAIDs) in patients taking narcotics for acute or chronic pain.
• Avoid prescribing aspirin-containing products.
• Examine for oral manifestation of opportunistic infection.
• This drug usually is administered in a hospital, a cancer treatment center, or possibly a home IV service. Dentists are involved in the management of oral mucositis associated with the chemotherapy.
• Chlorhexidine mouth rinse prior to and during chemotherapy may reduce severity of mucositis.
• Patient on chronic drug therapy may rarely present with symptoms of blood dyscrasias, which can include infection, bleeding and poor healing. If dyscrasia is present, caution patient to prevent oral tissue trauma when using oral hygiene aids.
• Palliative medication may be required for management of oral side effects.
• Consider local hemostasis measures to prevent excessive bleeding.
• Patient may be at risk of bleeding; check oral signs.
Consultations:
• Medical consultation should include routine blood counts including platelet counts and bleeding time.
• Consult physician; prophylactic or therapeutic antiinfectives may be indicated if surgery or periodontal treatment is required.
• Medical consultation may be required to assess immunologic status during cancer chemotherapy and determine safety risk, if any, posed by the required dental treatment.
• Medical consultation may be required to assess disease control and patient's ability to tolerate stress.
• In a patient with symptoms of blood dyscrasias, request a medical consultation for blood studies and postpone treatment until normal values are reestablished.
Teach Patient/Family to:
• Be aware of oral side effects
• Use effective oral hygiene to prevent soft tissue inflammation
• See dentist immediately if signs of secondary oral infection occur
• Prevent trauma when using oral hygiene aids
• Update health and medication history if physician makes any changes in evaluation or drug regimens; include OTC, herbal, and nonherbal remedies in the update

doxycycline
dox-ih-sye´-kleen
(Adoxa, Apo-Doxy[CAN], Doryx, Doxsig[AUS], Doxy-100, Doxycin[CAN], Doxyhexal[AUS], Doxylin[AUS], Monodox, Vibramycin, Vibra-Tabs)
Do not confuse doxycycline with Dicyclomine or doxylamine, or Monodox with Monopril.

CATEGORY AND SCHEDULE
Pregnancy Risk Category: D

Drug Class: Tetracycline, broad-spectrum antiinfective

MECHANISM OF ACTION
A tetracycline antibiotic that inhibits bacterial protein synthesis by binding to ribosomes. *Therapeutic Effect:* Bacteriostatic.

USES
Treatment of syphilis, *C. trachomatis*, gonorrhea, lymphogranuloma venereum, uncommon gram-negative and gram-positive organisms, necrotizing ulcerative

gingivostomatitis; cutaneous or inhalational anthrax exposure

PHARMACOKINETICS

PO: Peak 1.5–4 hr, *Half-life:* 15-22 hr; 25%–93% protein bound; excreted in bile.

INDICATIONS AND DOSAGES

▶ **Respiratory, Skin, and Soft-Tissue Infections; UTIs; Pelvic Inflammatory Disease (PID); Brucellosis; Trachoma; Rocky Mountain Spotted Fever; Typhus; Q Fever; Rickettsia; Severe Acne (Adoxa); Smallpox; Psittacosis; Ornithosis; Granuloma Inguinale; Lymphogranuloma Venereum; Intestinal Amebiasis (Adjunctive Treatment); Prevention of Rheumatic Fever**
PO
Adults, Elderly. Initially, 100 mg q12h, then 100 mg/day as single dose or 50 mg q12h for severe infections.
Children 8 yr and older and weighing more than 45 kg.
2–4 mg/kg/day divided q12–24h. Maximum: 200 mg/day.
IV
Adults, Elderly. Initially, 200 mg as 1–2 infusions; then 100–200 mg/day in 1–2 divided doses.
Children 8 yr and older. 2–4 mg/kg/day divided q12–24h. Maximum: 200 mg/day.
▶ **Acute Gonococcal Infections**
PO
Adults. Initially, 200 mg, then 100 mg at bedtime on first day; then 100 mg twice a day for 14 days.
▶ **Syphilis**
PO, IV
Adults. 200 mg/day in divided doses for 14–28 days.
▶ **Traveler's Diarrhea**
PO
Adults, Elderly. 100 mg/day during a period of risk (up to 14 days) and for 2 days after returning home.

▶ **Periodontitis**
PO
Adults. 20 mg twice a day as an adjunct to scaling and root planning; may be administered for up to 9 mo; exceeding the recommended dosage may increase risk of side effects, including the development of resistant organisms.

SIDE EFFECTS/ADVERSE REACTIONS

Frequent
Anorexia, nausea, vomiting, diarrhea, dysphagia, possibly severe photosensitivity
Occasional
Rash, urticaria

PRECAUTIONS AND CONTRAINDICATIONS

Children 8 yr and younger, hypersensitivity to tetracyclines or sulfites, last half of pregnancy, severe hepatic dysfunction
Caution
Hepatic disease, lactation.

DRUG INTERACTIONS OF CONCERN TO DENTISTRY

• No data reported for this dose form; see doxycycline hyclate monograph for drug interactions reported with tetracyclines

DRUG INTERACTIONS OF CONCERN TO DENTISTRY FOR SYSTEMIC FORM:

• Decreased absorption: $NaHCO_3$, other antacids
• Increased rate of metabolism: barbiturates, carbamazepine, hydantoins
• Decreased effect of penicillins, cephalosporins
• May increase the effectiveness of anticoagulants, methotrexate, digoxin
• Oral contraceptives: advise patient of a potential risk for decreased contraceptive action, to maintain compliance with oral contraceptive

use while using antibiotics, and to consider the use of additional nonhormonal contraception
• Contraindicated with isotretinoin (Accutane)

SERIOUS REACTIONS

! Superinfection (especially fungal) and benign intracranial hypertension (headache, visual changes) may occur.
! Hepatoxicity, fatty degeneration of the liver, and pancreatitis occur rarely.

DENTAL CONSIDERATIONS

Doxycycline Hyclate (Dental-Systemic)
General:
• Examine for oral manifestation of opportunistic infection.
• Should be administered at least 1 hr before or 2 hr after morning or evening meals.
Teach Patient/Family to:
• Avoid using ingestible sodium bicarbonate products, such as the Prophy-Jet air polishing system, within 2 hr of drug use

Doxycycline Hyclate/Doxycycline Calcium (Systemic Form)
General:
• Determine why the patient is taking tetracycline.
• Broad-spectrum antibiotics may promote oral or vaginal Candida infection.
Consultations:
• Medical consultation may be required to assess disease control.
Teach Patient/Family:
• That tetracycline can be taken with milk, food; take with a full glass of water
• To take tetracycline doses 1 hr before or 2 hr after air polishing device (Prophy-Jet), if used
• When used for dental infection, advise patient:

• To report sore throat, oral burning sensation, fever, and fatigue, any of which could indicate superinfection
• To take at prescribed intervals and complete dosage regimen
• To immediately notify the dentist if signs or symptoms of infection increase

doxycycline hyclate (dental-systemic)
dox-ih-sye′-kleen
(Periostat)

CATEGORY AND SCHEDULE
Pregnancy Risk Category: D

Drug Class: Tetracycline derivative for nonantibacterial use

MECHANISM OF ACTION
Reduces elevated collagenase activity in gingival crevicular fluid of patients with adult periodontitis; no antibacterial effect reported at this dose

USES
Adjunct to scaling and root planing to promote attachment level gain and reduce pocket depth in adult periodontitis

PHARMACOKINETICS
No data available

INDICATIONS AND DOSAGES
PO
Adult. 20 mg twice daily as an adjunct to scaling and root planing; may be administered for up to 9 mo; exceeding the recommended dosage may increase risk of side effects, including the development of resistant organisms.

SIDE EFFECTS/ADVERSE REACTIONS

Note: In a clinical study of 428 patients there was little to no difference in the incidence of side effects reported between this drug and a placebo. See doxycycline hyclate monograph for typical side effects associated with oral administration. Whether these side effects would occur at doses used in this product is unknown.

PRECAUTIONS AND CONTRAINDICATIONS

Hypersensitivity to tetracyclines
Caution
Children younger than 8 yr, pregnant and nursing mothers, predisposition to oral or vaginal candidiasis; not to be used for antimicrobial effect in periodontitis

DRUG INTERACTIONS OF CONCERN TO DENTISTRY

No data reported for this dose form; see doxycycline hyclate monograph for drug interactions reported with tetracyclines

SERIOUS REACTIONS

Pregnancy (permanent tooth discoloration), fetal toxicity

DENTAL CONSIDERATIONS

General:
• Examine for oral manifestation of opportunistic infection.
• Should be administered at least 1 hr before or 2 hr after morning or evening meals.
Teach Patient/Family to:
• Avoid using ingestible sodium bicarbonate products, such as the air polishing system ProphyJet, within 2 hr of drug use

doxycycline hyclate gel

dox-ih-sye′-kleen
(Atridox)

CATEGORY AND SCHEDULE
Pregnancy Risk Category: D

Drug Class: Tetracycline, antiinfective

MECHANISM OF ACTION
Inhibits bacterial protein synthesis by disruption of transfer RNA and messenger RNA

USES
Adjunctive treatment of chronic adult periodontitis to increase clinical attachment, reduce probing depth, and reduce bleeding on probing

PHARMACOKINETICS
Gingival crevicular fluid levels peak at 2 hr, sustained levels up to 18 hr and decline over 7 days; low serum levels not exceeding 0.1 g/ml.

INDICATIONS AND DOSAGES
Topical
Adult. Mix contents of syringes according to detailed instructions, completing 100 cycles; attach blunt cannula to syringe A and fill the pocket; after it becomes firm, the mixture may be packed further into the pocket with a dental instrument.

SIDE EFFECTS/ADVERSE REACTIONS
Oral: Gingival discomfort, pain, loss of attachment, toothache, periodontal abscess, exudate, infection, drainage, swelling, thermal tooth sensitivity, extreme mobility, localized allergic reaction
CNS: Headache
CV: High B/P
GI: Diarrhea
GU: PMS

EENT: Skin infection,
photosensitivity
MS: Muscle aches, backache
Misc: Common cold

PRECAUTIONS AND CONTRAINDICATIONS
Hypersensitivity
Caution
Children (tooth staining), lactation,
photosensitivity, predisposition to
candidiasis

DRUG INTERACTIONS OF CONCERN TO DENTISTRY
❗ None specifically identified for this
product; unknown whether typical
tetracycline interactions occur

SERIOUS REACTIONS
Pregnancy (permanent tooth
discoloration), fetal toxicity

DENTAL CONSIDERATONS

General:
• Examine for oral manifestation of
opportunistic infection.
Teach Patient/Family to:
• Be alert to the possibility of
secondary oral infection and the need
to see dentist immediately if signs of
infection occur
• Avoid oral hygiene procedures in
treated areas of mouth for 7 days to
avoid dislodging product

---

dronabinol
droe-nab´-ih-nol
(Marinol)
Do not confuse dronabinol with
droperidol.

CATEGORY AND SCHEDULE
Pregnancy Risk Category: C
Controlled Substance Schedule: III

Drug Class: Antiemetic, appetite
stimulant

MECHANISM OF ACTION
An antiemetic and appetite stimulant
that may act by inhibiting vomiting
control mechanisms in the medulla
oblongata. **Therapeutic Effect:** Inhibits
vomiting and stimulates appetite.

USES
Control of nausea, vomiting in
selected patients receiving
emetogenic cancer chemotherapy;
stimulate appetite in AIDS-
associated anorexia

PHARMACOKINETICS
Well absorbed after PO
administration. Protein binding: 97%.
Undergoes first-pass metabolism.
Is highly lipid soluble. Primarily
excreted in feces. **Half-life:** 4 hr.

INDICATIONS AND DOSAGES
▸ **Prevention of Chemotherapy-
Induced Nausea and Vomiting**
PO
Adults, Children. Initially, 5 mg/m^2
1–3 hr before chemotherapy, then
q2–4h after chemotherapy for total of
4–6 doses a day. May increase by
2.5 mg/m^2 up to 15 mg/m^2 per dose.
▸ **Appetite Stimulant**
PO
Adults. Initially, 2.5 mg twice a day
(before lunch and dinner). Range:
2.5–20 mg/day.

SIDE EFFECTS/ADVERSE REACTIONS
Frequent
Euphoria, dizziness, paranoid
reaction, somnolence
Occasional
Asthenia, ataxia, confusion,
abnormal thinking, depersonalization
Rare
Diarrhea, depression, nightmares,
speech difficulties, headache,
anxiety, tinnitus, flushed skin

PRECAUTIONS AND CONTRAINDICATIONS

Treatment of nausea and vomiting not caused by chemotherapy, hypersensitivity to sesame oil or tetrahydrocannabinol products

Caution

Lactation, children, elderly, cardiac disorders, drug abuse, alcoholism, hypertension, manic or depressive state, schizophrenia

DRUG INTERACTIONS OF CONCERN TO DENTISTRY

• Increased CNS depression: alcohol, CNS depressants, tricyclic antidepressants
• Additive hypertension, tachycardia, possible cardiotoxicity: tricyclic antidepressants, amphetamines, other sympathomimetics
• Additive tachycardia, drowsiness: atropine, scopolamine, antihistamines, anticholinergic drugs

SERIOUS REACTIONS

❗ Mild intoxication may produce increased sensory awareness (including taste, smell, and sound), altered time perception, reddened conjunctiva, dry mouth, and tachycardia.
❗ Moderate intoxication may produce memory impairment and urine retention.
❗ Severe intoxication may produce lethargy, decreased motor coordination, slurred speech, and orthostatic hypotension.

DENTAL CONSIDERATIONS

General:
• Monitor vital signs at every appointment because of cardiovascular side effects.
• After supine positioning, have patient sit upright for at least 2 min to avoid orthostatic hypotension.
• Patients taking opioids for acute or chronic pain should be given alternative analgesics for dental pain.

• Assess salivary flow as a factor in caries, periodontal disease, and candidiasis.
• Consider semisupine chair position for patient comfort if GI side effects occur.

Teach Patient/Family to:
• When chronic dry mouth occurs, advise patient to:
  • Avoid mouth rinses with high alcohol content because of drying effects
  • Use daily home fluoride products for anticaries effect
  • Use sugarless gum, frequent sips of water, or saliva substitutes

droperidol
droe-pear´-ih-dall
(Inapsine)

CATEGORY AND SCHEDULE
Pregnancy Risk Category: C

Drug Class: General anesthetic; anesthesia adjunct, antiemetic

MECHANISM OF ACTION

A general anesthetic and antiemetic agent that antagonizes dopamine neurotransmission at synapses by blocking postsynaptic dopamine receptor sites; partially blocks adrenergic receptor binding sites. *Therapeutic Effect:* Produces tranquilization, antiemetic effect.

USES

Treatment of nausea and vomiting associated with surgical and diagnostic procedures

PHARMACOKINETICS
Onset of action occurs within
30 min. Well absorbed. Metabolized
in liver. Excreted in urine and feces.
Half-life: 2.3 hr.

INDICATIONS AND DOSAGES
▶ **Preoperative**
IM/IV
*Adults, Elderly, Children 12 yr and
older.* 2.5–10 mg 30–60 min before
induction of general anesthesia.
Children 2–12 yr. 0.088–0.165 mg/kg.
▶ **Adjunct for Induction of General
Anesthesia**
IV
*Adults, Elderly, Children 12 yr and
older.* 0.22–0.275 mg/kg.
Children 2–12 yr. 0.088–0.165 mg/kg.
▶ **Adjunct for Maintenance of
General Anesthesia**
IV
Adults, Elderly. 1.25–2.5 mg.
▶ **Diagnostic Procedures without
General Anesthesia**
IM
Adults, Elderly. 2.5–10 mg 30–60 min
before procedure. If needed, may
give additional doses of 1.25–2.5 mg
(usually by IV injection).

SIDE EFFECTS/ADVERSE
REACTIONS
Frequent
Mild-to-moderate hypotension
Occasional
Tachycardia, postoperative drowsiness,
dizziness, chills, shivering
Rare
Postoperative nightmares, facial
sweating, bronchospasm

PRECAUTIONS AND
CONTRAINDICATIONS
Known or suspected QT prolongation,
hypersensitivity to droperidol or any
component of the formulation

DRUG INTERACTIONS OF
CONCERN TO DENTISTRY
• Increased frequency of nausea/
vomiting: propofol
• Increased CNS depression: all
CNS depressants
• Prolonged QT interval: intravenous
narcotics
• Increased hypotension: anesthetics,
systemic or local
• Risk of hypotension: epinephrine
• Orthostatic hypotension:
antihypertensive medications

SERIOUS REACTIONS
❗ Extrapyramidal symptoms may
appear as akathisia (motor restlessness)
and dystonias: torticollis (neck muscle
spasm), opisthotonos (rigidity of back
muscles), and oculogyric crisis (rolling
back of eyes).
❗ Overdosage includes symptoms of
hypotension, tachycardia, hallucinations, and extrapyramidal symptoms.
❗ Prolonged QT interval, seizures,
and arrhythmias have been reported.

DENTAL CONSIDERATIONS
General:
• Used in a hospital, emergency
room, or cancer treatment center for
acute need.
• Caution in the use of drugs that
prolong the QT interval.
• Use caution if sedation or general
anesthesia is required; risk of
hypotensive episode.
• After supine positioning, have
patient sit upright for at least 2 min
before standing to avoid orthostatic
hypotension.
• Monitor vital signs at every
appointment due to cardiovascular
side effects.
Consultations:
• Consultation with physician may
be necessary if sedation or general
anesthesia is required.

• Medical consultation may be required to assess disease control.

duloxetine
doo-lox'-eh-teen
(Cymbalta)

CATEGORY AND SCHEDULE
Pregnancy Risk Category: C

Drug class: Antidepressant

MECHANISM OF ACTION
Selectively inhibits the reuptake of serotonin (5-HT) and norepinephrine in the brain.

USES
Treatment of major depressive disorder; diabetic peripheral neuropathic pain

PHARMACOKINETICS
Peak 6 hr, plasma protein binding greater than 90%; metabolized in liver by CYP2D6 and CYP1A2 isoenzymes; excreted in urine (70%) and feces (30%) *Half-life 8–17 hr.*

INDICATIONS AND DOSAGES
▸ **Depression:**
PO
Adult: 40 mg per day (20 mg twice daily) to 60 mg/day (once daily or 30 mg twice daily).
▸ **Diabetic peripheral neuropathic pain**
PO
Adult: Up to a total dose of 60 mg per day (once a day).
▸ **Available forms include:**
Caplets 20, 30, and 60 mg.

SIDE EFFECTS/ADVERSE REACTIONS
Oral: Dry mouth

CNS: Insomnia, anxiety, decreased appetite, dizziness, somnolence, tremors, fatigue, decreased libido
CV: Hot flushes, elevated B/P
GI: Nausea, constipation, diarrhea, vomiting, dyspepsia
RESP: Cough, nasopharyngitis
GU: Erectile and ejaculation dysfunction, poliakiuria
EENT: Blurred vision, pharyngolaryngeal pain
INTEG: Sweating
MS: Muscle cramps, myalgia
SYST: Fatigue, asthenia, pyrexia

PRECAUTIONS AND CONTRAINDICATIONS
Hypersensitivity, MAOIs, uncontrolled narrow-angle glaucoma, hepatotoxicity, elevated B/P, psychiatric changes, seizures, glaucoma, physical and pyschological symptoms of withdrawal, renal impairment

DRUG INTERACTIONS OF CONCERN TO DENTISTRY
• Potentiation of anticholinergic effects by antisialogogues used in dentistry (e.g., atropine, glycopyrrolate)
• Increased fluoxetine blood levels and toxicity with some fluoroquinolone antibacterials
• Centrally-acting drugs (e.g., sedatives) may enhance CNS adverse effects
• Caution: can inhibit CYP2D6 isoenzymes, use phenothiazines with caution (see Appendix I)
• Avoid administration with alcohol or alcohol-containing agents (e.g., elixirs)

SERIOUS REACTIONS

DENTAL CONSIDERATIONS
General
• Monitor vital signs at every appointment because of cardiovascular side effects.

- Assess salivary flow as a factor in caries, periodontal disease, candidiasis, denture sore mouth.
- Assess salivary flow as a factor in reduced retention and/or increased irritation of removable prostheses.

Consultations
- Medical consultation may be required to assess disease control and patient's ability to tolerate stress.
- Inform physician of potential adverse effects of dry mouth and possible need to change medications if severe.

Teach Patient/Family to:
- Use effective oral hygiene measures to minimize effects of reduced salivary flow
- Avoid mouth rinses with high alcohol content because of drying effects
- Use daily home fluoride products for anticaries effect
- Use sugarless or xylitol chewing gums, frequent sips of water, and/or saliva substitutes if dry mouth occurs

dutasteride
do-tah-stir´-eyed
(Avodart)

CATEGORY AND SCHEDULE
Pregnancy Risk Category: X

Drug Class: Synthetic steroid

MECHANISM OF ACTION
An androgen hormone inhibitor that inhibits 5-alpha reductase, an intracellular enzyme that converts testosterone into dihydrotestosterone (DHT) in the prostate gland, reducing the serum DHT level.
Therapeutic Effect: Reduces size of the prostate gland.

USES
Treatment of benign prostate hyperplasia (BPH) in men to improve symptoms, reduce the risk of urinary retention, and reduce the need for BPH-related surgery

PHARMACOKINETICS

Route	Onset	Peak	Duration
PO	24 hr	N/A	3–8 wk

Moderately absorbed after PO administration. Widely distributed. Protein binding: 99%. Metabolized in the liver. Primarily excreted in feces. **Half-life:** Up to 5 wk.

INDICATIONS AND DOSAGES
▸ **BPH**
PO
Adults, Elderly. 0.5 mg once a day.

SIDE EFFECTS/ADVERSE REACTIONS
Occasional
Gynecomastia, sexual dysfunction (decreased libido, impotence, and decreased volume of ejaculate)

PRECAUTIONS AND CONTRAINDICATIONS
Females, physical handling of tablets by those who are or may be pregnant
Caution
Hepatic impairment, men cannot donate blood until at least 6 mo after last dose, drug also found in semen, no data on use in patients younger than 18 yr or in renal impairment, nursing mothers (not used in women)

DRUG INTERACTIONS OF CONCERN TO DENTISTRY
- No drug interaction studies have been conducted; however, caution should be observed when used in

combination with potent and chronically used CYP3A4 inhibitors
• Opioids and anticholinergic drugs may enhance urinary retention; use alternative analgesics (NSAIDs)

SERIOUS REACTIONS
! Toxicity may be manifested as rash, diarrhea, and abdominal pain.

DENTAL CONSIDERATIONS
General:
• Determine why patient is taking the drug.
Consultations:
• Medical consultation may be required to assess disease control.
Teach Patient/Family to:
• Update health and drug history if physician makes any changes in evaluation or drug regimens

dyphylline
die´-fih-lin
(Dilor, Lufyllin)
Do not confuse with Dilacor.

CATEGORY AND SCHEDULE
Pregnancy Risk Category: C

Drug Class: Xanthine derivative

MECHANISM OF ACTION
A xanthine derivative that acts as a bronchodilator by directly relaxing smooth muscle of the bronchial airway and pulmonary blood vessels similar to theophylline. **Therapeutic Effect:** Relieves bronchospasm, increases vital capacity, produces cardiac, and skeletal muscle stimulation.

USES
Treatment of bronchial asthma, bronchospasm in chronic bronchitis, COPD, emphysema

PHARMACOKINETICS
Rapid absorption after PO administration. Excreted in urine. **Half-life:** 2 hr.

INDICATIONS AND DOSAGES
▸ **Chronic Bronchospasm, Asthma**
PO
Adults, Elderly. 15 mg/kg 4 times a day.
IM
Adults, Elderly. 250–500 mg. Maximum: 15 mg/kg q6h.
Children. 4.4–6.6 mg/kg/day in divided doses.
▸ **Dosage in renal impairment**

Creatinine Clearance	Dosage Percent
50–80 ml/min	Administer 75% of dose
10–50 ml/min	Administer 50% of dose
Less than 10 ml/min	Administer 25% of dose

SIDE EFFECTS/ADVERSE REACTIONS
Frequent
Tachycardia, nervousness, restlessness
Occasional
Heartburn, vomiting, headache, mild diuresis, insomnia, nausea

PRECAUTIONS AND CONTRAINDICATIONS
Uncontrolled arrhythmias, hyperthyroidism, history of hypersensitivity to dyphylline,

related xanthine derivatives, or any component of the formulation

Caution

Elderly, CHF, cor pulmonale, hepatic disease, active peptic ulcer disease, diabetes mellitus, hyperthyroidism, hypertension, children, renal disease, glaucoma

DRUG INTERACTIONS OF CONCERN TO DENTISTRY

• Increased action: erythromycin, ciprofloxacin, tetracyclines
• Increased risk of cardiac dysrhythmia: halothane-inhalation anesthesia, CNS stimulants
• Decreased effect: barbiturates, carbamazepine, ketoconazole

• May decrease sedative effects of benzodiazepines

SERIOUS REACTIONS

! Ventricular arrhythmias, hypotension, circulatory failure, seizures, hyperglycemia, and syndrome of inappropriate antidiuretic hormone (SIADH) have been reported.

DENTAL CONSIDERATIONS

General:
• Monitor vital signs at every appointment because of cardiovascular and respiratory side effects.
• Consider semisupine chair position for patients with respiratory disease.

echothiophate iodide
ek-oh-thye´-oh-fate eye´-oh-dide
(Phospholine Iodide)

CATEGORY AND SCHEDULE
Pregnancy Risk Category: C

Drug Class: Antiglaucoma
agent, ophthalmic;
cyclostimulant, accommodative
esotropia; diagnostic aid,
accommodative esotropia

MECHANISM OF ACTION
A cholinesterase inhibitor that causes
acetylcholine to accumulate at
cholinergic receptor sites and
produce effects like excessive
stimulation of cholinergic receptors.
Therapeutic Effect: Causes
conjunctival hyperemia and constriction
of the sphincter pupillae and ciliary
muscles, which results in miosis and
paralysis of accommodation.

USES
Treatment certain types of glaucoma
and other eye conditions, such as
accommodative esotropia. They may
also be used in the diagnosis of
certain eye conditions, such as
accommodative esotropia.

PHARMACOKINETICS
None reported

INDICATIONS AND DOSAGES
▶ **Glaucoma**
Ophthalmic
Adults, Elderly. Instill 1 drop twice
daily into eyes with 1 dose prior to
bedtime.
▶ **Accommodative Esotropia,
Diagnosis**
Ophthalmic
Children. Instill 1 drop once daily
into both eyes at bedtime for 2–3 wk.

▶ **Accommodative Esotropia,
Treatment**
Ophthalmic
Children. Instill 1 drop once daily.

SIDE EFFECTS/ADVERSE REACTIONS
Occasional
Headache, browache, blurred vision,
burning and stinging of eyes,
decreased night vision, intraocular
pressure changes, iritis, uveitis

PRECAUTIONS AND CONTRAINDICATIONS
Active uveal inflammation, angle-
closure glaucoma, hypersensitivity
to echothiophate products

DRUG INTERACTIONS OF CONCERN TO DENTISTRY
• Avoid use of succinylcholine in
general anesthesia
• Possible inhibition of the
metabolism of ester-type local and
topical anesthetics
• Avoid use of anticholinergics, such
as systemic atropine or related drugs

SERIOUS REACTIONS
❗ Cardiac irregularities have been
reported.

DENTAL CONSIDERATIONS
General:
• Determine why patient is taking
the drug.
• Avoid drugs with anticholinergic
activity, such as antihistamines,
opioids, benzodiazepines,
propantheline, atropine, and
scopolamine.
• Avoid dental light in patient's
eyes; offer dark glasses for patient
comfort.
• Question glaucoma patient about
compliance with prescribed drug
regimen.

Consultations:
• Medical consultation may be required to assess disease control.
Teach Patient/Family to:
• Update health and medication history if physician makes any changes in evaluation or drug regimens; include OTC, herbal, and nonherbal remedies in the update

efalizumab
ef-ah-liz´-ewe-mab
(Raptiva)

CATEGORY AND SCHEDULE
Pregnancy Risk Category: C

Drug Class: Monoclonal antibody

MECHANISM OF ACTION
A monoclonal antibody that interferes with lymphocyte activation by binding to the lymphocyte antigen, inhibiting the adhesion of leukocytes to other cell types. *Therapeutic Effect:* Prevents the release of cytokines and the growth and migration of circulating total lymphocytes, predominant in psoriatic lesions.

USES
Treatment of chronic moderate to severe plaque psoriasis in patients (older than 18 yr) who are candidates for systemic therapy or phototherapy

PHARMACOKINETICS
Clearance is affected by body weight, not by gender or race, after subcutaneous injection. Serum concentration reaches steady state at 4 wk. Mean time to elimination: 25 days.

INDICATIONS AND DOSAGES
▸ **Psoriasis**
Subcutaneous
Adults, Elderly. Initially, 0.7 mg/kg followed by weekly doses of 1 mg/kg. Maximum: 200 mg (single dose).

SIDE EFFECTS/ADVERSE REACTIONS
Frequent
Headache, chills, nausea, injection site pain
Occasional
Myalgia, flu-like symptoms, fever
Rare
Back pain, acne

PRECAUTIONS AND CONTRAINDICATIONS
Concurrent use of immunosuppressive agents
Caution
Increased risk of infections, malignancies, worsening of psoriasis, use in elderly, safety and efficacy have not been established in lactation or children

DRUG INTERACTIONS OF CONCERN TO DENTISTRY
None reported

SERIOUS REACTIONS
! Hypersensitivity reaction, malignancies, serious infections (abscess, cellulitis, postoperative wound infection, pneumonia), thrombocytopenia, and worsening of psoriasis occur rarely.

DENTAL CONSIDERATIONS
General:
• Understand the disease and the patient's need to use this drug.
• Rarely oral lesions and geographic tongue may occur in patients with psoriasis.

efavirenz

eh-fahv´-er-ins
(Stocrin[AUS], Sustiva)
Do not confuse Sustiva with
Survanta.

CATEGORY AND SCHEDULE

Pregnancy Risk Category: C.

Drug Class: Antiviral
(nonnucleoside)

MECHANISM OF ACTION

A nonnucleoside reverse
transcriptase inhibitor that inhibits
the activity of HIV reverse
transcriptase of HIV-1 and the
transcription of HIV-1 RNA to DNA.
Therapeutic Effect: Interrupts HIV
replication, slowing the progression
of HIV infection.

USES

Treatment in HIV-1 infection, only
in combination with other HIV-1
antiretroviral agents

PHARMACOKINETICS

Rapidly absorbed after PO
administration. Protein binding: 99%.
Metabolized to major isoenzymes in
the liver. Eliminated in urine and
feces. **Half-life:** 40–55 hr.

INDICATIONS AND DOSAGES

▶ **HIV Infection (in combination with
other antiretrovirals)**
PO
*Adults, Elderly, Children 3 yr and
older weighing 40 kg or more.*
600 mg once a day at bedtime.
*Children 3 yr and older weighing
32.5 kg to less than 40 kg.* 400 mg
once a day.
*Children 3 yr and older weighing
25 kg to less than 32.5 kg.* 350 mg
once a day.

*Children 3 yr and older weighing 20 kg
to less than 25 kg.* 300 mg once a day.
*Children 3 yr and older weighing
15 kg to less than 20 kg.* 250 mg
once a day.
*Children 3 yr and older weighing 10 kg
to less than 15 kg.* 200 mg once a day.

SIDE EFFECTS/ADVERSE REACTIONS

Frequent
Mild to severe: Dizziness, vivid
dreams, insomnia, confusion,
impaired concentration, amnesia,
agitation, depersonalization,
hallucinations, euphoria, somnolence
(mild symptoms don't interfere with
daily activities; severe symptoms
interrupt daily activities)
Occasional
Mild to moderate: Maculopapular
rash; nausea, fatigue, headache,
diarrhea, fever, cough (moderate
symptoms may interfere with daily
activities)

PRECAUTIONS AND CONTRAINDICATIONS

Concurrent use with ergot
derivatives, midazolam, or triazolam;
efavirenz as monotherapy;
hypersensitivity to efavirenz
Caution
Must not be used as a single agent
for HIV, avoid pregnancy with use,
lactation, mental illness, substance
abuse, caution with alcohol or
psychotropic drugs, driving or other
hazardous tasks, monitor cholesterol,
hepatic impairment

DRUG INTERACTIONS OF CONCERN TO DENTISTRY

• Contraindicated drugs: midazolam,
triazolam
• Decreased plasma levels of
clarithromycin, carbamazepine,
St. John's wort (herb)

• Potential for increased levels with ketoconazole, itraconazole (no studies)
• Increased risk of CNS side effects with CNS depressants

SERIOUS REACTIONS
None known

General:
• Examine for oral manifestation of opportunistic infection.
• Monitor vital signs at every appointment because of cardiovascular and respiratory side effects.
• Consider semisupine chair position for patient comfort because of GI side effects of drug.
• Assess salivary flow as a factor in caries, periodontal disease, and candidiasis.
• Short appointments and a stress-reduction protocol may be required for anxious patients.
Consultations:
• Medical consultation may be required to assess disease control.
Teach Patient/Family to:
• Prevent trauma when using oral hygiene aids
• Use effective oral hygiene to prevent soft tissue inflammation
• Be alert for the possibility of secondary oral infection and to see dentist immediately if signs of infection occur
• When chronic dry mouth occurs, advise patient to:
   • Avoid mouth rinses with high alcohol content because of drying effects
   • Use daily home fluoride products for anticaries effect
   • Use sugarless gum, frequent sips of water, or saliva substitutes

eletriptan
el-eh-trip´-tan
(Relpax)

CATEGORY AND SCHEDULE
Pregnancy Risk Category: C

Drug Class: Serotonin receptor agonist

MECHANISM OF ACTION
A serotonin receptor agonist that binds selectively to vascular receptors, producing a vasoconstrictive effect on cranial blood vessels. *Therapeutic Effect:* Relieves migraine headache.

USES
Treatment of acute migraine with or without aura in adults

PHARMACOKINETICS
Well absorbed after PO administration. Metabolized by the liver to inactive metabolite. Eliminated in urine. *Half-life:* 4.4 hr (increased in hepatic impairment and the elderly [older than 65 yr]).

INDICATIONS AND DOSAGES
▸ **Acute Migraine Headache**
PO
Adults, Elderly. 20–40 mg. If headache improves but then returns, dose may be repeated after 2 hr. Maximum: 80 mg/day.

SIDE EFFECTS/ADVERSE REACTIONS
Occasional
Dizziness, somnolence, asthenia, nausea
Rare
Paresthesia, headache, dry mouth, warm or hot sensation, dyspepsia, dysphagia

PRECAUTIONS AND CONTRAINDICATIONS

Arrhythmias associated with conduction disorders, coronary artery disease, ischemic heart disease, severe hepatic impairment, uncontrolled hypertension

Caution

Do not use within 72 hr of treatment with strong CYP3A4 enzyme inhibitors, caution in lactation, safety and use in children younger than 18 yr has not been established

DRUG INTERACTIONS OF CONCERN TO DENTISTRY

• Avoid use of strong CYP3A4 drugs concurrently or within 72 hr of use of eletriptan: ketoconazole, itraconazole, erythromycin, clarithromycin, others

SERIOUS REACTIONS

! Cardiac reactions (including ischemia, coronary artery vasospasm, and MI) and noncardiac vasospasm-related reactions (such as hemorrhage and CVA) occur rarely, particularly in patients with hypertension, diabetes, or a strong family history of coronary artery disease; obese patients; smokers; males older than 40 yr; and postmenopausal women.

DENTAL CONSIDERATIONS

General:
• This is an acute-use drug; it is doubtful that patients will seek dental treatment during acute migraine attacks.
• Be aware of the patient's disease, its severity, and its frequency, when known.
• Monitor vital signs at every appointment because of cardiovascular side effects.
• Assess salivary flow as a factor in caries, periodontal disease, and candidiasis.

• Consider semisupine chair position for patient comfort if GI side effects occur.

Consultations:
• If treating chronic orofacial pain, consult with patient's physician.

Teach Patient/Family to:
• Be aware that oral symptoms will disappear when drug is discontinued

emedastine
eh-med´-ah-steen
(Emadine)

CATEGORY AND SCHEDULE
Pregnancy Risk Category: B

Drug Class: Ophthalmic antihistamine

MECHANISM OF ACTION
An ophthalmic H_1-receptor antagonist that inhibits histamine-stimulated vascular permeability in the conjunctiva. **Therapeutic Effect:** Relieves ocular itching associated with allergic conjunctivitis.

USES
Temporary relief of signs and symptoms of allergic conjunctivitis

PHARMACOKINETICS
Negligible absorption after ophthalmic administration. Metabolized into inactive metabolites. Excreted in urine. **Half-life:** 6.6 hr.

INDICATIONS AND DOSAGES
▶ **Allergic Conjunctivitis**
Ophthalmic
Adults, Elderly, Children 3 yr and older. 1–2 drops in affected eye(s) twice daily.

SIDE EFFECTS/ADVERSE REACTIONS

Frequent
Headache
Occasional
Abnormal dreams, asthenia (loss of strength, energy), bad taste, blurred vision, burning or stinging, dry eyes, foreign body sensation, tearing

PRECAUTIONS AND CONTRAINDICATIONS

Hypersensitivity to emedastine or any other component of the formulation
Caution
Avoid wearing contact lens if eye is red, wait at least 10 min after application to insert contact lens, lactation, no data for use in children younger than 3 yr

DRUG INTERACTIONS OF CONCERN TO DENTISTRY

None reported

SERIOUS REACTIONS

! Somnolence and malaise occurs rarely.

emtricitabine
em-trih-sit´-ah-bean
(Emtriva)

CATEGORY AND SCHEDULE
Pregnancy Risk Category: B

Drug Class: Antiviral, nucleoside reverse transcriptase inhibitor

MECHANISM OF ACTION

An antiretroviral that inhibits HIV-1 reverse transcriptase by incorporating itself into viral DNA, resulting in chain termination. **Therapeutic Effect:** Interrupts HIV replication, slowing the progression of HIV infection.

USES

Treatment of HIV-1 infection in adults; used in combination with other antiretroviral medications

PHARMACOKINETICS

Rapidly and extensively absorbed from the GI tract. Excreted primarily in urine (86%) and, to a lesser extent, in feces (14%); 30% removed by hemodialysis. Unknown if removed by peritoneal dialysis. **Half-life:** 10 hr.

INDICATIONS AND DOSAGES

▸ **HIV Infection (in combination with other antiretrovirals)**
PO
Adults, Elderly. 200 mg once a day.
▸ **Dosage in Renal Impairment**
Dosage and frequency are modified on the basis of creatinine clearance.

Creatinine Clearance	Dosage
30–49 ml/min	200 mg q48h
15–29 ml/min	200 mg q72h
Less than 15 ml/min, hemodialysis patients	200 mg q96h

SIDE EFFECTS/ADVERSE REACTIONS

Frequent
Headache, rhinitis, rash, diarrhea, nausea
Occasional
Cough, vomiting, abdominal pain, insomnia, depression, paresthesia, dizziness, peripheral neuropathy, dyspepsia, myalgia

Rare
Arthralgia, abnormal dreams

PRECAUTIONS AND CONTRAINDICATIONS

Hypersensitivity
Caution
Possible risk of lactic acidosis, severe hepatomegaly with steatosis, use not established in HIV/HBV infections, renal impairment (dose reduction required), avoid nursing when taking this drug, safety and efficacy in pediatric patients have not been established

DRUG INTERACTIONS OF CONCERN TO DENTISTRY

None reported

SERIOUS REACTIONS

! Lactic acidosis and hepatomegaly with steatosis occur rarely and may be severe.

DENTAL CONSIDERATIONS

General:
• Examine for oral manifestation of opportunistic infection.
• Consider semisupine chair position for patient comfort if GI side effects occur.
• Patient history should include all medications and herbal or nonherbal remedies taken by the patient.
Consultations:
• Medical consultation may be required to assess disease control and patient's ability to tolerate stress.
Teach Patient/Family to:
• Use effective oral hygiene to prevent soft tissue inflammation, infection
• Prevent trauma when using oral hygiene aids
• Update health and drug history, reporting changes in health status, drug regimen changes, or disease/treatment status

enalapril maleate

en-al´-ah-pril ma´-lee-ate
(Alphapril[AUS], Amprace[AUS], Apo-Enalapril[CAN], Auspril[AUS], Renitec[AUS], Vasotec)
Do not confuse enalapril with Anafranil, Eldepryl, or ramipril.

CATEGORY AND SCHEDULE

Pregnancy Risk Category: D (C if used in first trimester)

Drug Class: Angiotensin-converting enzyme (ACE) inhibitor

MECHANISM OF ACTION

This ACE inhibitor suppresses the renin-angiotensin-aldosterone system and prevents conversion of angiotensin I to angiotensin II, a potent vasoconstrictor; may inhibit angiotensin II at local vascular, renal sites. Decreases plasma angiotensin II, increases plasma renin activity, decreases aldosterone secretion.
Therapeutic Effect: In hypertension, reduces peripheral arterial resistance. In CHF, increases cardiac output; decreases peripheral vascular resistance, B/P, pulmonary capillary wedge pressure, heart size.

USES

Treatment of hypertension, heart failure adjunct, asymptomatic left ventricular dysfunction

PHARMACOKINETICS

Route	Onset	Peak	Duration
PO	1 hr	4–6 hr	24 hr
IV	15 min	1–4 hr	6 hr

Readily absorbed from the GI tract (not affected by food).

Protein binding: 50%–60%.
Converted to active metabolite.
Primarily excreted in urine. Removed by hemodialysis. *Half-life:* 11 hr (half-life is increased in those with impaired renal function).

INDICATIONS AND DOSAGES

▸ **Hypertension Alone or in Combination with Other Antihypertensives**

PO

Adults, Elderly. Initially, 2.5–5 mg/day. Range: 10–40 mg/day in 1–2 divided doses.

Children. 0.1 mg/kg/day in 1–2 divided doses. Maximum: 0.5 mg/kg/day.

Neonates. 0.1 mg/kg/day q24h.

IV

Adults, Elderly. 0.625–1.25 mg q6h up to 5 mg q6h.

Children, Neonates. 5–10 mcg/kg/dose q8–24h.

▸ **Adjunctive Therapy for CHF**

PO

Adults, Elderly. Initially, 2.5–5 mg/day. Range: 5–20 mg/day in 2 divided doses.

▸ **Dosage in Renal Impairment**

Dosage is modified on the basis of creatinine clearance.

Creatinine Clearance	% of Usual Dose
10–50 ml/min	75–100
Less than 10 ml/min	50

SIDE EFFECTS/ADVERSE REACTIONS

Frequent

Headache, dizziness

Occasional

Orthostatic hypotension, fatigue, diarrhea, cough, syncope

Rare

Angina, abdominal pain, vomiting, nausea, rash, asthenia (loss of strength, energy), syncope

PRECAUTIONS AND CONTRAINDICATIONS

History of angioedema from previous treatment with ACE inhibitors

Caution

Renal disease, hyperkalemia

DRUG INTERACTIONS OF CONCERN TO DENTISTRY

• Increased hypotension: alcohol, phenothiazines
• Decreased hypotensive effects: indomethacin, possibly other NSAIDs, sympathomimetics
• Suspected reduction in the antihypertensive and vasodilator effects by salicylates; monitor B/P if used concurrently

SERIOUS REACTIONS

! Excessive hypotension ("first-dose syncope") may occur in patients with CHF and in those who are severely salt or volume depleted.
! Angioedema (swelling of face, lips) and hyperkalemia occur rarely.
! Agranulocytosis and neutropenia may be noted in patients with collagen vascular diseases, including scleroderma and systemic lupus erythematosus, and impaired renal function.
! Nephrotic syndrome may be noted in those with history of renal disease.

DENTAL CONSIDERATIONS

General:

• Monitor vital signs at every appointment because of cardiovascular side effects.
• After supine positioning, have patient sit upright for at least 2 min before standing to avoid orthostatic hypotension.
• Patients on chronic drug therapy may rarely have symptoms of blood dyscrasias, which can include infection, bleeding, and poor healing.

• Assess salivary flow as a factor in caries, periodontal disease, and candidiasis.

• Limit use of sodium-containing products, such as saline IV fluids, for those patients with a dietary salt restriction.

• Use vasoconstrictors with caution, in low doses, and with careful aspiration.

• Stress from dental procedures may compromise cardiovascular function; determine patient risk.

• Short appointments and a stress-reduction protocol may be required for anxious patients.

Consultations:

• Medical consultation may be required to assess patient's ability to tolerate stress.

• In a patient with symptoms of blood dyscrasias, request a medical consultation for blood studies and postpone dental treatment until normal values are reestablished.

• Take precautions if dental surgery is anticipated and sedation or general anesthesia is required; risk of hypotensive episode.

Teach Patient/Family to:

• Use effective oral hygiene to prevent soft tissue inflammation

• When chronic dry mouth occurs, advise patient to:

• Avoid mouth rinses with high alcohol content because of drying effects

• Use daily home fluoride products for anticaries effect

• Use sugarless gum, frequent sips of water, or saliva substitutes

enfuvirtide
en-few´-vir-tide
(Fuzeon)
Do not confuse Fuzeon with Furoxone.

CATEGORY AND SCHEDULE
Pregnancy Risk Category: B

Drug Class: Antiviral

MECHANISM OF ACTION
A fusion inhibitor that interferes with the entry of HIV-1 into CD4+ cells by inhibiting the fusion of viral and cellular membranes. *Therapeutic Effect:* Impairs HIV replication, slowing the progression of HIV infection.

USES
Treatment, in combination with other antiretroviral agents, of HIV-1 infection in treatment-experienced patients with HIV-1 replication despite ongoing antiretroviral therapy

PHARMACOKINETICS
Comparable absorption when injected into subcutaneous tissue of abdomen, arm, or thigh. Protein binding: 92%. Undergoes catabolism to amino acids. *Half-life:* 3.8 hr.

INDICATIONS AND DOSAGES
▸ **HIV Infection (in combination with other antiretrovirals)**
Subcutaneous
Adults, Elderly. 90 mg (1 ml) twice a day.
Children 6–16 yr. 2 mg/kg twice a day. Maximum 90 mg twice a day.

Pediatric Dosing Guidelines

Weight: kg (lb)	Dose: mg (ml)
11–15.5 (24–34)	27 (0.3)
15.6–20 (35–44)	36 (0.4)
20.1–24.5 (45–54)	45 (0.5)
24.6–29 (55–64)	54 (0.6)
29.1–33.5 (65–74)	63 (0.7)
33.6–38 (75–84)	72 (0.8)
38.1–42.5 (85–94)	81 (0.9)
Greater than 42.5 (greater than 94)	90 (1)

SIDE EFFECTS/ADVERSE REACTIONS

Expected
Local injection site reactions (pain, discomfort, induration, erythema, nodules, cysts, pruritus, ecchymosis)
Frequent
Diarrhea, nausea, fatigue
Occasional
Insomnia, peripheral neuropathy, depression, cough, decreased appetite or weight loss, sinusitis, anxiety, asthenia, myalgia, cold sores
Rare
Constipation, influenza, upper abdominal pain, anorexia, conjunctivitis

PRECAUTIONS AND CONTRAINDICATIONS

Hypersensitivity; patients should be instructed in recognizing local injection site reactions and trained in aseptic technique, HIV-infected mothers must not nurse, use in children younger than 6 yr has not been established.

DRUG INTERACTIONS OF CONCERN TO DENTISTRY

None reported

SERIOUS REACTIONS

! Enfuvirtide use may potentiate bacterial pneumonia.
! Hypersensitivity (rash, fever, chills, rigors, hypotension), thrombocytopenia, neutropenia, and renal insufficiency or failure may occur rarely.

DENTAL CONSIDERATIONS

General:
• Patients taking this drug will be taking other antiviral drugs that may interact with some dental drugs. Be sure to take a complete drug history.
• Patients on chronic drug therapy may rarely have symptoms of blood dyscrasias, which can include infection, bleeding, and poor healing.
• Examine for oral manifestation of opportunistic infection.
Consultations:
• Medical consultation may be required to assess disease control in the patient.
• In a patient with symptoms of blood dyscrasias, request a medical consultation for blood studies and postpone treatment until normal values are reestablished.
Teach Patient/Family to:
• Use effective oral hygiene to prevent soft tissue inflammation
• Prevent trauma when using oral hygiene aids
• Update health and drug history if physician makes any changes in evaluation or drug regimens

enoxaparin sodium
eh-nox-ah-pair´-in soe´-dee-um
(Clexane[AUS], Klexane[CAN],
Lovenox)
Do not confuse Lovenox with
Lotronex.

CATEGORY AND SCHEDULE
Pregnancy Risk Category: B

Drug Class: Heparin-type
anticoagulant

MECHANISM OF ACTION
A low-molecular-weight heparin that
potentiates the action of antithrombin
III and inactivates coagulation factor
Xa. *Therapeutic Effect:* Produces
anticoagulation. Does not significantly
influence bleeding time, PT, or aPTT.

USES
Prevention and treatment of deep
vein thrombosis (DVT) following hip
or knee replacement surgery; also
used in abdominal and gynecologic
surgery; with aspirin in the
prevention of ischemic complications
of unstable angina and non–Q-wave
MI; in combination with warfarin for
DVT, with or without pulmonary
embolism

PHARMACOKINETICS

Route	Onset	Peak	Duration
Subcutaneous	N/A	3–5 hr	12 hr

Well absorbed after subcutaneous
administration. Eliminated primarily
in urine. Not removed by
hemodialysis. *Half-life:* 4.5 hr.

INDICATIONS AND DOSAGES
▶ **Prevention of DVT after Hip and Knee Surgery**
Subcutaneous

Adults, Elderly. 30 mg twice a day,
generally for 7–10 days.
▶ **Prevention of DVT After Abdominal Surgery**
Subcutaneous
Adults, Elderly. 40 mg a day for
7–10 days.
▶ **Prevention of Long-Term DVT in Nonsurgical Acute Illness**
Subcutaneous
Adults, Elderly. 40 mg once a day
for 3 wk.
▶ **Prevention of Ischemic Complications of Unstable Angina and Non–Q-Wave MI (with oral aspirin therapy)**
Subcutaneous
Adults, Elderly. 1 mg/kg q12h.
▶ **Acute DVT**
Subcutaneous
Adults, Elderly. 1 mg/kg q12h or
1.5 mg/kg once daily.
▶ **Usual Pediatric Dosage**
Subcutaneous
Children. 0.5 mg/kg q12h (prophylaxis);
1 mg/kg q12h (treatment).
▶ **Dosage in Renal Impairment**
Clearance of enoxaparin is decreased
when creatinine clearance is less than
30 ml/min. Monitor patient and adjust
dosage as necessary. When enoxaparin
is used in abdomonal, hip, or knee
surgery or acute illness, the dosage in
renal impairment is 30 mg once a day.
When enoxaparin is used to treat DVT,
angina, or MI the dosage in renal
impairment is 1 mg/kg once a day.

SIDE EFFECTS/ADVERSE REACTIONS
Occasional
Injection site hematoma, nausea,
peripheral edema

PRECAUTIONS AND CONTRAINDICATIONS
Active major bleeding, concurrent
heparin therapy, hypersensitivity to

heparin or pork products, thrombocytopenia associated with positive in vitro test for antiplatelet antibodies

Caution

Hemorrhage, thrombocytopenia, renal impairment, elderly, lactation, children, requires monitoring, GI bleeding

DRUG INTERACTIONS OF CONCERN TO DENTISTRY

- Avoid concurrent use of aspirin, NSAIDs, dipyridamole, sulfinpyrazone
- Use with caution in patients taking olanzapine

SERIOUS REACTIONS

❗ Overdose may lead to bleeding complications ranging from local ecchymoses to major hemorrhage. Antidote: Protamine sulfate (1% solution) equal to the dose of enoxaparin injected. One mg protamine sulfate neutralizes 1 mg enoxaparin. A second dose of 0.5 mg protamine sulfate per 1 mg enoxaparin may be given if aPTT tested 2–4 hr after first injection remains prolonged.

DENTAL CONSIDERATIONS

General:

- Determine why patient is taking the drug.
- Product may be used in outpatient therapy. Delay elective dental treatment until patient completes enoxaparin therapy.
- Consider local hemostasis measures to prevent excessive bleeding if dental treatment must be performed.
- Avoid products that affect platelet function, such as aspirin and NSAIDs.
- Antibiotic prophylaxis before dental treatment may be required for joint prosthesis.

Consultations:

- Medical consultation should include routine blood counts, including platelet counts and bleeding time.

Teach Patient/Family to:

- Use effective oral hygiene to prevent soft tissue inflammation
- Use caution to prevent trauma when using oral hygiene aids
- Report oral lesions, soreness, or bleeding to dentist

entacapone
en-tak´-ah-pone
(Comtan)

CATEGORY AND SCHEDULE
Pregnancy Risk Category: C

Drug Class: Antiparkinsonian

MECHANISM OF ACTION

An antiparkinson agent that inhibits the enzyme, catechol-O-methyltransferase (COMT), potentiating dopamine activity and increasing the duration of action of levodopa. *Therapeutic Effect:* Decreases signs and symptoms of Parkinson's disease.

USES

Adjunct to levodopa/carbidopa in the treatment of Parkinson's disease, not used alone

PHARMACOKINETICS

Rapidly absorbed after PO administration. Protein binding: 98%. Metabolized in the liver. Primarily eliminated by biliary excretion. Not removed by hemodialysis. *Half-life:* 2.4 hr.

INDICATIONS AND DOSAGES
▶ **Adjunctive Treatment of Parkinson's Disease**
PO
Adults, Elderly. 200 mg concomitantly with each dose of carbidopa and levodopa up to a maximum of 8 times a day (1600 mg).

SIDE EFFECTS/ADVERSE REACTIONS
Frequent
Dyskinesia, nausea, dark yellow or orange urine and sweat, diarrhea
Occasional
Abdominal pain, vomiting, constipation, dry mouth, fatigue, back pain
Rare
Anxiety, somnolence, agitation, dyspepsia, flatulence, diaphoresis, asthenia, dyspnea

PRECAUTIONS AND CONTRAINDICATIONS
Hypersensitivity, use within 14 days of MAOIs
Caution
Enhanced orthostatic hypotension with levodopa and carbidopa, hepatic impairment, caution in driving, lactation, children

DRUG INTERACTIONS OF CONCERN TO DENTISTRY
• Increased heart rate, arrhythmias, hypertension: epinephrine, norepinephrine, levonordefrin, other sympathomimetics metabolized by COMT
• Possible decrease in urinary excretion: erythromycin

SERIOUS REACTIONS
None known

DENTAL CONSIDERATIONS
General:
• Monitor vital signs at every appointment because of cardiovascular side effects.

• Short appointments and a stress-reduction protocol may be required for anxious patients.
• Consider semisupine chair position for patient comfort if GI side effects occur.
• Use vasoconstrictor with caution, in low doses and with careful aspiration. Avoid using gingival retraction cord containing epinephrine.
• Assess for presence of extrapyramidal motor symptoms, such as tardive dyskinesia and akathisia. Extrapyramidal motor activity may complicate dental treatment.
• After supine positioning, have patient sit upright for at least 2 min to avoid orthostatic hypotension.
• Assess salivary flow as a factor in caries, periodontal disease, and candidiasis.
Consultations:
• Medical consultation may be required to assess disease control and patient's ability to tolerate stress.
Teach Patient/Family to:
• Use electric tooth brush if patient has difficulty holding conventional devices
• Update health and drug history if physician makes any changes in evaluation or drug regimens
• When chronic dry mouth occurs, advise patient to:
   • Avoid mouth rinses with high alcohol content because of drying effects
   • Use daily home fluoride products for anticaries effect
   • Use sugarless gum, frequent sips of water, or saliva substitutes

ephedrine

eh-fed´-rin

(Pretz-D)

Do not confuse ephedrine with epinephrine.

CATEGORY AND SCHEDULE

Pregnancy Risk Category: C

Drug Class: Adrenergic, mixed direct and indirect effects

MECHANISM OF ACTION

A adrenergic agonist that stimulates alpha-adrenergic receptors causing vasoconstriction and pressor effects, β_1-adrenergic receptors, resulting in cardiac stimulation, and β_2-adrenergic receptors, resulting in bronchial dilation and vasodilation. *Therapeutic Effect:* Increases B/P and pulse rate, reduces nasal congestion.

USES

Treatment of shock, increased perfusion, hypotension, bronchodilation, nasal decongestant

PHARMACOKINETICS

Well absorbed after nasal and parenteral absorption. Metabolized in liver. Excreted in urine.
Half-life: 3–6 hr.

INDICATIONS AND DOSAGES
▶ **Asthma**

PO

Adults. 25–50 mg q3–4h as needed.
Children. 3 mg/kg/day in 4 divided doses.

▶ **Hypotension**

IM

Adults. 25–50 mg as a single dose. Maximum 150 mg/day.
Children. 0.2–0.3 mg/kg/dose q4–6h.

IV

Adults. 5 mg/dose slow IVP as prevention. 10–25 mg/dose slow IVP repeated q5–10 min as treatment. Maximum: 150 mg/day.
Children. 0.2–0.3 mg/kg/dose slow IVP q4–6h.

Subcutaneous

Adults. 25–50 q4–6h. Maximum 150 mg/day.
Children. 3 mg/kg/day q4–6h.

▶ **Nasal Congestion**

PO

Adults. 25–50 mg q6h as needed.
Children. 3 mg/kg/day in 4 divided doses.

Nasal

Adults, Children 12 yr and older. 2–3 sprays into each nostril q4h.
Children 6–12 yr. 1–2 sprays into each nostril q4h.

SIDE EFFECTS/ADVERSE REACTIONS

Frequent

Hypertension, anxiety

Occasional

Nausea, vomiting, palpitations, tremor

Nasal: Burning, stinging, runny nose

Rare

Psychosis, decreased urination, necrosis at injection site from repeated injections

PRECAUTIONS AND CONTRAINDICATIONS

Anesthesia with cyclopropane or halothane, diabetes (ephedrine injection), hypersensitivity to ephedrine or other sympathomimetic amines, hypertension or other cardiovascular disorders, pregnancy with maternal B/P above 130/80, thyrotoxicosis

Caution

Cardiac disorders, hyperthyroidism, diabetes mellitus, prostatic hypertrophy

DRUG INTERACTIONS OF CONCERN TO DENTISTRY

• Decreased pressor effect: haloperidol, phenothiazines, thioxanthenes
• Dysrhythmia: halogenated general anesthetics

SERIOUS REACTIONS

! Excessive doses may cause hypertension, intracranial hemorrhage, anginal pain, and fatal arrhythmias.
! Prolonged or excessive use may result in metabolic acidosis due to increased serum lactic acid concentrations.
! Observe for disorientation, weakness, hyperventilation, headache, nausea, vomiting, and diarrhea.

DENTAL CONSIDERATIONS

General:
• Monitor vital signs at every appointment because of cardiovascular side effects.
• Assess salivary flow as a factor in caries, periodontal disease, and candidiasis.
• Consider semisupine chair position for patients with respiratory disease.
• Consider short appointments and a stress reduction protocol for anxious patients.

Consultations:
• Medical consultation may be required to assess disease control and patient's tolerance for stress.

Teach Patient/Family:
• When chronic dry mouth occurs, advise patient to:
  • Avoid mouth rinses with high alcohol content because of drying effects
  • Use daily home fluoride products for anticaries effect
  • Use sugarless gum, frequent sips of water, or saliva substitutes

epinastine
eh-pin-ass´-teen
(Elestat)

CATEGORY AND SCHEDULE
Pregnancy Risk Category: C

Drug Class: Ophthalmic antihistamine

MECHANISM OF ACTION
An ophthalmic H_1 receptor antagonist that inhibits the release of histamine from the mast cell.
Therapeutic Effect: Prevents pruritus associated with allergic conjunctivitis.

USES
Prevention of itching associated with allergic conjunctivitis

PHARMACOKINETICS
Low systemic exposure. Protein binding: 64%. Less than 10% is metabolized. Excreted primarily in urine and, to a lesser extent, in feces.
Half-life: 12 hr.

INDICATIONS AND DOSAGES
▸ **Allergic Conjunctivitis**
Ophthalmic
Adults, Elderly, Children 3 yr and older. 1 drop in each eye twice a day. Continue treatment until period of exposure (pollen season, exposure to offending allergen) is over.

SIDE EFFECTS/ADVERSE REACTIONS
Occasional
Ocular (10%–1%): Burning sensation in the eye, hyperemia, pruritus
Non-ocular (10%): Cold symptoms, upper respiratory tract infection

Rare
Headache, rhinitis, sinusitis,
increased cough, pharyngitis

PRECAUTIONS AND CONTRAINDICATIONS
Hypersensitivity
Caution
Do not wear contact lens if the
eye is red, otherwise contact
may be placed in eye 10 min after
dosing; use in nursing and in
children younger than 3 yr has not
been established

DRUG INTERACTIONS OF CONCERN TO DENTISTRY
None reported

SERIOUS REACTIONS
None known

DENTAL CONSIDERATIONS
General:
• Avoid dental light in patient's eyes;
offer dark glasses for patient
comfort.

epinephrine
ep-ih-nef´-rin
(Adrenalin, Adrenaline
Injection[AUS], EpiPen, EpiPen Jr.
0.15 Adrenaline Autoinjector[AUS],
Primatene)
Do not confuse epinephrine with
ephedrine.

CATEGORY AND SCHEDULE
Pregnancy Risk Category: C

Drug Class: Adrenergic agonist,
catecholamine

MECHANISM OF ACTION
A sympathomimetic, adrenergic
agonist that stimulates alpha-
adrenergic receptors causing
vasoconstriction and pressor effects,
β_1-adrenergic receptors, resulting in
cardiac stimulation, and
β_2-adrenergic receptors, resulting in
bronchial dilation and vasodilation.
With ophthalmic form, increases
outflow of aqueous humor from
anterior eye chamber. ***Therapeutic
Effect:*** Relaxes smooth muscle of the
bronchial tree, produces cardiac
stimulation, and dilates skeletal
muscle vasculature. The ophthalmic
form dilates pupils and constricts
conjunctival blood vessels.

USES
Treatment of acute asthmatic attacks,
hemostasis, bronchospasm,
anaphylaxis, allergic reactions,
cardiac arrest, vasopressor, open-
angle glaucoma, nasal congestion

PHARMACOKINETICS

Route	Onset	Peak	Duration
IM	5–10 min	20 min	1–4 hr
Subcutaneous	5–10 min	20 min	1–4 hr
Inhalation	3–5 min	20 min	1–3 hr
Ophthalmic	1 hr	4–8 hr	12–24 hr

Well absorbed after parenteral
administration; minimally absorbed
after inhalation. Metabolized in the
liver, other tissues, and sympathetic
nerve endings. Excreted in urine.
The ophthalmic form may be
systemically absorbed as a result of
drainage into nasal pharyngeal
passages. Mydriasis occurs within
several min and persists several hr;
vasoconstriction occurs within 5 min,
and lasts less than 1 hr.

INDICATIONS AND DOSAGES
▸ **Asystole**
IV
Adults, Elderly. 1 mg q3–5 min up to 0.1 mg/kg q3–5 min.
Children. 0.01 mg/kg (0.1 ml/kg of 1:10,000 solution). May repeat q3–5 min. Subsequent doses of 0.1 mg/kg (0.1 ml/kg) of a 1:1000 solution q3–5 min.
▸ **Bradycardia**
IV Infusion
Adults, Elderly. 1–10 mcg/min titrated to desired effect.
IV
Children. 0.01 mg/kg (0.1 mg/kg of 1:10,000 solution) q3–5 min. Maximum: 1 mg/10 ml.
▸ **Bronchodilation**
IM, Subcutaneous
Adults, Elderly. 0.1–0.5 mg (1:1000) q10–15 min to 4 hr.
Subcutaneous
Children. 10 mcg/kg (0.01 ml/kg of 1:1,000) Maximum: 0.5 mg or suspension (1:200) 0.005 ml/kg/dose (0.025 mg/kg/dose) to a maximum of 0.15 ml (0.75 mg for single dose) q8–12h.
▸ **Hypersensitivity Reaction**
IM, Subcutaneous
Adults, Elderly. 0.3–0.5 mg q15–20 min.
Subcutaneous
Children. 0.01 mg/kg q15 min for 2 doses, then q4h. Maximum single dose: 0.5 mg.
Inhalation
Adults, Elderly, Children 4 yr and older. 1 inhalation, may repeat in at least 1 min. Give subsequent doses no sooner than 3 hr.
Nebulizer
Adults, Elderly, Children 4 yr and older. 1–3 deep inhalations. Give subsequent doses no sooner than 3 hr.
▸ **Glaucoma**
Ophthalmic
Adults, Elderly. 1–2 drops 1–2 times a day.

SIDE EFFECTS/ADVERSE REACTIONS
Frequent
Systemic: Tachycardia, palpitations, nervousness
Ophthalmic: Headache, eye irritation, watering of eyes
Occasional
Systemic: Dizziness, light-headedness, facial flushing, headache, diaphoresis, increased B/P, nausea, trembling, insomnia, vomiting, fatigue
Ophthalmic: Blurred or decreased vision, eye pain
Rare
Systemic: Chest discomfort or pain, arrhythmias, bronchospasm, dry mouth or throat

PRECAUTIONS AND CONTRAINDICATIONS
Cardiac arrhythmias, cerebrovascular insufficiency, hypertension, hyperthyroidism, ischemic heart disease, narrow-angle glaucoma, shock
Caution
Cardiac disorders, hyperthyroidism, diabetes mellitus, prostatic hypertrophy

DRUG INTERACTIONS OF CONCERN TO DENTISTRY
• Hypotension, tachycardia: haloperidol, loxapine, phenothiazines, thioxanthenes
• Ventricular dysrhythmia: hydrocarbon-inhalation anesthetics, CNS stimulants, tricyclic antidepressants
• With larger doses of epinephrine, risk of hypertension followed by bradycardia with β-adrenergic antagonists

SERIOUS REACTIONS
! Excessive doses may cause acute hypertension or arrhythmias.
! Prolonged or excessive use may result in metabolic acidosis due to increased serum lactic acid concentrations.

Metabolic acidosis may cause disorientation, fatigue, hyperventilation, headache, nausea, vomiting, and diarrhea.

DENTAL CONSIDERATIONS

General:
• Monitor vital signs at every appointment because of cardiovascular side effects.
• Assess salivary flow as a factor in caries, periodontal disease, and candidiasis.
• Consider semisupine chair position for patients with respiratory disease.
• Acute asthmatic episodes may be precipitated in the dental office. Sympathomimetic inhalants should be available for emergency use; a stress-reduction protocol may be required.

epinephryl borate
ep-ih-nef´-rill bor´-ate
(Epifrin, Epinal, Eppy/N)

CATEGORY AND SCHEDULE
Pregnancy Risk Category: C

Drug Class: Antiglaucoma agent, ophthalmic; surgical aid, ophthalmic

MECHANISM OF ACTION
A direct-acting sympathomimetic amine whose mechanism of action is unknown.
Therapeutic Effect:
Increases outflow of aqueous humor from anterior eye chamber.

USES
Treatment of certain types of glaucoma. It may also be used in eye surgery

PHARMACOKINETICS
May have systemic absorption from drainage into nasal pharyngeal passages. Mydriasis occurs within several min, persists several hr; vasoconstriction occurs within 5 min, lasts less than 1 hr.

INDICATIONS AND DOSAGES
▶ **Glaucoma**
Ophthalmic
Adults, Elderly. Instill 1 drop 1–2 times a day.

SIDE EFFECTS/ADVERSE REACTIONS
Frequent
Headache, stinging, burning or other eye irritation, watering of eyes
Occasional
Blurred or decreased vision, eye pain

PRECAUTIONS AND CONTRAINDICATIONS
Cardiac arrhythmias, cerebrovascular insufficiency, hypertension, hyperthyroidism, ischemic heart disease, narrow-angle glaucoma, shock, hypersensitivity to epinephryl borate or any component of the formulation

DRUG INTERACTIONS OF CONCERN TO DENTISTRY
• Risk of arrhythmias: halogenated hydrocarbon anesthetics, tricyclic antidepressants, amphetamine-like drugs

SERIOUS REACTIONS
! Systemic absorption occurs rarely. These effects include fast, irregular, or pounding heartbeat, feeling faint, increased sweating, paleness, trembling, and increased B/P.

DENTAL CONSIDERATIONS
General:
• Determine why patient is taking the drug.
• Avoid drugs with anticholinergic activity, such as antihistamines, opioids, benzodiazepines, propantheline, atropine, and scopolamine.
• Avoid dental light in patient's eyes; offer dark glasses for patient comfort.
• Question glaucoma patient about compliance with prescribed drug regimen.
Consultations:
• Medical consultation may be required to assess disease control.
Teach Patient/Family to:
• Update health and medication history if physician makes any changes in evaluation or drug regimens; include OTC, herbal, and nonherbal remedies in the update

epirubicin
eh-pea-rew´-bih-sin
(Ellence, Pharmorubicin)

CATEGORY AND SCHEDULE
Pregnancy Risk Category: D

Drug Class: Anthracycline antibiotic; antineoplastic

MECHANISM OF ACTION
An anthracycline antibiotic whose exact mechanism is unknown but may include formation of a complex with DNA and subsequent inhibition of DNA, RNA, and protein synthesis. Also inhibits DNA helicase activity, preventing enzymatic separation of double-stranded DNA and interfering with replication and transcription. **Therapeutic Effect:** Produces antiproliferative and cytotoxic activity.

USES
Treatment of some kinds of cancers of the breast, lung, lymph system, stomach, and ovaries

PHARMACOKINETICS
Widely distributed into tissues. Protein binding: 77%. Metabolized in the liver and RBCs. Primarily eliminated through biliary excretion. Not removed by hemodialysis. **Half-life:** 33 hr.

INDICATIONS AND DOSAGES
▸ **Breast Cancer**
IV
Adults. Initially, 100–120 mg/m² in repeated cycles of 3–4 wk, in combination with fluorouracil (5-FU) and Cytoxan. Total dose may be given on day 1 of each cycle or in equally divided doses on days 1 and 8 of each cycle.

SIDE EFFECTS/ADVERSE REACTIONS
Frequent
Nausea, vomiting alopecia, amenorrhea
Occasional
Stomatitis, diarrhea, hot flashes
Rare
Rash, pruritus, fever, lethargy, conjunctivitis

PRECAUTIONS AND CONTRAINDICATIONS
Baseline neutrophil count less than 1500/mm³, hypersensitivity to epirubicin, previous treatment with anthracyclines up to maximum cumulative dose, recent MI, severe hepatic impairment, severe myocardial insufficiency

DRUG INTERACTIONS OF CONCERN TO DENTISTRY
None reported

SERIOUS REACTIONS
❗ The risk of cardiotoxicity (either acute, manifested as transient ECG abnormalities, or chronic, manifested as CHF) increases when the total cumulative dose exceeds 900 mg/m^2.
❗ Extravasation during administration may result in severe local tissue necrosis.
❗ Myelosuppression may cause hematologic toxicity, manifested principally as leukopenia and, to a lesser extent, anemia and thrombocytopenia.

DENTAL CONSIDERATIONS
General:
• If additional analgesia is required for dental pain, consider alternative analgesics (NSAIDs) in patients taking narcotics for acute or chronic pain.
• Examine for oral manifestation of opportunistic infection.
• This drug may be used in the hospital or on an outpatient basis. Confirm the patient's disease and treatment status.
• Chlorhexidine mouth rinse prior to and during chemotherapy may reduce severity of mucositis.
• Patient on chronic drug therapy may rarely present with symptoms of blood dyscrasias, which can include infection, bleeding, and poor healing. If dyscrasia is present, caution patient to prevent oral tissue trauma when using oral hygiene aids.
• Palliative medication may be required for management of oral side effects.
• Patient may be at risk of bleeding; check oral signs.
• Patient may be at risk of infection.

Consultations:
• Medical consultation should include routine blood counts including platelet counts and bleeding time.
• In a patient with symptoms of blood dyscrasias, request a medical consultation for blood studies and postpone treatment until normal values are reestablished.
• Consult physician; prophylactic or therapeutic antiinfectives may be indicated if surgery or periodontal treatment is required.
• Medical consultation may be required to assess immunologic status during cancer chemotherapy and determine safety risk, if any, posed by the required dental treatment.
• Medical consultation may be required to assess disease control and patient's ability to tolerate stress.
Teach Patient/Family to:
• Be aware of oral side effects
• Use effective oral hygiene to prevent soft tissue inflammation
• Report oral lesions, soreness, or bleeding to dentist
• Prevent trauma when using oral hygiene aids
• Update health and medication history if physician makes any changes in evaluation or drug regimens; include OTC, herbal, and nonherbal remedies in the update

eplerenone
eh-plear´-ah-nown
(Inspra)

CATEGORY AND SCHEDULE
Pregnancy Risk Category: B

Drug Class: Antihypertensive, aldosterone antagonist

MECHANISM OF ACTION
An aldosterone receptor antagonist that binds to the mineralocorticoid receptors in the kidney, heart, blood vessels, and brain, blocking the binding of aldosterone. *Therapeutic Effect:* Reduces B/P.

USES
Treatment of hypertension as a single drug or in combination with other antihypertensive drugs; improved survival of CHF patients following an acute heart attack

PHARMACOKINETICS
Absorption unaffected by food. Protein binding: 50%. No active metabolites. Excreted in the urine with a lesser amount eliminated in the feces. Not removed by hemodialysis. *Half-life:* 4–6 hr.

INDICATIONS AND DOSAGES
▸ **Hypertension**
PO
Adults, Elderly. 50 mg once a day. If 50 mg once a day produces an inadequate B/P response, may increase dosage to 50 mg twice a day. If patient is concurrently receiving erythromycin, saquinavir, verapamil, or fluconazole, reduce initial dose to 25 mg once a day.
▸ **CHF Following MI**
PO
Adults, Elderly. Initially, 25 mg once a day. If tolerated, titrate up to 50 mg once a day within 4 wk.

SIDE EFFECTS/ADVERSE REACTIONS
Rare
Dizziness, diarrhea, cough, fatigue, flu-like symptoms, abdominal pain

PRECAUTIONS AND CONTRAINDICATIONS
Concurrent use of potassium supplements or potassium-sparing diuretics (such as amiloride, spironolactone, and triamterene), or strong inhibitors of the cytochrome P450 3A4 enzyme system (including ketoconazole and itraconazole), creatinine clearance less than 50 ml/min, serum creatinine level greater than 2 mg/dl in males or 1.8 mg/dl in females, serum potassium level greater than 5.5 mEq/L, type 2 diabetes mellitus with microalbuminuria
Caution
Hyperkalemia, monitor serum potassium periodically, impaired hepatic or renal function, angiotensin-converting enzyme (ACE) inhibitors, angiotensin II antagonists, lactation, use in children has not been established

DRUG INTERACTIONS OF CONCERN TO DENTISTRY
• See contraindications; use with caution in patients taking strong inhibitors of CYP3A4 isoenzymes (erythromycin)
• Monitor blood pressure if NSAIDs are required

SERIOUS REACTIONS
! Hyperkalemia may occur, particularly in patients with type 2 diabetes mellitus and microalbuminuria.

DENTAL CONSIDERATIONS
General:
• Monitor vital signs at every appointment because of cardiovascular side effects.
• Short appointments and a stress-reduction protocol may be required for anxious patients.

- Take precautions if dental surgery is anticipated and general anesthesia is required.

Consultations:
- Medical consultation may be required to assess disease control and patient's ability to tolerate stress.
- Consultation with physician may be necessary if sedation or general anesthesia is required.

Teach Patient/Family to:
- Update health and drug history if physician makes any changes in evaluation or drug regimens

epoetin alfa
eh-poh´-ee-tin al´-fa
(Epogen, Eprex[CAN], Procrit)
Do not confuse Epogen with Neupogen.

CATEGORY AND SCHEDULE
Pregnancy Risk Category: C

Drug Class: Hematinic, antianemic

MECHANISM OF ACTION
A glycoprotein that stimulates division and differentiation of erythroid progenitor cells in bone marrow. *Therapeutic Effect:* Induces erythropoiesis and releases reticulocytes from bone marrow.

USES
Anemia of chronic renal failure, end-stage renal disease, anemia in zidovudine-treated HIV patients, anemia in cancer patients on chemotherapy, reduction of allogenic blood transfusion in surgery patients

PHARMACOKINETICS
Well absorbed after subcutaneous administration. Following administration, an increase in reticulocyte count occurs within 10 days, and increases in Hgb, Hct, and RBC count are seen within 2–6 wk. *Half-life:* 4–13 hr.

INDICATIONS AND DOSAGES
▸ **Treatment of Anemia in Chemotherapy Patients**
IV, Subcutaneous
Adults, Elderly, Children.
150 units/kg/dose 3 times a wk.
Maximum: 1200 units/kg/wk.
▸ **Reduction of Allogenic Blood Transfusions in Elective Surgery**
Subcutaneous
Adults, Elderly. 300 units/kg/day 10 days before day of and 4 days after surgery.
▸ **Chronic Renal Failure**
IV Bolus, Subcutaneous
Adults, Elderly. Initially, 50–100 units/kg 3 times a wk. Target Hct range: 30%–36%. Adjust dosage no earlier than 1-mo intervals unless prescribed. Decrease dosage if Hct is increasing and approaching 36%. Plan to temporarily withhold doses if Hct continues to rise and to reinstate lower dosage when Hct begins to decrease. If Hct increases by more than 4 points in 2 wk, monitor Hct twice a wk for 2–6 wk. Increase dose if Hct does not increase 5–6 points after 8 wk (with adequate iron stores) and if Hct is below target range. Maintenance: For patients on dialysis: 75 units/kg 3 times a wk. Range: 12.5–525 units/kg. For patients not on dialysis: 75–150 units/kg/wk.
▸ **HIV Infection in Patients Treated with AZT**
IV, Subcutaneous
Adults. Initially, 100 units/kg 3 times a wk for 8 wk; may increase by

50–100 units/kg 3 times a wk.
Evaluate response q4–8wk thereafter.
Adjust dosage by 50–100 units/kg
3 times a wk. If dosages larger than
300 units/kg 3 times a wk are not
eliciting response, it is unlikely
patient will respond. Maintenance:
Titrate to maintain desired Hct.

SIDE EFFECTS/ADVERSE REACTIONS
Patients Receiving Chemotherapy
Frequent
Fever, diarrhea, nausea, vomiting,
edema
Occasional
Asthenia, shortness of breath,
paresthesia
Rare
Dizziness, trunk pain

Patients with Chronic Renal Failure
Frequent
Hypertension, headache, nausea,
arthralgia
Occasional
Fatigue, edema, diarrhea, vomiting,
chest pain, skin reactions at
administration site, asthenia,
dizziness

Patients with HIV Infection Treated with AZT
Frequent
Fever, fatigue, headache, cough,
diarrhea, rash, nausea
Occasional
Shortness of breath, asthenia,
skin reaction at injection site,
dizziness

PRECAUTIONS AND CONTRAINDICATIONS
History of sensitivity to
mammalian cell-derived products
or human albumin, uncontrolled
hypertension

Caution
Contains benzyl alcohol (risk of
complications in premature infants),
increased thrombosis risk in CHF,
ischemic heart disease, coronary
artery bypass, pure red cell aplasia,
monitor and control B/P, seizures in
CRF, thrombosis during
hemodialysis, porphyria, lactation,
safety and efficacy in children
younger than 1 mo have not been
established, monitor renal function,
monitor hematocrit

DRUG INTERACTIONS OF CONCERN TO DENTISTRY
None reported

SERIOUS REACTIONS
! Hypertensive encephalopathy,
thrombosis, cerebrovascular
accident, MI, and seizures have
occurred rarely.
! Hyperkalemia occurs occasionally
in patients with chronic renal failure,
usually in those who do not conform
to medication regimen, dietary
guidelines, and frequency of dialysis
regimen.

DENTAL CONSIDERATIONS
General:
• Patient's disease, treatment history,
and use of other drugs will affect
patient evaluation and management.
• Determine why patient is taking
the drug.
• Monitor vital signs at every
appointment because of
cardiovascular and respiratory
side effects.
• Take precautions if dental surgery
is anticipated and general anesthesia
is required.
• Patient history should include all
medications and herbal or nonherbal
remedies taken by the patient.

- Consider semisupine chair position for patient comfort if GI side effects occur.
- Place on frequent recall because of oral side effects, depending on chemotherapy regimen or HIV immunologic status.

Consultations:
- Medical consultation should include hematocrit and routine blood counts, including platelet counts and bleeding time.
- Consultation with physician may be necessary if sedation or general anesthesia is required.
- Medical consultation may be required to assess disease control and patient's ability to tolerate stress.

Teach Patient/Family to:
- Use effective oral hygiene to prevent soft tissue inflammation, infection

epoprostenol sodium, prostacyclin

eh-poe-pros´-ten-ol soe´-dee-um, pros-ta-sih´-klin
(Flolan)

CATEGORY AND SCHEDULE
Pregnancy Risk Category: B

Drug Class: Vasodilator; antihypertensive

MECHANISM OF ACTION
An antihypertensive that directly dilates pulmonary and systemic arterial vascular beds and inhibits platelet aggregation. ***Therapeutic Effect:*** Reduces right and left ventricular afterload; increases cardiac output and stroke volume.

USES
Treatment of the symptoms of primary pulmonary hypertension, or the high B/P that occurs in the main artery that carries blood from the right side of the heart (the ventricle) to the lungs

INDICATIONS AND DOSAGES
▶ **Long-term Treatment of New York Heart Association Class III and IV Primary Pulmonary Hypertension**
IV Infusion
Adults, Elderly. Procedure to determine dose range: Initially, 2 ng/kg/min, increased in increments of 2 ng/kg/min q15 min until dose-limiting adverse effects occur. Chronic infusion: Start at 4 ng/kg/min less than the maximum dose rate tolerated during acute dose ranging (or one-half of the maximum rate if rate was less than 5 ng/kg/min).

SIDE EFFECTS/ADVERSE REACTIONS
Frequent
Acute phase: Flushing, headache, nausea, vomiting, hypotension, anxiety, chest pain, dizziness
Chronic phase: Dyspnea, asthenia, dizziness, headache, chest pain, nausea, vomiting, palpitations, edema, jaw pain, tachycardia, flushing, myalgia, nonspecific muscle pain, paresthesia, diarrhea, anxiety, chills, fever, or flu-like symptoms
Occasional
Acute phase: Bradycardia, abdominal pain, muscle pain, dyspnea, back pain
Chronic phase: Rash, depression, hypotension, pallor, syncope, bradycardia, ascites
Rare
Acute phase: Paresthesia
Chronic phase: Diaphoresis, dyspepsia, tachycardia

PRECAUTIONS AND CONTRAINDICATIONS
Long-term use in patients with CHF (severe ventricular systolic dysfunction)

DRUG INTERACTIONS OF CONCERN TO DENTISTRY
• Increased risk of bleeding: drugs which interfere with coagulation or platelet function; such as NSAIDs and aspirin

SERIOUS REACTIONS
! Overdose may cause hyperglycemia or ketoacidosis manifested as increased urination, thirst, and fruitlike breath odor.
! Angina, MI, and thrombocytopenia occur rarely.
! Abrupt withdrawal, including a large reduction in dosage or interruption in drug delivery, may produce rebound pulmonary hypertension as evidenced by dyspnea, dizziness, and asthenia.

DENTAL CONSIDERATIONS
General:
• Continuous-use drug for patients with severe cardiovascular disease. Provide palliative emergency dental care as required.
• Determine why patient is taking the drug.
• Monitor vital signs at every appointment due to cardiovascular side effects.
• Avoid products that affect platelet function, such as aspirin and NSAIDs.
• Stress from dental procedures may compromise cardiovascular function, determine patient risk.
• Postpone elective dental treatment if patient shows signs of cardiac symptoms or respiratory distress.

• Use vasoconstrictor with caution, in low doses, and with careful aspiration. Avoid using gingival retraction cord containing epinephrine.
Consultations:
• Medical consultation may be required to assess disease control and patient's ability to tolerate stress.
• Medical consultation should include routine blood counts including platelet counts and bleeding time.
Teach Patient/Family to:
• Use effective oral hygiene to prevent soft tissue inflammation
• Prevent trauma when using oral hygiene aids
• Update health and medication history if physician makes any changes in evaluation or drug regimens; include OTC, herbal, and nonherbal remedies in the update

eprosartan
eh-pro-sar´-tan
(Teveten)

CATEGORY AND SCHEDULE
Pregnancy Risk Category: C (D if used in second or third trimester)

Drug Class: Antihypertensive, angiotensin II receptor (AT1) antagonist

MECHANISM OF ACTION
An angiotensin II receptor antagonist that blocks the vasoconstrictor and aldosterone-secreting effects of angiotensin II, inhibiting the binding of angiotensin II to the AT1 receptors. *Therapeutic Effect:* Causes vasodilation, decreases peripheral resistance, and decreases B/P.

USES

Treatment of hypertension as a single drug or in combination with other antihypertensive drugs

PHARMACOKINETICS

Rapidly absorbed after PO administration. Protein binding: 98%. Undergoes first-pass metabolism in the liver to active metabolites. Excreted in urine and biliary system. Minimally removed by hemodialysis. *Half-life:* 5–9 hr.

INDICATIONS AND DOSAGES

▸ **Hypertension**
PO
Adults, Elderly. Initially, 600 mg/day. Range: 400–800 mg/day.

SIDE EFFECTS/ADVERSE REACTIONS

Occasional
Headache, cough, dizziness
Rare
Muscle pain, fatigue, diarrhea, upper respiratory tract infection, dyspepsia

PRECAUTIONS AND CONTRAINDICATIONS

Bilateral renal artery stenosis, hyperaldosteronism
Caution
Renal impairment maximum daily dose is 600 mg, risk of renal impairment, pregnancy category C (first trimester) and pregnancy category D (second and third trimesters); safety and efficacy in lactation and patients younger than 18 yr have not been established

DRUG INTERACTIONS OF CONCERN TO DENTISTRY

None reported

SERIOUS REACTIONS

! Overdosage may manifest as hypotension and tachycardia. Bradycardia occurs less often.

DENTAL CONSIDERATIONS

General:
• Monitor vital signs at every appointment because of cardiovascular side effects.
• Stress from dental procedures may compromise cardiovascular function; determine patient risk.
• Limit use of sodium-containing products, such as saline IV fluids, for those patients with a dietary salt restriction.
• Short appointments and a stress reduction protocol may be required for anxious patients.
• Use precaution if sedation or general anesthesia is required; risk of hypotensive episode.
• Assess salivary flow as a factor in caries, periodontal disease, and candidiasis.
• After supine positioning, have patient sit upright for at least 2 min before standing to avoid orthostatic hypotension.
Consultations:
• Medical consultation may be required to assess disease control and patient's ability to tolerate stress.
Teach Patient/Family to:
• Update health and drug history if physician makes any changes in evaluation or drug regimens
• When chronic dry mouth occurs, advise patient to:
  • Avoid mouth rinses with high alcohol content because of drying effects
  • Use daily home fluoride products for anticaries effect
  • Use sugarless gum, frequent sips of water, or saliva substitutes

eptifibatide
ep-tih-fib´-ah-tide
(Integrilin)

CATEGORY AND SCHEDULE
Pregnancy Risk Category: B

Drug Class: Glycoprotein IIb/IIIa inhibitor; antiplatelet, antithrombotic

MECHANISM OF ACTION
A glycoprotein IIb/IIIa inhibitor that rapidly inhibits platelet aggregation by preventing binding of fibrinogen to receptor sites on platelets. **Therapeutic Effect:** Prevents closure of treated coronary arteries. Also prevents acute cardiac ischemic complications.

USES
Treatment of patients with acute coronary syndrome (ACS), including those managed medically and those undergoing percutaneous coronary intervention (PCI).

PHARMACOKINETICS
Half-life 2.5 hr, steady state 4–6 hr, metabolism limited, excretion via kidneys

INDICATIONS AND DOSAGES
▶ **Adjunct to Percutaneous Coronary Intervention**
IV Bolus, IV Infusion
Adults, Elderly. 180 mcg/kg before PCI initiation; then continuous drip of 2 mcg/kg/min and a second 180 mcg/kg bolus 10 min after the first. Maximum: 15 mg/h. Continue until hospital discharge or for up to 18–24 hr. Minimum 12 hr is recommended. Concurrent aspirin and heparin therapy is recommended.

▶ **Acute Coronary Syndrome**
IV Bolus, IV Infusion
Adults, Elderly. 180 mcg/kg bolus then 2 mcg/kg/min until discharge or coronary artery bypass graft, up to 72 hr. Maximum: 15 mg/h. Concurrent aspirin and heparin therapy is recommended.

▶ **Dosage in Renal Impairment**
Creatinine clearance less than 50 ml/min. Use 180 mcg/kg bolus (maximum 22.6 mg) and 1 mcg/kg/min infusion (maximum 7.5 mg/h).

SIDE EFFECTS/ADVERSE REACTIONS
Occasional
Hypotension

PRECAUTIONS AND CONTRAINDICATIONS
Active internal bleeding, AV malformation or aneurysm, history of cerebrovascular accident (CVA) within 2 yr or CVA with residual neurologic defect, history of vasculitis, intracranial neoplasm, oral anticoagulant use within last 7 days unless PT is less than 1.22 times the control, recent (6 wk) GI or GU bleeding, recent (6 wk) surgery or trauma, prior IV dextran use before or during PTCA, severe uncontrolled hypertension, thrombocytopenia (fewer than 100,000 cells/mcl)

DRUG INTERACTIONS OF CONCERN TO DENTISTRY
• Increased risk of bleeding: drugs that interfere with coagulation or platelet function, such as NSAIDs and aspirin

SERIOUS REACTIONS
! Minor to major bleeding complications may occur, most commonly at arterial access site for cardiac catheterization.

E

DENTAL CONSIDERATIONS
General:
• Monitor vital signs at every appointment due to cardiovascular side effects.
• Avoid products that affect platelet function, such as aspirin and NSAIDs.
• Consider local hemostasis measures to prevent excessive bleeding.
• For acute use in emergency rooms or hospitals.
• Provide palliative emergency dental care only during drug use.
• Patients may be at risk of bleeding, check for oral signs.
• Confirm patient's medical and drug history.
Consultations:
• Medical consultation may be required to assess disease control and patient's ability to tolerate stress.
• Medical consultation should include routine blood counts including platelet counts and bleeding time.
• Medical consultation should include PPT, PT, or INR
Teach Patient/Family to:
• Use effective oral hygiene to prevent soft tissue inflammation
• Prevent trauma when using oral hygiene aids
• Report oral lesions, soreness, or bleeding to dentist
• Update health and medication history if physician makes any changes in evaluation or drug regimens; include OTC, herbal, and nonherbal remedies in the update
• Use soft tooth brush to reduce risk of bleeding

ergoloid mesylates
ur´-go-loyd mess-ah-lates
(Gerimal, Hydergine, Hydergine[CAN])

CATEGORY AND SCHEDULE
Pregnancy Risk Category: C

Drug Class: Ergot alkaloids

MECHANISM OF ACTION
An ergot alkaloid that centrally acts on and decreases vascular tone, slows heart rate. Peripheral action blocks alpha adrenergic receptors. ***Therapeutic Effect:*** Improved O_2 uptake and improves cerebral metabolism.

USES
Senile dementia, Alzheimer's dementia, multiinfarct dementia, primary progressive dementia

PHARMACOKINETICS
Rapidly, incompletely absorbed from GI tract. Metabolized in liver. Eliminated primarily in feces. ***Half-life:*** 2–5 hr.

INDICATIONS AND DOSAGES
▶ **Age-Related Decline in Mental Capacity**
PO
Adults, Elderly. Initially, 1 mg 3 times a day. Range: 1.5–12 mg/day.

SIDE EFFECTS/ADVERSE REACTIONS
Occasional
GI distress, transient nausea, sublingual irritation

PRECAUTIONS AND CONTRAINDICATIONS
Acute or chronic psychosis (regardless or etiology),

hypersensitivity to ergoloid mesylates or any component of the formulation.
Caution
Acute intermittent porphyria

SERIOUS REACTIONS

! Overdose may produce blurred vision, dizziness, syncope, headache, flushed face, nausea, vomiting, decreased appetite, stomach cramps, and stuffy nose.

DENTAL CONSIDERATIONS

General:
• Monitor vital signs at every appointment because of cardiovascular side effects.
• After supine positioning, have patient sit upright for at least 2 min before standing to avoid orthostatic hypotension.
• Consider semisupine chair position for patient comfort because of GI effects of drug.
Teach Patient/Family to:
• Use electric tooth brush if patient is unable to carry out oral hygiene procedures

ergotamine tartrate/ dihydroergotamine

er-got´-ah-meen tahr´-treyt/dahy-hahy-droh-ur-got´-uh-meen
ergotamine tartrate:
(Cafergot[CAN], Ergodryl Mono[AUS], Ergomar, Ergostat, Gynergen)
dihyrdoergotamine:
(D.H.E. 45, Dihydergot[AUS], Dihydroergotamine Sandoz[CAN], Migranal)

CATEGORY AND SCHEDULE

Pregnancy Risk Category: X

Drug Class: α-adrenergic blocker

MECHANISM OF ACTION

An ergotamine derivative and alpha-adrenergic blocker that directly stimulates vascular smooth muscle, resulting in peripheral and cerebral vasoconstriction. May also have antagonist effects on serotonin.
Therapeutic Effect: Suppresses vascular headaches.

USES

Treatment of vascular headache (migraine or histamine), cluster headache

PHARMACOKINETICS

Slowly and incompletely absorbed from the GI tract; rapidly and extensively absorbed after rectal administration. Protein binding: greater than 90%. Undergoes extensive first-pass metabolism in the liver to active metabolite. Eliminated in feces by the biliary system.
Half-life: 21 hr.

INDICATIONS AND DOSAGES
▶ Vascular Headaches
PO (Cafergot [fixed-combination of ergotamine and caffeine])
Adults, Elderly. 2 mg at onset of headache, then 1–2 mg q30 min. Maximum: 6 mg/episode; 10 mg/wk.
PO, Sublingual
Children. 1 mg at onset of headache, then 1 mg q30 min. Maximum: 3 mg/episode.
IV
Adults, Elderly. 1 mg at onset of headache; may repeat hourly. Maximum: 2 mg/day; 6 mg/wk.
Sublingual
Adults, Elderly. 1 tablet at onset of headache, then 1 tablet q30 min. Maximum: 3 tablets/24 hr; 5 tablets/wk.
IM, Subcutaneous
(dihydroergotamine)

Adults, Elderly. 1 mg at onset of
headache; may repeat hourly.
Maximum: 3 mg/day; 6 mg/wk.
Intranasal
Adults, Elderly. 1 spray (0.5 mg) into
each nostril; may repeat in 15 min.
Maximum: 4 sprays/day;
8 sprays/wk.
Rectal
Adults, Elderly. 1 suppository at
onset of headache; may repeat dose
in 1 hr. Maximum: 2 suppositories/
episode; 5 suppositories/wk.

SIDE EFFECTS/ADVERSE REACTIONS

Occasional
Cough, dizziness
Rare
Myalgia, fatigue, diarrhea, upper
respiratory tract infection, dyspepsia

PRECAUTIONS AND CONTRAINDICATIONS

Coronary artery disease,
hypertension, impaired hepatic or
renal function, malnutrition,
peripheral vascular diseases (such as
thromboangiitis obliterans, syphilitic
arteritis, severe arteriosclerosis,
thrombophlebitis, and Raynaud's
disease), sepsis, severe pruritus
Caution
Lactation, children, anemia

DRUG INTERACTIONS OF CONCERN TO DENTISTRY

- Increased vasoconstriction:
vasoconstrictor in local anesthetics
- Suspected increased risk of
ergotism: erythromycin,
clarithromycin, troleandomycin
- Use anticholinergics with caution
in the elderly

SERIOUS REACTIONS

! Prolonged administration or
excessive dosage may produce
ergotamine poisoning, manifested as
nausea and vomiting; paresthesia,
muscle pain or weakness; precordial
pain; tachycardia or bradycardia; and
hypertension or hypotension.
Vasoconstriction of peripheral
arteries and arterioles may result in
localized edema and pruritus. Muscle
pain will occur when walking and
later, even at rest. Other rare effects
include confusion, depression,
drowsiness, seizures, and gangrene.

DENTAL CONSIDERATIONS

General:
- This is an acute-use drug; patients
are unlikely to seek dental treatment
while using this drug.
- Monitor vital signs at every
appointment because of
cardiovascular side effects.
Teach Patient/Family to:
- Use electric tooth brush if patient
has difficulty holding conventional
devices

erlotinib

er-low´-tih-nib
(Tarceva)

CATEGORY AND SCHEDULE

Pregnancy Risk Category: D

Drug Class: Antineoplastic

MECHANISM OF ACTION

A human epidermal growth factor
that inhibits tyrosine kinases (TK)
associated with transmembrane cell
surface receptors found on both
normal and cancer cells. One such
receptor is epidermal growth factor
receptor (EGFR). *Therapeutic
Effect:* TK activity appears to be
vitally important to cell proliferation
and survival.

USES
Treatment of non–small-cell lung cancer after the failure of other chemotherapy treatment. It is also used together with another medicine called gemcitabine (e.g., Gemzar) to treat cancer of the pancreas

PHARMACOKINETICS
Slowly absorbed, peak 3–7 hr, excreted in feces (86%), urine (less than 4%), metabolized by CYP3A4. *Terminal Half-Life:* 36 hr.

INDICATIONS AND DOSAGES
▸ **Overactive Bladder**
PO
Adults, Elderly. Initially, 7.5 mg once a day. If response is not adequate after a minimum of 2 wk, dosage may be increased to 15 mg once a day. Do not exceed 7.5 mg once a day in patients with moderate hepatic impairment.

SIDE EFFECTS/ADVERSE REACTIONS
Frequent
Dry mouth, constipation
Occasional
Dyspepsia, headache, nausea, abdominal pain
Rare
Asthenia, diarrhea, dizziness, ocular dryness

PRECAUTIONS AND CONTRAINDICATIONS
Pregnancy

DRUG INTERACTIONS OF CONCERN TO DENTISTRY
• Increased blood levels and effects: potent inhibitors of CYP3A4 isoenzymes (ketoconazole, itraconazole, erythromycin, clarithromycin, diclofenac, doxycycline, protease inhibitors)

• Decreased effects: potent inducers of CYP3A4 isoenzymes (carbamazepine, phenobarbital, St. John's wort [herb])

SERIOUS REACTIONS
! UTI occurs occasionally.

DENTAL CONSIDERATIONS
General:
• Note interactions with drugs commonly prescribed in dentistry.
• For longer dental appointments, offer patient frequent breaks.
• Consider semisupine chair position for patient comfort if GI side effects occur.
• Avoid dental light in patient's eyes; offer dark glasses for patient comfort.
• Examine for oral manifestation of opportunistic infection.
• Assess salivary flow as a factor in caries, periodontal disease, and candidiasis.
• Place on frequent recall due to oral side effects.
Consultations:
• Physician should be informed if significant xerostomic side effects occur (increased caries, sore tongue, problems eating or swallowing, difficulty wearing prosthesis) so that a medication change can be considered.
Teach Patient/Family to:
• Use effective oral hygiene to prevent soft tissue inflammation
• Update health and medication history if physician makes any changes in evaluation or drug regimens; include OTC, herbal, and nonherbal remedies in the update

- When chronic dry mouth occurs advise patient to:
  - Avoid mouth rinses with high alcohol content due to drying effects
  - Use daily home fluoride products for anticaries effect
  - Use sugarless gum, frequent sips of water, or saliva substitutes

ertapenem
er-ta-pen´-em
(Invanz)

CATEGORY AND SCHEDULE
Pregnancy Risk Category: B

Drug Class: Antinfective-miscellaneous; carbapenem

MECHANISM OF ACTION
A carbapenem that penetrates the bacterial cell wall of microorganisms and binds to penicillin-binding proteins, inhibiting cell wall synthesis. ***Therapeutic Effect:*** Produces bacterial cell death.

USES
Treatment of infections caused by bacteria

PHARMACOKINETICS
Almost completely absorbed after IM administration. Protein binding: 85%–95%. Widely distributed. Primarily excreted in urine with smaller amount eliminated in feces. Removed by hemodialysis. *Half-life:* 4 hr.

INDICATIONS AND DOSAGES
▸ **Intra-Abdominal Infection**
IV, IM
Adults, Elderly. 1 g/day for 5–14 days.

▸ **Skin and Skin Structure Infection**
IV, IM
Adults, Elderly. 1 g/day for 7–14 days.
▸ **Pneumonia, UTI**
IV, IM
Adults, Elderly. 1 g/day for 10–14 days.
▸ **Pelvic Infection**
IV, IM
Adults, Elderly. 1 g/day for 3–10 days.
▸ **Dosage in Renal Impairment**
For adults and elderly patients with creatinine clearance less than 30 ml/min, dosage is 500 mg once a day.

SIDE EFFECTS/ADVERSE REACTIONS
Frequent
Diarrhea, nausea, headache
Occasional
Altered mental status, insomnia, rash, abdominal pain, constipation, vomiting, edema, fever
Rare
Dizziness, cough, oral candidiasis, anxiety, tachycardia, phlebitis at IV site

PRECAUTIONS AND CONTRAINDICATIONS
History of hypersensitivity to beta-lactams (imipenem and cilastin, meropenem), hypersensitivity to amide-type local anesthetics (IM)

DRUG INTERACTIONS OF CONCERN TO DENTISTRY
- Increased or prolonged plasma levels: probenecid
- Dental drug interactions have not been studied

SERIOUS REACTIONS
❗ Antibiotic-associated colitis and other superinfections may occur.
❗ Anaphylactic reactions have been reported.

! Seizures may occur in those with CNS disorders (including patients with brain lesions or a history of seizures), bacterial meningitis, or severe renal impairment.

DENTAL CONSIDERATIONS
General:
• For selected infections in the hospital setting; provide palliative emergency dental treatment only.
• Examine for oral manifestation of opportunistic infection.
• Determine why patient is taking the drug.
• Caution regarding allergy to medication.
Consultations:
• Medical consultation may be required to assess disease control and patient's ability to tolerate stress.
Teach Patient/Family to:
• Use effective oral hygiene to prevent soft tissue inflammation
• Report sore throat, oral burning sensation, fever, or fatigue, any of which could indicate presence of a superinfection

erythromycin
er-ith-roe-mye´-sin
(A/T/S, Akne-Mycin, Apo-Erythro Base[CAN], EES, Emgel, Eryacne[AUS], Erybid[CAN], Eryc, Eryc LD[AUS], EryDerm, Erygel, EryPed, Ery-Tab, Erythra-Derm, Erythrocin, Erythromid[CAN], PCE)
Do not confuse erythromycin with azithromycin or Ethmozine, or Eryc with Emcyt.

CATEGORY AND SCHEDULE
Pregnancy Risk Category: B

Drug Class: Antiinfective

MECHANISM OF ACTION
A macrolide that reversibly binds to bacterial ribosomes, inhibiting bacterial protein synthesis.
Therapeutic Effect: Bacteriostatic.

USES
Treatment of infection of external eye, prophylaxis of neonatal conjunctivitis and ophthalmia neonatorum; acne vulgaris; infections caused by *N. gonorrhoeae;* mild-to-moderate respiratory tract, skin, soft tissue infections caused by *S. pneumoniae, M. pneumoniae, C. diphtheriae, B. pertussis, L. monocytogenes, S. pyogenes;* syphilis; legionnaires' disease; *C. trachomatis; H. influenzae;* endocarditis prophylaxis

PHARMACOKINETICS
Variably absorbed from the GI tract (depending on dosage form used). Protein binding: 70%–90%. Widely distributed. Metabolized in the liver. Primarily eliminated in feces by bile. Not removed by hemodialysis.
Half-life: 1.4–2 hr (increased in impaired renal function).

INDICATIONS AND DOSAGES
▸ **Mild-to-Moderate Infections of the Upper and Lower Respiratory Tract, Pharyngitis, Skin Infections**
PO
Adults, Elderly. 250 mg q6h, 500 mg q12h, or 333 mg q8h. Maximum: 4 g/day.
Children. 30–50 mg/kg/day in divided doses up to 60–100 mg/kg/day for severe infections.
Neonates. 20–40 mg/kg/day in divided doses q6–12h.
IV
Adults, Elderly, Children. 15–20 mg/kg/day in divided doses. Maximum: 4 g/day.

▶ **Preoperative Intestinal Antisepsis**
PO
Adults, Elderly. 1 g at 1 pm, 2 pm, and 11 pm on day before surgery (with neomycin).
Children. 20 mg/kg at 1pm, 2pm, and 11 pm on day before surgery (with neomycin).
▶ **Acne Vulgaris**
Topical
Adults. Apply thin layer to affected area twice a day.
▶ **Gonococcal Ophthalmia Neonatorum**
Ophthalmic
Neonates. 0.5–2 cm no later than 1 hr after delivery.

SIDE EFFECTS/ADVERSE REACTIONS

Frequent
IV: Abdominal cramping or discomfort, phlebitis or thrombophlebitis
Topical: Dry skin
Occasional
Nausea, vomiting, diarrhea, rash, urticaria
Rare
Ophthalmic: Sensitivity reaction with increased irritation, burning, itching, and inflammation
Topical: Urticaria

PRECAUTIONS AND CONTRAINDICATIONS

Administration of fixed-combination product, Pediazole, to infants younger than 2 mo; history of hepatitis due to macrolides; hypersensitivity to macrolides; preexisting hepatic disease.
Caution
Hepatic disease, lactation.

DRUG INTERACTIONS OF CONCERN TO DENTISTRY

● Increased duration of alfentanil, cyclosporine
● Increased serum levels: indinavir, digoxin
● Decreased action of clindamycin, penicillins, lincomycin
● Increased serum levels of alfentanil, carbamazepine, theophylline (and other methylxanthines) and felodipine (possibly with other calcium blockers in the dihydropyridine class), ergot alkaloids, oral anticoagulants, buspirone, tacrolimus
● Risk of rhabdomyolysis: HMG-CoA reductase inhibitors
● Oral contraceptives: advise patient of a low potential risk for decreased contraceptive action, to maintain compliance with oral contraceptive use while using antibiotics, and to consider the use of additional nonhormonal contraception
● May increase the effects of certain benzodiazepines: (e.g., midazolam, triazolam)
● Risk of prolonged QT interval; use with caution in patients taking gatifloxacin, moxifloxacin, pimozide, disopyramide
● Possible serotonin syndrome with SSRIs
● Suspected increase in plasma levels of repaglinide

SERIOUS REACTIONS

! Antibiotic-associated colitis and other superinfections may occur.
! High dosages in patients with renal impairment may lead to reversible hearing loss.
! Anaphylaxis and hepatotoxicity occur rarely.
! Ventricular arrhythmias and prolonged QT interval occur rarely with the IV drug form.

DENTAL CONSIDERATIONS

Erythromycin (Ophthalmic)
General:
• Avoid dental light in patient's eyes; offer dark glasses for patient comfort.

Erythromycin (Topical)
None indicated

Erythromycin Base/Erythromycin Estolate/Erythromycin Ethylsuccinate/Erythromycin Gluceptate/Erythromycin Lactobionate/Erythromycin Stearate
General:
• Alternative drug of choice for mild infection caused by a susceptible organism in patients who are allergic to penicillin.
• Determine why the patient is taking the drug.
• Estolate salt form is not indicated for adults because of risk of cholestatic jaundice.
Teach Patient/Family to:
• Take oral drug with full glass of water
• When used for dental infection, advise patient to:
  • Report sore throat, oral burning sensation, fever, and fatigue, any of which could indicate superinfection
  • Take at prescribed intervals and complete dosage regimen
  • Immediately notify the dentist if signs or symptoms of infection increase

escitalopram
es-sy-tal´-oh-pram
(Lexapro)

CATEGORY AND SCHEDULE
Pregnancy Risk Category: C

Drug Class: Antidepressant, selective serotonin reuptake inhibitor

MECHANISM OF ACTION
A selective serotonin reuptake inhibitor that blocks the uptake of the neurotransmitter serotonin at neuronal presynaptic membranes, increasing its availability at postsynaptic receptor sites. *Therapeutic Effect:* Relieves depression.

USES
Treatment of major depressive disorder; maintenance treatment of major depressive disorder

PHARMACOKINETICS
Well absorbed after PO administration. Primarily metabolized in the liver. Primarily excreted in feces with a lesser amount eliminated in urine. *Half-life:* 35 hr.

INDICATIONS AND DOSAGES
▶ **Depression, General Anxiety Disorder (GAD)**
PO
Adults. Initially, 10 mg once a day in the morning or evening. May increase to 20 mg after a minimum of 1 wk.
Elderly, Patients with hepatic impairment. 10 mg/day.

SIDE EFFECTS/ADVERSE REACTIONS

Frequent
Nausea, dry mouth, somnolence, insomnia, diaphoresis

Occasional
Tremor, diarrhea, abnormal ejaculation, dyspepsia, fatigue, anxiety, vomiting, anorexia

Rare
Sinusitis, sexual dysfunction, menstrual disorder, abdominal pain, agitation, decreased libido

PRECAUTIONS AND CONTRAINDICATIONS

Breast-feeding, use within 14 days of MAOIs

Caution
Hyponatremia, activation of mania/hypomania, seizures, suicide, hepatic impairment, renal impairment, concurrent use of citalopram, lactation, use in children has not been established

DRUG INTERACTIONS OF CONCERN TO DENTISTRY

- Increased sedation: alcohol, other CNS depressants
- Drugs that inhibit CYP3A4 or other CYP isoenzymes may or may not affect plasma levels; should be used with observation and caution
- Modest inhibitor of CYP2D6
- First-time users of SSRIs also taking NSAIDs may have a higher risk of GI side effects; until more data are available, it may be advisable to avoid use of NSAIDs in these patients (Br J Clin Pharmacol 55:591–595, 2003)

SERIOUS REACTIONS

! Overdose is manifested as dizziness, drowsiness, tachycardia, somnolence, confusion, and seizures.

DENTAL CONSIDERATIONS

General:
- Assess salivary flow as a factor in caries, periodontal disease, and candidiasis.
- Consider semisupine chair position for patient comfort if GI side effects occur.
- Question patient about tolerance of NSAIDs or aspirin related to GI disease.
- Evaluate respiration characteristics and rate.

Consultations:
- Medical consultation may be required to assess disease control and patient's ability to tolerate stress.
- Physician should be informed if significant xerostomia occurs (e.g., increased caries, sore tongue, problems eating or swallowing, difficulty wearing prosthesis) so that a medication change can be considered.

Teach Patient/Family to:
- Use effective oral hygiene to prevent soft tissue inflammation, infection
- When chronic dry mouth occurs, advise patient to:
  - Avoid mouth rinses with high alcohol content because of drying effects
  - Use daily home fluoride products for anticaries effect
  - Use sugarless gum, frequent sips of water, or saliva substitutes
- Comply with recommended regimens for oral care

esomeprazole
es-om-eh-pray´-zole
(Nexium, Nexium IV)

CATEGORY AND SCHEDULE
Pregnancy Risk Category: B

Drug Class: Antisecretory, proton pump inhibitor

MECHANISM OF ACTION
A proton pump inhibitor that is converted to active metabolites that irreversibly bind to and inhibit hydrogen-potassium adenosine triphosphates, an enzyme on the surface of gastric parietal cells. Inhibits hydrogen ion transport into gastric lumen. *Therapeutic Effect:* Increases gastric pH, reducing gastric acid production.

USES
Treatment of gastroesophageal reflux disease (GERD), healing and maintenance of erosive esophagitis and *H. pylori* eradication in combination with antibiotics

PHARMACOKINETICS
Well absorbed after oral administration. Protein binding: 97%. Extensively metabolized by the liver. Primarily excreted in urine. *Half-life:* 1–1.5 hr.

INDICATIONS AND DOSAGES
▸ **Erosive Esophagitis**
PO
Adults, Elderly. 20–40 mg once daily for 4–8 wk.
IV
Adults, Elderly. 20 or 40 mg once daily by IV injection over at least 3 min or IV infusion over 10–30 min.

▸ **To Maintain Healing of Erosive Esophagitis**
PO
Adults, Elderly. 20 mg/day.
▸ **GERD, to Reduce the Risk of NSAID-Induced Gastric Ulcer**
PO
Adults, Elderly. 20 mg once a day for 4 wk.
▸ **Duodenal Ulcer Caused by *H. Pylori***
PO
Adults, Elderly. 40 mg (esomeprazole) once a day, with amoxicillin 1,000 mg and clarithromycin 500 mg twice a day for 10 days.

SIDE EFFECTS/ADVERSE REACTIONS
Frequent
Headache
Occasional
Diarrhea, abdominal pain, nausea
Rare
Dizziness, asthenia or loss of strength, vomiting, constipation, rash, cough

PRECAUTIONS AND CONTRAINDICATIONS
Hypersensitivity to benzimidazoles
Caution
Presence of gastric malignancy, atrophic gastritis, lactation, use in pediatric patients has not been studied, severe hepatic impairment, allergic reactions to related proton pump inhibitors

DRUG INTERACTIONS OF CONCERN TO DENTISTRY
• May interfere with absorption of drugs where gastric pH is an important factor in bioavailability (e.g., iron products, ketoconazole, trovafloxacin, ampicillin)

SERIOUS REACTIONS
None known

DENTAL CONSIDERATIONS
General:
• Assess salivary flow as a factor in caries, periodontal disease, and candidiasis.
• Question patient about tolerance of NSAIDs or aspirin related to GI disease.
• Consider semisupine chair position for patient comfort because of GI side effects of disease.
• Patients on chronic drug therapy may rarely have symptoms of blood dyscrasias, which can include infection, bleeding, and poor healing.
• Place on frequent recall because of oral side effects and oral effects of reflux disease.
Consultations:
• In a patient with symptoms of blood dyscrasias, request a medical consult for blood studies and postpone treatment until normal values are reestablished.
Teach Patient/Family to:
• Be aware of oral side effects and potential sequelae
• Prevent trauma when using oral hygiene aids
• Use effective oral hygiene to prevent soft tissue inflammation, infection
• When chronic dry mouth occurs, advise patient to:
  • Avoid mouth rinses with high alcohol content because of drying effects
  • Use daily home fluoride products for anticaries effect
  • Use sugarless gum, frequent sips of water, or saliva substitutes

estazolam
es-tay´-zoe-lam
(ProSom)

CATEGORY AND SCHEDULE
Pregnancy Risk Category: X
Controlled Substance: Schedule IV

Drug Class: Benzodiazepine, sedativehypnotic

MECHANISM OF ACTION
A benzodiazepine that enhances action of gamma aminobutyric acid (GABA) neurotransmission in the CNS. *Therapeutic Effect:* Produces depressant effect at all levels of CNS, relieves insomnia.

USES
Treatment of insomnia

PHARMACOKINETICS
Rapidly absorbed from GI tract. Protein binding: 93%. Metabolized in liver. Primarily excreted in urine, minimal in feces. *Half-life:* 10–24 hr.

INDICATIONS AND DOSAGES
▶ **Insomnia**
PO
Adults (older than 18 yr). 1–2 mg at bedtime.
Elderly, debilitated, liver disease, low serum albumin. 0.5–1 mg at bedtime.

SIDE EFFECTS/ADVERSE REACTIONS
Frequent
Drowsiness, sedation, rebound insomnia (may occur for 1–2 nights after drug is discontinued), dizziness, confusion, euphoria
Occasional
Weakness, anorexia, diarrhea

Rare
Paradoxical CNS excitement,
restlessness (particularly noted
in elderly/debilitated)

PRECAUTIONS AND CONTRAINDICATIONS
Pregnancy, hypersensitivity to other
benzodiazepines
Caution
Hepatic disease, renal
disease, suicidal individuals,
drug abuse, elderly, psychosis,
children younger than 18 yr,
lactation, depression, pulmonary
insufficiency, narrow-angle
glaucoma

DRUG INTERACTIONS OF CONCERN TO DENTISTRY
• Increased CNS depression: alcohol,
all CNS depressants
• Increased serum levels and
prolonged effect of benzodiazepines:
ketoconazole, itraconazole,
fluconazole, miconazole (systemic),
indinavir
• Contraindicated with saquinavir
• Possible increase in CNS side
effects: kava kava (herb)
• Decreased plasma levels: St. John's
wort (herb)

SERIOUS REACTIONS
! Overdosage results in somnolence,
confusion, diminished reflexes, and
coma.

DENTAL CONSIDERATIONS
General:
• Psychologic and physical
dependence may occur with chronic
administration.
• Geriatric patients are more
susceptible to drug effects; use
lower dose.

• Avoid the use of this drug in a
patient with a history of drug abuse
or alcoholism.
Teach Patient/Family to:
• Avoid mouth rinses with high
alcohol content because of drying
effects

estradiol
ess-tra-dye´-ole
(Aerodil[AUS], Alora, Climara,
Delestrogen, Depo-Estradiol,
Esclim, Estrace, Estraderm,
Estraderm MX[AUS],
Estradot[CAN], Estrasorb, Estrogel,
Estring, Femring, Kliovance[AUS],
Menostar, Oesclim[CAN],
Primogyn Depot[AUS],
Progynova[AUS], Sandrena
Gel[AUS], Vagifem, Vivelle, Vivelle
Dot, Zumenon[AUS])
Do not confuse Estraderm with
Testoderm.

CATEGORY AND SCHEDULE
Pregnancy Risk Category: X

Drug Class: Estrogen

MECHANISM OF ACTION
An estrogen that increases synthesis
of DNA, RNA, and proteins in target
tissues; reduces release of
gonadotropin-releasing hormone
from the hypothalamus; and
reduces follicle-stimulating
hormone and luteinizing hormone
(LH) release from the pituitary.
Therapeutic Effect: Promotes
normal growth, promotes
development of female sex organs,
and maintains GU function and
vasomotor stability. Prevents
accelerated bone loss by inhibiting
bone resorption, restoring balance
of bone resorption and formation.

Inhibits LH and decreases serum testosterone concentration.

USES
Treatment of menopause, breast cancer, prostatic cancer, atrophic vaginitis, kraurosis vulvae, hypogonadism, ovariectomy, primary ovarian failure, prevention of osteoporosis and menopause-related vasomotor symptoms

PHARMACOKINETICS
Well absorbed from the GI tract. Widely distributed. Protein binding: 50%–80%. Metabolized in the liver. Primarily excreted in urine.
Half-life: Unknown.

INDICATIONS AND DOSAGES
▶ **Prostate Cancer**
IM (estradiol valerate)
Adults, Elderly. 30 mg or more q1–2wk.
PO
Adults, Elderly. 10 mg 3 times a day for at least 3 mo.
▶ **Breast Cancer**
PO
Adults, Elderly. 10 mg 3 times a day for at least 3 mo.
▶ **Osteoporosis Prophylaxis in Postmenopausal Females**
PO
Adults, Elderly. 0.5 mg/day cyclically (3 wk on, 1 wk off).
Transdermal (Climara)
Adults, Elderly. Initially, 0.025 mg/wk, adjust dose as needed.
Transdermal (Alora, Vivelle, Vivelle-Dot)
Adults, Elderly. Initially, 0.025 mg patch twice a wk, adjust dose as needed.
Transdermal (Estraderm)
Adults, Elderly. 0.05 mg twice a wk.
Transdermal (Menostar)
Adults, Elderly. 1 mg a wk.

▶ **Female Hypoestrogenism**
PO
Adults, Elderly. 1–2 mg/day, adjust dose as needed.
IM (cypionate)
Adults, Elderly. 1.5–2 mg/mo.
IM (estradiol valerate)
Adults, Elderly. 10–20 mg q4wk.
▶ **Vasomotor Symptoms Associated With Menopause**
PO
Adults, Elderly. 1–2 mg/day cyclically (3 wk on, 1 wk off), adjust dose as needed.
IM (estradiol cypionate)
Adults, Elderly. 1–5 mg q3–4wk.
IM (estradiol valerate)
Adults, Elderly. 10–20 mg q4wk.
Topical emulsion (Estrasorb)
Adults, Elderly. 3.84 g once a day in the morning.
Topical Gel (Estrogel)
Adults, Elderly. 1.25 g/day.
Transdermal (Climara)
Adults, Elderly. 0.025 mg/wk. Adjust dose as needed.
Transdermal (Alora, Esclim, Estrader, Vivelle-Dot)
Adults, Elderly. 0.05 mg twice a wk.
Transdermal (Vivelle)
Adults, Elderly. 0.0375 mg twice a wk.
Vaginal Ring (Femring)
Adults, Elderly. 0.05 mg. May increase to 0.1 mg if needed.
▶ **Vaginal Atrophy**
Vaginal Ring (Estring)
Adults, Elderly. 2 mg.
▶ **Atrophic Vaginitis**
Vaginal Tablet (Vagifem)
Adults, Elderly. Initially, 1 tablet/day for 2 wk. Maintenance: 1 tablet twice a wk.

SIDE EFFECTS/ADVERSE REACTIONS
Frequent
Anorexia, nausea, swelling of breasts, peripheral edema marked by swollen ankles and feet
Transdermal: Skin irritation, redness

Occasional
Vomiting, especially with high doses; headache that may be severe; intolerance to contact lenses; hypertension; glucose intolerance; brown spots on exposed skin
Vaginal: Local irritation, vaginal discharge, changes in vaginal bleeding, including spotting, and breakthrough or prolonged bleeding
Rare
Chorea or involuntary movements, hirsutism or abnormal hairiness, loss of scalp hair, depression

PRECAUTIONS AND CONTRAINDICATIONS

Abnormal vaginal bleeding, active arterial thrombosis, blood dyscrasias, estrogen-dependent cancer, known or suspected breast cancer, pregnancy, thrombophlebitis or thromboembolic disorders, thyroid dysfunction
Caution
Hypertension, asthma, blood dyscrasias, gallbladder disease, CHF, diabetes mellitus, bone disease, depression, migraine headache, convulsive disorders, hepatic disease, renal disease, family history of cancer of breast or reproductive tract

DRUG INTERACTIONS OF CONCERN TO DENTISTRY

• Increased action of corticosteroids

SERIOUS REACTIONS

❗ Estrogen therapy may increase the risk of developing coronary artery disease, hypercalcemia, gallbladder disease, cerebrovascular disease, and breast cancer.
❗ Prolonged administration increases the risk of gallbladder disease, thromboembolic disease, and breast, cervical, vaginal, endometrial, and hepatic carcinoma.
❗ Cholestatic jaundice occurs rarely.

DENTAL CONSIDERATIONS

General:
• Place on frequent recall to evaluate gingival condition.
• Monitor vital signs because of cardiovascular side effects.
Teach Patient/Family to:
• Use effective oral hygiene to prevent gingival inflammation

estramustine phosphate sodium
es-trah-mew´-steen foss´-fate
soe´-dee-um
(Emcyt)
Do not confuse Emcyt with Eryc.

CATEGORY AND SCHEDULE
Pregnancy Risk Category: C

Drug Class: Antineoplastic

MECHANISM OF ACTION
An alkylating agent, estrogen and nitrogen mustard that binds to microtubule-associated proteins, causing their disassembly. *Therapeutic Effect:* Reduces serum testosterone concentration.

USES
Treatment of metastatic prostate cancer

PHARMACOKINETICS

Well absorbed from the GI tract. Highly localized in prostatic tissue. Rapidly dephosphorylated during absorption into peripheral circulation. Metabolized in the liver. Primarily eliminated in feces by biliary system. *Half-life:* 20 hr.

INDICATIONS AND DOSAGES

▸ **Prostatic Carcinoma**

PO

Adults, Elderly. 10–16 mg/kg/day or 140 mg 4 times a day.

SIDE EFFECTS/ADVERSE REACTIONS

Frequent

Peripheral edema of lower extremities, breast tenderness or enlargement, diarrhea, flatulence, nausea

Occasional

Increase in B/P, thirst, dry skin, ecchymosis, flushing, alopecia, night sweats

Rare

Headache, rash, fatigue, insomnia, vomiting

PRECAUTIONS AND CONTRAINDICATIONS

Active thrombophlebitis or thromboembolic disorders (unless the tumor is the cause of the thromboembolic disorder and the benefits outweigh the risk), hypersensitivity to estradiol or nitrogen mustard

DRUG INTERACTIONS OF CONCERN TO DENTISTRY

• Increased risk of hepatoxicity: hepatoxic drugs
• Impaired absorption: calcium-containing products

SERIOUS REACTIONS

! Estramustine use may exacerbate CHF and increase the risk of pulmonary emboli, thrombophlebitis, and cerebrovascular accident.

DENTAL CONSIDERATIONS

General:

• Patients with prostate disease may experience urinary retention; caution with use of anticholinergic drugs that could aggravate urinary retention.
• Patients may have received other chemotherapy or radiation; confirm medical and drug history.
• Determine why patient is taking the drug.
• Monitor vital signs at every appointment due to cardiovascular side effects.
• Consider semisupine chair position for patient comfort if GI side effects occur.
• Patient may need assistance in getting into and out of dental chair. Adjust chair position for patient comfort.
• Short appointments and a stress-reduction protocol may be required for anxious patients.

Consultations:

• Consultation with physician may be needed if sedation or general anesthesia is required.
• Medical consultation may be required to assess disease control.

Teach Patient/Family to:

• Use effective oral hygiene to prevent soft tissue inflammation
• Update health and medication history if physician makes any changes in evaluation or drug regimens; include OTC, herbal, and nonherbal remedies in the update

estrogens, conjugated; medroxy-progesterone acetate

ess´-troe-jens, kon´-joo-gay-ted; me-drox´-ee-proe-jes´-ter-rone ass´-eh-tayte

(Premphase, Prempro, Prempro Low Dose)

CATEGORY AND SCHEDULE

Pregnancy Risk Category: X

Drug Class: Estrogens

MECHANISM OF ACTION

Conjugated estrogens are estrogens that increase synthesis of DNA, RNA, and various proteins in responsive tissues; reduces release of gonadotropin-releasing hormone, reducing follicle-stimulating hormone (FSH) and leuteinizing hormone (LH). Medroxy-progesterone acetate is a hormone that transforms endometrium from proliferative to secretory in an estrogen-primed endometrium; inhibits secretion of pituitary gonadotropins. *Therapeutic Effect:* Conjugated estrogens promote vasomotor stability, maintain GU function, normal growth, development of female sex organs; prevents accelerated bone loss by inhibiting bone resorption, restoring balance of bone resorption and formation; inhibits LH, decreases serum concentration of testosterone. Medroxyprogesterone acetate prevents follicular maturation and ovulation; stimulates growth of mammary alveolar tissue; relaxes uterine smooth muscle; restores hormonal imbalance.

USES

Treatment of symptoms associated with menopause, inoperable breast cancer, prostatic cancer, abnormal uterine bleeding, hypogonadism, primary ovarian failure, prevention of osteoporosis

PHARMACOKINETICS

Conjugated estrogens are well absorbed from the GI tract. Widely distributed. Protein binding: 50%–80%. Metabolized in liver. Primarily excreted in urine. *Half-life:* 4–10 hr. Medroxyprogesterone's absorption varies depending on the patient but is generally low. Binds mainly to albumin or other plasma proteins. Metabolized in liver. Primarily excreted in urine. *Half-life:* 2–4 hr.

INDICATIONS AND DOSAGES

▶ **Menopausal Symptoms, Osteoporosis, Vulvar/Vaginal Atrophy**

PO

(Prempro)Adults, Elderly. 1 tablet once daily.

▶ **Menopausal Symptoms, Osteoporosis, Vulvar or Vaginal Atrophy**

PO

(Premphase)Adults, Elderly. 1 maroon conjugated estrogen tablet on days 1–14 and 1 light blue conjugated estrogens/medroxyprogesterone tablet on days 15–28.

SIDE EFFECTS/ADVERSE REACTIONS

Frequent

Change in vaginal bleeding, such as spotting or breakthrough bleeding, breast pain or tenderness, gynecomastia

Occasional

Headache, increased B/P, intolerance to contact lenses, nausea, edema, weight change, breast tenderness, nervousness, insomnia, fatigue, dizziness

Rare

Loss of scalp hair, mental depression, dermatologic changes, headache, fever

PRECAUTIONS AND CONTRAINDICATIONS

Breast cancer with some exceptions, liver disease, thrombophlebitis, undiagnosed vaginal bleeding, estrogen-dependent neoplasia (known of suspected), pregnancy (known or suspected), hypersensitivity to conjugated estrogens, medroxyprogesterone acetate or any component of the formulation

Caution

Hypertension, asthma, blood dyscrasias, gallbladder disease, CHF, diabetes mellitus, bone disease, depression, migraine headache, convulsive disorders, hepatic disease, renal disease, family history of cancer of breast or reproductive tract

DRUG INTERACTIONS OF CONCERN TO DENTISTRY

• Increased action of corticosteroids

DRUG INTERACTIONS OF CONCERN TO DENTISTRY

None reported

SERIOUS REACTIONS

Estrogens A, Conjugated Synthetic

! Prolonged administration may increase risk of gallbladder, thromboembolic disease, or breast, cervical, vaginal, endometrial, and liver carcinoma.

DENTAL CONSIDERATIONS

Estrogens A, Conjugated Synthetic

General:

• Place on frequent recall to evaluate gingival condition.

• Monitor vital signs because of cardiovascular side effects.

• Consider semisupine chair position for patient comfort if GI side effects occur.

Teach Patient/Family to:

• Use effective oral hygiene to prevent gingival soft tissue inflammation

---

estropipate

es-tro-pip´-ate

(Genoral[AUS], Ogen, Ortho-Est)

CATEGORY AND SCHEDULE

Pregnancy Risk Category: X

Drug Class: Estrogen (piperazine estrone sulfate)

MECHANISM OF ACTION

An estrogen that increases synthesis of DNA, RNA, and proteins in target tissues; reduces release of gonadotropin-releasing hormone from the hypothalamus; and reduces follicle-stimulating hormone (FSH) and luteinizing hormone (LH) from the pituitary. *Therapeutic Effect:* Promotes normal growth, promotes development of female sex organs, and maintains GU function and vasomotor stability. Prevents accelerated bone loss by inhibiting bone resorption, restoring balance of bone resorption and formation. Inhibits LH and decreases serum testosterone concentration.

USES
Treatment of vasomotor symptoms of menopause, atrophic vaginitis, primary female hypogonadism, primary ovarian failure, estrogen imbalance, ovariectomy

PHARMACOKINETICS
PO: Well absorbed; moderate-to-high protein binding; hepatic metabolism with primary renal excretion

INDICATIONS AND DOSAGES
▶ **Vasomotor Symptoms, Atrophic Vaginitis, Kraurosis Vulvae**
PO
Adults, Elderly. 0.625–5 mg/day cyclically.
▶ **Atrophic Vaginitis, Kraurosis Vulvae**
Intravaginal
Adults, Elderly. 2–4 g/day cyclically.
▶ **Female Hypogonadism, Castration, Primary Ovarian Failure**
PO
Adults, Elderly. 1.25–7.5 mg/day for 21 days; then off for 8–10 days. Repeat if bleeding does not occur by end of off cycle.
▶ **Prevention of Osteoporosis**
PO
Adults, Elderly. 0.625 mg/day (25 days of 31-day cycle/mo).

SIDE EFFECTS/ADVERSE REACTIONS
Frequent
Anorexia, nausea, swelling of breasts, peripheral edema marked by swollen ankles and feet
Occasional
Vomiting, especially with high doses; headache that may be severe; intolerance to contact lenses; hypertension; glucose intolerance; brown spots on exposed skin

Vaginal: Local irritation, vaginal discharge, changes in vaginal bleeding, including spotting, and breakthrough or prolonged bleeding
Rare
Chorea or involuntary movements, hirsutism or abnormal hairiness, loss of scalp hair, depression

PRECAUTIONS AND CONTRAINDICATIONS
Abnormal vaginal bleeding, active arterial thrombosis, blood dyscrasias, estrogen-dependent cancer, known or suspected breast cancer, pregnancy, thrombophlebitis or thromboembolic disorders, thyroid dysfunction
Caution
Hypertension, asthma, blood dyscrasias, gallbladder disease, CHF, diabetes mellitus, bone disease, depression, migraine headache, convulsive disorders, hepatic disease, renal disease, family history of cancer of breast or reproductive tract

DRUG INTERACTIONS OF CONCERN TO DENTISTRY
• Increased action of corticosteroids

SERIOUS REACTIONS
❗ Prolonged administration increases the risk of gallbladder disease, thromboembolic disease and breast, cervical, vaginal, endometrial, and hepatic carcinoma.
❗ Cholestatic jaundice occurs rarely.

DENTAL CONSIDERATIONS
General:
• Place on frequent recall to evaluate gingival condition.
• Monitor vital signs because of cardiovascular side effects.
Teach Patient/Family to:
• Use effective oral hygiene to prevent gingival inflammation

eszopiclone
es-zoe´-pih-clone
(Lunesta)

CATEGORY AND SCHEDULE
Pregnancy Risk Category: C
Controlled Substance:
Schedule IV

Drug Class: Sedative-hypnotic

MECHANISM OF ACTION
A nonbenzodiazepine that enhances
the action of the inhibitory
neurotransmitter gamma-
aminobutyric acid (GABA).

USES
Treatment of insomnia

PHARMACOKINETICS
Rapidly absorbed, peak 1 hr.
Half-life: 6 hr, metabolized in liver
by CYP3A4 and CYP 2E1, weak
protein binding (52%–59%),
unchanged drug (10%) and
metabolites (75%) excreted in urine.

INDICATIONS AND DOSAGES
▶ **Insomnia:**
PO
Adult: 2 mg per day at bedtime.

SIDE EFFECTS/ADVERSE REACTIONS:
ORAL: Dry mouth, taste alterations
CNS: Somnolence, nervousness,
anxiety, confusion, depression,
dizziness, hallucinations, decreased
libido
GI: Dyspepsia, nausea, vomiting
RESP: Infection
GU: Dysmenorrhea (females),
gynecomastia (males)
INTEG: Rash
SYST: Headache, chest pain,
viral infection

PRECAUTIONS AND CONTRAINDICATIONS
Mental impairment, behavior and
mood changes (depression), use
lower doses in elderly and patients
with renal/hepatic impairment

DRUG INTERACTIONS OF CONCERN TO DENTISTRY:
• Increased CNS depression: all
CNS depressants, alcohol
• Inhibitors of CYP 3A4 (azole
antifungals, macrolide antibiotics,
e.g., erythromycin/clarithromycin):
increased blood levels and CNS
depression
• Use all necessary precautions when
prescribing for pre-operative
sedation
• Food: Effects delayed by taking
with or immediately after heavy/fatty
meal

DENTAL CONSIDERATIONS
General:
• Assess salivary flow as a factor
in caries, periodontal disease and
candiasis
• Differentiate taste changes due
to drug from those associated with
restorative materials
• Use all appropriate precautions if
prescribing for preoperative sedation
• After supine positioning, allow
patient to sit upright for 2 min before
standing to avoid dizziness
Consultations:
• Medical consultation may be
required to assess disease control
Teach Patient/Family to:
• Avoid mouth rinses with high
alcohol content because of drying
effect
• Use home fluoride products to
prevent caries

• Use sugarless chewing gum, frequent sips of water, or saliva substitutes if dry mouth occurs

etanercept
eh-tan´-er-cept
(Enbrel)

CATEGORY AND SCHEDULE
Pregnancy Risk Category: B

Drug Class: Antiinflammatory and immunomodulator; biologic response modifier

MECHANISM OF ACTION
A protein that binds to tumor necrosis factor (TNF), blocking its interaction with cell surface receptors. Elevated levels of TNF, which is involved in inflammatory and immune responses, are found in the synovial fluid of rheumatoid arthritis patients.
Therapeutic Effect: Relieves symptoms of rheumatoid arthritis.

USES
Reduction in signs and symptoms of moderately to severely active rheumatoid arthritis in patients with an inadequate response to one or more disease-modifying antirheumatic drugs; polyarticular-course juvenile rheumatoid arthritis; psoriatic arthritis; also approved for initial therapy

PHARMACOKINETICS
Well absorbed after subcutaneous administration. *Half-life:* 115 hr.

INDICATIONS AND DOSAGES
▶ **Rheumatoid Arthritis, Psoriatic Arthritis, Ankylosing Spondylitis**
Subcutaneous

Adults, Elderly. 25 mg twice weekly given 72–96 hr apart. Alternative weekly dosing: 0.8 mg/kg/dose once a wk. Maximum: 50 mg/wk. Maximum: 25 mg/dose.
▶ **Juvenile Rheumatoid Arthritis**
Subcutaneous
Children 4–17 yr. 0.4 mg/kg (Maximum: 25 mg dose) twice a wk given 72–96 hr apart. Alternative weekly dosing: 50 mg once a wk. Maximum: 25 mg/dose.
▶ **Plaque Psoriasis**
Subcutaneous
Adults, Elderly. 50 mg twice a wk (give 3–4 days apart) for 3 mo. Maintenance: 50 mg once a wk.

SIDE EFFECTS/ADVERSE REACTIONS
Frequent
Injection site erythema, pruritus, pain, and swelling; abdominal pain, vomiting (more common in children than adults)
Occasional
Headache, rhinitis, dizziness, pharyngitis, cough, asthenia, abdominal pain, dyspepsia
Rare
Sinusitis, allergic reaction

PRECAUTIONS AND CONTRAINDICATIONS
Serious active infection or sepsis
Caution
Risk of new malignancies and infrequent severe cardiovascular events, discontinue if serious infection occurs, immunosuppression risk, caution with preexisting demyelinating disorders, lactation, viral infections, children younger than 4 yr

DRUG INTERACTIONS OF CONCERN TO DENTISTRY
No studies have been conducted

E

SERIOUS REACTIONS

❗ Infections (such as pyelonephritis, cellulitis, osteomyelitis, wound infection, leg ulcer, septic arthritis, diarrhea, bronchitis, and pneumonia), occur in 38%–29% of patients.
❗ Rare adverse effects include heart failure, hypertension, hypotension, pancreatitis, GI hemorrhage, and dyspnea. The patient also may develop autoimmune antibodies.

DENTAL CONSIDERATIONS

General:
• Monitor vital signs at every appointment because of potential cardiovascular side effects.
• Consider semisupine chair position for patient comfort because of GI side effects of drug.
• If acute oral infection occurs, inform physician.
• Note elevated antinuclear antibody (ANA) levels if diagnosing Sögren's syndrome.
Consultations:
• Medical consultation if needed.
Teach Patient/Family to:
• Use effective oral hygiene to prevent soft tissue inflammation
• Use electric tooth brush if patient has difficulty holding conventional devices

ethambutol

eh-tham´-byoo-tole
(Etibi[CAN], Myambutol)
Do not confuse ethambutol or Myambutol with Nembutal.

CATEGORY AND SCHEDULE

Pregnancy Risk Category: B

Drug Class: Antitubercular

MECHANISM OF ACTION

An isonicotinic acid derivative that interferes with RNA synthesis.
Therapeutic Effect: Suppresses the multiplication of mycobacteria.

USES

Treatment of pulmonary tuberculosis (TB), as an adjunct

PHARMACOKINETICS

Rapidly and well absorbed from the GI tract. Protein binding: 20%–30%. Widely distributed. Metabolized in the liver. Primarily excreted in urine. Removed by hemodialysis.
Half-life: 3–4 hr (increased in impaired renal function).

INDICATIONS AND DOSAGES

▸ **TB**
PO
Adults, Elderly, Children. 15–25 mg/kg/day as a single dose or 50 mg/kg 2 times a wk. Maximum: 2.5 g/dose.
▸ **Atypical Mycobacterial Infections**
PO
Adults, Elderly, Children. 15 mg/kg/day. Maximum: 1 g/day.
▸ **Dosage in Renal Impairment**
Dosage interval is modified on the basis of creatinine clearance.

Creatinine Clearance	Dosage Interval
10–50 ml/ min	q24–36h
Less than 10 ml/min	q48h

SIDE EFFECTS/ADVERSE REACTIONS

Occasional
Acute gouty arthritis (chills, pain, swelling of joints with hot skin), confusion, abdominal pain, nausea, vomiting, anorexia, headache

Rare
Rash, fever, blurred vision, eye pain, red-green color blindness

PRECAUTIONS AND CONTRAINDICATIONS
Optic neuritis
Caution
Renal disease, diabetic retinopathy, cataracts, ocular defects, hepatic disorders, hematopoietic disorders

DRUG INTERACTIONS OF CONCERN TO DENTISTRY
None reported

SERIOUS REACTIONS
! Optic neuritis (more common with high-dosage or long-term ethambutol therapy), peripheral neuritis, thrombocytopenia, and an anaphylactoid reaction occur rarely.

DENTAL CONSIDERATIONS
General:
• Examine for evidence of oral signs of disease.
• Avoid dental light in patient's eyes; offer dark glasses for patient comfort.
• Determine why the patient is taking the drug.
Consultations:
• Medical consultation is required to assess patient's current status; avoid elective dental procedures in active infections.
• Determine that noninfectious status exists by ensuring the following:
• Anti-TB drugs have been taken for longer than 3 wk.
• Culture confirms antibiotic susceptibility to TB microorganisms.
• Patient has had three consecutive negative sputum smears.
• Patient is not in the coughing stage.

Teach Patient/Family to:
• Take medication for full length of prescribed therapy to ensure effectiveness of treatment and to prevent the emergence of resistant forms of microbes

ethionamide
eh-thye-on´-am-ide
(Trecator)
Do not confuse with Tricor.

CATEGORY AND SCHEDULE
Pregnancy Risk Category: C

Drug Class: Antitubercular

MECHANISM OF ACTION
An antitubercular agent that inhibits peptide synthesis. *Therapeutic Effect:* Suppresses mycobacterial multiplication. Bactericidal.

USES
Treatment of pulmonary, extrapulmonary tuberculosis (TB) when other antitubercular drugs have failed

PHARMACOKINETICS
Rapidly absorbed from the GI tract. Widely distributed. Protein binding: 10%. Metabolized in liver. Primarily excreted in urine. Removed by hemodialysis. *Half-life:* 2–3 hr (half-life is increased with impaired renal function).

INDICATIONS AND DOSAGES
▸ TB
PO
Adults, Elderly. 500–1000 mg/day as a single to 3 divided doses.

Children. 15–20 mg/kg/day.
Maximum 1 g/day.
▶ **Dosage in Renal Impairment**
*Creatinine clearance less than
50 ml/min.* Reduce dose by 50%.

SIDE EFFECTS/ADVERSE REACTIONS
Occasional
Abdominal pain, nausea, vomiting,
weakness, postural hypotension,
psychiatric disturbances, drowsiness,
dizziness, headache, confusion,
anorexia, headache, metallic taste,
anorexia, diarrhea, stomatitis,
peripheral neuritis
Rare
Rash, fever, blurred vision, optic
neuritis, seizures, hypothyroidism,
hypoglycemia, gynecomastia,
thrombocytopenia, jaundice

PRECAUTIONS AND CONTRAINDICATIONS
Severe hepatic impairment,
hypersensitivity to ethionamide
Caution
Lactation, renal disease, diabetic
retinopathy, cataracts, ocular defects,
children younger than 12 yr;
pyridoxine concurrent use is
recommended, resistance may
develop

DRUG INTERACTIONS OF CONCERN TO DENTISTRY
None reported

SERIOUS REACTIONS
! Peripheral neuropathy, anorexia,
and joint pain rarely occur.

DENTAL CONSIDERATIONS
General:
• Monitor vital signs at every
appointment because of
cardiovascular side effects.

• After supine positioning, have
patient sit upright for at least 2 min
before standing to avoid orthostatic
hypotension.
• Consider semisupine chair position
for patient comfort because of GI
effects of disease.
• Evaluate for clotting ability during
gingival instrumentation.
• Examine for evidence of oral
manifestations of blood dyscrasias
(infection, bleeding, poor healing).
• Palliative treatment may be
required for oral side effects.
• Examine for evidence of oral signs
of disease.
Consultations:
• Medical consultation for blood
studies (CBC); leukopenic or
thrombocytopenic side effects may
result in infection, delayed healing,
and excessive bleeding. Postpone
elective dental treatment until normal
values are maintained. Instruct
patient to take with meals to decrease
GI symptoms.
• Medical consultation may be
required to assess disease control
and determine infectious nature of
disease.
Teach Patient/Family to:
• Use effective oral hygiene to
prevent soft tissue inflammation
• Use caution in use of oral hygiene
aids to prevent injury

ethosuximide
eth-oh-sux´-ih-mide
(Zarontin)
Do not confuse with Zaroxolyn
or Neurontin.

CATEGORY AND SCHEDULE
Pregnancy Risk Category: C

Drug Class: Anticonvulsant

MECHANISM OF ACTION

An anticonvulsant that increases the seizure threshold and suppresses paroxysmal spike-and-wave pattern in absence seizures; depresses nerve transmission in the motor cortex. *Therapeutic Effect:* Produces anticonvulsant activity.

USES

Treatment of absence seizures (petit mal); unapproved: complex partial seizures

PHARMACOKINETICS

Well absorbed from the GI tract. Metabolized in liver. Excreted in urine. Removed by hemodialysis. *Half-life:* 50–60 hr (in adults); 30 hr (in children).

INDICATIONS AND DOSAGES

▶ **Absence Seizures**
PO
Adults, Elderly, Children older than 6 yr. Initially, 250 mg/day or 15 mg/kg/day in 2 divided doses. Maintenance: 15–40 mg/kg/day in 2 divided doses.
Children 3–6 yr. Initially, 250 mg in 2 divided doses, increased by 250 mg as needed every 4–7 days. Maintenance: 20–40 mg/kg/day in 2 divided doses.
Use with caution in patients with renal impairment.

SIDE EFFECTS/ADVERSE REACTIONS

Occasional
Dizziness, drowsiness, double vision, headache, ataxia, nausea, diarrhea, vomiting, somnolence, urticaria
Rare
Arganulocytosis, gum hypertrophy, leucopenia, myopia, swelling of the tongue, systemic lupus erythematosus, vaginal bleeding

PRECAUTIONS AND CONTRAINDICATIONS

Hypersensitivity to succinimides
Caution
Lactation, hepatic disease, renal disease

DRUG INTERACTIONS OF CONCERN TO DENTISTRY

• Enhanced CNS depression: CNS depressants, alcohol

SERIOUS REACTIONS

❗ Abrupt withdrawal may increase seizure frequency.
❗ Overdosage results in nausea, vomiting, and CNS depression including coma with respiratory depression.

DENTAL CONSIDERATIONS

General:
• Patients on chronic drug therapy may rarely have symptoms of blood dyscrasias, which can include infection, bleeding, and poor healing.
• Talk with patient to ascertain seizure frequency and how well seizures are controlled. A stress reduction protocol may be required.
Consultations:
• In a patient with symptoms of blood dyscrasias, request a medical consultation for blood studies and postpone dental treatment until normal values are reestablished.
• Medical consultation may be required to assess disease control and patient's ability to tolerate stress.
Teach Patient/Family to:
• Use effective oral hygiene to prevent gingival inflammation
• Avoid mouth rinses with high alcohol content because of drying effects

etidronate disodium

ee-tid´-roe-nate die-soe´-dee-um
(Didronel)
Do not confuse etidronate with
etidocaine or etomidate.

CATEGORY AND SCHEDULE
Pregnancy Risk Category: C
(parenteral), B (oral)

Drug Class: Antihypercalcemic

MECHANISM OF ACTION
A bisphosphonate that decreases
mineral release and matrix in bone
and inhibits osteocytic osteolysis.
Therapeutic Effect: Decreases bone
resorption.

USES
Treatment of Paget's disease,
heterotopic ossification,
hypercalcemia of malignancy

PHARMACOKINETICS
Therapeutic response: 1–3 mo; not
metabolized; excreted in urine.

INDICATIONS AND DOSAGES
▸ **Paget's Disease**
PO
Adults, Elderly. Initially,
5–10 mg/kg/day not to exceed 6 mo,
or 11–20 mg/kg/day not to exceed
3 mo. Repeat only after drug-free
period of at least 90 days.
▸ **Heterotopic Ossification Caused
by Spinal Cord Injury**
PO
Adult, Elderly. 20 mg/kg/day for
2 wk; then 10 mg/kg/day for 10 wk.
▸ **Heterotopic Ossification
Complicating Total Hip Replacement**
PO
Adults, Elderly. 20 mg/kg/day for
1 mo before surgery; then
20 mg/kg/day for 3 mo after surgery.

▸ **Hypercalcemia Associated With
Malignancy**
IV
Adults, Elderly. 7.5 mg/kg/day for
3 days. For retreatment, allow 7 days
between treatment courses. Follow
with oral therapy on day after last
infusion. Begin with 20 mg/kg/day
for 30 days; may extend up to
90 days.

SIDE EFFECTS/ADVERSE REACTIONS
Frequent
Nausea; diarrhea; continuing or more
frequent bone pain in patients with
Paget's disease
Occasional
Bone fractures, especially of the
femur
Parenteral: Metallic, altered taste
Rare
Hypersensitivity reaction

PRECAUTIONS AND CONTRAINDICATIONS
Clinically overt osteomalacia
Caution
Renal disease, lactation, adequate
intake of vitamin D and calcium,
safety and efficacy in children have
not been established

DRUG INTERACTIONS OF CONCERN TO DENTISTRY
• Possible increased risk of gastric
ulceration: NSAIDs

SERIOUS REACTIONS
! Nephrotoxicity, including
hematuria, dysuria, and proteinuria,
has occurred with parenteral route.

DENTAL CONSIDERATIONS
General:
• Be aware of oral manifestations of
Paget's disease (macrognathia,
alveolar pain).

Consultations:
• Medical consultation may be required to assess disease control.

etodolac
eh-toe-doe´-lak
(Apo-Etodolac[CAN], Lodine, Lodine XL, Ultradol[CAN])
Do not confuse Lodine with codeine or iodine.

CATEGORY AND SCHEDULE
Pregnancy Risk Category: C
(D if used in third trimester or near delivery)

Drug Class: Nonsteroidal antiinflammatory

MECHANISM OF ACTION
An NSAID that produces analgesic and antiinflammatory effects by inhibiting prostaglandin synthesis.
Therapeutic Effect: Reduces the inflammatory response and intensity of pain.

USES
Mild-to-moderate pain, osteoarthritis, rheumatoid arthritis

PHARMACOKINETICS

Route	Onset	Peak	Duration
PO (analgesic)	30 min	N/A	4–12 hr

Completely absorbed from the GI tract. Protein binding: greater than 99%. Widely distributed. Metabolized in the liver. Primarily excreted in urine. Not removed by hemodialysis.
Half-life: 6–7 hr.

INDICATIONS AND DOSAGES
▸ **Osteoarthritis, Rheumatoid Arthritis**
PO (Immediate-Release)
Adults, Elderly. Initially, 300 mg 2–3 times a day or 400–500 mg twice a day. Maintenance: 600–1000 mg/day in 2–4 divided doses.
PO (Extended-Release)
Adults, Elderly. 400–1000 mg once daily. Maximum: 1200 mg/day.
▸ **Juvenile Rheumatoid Arthritis**
PO (Extended-Release)
Children 6–16 yr. 1000 mg in children weighing more than 60 kg, 800 mg once daily in children weighing 46–60 kg, 600 mg once daily in children weighing 31–45 kg, 400 mg once daily in children weighing 20–30 kg.
▸ **Analgesia**
PO
Adults, Elderly. 200–400 mg q6–8h as needed. Maximum: 1200 mg/day.

SIDE EFFECTS/ADVERSE REACTIONS
Occasional
Dizziness, headache, abdominal pain or cramps, bloated feeling, diarrhea, nausea, indigestion
Rare
Constipation, rash, pruritus, visual disturbances, tinnitus

PRECAUTIONS AND CONTRAINDICATIONS
Active peptic ulcer disease, chronic inflammation of GI tract, GI bleeding or ulceration, history of hypersensitivity to aspirin or NSAIDs
Caution
Lactation, children, bleeding disorders, GI disorders, cardiac disorders, elderly, renal, hepatic disorders

E

DRUG INTERACTIONS OF CONCERN TO DENTISTRY
• GI ulceration, bleeding: aspirin, alcohol, corticosteroids, biphosphonates
• Decreased action: salicylates
• Nephrotoxicity: acetaminophen (prolonged use)
• Possible risk of decreased renal function: cyclosporine
• First-time users of SSRIs also taking NSAIDs may have a higher risk of GI side effects; until more data are available, it may be advisable to avoid use of NSAIDs in these patients (Br J Clin Pharmacol 55:591–595, 2003)
• When prescribed for dental pain:
  • Risk of increased effects: oral anticoagulants, oral antidiabetics, lithium, methotrexate
  • Decreased effects of diuretics
  • Increased risk of methotrexate toxicity

SERIOUS REACTIONS
! Overdose may result in acute renal failure.
! There is an increased risk of cardiovascular events (including MI and CVA) and serious and potentially life-threatening GI bleeding.
! Rare reactions with long-term use include peptic ulcer disease, GI bleeding, gastritis, severe hepatic reactions (jaundice), nephrotoxicity (hematuria, dysuria, proteinuria), and a severe hypersensitivity reaction (bronchospasm, angioedema).

DENTAL CONSIDERATIONS
General:
• Possible increase in adverse cardiovascular events in patients at risk for thromboembolism.
• Patients on chronic drug therapy may rarely have symptoms of blood dyscrasias, which can include infection, bleeding, and poor healing.
• Assess salivary flow as a factor in caries, periodontal disease, and candidiasis.
• Avoid prescribing for dental use in pregnancy.
• Avoid prescribing aspirin-containing products.
• Consider semisupine chair position for patients with arthritic disease.
Consultations:
• In a patient with symptoms of blood dyscrasias, request a medical consultation for blood studies and postpone dental treatment until normal values are reestablished.
• Medical consultation may be required to assess disease control.
Teach Patient/Family to:
• Avoid mouth rinses with high alcohol content because of drying effects

etoposide, VP-16
eh-toe´-poe-side
(Etopophos, Toposar, VePesid)
Do not confuse VePesid with Pepcid or Versed.

CATEGORY AND SCHEDULE
Pregnancy Risk Category: D

Drug Class: Antineoplastic-miscellaneous; semisynthetic podophyllotoxin

MECHANISM OF ACTION
An epipodophyllotoxin that induces single- and double-stranded breaks in DNA. Cell cycle-dependent and phase-specific; most effective in the S and G2 phases of cell division. *Therapeutic Effect:* Inhibits or alters DNA synthesis.

USES
Leukemias, testicular cancer, lymphomas, small cell carcinoma of the lung

PHARMACOKINETICS
Variably absorbed from the GI tract. Rapidly distributed, low concentrations in CSF. Protein binding: 97%. Metabolized in the liver. Primarily excreted in urine. Not removed by hemodialysis. *Half-life:* 3–12 hr.

INDICATIONS AND DOSAGES
▶ **Refractory Testicular Tumors**
IV
Adults. 50–100 mg/m^2/day on days 1–5, or 100 mg/m^2/day on days 1, 3, and 5 (as combination therapy).
▶ **Acute Myelocytic Leukemia**
IV
Children. 150 mg/m^2/day for 2–3 days and 2–3 cycles.
▶ **Brain Tumor**
IV
Children. 150 mg/m^2/day on days 2 and 3 of treatment course.
▶ **Neuroblastoma**
IV
Children. 100 mg/m^2/day on days 1–5 of treatment course; repeated q4wk.
▶ **Small-Cell Lung Carcinoma**
PO
Adults. Twice the IV dose rounded to nearest 50 mg. Give once a day for doses 400 mg or less, in divided doses for dosages greater than 400 mg.
IV
Adults. 35 mg/m^2/day for 4 consecutive days up to 50 mg/m^2/day for 5 consecutive days (as combination therapy).
Children. 60–150 mg/m^2/day for 2–5 days q3–6wk.

▶ **Dosage in Renal Impairment**
Creatinine clearance 10–50 ml/min. 75% of normal dose.
Creatinine clearance less than 10 ml/min. 50% of normal dose.

SIDE EFFECTS/ADVERSE REACTIONS
Frequent
Mild to moderate nausea and vomiting, alopecia
Occasional
Diarrhea, anorexia, stomatitis
Rare
Hypotension, peripheral neuropathy

PRECAUTIONS AND CONTRAINDICATIONS
Pregnancy

DRUG INTERACTIONS OF CONCERN TO DENTISTRY
None reported

SERIOUS REACTIONS
❗ Myelosuppression may result in hematologic toxicity, manifested as anemia, leukopenia (occurring 7–14 days after drug administration), thrombocytopenia (occurring 9–16 days after administration) and, to a lesser extent, pancytopenia. Bone marrow recovery occurs by day 20.
❗ Hepatotoxicity occurs occasionally.

DENTAL CONSIDERATIONS
General:
• Determine why patient is taking the drug.
• If additional analgesia is required for dental pain, consider alternative analgesics (NSAIDs) in patients taking narcotics for acute or chronic pain.
• Examine for oral manifestation of opportunistic infection.

- Avoid products that affect platelet function, such as aspirin and NSAIDs.
- This drug may be used in the hospital or on an outpatient basis. Confirm the patient's disease and treatment status.
- Chlorhexidine mouth rinse prior to and during chemotherapy may reduce severity of mucositis.
- Patient on chronic drug therapy may rarely present with symptoms of blood dyscrasias, which can include infection, bleeding, and poor healing. If dyscrasia is present, caution patient to prevent oral tissue trauma when using oral hygiene aids.
- Palliative medication may be required for management of oral side effects.
- Short appointments and a stress reduction protocol may be required for anxious patients.
- Consider semisupine chair position for patient comfort if GI side effects occur.
- Patients may be at risk of bleeding; check for oral signs.
- Oral infections should be eliminated and/or treated aggressively.

Consultations:
- Medical consultation should include routine blood counts including platelet counts and bleeding time.
- Consult physician; prophylactic or therapeutic antiinfectives may be indicated if surgery or periodontal treatment is required.
- Medical consultation may be required to assess immunologic status during cancer chemotherapy and determine safety risk, if any, posed by the required dental treatment.

- Medical consultation may be required to assess disease control and patient's ability to tolerate stress.

Teach Patient/Family to:
- Use effective oral hygiene to prevent soft tissue inflammation
- Report oral lesions, soreness, or bleeding to dentist
- Prevent trauma when using oral hygiene aids
- Update health and medication history if physician makes any changes in evaluation or drug regimens; include OTC, herbal, and nonherbal remedies in the update

exemestane
ex-eh-mess´-tane
(Aromasin)

CATEGORY AND SCHEDULE
Pregnancy Risk Category: D

Drug Class: Antineoplastic; aromatase inhibitor

MECHANISM OF ACTION
Inactivates aromatase, the principal enzyme that converts androgens to estrogens in both premenopausal and postmenopausal women, thereby lowering the circulating estrogen level. *Therapeutic Effect:* Inhibits the growth of breast cancers that are stimulated by estrogens.

USES
Treatment of advanced breast carcinoma not responsive to other therapy (postmenopausal)

PHARMACOKINETICS
Rapidly absorbed after PO administration. Protein binding: 90%. Distributed extensively into tissues.

Metabolized in the liver; eliminated in urine and feces. *Half-life:* 24 hr.

INDICATIONS AND DOSAGES
▶ **Breast Cancer**
PO
Adults, Elderly. 25 mg once a day after a meal.

SIDE EFFECTS/ADVERSE REACTIONS
Frequent
Fatigue, nausea, depression, hot flashes, pain, insomnia, anxiety, dyspnea
Occasional
Headache, dizziness, vomiting, peripheral edema, abdominal pain, anorexia, flu-like symptoms, diaphoresis, constipation, hypertension
Rare
Diarrhea

PRECAUTIONS AND CONTRAINDICATIONS
Hypersensitivity to exemestane

DRUG INTERACTIONS OF CONCERN TO DENTISTRY
• Data not available; however, possible reduction in plasma levels by inducers of CYP3A4 isoenzymes
• Ketoconazole had no significant effect

SERIOUS REACTIONS
None known

DENTAL CONSIDERATIONS
General:
• Monitor vital signs at every appointment due to cardiovascular side effects.
• If additional analgesia is required for dental pain, consider alternative analgesics (NSAIDs) in patients taking narcotics for acute or chronic pain.
• DHRDG
• Product may be used in outpatient therapy.
• If used in prostate cancer, consider urinary retention concern and avoid anticholinergic drugs that may aggravate retention.
Consultations:
• Medical consultation may be required to assess disease control and patient's ability to tolerate stress.
Teach Patient/Family to:
• Use effective oral hygiene to prevent soft tissue inflammation
• Prevent trauma when using oral hygiene aids
• Update health and medication history if physician makes any changes in evaluation or drug regimens; include OTC, herbal, and nonherbal remedies in the update

ezetimibe; simvastatin
ez-et´-ih-mib; sim-vah-stay´-tin (Vytorin)

CATEGORY AND SCHEDULE
Pregnancy Risk Category: X

Drug Class: Cholesterol-lowering agent

MECHANISM OF ACTION
Ezetimibe is an antihyperlipidemic that inhibits cholesterol absorption in the small intestine, leading to a decrease in the delivery of intestinal cholesterol to the liver. *Therapeutic Effect:* Reduces total cholesterol and low-density lipoprotein (LDL) cholesterol and triglyceride levels and increases high-density lipoprotein (HDL) cholesterol level.

E

Simvastatin is a 3-hydroxy-3-methylglutaryl coenzyme A (HMG-CoA) reductase inhibitor that interferes with cholesterol biosynthesis by inhibiting the conversion of the enzyme HMG-CoA to mevalonate. *Therapeutic Effect:* Decreases LDL cholesterol, very low density lipoprotein (VLDL) cholesterol, and plasma triglyceride levels; slightly increases HDL concentration.

USES
Adjunctive therapy to diet for reduction of cholesterol in patients with primary hypercholesterolemia

PHARMACOKINETICS
Ezetimibe: Well absorbed following oral administration. Protein binding: greater than 90%. Metabolized in the small intestine and liver. Excreted by the kidneys and bile. *Half-life:* 22 hr. Simvastatin: Well absorbed from the GI tract. Protein binding: 95%. Undergoes extensive first-pass metabolism. Hydrolyzed to active metabolite. Primarily eliminated in feces. Unknown if removed by hemodialysis.

INDICATIONS AND DOSAGES
▶ **Homozygous Familial Hypercholesterolemia**
PO
Adults. 10 mg/40 mg daily or 10 mg/80 mg daily.
▶ **Primary Hypercholesterolemia**
PO
Adults. Initially, 10 mg/20 mg daily. Initiate with a lower dose if the patient requires less aggressive LDL reductions. Initiate with a higher dose if the patient requires larger reduction in LDL.

SIDE EFFECTS/ADVERSE REACTIONS
Occasional
Headache, abdominal pain or cramps, constipation, upper respiratory tract infection, back pain, diarrhea, arthralgia, sinusitis
Rare
Cough, pharyngitis, fatigue, flatulence, asthenia (loss of strength and energy), nausea or vomiting

PRECAUTIONS AND CONTRAINDICATIONS
Active liver disease or unexplained, persistent elevations of liver function test results, age younger than 18 yr, pregnancy
Caution
When used with an HMG-CoA reductase inhibitor must follow all precautions for use (including pregnancy risk, risk of increased serum transaminase or myopathy); pregnancy, lactation, and children younger than 10 yr not established

DRUG INTERACTIONS OF CONCERN TO DENTISTRY
None reported

SERIOUS REACTIONS
! There is a potential for lens opacities.
! Hypersensitivity reaction and hepatitis occur rarely.

DENTAL CONSIDERATIONS
General:
• Consider semisupine chair position for patient comfort if GI, respiratory, or musculoskeletal side effects occur.
• Monitor vital signs at every appointment because of possible cardiovascular disease.
Teach Patient/Family to:
• Update health and drug history if physician makes any changes in evaluation, drug regimens

famciclovir
fam-si´-klo-veer
(Famvir)
Do not confuse Famvir with
Femhrt.

CATEGORY AND SCHEDULE
Pregnancy Risk Category: B

Drug Class: Antiviral

MECHANISM OF ACTION
A synthetic nucleoside that
inhibits viral DNA synthesis.
Therapeutic Effect: Suppresses
replication of herpes simplex virus
and varicella-zoster virus.

USES
Treatment of acute herpes zoster
(shingles) infection; recurrent genital
herpes; recurrent herpes simplex
virus infections in HIV-infected
patients

PHARMACOKINETICS
Rapidly and extensively absorbed
after PO administration. Protein
binding: 20%–25%. Rapidly
metabolized to penciclovir by
enzymes in the GI wall, liver, and
plasma. Eliminated unchanged in
urine. Removed by hemodialysis.
Half-life: 2 hr.

INDICATIONS AND DOSAGES
▸ **Herpes Zoster**
PO
Adults. 500 mg q8h for 7 days.
▸ **Recurrent Genital Herpes**
PO
Adults. 125 mg twice a day for 5 days.
▸ **Suppression of Recurrent Genital
Herpes**
PO
Adults. 250 mg twice a day for
up to 1 yr.

▸ **Recurrent Herpes Simplex**
PO
Adults. 500 mg twice a day for 7
days.
▸ **Dosage in Renal Impairment**
Dosage and frequency are modified
on the basis of creatinine clearance.

Creatinine Clearance	Herpes Zoster	Genital Herpes
40–59 ml/min	500 mg q12h	125 mg q12h
20–39 ml/min	500 mg q24h	125 mg q24h
Less than 20 ml/min	250 mg q24h	125 mg q24h

▸ **Dosage in Hemodialysis Patients**
For adults with herpes zoster, give
250 mg after each dialysis treatment;
for adults with genital herpes, give
125 mg after each dialysis treatment.

SIDE EFFECTS/ADVERSE REACTIONS
Frequent
Headache, nausea
Occasional
Dizziness, somnolence, numbness of
feet, diarrhea, vomiting, constipation,
decreased appetite, fatigue, fever,
pharyngitis, sinusitis, pruritus
Rare
Insomnia, abdominal pain,
dyspepsia, flatulence, back pain,
arthralgia

PRECAUTIONS AND CONTRAINDICATIONS
Hypersensitivity
Caution
Children younger than 18 yr,
lactation, elderly, hepatic and renal
function impairment

DRUG INTERACTIONS OF CONCERN TO DENTISTRY
None reported in otherwise
uncompromised patients

F

SERIOUS REACTIONS
None known

DENTAL CONSIDERATIONS
General:
• Determine why the patient is taking the drug.
• Consider semisupine chair position for patient comfort because of GI effects of drug.
• Be aware of general discomfort associated with shingles; acute symptoms may preclude patient's routine dental visit or mandate short dental appointments.
Consultations:
• Medical consultation may be required to assess disease control and patient's ability to tolerate stress.

---

famotidine
fam-oh´-tah-deen
(Amfamox[AUS], Novo-Famotidine[CAN] Pepcid, Pepcid AC, Pepcidine[AUS], Ulcidine[CAN])

CATEGORY AND SCHEDULE
Pregnancy Risk Category: B
OTC (10 mg tablets)

Drug Class: Histamine H$_2$-receptor antagonist

MECHANISM OF ACTION
An antiulcer agent and gastric acid secretion inhibitor that inhibits histamine action at H$_2$ receptors of parietal cells. ***Therapeutic Effect:*** Inhibits gastric acid secretion when fasting, at night, or when stimulated by food, caffeine, or insulin.

USES
Short-term treatment of active duodenal ulcer, maintenance therapy for duodenal ulcer, Zollinger-Ellison syndrome, multiple endocrine adenomas, benign gastric ulcers, gastroesophageal reflux disease (GERD); OTC: heartburn, acid indigestion

PHARMACOKINETICS

Route	Onset	Peak	Duration
PO	1 hr	1–4 hr	10–12 hr
IV	1 hr	0.5–3 hr	10–12 hr

Rapidly, incompletely absorbed from the GI tract. Protein binding: 15%–20%. Partially metabolized in the liver. Primarily excreted in urine. Not removed by hemodialysis. ***Half-life:*** 2.5–3.5 hr (increased with impaired renal function).

INDICATIONS AND DOSAGES
▸ **Acute Treatment of Duodenal and Gastric Ulcers**
PO
Adults, Elderly, Children 12 yr and older. 40 mg/day at bedtime.
Children 1–11 yr. 0.5 mg/kg/day at bedtime. Maximum: 40 mg/day.
▸ **Duodenal Ulcer Maintenance**
PO
Adults, Elderly. 20 mg/day at bedtime.
▸ **GERD**
PO
Adults, Elderly, Children 12 yr and older. 20 mg twice a day.
Children 1–11 yr. 1 mg/kg/day in 2 divided doses.
Children 3–11 mo. 0.5 mg/kg/dose twice a day.
Children younger than 3 mo. 0.5 mg/kg/dose once a day.
▸ **Esophagitis**
PO
Adults, Elderly, Children 12 yr and older. 2–40 mg twice a day.

▶ **Hypersecretory Conditions**
PO
Adults, Elderly, Children 12 yr and older. Initially, 20 mg q6h. May increase up to 160 mg q6h.
▶ **Acid Indigestion, Heartburn (OTC)**
PO
Adults, Elderly, Children 12 yr and older. 10–20 mg 15–60 min before eating. Maximum: 2 doses per day.
▶ **Usual Parenteral Dosage**
IV
Adults, Elderly, Children 12 yr and older. 20 mg q12h.
▶ **Dosage in Renal Impairment**
Dosing frequency is modified on the basis of creatinine clearance.

Creatinine Clearance	Dosage Interval
10–50 ml/min	q24h
Less than 10 ml/min	q36–48h

SIDE EFFECTS/ADVERSE REACTIONS
Occasional
Headache
Rare
Constipation, diarrhea, dizziness

PRECAUTIONS AND CONTRAINDICATIONS
Hypersensitivity
Caution
Lactation, children, severe renal disease, severe hepatic function, elderly, RPD tablets contain aspartame (caution: phenylketonuria)

DRUG INTERACTIONS OF CONCERN TO DENTISTRY
• Decreased absorption of ketoconazole or itraconazole (take doses 2 hr apart)

SERIOUS REACTIONS
None known

DENTAL CONSIDERATIONS
General:
• Avoid prescribing aspirin-containing products in patients with active GI disease.
• Consider semisupine chair position for patient comfort because of GI effects of disease.
• Assess salivary flow as a factor in caries, periodontal disease, and candidiasis.
Teach Patient/Family to:
• Use effective oral hygiene to prevent gingival inflammation
• When chronic dry mouth occurs, advise patient to:
   • Avoid mouth rinses with high alcohol content because of drying effects
   • Use daily home fluoride products for anticaries effect
   • Use sugarless gum, frequent sips of water, or saliva substitutes

felbamate
fel´-ba-mate
(Felbatol)

CATEGORY AND SCHEDULE
Pregnancy Risk Category: C

Drug Class: Anticonvulsant (carbamate derivative)

MECHANISM OF ACTION
An anticonvulsant, structurally similar to meprobamate, that weakly blocks repetitive, sustained firing of neurons by enhancing the ability of g-aminobutyric acid (GABA), and antagonizes the strychnine-insensitive glycine recognition site of the N-methyl-D-aspartate receptor-ionophore complex.
Therapeutic Effect: Decreases seizure activity.

USES
Used alone or as adjunct therapy in partial seizures; also for partial seizures associated with Lennox-Gastaut syndrome in children; because of severe side effects use only for severe seizures when other therapy is inadequate

PHARMACOKINETICS
Rapidly and almost completely absorbed after PO administration. Protein binding: 22%–25%, primarily to albumin. Partially excreted unchanged in the urine. *Half-life:* 20–23 hr.

INDICATIONS AND DOSAGES
▸ **Monotherapy or Adjunctive Therapy in the Treatment of Partial Seizures, with and without Generalization**
PO
Adults, Children older than 14 yr.
Initially, 1200 mg/day in divided doses 3–4 times a day. At wk 2, increase the felbamate dosage to 2400 mg/day while reducing the dosage of other antiepileptic drugs (AEDs) up to an additional one-third of their original dosage. At wk 3, increase the felbamate dosage up to 3600 mg/day and continue to reduce the dosage of other AEDs as clinically indicated.
▸ **Adjunctive Therapy in the Treatment of Partial Seizures, with and without Generalization**
PO
Adults, Children older than 14 yr.
Add 1200 mg/day in divided doses 3–4 times a day while reducing present AEDs by 20% in order-control plasma concentrations of concurrent phenytoin, valproic acid, and carbamazepine and its metabolites. Increase dosage by 1200 mg/day increments at weekly intervals to 3600 mg/day.

SIDE EFFECTS/ADVERSE REACTIONS
Frequent
Somnolence, dizziness, headache, fatigue, nausea, anorexia, vomiting, constipation
Occasional
Chest pain, palpitations, tachycardia, depression and behavioral changes, anxiety, nervousness, ataxia, malaise, agitation, rash, acne, pruritus, diarrhea, weight gain, tremors, abnormal vision, diplopia, sinusitis, difficulty with coordination, taste perversion
Rare
Delusion, bradycardia, hallucinations, urinary retention, acute renal failure

PRECAUTIONS AND CONTRAINDICATIONS
History of any blood dyscrasia or hepatic dysfunction, hypersensitivity to felbamate, its ingredients, or known sensitivity to other carbamates
Caution
Lactation, warning of increased risk of aplastic anemia, hepatic failure; safety and efficacy in children with other types of seizures has not been established

DRUG INTERACTIONS OF CONCERN TO DENTISTRY
● Decreased effects of carbamazepine
● Increased photosensitization: drugs causing photosensitivity (e.g., tetracyclines)

SERIOUS REACTIONS
ALERT
! Aplastic anemia has been reported during felbamate therapy.
! Hepatic failure resulting in death has been reported.

DENTAL CONSIDERATIONS

General:
• Examine for evidence of oral manifestations of blood dyscrasia (infection, bleeding, poor healing).
• Short appointments and a stress reduction protocol may be required for anxious patients.
• Determine type of epilepsy, seizure frequency, and quality of seizure control. A stress reduction protocol may be required.
• Assess salivary flow as a factor in caries, periodontal disease, and candidiasis.
• Monitor vital signs at every appointment because of cardiovascular side effects.
• Advise patient if dental drugs prescribed have a potential for photosensitivity.

Consultations:
• Medical consultation may be required to assess disease control and patient's ability to tolerate stress.

Teach Patient/Family to:
• Use effective oral hygiene to prevent soft tissue inflammation
• Use caution to prevent injury when using oral hygiene aids
• Use electric tooth brush if patient has difficulty holding conventional devices
• When chronic dry mouth occurs, advise patient to:
  • Avoid mouth rinses with high alcohol content because of drying effects
  • Use daily home fluoride products for anticaries effect
  • Use sugarless gum, frequent sips of water, or saliva substitutes

felodipine
fell-oh´-da-peen
(AGON SR[AUS], Felodur ER[AUS], Plendil, Plendil ER[AUS], Renedil[CAN])
Do not confuse Plendil with Pletal, or Renedil with Prinivil.

CATEGORY AND SCHEDULE
Pregnancy Risk Category: C

Drug Class: Calcium channel blocker

MECHANISM OF ACTION
An antihypertensive and antianginal agent that inhibits calcium movement across cardiac and vascular smooth-muscle cell membranes. Potent peripheral vasodilator (does not depress SA or AV nodes). ***Therapeutic Effect:*** Increases myocardial contractility, heart rate, and cardiac output; decreases peripheral vascular resistance and B/P.

USES
Essential hypertension, alone or with other antihypertensives, chronic angina pectoris

PHARMACOKINETICS

Route	Onset	Peak	Duration
PO	2–5 hr	N/A	N/A

Rapidly, completely absorbed from the GI tract. Protein binding: greater than 99%. Undergoes first-pass metabolism in the liver. Primarily excreted in urine. Not removed by hemodialysis.
Half-life: 11–16 hr.

INDICATIONS AND DOSAGES
▶ **Hypertension**
PO
Adults. Initially, 5 mg/day as single dose.
Elderly, Patients with impaired hepatic function. Initially, 2.5 mg/day. Adjust dosage at no less than 2-wk intervals. Maintenance: 2.5–10 mg/day.

SIDE EFFECTS/ADVERSE REACTIONS
Frequent
Headache, peripheral edema
Occasional
Flushing, respiratory infection, dizziness, light-headedness, asthenia (loss of strength, weakness)
Rare
Paresthesia, abdominal discomfort, nervousness, muscle cramping, cough, diarrhea, constipation

PRECAUTIONS AND CONTRAINDICATIONS
Hypersensitivity, sick sinus syndrome, second- or third-degree heart block
Caution
CHF, hypotension less than 90 mm Hg systolic, hepatic injury, lactation, children, renal disease, elderly

DRUG INTERACTIONS OF CONCERN TO DENTISTRY
• Decreased effect: NSAIDs, phenobarbital, carbamazepine
• Increased effect: parenteral and inhalational general anesthetics, other drugs with hypotensive actions
• Increased effects of nondepolarizing muscle relaxants, diazepam, midazolam
• Increased plasma levels: itraconazole, erythromycin, carbamazepine

SERIOUS REACTIONS
! Overdose produces nausea, somnolence, confusion, slurred speech, hypotension, and bradycardia.

DENTAL CONSIDERATIONS
General:
• Monitor cardiac status; take vital signs at each appointment because of cardiovascular side effects. Consider a stress reduction protocol to prevent stress-induced angina during the dental appointment.
• After supine positioning, have patient sit upright for at least 2 min before standing to avoid orthostatic hypotension at dismissal.
• Place on frequent recall to monitor gingival condition.
• Limit use of sodium-containing products, such as saline IV fluids, for patients with a dietary salt restriction.
• Assess salivary flow as a factor in caries, periodontal disease, and candidiasis.
• Use vasoconstrictors with caution, in low doses, and with careful aspiration. Avoid use of gingival retraction cord with epinephrine.
• Use precaution if sedation or general anesthesia is required; risk of hypotensive episode.
Consultations:
• Medical consultation may be required to assess disease control.
• Consultation with physician may be necessary if sedation or general anesthesia is required.
Teach Patient/Family to:
• Use effective oral hygiene to prevent gingival inflammation and minimize enlargement

- Schedule frequent oral prophylaxis if enlargement occurs
- When chronic dry mouth occurs, advise patient to:
  - Avoid mouth rinses with high alcohol content because of drying effects
  - Use daily home fluoride products for anticaries effect
  - Use sugarless gum, frequent sips of water, or saliva substitutes

fenofibrate
fee-no-fye´-brate
(Apo-Fenofibrate[CAN], Lafibra, Tricor)
Do not confuse Tricor with Tracleer.

CATEGORY AND SCHEDULE
Pregnancy Risk Category: C

Drug Class: Antihyperlipidemic

MECHANISM OF ACTION
An antihyperlipidemic that enhances synthesis of lipoprotein lipase and reduces triglyceride-rich lipoproteins and VLDLs. *Therapeutic Effect:* Increases VLDL catabolism and reduces total plasma triglyceride levels.

USES
Treatment of hyperlipidemia, types IV and V, as an adjunct to diet therapy

PHARMACOKINETICS
Well absorbed from the GI tract. Absorption increased when given with food. Protein binding: 99%. Rapidly metabolized in the liver to active metabolite. Excreted primarily in urine; lesser amount in feces. Not removed by hemodialysis.
Half-life: 20 hr.

INDICATIONS AND DOSAGES
▶ **Reduction of Very High Serum Triglyceride Levels in Patients at Risk for Pancreatitis**
PO
Adults, Elderly. Initially, 67 mg/day (capsule); may increase to 200 mg/day. Or initially, 48 mg/day (tablet); may increase to 145 mg/day.
▶ **Hypercholesterolemia**
PO
Adults, Elderly. 200 mg/day (capsule) with meals. Or 145 mg/day (tablet) with meals.

SIDE EFFECTS/ADVERSE REACTIONS
Frequent
Pain, rash, headache, asthenia or fatigue, flu symptoms, dyspepsia, nausea or vomiting, rhinitis
Occasional
Diarrhea, abdominal pain, constipation, flatulence, arthralgia, decreased libido, dizziness, pruritus
Rare
Increased appetite, insomnia, polyuria, cough, blurred vision, eye floaters, earache

PRECAUTIONS AND CONTRAINDICATIONS
Gallbladder disease, hypersensitivity to fenofibrate, severe renal or hepatic dysfunction (including primary biliary cirrhosis, unexplained persistent liver function abnormality)
Caution
Monitor liver function; may lead to cholelithiasis; can be associated with myositis, myopathy, or rhabdomyolysis; avoid if lactating; safe use in children unknown; discontinue use if no response in 2 mo; increased

anticoagulant effect with oral
anticoagulants

DRUG INTERACTIONS OF CONCERN TO DENTISTRY
None reported

SERIOUS REACTIONS
! Fenofibrate may increase excretion
of cholesterol into bile, leading to
cholelithiasis.
! Pancreatitis, hepatitis,
thrombocytopenia, and
agranulocytosis occur rarely.

DENTAL CONSIDERATIONS
General:
• Monitor vital signs at every
appointment because of
cardiovascular and respiratory side
effects.
• Consider semisupine chair
position for patient comfort
because of GI side effects
of drug.
• Patients on chronic drug
therapy may rarely have
symptoms of blood dyscrasias,
which can include infection,
bleeding, and poor healing.
• Avoid dental light in patient's
eyes; offer dark glasses for patient
comfort.
Consultations:
• In a patient with symptoms
of blood dyscrasias, request a
medical consultation for
blood studies and postpone
treatment until normal values
are reestablished.
Teach Patient/Family to:
• Use electric tooth
brush if patient has difficulty
holding conventional
devices
• Prevent trauma when
using oral hygiene aids

fenoprofen calcium
fen-oh-proe´-fen
(Nalfon)
Do not confuse Nalfon with
Naldecon.

CATEGORY AND SCHEDULE
Pregnancy Risk Category: B
(D if used in third trimester or near
delivery)

Drug Class: Nonsteroidal
antiinflammatory, propionic acid
derivative

MECHANISM OF ACTION
An NSAID that produces analgesic
and antiinflammatory effects by
inhibiting prostaglandin synthesis.
Therapeutic Effect: Reduces the
inflammatory response and intensity
of pain.

USES
Treatment of mild-to-moderate pain,
osteoarthritis, rheumatoid arthritis,
acute gout, arthritis, ankylosing
spondylitis, nonrheumatic
inflammation, dysmenorrhea

PHARMACOKINETICS
PO: Peak 2 hr. *Half-life:* 3–3.5 hr;
99% plasma protein binding;
metabolized in liver; excreted in
urine (metabolites), breast milk.

INDICATIONS AND DOSAGES
▸ **Mild-to-Moderate Pain**
PO
Adults, Elderly. 200 mg q4–6h as
needed.
▸ **Rheumatoid Arthritis, Osteoarthritis**
PO
Adults, Elderly. 300–600 mg
3–4 times a day.

SIDE EFFECTS/ADVERSE REACTIONS

Frequent
Headache, somnolence, dyspepsia, nausea, vomiting, constipation

Occasional
Dizziness, pruritus, nervousness, asthenia, diarrhea, abdominal cramps, flatulence, tinnitus, blurred vision, peripheral edema and fluid retention

PRECAUTIONS AND CONTRAINDICATIONS

Active peptic ulcer disease, chronic inflammation of GI tract, GI bleeding or ulceration, history of hypersensitivity to aspirin or NSAIDs, significant renal impairment

Caution
Lactation, children, bleeding disorders, GI disorders, cardiac disorders, hypersensitivity to other antiinflammatory agents

DRUG INTERACTIONS OF CONCERN TO DENTISTRY

• GI bleeding, ulceration: salicylates, alcohol, corticosteroids, other NSAIDs, bisphosphonates
• May decrease effects of fenoprofen: phenobarbital
• Nephrotoxicity: acetaminophen (prolonged use)
• Possible risk of decreased renal function: cyclosporine
• Probable increased bleeding risk: warfarin
• Suspected increased risk for methotrexate toxicity
• First-time users of SSRIs also taking NSAIDs may have a higher risk of GI side effects; until more data are

available, it may be advisable to avoid use of NSAIDs in these patients (Br J Clin Pharmacol 55:591–595, 2003)

SERIOUS REACTIONS

! Overdose may result in acute hypotension and tachycardia.
! Rare reactions with long-term use include peptic ulcer disease, GI bleeding, gastritis, severe hepatic reaction (jaundice), nephrotoxicity (hematuria, dysuria, proteinuria), and a severe hypersensitivity reaction (bronchospasm, angioedema).

DENTAL CONSIDERATIONS

General:
• Assess salivary flow as a factor in caries, periodontal disease, and candidiasis.
• Avoid prescribing for dental use in pregnancy.
• Possibility of cross-allergenicity when patient is allergic to aspirin.

Consultations:
• Medical consultation may be required to assess disease control.

Teach Patient/Family to:
• Use effective oral hygiene to prevent gingival inflammation
• Use caution to prevent injury when using oral hygiene aids
• When chronic dry mouth occurs, advise patient to:
  • Avoid mouth rinses with high alcohol content because of drying effects
  • Use daily home fluoride products for anticaries effect
  • Use sugarless gum, frequent sips of water, or saliva substitutes

fentanyl transdermal system

fen'-ta-nil trans-derr'-mal sis'-tem
(Dur.agesic 25, 50, 75, 100
Transdermal Patches, Fentanyl
oralet oral: transmucosal fentanyl
citrate: Actiq [lozenges])

CATEGORY AND SCHEDULE

Pregnancy Risk Category: C
Controlled Substance Schedule II

Drug Class: Narcotic analgesics

MECHANISM OF ACTION

Interacts with opioid receptors in the
CNS to alter pain perception.

USES

Management of chronic pain when
opioids are necessary; transmucosal
form: only for management of
breakthrough cancer pain in patients
with malignancies who are using or
tolerant to opioids; not appropriate
for acute postoperative pain

PHARMACOKINETICS

Transdermal: Dosage adjusted
according to opioid tolerance if patient
has been taking opioids (2.5 mg of
transdermal fentanyl is equivalent to
approximately 90 mg of oral morphine
in 24 hr); peak serum levels take up to
24 hr after applied; liver metabolism;
renal excretion of metabolites.

INDICATIONS AND DOSAGES
▶ **Chronic Pain**

Topical
Adult only. One patch every 72 hr;
dose depends on need for pain
control; titrate as required.
Transmucosal form
*Adult only (patch and lozenge on a
stick only [Actiq]).* Dose must be
titrated starting with lowest dose size
(must be kept secure from children).

▶ **Conscious Sedation or Anesthesia
(oralet only) in Hospital Setting:**
Adult. Doses must match patient,
usually no more than 5 μg/kg
(400 μg); doses for children must be
adjusted for weight; see package
insert directions for use.

SIDE EFFECTS/ADVERSE REACTIONS

ORAL: Dry mouth
CNS: Dizziness, delirium, euphoria
CV: Bradycardia, arrest, hypotension,
or hypertension
GI: Nausea, vomiting
RESP: Respiratory depression,
arrest, laryngospasm
EENT: Blurred vision, miosis
MS: Muscle rigidity

PRECAUTIONS AND CONTRAINDICATIONS

Hypersensitivity to opiates,
myasthenia gravis
Caution
Elderly, respiratory depression,
increased intracranial pressure,
seizure disorders, severe respiratory
disorders, cardiac dysrhythmias

DRUG INTERACTIONS OF CONCERN TO DENTISTRY

• Effects may be increased with
other CNS depressants: alcohol,
narcotics, sedative/hypnotics, skeletal
muscle relaxants, chlorpromazine
• Additive hypotension: nitrous oxide,
benzodiazepines, phenothiazines
• Increased anticholinergic effect:
anticholinergics
• Contraindication: MAOIs

SERIOUS REACTIONS

Life-threatening respiratory depression,
cardiorespiratory arrest, generalized
CNS depression, coma, death

DENTAL CONSIDERATIONS

General:
• Monitor vital signs at every
appointment because of

cardiovascular and respiratory side effects.
• After supine positioning, have patient sit upright for at least 2 min before standing to avoid orthostatic hypotension.
• Assess salivary flow as a factor in caries, periodontal disease, and candidiasis.
• Psychologic and physical dependence may occur with chronic administration.
• Determine why the patient is taking the drug.
• Consider alternative drugs to opioids and NSAIDs for management of dental pain.
Consultations:
• Medical consultation may be required to assess disease control.
Teach Patient/Family to:
• Use effective oral hygiene to prevent gingival inflammation
• Avoid mouth rinses with high alcohol content because of drying effects

ferrous fumarate/ ferrous gluconate/ ferrous sulfate

fer´-us fume´-ah-rate/fer´-us glue´-kuh-nate/fer´-us sul´-fate
ferrous fumarate
(Feostat, Femiron, Ferro-Sequels, Nephro-Fer, Palafer[CAN])
ferrous gluconate
(Apo-Ferrous Gluconate[CAN], Fergon)
ferrous sulfate
(Apo-Ferrous Sulfate[CAN], Fer-In-Sol, Fer-Iron, Ferro-Gradumet[AUS], Slow-Fe)

CATEGORY AND SCHEDULE
Pregnancy Risk Category: A
OTC

Drug Class: Hematinic, iron preparation

MECHANISM OF ACTION
An enzymatic mineral that is an essential component in the formation of Hgb, myoglobin, and enzymes. Promotes effective erythropoiesis and transport and utilization of oxygen (O_2). ***Therapeutic Effect:*** Prevents iron deficiency.

USES
Treatment of iron deficiency anemia, prophylaxis for iron deficiency in pregnancy

PHARMACOKINETICS
Absorbed in the duodenum and upper jejunum. Ten percent absorbed in patients with normal iron stores; increased to 20%–30% in those with inadequate iron stores. Primarily bound to serum transferrin. Excreted in urine, sweat, and sloughing of intestinal mucosa and by menses. ***Half-life:*** 6 hr.

INDICATIONS AND DOSAGES
▸ **Iron Deficiency Anemia**
Dosage is expressed in terms of milligrams of elemental iron, degree of anemia, patient weight, and presence of any bleeding. Expect to use periodic hematologic determinations as guide to therapy.
PO (ferrous fumarate)
Adults, Elderly. 60–100 mg twice a day.
Children. 3–6 mg/kg/day in 2–3 divided doses.
PO (ferrous gluconate)
Adults, Elderly. 60 mg 2–4 times a day.
Children. 3–6 mg/kg/day in 2–3 divided doses.
PO (ferrous sulfate)
Adults, Elderly. 325 mg 2–4 times a day.
Children. 3–6 mg/kg/day in 2–3 divided doses.

▶ **Prevention of Iron Deficiency**
PO (ferrous fumarate)
Adults, Elderly. 60–100 mg/day.
Children. 1–2 mg/kg/day.
PO (ferrous gluconate)
Adults, Elderly. 60 mg/day.
Children. 1–2 mg/kg/day.
PO (ferrous sulfate)
Adults, Elderly. 325 mg/day.
Children. 1–2 mg/kg/day.

SIDE EFFECTS/ADVERSE REACTIONS
Occasional
Mild, transient nausea
Rare
Heartburn, anorexia, constipation, diarrhea

PRECAUTIONS AND CONTRAINDICATIONS
Hemochromatosis, hemosiderosis, hemolytic anemias, peptic ulcer disease, regional enteritis, ulcerative colitis
Caution
Long-term anemia

DRUG INTERACTIONS OF CONCERN TO DENTISTRY
• Decreased absorption of tetracycline, zinc, ciprofloxacin

SERIOUS REACTIONS
! Large doses may aggravate existing GI tract disease, such as peptic ulcer disease, regional enteritis, and ulcerative colitis.
! Severe iron poisoning occurs most often in children and is manifested as vomiting, severe abdominal pain, diarrhea, and dehydration, followed by hyperventilation, pallor or cyanosis, and cardiovascular collapse.

DENTAL CONSIDERATIONS
Teach Patient/Family to:
• Avoid frequent use if patient is using hydrogen peroxide as a dentifrice to remove extrinsic stain

so that peroxide-related soft tissue injury does not occur
• That liquid iron preparation taken through straw followed by rinsing mouth can reduce staining

fexofenadine hydrochloride
fex-oh-fen´-eh-deen
hi-droh-klor´-ide
(Allegra, Telfast[AUS])

CATEGORY AND SCHEDULE
Pregnancy Risk Category: C

Drug Class: Antihistamine, nonsedating

MECHANISM OF ACTION
A piperidine that competes with histamine for H1-receptor sites on effector cells. *Therapeutic Effect:* Relieves allergic rhinitis symptoms.

USES
Treatment of seasonal allergic rhinitis, chronic idiopathic urticaria

PHARMACOKINETICS
Rapidly absorbed after PO administration. Protein binding: 60%–70%. Does not cross the blood-brain barrier. Minimally metabolized. Eliminated in feces and urine. Not removed by hemodialysis. *Half-life:* 14.4 hr (increased in renal impairment).

INDICATIONS AND DOSAGES
▶ **Allergic Rhinitis, Urticaria**
PO
Adults, Elderly, Children 12 yr and older. 60 mg twice a day or 180 mg once a day.
Children 6–11 yr. 30 mg twice a day.
▶ **Dosage in Renal Impairment**
Adults, Elderly, and Children 12 yr and older. Dosage is reduced to 60 mg once a day.

Children 6–11 yr. Dosage is reduced to 30 mg once a day.

SIDE EFFECTS/ADVERSE REACTIONS
Rare
Somnolence, headache, fatigue, nausea, vomiting, abdominal distress, dysmenorrhea

PRECAUTIONS AND CONTRAINDICATIONS
Hypersensitivity; troglitazone
Caution
Reduce dose in elderly, renally impaired, lactation, children younger than 12 yr

DRUG INTERACTIONS OF CONCERN TO DENTISTRY
• Elevated plasma levels with erythromycin, ketoconazole
• Decreased absorption: grapefruit juice
• Suspected decreased antihistaminic effects: rifampin

SERIOUS REACTIONS
None known

DENTAL CONSIDERATIONS
General:
• Consider semisupine chair position for patient comfort because of GI effects of drug.

filgrastim
fill-grass´-tim
(Neupogen)
Do not confuse Neupogen with Epogen or Nutramigen.

CATEGORY AND SCHEDULE
Pregnancy Risk Category: C

Drug Class: Biologic modifier; granulocyte colony-stimulating factor

MECHANISM OF ACTION
A biologic modifier that stimulates production, maturation, and activation of neutrophils to increase their migration and cytotoxicity. ***Therapeutic Effect:*** Decreases incidence of infection.

USES
Help the bone marrow to make new white blood cells

PHARMACOKINETICS
Readily absorbed after subcutaneous administration. Not removed by hemodialysis. ***Half-life:*** 3.5 hr.

INDICATIONS AND DOSAGES
▸ **Myelosuppression**
IV or Subcutaneous Infusion, Subcutaneous Injection
Adults, Elderly. Initially, 5 mcg/kg/day. May increase by 5 mcg/kg for each chemotherapy cycle on the basis of duration or severity of absolute neutrophil count nadir.
▸ **Bone Marrow Transplant**
IV or Subcutaneous Infusion
Adults, Elderly. 5–10 mcg/kg/day. Adjust dosage daily during period of neutrophil recovery on the basis of neutrophil response.
▸ **Mobilization Progenitor Cells**
IV or Subcutaneous Infusion
Adults. 10 mcg/kg/day beginning at least 4 days before first leukapheresis and continuing until last leukapheresis.
▸ **Chronic Neutropenia, Congenital Neutropenia**
Subcutaneous
Adults, Children. 6 mcg/kg/dose twice a day.
▸ **Idiopathic or Cyclic Neutropenia**
Subcutaneous
Adults, Children. 5 mcg/kg/dose once a day.

SIDE EFFECTS/ADVERSE REACTIONS

Frequent

Nausea or vomiting, mild to severe bone pain that occurs more frequently with high-dose IV form and less frequently with low-dose subcutaneous form; alopecia, diarrhea, fever, fatigue

Occasional

Anorexia, dyspnea, headache, cough, rash

Rare

Psoriasis, hematuria or proteinuria, osteoporosis

PRECAUTIONS AND CONTRAINDICATIONS

Hypersensitivity to *Escherichia coli*–derived proteins, 24 hr before or after cytotoxic chemotherapy, concurrent use of other drugs that may result in lowered platelet count

DRUG INTERACTIONS OF CONCERN TO DENTISTRY

• Dental drug interactions have not been studied

SERIOUS REACTIONS

! Long-term administration occasionally produces chronic neutropenia and splenomegaly.

! Thrombocytopenia, MI, and arrhythmias occur rarely.

! Adult respiratory distress syndrome may occur in patients with sepsis.

DENTAL CONSIDERATIONS

General:

• Determine why patient is taking the drug.

• Examine for oral manifestation of opportunistic infection.

• Monitor vital signs at every appointment due to cardiovascular side effects.

• Patient may need assistance in getting into and out of dental chair. Adjust chair position for patient comfort.

• Patients are at risk for infection.

• Oral infections should be eliminated and/or treated aggressively.

• Patients may have been treated with radiation and/or chemotherapy; confirm medical and drug history.

Consultations:

• Medical consultation may be required to assess disease control and patient's ability to tolerate stress.

• In a patient with symptoms of blood dyscrasias, request a medical consultation for blood studies and postpone treatment until normal values are reestablished.

• Medical consultation should include routine blood counts including platelet counts and bleeding time.

Teach Patient/Family to:

• Use effective oral hygiene to prevent soft tissue inflammation

• Prevent trauma when using oral hygiene aids

• Update health and medication history if physician makes any changes in evaluation or drug regimens; include OTC, herbal, and nonherbal remedies in the update

finasteride

feen-as´-ter-ide
(Propecia, Proscar)
Do not confuse Proscar with
Posicor, ProSom, Prozac, or
Psorcon.

CATEGORY AND SCHEDULE

Pregnancy Risk Category: X

Drug Class: Synthetic steroid

MECHANISM OF ACTION

An androgen hormone inhibitor that
inhibits 5-alpha reductase, an
intracellular enzyme that converts
testosterone into dihydrotestosterone
(DHT) in the prostate gland,
resulting in a decreased serum DHT
level. *Therapeutic Effect:* Reduces
size of the prostate gland.

USES

Proscar: Treatment of symptomatic
benign prostatic hyperplasia (BPH),
reduce risk for acute urinary
retention and surgery
Propecia: Treatment of male pattern
baldness (androgenic alopecia) in
men 18–41 yr

PHARMACOKINETICS

Route	Onset	Peak	Duration
PO	24 hr	1–2 days	5–7 days

Rapidly absorbed from the GI tract.
Protein binding: 90%. Widely
distributed. Metabolized in the liver.
Half-life: 6–8 hr. Onset of clinical
effect: 3–6 mo of continued therapy.

INDICATIONS AND DOSAGES
▸ BPH
PO
Adults, Elderly. 5 mg once a day
(for a minimum of 6 mo).

▸ Hair Loss
PO
Adults. 1 mg/day.

SIDE EFFECTS/ADVERSE REACTIONS
Rare
Gynecomastia, sexual
dysfunction (impotence,
decreased libido, decreased volume
of ejaculate)

PRECAUTIONS AND CONTRAINDICATIONS

Exposure to the patient's
semen or handling of finasteride
tablets by those who are or
may be pregnant
Caution
Lactation, lower PSA levels
do not suggest absence of
prostate cancer; women should
avoid drug or semen contact,
hepatic impairment

DRUG INTERACTIONS OF CONCERN TO DENTISTRY

• Opioids and anticholinergic
drugs may enhance urinary
retention; use alternative
analgesics (NSAIDs)

SERIOUS REACTIONS

None known

DENTAL CONSIDERATIONS

Consultations:
• Determine why patient is
taking the drug (for prostatic
hyperplasia or male pattern
baldness).
• Medical consultation
may be required to assess
disease control.

flavocoxid
flay-vox´-ah-sid
(Limbrel)

CATEGORY AND SCHEDULE
Pregnancy Risk Category:
Not classified.

Drug Class: Oral nutritional
supplement

MECHANISM OF ACTION
An oral nutritional supplement that
inhibits prostaglandin synthesis and
arachidonic acid metabolism, reducing
the production of leukotrienes. Also
acts through an antioxidant
mechanism. ***Therapeutic Effect:***
Produces antiinflammatory and
analgesic effects and increases
mobility.

USES
Dietary management of osteoarthritis

PHARMACOKINETICS
Undergoes hydrolysis at the gut
mucosal border. Food decreases
absorption. Little hepatic
metabolism.

INDICATIONS AND DOSAGES
▸ **Osteoarthritis**
PO
Adults 18 yr and older, Elderly. One
250-mg capsule q12h.

SIDE EFFECTS/ADVERSE
REACTIONS
Rare
Increase in varicose veins, psoriasis,
mild hypertension

PRECAUTIONS AND
CONTRAINDICATIONS
History of peptic ulcer

DRUG INTERACTIONS OF
CONCERN TO DENTISTRY
None reported

SERIOUS REACTIONS
! GI bleeding, perforation,
and ulceration occur rarely
in patients currently or
previously treated with
NSAIDs or COX-2 inhibitors.

DENTAL CONSIDERATIONS
General:
• Determine why patient is taking
the drug.
• Patient may need assistance in
getting into and out of dental chair.
Adjust chair position for patient
comfort.
• Patients presenting with a
history of osteoarthritis will be
taking other agents; confirm
medical and drug/herbal and
nonherbal history.
Consultations:
• Medical consultation may be
required to assess disease
control and patient's ability to
tolerate stress
Teach Patient/Family to:
• Use electric tooth brush if patient
has difficulty holding conventional
devices
• Use effective oral
hygiene to prevent soft tissue
inflammation
• Prevent trauma when using oral
hygiene aids
• Update health and
medication history if
physician makes any changes
in evaluation or drug regimens;
include OTC, herbal, and
nonherbal remedies in the
update

flavoxate
fla-vox´-ate
(Urispas)
Do not confuse Urispas with
Urised.

CATEGORY AND SCHEDULE
Pregnancy Risk Category: B

Drug Class: Antispasmodic

MECHANISM OF ACTION
An anticholinergic that relaxes
detrusor and other smooth
muscle by cholinergic
blockade, counteracting
muscle spasm in the urinary tract.
Therapeutic Effect: Produces
anticholinergic, local anesthetic, and
analgesic effects, relieving urinary
symptoms.

USES
Relief of nocturia, incontinence,
suprapubic pain, dysuria, frequency
associated with urologic conditions
(symptomatic only)

PHARMACOKINETICS
Excreted in urine.

INDICATIONS AND DOSAGES
▶ **To Relieve Symptoms of Cystitis,
Prostatitis, Urethritis,
Urethrocystitis, or Urethrotrigonitis**
PO
Adults, Elderly, Adolescents.
100–200 mg 3–4 times a day.

SIDE EFFECTS/ADVERSE REACTIONS
Frequent
Somnolence, dry mouth
and throat
Occasional
Constipation, difficult urination,
blurred vision, dizziness, headache,
increased light sensitivity,
nausea, vomiting, abdominal
pain
Rare
Confusion (primarily in
elderly), hypersensitivity,
increased intraocular pressure,
leukopenia

PRECAUTIONS AND CONTRAINDICATIONS
Duodenal or pyloric obstruction,
GI hemorrhage or obstruction,
ileus, lower urinary tract
obstruction
Caution
Lactation, suspected glaucoma,
children younger than 12 yr

DRUG INTERACTIONS OF CONCERN TO DENTISTRY
• Increased anticholinergic effect:
anticholinergic drugs
• Drug may cause drowsiness
or blurred vision: advise
patients when other CNS depressants
are used

SERIOUS REACTIONS
! Overdose may produce
anticholinergic effects, including
unsteadiness, severe dizziness,
somnolence, fever, facial flushing,
dyspnea, nervousness, and
irritability.

DENTAL CONSIDERATIONS
General:
• Assess salivary flow as a factor in
caries, periodontal disease, and
candidiasis.
Teach Patient/Family to:
• Use effective oral hygiene to
prevent gingival inflammation
• Avoid mouth rinses with high
alcohol content because of drying
effects

flecainide
fle´-kah-nide
(Flecatab[AUS], Tambocor)

CATEGORY AND SCHEDULE
Pregnancy Risk Category: C

Drug Class: Antidysrhythmic
(Class IC)

MECHANISM OF ACTION
An antiarrhythmic that slows atrial,
AV, His-Purkinje, and intraventricular
conduction. Decreases excitability,
conduction velocity, and
automaticity. ***Therapeutic Effect:***
Controls atrial, supraventricular, and
ventricular arrhythmias.

USES
Prevention of life-threatening
ventricular dysrhythmias, sustained
supraventricular tachycardia;
prevention of paroxysmal atrial
flutter (PAF), fibrillation, or
paroxysmal atrial tachycardia

PHARMACOKINETICS
PO: Peak 3 hr. ***Half-life:*** 12–27 hr;
metabolized by liver; excreted
unchanged by kidneys (10%);
excreted in breast milk.

INDICATIONS AND DOSAGES
▸ **Life-Threatening Ventricular
Arrhythmias, Sustained Ventricular
Tachycardia**
PO
Adults, Elderly. Initially, 100 mg q12h,
increased by 100 mg (50 mg twice a
day) every 4 days until effective dose or
maximum of 400 mg/day is attained.
▸ **Paroxysmal Supraventricular
Tachycardias (PSVT), PAF**
PO
Adults, Elderly. Initially, 50 mg q12h,
increased by 100 mg (50 mg twice a day)

every 4 days until effective dose or
maximum of 300 mg/day is attained.

SIDE EFFECTS/ADVERSE REACTIONS
Frequent
Dizziness, dyspnea, headache
Occasional
Nausea, fatigue, palpitations, chest
pain, asthenia (loss of strength,
energy), tremors, constipation

PRECAUTIONS AND CONTRAINDICATIONS
Cardiogenic shock, preexisting
second- or third-degree AV block,
right bundle-branch block (without
presence of a pacemaker).
Caution
Lactation, children, renal disease,
liver disease, CHF, respiratory
depression, myasthenia gravis

DRUG INTERACTIONS OF CONCERN TO DENTISTRY
● No specific interactions are
reported with dental drugs; however,
any drug that could affect the cardiac
action of flecainide (e.g., other local
anesthetics, vasoconstrictors,
anticholinergics) should be used in
the lowest effective dose

SERIOUS REACTIONS
❗ Flecainide may worsen existing
arrhythmias or produce new ones.
❗ CHF may occur or existing CHF
may worsen.
❗ Overdose may increase QRS
duration, prolong QT interval, cause
conduction disturbances, reduce
myocardial contractility, and cause
hypotension.

DENTAL CONSIDERATIONS
General:
● Monitor vital signs at every
appointment because of

cardiovascular and respiratory side effects.

• Assess salivary flow as a factor in caries, periodontal disease, and candidiasis.

• Stress from dental procedures may compromise cardiovascular function; determine patient risk.

• Use vasoconstrictors with caution, in low doses, and with careful aspiration. Avoid use of gingival retraction cord with epinephrine.

Consultations:

• Medical consultation may be required to assess disease control and patient's ability to tolerate stress.

Teach Patient/Family to:

• Use effective oral hygiene to prevent gingival inflammation

• Avoid mouth rinses with high alcohol content because of drying effects

fluconazole
floo-con´-ah-zole
(Apo-Fluconazole[CAN], Diflucan)
Do not confuse Diflucan with diclofenac.

CATEGORY AND SCHEDULE
Pregnancy Risk Category: C

Drug Class: Antifungal

MECHANISM OF ACTION
A fungistatic antifungal that interferes with cytochrome P-450, an enzyme necessary for ergosterol formation. *Therapeutic Effect:* Directly damages fungal membrane, altering its function.

USES
Treatment of oropharyngeal candidiasis, chronic mucocutaneous candidiasis, vaginal candidiasis, cryptococcal meningitis, esophageal candidiasis and prophylaxis in patients receiving bone marrow transplants with chemotherapy or radiation

PHARMACOKINETICS
Well absorbed from GI tract. Widely distributed, including to CSF. Protein binding: 11%. Partially metabolized in liver. Excreted unchanged primarily in urine. Partially removed by hemodialysis. *Half-life:* 20–30 hr (increased in impaired renal function).

INDICATIONS AND DOSAGES
▸ **Oropharyngeal Candidiasis**
PO, IV
Adults, Elderly. 200 mg once, then 100 mg/day for at least 14 days.
Children. 6 mg/kg/day once, then 3 mg/kg/day.
▸ **Esophageal Candidiasis**
PO, IV
Adults, Elderly. 200 mg once, then 100 mg/day (up to 400 mg/day) for 21 days and at least 14 days following resolution of symptoms.
Children. 6 mg/kg/day once, then 3 mg/kg/day (up to 12 mg/kg/day) for 21 days at least 14 days following resolution of symptoms.
▸ **Vaginal Candidiasis**
PO
Adults. 150 mg once.
▸ **Prevention of Candidiasis in Patients Undergoing Bone Marrow Transplantation**
PO
Adults. 400 mg/day.
▸ **Systemic Candidiasis**
PO, IV
Adults, Elderly. 400 mg once, then 200 mg/day (up to 400 mg/day) for at least 28 days and at least

14 days following resolution of symptoms.
Children. 6–12 mg/kg/day.

▶ **Cryptococcal Meningitis**
PO, IV
Adults, Elderly. 400 mg once, then 200 mg/day (up to 800 mg/day) for 10–12 wk after CSF becomes negative (200 mg/day for suppression of relapse in patients with AIDS).
Children. 12 mg/kg/day once, then 6–12 mg/kg/day (6 mg/kg/day for suppression of relapse in patients with AIDS).

▶ **Onychomycosis**
PO
Adults. 150 mg/wk.

▶ **Dosage in Renal Impairment**
After a loading dose of 400 mg, the daily dosage is based on creatinine clearance:

Creatinine Clearance	% of Recommended Dose
Greater than 50 ml/min	100
21–50 ml/min	50
11–20 ml/min	25
Dialysis	Dose after dialysis

SIDE EFFECTS/ADVERSE REACTIONS
Occasional
Hypersensitivity reaction (including chills, fever, pruritus, and rash), dizziness, drowsiness, headache, constipation, diarrhea, nausea, vomiting, abdominal pain

PRECAUTIONS AND CONTRAINDICATIONS
Hypersensitivity
Caution
Renal disease

DRUG INTERACTIONS OF CONCERN TO DENTISTRY
• Caution: potent inhibitor of cytochrome P450 3A4 isoenzymes

• Increased plasma levels of oral hypoglycemics: theophylline, cyclosporine, tacrolimus, corticosteroids
• Inhibits metabolism of certain benzodiazepines: alprazolam, chlordiazepoxide, clonazepam, clorazepate, diazepam, estazolam, flurazepam, halazepam, midazolam, triazolam, quazepam, zolpidem
• Increased anticoagulant effect: may inhibit metabolism of warfarin
• Suspected risk of increased neurologic side effects: haloperidol, tricyclic antidepressants
• May increase levels and side effects of HMG-CoA reductase inhibitors
• Suspected increase in antihypertensive effects of losartan; monitor blood pressure if used concurrently
• Decreased renal clearance: hydrochlorothiazide
• Suspected decrease in oral contraceptive effectiveness; may want to suggest additional contraception

SERIOUS REACTIONS
❗ Exfoliative skin disorders, serious hepatic effects, and blood dyscrasias (such as eosinophilia, thrombocytopenia, anemia, and leukopenia) have been reported rarely.

DENTAL CONSIDERATIONS
General:
• Culture may be required to confirm fungal organism.
• Patients on chronic drug therapy may rarely have symptoms of blood dyscrasias, which can include infection, bleeding, and poor healing.
Consultations:
• In a patient with symptoms of blood dyscrasias, request a medical consultation for blood studies and postpone treatment until normal values are reestablished.

Teach Patient/Family to:
• Be aware that long-term therapy may be necessary to clear infection
• Prevent revinoculation of *Candida* infection by disposing of toothbrush or other contaminated oral hygiene devices used during period of infection

flucytosine
floo-sye´-toe-seen
(Ancobon)

CATEGORY AND SCHEDULE
Pregnancy Risk Category: C

Drug Class: Antifungal

MECHANISM OF ACTION
An antifungal that penetrates fungal cells and is converted to fluorouracil which competes with uracil interfering with fungal RNA and protein synthesis. *Therapeutic Effect:* Damages fungal membrane.

USES
Treatment of *Candida* infections (septicemia, endocarditis, pulmonary and UTIs), *Cryptococcus* (meningitis, pulmonary and urinary tract infections)

PHARMACOKINETICS
Well absorbed from GI tract. Widely distributed, including CSF. Protein binding: 2–4%. Metabolized in liver. Partially removed by hemodialysis. *Half-life:* 3–8 hr (half-life is increased with impaired renal function).

INDICATIONS AND DOSAGES
▶ **Fungal Infections, Candidiasis, Cryptococcosis**
PO
Adults, Elderly, Children. 50 to 150 mg/kg/day in 4 equally divided doses.

▶ **Dosage in Renal Function Impairment**
Based on creatinine clearance:

Creatinine Clearance	Dosage Interval
20–40 ml/min	q12h
10–20 ml/min	q24h
0–10 ml/min	q24–48h

SIDE EFFECTS/ADVERSE REACTIONS
Occasional
Pruritus, rash, photosensitivity, dizziness, drowsiness, headache, diarrhea, nausea, vomiting, abdominal pain, increased liver enzymes, jaundice, increased BUN and creatinine, weakness, hearing loss

PRECAUTIONS AND CONTRAINDICATIONS
Hypersensitivity to flucytosine
Caution
Renal disease, bone marrow depression, blood dyscrasias, radiation therapy or chemotherapy

DRUG INTERACTIONS OF CONCERN TO DENTISTRY
None reported

SERIOUS REACTIONS
❗ Hepatic dysfunction and severe bone marrow suppression occur rarely.

DENTAL CONSIDERATIONS
General:
• Patients on chronic drug therapy may rarely have symptoms of blood dyscrasias, which can include infection, bleeding, and poor healing.

- Examine for evidence of oral *Candida* infection.
Consultations:
- Medical consultation may be required to assess disease control.
- In a patient with symptoms of blood dyscrasias, request a medical consultation for blood studies and postpone dental treatment until normal values are reestablished.
Teach Patient/Family to:
- Use effective oral hygiene to prevent gingival inflammation

fludarabine phosphate

flew-dare´-ah-bean foss´-fate
(Fludara)
Do not confuse Fludara with FUDR.

CATEGORY AND SCHEDULE
Pregnancy Risk Category: D

Drug Class: Antineoplastic, antimetabolite

MECHANISM OF ACTION
An antimetabolite that inhibits DNA synthesis by interfering with DNA polymerase alpha, ribonucleotide reductase, and DNA primase.
Therapeutic Effect: Induces cell death.

USES
Treatment of chronic lymphocyte leukemia, non-Hodgkin's lymphoma

PHARMACOKINETICS
Rapidly dephosphorylated in serum, then phosphorylated intracellularly to active triphosphate. Primarily excreted in urine. *Half-life:* 7–20 hr.

INDICATIONS AND DOSAGES
▸ **Chronic Lymphocytic Leukemia**

IV
Adults. 25 mg/m^2 daily for 5 consecutive days. Continue for up to 3 additional cycles. Begin each course of treatment every 28 days.
▸ **Non-Hodgkin's Lymphoma**
IV
Adults, Elderly. Initially, 20 mg/m^2, then 30 mg/m^2/day for 48 hr.
▸ **Dosage in Renal Impairment**

Creatinine Clearance	Dosage
30–70 ml/min	Decrease dose by 20%
Less than 30 ml/min	Not recommended

SIDE EFFECTS/ADVERSE REACTIONS
Frequent
Fever, nausea, and vomiting
Occasional
Chills, fatigue, generalized pain, rash, diarrhea, cough, asthenia, stomatitis, dyspnea, peripheral edema
Rare
Anorexia, sinusitis, dysuria, myalgia, paresthesia, headaches, visual disturbances

PRECAUTIONS AND CONTRAINDICATIONS
Concurrent use with pentostatin

DRUG INTERACTIONS OF CONCERN TO DENTISTRY
None reported

SERIOUS REACTIONS
! Pneumonia occurs frequently.
! Severe hematologic toxicity (as evidenced by anemia, thrombocytopenia, and neutropenia) and GI bleeding may occur.

! Tumor lysis syndrome may start with flank pain and hematuria and may include hypercalcemia, hyperphosphatemia, hyperuricemia and renal failure.

! High-dosage therapy may produce acute leukemia, blindness, and coma.

DENTAL CONSIDERATIONS

General:

• Monitor vital signs at every appointment because of cardiovascular side effects.

• If additional analgesia is required for dental pain, consider alternative analgesics in patients taking narcotics for acute or chronic pain.

• Examine for oral manifestation of opportunistic infection.

• Avoid products that affect platelet function, such as aspirin and NSAIDs.

• This drug may be used in the hospital or on an outpatient basis. Confirm the patient's disease and treatment status.

• Chlorhexidine mouth rinse prior to and during chemotherapy may reduce severity of mucositis.

• Patient on chronic drug therapy may rarely present with symptoms of blood dyscrasias, which can include infection, bleeding and poor healing. If dyscrasia is present, caution patient to prevent oral tissue trauma when using oral hygiene aids.

• Palliative medication may be required for management of oral side effects.

• Patients may be at risk of infection.

• Patients may be at risk of bleeding; check for oral signs.

• Oral infections should be eliminated and/or treated aggressively.

Consultations:

• Medical consultation should include routine blood counts including platelet counts and bleeding time.

• Consult physician; prophylactic or therapeutic antiinfectives may be indicated if surgery or periodontal treatment is required.

• Medical consultation may be required to assess immunologic status during cancer chemotherapy and determine safety risk, if any, posed by the required dental treatment.

• Medical consultation may be required to assess disease control and patient's ability to tolerate stress.

Teach Patient/Family to:

• Be aware of oral side effects

• Use effective oral hygiene to prevent soft tissue inflammation

• Report oral lesions, soreness, or bleeding to dentist

• Prevent trauma when using oral hygiene aids

• Update health and medication history if physician makes any changes in evaluation or drug regimens; include OTC, herbal, and nonherbal remedies in the update

fludrocortisone

floo-droe-kor´-ti-sone
(Florinef)
Do not confuse Florinef with Fioricet or Florinal.

CATEGORY AND SCHEDULE

Pregnancy Risk Category: C

Drug Class: Glucocorticoid and mineralocorticoid

MECHANISM OF ACTION

A mineralocorticoid that acts at distal tubules. ***Therapeutic Effect:*** Increases potassium and hydrogen ion excretion. Replaces sodium loss and raises blood pressure (with low dosages). Inhibits endogenous adrenal cortical secretion, thymic activity, and secretion of corticotropin by pituitary gland (with higher dosages).

USES

Treatment of adrenal insufficiency (Addison's disease), salt-losing adrenogenital syndrome

PHARMACOKINETICS

Well absorbed from the GI tract. Protein binding: 42%. Widely distributed. Metabolized in the liver and kidney. Primarily excreted in urine. *Half-life:* 3.5 hr.

INDICATIONS AND DOSAGES

▶ **Addison's Disease**
PO
Adults, Elderly. 0.05–0.1 mg/day. Range: 0.1 mg 3 times a wk to 0.2 mg/day. Administration with cortisone or hydrocortisone preferred.
▶ **Salt-Losing Adrenogenital Syndrome**
PO
Adults, Elderly. 0.1–0.2 mg/day.
▶ **Usual Pediatric Dosage**
Children. 0.05–0.1 mg/day.

SIDE EFFECTS/ADVERSE REACTIONS

Frequent
Increased appetite, exaggerated sense of well-being, abdominal distention, weight gain, insomnia, mood swings
High dosages, prolonged therapy, too rapid withdrawal: Increased susceptibility to infection with masked signs and symptoms, delayed wound healing, hypokalemia, hypocalcemia, GI distress, diarrhea or constipation, hypertension

Occasional
Headache, dizziness, menstrual difficulty or amenorrhea, gastric ulcer development
Rare
Hypersensitivity reaction

PRECAUTIONS AND CONTRAINDICATIONS

CHF, systemic fungal infection
Caution
Lactation, osteoporosis, CHF, safety and use in children has not been established

DRUG INTERACTIONS OF CONCERN TO DENTISTRY

• Decreased action: barbiturates
• Increased side effects: sodium-containing food, sodium-containing polishing devices
• Decreased effects of salicylates

SERIOUS REACTIONS

! Long-term therapy may cause muscle wasting (especially in the arms and legs), osteoporosis, spontaneous fractures, amenorrhea, cataracts, glaucoma, peptic ulcer disease, and CHF.
! Abruptly withdrawing the drug after long-term therapy may cause anorexia, nausea, fever, headache, joint pain, rebound inflammation, fatigue, weakness, lethargy, dizziness, and orthostatic hypotension.

DENTAL CONSIDERATIONS

General:
• Patients with Addison's disease are more susceptible to stress and may require supplemental systemic glucocorticoids before dental treatment.
• Patients who have been or are currently on chronic steroid therapy (longer than 2 wk) may require supplemental steroids for dental treatment.

- Monitor vital signs at every appointment because of nature of disease.
- Short appointments and a stress-reduction protocol may be required for anxious patients.
- Patients with Addison's disease must be evaluated closely for presence of oral infection.
- Do not use ingestible sodium bicarbonate products, such as the Prophy-Jet air polishing system, or IV saline fluids for patients on a salt-restricted regimen.
- Use precautions if dental surgery is anticipated and conscious sedation or general anesthesia is required.
- Monitor patient for any signs of inadequate management of disease, such as potassium depletion, muscle weakness, paresthesia, fatigue, nausea, depression, polyuria, and edema.

Consultations:
- Medical consultation is required to assess disease control and patient's ability to tolerate stress.
- Consultation may be required to confirm steroid dose and duration of use.

Teach Patient/Family to:
- Carry identification as a steroid user
- Report to the dental office any signs that might indicate an oral infection

flumazenil
flew-maz´-ah-nil
(Anexate[CAN], Romazicon)

CATEGORY AND SCHEDULE
Pregnancy Risk Category: C

Drug Class: Benzodiazepine receptor antagonist

MECHANISM OF ACTION
An antidote that antagonizes the effect of benzodiazepines on the gamma-aminobutyric acid receptor complex in the CNS. **Therapeutic Effect:** Reverses sedative effect of benzodiazepines.

USES
Reversal of the sedative effects of benzodiazepines

PHARMACOKINETICS

Route	Onset	Peak	Duration
IV	1–2 min	6–10 min	Less than 1 hr

Duration and degree of benzodiazepine reversal depend on dosage and plasma concentration. Protein binding: 50%. Metabolized by the liver; excreted in urine.

INDICATIONS AND DOSAGES
▶ **Reversal of Conscious Sedation or General Anesthesia**
IV
Adults, Elderly. Initially, 0.2 mg (2 ml) over 15 sec; may repeat dose in 45 sec; then at 60-sec intervals. Maximum: 1 mg (10-ml) total dose.
Children, Neonates. Initially, 0.01 mg/kg; may repeat in 45 sec, then at 60-sec intervals. Maximum: 0.2 mg single dose; 0.05 mg/kg or 1 mg cumulative dose.
▶ **Benzodiazepine Overdose**
IV
Adults, Elderly. Initially, 0.2 mg (2 ml) over 30 sec; if desired LOC is not achieved after 30 sec, 0.3 mg (3 ml) may be given over 30 sec. Further doses of 0.5 mg (5 ml) may be administered over 30 sec at 60-sec intervals. Maximum: 3 mg (30 ml) total dose.
Children, Neonates. Initially, 0.01 mg/kg; may repeat in

45 sec, then at 60-sec intervals.
Maximum: 0.2 mg single dose;
1 mg cumulative dose.

SIDE EFFECTS/ADVERSE REACTIONS

Frequent
Agitation, anxiety, dry mouth,
dyspnea, insomnia, palpitations,
tremors, headache, blurred vision,
dizziness, ataxia, nausea, vomiting,
pain at injection site, diaphoresis
Occasional
Fatigue, flushing, auditory
disturbances, thrombophlebitis, rash
Rare
Urticaria, pruritus, hallucinations

PRECAUTIONS AND CONTRAINDICATIONS

Anticholinergic signs (such as
mydriasis, dry mucosa, and
hypoperistalsis), arrhythmias,
cardiovascular collapse, history of
hypersensitivity to benzodiazepines,
patients with signs of serious cyclic
antidepressant overdose (such as
motor abnormalities), patients who
have been given a benzodiazepine for
control of a potentially life-
threatening condition (such as
control of status epilepticus or
increased intracranial pressure)
Caution
Lactation, elderly, renal disease,
seizure disorders, head injury, labor
and delivery, hepatic disease,
hypoventilation, panic disorder, drug
and alcohol dependency, ambulatory
patients; no risk-benefits have been
established for children

DRUG INTERACTIONS OF CONCERN TO DENTISTRY

• May not be effective: mixed drug
overdosage

SERIOUS REACTIONS

! Toxic effects, such as seizures and
arrhythmias, of other drugs taken in
overdose, especially tricyclic
antidepressants, may emerge with
reversal of sedative effect of
benzodiazepines.
! Flumazenil may provoke a panic
attack in those with a history of
panic disorder.

DENTAL CONSIDERATIONS

General:
• Monitor vital signs at every
appointment because of
cardiovascular side effects.
• Monitor for resedation; duration of
antagonism is short compared with
benzodiazepines.
Teach Patient/Family to:
• Be alert for possible resedation
when discharged from office

flunisolide
floo-niss´-oh-lide
(AeroBid, Nasalide, Nasarel,
Rhinalar[CAN])
Do not confuse flunisolide with
fluocinonide, or Nasalide with
Nasalcrom.

CATEGORY AND SCHEDULE
Pregnancy Risk Category: C

Drug Class: Synthetic
glucocorticoid

MECHANISM OF ACTION
An adrenocorticosteroid that controls
the rate of protein synthesis,
depresses migration of
polymorphonuclear leukocytes,
reverses capillary permeability, and
stabilizes lysosomal membranes.
Therapeutic Effect: Prevents or
controls inflammation.

USES
Oral inhalation for prophylaxis or maintenance treatment of chronic asthma; nasal solution for seasonal or perennial rhinitis

PHARMACOKINETICS
Aerosol: Effective response time 1–4 wk; metabolized in liver; excreted in urine and feces.

INDICATIONS AND DOSAGES
▶ **Long-Term Control of Bronchial Asthma, Assists in Reducing or Discontinuing Oral Corticosteroid Therapy**
Inhalation
Adults, Elderly. 2 inhalations twice a day, morning and evening.
Maximum: 4 inhalations twice a day.
Children 6–15 yr. 2 inhalations twice a day.
▶ **Relief of Symptoms of Perennial and Seasonal Rhinitis**
Intranasal
Adults, Elderly. Initially, 2 sprays each nostril twice a day, may increase at 4–7 day intervals to 2 sprays 3 times a day. Maximum: 8 sprays in each nostril daily.
Children 6–14 yr. Initially, 1 spray 3 times a day or 2 sprays twice a day. Maximum: 4 sprays in each nostril daily. Maintenance: 1 spray into each nostril each day.

SIDE EFFECTS/ADVERSE REACTIONS
Frequent
Inhalation: Unpleasant taste, nausea, vomiting, sore throat, diarrhea, upset stomach, cold symptoms, nasal congestion
Occasional
Inhalation: Dizziness, irritability, nervousness, tremors, abdominal pain, heartburn, oropharynx candidiasis, edema

Nasal: Mild nasopharyngeal irritation or dryness, rebound congestion, bronchial asthma, rhinorrhea, altered taste

PRECAUTIONS AND CONTRAINDICATIONS
Hypersensitivity to any corticosteroid, persistently positive sputum cultures for *C. albicans,* primary treatment of status asthmaticus, systemic fungal infections
Caution
Lactation; warning: switching patients from systemic steroids to inhalation must be done carefully to avoid severe adrenal insufficiency

SERIOUS REACTIONS
❗ An acute hypersensitivity reaction, marked by urticaria, angioedema, and severe bronchospasm, occurs rarely.
❗ A transfer from systemic to local steroid therapy may unmask previously suppressed bronchial asthma condition.

DENTAL CONSIDERATIONS
General:
• Examine oral cavity for evidence of drug side effects.
• Assess salivary flow as a factor in caries, periodontal disease, and candidiasis.
• Evaluate respiration characteristics and rate.
• Consider semisupine chair position for patients with respiratory disease.
• Determine dose and duration of steroid therapy for each patient to assess risk for stress tolerance and immunosuppression.
• Acute asthmatic episodes may be precipitated in the dental office. Sympathomimetic inhalants should be available for emergency use.

A stress reduction protocol may be required.
• Consider the drug in the diagnosis of taste alterations.
Consultations:
• Medical consultation may be required to assess disease control.
Teach Patient/Family to:
• Use effective oral hygiene to prevent soft tissue inflammation
• Use caution to prevent injury when using oral hygiene aids
• Gargle, rinse mouth with water, and expectorate after each aerosol dose
• When chronic dry mouth occurs, advise patient to:
   • Use daily home fluoride products for anticaries effect
   • Avoid mouth rinses with high alcohol content because of drying effects
   • Use sugarless gum, frequent sips of water, or saliva substitutes

fluocinolone acetonide

floo-oh-sin´-oh-lone
ah-seat´-oh-nide
(Capex, Derma-Smooth/FS, Fluoderm[CAN], Synalar)

CATEGORY AND SCHEDULE

Pregnancy Risk Category: C

Drug Class: Antiinflammatory, steroidal, topical; corticosteroid, topical

MECHANISM OF ACTION

A fluorinated topical corticosteroid that controls the rate of protein synthesis; depresses migration of polymorphonuclear leukocytes and fibroblasts; reduces capillary permeability; prevents or controls inflammation. *Therapeutic Effect:* Decreases tissue response to inflammatory process.

USES

Relief of redness, swelling, itching, and discomfort of many skin problems

PHARMACOKINETICS

Use of occlusive dressings may increase percutaneous absorption. Protein binding: more than 90%. Excreted in urine. *Half-life:* Unknown.

INDICATIONS AND DOSAGES
▶ **Atopic Dermatitis**
Topical
Adults, Elderly. Apply 3 times a day.
Children 2 yr and older. Apply 2 times a day.
▶ **Scalp Psoriasis**
Topical
Adults, Elderly. Apply to damp or wet hair and leave on overnight or for at least 4 hr. Remove by washing hair with shampoo.
▶ **Seborrheic Dermatitis, Scalp**
Shampoo
Adults, Elderly. Apply once daily, allow to remain on scalp for at least 5 min.

SIDE EFFECTS/ADVERSE REACTIONS

Occasional
Burning, dryness, itching, stinging
Rare
Allergic contact dermatitis, purpura or blood-containing blisters, thinning of skin with easy bruising, telangiectasis or raised dark red spots on skin

PRECAUTIONS AND CONTRAINDICATIONS

Hypersensitivity to fluocinolone or other corticosteroids

DRUG INTERACTIONS OF CONCERN TO DENTISTRY

None reported

SERIOUS REACTIONS

! When taken in excessive quantities, systemic hypercorticism and adrenal suppression may occur.

DENTAL CONSIDERATIONS

General:
• Determine why patient is taking the drug.
Teach Patient/Family to:
• Avoid use on oral herpetic ulcerations

fluocinonide

floo-oh-sin´-oh-nide
(Lidex, Lidex-E)

CATEGORY AND SCHEDULE

Pregnancy Risk Category: C

Drug Class: Topical corticosteroid, synthetic fluorinated agent, group II potency

MECHANISM OF ACTION

A topical corticosteroid that has antiinflammatory, antipruritic, and vasoconstrictive properties. The exact mechanism of the antiinflammatory process is unclear. **Therapeutic Effect:** Reduces or prevents tissue response to the inflammatory process.

USES

Treatment of psoriasis, eczema, contact dermatitis, pruritus, oral lichen planus lesions

PHARMACOKINETICS

Well absorbed systemically. Large variation in absorption among sites. Protein binding: varies. Metabolized in liver. Primarily excreted in urine.

INDICATIONS AND DOSAGES

▶ **Dermatoses**
Topical
Adults, Elderly. Apply sparingly 2–4 times a day.

SIDE EFFECTS/ADVERSE REACTIONS

Occasional
Itching, redness, irritation, burning at site of application, dryness, folliculitis, acneiform eruptions, hypopigmentation
Rare
Allergic contact dermatitis, maceration of the skin, secondary infection, skin atrophy

PRECAUTIONS AND CONTRAINDICATIONS

History of hypersensitivity to fluocinonide or other corticosteroids.
Caution
Lactation, viral infections, bacterial infections

DRUG INTERACTIONS OF CONCERN TO DENTISTRY

• None reported

SERIOUS REACTIONS

! The serious reactions of long-term therapy and the addition of occlusive dressings are reversible hypothalamic-pituitary-adrenal (HPA) axis suppression, manifestations of Cushing's syndrome, hyperglycemia, and glucosuria.

DENTAL CONSIDERATIONS

General:
• Place on frequent recall to evaluate healing response.

Teach Patient/Family to:
• Return for oral evaluation if response of oral tissues has not occurred in 7–14 days
• Avoid use on oral herpetic ulcerations
• Use effective oral hygiene to prevent soft tissue inflammation
• Apply at bedtime or after meals for maximum effect
• Apply with cotton-tipped applicator by pressing, not rubbing, paste on lesion

fluorometholone

flure-oh-meth′-oh-lone
(Eflone, Flarex, Fluor-Op, FML Forte Liquifilm, FML Liquifilm, FML S.O.P.)

CATEGORY AND SCHEDULE

Pregnancy Risk Category: C

Drug Class: Antiinflammatory, steroidal, ophthalmic; corticosteroid, ophthalmic

MECHANISM OF ACTION

An ophthalmic corticosteroid that decreases inflammation by suppression of migration of polymorphonuclear leukocytes and reversal of increased capillary permeability. **Therapeutic Effect:** Decreased ocular inflammation.

USES

Prevention of permanent damage to the eye, which may occur with certain eye problems. They also provide relief from redness, irritation, and other discomfort.

PHARMACOKINETICS

Absorbed into aqueous humor with slight systemic absorption.

INDICATIONS AND DOSAGES

▸ **Treatment of Steroid-Responsive Inflammatory Conditions of the Eye**
Ophthalmic Ointment
Adults, Elderly. Apply thin strip to conjunctival sac every 4 hr in severe cases or 1–3 times a day in mild to moderate cases.
Ophthalmic Solution
Adults, Elderly, Children 2 yr and older. Instill 1–2 drops into conjunctival sac every hour during the day, every 2 hr at night until favorable response is obtained. Then use 1 drop every 4 hr. For mild to moderate inflammation, instill 1–2 drops into conjunctival sac 2–4 times a day.

SIDE EFFECTS/ADVERSE REACTIONS

Occasional
Burning, tearing, itching, blurred vision
Rare
Cataract formation, corneal ulcers, glaucoma with optic nerve damage

PRECAUTIONS AND CONTRAINDICATIONS

Viral diseases of the cornea and conjunctiva, mycobacterial or fungal infections of the eye, untreated eye infections which may be masked or enhanced by steroids, hypersensitivity to fluorometholone or any component of the formulation

DRUG INTERACTIONS OF CONCERN TO DENTISTRY

None reported

SERIOUS REACTIONS

! Hypercorticoidism and taste perversion occurs rarely.

! Superinfections, particularly with fungi, may result from bacterial imbalance via any route of administration.

DENTAL CONSIDERATIONS

General:

• Determine why patient is taking the drug.

• Avoid dental light in patient's eyes; offer dark glasses for patient comfort.

• Protect patient's eyes from accidental spatter during dental treatment.

fluorouracil, 5FU

flure-oh-yoor´-ah-sill
(Adrucil, Carac, Efudex, Efudix[AUS], Fluoroplex)
Do not confuse Efudex with Efidac.

CATEGORY AND SCHEDULE

Pregnancy Risk Category: D

Drug Class: Topical antineoplastic

MECHANISM OF ACTION

An antimetabolite that blocks formation of thymidylic acid. Cell cycle-specific for S phase of cell division. ***Therapeutic Effect:*** Inhibits DNA and RNA synthesis. Topical form destroys rapidly proliferating cells.

USES

Treatment of keratosis (multiple/actinic), basal cell carcinoma; unapproved: condyloma acuminatum

PHARMACOKINETICS

Widely distributed. Crosses the blood-brain barrier. Rapidly metabolized in tissues to active metabolite, which is localized intracellularly. Primarily excreted by lungs as carbon dioxide. Removed by hemodialysis. *Half-life:* 20 hr.

INDICATIONS AND DOSAGES

▸ **Carcinoma of Breast, Colon, Pancreas, Rectum, and Stomach; in Combination with Levamisole after Surgical Resection in Patients with Duke's Stage C Colon Cancer**
IV
Adults, Elderly, Children. Initially, 12 mg/kg/day for 4–5 days. Maximum: 800 mg/day. Maintenance: 6 mg/kg every other day for 4 doses repeated in 4 wk; or 15 mg/kg as a single bolus dose; or 5–15 mg/kg/wk as a single dose, not to exceed 1 g.
▸ **Multiple Actinic or Solar Keratoses**
Topical (Carac)
Adults, Elderly. Apply once a day.
Topical (Efudex, Fluoroplex)
Adults, Elderly. Apply twice a day.
▸ **Basal Cell Carcinoma**
Topical (Efudex)
Adult, Elderly. Apply twice a day.

SIDE EFFECTS/ADVERSE REACTIONS

Occasional
Parenteral: Anorexia, diarrhea, minimal alopecia, fever, dry skin, skin fissures, scaling, erythema
Topical: Pain, pruritus, hyperpigmentation, irritation, inflammation, and burning at application site; photosensitivity
Rare
Nausea, vomiting, anemia, esophagitis, proctitis, GI ulcer, confusion, headache, lacrimation,

visual disturbances, angina, allergic reactions

PRECAUTIONS AND CONTRAINDICATIONS

Major surgery within previous month, myelosuppression, poor nutritional status, potentially serious infections

Caution

Occlusive dressings, lactation, children, excessive exposure to sunlight

DRUG INTERACTIONS OF CONCERN TO DENTISTRY

• None reported, but limit drugs that may also produce photosensitivity reaction

SERIOUS REACTIONS

! The earliest sign of toxicity, which may occur 4–8 days after beginning therapy, is stomatitis (as evidenced by dry mouth, burning sensation, mucosal erythema, and ulceration at inner margin of lips).

! Hematologic toxicity may be manifested as leukopenia (generally within 9–14 days after drug administration, but possibly as late as the 25th day), thrombocytopenia (within 7–17 days after administration), pancytopenia, or agranulocytosis.

! The most common dermatologic toxicity is a pruritic rash on the extremities or, less frequently, the trunk.

DENTAL CONSIDERATIONS

General:

• Be aware of patient's disease and avoid treated areas to prevent further irritation.

fluoxetine hydrochloride

floo-ox´-eh-teen hi-droh-klor´-ide (Auscap[AUS], Fluohexal[AUS], Lovan[AUS], Novo-Fluoxetine[CAN], Prozac, Prozac Weekly, Sarafem, Zactin[AUS])

Do not confuse fluoxetine with fluvastatin, Prozac with Prilosec, Proscar, or ProSom; or Sarafem with Serophene.

CATEGORY AND SCHEDULE

Pregnancy Risk Category: C

Drug Class: Antidepressant

MECHANISM OF ACTION

A psychotherapeutic agent that selectively inhibits serotonin uptake in the CNS, enhancing serotonergic function. *Therapeutic Effect:* Relieves depression; reduces obsessive-compulsive and bulimic behavior.

USES

Treatment of major depressive disorder, bulimia, obsessive-compulsive disorder, premenstrual tension, geriatric depression in patients older than 65 yr, panic disorder with or without agoraphobia; premenstrual dysphoric disorder (Sarafem)

PHARMACOKINETICS

Well absorbed from the GI tract. Crosses the blood-brain barrier. Protein binding: 94%. Metabolized in the liver to active metabolite. Primarily excreted in urine. Not removed by hemodialysis. *Half-life:* 2–3 days; metabolite 7–9 days.

INDICATIONS AND DOSAGES
▶ **Depression, Obsessive-Compulsive Disorder**
PO
Adults. Initially, 20 mg each morning. If therapeutic improvement does not occur after 2 wk, gradually increase to maximum of 80 mg/day in 2 equally divided doses in morning and at noon. Prozac Weekly: 90 mg/wk, begin 7 days after last dose of 20 mg.
Elderly. Initially, 10 mg/day. May increase by 10–20 mg q2wk.
Children 7–17 yr. Initially, 5–10 mg/day. Titrate upward as needed. Usual dosage is 20 mg/day.
▶ **Panic Disorder**
PO
Adults, Elderly. Initially, 10 mg/day. May increase to 20 mg/day after 1 wk. Maximum: 60 mg/day.
▶ **Bulimia Nervosa**
PO
Adults. 60 mg each morning.
▶ **Premenstrual Dysphoric Disorder**
PO
Adults. 20 mg/day.

SIDE EFFECTS/ADVERSE REACTIONS
Frequent
Headache, asthenia, insomnia, anxiety, nervousness, somnolence, nausea, diarrhea, decreased appetite
Occasional
Dizziness, tremors, fatigue, vomiting, constipation, dry mouth, abdominal pain, nasal congestion, diaphoresis, rash
Rare
Flushed skin, light-headedness, impaired concentration

PRECAUTIONS AND CONTRAINDICATIONS
Use within 14 days of MAOIs
Caution
Lactation, children, elderly; treatment-emergent adverse effects, hepatic impairment, interference with cognitive or motor performance

DRUG INTERACTIONS OF CONCERN TO DENTISTRY
• Increased CNS depression: alcohol, all CNS depressants, tricyclic antidepressants, benzodiazepines, St. John's wort (herb)
• Increased side effects: highly protein-bound drugs (aspirin)
• Caution: can inhibit cytochrome P4502D6 isoenzymes
• Increased serum levels of carbamazepine
• Possible "serotonin syndrome" with macrolide antibiotics
• First-time users of SSRIs also taking NSAIDs may have a higher risk of GI side effects; until more data are available, it may be advisable to avoid use of NSAIDs in these patients (Br J Clin Pharmacol 55:591–595, 2003)

SERIOUS REACTIONS
❗ Overdose may produce seizures, nausea, vomiting, agitation, and restlessness.

DENTAL CONSIDERATIONS
General:
• Monitor vital signs at every appointment because of cardiovascular side effects.
• Assess salivary flow as a factor in caries, periodontal disease, and candidiasis.
Consultations:
• Medical consultation may be required to assess disease control and patient's ability to tolerate stress.
• Physician should be informed if significant xerostomic side effects occur (e.g., increased caries, sore tongue, problems eating or swallowing, difficulty wearing prosthesis) so that a medication change can be considered.

Teach Patient/Family to:
• Use electric tooth brush if patient has difficulty holding conventional devices
• When chronic dry mouth occurs, advise patient to:
  • Avoid mouth rinses with high alcohol content because of drying effects
  • Use daily home fluoride products for anticaries effect
  • Use sugarless gum, frequent sips of water, or saliva substitutes

---

fluoxymesterone
floo-ox-ih-meś-teh-rone
(Android-F, Halotestin, Halotestin[CAN])

CATEGORY AND SCHEDULE
Pregnancy Risk Category: X
Controlled substance: Schedule III

Drug Class: Androgenic anabolic steroid

MECHANISM OF ACTION
An androgen that suppresses gonadotropin-releasing hormone, leutenizing hormone (LH), and follicle-stimulating hormone (FSH). *Therapeutic Effect:* Stimulates spermatogenesis, development of male secondary sex characteristics, and sexual maturation at puberty. Stimulates production of red blood cells (RBCs).

USES
Treatment of impotence from testicular deficiency, hypogonadism, palliative treatment of female breast cancer

PHARMACOKINETICS
Rapidly absorbed from the GI tract. Protein binding: 98%. Metabolized in liver. Excreted in urine.
Half-life: 9.2 hr.

INDICATIONS AND DOSAGES
▶ **Males (hypogonadism)**
PO
Adults. 5–20 mg/day.
▶ **Males (delayed puberty)**
PO
Adults. 2.5–20 mg/day for 4–6 mo.
▶ **Females (inoperable breast cancer)**
PO
Adults. 10–40 mg/day in divided doses for 1–3 mo.
▶ **Females (prevent postpartum breast pain/engorgement)**
PO
Adults. Initially, 2.5 mg shortly after delivery, then 5–10 mg/day in divided doses for 4–5 days.

SIDE EFFECTS/ADVERSE REACTIONS
Frequent
Females: Amenorrhea, virilism (e.g., acne, decreased breast size, enlarged clitoris, male pattern baldness), deepening voice
Males: UTI, breast soreness, gynecomastia, priapism, virilism (e.g., acne, early pubic hair growth)
Occasional
Edema, nausea, vomiting, mild acne, diarrhea, stomach pain
Males: Impotence, testicular atrophy

PRECAUTIONS AND CONTRAINDICATIONS
Serious cardiac, renal, or hepatic dysfunction, men with carcinomas of the breast or prostate, hypersensitivity to fluoxymesterone or any component of the formulation including tartrazine
Caution
Diabetes mellitus, CV disease, MI

DRUG INTERACTIONS OF CONCERN TO DENTISTRY
* Edema: corticosteroids

SERIOUS REACTIONS
! Peliosis hepatitis (liver, spleen replaced with blood-filled cysts), hepatic neoplasms, and hepatocellular carcinoma have been associated with prolonged high dosage.

DENTAL CONSIDERATIONS
General:
* Monitor vital signs at every appointment because of cardiovascular side effects.
* Patients receiving chemotherapy may require palliative treatment for stomatitis.
Teach Patient/Family to:
* Use effective oral hygiene to prevent soft tissue inflammation
* Prevent trauma when using oral hygiene aids

fluphenazine decanoate
floo-fen′-ah-zeen
(Apo-Fluphenazie[CAN], Modecate[AUS], Prolixin); fluphenazine enanthate (Moditen[CAN], Prolixin); fluphenazine hydrochloride (Prolixin, Permitil)

CATEGORY AND SCHEDULE
Pregnancy Risk Category: C

Drug Class: Phenothiazine antipsychotic

MECHANISM OF ACTION
A phenothiazine that blocks dopamine at postsynaptic receptor sites. Possesses weak anticholinergic, sedative and entimetic effects and strong extrapyramidal activity. *Therapeutic Effect:* Decreases psychotic behavior.

USES
Treatment of psychotic disorders, schizophrenia

PHARMACOKINETICS
Erratic and variable absorption from the GI tract. Widely distributed. Metabolized in liver. Primarily excreted in urine. *Half-life:* 16.3-23.2 hr.

INDICATIONS AND DOSAGES
▸ Psychotic Disorders
PO
Adults. Initially, 0.5–10 mg/day fluphenazine HCl in divided doses q6–8h. Increase gradually until therapeutic response is achieved (usually under 20 mg daily); decrease gradually to maintenance level (1–5 mg/day).
Elderly. Initially, 1–2.5 mg/day.
IM
Adults. Initially, 1.25 mg, followed by 2.5–10 mg/day in divided doses q6–8h.
▸ Chronic Schizophrenic Disorder
IM
Adults. Initially, 12.5–25 mg of fluphenazine decanoate q1–6wk, or 25 mg fluphenazine enanthate q2wk.
▸ Usual Elderly Dosage (nonpsychotic)
PO
Initially, 1–2.5 mg/day. May increase by 1–2.5 mg/day q4–7 days. Maximum: 20 mg/day.

SIDE EFFECTS/ADVERSE REACTIONS
Frequent
Hypotension, dizziness, and fainting occur frequently after first injection,

occasionally after subsequent injections, and rarely with oral dosage

Occasional
Drowsiness during early therapy, dry mouth, blurred vision, lethargy, constipation or diarrhea, nasal congestion, peripheral edema, urinary retention

Rare
Ocular changes, skin pigmentation (those on high doses for prolonged periods)

PRECAUTIONS AND CONTRAINDICATIONS
Severe CNS depression, comatose states, severe cardiovascular disease, bone marrow depression, subcortical brain damage, hypersensitivity to fluphenazine or any component of the formulation including tartrazine

Caution
lactation, seizure disorders, hypertension, hepatic disease, cardiac disease

DRUG INTERACTIONS OF CONCERN TO DENTISTRY
• Increased sedation: other CNS depressants, alcohol, barbiturate anesthetics, opioid analgesics
• Hypotension, tachycardia: epinephrine
• Increased extrapyramidal effects: phenothiazines and related drugs (haloperidol, droperidol), metoclopramide
• Additive photosensitization: tetracyclines
• Increased anticholinergic effects: anticholinergics

SERIOUS REACTIONS
! Extrapyramidal symptoms appear dose related (particularly high dosage), divided into 3 categories: akathisia (inability to sit still, tapping of feet, urge to move around); parkinsonian symptoms (mask-like face, tremors, shuffling gait, hypersalivation); and acute dystonias: torticollis (neck muscle spasm), opisthotonos (rigidity of back muscles), and oculogyric crisis (rolling back of eyes).
! Dystonic reaction may also produce profuse sweating, and pallor.
! Tardive dyskinesia (protrusion of tongue, puffing of cheeks, chewing/puckering of the mouth) occurs rarely (may be irreversible).
! Abrupt withdrawal after long-term therapy may precipitate nausea, vomiting, gastritis, dizziness, and tremors.
! Blood dyscrasias, particularly agranulocytosis, or mild leukopenia (sore mouth/gums/throat) may occur.
! May lower seizure threshold.

DENTAL CONSIDERATIONS
General:
• Monitor vital signs at every appointment because of cardiovascular side effects.
• Patients on chronic drug therapy may rarely have symptoms of blood dyscrasias, which can include infection, bleeding, and poor healing.
• After supine positioning, have patient sit upright for at least 2 min before standing to avoid orthostatic hypotension.
• Assess salivary flow as a factor in caries, periodontal disease, and candidiasis.
• Avoid dental light in patient's eyes; offer dark glasses for patient comfort.
• Assess for presence of extrapyramidal motor symptoms, such as tardive dyskinesia and akathisia. Extrapyramidal motor activity may complicate dental treatment.

• Geriatric patients are more susceptible to drug effects; use a lower dose.
• Use vasoconstrictors with caution, in low doses, and with careful aspiration.
Consultations:
• In a patient with symptoms of blood dyscrasias, request a medical consultation for blood studies and postpone dental treatment until normal values are reestablished.
• Take precautions if dental surgery is anticipated and anesthesia is required.
• If signs of tardive dyskinesia or akathisia are present, refer to physician.
• Physician should be informed if significant xerostomic side effects occur (e.g., increased caries, sore tongue, problems eating or swallowing, difficulty wearing prosthesis) so that a medication change can be considered.
Teach Patient/Family to:
• Use effective oral hygiene to prevent soft tissue inflammation
• Prevent injury when using oral hygiene aids
• Use electric tooth brush if patient has difficulty holding conventional devices
• When chronic dry mouth occurs, advise patient to:
  • Avoid mouth rinses with high alcohol content because of drying effects
  • Use daily home fluoride products for anticaries effect
  • Use sugarless gum, frequent sips of water, or saliva substitutes

flurandrenolide
flure-an-dren´-oh-lide
(Cordran, Cordran SP)

CATEGORY AND SCHEDULE
Pregnancy Risk Category: C

Drug Class: Topical corticosteroid, group III medium potency

MECHANISM OF ACTION
A fluorinated orticosteroid that decreases inflammation by suppressing the migration of polymorphonuclear leukocytes and reversal of increased capillary permeability. **Therapeutic Effect:** Decreases tissue response to inflammatory process.

USES
Treatment of corticosteroid-responsive dermatoses, pruritus

PHARMACOKINETICS
Repeated applications may lead to percutaneous absorption. Absorption is about 36% from scrotal area, 7% from the forehead, 4% from scalp, and 1% from forearm. Metabolized in liver. Excreted in urine.
Half-life: Unknown.

INDICATIONS AND DOSAGES
▶ **Antiinflammatory, Immunosuppressant, Corticosteroid Replacement Therapy**
Topical
Adults, Elderly. Apply 2–3 times a day.
Children. Apply 1–2 times a day.

SIDE EFFECTS/ADVERSE REACTIONS
Occasional
Itching, dry skin, folliculitis

Rare
Intracranial hemorrhage, acne, striae, miliaria, allergic contact dermatitis, telangiectasis or raised dark red spots on skin

PRECAUTIONS AND CONTRAINDICATIONS

Hypersensitivity to flurandrenolide or any component of the formulation, viral, fungal, or tubercular skin lesions
Caution
Lactation, viral infections, bacterial infections

DRUG INTERACTIONS OF CONCERN TO DENTISTRY

• None reported

SERIOUS REACTIONS

! When taken in excessive quantities, systemic hypercorticism and adrenal suppression may occur.

DENTAL CONSIDERATIONS

General:
• Determine why the patient is taking the drug.
• Apply lubricant to dry lips for patient comfort before dental procedures.
• Place on frequent recall to evaluate healing response when used on chronic basis.

flurazepam hydrochloride

flure-az´-eh-pam hi-droh-klor´-ide
(Apo-Flurazepam[can], Dalmane)
Do not confuse Dalmane with Dialume.

CATEGORY AND SCHEDULE

Pregnancy Risk Category: X
Controlled Substance: Schedule IV

Drug Class: Benzodiazepine, sedative-hypnotic

MECHANISM OF ACTION

A benzodiazepine that enhances action of inhibitory neurotransmitter gamma-aminobutyric acid (GABA). ***Therapeutic Effect:*** Produces hypnotic effect due to CNS depression.

USES

Treatment of insomnia

PHARMACOKINETICS

Route	Onset	Peak	Duration
PO	15–20 min	3–6 hr	7–8 hr

Well absorbed from the GI tract. Protein binding: 97%. Crosses the blood-brain barrier. Widely distributed. Metabolized in liver to active metabolite. Primarily excreted in urine. Not removed by hemodialysis. ***Half-life:*** 2.3 hr; metabolite: 40–114 hr.

INDICATIONS AND DOSAGES

▸ **Insomnia**
PO
Adults. 15–30 mg at bedtime.
Elderly, debilitated, liver disease, low serum albumin, Children 15 yr and older. 15 mg at bedtime.

SIDE EFFECTS/ADVERSE REACTIONS

Frequent
Drowsiness, dizziness, ataxia, sedation
Morning drowsiness may occur initially.
Occasional
GI disturbances, nervousness, blurred vision, dry mouth, headache, confusion, skin rash, irritability, slurred speech
Rare
Paradoxical CNS excitement or restlessness, particularly noted in elderly or debilitated

PRECAUTIONS AND CONTRAINDICATIONS
Acute alcohol intoxication, acute angle-closure glaucoma, pregnancy or breast-feeding
Caution
Anemia, hepatic disease, renal disease, suicidal individuals, drug abuse, elderly, psychosis, children younger than 15 yr

DRUG INTERACTIONS OF CONCERN TO DENTISTRY
• Increased sedation: alcohol, CNS depressants
• Increased serum levels and prolonged effect of benzodiazepines: ketoconazole, itraconazole, fluconazole, miconazole (systemic), indinavir
• Contraindicated with saquinavir
• Possible increase in CNS side effects: kava kava (herb)

SERIOUS REACTIONS
! Abrupt or too-rapid withdrawal after long-term use may result in pronounced restlessness and irritability, insomnia, hand tremors, abdominal or muscle cramps, vomiting, diaphoresis, and seizures.
! Overdose results in somnolence, confusion, diminished reflexes, and coma.

DENTAL CONSIDERATIONS
General:
• Assess salivary flow as a factor in caries, periodontal disease, and candidiasis.
• Psychologic and physical dependence may occur with chronic administration.
• Geriatric patients are more susceptible to drug effects; use lower dose.
Consultations:
• Medical consultation may be required to assess disease control.
Teach Patient/Family to:
• Avoid mouth rinses with high alcohol content because of drying effects

flurbiprofen
flure-bi´-proe-fen
(Ansaid, Froben[CAN], Ocufen, Strepfen[AUS])
Do not confuse Ocufen with Ocuflox.

CATEGORY AND SCHEDULE
Pregnancy Risk Category: B
(D if used in third trimester or near delivery; C for ophthalmic solution)

Drug Class: Nonsteroidal antiinflammatory

MECHANISM OF ACTION
A phenylalkanoic acid that produces analgesic and antiinflammatory effect by inhibiting prostaglandin synthesis. Also relaxes the iris sphincter. *Therapeutic Effect:* Reduces the inflammatory response and intensity of pain. Prevents or decreases miosis during cataract surgery.

USES
Acute, long-term treatment of rheumatoid arthritis, osteoarthritis

PHARMACOKINETICS
Well absorbed from the GI tract; ophthalmic solution penetrates cornea after administration, and may be systemically absorbed. Protein binding: 99%. Widely distributed. Metabolized in the liver. Primarily excreted in urine. *Half-life:* 3–4 hr.

INDICATIONS AND DOSAGES
▶ **Rheumatoid Arthritis, Osteoarthritis**
PO
Adults, Elderly. 200–300 mg/day in 2–4 divided doses. Maximum: 100 mg/dose or 300 mg/day.

▶ **Dysmenorrhea, Pain**
PO
Adults. 50 mg 4 times a day
▶ **Usual Ophthalmic Dosage**
Adults, Elderly, Children. Apply
1 drop q30min starting 2 hr before
surgery for total of 4 doses.

SIDE EFFECTS/ADVERSE REACTIONS
Occasional
PO: Headache, abdominal pain,
diarrhea, indigestion, nausea, fluid
retention
Ophthalmic: Burning or stinging on
instillation, keratitis, elevated
intraocular pressure
Rare
PO: Blurred vision, flushed skin,
dizziness, somnolence, nervousness,
insomnia, unusual fatigue,
constipation, decreased appetite,
vomiting, confusion

PRECAUTIONS AND CONTRAINDICATIONS
Active peptic ulcer, chronic
inflammation of GI tract, GI bleeding
or ulceration, history of
hypersensitivity to aspirin or
NSAIDs
Caution
Lactation, children, bleeding
disorders, GI disorders, cardiac
disorders, severe renal disease,
severe hepatic disease

DRUG INTERACTIONS OF CONCERN TO DENTISTRY
• GI ulceration, bleeding: aspirin,
alcohol, corticosteroids
• Decreased action: salicylates
• Nephrotoxicity: acetaminophen
(prolonged use)
• When prescribed for dental pain:
   • Risk of increased effects: oral
   anticoagulants, oral antidiabetics,
   lithium, methotrexate
   • Decreased effects of diuretics

• First-time users of SSRIs also
taking NSAIDs may have a higher
risk of GI side effects; until more
data are available, it may be
advisable to avoid use of NSAIDs
in these patients (Br J Clin
Pharmacol 55:591–595, 2003)

SERIOUS REACTIONS
! Overdose may result in acute renal
failure.
! Rare reactions with long-term use
include peptic ulcer disease, GI
bleeding, gastritis, severe hepatic
reaction (jaundice), nephrotoxicity
(hematuria, dysuria, proteinuria), a
severe hypersensitivity reaction
(angioedema, bronchospasm), and
cardiac arrhythmias.

DENTAL CONSIDERATIONS
General:
• Patients on chronic drug therapy
may rarely have symptoms of blood
dyscrasias, which can include
infection, bleeding, and poor healing.
• Assess salivary flow as a factor in
caries, periodontal disease, and
candidiasis.
• Avoid prescribing for dental use in
last trimester of pregnancy.
• Avoid prescribing aspirin-
containing products.
• Consider semisupine chair position
for patients with arthritic disease.
Consultations:
• Medical consultation may be
required to assess disease control.
• In a patient with symptoms of
blood dyscrasias, request a medical
consultation for blood studies and
postpone dental treatment until
normal values are reestablished.
Teach Patient/Family to:
• Use effective oral hygiene to
prevent soft tissue inflammation
• Prevent injury when using oral
hygiene aids

- When chronic dry mouth occurs, advise patient to:
  - Avoid mouth rinses with high alcohol content because of drying effects
  - Use daily home fluoride products for anticaries effect
  - Use sugarless gum, frequent sips of water, or saliva substitutes

Flurbiprofen Sodium
General:
- Avoid dental light in patient's eyes; offer dark glasses for patient comfort.

flutamide
flew´-tah-myd
(Euflex[CAN], Eulexin, Flugerel[AUS], Flutamin[AUS], Fugerel[AUS], Novo-Flutamide[CAN])
Do not confuse flutamide with Flumadine.

CATEGORY AND SCHEDULE
Pregnancy Risk Category: D

Drug Class: Antineoplastic

MECHANISM OF ACTION
An antiandrogen hormone that inhibits androgen uptake and prevents androgen from binding to androgen receptors in target tissue. Used in conjuction with leuprolide to inhibit the stimulant effects of flutamide on serum testosterone levels.
Therapeutic Effect: Suppresses testicular androgen production and decreases growth of prostate carcinoma.

USES
Treatment of metastatic prostatic carcinoma, stage D2; early-stage prostate cancer, stages B2 and C, in combination with LHRH agonistic analogs (leuprolide) and radiation

PHARMACOKINETICS
Completely absorbed from the GI tract. Protein binding: 94%–96%. Metabolized in the liver to active metabolite. Primarily excreted in urine. Not removed by hemodialysis. *Half-life:* 6 hr (increased in elderly).

INDICATIONS AND DOSAGES
▶ **Prostatic Carcinoma (in combination with leuprolide)**
PO
Adults, Elderly. 250 mg q8h.

SIDE EFFECTS/ADVERSE REACTIONS
Frequent
Hot flashes; decreased libido, diarrhea; generalized pain; asthenia; constipation; nausea, nocturia
Occasional
Dizziness, paresthesia, insomnia, impotence, peripheral edema, gynecomastia
Rare
Rash, diaphoresis, hypertension, hematuria, vomiting, urinary incontinence, headache, flu-like syndromes, photosensitivity

PRECAUTIONS AND CONTRAINDICATIONS
Severe hepatic impairment
Caution
Liver toxicity, monitoring requirements for hepatic injury, women

SERIOUS REACTIONS
❗ Hepatoxicity, including hepatic encephalopathy, and hemolytic anemia may be noted.

DENTAL CONSIDERATIONS

General:

• Possible increase in adverse cardiovascular events in patients at risk for thromboembolism.

• Talk with patient about any pain medication being taken.

• Avoid drugs (anticholinergics) that could exacerbate urinary retention (if present).

fluticasone propionate

flu-tic´-ah-zone proh´-pee-uh-neyt
(Beconase Allergy 24 Hour[AUS], Beconase Hayfever[AUS], Cutivate, Flixotide Disks[AUS], Flixotide Inhaler[AUS], Flonase, Flovent, Flovent Diskus, Flovent HFA)

CATEGORY AND SCHEDULE

Pregnancy Risk Category: C

Drug Class: Synthetic corticosteroid, medium potency

MECHANISM OF ACTION

A corticosteroid that controls the rate of protein synthesis, depresses migration of polymorphonuclear leukocytes, reverses capillary permeability, and stabilizes lysosomal membranes. **Therapeutic Effect:** Prevents or controls inflammation.

USES

Nasal spray: Management of nasal symptoms of seasonal and perennial allergic and nonallergic rhinitis in adults and pediatric patient 4 yr and older
Oral: inhalation: For maintenance treatment of asthma as prophylactic therapy; also indicated for patients requiring oral glucocorticoid therapy

PHARMACOKINETICS

Inhalation/intranasal: Protein binding: 91%. Undergoes extensive first-pass metabolism in liver. Excreted in urine. **Half-life:** 3–7.8 hr.
Topical: Amount absorbed depends on affected area and skin condition (absorption increased with fever, hydration, inflamed or denuded skin).

INDICATIONS AND DOSAGES

▶ **Allergic Rhinitis**

Intranasal

Adults, Elderly. Initially, 200 mcg (2 sprays in each nostril once daily or 1 spray in each nostril q12h). Maintenance: 1 spray in each nostril once daily. Maximum: 200 mcg/day. *Children 4 yr and older.* Initially, 100 mcg (1 spray in each nostril once daily). Maximum: 200 mcg/day.

▶ **Relief of Inflammation and Pruritus Associated with Steroid-Responsive Disorders, Such as Contact Dermatitis and Eczema**

Topical

Adults, Elderly, Children 3 mo and older. Apply sparingly to affected area once or twice a day.

▶ **Maintenance Treatment for Asthma for Those Previously Treated with Bronchodilators**

Inhalation Powder (Flovent Diskus)
Adults, Elderly, Children 12 yr and older. Initially, 100 mcg q12h. Maximum: 500 mcg/day.
Inhalation (Oral [Flovent])
Adults, Elderly, Children 12 yr and older. 88 mcg twice a day. Maximum: 440 mcg twice a day.

▶ **Maintenance Treatment for Asthma for Those Previously Treated with Inhaled Steroids**

Inhalation Powder (Flovent Diskus)
Adults, Elderly, Children 12 yr and older. Initially, 100–250 mcg q12h. Maximum: 500 mcg q12h.
Inhalation (Oral [Flovent])

Adults, Elderly, Children 12 yr and older. 88–220 mcg twice a day. Maximum: 440 mcg twice a day.
▶ **Maintenance Treatment for Asthma for Those Previously Treated with Oral Steroids**
Inhalation Powder (Flovent Diskus)
Adults, Elderly, Children 12 yr and older. 500–1000 mcg twice a day.
Inhalation (Oral [Flovent])
Adults, Elderly, Children 12 yr and older. 880 mcg twice a day.

SIDE EFFECTS/ADVERSE REACTIONS

Frequent
Inhalation: Throat irritation, hoarseness, dry mouth, cough, temporary wheezing, oropharyngeal candidiasis (particularly if mouth is not rinsed with water after each administration)
Intranasal: Mild nasopharyngeal irritation; nasal burning, stinging, or dryness; rebound congestion; rhinorrhea; loss of taste
Occasional
Inhalation: Oral candidiasis
Intranasal: Nasal and pharyngeal candidiasis, headache
Topical: Skin burning, pruritus

PRECAUTIONS AND CONTRAINDICATIONS

Primary treatment of status asthmaticus or other acute asthma episodes (inhalation); untreated localized infection of nasal mucosa
Caution
Suppression of hypothalamic-pituitary-adrenal axis, warning of manifestation of HPA suppression when switching drug from oral to inhaled steroids, suppression of growth in children younger than 4 yr; use is restricted for some dose forms to children older than 12 yr; lactation

DRUG INTERACTIONS OF CONCERN TO DENTISTRY

● No specific interactions reported, but use CYP3A4 inhibitors with caution

SERIOUS REACTIONS

! Deaths due to adrenal insufficiency have occurred in asthma patients during and after transfer from use of long-term systemic corticosteroids to less systemically available inhaled corticosteroids.

DENTAL CONSIDERATIONS

General:
● Examine oral cavity for evidence of opportunistic candidiasis in patients using the inhaler.
● Allergic rhinitis may be a factor in mouth breathing and drying of oral tissues.
● Be aware that aspirin or sulfite preservatives in vasoconstrictor-containing products can exacerbate asthma.
● Acute asthmatic episodes may be precipitated in the dental office. Rapid-acting sympathomimetic inhalants should be available for emergency use. A stress reduction protocol may be required.
● Consider semisupine chair position for patients with respiratory disease.
Consultations:
● Consultation may be required to confirm steroid dose and duration of use.
Teach Patient/Family to:
● Update health and drug history if physician makes any changes in drug regimens
● Gargle, rinse mouth with water, and expectorate after each aerosol use

Fluticasone propionate

Teach Patient/Family to:
● Avoid use of topical preparations on fungal or herpetic lesions

fluvastatin

floo´-va-sta-tin
(Lescol, Lescol XL, Vastin[aus])
Do not confuse fluvastatin with
fluoxetine.

CATEGORY AND SCHEDULE

Pregnancy Risk Category: X

Drug Class: Cholesterol-
lowering agent, antihyperlipidemic

MECHANISM OF ACTION

An antihyperlipidemic that
inhibits HMG-CoA reductase, the
enzyme that catalyzes the early step
in cholesterol synthesis.
Therapeutic Effect: Decreases
low-density lipoproteins (LDL)
cholesterol, very low-density
lipoproteins (VLDL), and
plasma triglyceride levels.
Slightly increases high-density
lipoproteins (HDL) cholesterol
concentration.

USES

As an adjunct in homozygous
familial hypercholesterolemia,
mixed hyperlipidemia, elevated
serum triglyceride levels and
type IV hyperproteinemia, also
reduces total cholesterol
LDL-C, apo B and triglyceride
levels; patient should first
be placed on cholesterol-
lowering diet; to reduce risk in
coronary artery revascularization
procedures; prevention of secondary
coronary events

PHARMACOKINETICS

Well absorbed from the GI tract
and is unaffected by food. Does
not cross the blood-brain barrier.
Protein binding: greater than 98%.
Primarily eliminated in feces. *Half-
life:* 1.2 hr.
Tablets (Extended-Release [Lescol
XL]): 80 mg.

INDICATIONS AND DOSAGES
▶ **Hyperlipoproteinemia**
PO
Adults, Elderly. Initially, 20 mg/day
(capsule) in the evening. May
increase up to 40 mg/day.
Maintenance: 20–40 mg/day in a
single dose or divided doses.
*Patients requiring more than a 25%
decrease in LDL cholesterol.* 40 mg
(capsule) 1–2 times a day, or 80 mg
tablet once a day.

SIDE EFFECTS/ADVERSE
REACTIONS
Frequent
Headache, dyspepsia, back pain,
myalgia, arthralgia, diarrhea,
abdominal cramping, rhinitis
Occasional
Nausea, vomiting, insomnia,
constipation, flatulence, rash,
pruritus, fatigue, cough,
dizziness

PRECAUTIONS AND
CONTRAINDICATIONS
Active hepatic disease, unexplained
increased serum transaminase
levels
Caution
Liver dysfunction; alcoholism;
severe acute infection; metabolic,
endocrine, or electrolyte disorders;
uncontrolled seizures; alterations in
liver function tests may be observed
with use

DRUG INTERACTIONS OF
CONCERN TO DENTISTRY
• Increased plasma levels: alcohol,
fluconazole, itraconazole,
ketoconazole, erythromycin

SERIOUS REACTIONS

! Myositis (inflammation of voluntary muscle) with or without increased CK, and muscle weakness, occur rarely. These conditions may progress to frank rhabdomyolysis and renal impairment.

DENTAL CONSIDERATIONS
General:
• Consider semisupine chair position for patient comfort because of GI, musculoskeletal, and respiratory side effects.

fluvoxamine maleate
floo-vox´-ah-meen mal-ee-ate
(Faverin[AUS], Luvox)

CATEGORY AND SCHEDULE
Pregnancy Risk Category: C

Drug Class: Selective serotonin reuptake inhibitor, antidepressant

MECHANISM OF ACTION

An antidepressant and antiobsessive agent that selectively inhibits neuronal reuptake of serotonin.
Therapeutic Effect: Relieves depression and symptoms of obsessive-compulsive disorder.

USES

Obsessive-compulsive disorder and panic disorder

PHARMACOKINETICS

PO: Rapid absorption, peak plasma levels 5 hr; plasma protein binding 77%; hepatic metabolism; urinary excretion.

INDICATIONS AND DOSAGES
▶ **Obsessive-Compulsive Disorder**
PO
Adults. 50 mg at bedtime; may increase by 50 mg every 4–7 days. Dosages greater than 100 mg/day given in 2 divided doses. Maximum: 300 mg/day.
Children 8–17 yr. 25 mg at bedtime; may increase by 25 mg every 4–7 days. Dosages greater than 50 mg/day given in 2 divided doses. Maximum: 200 mg/day.

SIDE EFFECTS/ADVERSE REACTIONS
Frequent
Nausea, headache, somnolence, insomnia
Occasional
Dizziness, diarrhea, dry mouth, asthenia, weakness, dyspepsia, constipation, abnormal ejaculation
Rare
Anorexia, anxiety, tremors, vomiting, flatulence, urinary frequency, sexual dysfunction, altered taste

PRECAUTIONS AND CONTRAINDICATIONS
Use within 14 days of MAOIs
Caution
Lactation, renal and hepatic impairment, epilepsy, elderly

DRUG INTERACTIONS OF CONCERN TO DENTISTRY
• Increased plasma levels of tricyclic antidepressants, carbamazepine, benzodiazepine; reduce doses of alprazolam, diazepam, midazolam, triazolam by half
• Risk of serotonin syndrome: SSRIs
• First-time users of SSRIs also taking NSAIDs may have a higher risk of GI side effects; until

more data are available, it may be advisable to avoid use of NSAIDs in these patients (Br J Clin Pharmacol 55: 591–595, 2003)

SERIOUS REACTIONS

! Overdose may produce seizures, nausea, vomiting, and extreme agitation and restlessness.

DENTAL CONSIDERATIONS

General:
• After supine positioning, have patient sit upright for at least 2 min to avoid orthostatic hypotension.
• Assess salivary flow as a factor in caries, periodontal disease, and candidiasis.
• Consider semisupine chair position for patient comfort because of GI effects of drug.

Consultations:
• Medical consultation may be required to assess patient's ability to tolerate stress.
• Physician should be informed if significant xerostomic side effects occur (e.g., increased caries, sore tongue, problems eating or swallowing, difficulty wearing prosthesis) so that a medication change can be considered.

Teach Patient/Family:
• When chronic dry mouth occurs, advise patient to:
  • Avoid mouth rinses with high alcohol content because of drying effects
  • Use daily home fluoride products for anticaries effect
  • Use sugarless gum, frequent sips of water, or saliva substitutes

folic acid/sodium folate (vitamin B9)

foe´-lik ass´-id/soe´-dee-um foe´-late
folic acid
(Apo-Folic[CAN], Folvite, Megafol[AUS])
sodium folate
(Folvite-parenteral)
Do not confuse Folvite with Florvite.

CATEGORY AND SCHEDULE

Pregnancy Risk Category: A (C if used in doses above the recommended daily allowance)
OTC (0.4-mg and 0.8-mg tablets only)

Drug Class: Water-soluble B vitamin

MECHANISM OF ACTION

A coenzyme that stimulates production of platelets, RBCs, and WBCs. *Therapeutic Effect:* Essential for nucleoprotein synthesis and maintenance of normal erythropoiesis.

USES

Treatment of megaloblastic or macrocytic anemia caused by folic acid deficiency, liver disease, alcoholism, hemolysis, intestinal obstruction, pregnancy

PHARMACOKINETICS

PO form almost completely absorbed from the GI tract (upper duodenum). Protein binding: High. Metabolized in the liver and plasma to active form. Excreted in urine. Removed by hemodialysis.

INDICATIONS AND DOSAGES
▸ **Vitamin B9 Deficiency**
PO, IV, IM, Subcutaneous
Adults, Elderly, Children 12 yr and older. Initially, 1 mg/day.
Maintenance: 0.5 mg/day.
Children 1–11 yr. Initially
1 mg/day. Maintenance:
0.1–0.4 mg/day.
Infants. 50 mcg/day.
▸ **Dietary Supplement**
PO, IV, IM, Subcutaneous
Adults, Elderly, Children 4 yr and older. 0.4 mg/day.
Children 1–younger than 4 yr.
0.3 mg/day.
Children younger than 1 yr.
0.1 mg/day.
Pregnant women. 0.8 mg/day.

SIDE EFFECTS/ADVERSE REACTIONS
None known

PRECAUTIONS AND CONTRAINDICATIONS
Anemias (aplastic, normocytic, pernicious, refractory)

DRUG INTERACTIONS OF CONCERN TO DENTISTRY
• Increased metabolism of phenobarbital

SERIOUS REACTIONS
! Allergic hypersensitivity occurs rarely with parenteral form. Oral folic acid is nontoxic.

DENTAL CONSIDERATIONS
General:
• Deficiency in folic acid; glossitis may be a symptom of folic acid deficiency.

fondaparinux sodium
fawn-da-pear´-ih-nux soe´-dee-um
(Arixtra)

CATEGORY AND SCHEDULE
Pregnancy Risk Category: B

Drug Class: Synthetic anticoagulant

MECHANISM OF ACTION
A factor Xα inhibitor and pentasaccharide that selectively binds to antithrombin, and increases its affinity for factor Xα, thereby inhibiting factor Xα and stopping the blood coagulation cascade.
Therapeutic Effect: Indirectly prevents formation of thrombin and subsequently the fibrin clot.

USES
Prophylaxis of deep vein thrombosis (DVT) in patients undergoing hip fracture surgery, hip replacement surgery, or knee replacement surgery

PHARMACOKINETICS
Well absorbed after subcutaneous administration. Undergoes minimal, if any, metabolism. Highly bound to antithrombin III. Distributed mainly in blood and to a minor extent in extravascular fluid. Excreted unchanged in urine. Removed by hemodialysis. *Half-life:* 17–21 hr (prolonged in patients with impaired renal function).

INDICATIONS AND DOSAGES
▸ **Prevention of Venous Thromboembolism**
Subcutaneous
Adults. 2.5 mg once a day for 5–9 days after surgery. Initial dose should be given 6–8 hr after surgery.

Dosage should be adjusted in the elderly and in those with renal impairment.

SIDE EFFECTS/ADVERSE REACTIONS
Occasional
Fever
Rare
Injection site hematoma, nausea, peripheral edema

PRECAUTIONS AND CONTRAINDICATIONS
Active major bleeding, bacterial endocarditis, severe renal impairment (with creatinine clearance less than 30 ml/min), thrombocytopenia associated with antiplatelet antibody formation in the presence of fondaparinux, body weight less than 50 kg
Caution
Neuroaxial (spinal/ epidural) anesthesia, avoid IM use, anticoagulant effects persist for 2–4 days after administration, elderly patients, no data available for nursing mothers, use in children has not been established

DRUG INTERACTIONS OF CONCERN TO DENTISTRY
• Avoid concurrent use of aspirin and NSAIDs

SERIOUS REACTIONS
! Accidental overdose may lead to bleeding complications ranging from local ecchymoses to major hemorrhage.
! Thrombocytopenia occurs rarely.

DENTAL CONSIDERATIONS
General:
• Determine why patient is taking the drug.

• Monitor vital signs at every appointment because of cardiovascular side effects.
• Consider local hemostasis measures to prevent excessive bleeding.
• Antibiotic prophylaxis before dental treatment may be required for joint prosthesis (see 2003 ADA guidelines).
• Delay elective dental treatment until patient completes anticoagulant therapy.
Consultations:
• Medical consultation should include routine blood counts, including platelet counts and bleeding time.
Teach Patient/Family to:
• Use effective oral hygiene to prevent soft tissue inflammation, infection
• Prevent injury when using oral hygiene aids
• Report oral lesions, soreness, or bleeding to dentist

formoterol fumarate
for-moe´-ter-ol fyoo´-muh-reyt
(Foradil Aerolizer, Foradile[AUS], Oxis[AUS])

CATEGORY AND SCHEDULE
Pregnancy Risk Category: C

Drug Class: Selective β_2-adrenergic bronchodilator

MECHANISM OF ACTION
A long-acting bronchodilator that stimulates β_2-adrenergic receptors in the lungs, resulting in relaxation of bronchial smooth muscle. Also inhibits release of mediators from various cells in the lungs, including mast cells, with little effect on heart rate.

Therapeutic Effect: Relieves bronchospasm, reduces airway resistance. Improves bronchodilation, nighttime asthma control, and peak flow rates.

USES

Long-term treatment of asthma and prevention of bronchospasm in adults and children older than 5 yr; prevention of exercise-induced bronchospasm in adults and children older than 12 yr; maintenance treatment of COPD

PHARMACOKINETICS

Route	Onset	Peak	Duration
Inhalation	1–3 min	0.5–1 hr	12 hr

Absorbed from bronchi after inhalation. Metabolized in the liver. Primarily excreted in urine. Unknown if removed by hemodialysis. *Half-life:* 10 hr.

INDICATIONS AND DOSAGES
▶ **Asthma, COPD**
Inhalation
Adults, Elderly, Children 5 yr and older. 12 mcg capsule q12h.
▶ **Exercise-Induced Bronchospasm**
Inhalation
Adults, Elderly, Children 5 yr and older. 12 mcg capsule at least 15 min before exercise. Do not repeat for another 12 hr.

SIDE EFFECTS/ADVERSE REACTIONS
Occasional
Tremors, muscle cramps, tachycardia, insomnia, headache, irritability, irritation of mouth or throat

PRECAUTIONS AND CONTRAINDICATIONS
Hypersensitivity

Caution
Not for acute asthma symptoms, not for use in life-threatening situations; paradoxic bronchospasm may occur with use; not a substitute for corticosteroids; cardiovascular disease (coronary insufficiency, cardiac arrhythmias, hypertension), hyperthyroidism, seizures, hypokalemia, lactation

DRUG INTERACTIONS OF CONCERN TO DENTISTRY
• Avoid MAOIs, tricyclic antidepressants, and drugs that prolong the QT interval (phenothiazines, procainamide)
• Adrenergic agents/ sympathomimetics may potentiate effects
• β-Adrenergic blockers may antagonize sympathomimetic effects

SERIOUS REACTIONS
! Excessive sympathomimetic stimulation may produce palpitations, extrasystole, and chest pain.

DENTAL CONSIDERATIONS
General:
• Monitor vital signs at every appointment because of cardiovascular side effects.
• Assess salivary flow as a factor in caries, periodontal disease, and candidiasis.
• Consider semisupine chair position for patient comfort because of respiratory side effects of disease.
• Short midday appointments and a stress reduction protocol may be required for anxious patients.
• Have patient bring personal short-acting bronchodilator to appointment for use in emergency.
• Acute asthmatic episodes may be precipitated in the dental office.

Rapid-acting sympathomimetic inhalants should be available for emergency use.
• Avoid prescribing aspirin-containing products.

Consultations:
• Medical consultation may be required to assess disease control and patient's ability to tolerate stress.

Teach Patient/Family to:
• Gargle, rinse mouth with water, and expectorate after each aerosol dose
• When chronic dry mouth occurs, advise patient to:
  • Avoid mouth rinses with high alcohol content because of drying effects
  • Use daily home fluoride products for anticaries effect
  • Use sugarless gum, frequent sips of water, or saliva substitutes

fosamprenavir
foss-am-pren´-ah-vur
(Lexiva)

CATEGORY AND SCHEDULE
Pregnancy Risk Category: C

Drug Class: Antiretroviral; protease inhibitor

MECHANISM OF ACTION
An antiretroviral that is rapidly converted to amprenavir, which inhibits HIV-1 protease by binding to the enzyme's active site, thus preventing the processing of viral precursors and resulting in the formation of immature, noninfectious viral particles. *Therapeutic Effect:* Impairs HIV replication and proliferation.

USES
Treatment of HIV-1 infection in combination with antiretrovirals

PHARMACOKINETICS
Rapidly absorbed after PO administration. Protein binding: 90%. Metabolized in the liver. Excreted in urine and feces. *Half-life:* 7.7 hr.

INDICATIONS AND DOSAGES
▸ **HIV Infection in Patients Who Have Not Had Previous Protease Inhibitor Therapy**
PO
Adults, Elderly. 1400 mg twice daily without ritonavir; or 1400 mg twice daily plus ritonavir 200 mg once daily; or 700 mg twice daily plus ritonavir 100 mg twice daily.
▸ **HIV Infection in Patients Who Have Had Previous Protease Inhibitor Therapy**
PO
Adults, Elderly. 700 mg twice daily plus ritonavir 100 mg twice daily.
▸ **Concurrent Therapy with Efavirenz**
PO
Adults, Elderly. In patients receiving fosamprenavir plus once-daily ritonavir in combination with efavirenz, an additional 100 mg/day ritonavir (300 mg total/day) should be given.

SIDE EFFECTS/ADVERSE REACTIONS
Frequent
Nausea, rash, diarrhea
Occasional
Headache, vomiting, fatigue, depression
Rare
Pruritus, abdominal pain, perioral paresthesia

PRECAUTIONS AND CONTRAINDICATIONS

Concurrent use of amprenavir, dihydroergotamine, ergonovine, ergotamine, methylergonovine, pimozide, midazolam, or triazolam. If fosamprenavir is given concurrently with ritonavir, flecainide and propafenone are also contraindicated.

DRUG INTERACTIONS OF CONCERN TO DENTISTRY

• Contraindicated with midazolam, triazolam
• Increased plasma levels of: tricyclic antidepressants, lidocaine, alprazolam, chlorazepate, diazepam, flurazepam, ketoconazole, itraconazole, sildenafil, vardenafil
• Reduced absorption: antacids, carbamazepine, phenobarbital, St. John's wort (herb).

SERIOUS REACTIONS

❗ Severe and possibly life-threatening dermatologic reactions occur rarely.

DENTAL CONSIDERATIONS

General:
• Caution significant drug interactions with drugs used in dentistry.
• Question patient about other drugs or herbals they may be taking.
• Patient on chronic drug therapy may rarely present with symptoms of blood dyscrasias, which can include infection, bleeding, and poor healing. If dyscrasia is present, caution patient to prevent oral tissue trauma when using oral hygiene aids.
• Consider semisupine chair position for patient comfort if GI side effects occur.
Consultations:
• In a patient with symptoms of blood dyscrasias, request a medical consultation for blood studies and postpone treatment until normal values are reestablished.
• Medical consultation may be required to assess disease control and patient's ability to tolerate stress.
Teach Patient/Family to:
• Use effective soft tissue inflammation
• Prevent trauma when using oral hygiene aids
• Update health and medication history if physician makes any changes in evaluation or drug regimens; include OTC, herbal, and nonherbal remedies in the update

---

foscarnet sodium
foss-car´-net soe´-dee-um
(Foscavir)

CATEGORY AND SCHEDULE
Pregnancy Risk Category: C

Drug Class: Antiviral

MECHANISM OF ACTION
An antiviral that selectively inhibits binding sites on virus-specific DNA polymerase and reverse transcriptase. **Therapeutic Effect:** Inhibits replication of herpes virus.

USES
Treatment of cytomegalovirus (CMV) retinitis in AIDS, acyclovirresistant herpes simplex I mucocutaneous diseases, and acyclovirresistant HSV in immunocompromised patients

PHARMACOKINETICS
Sequestered into bone and cartilage. Protein binding: 14%–17%. Primarily excreted unchanged in urine. Removed by hemodialysis. **Half-life:** 3.3–6.8 hr (increased in impaired renal function).

F

INDICATIONS AND DOSAGES
▶ **CMV Retinitis**
IV
Adults, Elderly. Initially, 60 mg/kg q8h or 100 mg/kg q12h for 2–3 wk. Maintenance: 90–120 mg/kg/day as a single IV infusion.
▶ **Herpes Infection**
IV
Adults. 40 mg/kg q8–12h for 2–3 wk or until healed.
▶ **Dosage in Renal Impairment**
Dosages are individualized on the basis of creatinine clearance. Refer to the dosing guide provided by the manufacturer.

SIDE EFFECTS/ADVERSE REACTIONS
Frequent
Fever, nausea, vomiting, diarrhea
Occasional
Anorexia, pain and inflammation at injection site, fever, rigors, malaise, headache, paresthesia, dizziness, rash, diaphoresis, abdominal pain
Rare
Back or chest pain, edema, flushing, pruritus, constipation, dry mouth

PRECAUTIONS AND CONTRAINDICATIONS
Hypersensitivity
Caution
Lactation, children, elderly, renal disease, seizure disorders, electrolyte/ mineral imbalances, severe anemia; monitor for renal impairment

DRUG INTERACTIONS OF CONCERN TO DENTISTRY
• Avoid nephrotoxic drugs (amphotericin B)
• Possible increased risk of seizures: fluoroquinolones

SERIOUS REACTIONS
❗ Nephrotoxicity occurs to some extent in most patients.
❗ Seizures and serum mineral or electrolyte imbalances may be life-threatening.

DENTAL CONSIDERATIONS
General:
• Examine for oral manifestations of opportunistic infections.
• Examine for evidence of oral manifestations of blood dyscrasias (infection, bleeding, poor healing).
• Consider local hemostasis measures to prevent excessive bleeding.
• Assess salivary flow as a factor in caries, periodontal disease, and candidiasis.
• Monitor vital signs at every appointment because of cardiovascular and respiratory side effects.
• Place on frequent recall to evaluate healing response.
Consultations:
• Medical consultation for blood studies (CBC); leukopenic or thrombocytopenic side effects may result in infection, delayed healing, and excessive bleeding. Postpone elective dental treatment until normal values are maintained.
• Medical consultation may be required to assess disease control.
Teach Patient/Family to:
• Use oral hygiene aids carefully to prevent injury
• See dentist immediately if secondary oral infection occurs
• Use effective oral hygiene to prevent soft tissue inflammation
• Use electric tooth brush if patient has difficulty holding conventional devices because of extrapyramidal side effects

• When chronic dry mouth occurs, advise patient to:
  • Avoid mouth rinses with high alcohol content because of drying effects
  • Use daily home fluoride products for anticaries effect
  • Use sugarless gum, frequent sips of water, or saliva substitutes

fosfomycin tromethamine

foss-fo-mye´-sin troe-meth´-a-mine (Monurol)
Do not confuse Monurol with Monopril.

CATEGORY AND SCHEDULE

Pregnancy Risk Category: B

Drug Class: Antiinfective (phosphonic acid derivative)

MECHANISM OF ACTION

An antibiotic that prevents bacterial cell wall formation by inhibiting the synthesis of peptidoglycan.
Therapeutic Effect: Bactericidal.

USES

Treatment of uncomplicated UTIs in women caused by susceptible strains of *E. coli* and *Enterococcus faecalis*

PHARMACOKINETICS

PO: Peak plasma levels after 2 hr; not plasma protein bound; widely distributed to GU tissues; excreted unchanged in urine and feces.

INDICATIONS AND DOSAGES
▸ **Uncomplicated UTIs**
PO
Females. 3 g mixed in 4 oz water as a single dose.
Males. 3 g/day for 2–3 days.

SIDE EFFECTS/ADVERSE REACTIONS

Occasional
Diarrhea, nausea, headache, back pain
Rare
Dysmenorrhea, pharyngitis, abdominal pain, rash

PRECAUTIONS AND CONTRAINDICATIONS

Hypersensitivity
Caution
Renal impairment, one dose per single episode of cystitis, lactation, children younger than 12 yr

DRUG INTERACTIONS OF CONCERN TO DENTISTRY

• Lowered serum concentrations: metoclopramide

SERIOUS REACTIONS

None known

DENTAL CONSIDERATIONS

General:
• Determine why patient is taking the drug.
• Consider semisupine chair position for patient comfort if GI side effects occur.
Teach Patient/Family:
• When chronic dry mouth occurs, advise patient to:
  • Avoid mouth rinses with high alcohol content because of drying effects
  • Use daily home fluoride products for anticaries effect
  • Use sugarless gum, frequent sips of water, or saliva substitutes

fosinopril
fo-sin´-oh-pril
(Monopril)
Do not confuse Monopril with
Monurol.

CATEGORY AND SCHEDULE
Pregnancy Risk Category: C
(D if used in second or third
trimester)

Drug Class: Angiotension-
converting enzyme (ACE) inhibitor

MECHANISM OF ACTION
An ACE inhibitor that suppresses the
renin-angiotensin-aldosterone system
and prevents conversion of
angiotensin I to angiotensin II, a
potent vasoconstrictor; may also
inhibit angiotensin II at local
vascular and renal sites. Decreases
plasma angiotensin II, increases
plasma renin activity, and decreases
aldosterone secretion. *Therapeutic
Effect:* Reduces peripheral arterial
resistance, pulmonary capillary
wedge pressure; improves cardiac
output, and exercise tolerance.

USES
Treatment of hypertension, alone or
in combination with thiazide
diuretics, management of heart
failure

PHARMACOKINETICS

Route	Onset	Peak	Duration
PO	1 hr	2–6 hr	24 hr

Slowly absorbed from the GI tract.
Protein binding: 97%–98%.
Metabolized in the liver and GI
mucosa to active metabolite.
Primarily excreted in urine.

Minimal removal by hemodialysis.
Half-life: 11.5 hr.

INDICATIONS AND DOSAGES
▸ **Hypertension (monotherapy)**
PO
Adults, Elderly. Initially, 10 mg/day.
Maintenance: 20–40 mg/day.
Maximum: 80 mg/day.
▸ **Hypertension (with diuretic)**
PO
Adults, Elderly. Initially, 10 mg/day
titrated to patient's needs.
▸ **Heart Failure**
PO
Adults, Elderly. Initially, 5–10 mg.
Maintenance: 20–40 mg/day.

SIDE EFFECTS/ADVERSE REACTIONS
Frequent
Dizziness, cough
Occasional
Hypotension, nausea, vomiting,
upper respiratory tract infection

PRECAUTIONS AND CONTRAINDICATIONS
History of angioedema from
previous treatment with ACE
inhibitors
Caution
Impaired liver function,
hypovolemia, blood dyscrasias, CHF,
COPD, asthma, elderly

DRUG INTERACTIONS OF CONCERN TO DENTISTRY
• Increased hypotension: alcohol,
phenothiazines
• Decreased hypotensive effects:
indomethacin, possibly other
NSAIDs, sympathomimetics
• Suspected reduction in the
antihypertensive and vasodilator
effects by salicylates;
monitor B/P if used
concurrently

SERIOUS REACTIONS

! Excessive hypotension ("first-dose syncope") may occur in patients with CHF and in those who are severely salt and volume depleted.

! Angioedema (swelling of face and lips) and hyperkalemia occur rarely.

! Agranulocytosis and neutropenia may be noted in those with collagen vascular disease, including scleroderma and systemic lupus erythematosus, and impaired renal function.

! Nephrotic syndrome may be noted in those with history of renal disease.

DENTAL CONSIDERATIONS

General:

• Monitor vital signs at every appointment because of cardiovascular and respiratory side effects.

• After supine positioning, have patient sit upright for at least 2 min before standing to avoid orthostatic hypotension.

• Patients on chronic drug therapy may rarely have symptoms of blood dyscrasias, which can include infection, bleeding, and poor healing.

• Assess salivary flow as a factor in caries, periodontal disease, and candidiasis.

• Limit use of sodium-containing products, such as saline IV fluids, for patients with a dietary salt restriction.

• Stress from dental procedures may compromise cardiovascular function; determine patient risk.

• Short appointments and a stress-reduction protocol may be required for anxious patients.

Consultations:

• Medical consultation may be required to assess disease control and patient's ability to tolerate stress.

• In a patient with symptoms of blood dyscrasias, request a medical consultation for blood studies and postpone dental treatment until normal values are reestablished.

• Take precautions if dental surgery is anticipated and sedation or general anesthesia is required; risk of hypotensive episode.

Teach Patient/Family to:

• Use effective oral hygiene to prevent soft tissue inflammation

• Use caution to prevent injury when using oral hygiene aids

• When chronic dry mouth occurs, advise patient to:

 • Avoid mouth rinses with high alcohol content because of drying effects

 • Use daily home fluoride products for anticaries effect

 • Use sugarless gum, frequent sips of water, or saliva substitutes

fosphenytoin
fos-phen´-ih-toyn
(Cerebyx)
Do not confuse Cerebyx with Celebrex or Celexa.

CATEGORY AND SCHEDULE
Pregnancy Risk Category: D

Drug Class:
Hydantoin-anticonvulsant

MECHANISM OF ACTION
A hydantoin-anticonvulsant that stabilizes neuronal membranes by decreasing sodium and calcium ion influx into the neurons. Also decreases post-tetanic potentiation and repetitive discharge.
Therapeutic Effect: Decreases seizure activity.

USES

Control of generalized convulsive status epilepticus; prevention and treatment of seizures during neurosurgery; short-term substitute for oral phenytoin

PHARMACOKINETICS

Completely absorbed after IM administration. Protein binding: 95%–99%. Rapidly and completely hydrolyzed to phenytoin after IM or IV administration. Time of complete conversion to phenytoin: 4 hr after IM injection; 2 hr after IV infusion. *Half-life:* 8–15 min (for conversion to phenytoin).

INDICATIONS AND DOSAGES

▶ **Status Epilepticus**
IV
Adults. Loading dose: 15–20 mg phenytoin equivalent (PE)/kg infused at rate of 100–150 mg PE/min.
▶ **Nonemergent Seizures**
IV, IM
Adults. Loading dose: 10–20 mg PE/kg. Maintenance: 4–6 mg PE/kg/day.
▶ **Short-Term Substitution for Oral Phenytoin**
IV, IM
Adults. May substitute for oral phenytoin at same total daily dose.

SIDE EFFECTS/ADVERSE REACTIONS

Frequent
Dizziness, paresthesia, tinnitus, pruritus, headache, somnolence
Occasional
Morbilliform rash

PRECAUTIONS AND CONTRAINDICATIONS

Adams-Stokes syndrome, hypersensitivity to fosphenytoin or phenytoin, second- or third-degree AV block, severe bradycardia, sinoatrial block

Caution
IV: Do not exceed injection rate of 150 mg PE/min, risk of seizures with abrupt withdrawal; hypotension, severe myocardial insufficiency, phosphate restriction; thyroid, renal, or hepatic disease; elderly, lactation, pediatric use

DRUG INTERACTIONS OF CONCERN TO DENTISTRY

• Increased phenytoin levels: benzodiazepines (chlordiazepoxide, diazepam), halothane, salicylates
• Increased CNS depression: benzodiazepines, H1-blocker antihistamines, opiate agonists
• Decreased phenytoin levels: carbamazepine, ciprofloxacin
• Decreased effectiveness of corticosteroids
• Suspected risk of hepatic toxicity: chronic use of acetaminophen and phosphenytoin

SERIOUS REACTIONS

❗ An elevated fosphenytoin blood concentration may produce ataxia, nystagmus, diplopia, lethargy, slurred speech, nausea, vomiting, and hypotension. As the drug level increases, extreme lethargy may progress to coma.
▶ **Dental Considerations**
General:
• This drug is intended for short-term use in an emergency department or hospital setting. Patient probably will return to oral phenytoin or other anticonvulsant after hospital care.
• Use precaution if sedation or general anesthesia is required; risk of hypotensive episode.
Consultations:
• Determine type of epilepsy, seizure frequency, and quality of seizure control. A stress reduction protocol may be required.

• Medical consultation may be required to assess disease control and patient's ability to tolerate stress.
Teach Patient/Family to:
• Update health and drug history if physician makes any changes in evaluation or drug regimens

frovatriptan
fro-va-trip´-tan
(Frovan)

CATEGORY AND SCHEDULE
Pregnancy Risk Category: C

Drug Class: Antimigraine agent; 5HT$_1$-receptor agonist

MECHANISM OF ACTION
A serotonin receptor agonist that binds selectively to vascular receptors, producing a vasoconstrictive effect on cranial blood vessels. *Therapeutic Effect:* Relieves migraine headache.

USES
Acute treatment of migraine with or without aura

PHARMACOKINETICS
Well absorbed after PO administration. Metabolized by the liver to inactive metabolite. Eliminated in urine. *Half-life:* 26 hr (increased in hepatic impairment).

INDICATIONS AND DOSAGES
▶ **Acute Migraine Attack**
PO
Adults, Elderly. Initially 2.5 mg. If headache improves but then returns, dose may be repeated after 2 hr. Maximum: 7.5 mg/day.

SIDE EFFECTS/ADVERSE REACTIONS
Occasional
Dizziness, paresthesia, fatigue, flushing
Rare
Hot or cold sensation, dry mouth, dyspepsia

PRECAUTIONS AND CONTRAINDICATIONS
Basilar or hemiplegic migraine, cerebrovascular or peripheral vascular disease, coronary artery disease, ischemic heart disease (including angina pectoris, history of MI, silent ischemia, and Prinzmetal's angina), severe hepatic impairment (Child-Pugh grade C), uncontrolled hypertension, use within 24 hr of ergotamine-containing preparations or another serotonin receptor agonist, use within 14 days of MAOIs

DRUG INTERACTIONS OF CONCERN TO DENTISTRY
• Potential serotonin crisis: SSRIs, ergot-containing drugs (avoid use within 24 hr of taking this drug)
• Decreased plasma levels: cimetidine

SERIOUS REACTIONS
! Cardiac reactions (including ischemia, coronary artery vasospasm, and MI), and noncardiac vasospasm-related reactions (such as hemorrhage and CVA), occur rarely, particularly in patients with hypertension, diabetes, or a strong family history of coronary artery disease; obese patients; smokers; males older than 40 yr; and postmenopausal women.

DENTAL CONSIDERATIONS
General:
• This is an acute-use drug; it is doubtful that patients will seek

dental treatment during acute migraine attacks.

• Be aware of patient's disease, its severity, and its frequency, when known.

• Advise patient if dental drugs prescribed have a potential for photosensitivity.

Consultations:

• If treating chronic orofacial pain, consult with physician of record.

• Medical consultation may be required to assess disease control and patient's ability to tolerate stress.

Teach Patient/Family to:

• Avoid mouth rinses with high alcohol content because of additional drying effects

• Update health and drug history if physician makes any changes in evaluation or drug regimens

furosemide

fur-oh´-se-mide
(Apo-Furosemide[CAN],
Frusehexal[AUS], Frusid[AUS],
Lasix, Uremide[AUS],
Urex-M[AUS])
Do not confuse Lasix with Lidex,
Luvox, or Luxiq, or furosemide
with Torsemide.

CATEGORY AND SCHEDULE

Pregnancy Risk Category: C
(D if used in pregnancy-induced hypertension)

Drug Class: Loop diuretic

MECHANISM OF ACTION

A loop diuretic that enhances excretion of sodium, chloride, and potassium by direct action at the ascending limb of the loop of Henle.

Therapeutic Effect: Produces diuresis and lower B/P.

USES

Pulmonary edema, edema in CHF, liver disease, nephrotic syndrome, ascites, hypertension

PHARMACOKINETICS

Route	Onset	Peak	Duration
PO	30–60 min	1–2 hr	6–8 hr
IV	5 min	20–60 min	2 hr
IM	30 min	N/A	N/A

Well absorbed from the GI tract. Protein binding: 91%–97%. Partially metabolized in the liver. Primarily excreted in urine (nonrenal clearance increases in severe renal impairment). Not removed by hemodialysis. **Half-life:** 30–90 min (increased in renal or hepatic impairment, and in neonates).

INDICATIONS AND DOSAGES

▸ **Edema, Hypertension**

PO

Adults, Elderly. Initially, 20–80 mg/dose; may increase by 20–40 mg/dose q6–8h. May titrate up to 600 mg/day in severe edematous states.

Children. 1–6 mg/kg/day in divided doses q6–12h.

IV, IM

Adults, Elderly. 20–40 mg/dose; may increase by 20 mg/dose q1–2h.

Children. 1–2 mg/kg/dose q6–12h.

Neonates. 1–2 mg/kg/dose q12–24h.

IV Infusion

Adults, Elderly. Bolus of 0.1 mg/kg, followed by infusion of 0.1 mg/kg/hr; may double q2h. Maximum: 0.4 mg/kg/hr.

Children. 0.05 mg/kg/hr; titrate to desired effect.

SIDE EFFECTS/ADVERSE REACTIONS
Expected
Increased urinary frequency and urine volume
Frequent
Nausea, dyspepsia, abdominal cramps, diarrhea or constipation, electrolyte disturbances
Occasional
Dizziness, light-headedness, headache, blurred vision, paresthesia, photosensitivity, rash, fatigue, bladder spasm, restlessness, diaphoresis
Rare
Flank pain

PRECAUTIONS AND CONTRAINDICATIONS
Anuria, hepatic coma, severe electrolyte depletion
Caution
Diabetes mellitus, dehydration, ascites, severe renal disease

DRUG INTERACTIONS OF CONCERN TO DENTISTRY
• Increased electrolyte imbalance: corticosteroids
• Masked ototoxicity: phenothiazines
• Decreased antihypertensive effect: NSAIDs, especially indomethacin

SERIOUS REACTIONS
! Vigorous diuresis may lead to profound water loss and electrolyte depletion, resulting in hypokalemia, hyponatremia, and dehydration.
! Sudden volume depletion may result in increased risk of thrombosis, circulatory collapse, and sudden death.
! Acute hypotensive episodes may occur, sometimes several days after beginning therapy.
! Ototoxicity—manifested as deafness, vertigo, or tinnitus—may occur, especially in patients with severe renal impairment.
! Furosemide use can exacerbate diabetes mellitus, systemic lupus erythematosus, gout, and pancreatitis.
! Blood dyscrasias have been reported.

DENTAL CONSIDERATIONS
General:
• Monitor vital signs at every appointment because of cardiovascular side effects.
• Patients on chronic drug therapy may rarely have symptoms of blood dyscrasias, which can include infection, bleeding, and poor healing.
• Assess salivary flow as a factor in caries, periodontal disease, and candidiasis.
• After supine positioning, have patient sit upright for at least 2 min before standing to avoid orthostatic hypotension.
• Patients on high-potency diuretics should be monitored for serum K levels.
Consultations:
• In a patient with symptoms of blood dyscrasias, request a medical consultation for blood studies and postpone dental treatment until normal values are reestablished.
• Medical consultation may be required to assess disease control.
Teach Patient/Family to:
• Use effective oral hygiene to prevent soft tissue inflammation
• Use caution to prevent injury when using oral hygiene aids
• When chronic dry mouth occurs, advise patient to:
  • Use daily home fluoride products for anticaries effect
  • Avoid mouth rinses with high alcohol content because of drying effects
  • Use sugarless gum, frequent sips of water, or saliva substitutes

gabapentin
ga´-ba-pen-tin
(Neurontin, Pendine[AUS])
Do not confuse Neurontin with
Noroxin.

CATEGORY AND SCHEDULE
Pregnancy Risk Category: C

Drug Class: Anticonvulsant,
analgesic

MECHANISM OF ACTION
An anticonvulsant and antineuralgic
agent whose exact mechanism
unknown. May increase the
synthesis or accumulation of
gamma-aminobutyric acid (GABA)
by binding to as-yet-undefined
receptor sites in brain tissue.
Therapeutic Effect: Reduces seizure
activity and neuropathic pain.

USES
Adjunctive therapy in patients 12 yr
or older with partial seizures with or
without secondary generalization and
as adjunctive therapy for partial
seizures in children 3–12 yr;
postherpetic neuralgia in adults

PHARMACOKINETICS
Well absorbed from the GI tract (not
affected by food). Protein binding: less
than 5%. Widely distributed. Crosses
the blood-brain barrier. Primarily
excreted unchanged in urine. Removed
by hemodialysis. *Half-life:* 5–7 hr
(increased in impaired renal function
and the elderly).

INDICATIONS AND DOSAGES
▶ **Adjunctive Therapy for Seizure
Control**
PO
*Adults, Elderly, Children older than
12 yr.* Initially, 300 mg 3 times a day.
May titrate dosage. Range:
900–1800 mg/day in 3 divided doses.
Maximum: 3600 mg/day.
Children 3–12 yr. Initially,
10–15 mg/kg/day in 3 divided doses.
May titrate up to 25–35 mg/kg/day
(for children 5–12 yr) and 40 mg/kg/
day (for children 3–4 yr) Maximum:
50 mg/kg/day.
▶ **Adjunctive Therapy for
Neuropathic Pain**
PO
Adults, Elderly. Initially, 100 mg
3 times a day; may increase by
300 mg/day at weekly intervals.
Maximum: 3600 mg/day in
3 divided doses.
Children. Initially, 5 mg/kg/dose
at bedtime, followed by
5 mg/kg/dose for 2 doses on
day 2, then 5 mg/kg/dose for
3 doses on day 3. Range:
8–35 mg/kg/day in 3 divided
doses.
▶ **Postherpetic Neuralgia**
PO
Adults, Elderly. 300 mg on
day 1300 mg twice a day
on day 2, and 300 mg 3 times
a day on day 3. Titrate up to
1800 mg/day.
▶ **Dosage in Renal Impairment**
Dosage and frequency are
modified on the basis of creatinine
clearance:

Creatinine Clearance	Dosage
60 ml/min or higher	400 mg q8h
30–59 ml/min	300 mg q12h
16–29 ml/min	300 mg daily
Less than 16 ml/min	300 mg every other day
Hemodialysis	200–300 mg after each 4-hr hemodialysis session

SIDE EFFECTS/ADVERSE REACTIONS
Frequent
Fatigue, somnolence, dizziness, ataxia
Occasional
Nystagmus, tremors, diplopia, rhinitis, weight gain
Rare
Nervousness, dysarthria, memory loss, dyspepsia, pharyngitis, myalgia

PRECAUTIONS AND CONTRAINDICATIONS
Hypersensitivity
Caution
Lactation, renal function impairment, children younger than 12 yr, elderly

DRUG INTERACTIONS OF CONCERN TO DENTISTRY
• None reported at this time, but, because CNS side effects are common, the use of anxiolytic sedative drugs may potentially increase the CNS side effects.

SERIOUS REACTIONS
! Abrupt withdrawal may increase seizure frequency.
! Overdosage may result in diplopia, slurred speech, drowsiness, lethargy, and diarrhea.

DENTAL CONSIDERATIONS
General:
• Early-morning appointments and a stress reduction protocol may be required for anxious patients.
• Place on frequent recall because of oral side effects.
• Monitor vital signs at every appointment because of cardiovascular side effects.
• Assess salivary flow as a factor in caries, periodontal disease, and candidiasis.

• Determine type of epilepsy and quality of seizure control.
Consultations:
• Medical consultation may be required to assess disease control and patient's ability to tolerate stress.
Teach Patient/Family to:
• Use effective oral hygiene to prevent soft tissue inflammation
• Use caution with oral hygiene aids to prevent injury
• When chronic dry mouth occurs, advise patient to:
  • Avoid mouth rinses with high alcohol content because of drying effects
  • Use daily home fluoride products for anticaries effect
  • Use sugarless gum, frequent sips of water, or saliva substitutes

galantamine
ga-lan´-ta-mene
(Reminyl)
Do not confuse Reminyl with Remeron, Remicade, or Robinul.

CATEGORY AND SCHEDULE
Pregnancy Risk Category: B

Drug Class: Cholinesterase inhibitor

MECHANISM OF ACTION
A cholinesterase inhibitor that inhibits the enzyme acetylcholinesterase, thus increasing the concentration of acetylcholine at cholinergic synapses and enhancing cholinergic function in the CNS.
Therapeutic Effect: Slows the progression of Alzheimer's disease.

USES
Treatment of mild-to-moderate dementia of Alzheimer's disease

PHARMACOKINETICS

Rapidly absorbed from the GI tract. Protein binding: 18%. Distributed to blood cells; binds to plasma proteins, mainly albumin. Metabolized in the liver. Excreted in urine. *Half-life:* 7 hr.

INDICATIONS AND DOSAGES

▸ **Alzheimer's Disease**

PO

Adults, Elderly. Initially, 4 mg twice a day (8 mg/day). After a minimum of 4 wk (if well tolerated), may increase to 8 mg twice a day (16 mg/day). After another 4 wk, may increase to 12 mg twice daily (24 mg/day). Range: 16–24 mg/day in 2 divided doses.

▸ **Dosage in Renal Impairment**

For moderate impairment, maximum dosage is 16 mg/day. Drug is not recommended for patients with severe impairment.

SIDE EFFECTS/ADVERSE REACTIONS

Frequent

Nausea, vomiting, diarrhea, anorexia, weight loss

Occasional

Abdominal pain, insomnia, depression, headache, dizziness, fatigue, rhinitis

Rare

Tremors, constipation, confusion, cough, anxiety, urinary incontinence

PRECAUTIONS AND CONTRAINDICATIONS

Severe hepatic or renal impairment

Caution

Potentiation of succinylcholine-like neuromuscular blocking drugs, obstructive GI disease, Parkinson's disease, epilepsy, cardiac conduction disorders, AV block, bradycardia, history of GI ulcer, hypersecretory disorders (gastric), bladder outflow obstruction, COPD, asthma, moderate hepatic impairment, moderate renal impairment, lactation, pediatric use

DRUG INTERACTIONS OF CONCERN TO DENTISTRY

• Increased plasma levels: ketoconazole
• Increased bioavailability: cimetidine, paroxetine
• Enhanced succinylcholine muscle relaxation during anesthesia
• Action may be inhibited by anticholinergic drugs or enhanced by cholinergic agonists

SERIOUS REACTIONS

! Overdose may cause cholinergic crisis, characterized by increased salivation, lacrimation, severe nausea and vomiting, bradycardia, respiratory depression, hypotension, and increased muscle weakness. Treatment usually consists of supportive measures and an anticholinergic such as atropine.

DENTAL CONSIDERATIONS

General:

• Monitor vital signs at every appointment because of cardiovascular side effects.
• After supine positioning, have patient sit upright for at least 2 min to avoid orthostatic hypotension.
• Drug is used early in the disease; ensure that patient or caregiver understands informed consent.
• Place on frequent recall because early attention to dental health is important for Alzheimer's patients.
• Consider semisupine chair position for patient comfort if GI side effects occur.

Consultations:
• Consultation with physician may be necessary if sedation or general anesthesia is required.
• Medical consultation may be required to assess disease control and patient's ability to tolerate stress.
Teach Patient/Family to:
• Use effective oral hygiene to prevent soft tissue inflammation
• Have caregiver assist patient with oral home-care regimen as cognitive ability declines
• Use electric tooth brush if patient has difficulty holding conventional devices
• Update health and drug history if physician makes any changes in evaluation or drug regimens

galsulfase
gal-sul´-face
(Naglazyme)

CATEGORY AND SCHEDULE
Pregnancy Risk Category: B

Drug Class: Enzyme

MECHANISM OF ACTION
A recombinant normal variant form of a polymorphic enzyme (N-acetylgalactosamine 4-sulfatase), produced in Chinese hamster cells, that is taken up into lysosomes and increases the catabolism of glycosaminoglycans. *Therapeutic Effect:* Replaces enzyme (N-acetylgalactosamine 4-sulfatase).

USES
Treatment of Maroteaux-Lamy syndrome

PHARMACOKINETICS
Half-life: wk 1: 6–21 hr; wk 24: 8–40 hr.

INDICATIONS AND DOSAGES
▶ Maroteaux-Lamy Syndrome
IV
Adults. 1 mg/kg once a wk.
Children (5 yr and older). 1 mg/kg once a wk.

SIDE EFFECTS/ADVERSE REACTIONS:
Frequent
Antibody development, abdominal pain, ear pain, headache, fever, arthralgia, vomiting, upper respiratory infections, diarrhea, cough, otitis media, infusion-related reactions, pain, rigors, conjunctivitis, dyspnea, chest pain, pharyngitis, facial edema, hypertension, malaise, gastroenteritis, areflexia, corneal opacification, nasal congestion, umbilical hernia
Less frequent adverse effects were not described

PRECAUTIONS AND CONTRAINDICATIONS
Hypersensitivity to galsulfase or its components
Caution
Respiratory illness

DRUG INTERACTIONS OF CONCERN TO DENTISTRY
None reported

SERIOUS REACTIONS
! Respiratory distress has been reported.

DENTAL CONSIDERATIONS
General
• Monitor vital signs at every appointment due to cardiovascular side effects

• Consider semisupine chair position for patient comfort due to respiratory complications
• Avoid aspirin and NSAIDs
• Consider visual disturbances when presenting instructions to patients
Consultations:
• Consult physician to determine disease control and ability of patient to tolerate dental procedures
Teach Patient/Family to:
• Update medication/health history whenever symptoms of disease or medication regimen is changed
• Use effective, atraumatic oral hygiene measures to reduce soft-tissue inflammation
• Use home fluoride products for anticaries effect

ganciclovir sodium
gan-sy´-clo-ver soe´-dee-um
(Cymevene[AUS], Cytovene, Vitrasert)
Do not confuse Cytovene with Cytosar.

CATEGORY AND SCHEDULE
Pregnancy Risk Category: C

Drug Class: Antiviral, nucleoside analog

MECHANISM OF ACTION
This synthetic nucleoside competes with viral DNA polymerase and is incorporated into growing viral DNA chains. **Therapeutic Effect:** Interferes with synthesis and replication of viral DNA.

USES
Prevention and treatment of cytomegalovirus (CMV) retinitis in patients with AIDS or organ transplants; life-threatening CMV disease

PHARMACOKINETICS
Widely distributed. Protein binding: 1%–2%. Undergoes minimal metabolism. Excreted unchanged primarily in urine. Removed by hemodialysis. **Half-life:** 2.5–3.6 hr (increased in impaired renal function).

INDICATIONS AND DOSAGES
▶ **CMV Retinitis**
IV
Adults, Children 3 mo and older.
10 mg/kg/day in divided doses q12h for 14–21 days, then 5 mg/kg/day as a single daily dose.
▶ **Prevention of CMV Disease in Transplant Patients**
IV
Adults, Children. 10 mg/kg/day in divided doses q12h for 7–14 days, then 5 mg/kg/day as a single daily dose.
▶ **Other CMV Infections**
IV
Adults. Initially, 10 mg/kg/day in divided doses q12h for 14–21 days, then 5 mg/kg/day as a single daily dose. Maintenance: 1000 mg 3 times a day or 500 mg q3h (6 times a day).
Children. Initially, 10 mg/kg/day in divided doses q12h for 14–21 days, then 5 mg/kg/day as a single daily dose. Maintenance: 30 mg/kg/dose q8h.
▶ **Intravitreal implant**
Adults. 1 implant q6–9mo plus oral ganciclovir.
Children 9 yr and older. 1 implant q6–9mo plus oral ganciclovir (30 mg/dose q8h).
▶ **Adult Dosage in Renal Impairment**
Dosage and frequency are modified on the basis of CrCl.

CrCl	Induction Dosage	Mainte-nance Dosage	Oral
50–69 ml/min	2.5 mg/kg q12h	2.5 mg/kg q24h	1500 mg/day
25–49 ml/min	2.5 mg/kg q24h	1.25 mg/kg q24h	1000 mg/day
10–24 ml/min	1.25 mg/kg q24h	0.625 mg/ kg q24h	500 mg/day
Less than 10 ml/mn	1.25 mg/kg 3 times a wk	0.625 mg/kg 3 times a wk	500 mg 3 times a wk

CrCl = creatinine clearance

SIDE EFFECTS/ADVERSE REACTIONS

Frequent
Diarrhea, fever, nausea, abdominal pain, vomiting
Occasional
Diaphoresis, infection, paresthesia, flatulence, pruritus
Rare
Headache, stomatitis, dyspepsia, phlebitis

PRECAUTIONS AND CONTRAINDICATIONS

Hypersensitivity to acyclovir or ganciclovir
Caution
Preexisting cytopenia, renal function impairment, lactation, children younger than 6 mo, elderly, platelet count less than 25,000/mm^3

DRUG INTERACTIONS OF CONCERN TO DENTISTRY

• Increased risk of blood dyscrasias: dapsone, carbamazepine, phenothiazines
• Increased risk of seizures: imipenem/cilastatin (Primaxin)
• Low platelet counts may prevent the use of aspirin, NSAIDs

SERIOUS REACTIONS

! Hematologic toxicity occurs commonly: leukopenia in 41%–29% of patients and anemia in 25%–19%.
! Intraocular insertion occasionally results in visual acuity loss, vitreous hemorrhage, and retinal detachment.
! GI hemorrhage occurs rarely.

DENTAL CONSIDERATIONS

G

General:
• Examine for oral manifestations of opportunistic infection.
• Examine for evidence of oral manifestations of blood dyscrasias (infection, bleeding, poor healing).
• Place on frequent recall to evaluate healing response.
• Consider local hemostasis measures to prevent excessive bleeding.
• Monitor vital signs at every appointment because of cardiovascular and respiratory side effects.
Consultations:
• Medical consultation for blood studies (CBC); leukopenic or thrombocytopenic side effects may result in infection, delayed healing, and excessive bleeding. Postpone elective dental treatment until normal values are maintained.
• Medical consultation may be required to assess disease control.
Teach Patient/Family to:
• Use caution in use of oral hygiene aids to prevent injury
• See dentist immediately if secondary oral infection occurs
• Use effective oral hygiene to prevent soft tissue inflammation

gatifloxacin

gah-tee-floks´-ah-sin
(Tequin, Zymar)

CATEGORY AND SCHEDULE

Pregnancy Risk Category: C

Drug Class: Fluoroquinolone
antiinfective

G

MECHANISM OF ACTION

A fluoroquinolone that inhibits two
enzymes, topoisomerase II and IV, in
susceptible microorganisms.
Therapeutic Effect: Interferes with
bacterial DNA replication. Prevents
or delays resistance emergence.
Bactericidal.

USES

Treatment of acute bacterial
exacerbation of chronic bronchitis
caused by *S. pneumoniae,
H. influenzae, H. parainfluenzae,
M. catarrhalis, or S. aureus;* acute
sinusitis (*S. pneumoniae,
H. influenzae*); community-acquired
pneumonia (*S. pneumoniae,
H. influenzae, H. para-influenzae,
M. catarrhalis, M. pneumoniae,
C. pneumoniae, L. pneumoniae,* or
S. aureus; complicated or
uncomplicated UTI (*E. coli,
K. pneumoniae, P. mirabilis*);
pyelonephritis (*E. coli*), acute
uncomplicated rectal infections in
women or uncomplicated urethral or
cervical gonorrhea (*N. gonorrhoeae*);
uncomplicated skin and skin-
structure infections

PHARMACOKINETICS

Well absorbed from the GI tract after
PO administration. Protein binding:
20%. Widely distributed.
Metabolized in liver. Primarily
excreted in urine. ***Half-life:*** 7–14 hr.

INDICATIONS AND DOSAGES

▶ **Chronic Bronchitis, Complicated
UTIs, Pyelonephritis, Skin Infections**
PO, IV
Adults, Elderly. 400 mg/day for
7–10 days (5 days for chronic
bronchitis).
▶ **Sinusitis**
PO, IV
Adults, Elderly. 400 mg/day for
10 days.
▶ **Pneumonia**
PO, IV
Adults, Elderly. 400 mg/day for
7–14 days.
▶ **Cystitis**
PO, IV
Adults, Elderly. 400 mg as a
single dose or 200 mg/day for
3 days.
▶ **Urethral Gonorrhea in Men and
Women, Endocervical and Rectal
Gonorrhea in Women**
PO, IV
Adults, Elderly. 400 mg as a single
dose.
▶ **Topical Treatment of Bacterial
Conjunctivitis Caused by
Susceptible Strains of Bacteria**
Ophthalmic
*Adults, Elderly, Children 1 yr and
older.* 1 drop q2h while awake for
2 days, then 1 drop up to 4 times a
day for days 3–7.
▶ **Dosage in Renal Impairment**

Creatinine Clearance	Dosage
40 ml/min	400 mg/day
Less than 40 ml/min	Initially, 400 mg/day then 200 mg/day
Hemodialysis	Initially, 400 mg/day then 200 mg/day
Peritoneal dialysis	Initially, 400 mg/day then 200 mg/day

SIDE EFFECTS/ADVERSE REACTIONS

Occasional

Nausea, vaginitis, diarrhea, headache, dizziness
Ophthalmic: conjunctival irritation, increased tearing, corneal inflammation

Rare

Abdominal pain, constipation, dyspepsia, stomatitis, edema, insomnia, abnormal dreams, diaphoresis, altered taste, rash
Ophthalmic: corneal swelling, dry eye, eye pain, eyelid swelling, headache, red eye, reduced visual acuity, altered taste

PRECAUTIONS AND CONTRAINDICATIONS

Hypersensitivity to quinolones.

Caution

Reduce dose with creatinine clearance less than 40 ml/min; probenecid increases half life; children younger than 18 yr, lactation, seizure history, avoid use with class IA and III antiarrhythmics; many prolong QT interval; cross resistance with other fluoroquinolones, monitor blood glucose in diabetes

DRUG INTERACTIONS OF CONCERN TO DENTISTRY

• Use caution with erythromycin and tricyclic antidepressants (no data, risk of prolonged QT interval)
• Decreased absorption: divalent and trivalent cations, iron and zinc salts
• Increased risk of CNS stimulation and seizures: NSAIDs

SERIOUS REACTIONS

❗ Pseudomembranous colitis as evidenced by severe abdominal pain and cramps, severe watery diarrhea, and fever, may occur.

❗ Superinfection manifested as genital or anal pruritus, ulceration or changes in oral mucosa, and moderate to severe diarrhea, may occur.

DENTAL CONSIDERATIONS

General:
• Determine why patient is taking the drug.
• Monitor vital signs at every appointment because of cardiovascular side effects.
• Examine for oral manifestation of opportunistic infection.
• Advise patient if dental drugs prescribed have a potential for photosensitivity.
• Ruptures of the shoulder, hand, and Achilles tendons requiring surgical repair or resulting in prolonged disability have been reported with use of fluoroquinolones. Question patient about history of side effects associated with fluoroquinolone use.

Consultations:
• Physician consultation is advised in the presence of an acute dental infection requiring another antibiotic.

Teach Patient/Family to:
• Minimize exposure to sunlight and wear sunscreen if sun exposure is planned
• Discontinue treatment and inform dentist immediately if patient experiences pain or inflammation of a tendon, and to rest and refrain from exercise

Gatifloxacin Ophthalmic
General:
• Avoid dental light in patient's eyes; offer dark glasses for patient comfort.

gefitinib
geh-fih´-tih-nib
(Iressa)

CATEGORY AND SCHEDULE
Pregnancy Risk Category: D

Drug Class: Antineoplastic-miscellaneous; epidermal growth factor receptor inhibitor

MECHANISM OF ACTION
Blocks the signaling pathway that binds to the epidermal growth factor receptor (EGFR) on the surface of normal and cancer cells. EGFR activates the enzyme tyrosine kinase, which sends signals instructing the cells to grow. *Therapeutic Effect:* Inhibits the growth of cancer cells.

USES
Treatment of advanced/metastatic non–small-cell lung cancer in those that have not responded to platinum or docetaxel products

PHARMACOKINETICS
Slowly absorbed and extensively distributed throughout the body. Protein binding: 90%. Undergoes extensive metabolism in the liver. Excreted in the feces. *Half-life:* 48 hr.

INDICATIONS AND DOSAGES
▸ **Non–Small-Cell Lung Cancer**
PO
Adults, Elderly. 250 mg/day; may increase to 500 mg/day for patients receiving drugs that may decrease gefitinib blood concentrations, such as rifampin and phenytoin

SIDE EFFECTS/ADVERSE REACTIONS
Frequent
Diarrhea, rash, acne

Occasional
Dry skin, nausea, vomiting, pruritus
Rare
Anorexia, asthenia, weight loss, peripheral edema, eye pain

PRECAUTIONS AND CONTRAINDICATIONS
None known

DRUG INTERACTIONS OF CONCERN TO DENTISTRY
- Decreased plasma levels: sodium bicarbonate
- Decreased metabolism: potent inhibitors of CYP3A4 isoenzymes (ketoconazole, itraconazole, erythromycin, clarithromycin)

SERIOUS REACTIONS
❗ Pancreatitis and ocular hemorrhage occur rarely.
❗ Hypersensitivity reaction produces angioedema and urticaria.

DENTAL CONSIDERATIONS
General:
- If additional analgesia is required for dental pain, consider alternative analgesics (NSAIDs) in patients taking narcotics for acute or chronic pain.
- This drug may be used in the hospital or on an outpatient basis. Confirm the patient's disease and treatment status.
- Consider semisupine chair position for patients with respiratory disease.
- Examine for oral manifestation of opportunistic infection.
- Patients may have received other chemotherapy or radiation: confirm medical and drug history.
- Caution: drug interactions with drugs used in dentistry.

Consultations:
- Medical consultation may be required to assess disease control and patient's ability to tolerate stress.

• Medical consultation may be required to assess immunologic status during cancer chemotherapy and determine safety risk, if any, posed by the required dental treatment.

Teach Patient/Family to:
• Use effective oral hygiene to prevent soft tissue inflammation
• Use caution to prevent trauma when using oral hygiene aids
• Update health and medication history if physician makes any changes in evaluation or drug regimens; include OTC, herbal, and nonherbal remedies in the update

gemcitabine hydrochloride
jem-cih´-tah-bean hi-droh-klor´-ide
(Gemzar)

CATEGORY AND SCHEDULE
Pregnancy Risk Category: D

Drug Class: Antineoplastic-miscellaneous; nucleoside analog

MECHANISM OF ACTION
An antimetabolite that inhibits ribonucleotide reductase, the enzyme necessary for catalyzing DNA synthesis. *Therapeutic Effect:* Produces death in cells undergoing DNA synthesis.

USES
Treatment of cancer of the breast, pancreas, and lung

PHARMACOKINETICS
Not extensively distributed after IV infusion (increased with length of infusion). Protein binding: less than 10%. Excreted primarily in urine as metabolite. *Half-life:* 42–94 min

(influenced by gender of patient and duration of infusion).

INDICATIONS AND DOSAGES
▶ **Non–Small-Cell Lung Cancer (in combination with cisplatin)**
IV
Adults, Elderly, Children. 1000 mg/m² on days 1, 8, and 15, repeated every 28 days; or 1250 mg/m² on days 1 and 8. Repeat every 21 days.
▶ **Pancreatic Cancer**
IV
Adults. 1000 mg/m² once weekly for up to 7 wk or until toxicity necessitates decreasing dosage or withholding the dose, followed by 1 wk of rest. Subsequent cycles should consist of once-weekly dose for 3 consecutive wk out of every 4 wk. For patients completing cycles at 1000 mg/m², increase dose to 1250 mg/m² as tolerated. Dose for next cycle may be increased to 1500 mg/m².
▶ **Dosage Reduction Guidelines**
Dosage adjustments should be on the basis of granulocyte count and platelet count, as follows:

Absolute Granulocyte Counts (cells/mm³)	Platelet Count (cells/mm³)	% of Full Dose
1000	100,000	100
500–999	50,000–99,000	75
Fewer than 500	Less than 50,000	Hold

SIDE EFFECTS/ADVERSE REACTIONS
Frequent
Nausea and vomiting, generalized pain, fever, mild to moderate pruritic rash, mild to moderate dyspnea, constipation, peripheral edema

Occasional
Diarrhea, petechiae, alopecia, stomatitis, infection, somnolence, paresthesia
Rare
Diaphoresis, rhinitis, insomnia, malaise

PRECAUTIONS AND CONTRAINDICATIONS
None known

DRUG INTERACTIONS OF CONCERN TO DENTISTRY
None reported

SERIOUS REACTIONS
! Severe myelosuppression, as evidenced by anemia, thrombocytopenia, and leukopenia, is a common reaction

DENTAL CONSIDERATIONS
General:
• Monitor vital signs at every appointment because of cardiovascular side effects.
• Consider semisupine chair position for patients with respiratory disease.
• If additional analgesia is required for dental pain, consider alternative analgesics in patients taking narcotics for acute or chronic pain.
• Examine for oral manifestation of opportunistic infection.
• Avoid products that affect platelet function, such as aspirin and NSAIDs.
• This drug may be used in the hospital or on an outpatient basis. Confirm the patient's disease and treatment status.
• Chlorhexidine mouth rinse prior to and during chemotherapy may reduce severity of mucositis.
• Patient on chronic drug therapy may rarely present with symptoms of

blood dyscrasias, which can include infection, bleeding and poor healing. If dyscrasia is present, caution patient to prevent oral tissue trauma when using oral hygiene aids.
• Palliative medication may be required for management of oral side effects.
• Short appointments and a stress reduction protocol may be required for anxious patients.
• Patients may be at risk of bleeding; check for oral signs.
• Oral infections should be eliminated and/or treated aggressively.
Consultations:
• Medical consultation should include routine blood counts including platelet counts and bleeding time.
• Consult physician; prophylactic or therapeutic antiinfectives may be indicated if surgery or periodontal treatment is required.
• Medical consultation may be required to assess immunologic status during cancer chemotherapy and determine safety risk, if any, posed by the required dental treatment.
• Medical consultation may be required to assess disease control and patient's ability to tolerate stress.
Teach Patient/Family to:
• Be aware of oral side effects
• Use effective, atraumatic oral hygiene to prevent soft tissue inflammation
• Report oral lesions, soreness, or bleeding to dentist
• Prevent trauma when using oral hygiene aids
• Update health and medication history if physician makes any changes in evaluation or drug regimens; include OTC, herbal, and nonherbal remedies in the update

gemfibrozil

jem-fi´-broe-zil
(Apo-Gemfibrozil[CAN],
Ausgem[AUS], Gemfibromax[AUS],
Jezil[AUS], Lipazil[AUS], Lopid,
Novo-Gemfibrozil[CAN])
Do not confuse Lopid with Lorabid
or Levbid.

CATEGORY AND SCHEDULE

Pregnancy Risk Category: C

Drug Class: Antihyperlipidemic

MECHANISM OF ACTION

A fibric acid derivative that inhibits
lipolysis of fat in adipose tissue;
decreases liver uptake of free fatty
acids and reduces hepatic triglyceride
production. Inhibits synthesis of very
low-density lipoproteins (VLDL)
carrier apolipoprotein B.
Therapeutic Effect: Lowers serum
cholesterol and triglycerides
(decreases VLDL, low-density
lipoproteins [LDL]; increases
high-density lipoproteins
[HDL]).

USES

Treatment of type IIb, IV, and V
hyperlipidemia

PHARMACOKINETICS

Well absorbed from the GI tract.
Protein binding: 99%. Metabolized
in liver. Primarily excreted in urine.
Not removed by hemodialysis.
Half-life: 1.5 hr.

INDICATIONS AND DOSAGES

▶ **Hyperlipidemia**
PO
Adults, Elderly. 1200 mg/day in 2
divided doses 30 min before
breakfast and dinner.

SIDE EFFECTS/ADVERSE REACTIONS

Frequent
Dyspepsia
Occasional
Abdominal pain, diarrhea, nausea,
vomiting, fatigue
Rare
Constipation, acute appendicitis,
vertigo, headache, rash, pruritus,
altered taste

PRECAUTIONS AND CONTRAINDICATIONS

Liver dysfunction (including primary
biliary cirrhosis), preexisting
gallbladder disease, severe renal
dysfunction
Caution
Monitor hematologic and hepatic
function, lactation

DRUG INTERACTIONS OF CONCERN TO DENTISTRY

None reported

SERIOUS REACTIONS

! Cholelithiasis, cholecystitis,
acute appendicitis, pancreatitis, and
malignancy occur rarely.

DENTAL CONSIDERATIONS

General:
• Patients on chronic drug therapy
may rarely have symptoms of
blood dyscrasias, which can include
infection, bleeding, and poor
healing.
Consultations:
• In a patient with symptoms
of blood dyscrasias, request a
medical consultation for blood
studies and postpone dental
treatment until normal values
are reestablished.

gemifloxacin mesylate
jem-ih-flocks´-ah-sin mess-ah-late
(Factive)

CATEGORY AND SCHEDULE
Pregnancy Risk Category: C

Drug Class: Fluoroquinolone antiinfective

MECHANISM OF ACTION
A fluoroquinolone that inhibits the enzyme DNA gyrase in susceptible microorganisms, interfering with bacterial cell replication and repair. **Therapeutic Effect:** Bactericidal.

USES
Treatment of acute bacterial exacerbation of chronic bronchitis caused by susceptible strains of *S. pneumoniae, H. influenzae, H. parainfluenzae*, or *M. catarrhalis;* community-acquired pneumonia caused by susceptible strains of *S. pneumoniae* (except drug-resistant strains), *H. influenzae, M. catarrhalis, M. pneumoniae, C. pneumoniae*, or *K. pneumoniae*

PHARMACOKINETICS
Rapidly and well absorbed from the GI tract. Protein binding: 70%. Widely distributed. Penetrates well into lung tissue and fluid. Undergoes limited metabolism in the liver. Primarily excreted in feces; lesser amount eliminated in urine. Partially removed by hemodialysis. **Half-life:** 4–12 hr.

INDICATIONS AND DOSAGES
▶ **Acute Bacterial Exacerbation of Chronic Bronchitis**
PO
Adults, Elderly. 320 mg once a day for 5 days.

▶ **Community-Acquired Pneumonia**
PO
Adults, Elderly. 320 mg once a day for 7 days.
▶ **Dosage in Renal Impairment**
Dosage and frequency are modified on the basis of creatinine clearance.

Creatinine Clearance	Dosage
Greater than 40 ml/min	320 mg once a day
40 ml/min or less	160 mg once a day

SIDE EFFECTS/ADVERSE REACTIONS
Occasional
Diarrhea, rash, nausea
Rare
Headache, abdominal pain, dizziness

PRECAUTIONS AND CONTRAINDICATIONS
Concurrent use of amiodarone, quinidine, procainamide, or sotalol; history of prolonged QT interval; hypersensitivity to fluoroquinolones; uncorrected electrolyte disorders (such as hypokalemia and hypomagnesemia)
Caution
Safety and efficacy in children younger than 18 yr, pregnancy and nursing not established; may prolong QT interval, risk of tendinitis and tendon rupture, epilepsy, cerebral arteriosclerosis, renal dysfunction

DRUG INTERACTIONS OF CONCERN TO DENTISTRY
• Decreased absorption: divalent or trivalent antacids, iron or zinc salts
• Use with caution or avoid drugs that affect QT interval: erythromycin, antipsychotics, tricyclic antidepressants

SERIOUS REACTIONS

! Antibiotic-associated colitis may result from altered bacterial balance. Hypersensitivity reactions, including photosensitivity (as evidenced by rash, pruritus, blisters, edema, and burning skin), have occurred in patients receiving fluoroquinolones.

DENTAL CONSIDERATIONS

General:
• Determine why patient is taking the drug.
• Avoid dental light in patient's eyes; offer dark glasses for patient comfort.
• Examine for oral manifestation of opportunistic infection.
• Advise patient if dental drugs prescribed have a potential for photosensitivity.
• As with other fluoroquinolones there is a risk of tendinitis and tendon rupture.
• Consider semisupine chair position for patient comfort if GI side effects occur.
Consultations:
• Consult with patient's physician if an acute dental infection occurs and another antiinfective is required.
Teach Patient/Family:
• When chronic dry mouth occurs, advise patient to:
  • Avoid mouth rinses with high alcohol content because of drying effects
  • Use daily home fluoride products for anticaries effect
  • Use sugarless gum, frequent sips of water, or saliva substitutes

gentamicin sulfate

jen-ta-mye´-sin suhl´-feyt
(Alcomicin[CAN], Cidomycin[CAN], Garamycin, Genoptic, Gentak, Gentacidin)

CATEGORY AND SCHEDULE
Pregnancy Risk Category: C

Drug Class: Aminoglycoside antiinfective ophthalmic

MECHANISM OF ACTION
An aminoglycoside antibiotic that irreversibly binds to the protein of bacterial ribosomes. **Therapeutic Effect:** Interferes with protein synthesis of susceptible microorganisms. Bactericidal.

USES
Treatment of external eye infection

PHARMACOKINETICS
Rapid, complete absorption after IM administration. Protein binding: less than 30%. Widely distributed (does not cross the blood-brain barrier, low concentrations in CSF). Excreted unchanged in urine. Removed by hemodialysis.
Half-life: 2–4 hr (increased in impaired renal function and neonates; decreased in cystic fibrosis and burn or febrile patients).

INDICATIONS AND DOSAGES
▸ **Acute Pelvic, Bone, Intraabdominal, Joint, Respiratory Tract, Burn Wound, Postoperative, and Skin or Skin-Structure Infections; Complicated UTIs; Septicemia; Meningitis**
IV, IM
Adults, Elderly. Usual dosage, 3–6 mg/kg/day in divided doses q8h or 4–6.6 mg/kg once a day.

Children 5–12 yr. Usual dosage
2–2.5 mg/kg/dose q8h.
Children younger than 5 yr.
Usual dosage, 2.5 mg/kg/dose q8h.
Neonates. Usual dosage 2.5–3.5 mg/
kg/dose q8–12h.

▸ **Hemodialysis**
IV, IM
Adults, Elderly. 0.5–0.7 mg/kg/dose
after dialysis.
Children. 1.25–1.75 mg/kg/dose after
dialysis.

▸ **Intrathecal**
Adults. 4–8 mg/day.
Children 3 mo–12 yr. 1–2 mg/day.
Neonates. 1 mg/day.

▸ **Superficial Eye Infections**
Ophthalmic Ointment
Adults, Elderly. Usual dosage, apply
thin strip to conjunctiva 2–3 times a
day.
Ophthalmic Solution
Adults, Elderly, Children. Usual
dosage, 1–2 drops q2–4h up to
2 drops/hr.

▸ **Superficial Skin Infections**
Topical
Adults, Elderly. Usual dosage, apply
3–4 times a day.

▸ **Dosage in Renal Impairment**
*Creatinine clearance greater than
41–60 ml/min.* Dosage interval q12h.
Creatinine clearance 20–40 ml/min.
Dosage interval q24h.
*Creatinine clearance less than 20 ml/
min.* Monitor levels to determine
dosage interval.

SIDE EFFECTS/ADVERSE REACTIONS
Occasional
IM: Pain, induration
IV: Phlebitis, thrombophlebitis,
hypersensitivity reactions
(fever, pruritus, rash, urticaria)
Ophthalmic: Burning, tearing,
itching, blurred vision
Topical: Redness, itching

Rare
Alopecia, hypertension, weakness
EENT: Poor corneal wound healing,
temporary visual haze, overgrowth of
nonsusceptible organisms

PRECAUTIONS AND CONTRAINDICATIONS
Hypersensitivity to gentamicin, other
aminoglycosides (cross-sensitivity),
or their components; sulfite
sensitivity may result in anaphylaxis,
especially in asthmatic patients.
Caution
Antibiotic hypersensitivity

DRUG INTERACTIONS OF CONCERN TO DENTISTRY
• Increased risk of nephrotoxicity:
cephalsporins, vancomycin,
enflurane
• Increased neuromuscular
blockade: neuromuscular-blocking
drugs

SERIOUS REACTIONS
! Nephrotoxicity (as evidenced by
increased BUN and serum creatinine
levels and decreased creatinine
clearance) may be reversible if the
drug is stopped at the first sign of
symptoms.
! Irreversible ototoxicity (manifested
as tinnitus, dizziness, ringing
or roaring in the ears, and
diminished hearing), and
neurotoxicity (as evidenced by
headache, dizziness, lethargy,
tremors, and visual disturbances)
occur occasionally. The risk of these
effects increases with higher dosages
or prolonged therapy and when the
solution is applied directly to the
mucosa.
! Superinfections, particularly
with fungal infections, may result
from bacterial imbalance no matter
which administration route is used.

❗ Ophthalmic application may cause paresthesia of conjunctiva or mydriasis.

DENTAL CONSIDERATIONS

General:
• For selected infections in the hospital setting; provide emergency dental treatment only.
• Examine for oral manifestation of opportunistic infection.
• Determine why patient is taking the drug.
• Caution patient regarding allergy to medication.

Consultations:
• Medical consultation may be required to assess disease control and patient's ability to tolerate stress.

Teach Patient/Family to:
• Use effective oral hygiene to prevent soft tissue inflammation
• Prevent trauma when using oral hygiene aids
• Report oral lesions, soreness, or bleeding to dentist

gentamicin sulfate; prednisolone acetate

jen-ta-mye´sin suhl´-feyt;
pred-nis´-oh-lone ass´-eh-tayte
(Pred-G, Pred-G S.O.P.)

CATEGORY AND SCHEDULE

Pregnancy Risk Category: C

Drug Class: Aminoglycoside antiinfective ophthalmic

MECHANISM OF ACTION

Gentamicin is an aminoglycoside that irreversibly binds to the protein of bacterial ribosomes. Prednisolone is an adrenal corticosteroid that inhibits accumulation of inflammatory cells at inflammation sites, phagocytosis, lysosomal enzyme release and synthesis, and release of mediators of inflammation. ***Therapeutic Effect:*** Interferes in protein synthesis of susceptible microorganisms. Prevents or suppresses cell-mediated immune reactions; decreases or prevents tissue response to inflammatory process.

USES

Treatment of external eye infection

PHARMACOKINETICS

None reported

INDICATIONS AND DOSAGES

▸ **Treatment of Steroid Responsive Inflammatory Conditions, Superficial Ocular Infections**

Ophthalmic Ointment
Adults, Elderly. Apply 1/2 inch ribbon in the conjunctival sac 1–3 times a day.
Ophthalmic Suspension
Adults, Elderly. Instill 1 drop 2–4 times a day. During the initial 24–48 hr, the dosing frequency may be increased if necessary up to 1 drop/hr.

SIDE EFFECTS/ADVERSE REACTIONS

Occasional
Burning, tearing, itching, blurred vision
Rare
Delayed wound healing, secondary infection, intraocular pressure increased, glaucoma

PRECAUTIONS AND CONTRAINDICATIONS

Viral disease of the cornea and conjunctiva (including epithelia herpes simplex keratitis, vaccinia, varicella), mycobacterial or fungal infection of the eye, uncomplicated removal of a corneal foreign body, hypersensitivity to gentamicin, prednisolone, other aminoglycosides or corticosteroids, or any component of the formulation

SERIOUS REACTIONS
! Optic nerve damage occurs rarely.

DENTAL CONSIDERATIONS
General:
• Avoid dental light in patient's eyes; offer dark glasses for patient comfort.

glatiramer
gla-teer´-ah-mer
(Copaxone)
Do not confuse Copaxone with Compazine.

CATEGORY AND SCHEDULE
Pregnancy Risk Category: B

Drug Class: Multiple sclerosis agent

MECHANISM OF ACTION
An immunosuppressive whose exact mechanism is unknown. May act by modifying immune processes thought to be responsible for the pathogenesis of multiple sclerosis. **Therapeutic Effect:** Slows progression of multiple sclerosis.

USES
Reduction of the frequency of relapses in patients with relapsing-remitting multiple sclerosis

PHARMACOKINETICS
Substantial fraction of glatiramer is hydrolyzed locally. Some fraction of injected material enters lymphatic circulation, reaching regional lymph nodes; some may enter systemic circulation intact.

INDICATIONS AND DOSAGES
▶ **Multiple Sclerosis**
Subcutaneous
Adults, Elderly. 20 mg once a day.

SIDE EFFECTS/ADVERSE REACTIONS
Expected
Pain, erythema, inflammation, or pruritus at injection site; asthenia
Frequent
Arthralgia, vasodilation, anxiety, hypertonia, nausea, transient chest pain, dyspnea, flu-like symptoms, rash, pruritus
Occasional
Palpitations, back pain, diaphoresis, rhinitis, diarrhea, urinary urgency
Rare
Anorexia, fever, neck pain, peripheral edema, ear pain, facial edema, vertigo, vomiting

PRECAUTIONS AND CONTRAINDICATIONS
Hypersensitivity to glatiramer or mannitol

DRUG INTERACTIONS OF CONCERN TO DENTISTRY
Dental drug interactions have not been studied

SERIOUS REACTIONS
! Infection is a common effect.
! Lymphadenopathy occurs occasionally.

DENTAL CONSIDERATIONS
General:
• Monitor vital signs at every appointment because of cardiovascular side effects.

- Protect patient's eyes from accidental spatter during dental treatment.
- Avoid dental light in patient's eyes; offer dark glasses for patient comfort.
- Short appointments may be required because of effects of disease on musculature.
- Short appointments and a stress-reduction protocol may be required for anxious patients.
- Advise patient if dental drugs prescribed have a potential for photosensitivity.
- Inquire about history of disease, any physical limitations, and other drugs the patient may be taking.
- For longer dental appointments, offer patient frequent breaks.

Consultations:
- Consultation with physician may be necessary if sedation or general anesthesia is required.
- Medical consultation may be required to assess disease control and patient's ability to tolerate stress.

Teach Patient/Family to:
- Use effective oral hygiene to prevent soft tissue inflammation
- Prevent trauma when using oral hygiene aids
- Update health and medication history if physician makes any changes in evaluation or drug regimens; include OTC, herbal, and nonherbal remedies in the update

glimepiride
gly-mep´-er-ide
(Amaryl)
Do not confuse glimepiride with glipizide or glyburide.

CATEGORY AND SCHEDULE
Pregnancy Risk Category: C

Drug Class: Oral antidiabetic (second generation)

MECHANISM OF ACTION
A second-generation sulfonylurea that promotes release of insulin from beta cells of the pancreas and increases insulin sensitivity at peripheral sites. **Therapeutic Effect:** Lowers blood glucose concentration.

USES
Stable adult-onset diabetes mellitus (type II); may also be used with insulin or metformin where diet and exercise are not effective in controlling hyperglycemia

PHARMACOKINETICS

Route	Onset	Peak	Duration
PO	N/A	2–3 hr	24 hr

Completely absorbed from the GI tract. Protein binding: greater than 99%. Metabolized in the liver. Excreted in urine and eliminated in feces. **Half-life:** 5–9.2 hr.

INDICATIONS AND DOSAGES
▶ **Diabetes Mellitus**
PO
Adults, Elderly. Initially, 1–2 mg once a day, with breakfast or first main meal. Maintenance: 1–4 mg once a day. After dose of 2 mg is reached, dosage should be increased in increments of up to 2 mg q1–2wk, on the basis of blood glucose response. Maximum: 8 mg/day.
▶ **Dosage in Renal Impairment**
PO
Adults. 1 mg once a day.

SIDE EFFECTS/ADVERSE REACTIONS
Frequent
Altered taste sensation, dizziness, somnolence, weight gain, constipation, diarrhea, heartburn,

nausea, vomiting, stomach fullness, headache

Occasional

Increased sensitivity of skin to sunlight, peeling of skin, itching, rash

PRECAUTIONS AND CONTRAINDICATIONS

Diabetic complications, such as ketosis, acidosis, and diabetic coma; severe hepatic or renal impairment; monotherapy for type 1 diabetes mellitus; stress situations, including severe infection, trauma, and surgery

Caution

Malnourished; adrenal, pituitary, or hepatic insufficiency; hypoglycemia recognition in elderly or in those taking β-blockers; increased risk of cardiovascular mortality has been reported in patients using oral hypoglycemics; alcohol use; lactation; children

DRUG INTERACTIONS OF CONCERN TO DENTISTRY

• Risk of potentiation of hypoglycemic effects: NSAIDs, salicylates, sulfonamides, β-adrenergic blockers, ketoconazole

SERIOUS REACTIONS

! Overdose or insufficient food intake may produce hypoglycemia, especially with increased glucose demands.

! GI hemorrhage, cholestatic hepatic jaundice, leukopenia, thrombocytopenia, pancytopenia, agranulocytosis, and aplastic or hemolytic anemia occur rarely.

DENTAL CONSIDERATIONS

General:

• Short appointments and a stress-reduction protocol may be required for anxious patients.

• Question patient about self-monitoring of drug's antidiabetic effect, including blood glucose values or finger-stick records.

• Ensure that patient is following prescribed diet and regularly takes medication.

• Patients on chronic drug therapy may rarely have symptoms of blood dyscrasias, which can include infection, bleeding, and poor healing.

• Diabetics may be more susceptible to infection and have delayed wound healing.

• Place on frequent recall to evaluate healing response.

• Advise patient if dental drugs prescribed have a potential for photosensitivity.

Consultations:

• Medical consultation may be required to assess disease control.

• In a patient with symptoms of blood dyscrasias, request a medical consultation for blood studies and postpone treatment until normal values are reestablished.

• Medical consultation may include data from patient's blood glucose monitoring, including glycosylated hemoglobin or HbA1c testing.

Teach Patient/Family to:

• Use effective oral hygiene to prevent soft tissue inflammation

• Use caution to prevent trauma when using oral hygiene aids

• Update health and drug history if physician makes any changes in evaluation or drug regimens

glipizide
glip´-ih-zide
(Glucotrol, Glucotrol XL,
Melizide[AUS], Minidiab[AUS])
Do not confuse glipizide with
glimepiride or glyburide.

CATEGORY AND SCHEDULE
Pregnancy Risk Category: C

Drug Class: Oral antidiabetic
(second generation)

MECHANISM OF ACTION
A second-generation sulfonylurea
that promotes the release of insulin
from beta cells of the pancreas and
increases insulin sensitivity at
peripheral sites. *Therapeutic Effect:*
Lowers blood glucose concentration.

USES
Stable adult-onset diabetes mellitus
(type II)

PHARMACOKINETICS

Route	Onset	Peak	Duration
PO	15–30 min	2–3 hr	12–24 hr
Extended release	2–3 hr	6–12 hr	24 hr

Well absorbed from the GI tract.
Protein binding: 99%. Metabolized
in the liver. Excreted in urine.
Half-life: 2–4 hr.

INDICATIONS AND DOSAGES
▸ **Diabetes Mellitus**
PO
Adults. Initially, 5 mg/day or 2.5 mg
in the elderly or those with hepatic
disease. Adjust dosage in 2.5- to
5-mg increments at intervals of
several days. Maximum single dose:
15 mg. Maximum dose/day: 40 mg.

Maintenance (extended-release
tablet): 20 mg/day.
Elderly. Initially, 2.5–5 mg/day.
May increase by 2.5–5 mg/day
q1–2wk.

SIDE EFFECTS/ADVERSE REACTIONS
Frequent
Altered taste sensation, dizziness,
somnolence, weight gain,
constipation, diarrhea, heartburn,
nausea, vomiting, stomach fullness,
headache
Occasional
Increased sensitivity of skin to
sunlight, peeling of skin, itching,
rash

PRECAUTIONS AND CONTRAINDICATIONS
Diabetic ketoacidosis with or without
coma, type 1 diabetes mellitus
Caution
Elderly, cardiac disease, severe renal
disease, severe hepatic disease,
thyroid disease

DRUG INTERACTIONS OF CONCERN TO DENTISTRY
• Increased hypoglycemic effects:
salicylates, ketoconazole
• Decreased action of glipizide:
corticosteroids
• Disulfiram-like reaction:
alcohol

SERIOUS REACTIONS
! Overdose or insufficient food
intake may produce hypoglycemia,
especially with increased glucose
demands.
! GI hemorrhage, cholestatic
hepatic jaundice, leukopenia,
thrombocytopenia, pancytopenia,
agranulocytosis, and aplastic or
hemolytic anemia occurs rarely.

DENTAL CONSIDERATIONS

General:
- Monitor vital signs at every appointment because of cardiovascular side effects.
- Patients on chronic drug therapy may rarely have symptoms of blood dyscrasias, which can include infection, bleeding, and poor healing.
- Short appointments and a stress-reduction protocol may be required for anxious patients.
- Place on frequent recall to evaluate healing response.
- Diabetics may be more susceptible to infection and have delayed wound healing.
- Question patient about self-monitoring of drug's antidiabetic effect, including blood glucose values or finger-stick records.
- Ensure that patient is following prescribed diet and regularly takes medication.
- Avoid prescribing aspirin-containing products.

Consultations:
- In a patient with symptoms of blood dyscrasias, request a medical consultation for blood studies and postpone dental treatment until normal values are reestablished.
- Medical consultation may be required to assess disease control.
- Medical consultation may include data from patient's blood glucose monitoring, including glycosylated hemoglobin or HbA1c testing.

Teach Patient/Family to:
- Use effective oral hygiene to prevent soft tissue inflammation
- Use caution to prevent injury when using oral hygiene aids
- Avoid mouth rinses with high alcohol content because of drying effects

glucagon hydrochloride

glue´-ka-gon hi-droh-klor´-ide
(GlucaGen, GlucaGen Diagnostic Kit, Glucagen[AUS], Glucagon, Glucagon Diagnostic Kit, Glucagon Emergency Kit)
Do not confuse glucagon with Glaucon.

CATEGORY AND SCHEDULE
Pregnancy Risk Category: B

Drug Class: Antihypoglycemic, hormone

MECHANISM OF ACTION
A glucose-elevating agent that promotes hepatic glycogenolysis, gluconeogenesis. Stimulates production of cyclic adenosine monophosphate (cAMP), which results in increased plasma glucose concentration, smooth muscle relaxation, and an inotropic myocardial effect.
Therapeutic Effect: Increases plasma glucose level.

USES
Severe hypoglycemia; as a diagnostic aid to facilitate in the radiologic examination of the GI tract by relaxing smooth muscle

PHARMACOKINETICS
Parenteral: Peak levels in 20 min (subcutaneous) or 13 min (IM); extensively metabolized in liver, kidney, and plasma

INDICATIONS AND DOSAGES
▸ **Hypoglycemia**
IV, IM, Subcutaneous
Adults, Elderly, Children weighing more than 20 kg. 0.5–1 mg. May give

1 or 2 additional doses if response is delayed.
Children weighing 20 kg or less.
0.5 mg.

▶ **Diagnostic Aid**
IV, IM
Adults, Elderly. 0.25–2 mg 10 min prior to procedure.

SIDE EFFECTS/ADVERSE REACTIONS
Occasional
Nausea, vomiting
Rare
Allergic reaction, such as urticaria, respiratory distress, and hypotension

PRECAUTIONS AND CONTRAINDICATIONS
Hypersensitivity to glucagon or beef or pork proteins, known pheochromocytoma.
Caution
For Type 1 diabetes give supplemental carbohydrates as soon as possible; insulinoma, starvation, glycogen depletion, adrenal insufficiency, chronic hypoglycemia, lactation

DRUG INTERACTIONS OF CONCERN TO DENTISTRY
• Patients taking β-adrenergic blockers: may be expected to have a transient but greater increase in B/P and pulse

SERIOUS REACTIONS
! Overdose may produce persistent nausea and vomiting and hypokalemia, marked by severe weakness, decreased appetite, irregular heartbeat, and muscle cramps.

DENTAL CONSIDERATIONS
General:
• Glucagon may be used as an emergency drug for severe

hypoglycemia. Patients should be closely monitored and referred immediately for evaluation.
• IV glucose may be required for patients nonresponsive to glucagon.
• Unconscious patients should awaken within 15 min or less.

glyburide
glye´-byoor-ide
(Daonil[CAN], DiaBeta, Euglucon[CAN], Glimel[AUS], Glynase, Micronase, Semi-Daonil[AUS], Semi-Euglucon[AUS])
Do not confuse glyburide with glimepiride or glipizide, or Micronase with Micro-K or Micronor.

CATEGORY AND SCHEDULE
Pregnancy Risk Category: C

Drug Class: Oral antidiabetic (second generation)

MECHANISM OF ACTION
A second-generation sulfonylurea that promotes release of insulin from beta cells of the pancreas and increases insulin sensitivity at peripheral sites. *Therapeutic Effect:* Lowers blood glucose concentration.

USES
Treatment of stable adult-onset diabetes mellitus (type II)

PHARMACOKINETICS

Route	Onset	Peak	Duration
PO	0.25–1 hr	1–2 hr	12–24 hr

Well absorbed from the GI tract. Protein binding: 99%. Metabolized in the liver to weakly active metabolite. Primarily excreted in urine.

Not removed by hemodialysis.
Half-life: 1.4–1.8 hr.

INDICATIONS AND DOSAGES
▸ **Diabetes Mellitus**
PO
Adults. Initially 2.5–5 mg. May
increase by 2.5 mg/day at weekly
intervals. Maintenance: 1.25–20 mg/
day. Maximum: 20 mg/day.
Elderly. Initially, 1.25–2.5 mg/day.
May increase by 1.25–2.5 mg/day at
1- to 3-wk intervals.
PO (micronized tablets [Glynase])
Adults, Elderly. Initially 0.75–3 mg/
day. May increase by 1.5 mg/day at
weekly intervals. Maintenance:
0.75–12 mg/day as a single dose or
in divided doses.
▸ **Dosage in Renal Impairment**
Glyburide is not recommended in
patients with creatinine clearance
less than 50 ml/min.

SIDE EFFECTS/ADVERSE REACTIONS
Frequent
Altered taste sensation, dizziness,
somnolence, weight gain,
constipation, diarrhea, heartburn,
nausea, vomiting, stomach fullness,
headache
Occasional
Increased sensitivity of skin
to sunlight, peeling of skin,
itching, rash

PRECAUTIONS AND CONTRAINDICATIONS
Diabetic ketoacidosis with or without
coma, monotherapy for type 1
diabetes mellitus
Caution
Elderly, cardiac disease, severe renal
disease, severe hepatic disease,
thyroid disease, severe hypoglycemia
reactions

DRUG INTERACTIONS OF CONCERN TO DENTISTRY
● Increased hypoglycemic effects:
NSAIDs, salicylates, ketoconazole
● Decreased action of glyburide:
corticosteroids
● Disulfiram-like reaction: alcohol

SERIOUS REACTIONS
! Overdose or insufficient food
intake may produce hypoglycemia,
especially in patients with increased
glucose demands.
! Cholestatic jaundice, leukopenia,
thrombocytopenia, pancytopenia,
agranulocytosis, and aplastic or
hemolytic anemia occur rarely.

DENTAL CONSIDERATIONS
General:
● Monitor vital signs at every
appointment because of
cardiovascular side effects.
● Patients on chronic drug therapy
may rarely have symptoms of blood
dyscrasias, which can include
infection, bleeding, and poor healing.
● Place on frequent recall to evaluate
healing response.
● Ensure that patient is following
prescribed diet and regularly takes
medication.
● Short appointments and stress-
reduction protocol may be required
for anxious patients.
● Patients with diabetes may be more
susceptible to infection and have
delayed wound healing.
● Question patient about self-
monitoring of drug's antidiabetic
effect, including blood glucose
values or finger-stick records.
● Avoid prescribing aspirin-
containing products.
Consultations:
● In a patient with symptoms of
blood dyscrasias, request a medical
consultation for blood studies and

postpone dental treatment until normal values are reestablished.
• Medical consultation may be required to assess disease control.
• Medical consultation may include data from patient's blood glucose monitoring, including glycosylated hemoglobin or HbA1c testing.

Teach Patient/Family to:
• Use effective oral hygiene to prevent soft tissue inflammation
• Use caution to prevent injury when using oral hygiene aids
• Avoid mouth rinses with high alcohol content because of drying effects

glycopyrrolate
glye-koe-pye´-roe-late
(Robinul, Robinul Forte, Robinul Injection[AUS])
Do not confuse Robinul with Reminyl.

CATEGORY AND SCHEDULE
Pregnancy Risk Category: B

Drug Class: Anticholinergic

MECHANISM OF ACTION
A quaternary anticholinergic that inhibits action of acetylcholine at postganglionic parasympathetic sites in smooth muscle, secretory glands, and CNS. ***Therapeutic Effect:*** Reduces salivation and excessive secretions of respiratory tract; reduces gastric secretions and acidity.

USES
Decreased secretions before surgery, reversal of neuromuscular blockade, peptic ulcer disease, irritable bowel syndrome

PHARMACOKINETICS
Poorly and irregularly absorbed from GI tract after oral administration. Metabolized in the liver. Primarily excreted in urine. ***Half-life:*** 1.7 hr.

INDICATIONS AND DOSAGES
▶ **Preoperative Inhibition of Salivation and Excessive Respiratory Tract Secretions**
IM
Adults, Elderly. 4 mcg/kg 30–60 min before procedure.
Children 2 yr and older. 4 mcg/kg.
Children younger than 2 yr. 4–9 mcg/kg.
▶ **To Block Effects of Anticholinesterase Agents**
IV
Adults, Elderly. 0.2 mg for each 1 mg neostigmine or 5 mg pyridostigmine.
▶ **Peptic Ulcer Disease, Adjunct**
IV, IM
Adults, Elderly. 0.1 mg IV or IM 3–4 times a day.
PO
Adults, Elderly. 1–2 mg 2–3 times a day. Maximum: 8 mg/day.

SIDE EFFECTS/ADVERSE REACTIONS
Frequent
Dry mouth, decreased sweating, constipation
Occasional
Blurred vision, gastric bloating, urinary hesitancy, somnolence (with high dosage), headache, intolerance to light, loss of taste, nervousness, flushing, insomnia, impotence, mental confusion or excitement (particularly in the elderly and children), temporary light-headedness (with parenteral form), local irritation (with parenteral form)
Rare
Dizziness, faintness

PRECAUTIONS AND CONTRAINDICATIONS

Acute hemorrhage, myasthenia gravis, narrow-angle glaucoma, obstructive uropathy, paralytic ileus, tachycardia, ulcerative colitis

Caution

Elderly, lactation, prostatic hypertrophy, renal disease, CHF, pulmonary disease, hyperthyroidism

DRUG INTERACTIONS OF CONCERN TO DENTISTRY

• Increased anticholinergic effect: antihistamines, phenothiazines, meperidine, haloperidol, scopolamine, atropine
• Do not mix with diazepam, pentobarbital, in syringe or solution
• Constipation, urinary retention: opioid analgesics
• Reduced absorption of ketoconazole

SERIOUS REACTIONS

! Overdose may produce temporary paralysis of ciliary muscle; pupillary dilation; tachycardia; palpitations; hot, dry, or flushed skin; absence of bowel sounds; hyperthermia; increased respiratory rate; ECG abnormalities; nausea; vomiting; rash over face or upper trunk; CNS stimulation; and psychosis (marked by agitation, restlessness, rambling speech, visual hallucinations, paranoid behavior, and delusions, followed by depression).

DENTAL CONSIDERATIONS

General:

• Avoid dental light in patient's eyes; offer dark glasses for patient comfort.
• Assess salivary flow as a factor in caries, periodontal disease, and candidiasis.

Consultation:

• Physician should be informed if significant xerostomic side effects occur (e.g., increased caries, sore tongue, problems eating or swallowing, difficulty wearing prosthesis) so that a medication change can be considered.

Teach Patient/Family:

• When chronic dry mouth occurs, advise patient to:
  • Avoid mouth rinses with high alcohol content because of drying effects
  • Use daily home fluoride products for anticaries effect
  • Use sugarless gum, frequent sips of water, or saliva substitutes

goserelin acetate

gos-er´-ah-lin ass´-eh-tayte
(Zoladex, Zoladex Implant[AUS], Zoladex LA)

CATEGORY AND SCHEDULE

Pregnancy Risk Category:
D (advanced breast cancer),
X (endometriosis, endometrial thinning)

Drug Class: Gonadotropin-releasing hormone, antineoplastic (hormone); synthetic decapeptide analog of LHRH

MECHANISM OF ACTION

A gonadotropin-releasing hormone analog and antineoplastic agent that stimulates the release of luteinizing hormone (LH) and follicle-stimulating hormone (FSH) from the anterior pituitary gland. In males, increases testosterone concentrations initially, then suppresses secretion of LH and FSH, resulting in decreased testosterone levels.

Therapeutic Effect: In females, causes a reduction in ovarian size and function, reduction in uterine and mammary gland size, and regression of sex-hormone-responsive tumors. In males, produces pharmacologic castration and decreases the growth of abnormal prostate tissue.

USES

Treatment of advanced prostate cancer stage B2-C (10.8 mg), endometriosis, advanced breast cancer, endometrial thinning (3.6 mg)

PHARMACOKINETICS

Peak serum concentrations in 14–28 days. ***Half-life*** 4.5 hr.

INDICATIONS AND DOSAGES
▶ **Prostatic Carcinoma**
Implant
Adults older than 18 yr, Elderly. 3.6 mg every 28 days or 10.8 mg q12wk subcutaneously into upper abdominal wall.
▶ **Breast Carcinoma, Endometriosis**
Implant
Adults. 3.6 mg every 28 days subcutaneously into upper abdominal wall.
▶ **Endometrial Thinning**
Implant
Adults. 3.6 mg subcutaneously into upper abdominal wall as a single dose or in 2 doses 4 wk apart.

SIDE EFFECTS/ADVERSE REACTIONS
Frequent
Headache, hot flashes, depression, diaphoresis, sexual dysfunction, decreased erection, lower urinary tract symptoms
Occasional
Pain, lethargy, dizziness, insomnia, anorexia, nausea, rash, upper respiratory tract infection, hirsutism, abdominal pain

Rare
Pruritus

PRECAUTIONS AND CONTRAINDICATIONS
Pregnancy

DRUG INTERACTIONS OF CONCERN TO DENTISTRY
None reported

SERIOUS REACTIONS
❗ Arrhythmias, CHF, and hypertension occur rarely.
❗ Ureteral obstruction and spinal cord compression have been observed. An immediate orchiectomy may be necessary if these conditions occur.

DENTAL CONSIDERATIONS
General:
• Monitor vital signs at every appointment due to cardiovascular side effects.
• Determine why patient is taking the drug.
• If additional analgesia is required for dental pain, consider alternative analgesics (NSAIDs) in patients taking narcotics for acute or chronic pain.
• Consider semisupine chair position for patient comfort if GI side effects occur.
• Assess salivary flow as a factor in caries, periodontal disease, and candidiasis.
• If used in prostate cancer, consider urinary retention concern and avoid anticholinergic drugs that may aggravate retention.
• Patients may be taking other medications; see complete drug and herbal history.

Consultations:
• Medical consultation may be required to assess immunologic status during cancer chemotherapy and determine safety risk, if any, posed by the required dental treatment.
• Medical consultation may be required to assess disease control and patient's ability to tolerate stress.
Teach Patient/Family to:
• When chronic dry mouth occurs advise patient to:
  • Avoid mouth rinses with high alcohol content due to drying effects
  • Use daily home fluoride products for anticaries effect
  • Use sugarless gum, frequent sips of water, or saliva substitutes
• Use effective oral hygiene to prevent soft tissue inflammation
• Report oral lesions, soreness, or bleeding to dentist
• Prevent trauma when using oral hygiene aids
• Update health and medication history if physician makes any changes in evaluation or drug regimens; include OTC, herbal, and nonherbal remedies in the update

granisetron
gra-nih´-se-tron
(Kytril)

CATEGORY AND SCHEDULE
Pregnancy Risk Category: B

Drug Class: Antiemetic; 5-HT$_3$ receptor antagonist

MECHANISM OF ACTION
A 5-HT$_3$ receptor antagonist that acts centrally in the chemoreceptor trigger zone or peripherally at the vagal nerve terminals. ***Therapeutic Effect:*** Prevents nausea and vomiting.

USES
Prevention of nausea, vomiting associated with cancer chemotherapy including high-dose cisplatin

PHARMACOKINETICS

Route	Onset	Peak	Duration
IV	1–3 min	N/A	24 hr

Rapidly and widely distributed to tissues. Protein binding: 65%. Metabolized in the liver to active metabolite. Eliminated in urine and feces. ***Half-life:*** 10–12 hr (increased in the elderly).

INDICATIONS AND DOSAGES
▸ **Prevention of Chemotherapy-Induced Nausea and Vomiting**
PO
Adults, Elderly. 2 mg once a day up to 1 hr before chemotherapy or 1 mg twice a day.
IV
Adults, Elderly, Children 2 yr and older. 10 mcg/kg/dose (or 1 mg/dose) within 30 min of chemotherapy.
▸ **Prevention of Radiation-Induced Nausea and Vomiting**
PO
Adults, Elderly. 2 mg once a day given 1 hr before radiation therapy.
▸ **Postoperative Nausea or Vomiting**
PO
Adults, Elderly, Children 4 yr and older. 20–40 mcg/kg as a single postoperative dose.
IV
Adults, Elderly. 1 mg as a single postoperative dose.
Children older than 4 yr. 20–40 mcg/kg. Maximum: 1 mg.

SIDE EFFECTS/ADVERSE REACTIONS
Frequent
Headache, constipation, asthenia
Occasional
Diarrhea, abdominal pain
Rare
Altered taste, hypersensitivity reaction

PRECAUTIONS AND CONTRAINDICATIONS
None known

DRUG INTERACTIONS OF CONCERN TO DENTISTRY
• Possible decreased effects: strong inducers of CYP3A4 isoenzymes
• Possible increased effects: strong inhibitors of CYP3A4 isoenzymes

SERIOUS REACTIONS
None known

DENTAL CONSIDERATIONS
General:
• When used in anesthesia, monitor patients to prevent untoward events.
Teach Patient/Family to:
• Be aware of possible oral side effects from concurrent cancer chemotherapy.
• Report troublesome nausea and vomiting to dentist for patients recovering from anesthesia after dental treatment.
• Understand that alteration in taste is temporary.

griseofulvin
griz-ee-oh-full´-vin
(Fulvicin P/G, Fulvicin U/F, Grifulvin V, Gris-PEG, Grisovin[AUS])

CATEGORY AND SCHEDULE
Pregnancy Risk Category: C

Drug Class: Antifungal

MECHANISM OF ACTION
An antifungal that inhibits fungal cell mitosis by disrupting mitotic spindle structure. ***Therapeutic Effect:*** Fungistatic.

PHARMACOKINETICS
Variable GI absorption after oral administration; fatty meals may enhance absorption. Peak blood levels: 4 hr. Deposited in keratinized cells.

USES
Myotic infections: tinea corporis, tinea pedis, tinea cruris, tinea barbae, tinea capitis, tinea unguium if caused by *Epidermophyton, Microsporum,* or *Trichophyton*

INDICATIONS AND DOSAGES
▶ **Tinea Capitis, Tinea Corporis, Tinea Cruris, Tinea Pedis, Tinea Unguium**
PO (Microsize Tablets, Oral Suspension)
Adults. Usual dosage, 500–1000 mg as a single dose or in divided doses.
Children 2 yr and older. Usual dosage, 10–20 mg/kg/day.
PO (Ultramicrosize Tablets)
Adults. Usual dosage, 330–750 mg/day as a single dose or in divided doses.
Children 2 yr and older.
5–10 mg/kg/day.

SIDE EFFECTS/ADVERSE REACTIONS
Occasional
Hypersensitivity reaction (including pruritus, rash, and urticaria), headache, nausea, diarrhea, excessive thirst, flatulence, oral thrush, dizziness, insomnia
Rare
Paresthesia of hands or feet, proteinuria, photosensitivity reaction

PRECAUTIONS AND CONTRAINDICATIONS
Hepatocellular failure, porphyria

DRUG INTERACTIONS OF CONCERN TO DENTISTRY
• Possible decreased effects: phenobarbital

SERIOUS REACTIONS
! Granulocytopenia occurs rarely.

DENTAL CONSIDERATIONS
General:
• Determine why patient is taking the drug.
• Assess salivary flow as a factor in caries, periodontal disease, and candidiasis.
• Examine for oral manifestation of opportunistic infection.
• Advise patient if dental drugs prescribed have a potential for photosensitivity.
Teach Patient/Family to:
• Report oral lesions, soreness, or bleeding to dentist
• Use effective oral hygiene to prevent soft tissue inflammation
• Report sore throat, oral burning sensation, fever, or fatigue, any of which could indicate presence of a superinfection
• Update health and medication history if physician makes any changes in evaluation or drug regimens; include OTC, herbal, and nonherbal remedies in the update
• Avoid concurrent use of alcohol
• When chronic dry mouth occurs advise patient to:
  • Avoid mouth rinses with high alcohol content due to drying effects
  • Use daily home fluoride products for anticaries effect
  • Use sugarless gum, frequent sips of water, or saliva substitutes

guaifenesin
gwye-fen´-eh-sin
(Balminil[CAN], Benylin E[CAN], Guiatuss, Humibid LA, Mucinex, Organidin, Robitussin, Tussin)
Do not confuse guaifenesin with guanfacine.

CATEGORY AND SCHEDULE
Pregnancy Risk Category: C
OTC

Drug Class: Expectorant, glyceryl guaiacolate

MECHANISM OF ACTION
An expectorant that stimulates respiratory tract secretions by decreasing adhesiveness and viscosity of phlegm. ***Therapeutic Effect:*** Promotes removal of viscous mucus.

USES
Treatment of dry, nonproductive cough

PHARMACOKINETICS
Well absorbed from the GI tract. Metabolized in the liver. Excreted in urine.

INDICATIONS AND DOSAGES
▸ **Expectorant**
PO
Adults, Elderly, Children older than 12 yr. 200–400 mg q4h.
Children 6–12 yr. 100–200 mg q4h.
Maximum: 1.2 g/day.
Children 2–5 yr. 50–100 mg q4h.
Children younger than 2 yr. 12 mg/kg/day in 6 divided doses.
PO (Extended-Release)
Adults, Elderly, Children older than 12 yr. 600–1200 mg q12h.
Maximum: 2.4 g/day.

Children 2–5 yr. 600 mg q12h.
Maximum: 600 mg/day.

SIDE EFFECTS/ADVERSE REACTIONS
Rare
Dizziness, headache, rash, diarrhea, nausea, vomiting, abdominal pain

PRECAUTIONS AND CONTRAINDICATIONS
Hypersensitivity, persistent cough

SERIOUS REACTIONS
! Overdose may produce nausea and vomiting.

DENTAL CONSIDERATIONS
General:
• Consider semisupine chair position for patients with respiratory disease.
• Elective dental treatment may be precluded by significant coughing episodes.

guanabenz
gwan´-ah-benz
(Wytensin)

CATEGORY AND SCHEDULE
Pregnancy Risk Category: C

Drug Class: Centrally acting antihypertensive

MECHANISM OF ACTION
An alpha-adrenergic agonist that stimulates α_2-adrenergic receptors. Inhibits sympathetic cardioaccelerator and vasoconstrictor center to heart, kidneys, peripheral vasculature. *Therapeutic Effect:* Decreases systolic, diastolic B/P. Chronic use decreases peripheral vascular resistance.

USES
Treatment of hypertension

PHARMACOKINETICS
Well absorbed from GI tract. Widely distributed. Protein binding: 90%. Metabolized in liver. Excreted in urine and feces. Not removed by hemodialysis. *Half-life:* 6 hr.

INDICATIONS AND DOSAGES
▸ **Hypertension**
PO
Adults. Initially, 4 mg 2 times a day. Increase by 4–8 mg at 1–2 wk intervals.
Elderly. Initially, 4 mg/day. May increase q1–2 wk.
Maintenance: 8–16 mg/day.
Maximum: 32 mg/day.

SIDE EFFECTS/ADVERSE REACTIONS
Frequent
Drowsiness, dry mouth, dizziness
Occasional
Weakness, headache, nausea, decreased sexual ability
Rare
Ataxia, sleep disturbances, rash, itching, diarrhea, constipation, altered taste, muscle aches

PRECAUTIONS AND CONTRAINDICATIONS
History of hypersensitivity to guanabenz or any component of the formulation
Caution
Lactation, children younger than 12 yr, severe coronary insufficiency, recent MI, cerebrovascular disease, severe hepatic or renal failure

DRUG INTERACTIONS OF CONCERN TO DENTISTRY
• Increased CNS depression: alcohol, all CNS depressants

• Decreased hypotensive effects: NSAIDs, especially indomethacin, sympathomimetics

SERIOUS REACTIONS

! Abrupt withdrawal may result in rebound hypertension manifested as nervousness, agitation, anxiety, insomnia, hand tingling, tremors, flushing, and sweating.

! Overdosage produces hypotension, somnolence, lethargy, irritability, bradycardia, and miosis (pupillary constriction).

DENTAL CONSIDERATIONS

General:
• Monitor vital signs at every appointment because of cardiovascular side effects.
• Limit use of sodium-containing products, such as saline IV fluids, for patients with a dietary salt restriction.
• Assess salivary flow as a factor in caries, periodontal disease, and candidiasis.
• Stress from dental procedures may compromise cardiovascular function; determine patient risk.
• Short appointments and a stress reduction protocol may be required for anxious patients.
Consultations:
• Medical consultation may be required to assess disease control and patient's ability to tolerate stress.
Teach Patient/Family:
• When chronic dry mouth occurs, advise patient to:
    • Avoid mouth rinses with high alcohol content because of drying effects
    • Use daily home fluoride products for anticaries effect
    • Use sugarless gum, frequent sips of water, or saliva substitutes

guanadrel sulfate

gwahn´-ah-drel sull´-fate
(Hylorel)

CATEGORY AND SCHEDULE

Pregnancy Risk Category: C

Drug Class: Antihypertensive

MECHANISM OF ACTION

An adrenergic blocking agent that depletes norepinephrine from adrenergic nerve endings. Prevents release of norepinephrine normally produced by nerve stimulation. *Therapeutic Effect:* Reduces B/P.

USES

Treatment of hypertension

PHARMACOKINETICS

Rapidly and well absorbed from GI tract. Widely distributed. Protein binding: 20%. Primarily excreted in urine. *Half-life:* 10 hr.

INDICATIONS AND DOSAGES

▸ **Hypertension**
PO
Adults. Initially, 5 mg 2 times a day. Increase at 1–4 wk intervals. Maintenance: 20–75 mg/day in 2 divided doses. Maximum: 400 mg/day.
Elderly. Initially, 5 mg/day. May gradually increase at 1–4 wk intervals. Maintenance: 20–75 mg/day in 2 divided doses.

SIDE EFFECTS/ADVERSE REACTIONS

Frequent
Fatigue, headache, faintness, drowsiness, nocturia, urinary frequency, change in weight, aching limbs, shortness of breath (resting)

Occasional
Cough, change in vision, paresthesia, confusion, indigestion, constipation, anorexia, peripheral edema, leg cramps
Rare
Depression, altered sleep, nausea, vomiting, dry mouth, throat, impotence, backache

PRECAUTIONS AND CONTRAINDICATIONS
Frank CHF, pheochromocytoma, hypersensitivity to guanadrel or any component of the formulation
Caution
Elderly, bronchial asthma, peptic ulcer, electrolyte imbalances, vascular disease

DRUG INTERACTIONS OF CONCERN TO DENTISTRY
• Increased orthostatic hypotension: alcohol, opioid analgesics, barbiturates, phenothiazines, haloperidol
• Decreased hypotensive effect: ephedrine, sympathomimetics, NSAIDs, indomethacin, tricyclic antidepressants

SERIOUS REACTIONS
! Overdose may produce blurred vision, severe dizziness/faintness.

DENTAL CONSIDERATIONS
General:
• Monitor vital signs at every appointment because of cardiovascular side effects.
• After supine positioning, have patient sit upright for at least 2 min before standing to avoid orthostatic hypotension.
• Limit use of sodium-containing products, such as saline IV fluids, for patients with a dietary salt restriction.

• Stress from dental procedures may compromise cardiovascular function; determine patient risk.
• Short appointments and a stress-reduction protocol may be required for anxious patients.
• Assess salivary flow as a factor in caries, periodontal disease, and candidiasis.
Consultations:
• Medical consultation may be required to assess disease control and patient's ability to tolerate stress.
Teach Patient/Family:
• When chronic dry mouth occurs, advise patient to:
  • Avoid mouth rinses with high alcohol content because of drying effects
  • Use daily home fluoride products for anticaries effect
  • Use sugarless gum, frequent sips of water, or saliva substitutes

guanethidine monosulfate
gwahn-eth´-ih-deen
mah-no-sull´-fate
(Ismelin)

CATEGORY AND SCHEDULE
Pregnancy Risk Category: C

Drug Class: Antihypertensive

MECHANISM OF ACTION
An adrenergic blocker that inhibits the release of catecholamines produced by sympathetic nerve stimulation, thus suppressing peripheral sympathetic vasoconstriction. *Therapeutic Effect:* Decreases B/P.

USES
Treatment of moderate-to-severe hypertension

PHARMACOKINETICS
Absorption is highly variable among patients. Protein binding: 26%. Metabolized in liver. Excreted in urine and feces. *Half-life:* 5–10 days.

INDICATIONS AND DOSAGES
▸ **Hypertension**
PO
Adults. Initially, 10 mg/day. May increase in 10–25 mg increments at 5–7 day intervals. Maximum: 100 mg/day. Lower initial doses are recommended for the elderly.

SIDE EFFECTS/ADVERSE REACTIONS
Frequent
Bradycardia, dizziness, blurred vision, orthostatic hypotension, fluid retention
Occasional
Impotence, inhibition of ejaculation, nasal stuffiness
Rare
Apnea, hypertension, renal dysfunction

PRECAUTIONS AND CONTRAINDICATIONS
MAOI therapy within 1 wk, overt CHF, pheochromocytoma, hypersensitivity to guanethidine or any component of the formulation
Caution
Lactation, children; peptic ulcer, asthma, frequent orthostatic hypotension, fever, renal impairment

DRUG INTERACTIONS OF CONCERN TO DENTISTRY
• Increased orthostatic hypotension: alcohol, opioid analgesics, barbiturates, phenothiazines, haloperidol
• Decreased hypotensive effect: ephedrine, NSAIDs, indomethacin, sympathomimetics, tricyclic antidepressants

SERIOUS REACTIONS
! Arrhythmias, angina, and pulmonary edema have been reported.
! Overdosage may produce bradycardia, diarrhea, nausea, orthostatic hypotension, and shock.

DENTAL CONSIDERATIONS
General:
• Monitor vital signs at every appointment because of cardiovascular and respiratory side effects.
• Patients on chronic drug therapy may rarely have symptoms of blood dyscrasias, which can include infection, bleeding, and poor healing.
• Assess salivary flow as a factor in caries, periodontal disease, and candidiasis.
• After supine positioning, have patient sit upright for at least 2 min before standing to avoid orthostatic hypotension.
• Limit use of sodium-containing products, such as saline IV fluids, for patients with a dietary salt restriction.
• Stress from dental procedures may compromise cardiovascular function; determine patient risk.
• Short appointments and a stress-reduction protocol may be required for anxious patients.
• Use vasoconstrictors with caution, in low doses, and with careful aspiration. Avoid using gingival retraction cord with epinephrine.
• Consider semisupine chair position for patients with respiratory distress.

Consultations:
• Medical consultation may be required to assess disease control and patient's ability to tolerate stress.
• In a patient with symptoms of blood dyscrasias, request a medical consultation for blood studies and postpone dental treatment until normal values are reestablished.
Teach Patient/Family to:
• Use effective oral hygiene to prevent soft tissue inflammation
• Use caution to prevent injury when using oral hygiene aids
• When chronic dry mouth occurs, advise patient to:
  • Avoid mouth rinses with high alcohol content because of drying effects
  • Use daily home fluoride products for anticaries effect
  • Use sugarless gum, frequent sips of water, or saliva substitutes

guanfacine
gwan´-fa-seen
(Tenex)

CATEGORY AND SCHEDULE
Pregnancy Risk Category: B

Drug Class: Antihypertensive

MECHANISM OF ACTION
An alpha-adrenergic agonist that stimulates α_2-adrenergic receptors and inhibits sympathetic cardioaccelerator and vasoconstrictor center to heart, kidneys, peripheral vasculature. *Therapeutic Effect:* Decreases systolic, diastolic B/P. Chronic use decreases peripheral vascular resistance.

USES
Treatment of hypertension in individual using a thiazide diuretic or other antihypertensive

PHARMACOKINETICS
Well absorbed from GI tract. Widely distributed. Protein binding: 71%. Metabolized in liver. Excreted in urine and feces. Not removed by hemodialysis. *Half-life:* 17 hr.

INDICATIONS AND DOSAGES
▶ **Hypertension**
PO
Adults, Elderly. Initially, 1 mg/day. Increase by 1 mg/day at intervals of 3–4 wk up to 3 mg/day in single or divided doses.

SIDE EFFECTS/ADVERSE REACTIONS
Frequent
Dry mouth, somnolence
Occasional
Fatigue, headache, asthenia (loss of strength, energy), dizziness

PRECAUTIONS AND CONTRAINDICATIONS
History of hypersensitivity to guanfacine or any component of the formulation

DRUG INTERACTIONS OF CONCERN TO DENTISTRY
• Possible increase in CNS depression: alcohol and all CNS depressants
• Possible reduced antihypertensive effect: indomethacin and perhaps other NSAIDs
• Possible increase in antihypertensive effects: other antihypertensive drugs

SERIOUS REACTIONS

! Overdosage may produce difficult breathing, dizziness, faintness, severe drowsiness, bradycardia.

DENTAL CONSIDERATIONS

General:
• Monitor vital signs at every appointment because of cardiovascular side effects.
• Limit use of sodium-containing products, such as saline IV fluids, for patients with a dietary salt restriction.
• Assess salivary flow as a factor in caries, periodontal disease, and candidiasis.
• Short appointments and a stress-reduction protocol may be required for anxious patients.
• Stress from dental procedures may compromise cardiovascular function; determine patient risk.
• Use precaution if sedation or general anesthesia is required; risk of hypotensive episode.

Consultations:
• Medical consultation may be required to assess disease control and patient's ability to tolerate stress.

Teach Patient/Family to:
• Update health and medication history if physician makes any changes in evaluation or drug regimens; include OTC, herbal, and nonherbal remedies in the update
• Use caution when driving or performing other tasks requiring mental alertness; avoid if drowsiness occurs.
• When chronic dry mouth occurs advise patient to:
  • Avoid mouth rinses with high alcohol content due to drying effects
  • Use daily home fluoride products for anticaries effect
  • Use sugarless gum, frequent sips of water, or saliva substitutes

halcinonide

hal-sin´-oh-nide
(Halog, Halog-E)

CATEGORY AND SCHEDULE

Pregnancy Risk Category: C

Drug Class: Corticosteroid,
synthetic topical

MECHANISM OF ACTION

A topical corticosteroid that has
antiinflammatory, antipruritic, and
vasoconstrictive properties.
The exact mechanism of the
antiinflammatory process is unclear.
Therapeutic Effect: Reduces or
prevents tissue response to the
inflammatory process.

USES

Treatment of inflammation of
corticosteroid-responsive dermatoses

PHARMACOKINETICS

Well absorbed systemically. Large
variation in absorption among sites.
Protein binding: varies. Metabolized
in liver. Primarily excreted in urine.

INDICATIONS AND DOSAGES

▶ **Dermatoses**
Topical
Adults, Elderly. Apply sparingly
1–3 times a day.

SIDE EFFECTS/ADVERSE REACTIONS

Occasional
Itching, redness, irritation, burning at
site of application, dryness,
folliculitis, acneiform eruptions,
hypopigmentation
Rare
Allergic contact dermatitis,
maceration of the skin, secondary
infection, skin atrophy

PRECAUTIONS AND CONTRAINDICATIONS

History of hypersensitivity to
halcinonide or other corticosteroids

SERIOUS REACTIONS

! The serious reactions of long-term
therapy and the addition of occlusive
dressings are reversible
hypothalamic-pituitary-adrenal
(HPA) axis suppression,
manifestations of Cushing's
syndrome, hyperglycemia, and
glucosuria.

DENTAL CONSIDERATIONS

General:
• Place on frequent recall to evaluate
healing response when used on
chronic basis.
Teach Patient/Family to:
• Use effective oral hygiene to
prevent soft tissue inflammation
• Return for oral evaluation if
response of oral tissues has not
occurred in 7–14 days
• Apply at bedtime or after meals for
maximum effect
• Apply with cotton-tipped
applicator by pressing, not rubbing,
paste on lesion
• Avoid use on oral herpetic
ulcerations

halobetasol

hal-oh-bay´-ta-sol
(Ultravate)

CATEGORY AND SCHEDULE

Pregnancy Risk Category: C

Drug Class: Topical
corticosteroid, group VI potency

MECHANISM OF ACTION
A corticosteroid that inhibits accumulation of inflammatory cells at inflammation sites, phagocytosis, lysosomal enzyme release, and synthesis or release of mediators of inflammation. *Therapeutic Effect:* Decreases or prevents tissue response to inflammatory process.

USES
Treatment of psoriasis, eczema, contact dermatitis, pruritus

PHARMACOKINETICS
Variation in absorption among individuals and sites: scrotum 36%, forehead 7%, scalp 4%, forearm 1%.

INDICATIONS AND DOSAGES
▸ **Dermatoses, Corticosteroid-Unresponsive**
Topical
Adults, Elderly, Children 12 yr and older. Apply 1–2 times a day. Maximum: 50 g for 2 wk.

SIDE EFFECTS/ADVERSE REACTIONS
Frequent
Burning, stinging, pruritus
Rare
Cushing's syndrome, hyperglycemia, glucosuria, hypothalamic-pituitary-adrenal axis suppression

PRECAUTIONS AND CONTRAINDICATIONS
Hypersensitivity to halobetasol or other corticosteroids
Caution
Lactation, viral infections, bacterial infections

SERIOUS REACTIONS
! Overdosage can occur from topically applied halobetasol absorbed in sufficient amounts to produce systemic effects producing reversible adrenal suppression, manifestations of Cushing's syndrome, hyperglycemia, and glucosuria in some patients.

DENTAL CONSIDERATIONS
Teach Patient/Family to:
• Avoid use on oral herpetic ulcerations

haloperidol
ha-loe-per´-ih-dole
(Apo-Haloperidol[CAN], Haldol, Haldol Decanoate, Novoperidol[CAN], Peridol[CAN], Serenace[AUS])
Do not confuse Haldol with Halcion, Halog, or Stadol.

CATEGORY AND SCHEDULE
Pregnancy Risk Category: C

Drug Class:
Antipsychotic/butyrophenone

MECHANISM OF ACTION
An antipsychotic, antiemetic, and antidyskinetic agent that competitively blocks postsynaptic dopamine receptors, interrupts nerve impulse movement, and increases turnover of dopamine in the brain. Has strong extrapyramidal and antiemetic effects; weak anticholinergic and sedative effects. *Therapeutic Effect:* Produces tranquilizing effect.

USES
Treatment of psychotic disorders, control of tics and vocal utterances in Tourette's syndrome, short-term treatment of hyperactive children showing excessive motor activity

PHARMACOKINETICS

Readily absorbed from the GI tract. Protein binding: 92%. Extensively metabolized in the liver. Primarily excreted in urine. Not removed by hemodialysis. *Half-life:* 12–37 hr PO; 10–19 hr IV; 17–25 hr IM.

INDICATIONS AND DOSAGES

▸ **Treatment of Psychotic Disorders**
PO
Adults, Children 12 yr and older. Initially, 0.5–5 mg 2–3 times a day. Dosage gradually adjusted as needed.
Elderly. 0.5–2 mg 2–3 times a day. Dosage gradually adjusted as needed.
Children 3–12 yr or weighing 15–40 kg. Initially, 0.05 mg/kg/day in 2–3 divided doses. May increase by 0.5 mg increments at 5–7 day intervals. Maximum: 0.15 mg/kg/day in divided doses.
IM
Adults, Elderly, Children 12 yr and older. Initially, 2–5. May repeat at 1-hr intervals as needed. Maximum: 100 mg/day.
IM (Decanoate)
Adults, Elderly, Children 12 yr and older. Initially, 10–15 times previous daily oral dose up to maximum initial dose of 100 mg. Maximum: 300 mg/mo.
▸ **Treatment of Non-Psychotic Disorders, Tourette's Syndrome**
PO
Children 3–12 yr or weighing 15–40 kg. Initially, 0.05 mg/kg/day in 2–3 divided doses. May increase by 0.5 mg at 5–7 day intervals. Maximum: 0.075 mg/kg/day.

SIDE EFFECTS/ADVERSE REACTIONS

Frequent
Blurred vision, constipation, orthostatic hypotension, dry mouth, swelling or soreness of female breasts, peripheral edema
Occasional
Allergic reaction, difficulty urinating, decreased thirst, dizziness, decreased sexual function, drowsiness, nausea, vomiting, photosensitivity, lethargy

PRECAUTIONS AND CONTRAINDICATIONS

Angle-closure glaucoma, CNS depression, myelosuppression, Parkinson's disease, severe cardiac or hepatic disease
Caution
Lactation, seizure disorders, hypertension, hepatic disease, cardiac disease

DRUG INTERACTIONS OF CONCERN TO DENTISTRY

• Increased sedation: other CNS depressants, alcohol, barbiturate anesthetics, opioid analgesics
• Hypotension, tachycardia: epinephrine
• Increased extrapyramidal effects: phenothiazines and related drugs (haloperidol, droperidol), metoclopramide
• Additive photosensitization: tetracyclines
• Increased anticholinergic effects: anticholinergics
• Suspected increase in neurologic side effects: fluconazole, itraconazole, ketoconazole

SERIOUS REACTIONS

! Extrapyramidal symptoms appear to be dose related and typically occur in the first few days of therapy. Marked drowsiness and lethargy, excessive salivation, and fixed stare occur frequently. Less common reactions include severe akathisia (motor restlessness) and acute dystonias (such as torticollis, opisthotonos, and oculogyric crisis). ! Tardive dyskinesia (tongue protrusion, puffing of the cheeks, chewing or puckering of the mouth) may occur during long-term therapy or after discontinuing the drug and may be irreversible. Elderly female patients have a greater risk of developing this reaction.

DENTAL CONSIDERATIONS

General:
• Monitor vital signs at every appointment because of cardiovascular side effects.
• After supine positioning, have patient sit upright for at least 2 min before standing to avoid orthostatic hypotension.
• Assess salivary flow as a factor in caries, periodontal disease, and candidiasis.
• Avoid dental light in patient's eyes; offer dark glasses for patient comfort.
• Assess for presence of extrapyramidal motor symptoms, such as tardive dyskinesia and akathisia. Extrapyramidal motor activity may complicate dental treatment.
• Geriatric patients are more susceptible to drug effects; use lower dose.
• Use vasoconstrictors with caution, in low doses, and with careful aspiration. Avoid use of gingival retraction cord with epinephrine.
Consultations:
• Take precautions if dental surgery is anticipated and anesthesia is required.
• Refer to physician if signs of tardive dyskinesia or akathisia are present.
• Physician should be informed if significant xerostomic side effects occur (e.g., increased caries, sore tongue, problems eating or swallowing, difficulty wearing prosthesis) so that a medication change can be considered.
Teach Patient/Family to:
• Use effective oral hygiene to prevent soft tissue inflammation
• Use caution to prevent injury when using oral hygiene aids
• Use electric tooth brush if patient has difficulty holding conventional devices
• When chronic dry mouth occurs, advise patient to:
  • Avoid mouth rinses with high alcohol content because of drying effects
  • Use daily home fluoride products for anticaries effect
  • Use sugarless gum, frequent sips of water, or saliva substitutes

heparin sodium

hep´-ah-rin soe´-dee-um
(Hepalean[CAN], Heparin injection B.P.[AUS], Heparin Leo, Uniparin[AUS])
Do not confuse heparin with Hespan.

CATEGORY AND SCHEDULE
Pregnancy Risk Category: C

Drug Class: Anticoagulant

MECHANISM OF ACTION
A blood modifier that interferes with blood coagulation by blocking conversion of prothrombin to thrombin and fibrinogen to fibrin. *Therapeutic Effect:* Prevents further extension of existing thrombi or new clot formation. Has no effect on existing clots.

USES
Anticoagulant in thrombosis, embolism (both prevention and treatment), coagulopathies, deep vein thrombosis (DVT), prevention of clotting when extracorporeal circulation is required (cardiac surgery), dialysis, maintenance of patency of indwelling IV lines

PHARMACOKINETICS
Well absorbed following subcutaneous administration. Protein binding: Very high. Metabolized in the liver. Removed from the circulation via uptake by the reticuloendothelial system. Primarily excreted in urine. Not removed by hemodialysis. *Half-life:* 1–6 hr.

INDICATIONS AND DOSAGES
▶ **Line Flushing**
IV
Adults, Elderly, Children. 100 units q6–8h.
Infants weighing less than 10 kg. 10 units q6–8h.
▶ **Treatment of Venous Thrombosis, Pulmonary Embolism, Peripheral Arterial Embolism, Atrial Fibrillation with Embolism**
Intermittent IV
Adults, Elderly. Initially, 10,000 units, then 50–70 units/kg (5000–10,000 units) q4–6h.
Children 1 yr and older. Initially, 50–100 units/kg, then 50–100 units q4h.
IV Infusion
Adults, Elderly. Loading dose: 80 units/kg, then 18 units/kg/hr, with adjustments based on aPTT. Range: 10–30 units/kg/hr.
Children 1 yr and older. Loading dose: 75 units/kg, then 20 units/kg/hr with adjustments based on aPTT.
Children younger than 1 yr. Loading dose: 75 units/kg, then 28 units/kg/hr.

▶ **Prevention of Venous Thrombosis, Pulmonary Embolism, Peripheral Arterial Embolism, Atrial Fibrillation with Embolism**
Subcutaneous
Adult, Elderly. 5000 units q8–12h.

SIDE EFFECTS/ADVERSE REACTIONS
Occasional
Itching, burning (particularly on soles of feet) caused by vasospastic reaction
Rare
Pain, cyanosis of extremity 6–10 days after initial therapy lasting 4–6 hr; hypersensitivity reaction, including chills, fever, pruritus, urticaria, asthma, rhinitis, lacrimation, and headache

PRECAUTIONS AND CONTRAINDICATIONS
Intracranial hemorrhage, severe hypotension, severe thrombocytopenia, subacute bacterial endocarditis, uncontrolled bleeding
Caution
Hematoma (IM); elderly; lactation; hyperkalemia; monitor aPTT, PTT, WBC, ACT; endocarditis; trauma; alcoholism; prolongs intrinsic clotting pathway approximately 4–6 hr after each dose

DRUG INTERACTIONS OF CONCERN TO DENTISTRY
• Increased risk of bleeding: salicylates, NSAIDs, parenteral penicillins, glucocorticoids, certain cephalosporins (cefamandole, cefoperazone, cefotetan)

SERIOUS REACTIONS
! Bleeding complications ranging from local ecchymoses to major hemorrhage occur more frequently in high-dose therapy, intermittent IV

infusion, and in women 60 yr and older.

! Antidote: Protamine sulfate 1–1.5 mg, IV, for every 100 units heparin subcutaneous within 30 min of overdose, 0.5–0.75 mg for every 100 units heparin subcutaneous if within 30–60 min of overdose, 0.25–0.375 mg for every 100 units heparin subcutaneous if 2 hr have elapsed since overdose, 25–50 mg if heparin was given by IV infusion.

DENTAL CONSIDERATIONS

General:
• Heparin is used only in hospitalized patients or during dialysis. A medical consultation is necessary if oral and maxillofacial surgery or trauma treatment is required. May need to defer treatment.
• Avoid products that affect platelet function, such as aspirin and NSAIDs.
• Consider local hemostasis measures to prevent excessive bleeding.
• Take precautions if dental surgery or intubation for general anesthesia is anticipated.

Consultations:
• Medical consultation may be required to assess disease control and patient's ability to tolerate stress.
• Medical consultation should include ACT, partial prothrombin, and PT.

Teach Patient/Family to:
• Use caution to prevent trauma when using oral hygiene aids
• Use effective, atraumatic oral hygiene to prevent soft tissue inflammation
• Report oral lesions, soreness, or bleeding

homatropine hydrobromide

hoe-ma´-troe-peen
high-droh-broh´-mide
(Isopto Homatropine, Minims Homatropine[CAN])

CATEGORY AND SCHEDULE
Pregnancy Risk Category: C

Drug Class: Mydriatic (topical)

MECHANISM OF ACTION
An ophthalmic agent that blocks response of iris sphincter muscle and the accommodative muscle of the ciliary body to cholinergic stimulation, resulting in dilation and loss of accommodation.
Therapeutic Effect: Produces cycloplegia and mydriasis for refraction.

USES
Treatment of cycloplegic refraction, uveitis, mydriatic lens opacities

PHARMACOKINETICS
Maximum mydriatic effect occurs within 10–30 min; maximum cycloplegic effect occurs within 30–90 min. Duration of mydriasis is 6 hr–4 days; duration of cycloplegia is 10–48 hr.

INDICATIONS AND DOSAGES
▸ **Mydriasis and Cycloplegia for Refraction**
Ophthalmic
Adults, Elderly. Instill 1–2 drops of 2% solution or 1 drop of 5% solution before the procedure. Repeat at 5- to 10-min intervals as needed. Maximum: 3 doses for refraction.
Children. Instill 1 drop of 2% solution immediately before

the procedure. Repeat at 10-min
intervals as needed.
▶ **Uveitis**
Ophthalmic
Adults, Elderly. Instill 1–2 drops of
2% or 5% solution 2–3 times a day
up to every 3–4 hr as needed.
Children. Instill 1 drop of 2%
solution 2–3 times a day.

SIDE EFFECTS/ADVERSE REACTIONS
Frequent
Blurred vision, photophobia
Occasional
Irritation, increased intraocular
pressure, congestion
Rare
Eczematoid dermatitis, edema,
exudates, follicular conjunctivitis,
somnolence, vascular congestion

PRECAUTIONS AND CONTRAINDICATIONS
Narrow-angle glaucoma, acute
hemorrhage, hypersensitivity to
homatropine or any component of
the formulation
Caution
Children, elderly, hypertension,
hyperthyroidism, diabetes

DRUG INTERACTIONS OF CONCERN TO DENTISTRY
• Avoid concurrent use with
pilocarpine
• Increased anticholinergic effects
with other anticholinergic drugs
(when significant absorption from
the eye occurs)

SERIOUS REACTIONS
! Overdosage may produce
symptoms of blurred vision, urinary
retention, and tachycardia.
Anticholinergic toxicity is caused by
strong binding of the drug to
cholinergic receptors.

DENTAL CONSIDERATIONS
General:
• Avoid dental light in patient's eyes;
offer dark glasses for patient
comfort.

---

hydralazine hydrochloride
high-dral´-ah-zeen
high-droh-klor´-ide
(Alphapress[AUS], Apresoline,
Novohylazin[CAN])
Do not confuse hydralazine with
hydroxyzine.

CATEGORY AND SCHEDULE
Pregnancy Risk Category: C

Drug Class: Antihypertensive,
direct-acting peripheral vasodilator

MECHANISM OF ACTION
An antihypertensive with direct
vasodilating effects on arterioles.
Therapeutic Effect: Decreases
B/P and systemic resistance.

USES
Treatment of essential hypertension;
parenteral: treatment of severe
essential hypertension

PHARMACOKINETICS

Route	Onset	Peak	Duration
PO	20–30 min	N/A	2–4 hr
IV	5–20 min	N/A	2–6 hr

Well absorbed from the GI tract.
Widely distributed. Protein
binding: 85%–90%. Metabolized
in the liver to active metabolite.

Primarily excreted in urine. Not removed by hemodialysis. *Half-life:* 3–7 hr (increased with impaired renal function).

INDICATIONS AND DOSAGES
▶ **Moderate to Severe Hypertension**
PO
Adults. Initially, 10 mg 4 times a day. May increase by 10–25 mg/dose q2–5 days. Maximum: 300 mg/day.
Children. Initially, 0.75–1 mg/kg/day in 2–4 divided doses, not to exceed 25 mg/dose. May increase over 3–4 wk. Maximum: 7.5 mg/kg/day (5 mg/kg/day in infants).
IV, IM
Adults, Elderly. Initially, 10–20 mg/dose q4–6h. May increase to 40 mg/dose.
Children. Initially, 0.1–0.2 mg/kg/dose (maximum: 20 mg) q4–6h, as needed, up to 1.7–3.5 mg/kg/day in divided doses q4–6h.
▶ **Dosage in Renal Impairment**
Dosage interval is based on creatinine clearance.

Creatinine Clearance	Dosage Interval
10–50 ml/min	q8h
Less than 10 ml/min	q8–24h

SIDE EFFECTS/ADVERSE REACTIONS
Frequent
Headache, palpitations, tachycardia (generally disappears in 7–10 days)
Occasional
GI disturbance (nausea, vomiting, diarrhea), paraesthesia, fluid retention, peripheral edema, dizziness, flushed face, nasal congestion

PRECAUTIONS AND CONTRAINDICATIONS
Coronary artery disease, lupus erythematosus, rheumatic heart disease.
Caution
CVA, advanced renal disease

DRUG INTERACTIONS OF CONCERN TO DENTISTRY
• Reduced effects: NSAIDs, indomethacin, sympathomimetics

SERIOUS REACTIONS
! High dosage may produce lupus erythematosus-like reaction, including fever, facial rash, muscle and joint aches, and splenomegaly.
! Severe orthostatic hypotension, skin flushing, severe headache, myocardial ischemia, and cardiac arrhythmias may develop.
! Profound shock may occur with severe overdosage.

DENTAL CONSIDERATIONS
General:
• Monitor vital signs at every appointment because of cardiovascular side effects.
• Patients on chronic drug therapy may rarely have symptoms of blood dyscrasias, which can include infection, bleeding, and poor healing.
• Limit use of sodium-containing products, such as saline IV fluids, for patients with a dietary salt restriction.
• After supine positioning, have patient sit upright for at least 2 min to avoid orthostatic hypotension.
Consultations:
• In a patient with symptoms of blood dyscrasias, request a medical consultation for blood studies and postpone dental treatment until normal values are reestablished.

• Medical consultation may be required to assess disease control and patient's ability to tolerate stress.
Teach Patient/Family to:
• Use effective oral hygiene to prevent soft tissue inflammation
• Use caution to prevent injury when using oral hygiene aids

hydrochlorothiazide

high-droe-klor-oh-thye´-ah-zide
(Apo-Hydro[CAN], Aquazide H, Dichlotride[AUS], Dithiazide[AUS], Esidrix, HydroDIURIL, Microzide, Oretic)

CATEGORY AND SCHEDULE

Pregnancy Risk Category: B
(D if used in pregnancy-induced hypertension)

Drug Class: Thiazide diuretic

MECHANISM OF ACTION

A sulfonamide derivative that acts as a thiazide diuretic and antihypertensive. As a diuretic blocks reabsorption of water, sodium, and potassium at the cortical diluting segment of the distal tubule. As an antihypertensive reduces plasma, extracellular fluid volume, and peripheral vascular resistance by direct effect on blood vessels.
Therapeutic Effect: Promotes diuresis; reduces B/P.

USES

Treatment of edema, hypertension, diuresis, CHF

PHARMACOKINETICS

Route	Onset	Peak	Duration
PO (diuretic)	2 hr	4–6 hr	6–12 hr

Variably absorbed from the GI tract. Primarily excreted unchanged in urine. Not removed by hemodialysis.
Half-life: 5.6–14.8 hr.

INDICATIONS AND DOSAGES
▸ **Edema, Hypertension**
PO
Adults. 12.5–100 mg/day. Maximum: 200 mg/day.
▸ **Usual Pediatric Dosage**
PO
Children 6 mo–12 yr. 2 mg/kg/day in 2 divided doses. Maximum: 200 mg/day.
Children younger than 6 mo. 2–4 mg/kg/day in 2 divided doses. Maximum: 37.5 mg/day.

SIDE EFFECTS/ADVERSE REACTIONS

Expected
Increase in urinary frequency and urine volume
Frequent
Potassium depletion
Occasional
Orthostatic hypotension, headache, GI disturbances, photosensitivity

PRECAUTIONS AND CONTRAINDICATIONS

Anuria, history of hypersensitivity to sulfonamides or thiazide diuretics, renal decompensation
Caution
Hypokalemia, renal disease, hepatic disease, gout, COPD, lupus erythematosus, diabetes mellitus

DRUG INTERACTIONS OF CONCERN TO DENTISTRY
• Decreased hypotensive response: NSAIDs, especially indomethacin

SERIOUS REACTIONS
! Vigorous diuresis may lead to profound water and electrolyte

depletion, resulting in hypokalemia, hyponatremia, and dehydration.
! Acute hypotensive episodes may occur.
! Hyperglycemia may occur during prolonged therapy.
! Pancreatitis, blood dyscrasias, pulmonary edema, allergic pneumonitis, and dermatologic reactions occur rarely.
! Overdose can lead to lethargy and coma without changes in electrolytes or hydration.

DENTAL CONSIDERATIONS

General:
• Monitor vital signs at every appointment because of cardiovascular side effects.
• Patients on chronic drug therapy may rarely have symptoms of blood dyscrasias, which can include infection, bleeding, and poor healing.
• After supine positioning, have patient sit upright for at least 2 min before standing to avoid orthostatic hypotension.
• Assess salivary flow as a factor in caries, periodontal disease, and candidiasis.
• Limit use of sodium-containing products, such as saline IV fluids, for patients with a dietary salt restriction.
• Stress from dental procedures may compromise cardiovascular function; determine patient risk.
• Short appointments and a stress reduction protocol may be required for anxious patients.
• Patients taking diuretics should be monitored for serum K^+ levels.
Consultations:
• In a patient with symptoms of blood dyscrasias, request a medical consultation for blood studies and postpone dental treatment until normal values are reestablished.

• Medical consultation may be required to assess disease control and patient's ability to tolerate stress.
• Physician should be informed if significant xerostomic side effects occur (e.g., increased caries, sore tongue, problems eating or swallowing, difficulty wearing prosthesis) so that a medication change can be considered.
Teach Patient/Family to:
• Use effective oral hygiene to prevent soft tissue inflammation
• Use caution to prevent injury when using oral hygiene aids
• When chronic dry mouth occurs, advise patient to:
  • Avoid mouth rinses with high alcohol content because of drying effects
  • Use daily home fluoride products for anticaries effect
  • Use sugarless gum, frequent sips of water, or saliva substitutes

hydrocodone bitartrate

high-drough-koe´-doan
bye-tar´-trate
(Hycodan [CAN], Robidone [CAN])

CATEGORY AND SCHEDULE
Pregnancy Risk Category: C
Controlled Substance: Schedule III

Drug Class: Narcotic analgesic

MECHANISM OF ACTION
A narcotic analgesic and antitussive that binds with opioid receptors in the CNS. ***Therapeutic Effect:*** Alters the perception of and emotional response to pain; suppresses cough reflex.

USES
Treatment of hyperactive and nonproductive cough; mild-to-moderate pain; normally used in combination with aspirin or acetaminophen for post-treatment pain control

PHARMACOKINETICS

Route	Onset	Peak	Duration
PO (analgesic)	10–20 min	30–60 min	4–6 hr
PO (antitussive)	N/A	N/A	4–6 hr

Well absorbed from the GI tract. Metabolized in the liver. Primarily excreted in urine. *Half-life:* 3.8 hr (increased in elderly).

INDICATIONS AND DOSAGES
▸ **Analgesia**
PO
Adults, Children older than 12 yr. 5–10 mg q4–6h.
Elderly. 2.5–5 mg q4–6h.
▸ **Cough**
PO
Adults. 5–10 mg q4–6h as needed. Maximum: 15 mg/dose.
Children. 0.6 mg/kg/day in 3–4 divided doses at intervals of at least 4 hr. Maximum single dose: 5 mg (children 2–12 yr), 1.25 mg (children younger than 2 yr).
PO (Extended-Release)
Adults. 10 mg q12h.
Children 6–12 yr. 5 mg q12h.

SIDE EFFECTS/ADVERSE REACTIONS
Frequent
Sedation, hypotension, diaphoresis, facial flushing, dizziness, somnolence
Occasional
Urine retention, blurred vision, constipation, dry mouth, headache, nausea, vomiting, difficult or painful urination, euphoria, dysphoria

PRECAUTIONS AND CONTRAINDICATIONS
Hypersensitivity, addiction (narcotic)
Caution
Addictive personality, lactation, increased intracranial pressure, MI (acute), severe heart disease, respiratory depression, hepatic disease, renal disease, children younger than 18 yr

DRUG INTERACTIONS OF CONCERN TO DENTISTRY
• Increased CNS depression: alcohol, other opioids, phenothiazines, sedative/hypnotics, skeletal muscle relaxants, general anesthetics
• Contraindication: MAOIs
• Increased effects of anticholinergics

SERIOUS REACTIONS
! Overdose results in respiratory depression, skeletal muscle flaccidity, cold or clammy skin, cyanosis, and extreme somnolence progressing to seizures, stupor, and coma.
! The patient who uses hydrocodone repeatedly may develop a tolerance to the drug's analgesic effect, as well as physical dependence.
! The drug may have a prolonged duration of action and cumulative effect in patients with hepatic or renal impairment.

DENTAL CONSIDERATIONS
General:
• Monitor vital signs at every appointment because of cardiovascular and respiratory side effects.

• After supine positioning, have patient sit upright for at least 2 min to avoid orthostatic hypotension.
• Psychologic and physical dependence may occur with chronic administration.
• Determine why the patient is taking the drug.
Teach Patient/Family to:
• Avoid mouth rinses with high alcohol content because of drying effects

H

hydrocodone
high-droe-koe-done
Hydrocodone and acetaminophen (Anexsia, Bancap HC, Ceta-Plus, Co-Gesic, Hydrocet, Hydrogesic, Lorcet 10/650, Lorcet-HD Lorcet Plus, Lortab, Margesic H, Maxidone, Norco, Stagesic, Vicodin, Vicodin ES, Vicodin HP, Zydone); hydrocodone and aspirin (Damason-P); hydrocodone and chlorpheniramine (Tussionex) hydrocodone and guaifenesin (Codiclear DH, Hycosin, Hycotuss, Kwelcof, Pneumotussin, Vicoden Tuss, Vitussin); hydrocodone and homatropin (Hycodan and Hydromet, Hydropane, Tussigon); hydrocodone and ibuprofen, (Vicoprofen); hydrocodone and pseudoephedrine (Detussin, Histussin D, P-V Tussin); hydrocodone, chlorpheniramine, phenylephrine, acetaminophen, and caffeine (Hycomine Compound)

CATEGORY AND SCHEDULE
Pregnancy Risk Category: C
Controlled substance: Schedule III

Drug Class: Antitussive opioid analgesic, nonopioid analgesic

MECHANISM OF ACTION
Hydrocodone blocks pain perception in the cerebral cortex by binding to specific opiate receptors' (μ and κ) neuronal membranes of synapses. This binding results in a decreased synaptic chemical transmission throughout the CNS, thus inhibiting the flow of pain sensations into the higher centers and causing analgesia. **Therapeutic Effect:** Alters perception of pain and produces analgesic effect.

USES
Treatment of hyperactive and nonproductive cough, mild pain

PHARMACOKINETICS
Well absorbed. Metabolized in liver. Excreted in urine. **Half-life:** 3.3–3.4 hr.

INDICATIONS AND DOSAGES
Hydrocodone and Acetaminophen
▶ **Analgesia**
PO
Adults, Children older than 13 yr or weighing more than 50 kg. 2.5–10 mg q4–6h. Maximum: 60 mg/day hydrocodone. Maximum dose of acetaminophen: 4 g/day.
Elderly. 2.5–5 mg hydrocodone q4–6h. Titrate dose to appropriate analgesic effect. Maximum: 4 g/day acetaminophen.
Children 2–13 yr or weighing less than 50 kg. 0.135 mg/kg/dose hydrocodone q4–6h. Maximum: 6 doses/day of hydrocodone or maximum recommended dose of acetaminophen.
Hydrocodone and Aspirin
PO
Adults. 2.5–10 mg q4–6h. Maximum: 60 mg/day hydrocodone.
Elderly. 2.5–5 mg hydrocodone q4–6h. Titrate dose to appropriate analgesic effect.

Children 2–13 yr or weighing less than 50 kg. 0.135 mg/kg/dose hydrocodone q4–6h.

Hydrocodone and Chlorpheniramine
Adults, Elderly, Children 12 yr and older. 5 ml q12h. Maximum: 10 ml/24h.
Children 6–12 yr. 2.5 ml q12h. Maximum: 5 ml/24h.

Hydrocodone and Guaifenesin
Adults, Elderly, Children 12 yr and older. 5 ml q4h. Maximum: 30 ml/24h.
Children 2–12 yr. 2.5 ml q4h.
Children younger than 2 yr. 0.3 mg/kg/day (hydrocodone) in 4 divided doses.

Hydrocodone and Homatropine
Adults, Elderly. 10 mg (hydrocodone) q4–6h. A single dose should not exceed 15 mg and should not be administered more frequently than q4h.
Children. 0.6 mg/kg/day (hydrocodone) in 3–4 divided doses. Do not administer more frequently than q4h.

Hydrocodone and Ibuprofen
Adults. 7.5–15 mg (hydrocodone) q4–6h as needed for pain. Maximum: 5 tablets/day.

Hydrocodone & Pseudoephedrine
Adults, Elderly. 5 ml 4 times a day.

Hydrocodone, Chlorpheniramine, Phenylephrine, Acetaminophen, and Caffeine
Adults, Elderly. 1 tablet q4h up to 4 times a day.

SIDE EFFECTS/ADVERSE REACTIONS

Frequent
Dizziness, sedation, drowsiness, bradycardia
Occasional
Anxiety, dysphoria, euphoria, fear, lethargy, lightheadedness, malaise, mental clouding, mental impairment, mood changes, physiological dependence, sedation, somnolence, constipation, bradycardia, heartburn, nausea, vomiting
Rare
Hypersensitivity reaction, rash

PRECAUTIONS AND CONTRAINDICATIONS

CNS depression, severe respiratory depression, hypersensitivity to hydrocodone, or any component of the formulation

DRUG INTERACTIONS OF CONCERN TO DENTISTRY

• Increased CNS depression: alcohol, local anesthetics, other opioids, phenothiazines, sedative/hypnotics, skeletal muscle relaxants, general anesthetics
• Contraindication: MAOIs
• Increased effects of anticholinergics

SERIOUS REACTIONS

! Cardiac arrest, circulatory collapse, coma, hypotension, hypoglycemic coma, ureteral spasm, urinary retention, vesical sphincter spasm, agranulocytosis, bleeding time prolonged, hemolytic anemia, iron deficiency anemia, occult blood loss, thrombocytopenia, hepatic necrosis, hepatitis, skeletal muscle rigidity, renal toxicity, renal tubular necrosis have been reported.
! Hearing impairment or loss have been reported with chronic overdose.
! Acute airway obstruction, apnea, dyspnea, and respiratory depression occur rarely and are usually dose related.

DENTAL CONSIDERATIONS

General:
• Monitor vital signs at every appointment because of

cardiovascular and respiratory side effects.
- After supine positioning, have patient sit upright for at least 2 min to avoid orthostatic hypotension.
- Psychologic and physical dependence may occur with chronic administration.
- Determine why the patient is taking the drug.

Teach Patient/Family to:
- Avoid mouth rinses with high alcohol content because of drying effects

hydrocortisone

high-droh-kor´-tih-sone
(A-HydroCort, Anusol-HC, Colifoam[AUS], Cortaid, Cortef cream[AUS], Cortic cream[AUS], Cortic DS[AUS], Cortifoam, Cortizone-5, Cortizone-10, Derm-Aid cream[AUS], Dermaid[AUS], Dermaid soft cream[AUS], Egocort cream[AUS], Emcort, Hycor[AUS], Hycor Eye Oinment[AUS], Hysone[AUS], Hytone, Locoid, Nupercainal Hydrocortisone Cream, Preparation H Hydrocortisone, Protocort, Siquent Hycor[AUS], Solu-Cortef, Squibb HC[AUS], WestCort)

CATEGORY AND SCHEDULE
Pregnancy Risk Category: C
OTC (Hydrocortisone 0.5% and 1% Cream, Gel, and Ointment)

Drug Class: Topical corticosteroid

MECHANISM OF ACTION
An adrenocortical steroid that inhibits accumulation of inflammatory cells at inflammation sites, phagocytosis, lysosomal enzyme release and synthesis and release of mediators of inflammation. ***Therapeutic Effect:*** Prevents or suppresses cell-mediated immune reactions. Decreases or prevents tissue response to inflammatory process.

USES
Treatment of psoriasis, eczema, contact dermatitis, pruritus

PHARMACOKINETICS

Route	Onset	Peak	Duration
IV	N/A	4–6 hr	8–12 hr

Well absorbed after IM administration. Widely distributed. Metabolized in the liver. ***Half-life:*** Plasma, 1.5–2 hr; biologic, 8–12 hr.

INDICATIONS AND DOSAGES
▸ **Acute Adrenal Insufficiency**
IV
Adults, Elderly. 100 mg IV bolus; then 300 mg/day in divided doses q8h.
Children. 1–2 mg/kg IV bolus; then 150–250 mg/day in divided doses q6–8h.
Infants. 1–2 mg/kg/dose IV bolus; then 25–150 mg/day in divided doses q6–8h.
▸ **Antiinflammation, Immunosuppression**
IV, IM
Adults, Elderly. 15–240 mg q12h.
Children. 1–5 mg/kg/day in divided doses q12h.
▸ **Physiologic Replacement**
PO
Children. 0.5–0.75 mg/kg/day in divided doses q8h.
IM
Children. 0.25–0.35 mg/kg/day as a single dose.

▸ **Status Asthmaticus**
IV
Adults, Elderly. 100–500 mg q6h.
Children. 2 mg/kg/dose q6h.
▸ **Shock**
IV
Adults, Elderly, Children 12 yr and older. 100–500 mg q6h.
Children younger than 12 yr.
50 mg/kg. May repeat in 4 hr, then q24h as needed.
▸ **Adjunctive Treatment of Ulcerative Colitis**
Rectal
Adults, Elderly. 100 mg at bedtime for 21 nights or until clinical and proctologic remission occurs (may require 2–3 mo of therapy).
Rectal (Cortifoam)
Adults, Elderly. 1 applicator 1–2 times a day for 2–3 wk, then every second day until therapy ends.
Topical
Adults, Elderly. Apply sparingly 2–4 times a day.

SIDE EFFECTS/ADVERSE REACTIONS
Frequent
Insomnia, heartburn, nervousness, abdominal distention, diaphoresis, acne, mood swings, increased appetite, facial flushing, delayed wound healing, increased susceptibility to infection, diarrhea or constipation
Occasional
Headache, edema, change in skin color, frequent urination
Topical: Itching, redness, irritation
Rare
Tachycardia, allergic reaction (such as rash and hives), psychological changes, hallucinations, depression
Topical: Allergic contact dermatitis, purpura
Systemic: Absorption more likely with use of occlusive dressings or extensive application in young children

PRECAUTIONS AND CONTRAINDICATIONS
Fungal, tuberculosis, or viral skin lesions; serious infections
Caution
Lactation, viral infections, bacterial infections

DRUG INTERACTIONS OF CONCERN TO DENTISTRY
• Inhibitors of CYP hepatic isoenzymes (e.g., azole antifungals, macrolide antibiotics): potential increased blood levels of hydrocortisone and increased hydrocortisone toxicity
• Aspirin, salicylates: potentially increased salicylate GI irritation and toxicity
• Anticoagulants: variable effects on coagulation levels, potentially increased bleeding

SERIOUS REACTIONS
! Long-term therapy may cause hypocalcemia, hypokalemia, muscle wasting (especially in arms and legs), osteoporosis, spontaneous fractures, amenorrhea, cataracts, glaucoma, peptic ulcer disease, and CHF.
! Abruptly withdrawing the drug after long-term therapy may cause anorexia, nausea, fever, headache, sudden severe joint pain, rebound inflammation, fatigue, weakness, lethargy, dizziness, and orthostatic hypotension.

DENTAL CONSIDERATIONS

Topical Form
General:
• Place on frequent recall to evaluate healing response if used on a chronic basis.
Teach Patient/Family to:
• Use effective oral hygiene to prevent soft tissue inflammation
• Apply at bedtime or after meals for maximum effect

• Avoid use on oral herpetic ulcerations
• Apply with cotton-tipped applicator by pressing, not rubbing, paste on lesion
• Return for oral evaluation if response of oral tissues has not occurred in 7–14 days

hydroflumethiazide
high-droh-floo-meth-eye´-ah-zide
(Diucardin, Saluron)

CATEGORY AND SCHEDULE
Pregnancy Risk Category: C, D if used in pregnancy-induced hypertension

Drug Class: Antidiuretic, central and nephrogenic diabetes insipidus; antihypertensive; antiurolithic, calcium calculi; diuretic

MECHANISM OF ACTION
A diuretic that blocks reabsorption of water and the electrolytes sodium and potassium at cortical diluting segment of distal tubule. As an antihypertensive it reduces plasma and extracellular fluid volume and decreases peripheral vascular resistance (PVR) by direct effect on blood vessels. *Therapeutic Effect:* Promotes diuresis, reduces B/P.

USES
Treatment of high B/P (hypertension)

PHARMACOKINETICS
Rapidly but incompletely absorbed from the GI tract. Metabolized to metabolite that is extensively bound to red blood cells and has a longer half-life than parent compound. Primarily excreted in urine. Not removed by hemodialysis.
Half-life: 2–17 hr.

INDICATIONS AND DOSAGES
▶ **Edema**
PO
Adults, Elderly. Initially, 50 mg 2 times a day. Maintenance: 25–200 mg/day.
▶ **Hypertension**
Adults, Elderly, Children.
1 mg/kg/day.
Initially, 50 mg 2 times a day.
Maintenance: 50–100 mg/day.

SIDE EFFECTS/ADVERSE REACTIONS
Expected
Increase in urine frequency and volume
Frequent
Potassium depletion
Occasional
Postural hypotension, headache, GI disturbances, photosensitivity reaction

PRECAUTIONS AND CONTRAINDICATIONS
Anuria, history of hypersensitivity to sulfonamides or thiazide diuretics, renal decompensation, pregnancy

DRUG INTERACTIONS OF CONCERN TO DENTISTRY
• Decreased hypotensive response: NSAIDs, especially indomethacin

SERIOUS REACTIONS
! Vigorous diuresis may lead to profound water loss and electrolyte depletion, resulting in hypokalemia, hyponatremia, and dehydration.
! Acute hypotensive episodes may occur.
! Hyperglycemia may be noted during prolonged therapy.
! GI upset, pancreatitis, dizziness, paresthesias, headache, blood dyscrasias, pulmonary edema, allergic pneumonitis, and dermatologic reactions occur rarely.

! Overdosage can lead to lethargy and coma without changes in electrolytes or hydration.

DENTAL CONSIDERATIONS

General:
• Monitor vital signs at every appointment due to cardiovascular side effects.
• Patient on chronic drug therapy may rarely present with symptoms of blood dyscrasias, which can include infection, bleeding, and poor healing. If dyscrasia is present, caution patient to prevent oral tissue trauma when using oral hygiene aids.
• After supine positioning, have patient sit upright for at least 2 min before standing to avoid orthostatic hypotension.
• Assess salivary flow as a factor in caries, periodontal disease, and candidiasis.
• Limit use of sodium-containing products, such as saline IV fluids, for patients with a dietary salt restriction.
• Stress from dental procedures may compromise cardiovascular function, determine patient risk.
• Patients taking diuretics should be monitored for serum K+ levels.

Consultations:
• In a patient with symptoms of blood dyscrasias, request a medical consultation for blood studies and postpone treatment until normal values are reestablished.
• Medical consultation may be required to assess disease control and patient's ability to tolerate stress.
• Physician should be informed if significant xerostomic side effects occur (increased caries, sore tongue, problems eating or swallowing, difficulty wearing prosthesis) so that a medication change can be considered.

Teach Patient/Family to:
• Use effective oral hygiene to prevent soft tissue inflammation
• Prevent trauma when using oral hygiene aids
• When chronic dry mouth occurs advise patient to:
  • Avoid mouth rinses with high alcohol content due to drying effects
  • Use daily home fluoride products for anticaries effect
  • Use sugarless gum, frequent sips of water, or saliva substitutes
• Update health and medication history if physician makes any changes in evaluation or drug regimens; include OTC, herbal, and nonherbal remedies in the update

hydromorphone hydrochloride

high-droe-mor´-fone
high-droh-klor´-ide
(Dilaudid, Dilaudid HP, Hydromorph Contin[CAN], Palladone)
Do not confuse with morphine or Dilantin.

CATEGORY AND SCHEDULE

Pregnancy Risk Category: C
Controlled Substance: Schedule II

Drug Class: Synthetic narcotic analgesic

MECHANISM OF ACTION

An opioid agonist that binds to opioid receptors in the CNS, reducing the intensity of pain stimuli from sensory nerve endings. **Therapeutic Effect:** Alters the perception of and emotional response to pain; suppresses cough reflex.

USES
Treatment of moderate-to-severe pain

PHARMACOKINETICS

Route	Onset	Peak	Duration
PO	30 min	90–120 min	4 hr
IV	10–15 min	15–30 min	2–3 hr
IM	15 min	30–60 min	4–5 hr
Subcutaneous	15 min	30–90 min	4 hr
Rectal	15–30 min	N/A	N/A

Well absorbed from the GI tract after IM administration. Widely distributed. Metabolized in the liver. Excreted in urine. *Half-life:* 1–3 hr.

INDICATIONS AND DOSAGES
▶ **Analgesia**
PO
Adults, Elderly, Children weighing 50 kg and more. 2–4 mg q3–4h. Range: 2–8 mg/dose.
Children older than 6 mo and weighing less than 50 kg. 0.03–0.08 mg/kg/dose q3–4h.
PO (Extended-Release)
Adults, Elderly. 12–32 mg once a day.
IV
Adults, Elderly, Children weighing more than 50 kg. 0.2–0.6 mg q2–3h.
Children weighing 50 kg or less. 0.015 mg/kg/dose q3–6h as needed.
Rectal
Adults, Elderly. 3 mg q4–8h.
▶ **Patient-Controlled Analgesia (PCA)**
IV
Adults, Elderly. 0.05–0.5 mg at 5–15 min lockout. Maximum (4 hr): 4–6 mg.
Epidural

Adults, Elderly. Bolus dose of 1–1.5 mg at rate of 0.04–0.4 mg/hr. Demand dose of 0.15 mg at 30 min lockout.
▶ **Cough**
PO
Adults, Elderly, Children older than 12 yr. 1 mg q3–4h.
Children 6–12 yr. 0.5 mg q3–4h.

SIDE EFFECTS/ADVERSE REACTIONS
Frequent
Somnolence, dizziness, hypotension (including orthostatic hypotension), decreased appetite
Occasional
Confusion, diaphoresis, facial flushing, urine retention, constipation, dry mouth, nausea, vomiting, headache, pain at injection site
Rare
Allergic reaction, depression

PRECAUTIONS AND CONTRAINDICATIONS
Hypersensitivity, addiction (narcotic), MAOIs
Caution
Addictive personality, lactation, increased intracranial pressure, MI (acute), severe heart disease, respiratory depression, hepatic disease, renal disease, children younger than 18 yr

DRUG INTERACTIONS OF CONCERN TO DENTISTRY
• Effects may be increased with other CNS depressants: alcohol, narcotics, sedative/hypnotics, skeletal muscle relaxants
• Increased effects of anticholinergic drugs

SERIOUS REACTIONS

! Overdose results in respiratory depression, skeletal muscle flaccidity, cold or clammy skin, cyanosis, and extreme somnolence progressing to seizures, stupor, and coma.

! The patient who uses hydromorphone repeatedly may develop a tolerance to the drug's analgesic effect, as well as physical dependence.

! This drug may have a prolonged duration of action and cumulative effect in patients with hepatic or renal impairment.

DENTAL CONSIDERATIONS

General:
• Monitor vital signs at every appointment because of cardiovascular and respiratory side effects.
• After supine positioning, have patient sit upright for at least 2 min to avoid orthostatic hypotension.
• Assess salivary flow as a factor in caries, periodontal disease, and candidiasis.
• Psychologic and physical dependence may occur with chronic administration.
• Determine why the patient is taking the drug.
• Avoid use in patients with chronic obstructive pulmonary disease.
Teach Patient/Family to:
• Avoid mouth rinses with high alcohol content because of drying effects

hydroxychloroquine sulfate

high-drox-ee-klor′-oh-kwin sull′-fate
(Apo-Hydroxyquine[CAN], Plaquenil)
Do not confuse hydroxychloroquine with hydrocortisone or hydroxyzine.

CATEGORY AND SCHEDULE
Pregnancy Risk Category: C

Drug Class: Antimalarial

MECHANISM OF ACTION

An antimalarial and antirheumatic that concentrates in parasite acid vesicles, increasing the pH of the vesicles and interfering with parasite protein synthesis. Antirheumatic action may involve suppressing formation of antigens responsible for hypersensitivity reactions. *Therapeutic Effect:* Inhibits parasite growth.

USES

Treatment of malaria caused by *P. vivax, P. malariae, P. ovale, P. falciparum* (some strains); lupus erythematosus; rheumatoid arthritis

PHARMACOKINETICS

PO: Peak 1–2 hr. *Half-life:* 3–5 days; metabolized in liver; excreted in urine, feces, breast milk; crosses placenta

INDICATIONS AND DOSAGES
▶ **Treatment of Acute Attack of Malaria (dosage in mg base)**
PO

Dose	Times	Adults	Children
Initial	Day 1	620 mg	10 mg/kg
Second	6 hr later	310 mg	5 mg/kg
Third	Day 2	310 mg	5 mg/kg
Fourth	Day 3	310 mg	5 mg/kg

▶ **Suppression of Malaria**

PO

Adults. 310 mg base weekly on same day each wk, beginning 2 wk before entering an endemic area and continuing for 4–6 wk after leaving the area.

Children. 5 mg base/kg/wk, beginning 2 wk before entering an endemic area and continuing for 4–6 wk after leaving the area. If therapy is not begun before exposure, administer a loading dose of 10 mg base/kg in 2 equally divided doses 6 hr apart, followed by the usual dosage regimen.

▶ **Rheumatoid Arthritis**

PO

Adults. Initially, 400–600 mg (310–465 mg base) daily for 5–10 days, gradually increased to optimum response level. Maintenance (usually within 4–12 wk): Dosage decreased by 50% and then continued at maintenance dose of 200–400 mg/day. Maximum effect may not be seen for several months.

▶ **Lupus Erythematosus**

PO

Adults. Initially, 400 mg once or twice a day for several wk or mo. Maintenance: 200–400 mg/day.

SIDE EFFECTS/ADVERSE REACTIONS

Frequent

Mild, transient headache; anorexia; nausea; vomiting

Occasional

Visual disturbances, nervousness, fatigue, pruritus (especially of palms, soles, and scalp), irritability, personality changes, diarrhea

Rare

Stomatitis, dermatitis, impaired hearing

PRECAUTIONS AND CONTRAINDICATIONS

Long-term therapy for children, porphyria, psoriasis, retinal or visual field changes

Caution

Blood dyscrasias, severe GI disease, neurologic disease, alcoholism, hepatic disease, G6PD deficiency, psoriasis, eczema

DRUG INTERACTIONS OF CONCERN TO DENTISTRY

None reported

SERIOUS REACTIONS

! Ocular toxicity, especially retinopathy, may occur and may progress even after drug is discontinued.

! Prolonged therapy may result in peripheral neuritis, neuromyopathy, hypotension, ECG changes, agranulocytosis, aplastic anemia, thrombocytopenia, seizures, and psychosis.

! Overdosage may result in headache, vomiting, visual disturbances, drowsiness, seizures, and hypokalemia followed by cardiovascular collapse and death.

DENTAL CONSIDERATIONS

General:

• Patients on chronic drug therapy may rarely have symptoms of blood dyscrasias, which can include infection, bleeding, and poor healing.

• Avoid dental light in patient's eyes; offer dark glasses for patient comfort.

• Determine why the patient is taking the drug.

Consultations:

• In a patient with symptoms of blood dyscrasias, request a medical consultation for blood studies and

postpone dental treatment until normal values are reestablished.
Teach Patient/Family to:
• Use effective oral hygiene to prevent soft tissue inflammation
• Avoid mouth rinses with high alcohol content because of drying effects

hydroxyurea
high-drocks´-ee-your-ee-ah
(Droxia, Hydrea, Mylocel)

CATEGORY AND SCHEDULE
Pregnancy Risk Category: D

Drug Class: Antineoplastic

MECHANISM OF ACTION
A synthetic urea analog that inhibits DNA synthesis without interfering with RNA synthesis or protein. *Therapeutic Effect:* Interferes with the normal repair process of cancer cells damaged by irradiation.

USES
Treatment of melanoma, chronic myelocytic leukemia (CML), recurrent or metastatic ovarian cancer, in combination with irradiation therapy for carcinomas of the head and neck (except the lip); sickle cell anemia

PHARMACOKINETICS
PO: Readily absorbed with PO use, peak level in 2 hr; 80% excreted in urine.

INDICATIONS AND DOSAGES
▸ **Melanoma; Recurrent, Metastatic, or Inoperable Ovarian Carcinoma**
PO
Adults, Elderly. 80 mg/kg every 3 days or 20–30 mg/kg/day as a single dose.

▸ **Control of Primary Squamous Cell Carcinoma of the Head and Neck, Excluding Lips (in combination with radiation therapy)**
PO
Adults, Elderly. 80 mg/kg every 3 days, beginning at least 7 days before starting radiation therapy.
▸ **Resistant CML**
PO
Adults, Elderly. 20–30 mg/kg once a day.
Children. 10–20 mg/kg once a day.
▸ **HIV Infection**
PO
Adults, Elderly. 500 mg twice a day with didanosine.
▸ **Sickle Cell Anemia**
PO
Adults, Elderly, Children. Initially, 15 mg/kg once a day. May increase by 5 mg/kg/day. Maximum: 35 mg/kg/day.

SIDE EFFECTS/ADVERSE REACTIONS
Frequent
Nausea, vomiting, anorexia, constipation or diarrhea
Occasional
Mild, reversible rash; facial flushing; pruritus; fever; chills; malaise
Rare
Alopecia, headache, drowsiness, dizziness, disorientation

PRECAUTIONS AND CONTRAINDICATIONS
WBC count less than 2500/mm^3 or platelet count less than 100,000/mm^3
Caution
Monitor blood counts and hemoglobin, renal impairment, elderly

DRUG INTERACTIONS OF CONCERN TO DENTISTRY
None reported

SERIOUS REACTIONS
! Myelosuppression may cause hematologic toxicity (manifested as leukopenia and, to a lesser extent, thrombocytopenia and anemia).

DENTAL CONSIDERATIONS
General:
• Patients receiving chemotherapy may be taking chronic opioids for pain. Consider NSAIDs for dental pain management.
• Patients receiving chemotherapy may require palliative therapy for stomatitis.
• Patients on chronic drug therapy may rarely have symptoms of blood dyscrasias, which can include infection, bleeding, and poor healing.
Consultations:
• Medical consultation may be required to assess disease control.
• In a patient with symptoms of blood dyscrasias, request a medical consultation for blood studies and postpone dental treatment until normal values are reestablished.
Teach Patient/Family to:
• See dentist immediately if secondary oral infection occurs
• When chronic dry mouth occurs, advise patient to:
 • Avoid mouth rinses with high alcohol content because of drying effects
 • Use sugarless gum, frequent sips of water, or saliva substitutes
 • Use daily home fluoride products for anticaries effect

hydroxyzine
high-drox´-ih-zeen
(Apo-Hydroxyzine[CAN], Atarax, Novohydroxyzin[CAN], Vistaril)
Do not confuse hydroxyzine with hydralazine or hydroxyurea.

CATEGORY AND SCHEDULE
Pregnancy Risk Category: C

Drug Class: Antianxiety, antihistamine

MECHANISM OF ACTION
A piperazine derivative that competes with histamine for receptor sites in the GI tract, blood vessels, and respiratory tract. May exert CNS depressant activity in subcortical areas. Diminishes vestibular stimulation and depresses labyrinthine function. ***Therapeutic Effect:*** Produces anxiolytic, anticholinergic, antihistaminic, and analgesic effects; relaxes skeletal muscle; controls nausea and vomiting.

USES
Treatment of anxiety, preoperatively or postoperatively to prevent nausea and vomiting, to potentiate narcotic analgesics, sedation, pruritus

PHARMACOKINETICS

Route	Onset	Peak	Duration
PO	15–30 min	N/A	4–6 hr

Well absorbed from the GI tract and after parenteral administration. Metabolized in the liver. Primarily excreted in urine. Not removed by hemodialysis. ***Half-life:*** 20–25 hr (increased in the elderly).

INDICATIONS AND DOSAGES
▶ **Anxiety**
PO
Adults, Elderly. 25–100 mg
4 times a day. Maximum:
600 mg/day.
▶ **Nausea and Vomiting**
IM
Adults, Elderly. 25–100 mg/dose
q4–6h.
▶ **Pruritus**
PO
Adults, Elderly. 25 mg 3–4 times
a day.
▶ **Preoperative Sedation**
PO
Adults, Elderly. 50–100 mg.
IM
Adults, Elderly. 25–100 mg.
▶ **Usual Pediatric Dosage**
PO
Children. 2 mg/kg/day in divided
doses q6–8h.
IM
Children. 0.5–1 mg/kg/dose
q4–6h.

SIDE EFFECTS/ADVERSE REACTIONS
Side effects are generally mild and
transient.
Frequent
Somnolence, dry mouth, marked
discomfort with IM injection
Occasional
Dizziness, ataxia, asthenia, slurred
speech, headache, agitation,
increased anxiety
Rare
Paradoxical CNS reactions,
such as hyperactivity or
nervousness in children and
excitement or restlessness in
elderly or debilitated patients
(generally noted during first
2 wk of therapy, particularly in
presence of uncontrolled pain)

PRECAUTIONS AND CONTRAINDICATIONS
Hypersensitivity, avoid in
pregnancy
Caution
Elderly, debilitated, hepatic disease,
renal disease

DRUG INTERACTIONS OF CONCERN TO DENTISTRY
• Increased CNS depressant effect:
alcohol, all CNS depressants
• Increased anticholinergic effects:
other antihistamines,
anticholinergics, opioid analgesics

SERIOUS REACTIONS
! A hypersensitivity reaction,
including wheezing, dyspnea, and
chest tightness, may occur.

DENTAL CONSIDERATIONS
General:
• Potentiates other CNS depressant
drugs. When used in combination,
the dose of other CNS depressants
should be reduced by half.
• Assess salivary flow as a factor in
caries, periodontal disease, and
candidiasis.
• Geriatric patients are more
susceptible to drug effects; use lower
dose.
• Have someone drive patient to
and from dental appointment
if the drug is prescribed for dental
therapy.
Teach Patient/Family:
• When chronic dry mouth occurs,
advise patient to:
  • Avoid mouth rinses with high
  alcohol content because of drying
  effects
  • Use sugarless gum, frequent sips
  of water, or saliva substitutes
  • Use daily home fluoride products
  for anticaries effect

H

hyoscyamine
high-oh-sye´-ah-meen
(Anaspaz, Buscopan[CAN],
Cystospaz, Cystospaz-M, Hyosine,
Levbid, Levsin, Levsin S/L,
Levsinex, NuLev, Spacol, Spacol T/S,
Symax SL, Symax SR)
Do not confuse Anaspaz with
Anaprox.

CATEGORY AND SCHEDULE
Pregnancy Risk Category: C

Drug Class: Anticholinergic

MECHANISM OF ACTION
A GI antispasmodic and
anticholinergic agent that inhibits the
action of acetylcholine at postganglionic (muscarinic) receptor
sites. *Therapeutic Effect:* Decreases
secretions (bronchial, salivary, sweat
gland) and gastric juices and reduces
motility of GI and urinary tract.

USES
Treatment of peptic ulcer disease in
combination with other drugs, other
GI disorders, other spastic disorders
such as parkinsonism, preoperatively
to reduce secretions, GU disorders
(cystitis, renal colic), partial heart
block

PHARMACOKINETICS
PO: Duration 4–6 hr; metabolized by
liver, excreted in urine. *Half-life:*
3.5 hr.

INDICATIONS AND DOSAGES
▶ **GI Tract Disorders**
PO
*Adults, Elderly, Children 12 yr and
older.* 0.125–0.25 mg q4h as needed.
Extended-release: 0.375–0.75 mg
q12h. Maximum: 1.5 mg/day.
Children 2–11 yr. 0.0625–0.125 mg
q4h as needed. Extended-release:

0.375 mg q12h. Maximum:
0.75 mg/day.
IV, IM
*Adults, Elderly, Children 12 yr
and older.* 0.25–0.5 mg q4h for
1–4 doses.
▶ **Hypermotility of Lower Urinary
Tract**
PO, Sublingual
Adults, Elderly. 0.15–0.3 mg 4 times
a day; or extended-release 0.375 mg
q12h.
▶ **Infant Colic**
PO
Infants. Individualized drops dosed
q4h as needed.

SIDE EFFECTS/ADVERSE
REACTIONS
Frequent
Dry mouth (sometimes severe),
decreased sweating, constipation
Occasional
Blurred vision, bloated feeling,
urinary hesitancy, somnolence (with
high dosage), headache, intolerance
to light, loss of taste, nervousness,
flushing, insomnia, impotence,
mental confusion or excitement
(particularly in the elderly and
children), temporary light-
headedness (with parenteral form),
local irritation (with parenteral form)
Rare
Dizziness, faintness

PRECAUTIONS AND
CONTRAINDICATIONS
GI or GU obstruction, myasthenia
gravis, narrow-angle glaucoma,
paralytic ileus, severe ulcerative
colitis
Caution
Hyperthyroidism, CAD,
dysrhythmias, CHF, ulcerative colitis,
hypertension, hiatal hernia, hepatic
disease, renal disease, urinary
retention

DRUG INTERACTIONS OF CONCERN TO DENTISTRY

• Increased anticholinergic effect: other anticholinergics, opioid analgesics
• Decreased effect of phenothiazines

SERIOUS REACTIONS

! Overdose may produce temporary paralysis of ciliary muscle; pupillary dilation; tachycardia; palpitations; hot, dry, or flushed skin; absence of bowel sounds; hyperthermia; increased respiratory rate; ECG abnormalities; nausea; vomiting; rash over face or upper trunk; CNS stimulation; and psychosis (marked by agitation, restlessness, rambling speech, visual hallucinations, paranoid behavior, and delusions, followed by depression).

DENTAL CONSIDERATIONS

General:
• After supine positioning, have patient sit upright for at least 2 min to avoid orthostatic hypotension.

• Assess salivary flow as a factor in caries, periodontal disease, and candidiasis.
• Avoid dental light in patient's eyes; offer dark glasses for patient comfort.

Consultation:
• Physician should be informed if significant xerostomic side effects occur (e.g., increased caries, sore tongue, problems eating or swallowing, difficulty wearing prosthesis) so that a medication change can be considered.

Teach Patient/Family to:
• Use effective oral hygiene to prevent soft tissue inflammation
• When chronic dry mouth occurs, advise patient to:
  • Avoid mouth rinses with high alcohol content because of drying effects
  • Use sugarless gum, frequent sips of water, or artificial saliva substitutes
  • Use daily home fluoride products for anticaries effect

ibandronate sodium

eye-band´-droh-nate soe´-dee-um
(Boniva)

CATEGORY AND SCHEDULE

Pregnancy Risk Category: C

Drug Class: Bisphosphonate;
calcium regulator

MECHANISM OF ACTION

A bisphosphonate that binds to bone
hydroxyapatite (part of the mineral
matrix of bone) and inhibits
osteoclast activity. ***Therapeutic
Effect:*** Reduces rate of bone
turnover and bone resorption,
resulting in a net gain in bone
mass.

USES

Treatment and prevention of
osteoporosis in postmenopausal
women

PHARMACOKINETICS

Absorbed in the upper GI tract.
Extent of absorption impaired by
food or beverages (other than plain
water). Rapidly binds to bone.
Unabsorbed portion is eliminated in
urine. Protein binding: 90%.
Half-life: 10–60 hr.

INDICATIONS AND DOSAGES

▸ **Osteoporosis**
PO
Adults, Elderly. 2.5 mg daily.

SIDE EFFECTS/ADVERSE REACTIONS

Frequent (13%–6%)
Back pain; dyspepsia, including
epigastric distress and heartburn;
peripheral discomfort; diarrhea;
headache; myalgia
Occasional (4%–3%)
Dizziness, arthralgia, asthenia

Rare (less than 2%)
Vomiting, hypersensitivity reaction

PRECAUTIONS AND CONTRAINDICATIONS

Hypersensitivity to other
bisphosphonates, including
alendronate, etidronate, pamidronate,
risedronate, and tiludronate; inability
to stand or sit upright for at least
60 min; severe renal impairment with
creatinine clearance less than 30 ml/
min; uncorrected hypocalcemia

DRUG INTERACTIONS OF CONCERN TO DENTISTRY

● Decreased absorption: antacids
containing aluminum, calcium, or
magnesium salts, vitamin D
● Use with monitoring, risk of
increased GI side effects: aspirin and
NSAIDs

SERIOUS REACTIONS

! Upper respiratory tract infection
occurs occasionally.
! Overdose causes hypocalcemia,
hypophosphatemia, and significant
GI disturbances.

DENTAL CONSIDERATIONS

General:
● Potential for osteochemonecrosis
of jaws.
● Consider semisupine chair position
for patient comfort if GI side effects
occur.
● Patient may need assistance in
getting into and out of dental chair.
Adjust chair position for patient
comfort.
● Emphasize importance of caries
prevention.
Consultations:
● Medical consultation may be
required to assess disease control and
patient's ability to tolerate stress.
Teach Patient/Family to:
● Update health and medication
history if physician makes any

changes in evaluation or drug regimens; include OTC, herbal, and nonherbal remedies in the update
• Use effective, atraumatic oral hygiene measures to reduce risk of osteochemonecrosis

ibuprofen
eye-byoo-pró-fen
(Act-3[AUS], Advil, Apo-Ibuprofen, Brufen[AUS], Codral Period Pain[AUS], Motrin, Novoprofen[CAN], Nurofen[AUS], Rafen[AUS])

CATEGORY AND SCHEDULE
Pregnancy Risk Category: B
(D if used in third trimester or near delivery)
OTC (Tablets: 200 mg, Oral Suspension: 100 mg/5 ml)

Drug Class: Nonsteroidal antiinflammatory

MECHANISM OF ACTION
An NSAID that inhibits prostaglandin synthesis. Also produces vasodilation by acting centrally on the heat-regulating center of the hypothalamus.
Therapeutic Effect: Produces analgesic and antiinflammatory effects and decreases fever.

USES
Treatment of rheumatoid arthritis, osteoarthritis, primary dysmenorrhea, gout, mild to moderate pain, fever

PHARMACOKINETICS

Route	Onset	Peak	Duration
PO (analgesic)	0.5 hr	N/A	4–6 hr
PO (antirheumatic)	2 days	1–2 wk	N/A

Rapidly absorbed from the GI tract. Protein binding: greater than 90%. Metabolized in the liver. Primarily excreted in urine. Not removed by hemodialysis. **Half-life:** 2–4 hr.

INDICATIONS AND DOSAGES
▶ **Acute or Chronic Rheumatoid Arthritis, Osteoarthritis, Migraine Pain, Gouty Arthritis**
PO
Adults, Elderly. 400–800 mg 3–4 times a day. Maximum: 3.2 g/day.
▶ **Mild-to-Moderate Pain, Primary Dysmenorrhea**
PO
Adults, Elderly. 200–400 mg q4–6h as needed. Maximum: 1.6 g/day.
▶ **Fever, Minor Aches or Pain**
PO
Adults, Elderly. 200–400 mg q4–6h. Maximum: 1.6 g/day.
Children. 5–10 mg/kg/dose q6–8h. Maximum: 40 mg/kg/day. OTC: 7.5 mg/kg/dose q6–8h. Maximum: 30 mg/kg/day.
▶ **Juvenile Arthritis**
PO
Children. 30–70 mg/kg/day in 3–4 divided doses. Maximum: 400 mg/day in children weighing less than 20 kg, 600 mg/day in children weighing 20–30 kg, 800 mg/day in children weighing greater than 30–40 kg.

SIDE EFFECTS/ADVERSE REACTIONS
Occasional (9%–3%)
Nausea with or without vomiting, dyspepsia, dizziness, rash
Rare (less than 3%)
Diarrhea or constipation, flatulence, abdominal cramps or pain, pruritus

PRECAUTIONS AND CONTRAINDICATIONS
• Active peptic ulcer, chronic inflammation of GI tract, GI bleeding disorders or ulceration, history of

hypersensitivity to aspirin or NSAIDs
• Possible increased risk for adverse cardiovascular events in patients at risk for thromboembolism

Caution
Lactation, children, bleeding disorders, GI disorders, cardiac disorders, hypersensitivity to other antiinflammatory agents

DRUG INTERACTIONS OF CONCERN TO DENTISTRY

• GI ulceration, bleeding: aspirin, alcohol (three or more drinks per day), corticosteroids
• Decreased action: salicylates
• Nephrotoxicity: acetaminophen (prolonged use)
• Possible risk of decreased renal function: cyclosporine
• First-time users of SSRIs also taking NSAIDs may have a higher risk of GI side effects; until more data are available, it may be advisable to avoid use of NSAIDs in these patients (Br J Clin Pharmacol 55:591–595, 2003)
• When prescribed for dental pain:
  • Risk of increased effects: oral anticoagulants, oral antidiabetics, lithium, methotrexate
  • Decreased antihypertensive effects of diuretics, β-adrenergic blockers, and ACE inhibitors

SERIOUS REACTIONS

! Acute overdose may result in metabolic acidosis.
! Rare reactions with long-term use include peptic ulcer disease, GI bleeding, gastritis, a severe hepatic reaction (cholestasis, jaundice), nephrotoxicity (dysuria, hematuria, proteinuria, nephrotic syndrome), and a severe hypersensitivity reaction (particularly in patients with systemic lupus erythematosus or other collagen diseases).

General:
• Patients on chronic drug therapy may rarely have symptoms of blood dyscrasias, which can include infection, bleeding, and poor healing.
• Assess salivary flow as a factor in caries, periodontal disease, and candidiasis.
• Avoid prescribing aspirin-containing products.
• Consider semisupine chair position for patients with arthritic disease.

Consultations:
• In a patient with symptoms of blood dyscrasias, request a medical consultation for blood studies and postpone dental treatment until normal values are reestablished.
• Medical consultation may be required to assess disease control.

Teach Patient/Family to:
• Follow labeled directions for OTC products
• Use effective oral hygiene to prevent soft tissue inflammation
• Use caution to prevent injury when using oral hygiene aids
• When chronic dry mouth occurs, advise patient to:
  • Avoid mouth rinses with high alcohol content because of drying effects
  • Use sugarless gum, frequent sips of water, or saliva substitutes
  • Use daily home fluoride products for anticaries effect

ibutilide fumarate
eye-byoo´-ti-lide fyoo´-muh-reyt
(Corvert)

CATEGORY AND SCHEDULE
Pregnancy Risk Category: C

Drug Class: Antidysrhythmic

MECHANISM OF ACTION

An antiarrhythmic that prolongs both atrial and ventricular action potential duration and increases the atrial and ventricular refractory period. Activates slow, inward current (mostly of sodium), produces mild slowing of sinus node rate and AV conduction, and causes dose-related prolongation of QT interval. *Therapeutic Effect:* Converts arrhythmias to sinus rhythm.

USES

For rapid conversion of atrial fibrillation/flutter occurring within 1 wk of coronary artery bypass or valve surgery

PHARMACOKINETICS

After IV administration, highly distributed, rapidly cleared. Protein binding: 40%. Primarily excreted in urine as metabolite. *Half-life:* 2–12 hr (average: 6 hr).

INDICATIONS AND DOSAGES

▶ **Rapid Conversion of Atrial Fibrillation or Flutter of Recent Onset to Normal Sinus Rhythm**
IV Infusion
Adults, Elderly weighing 60 kg and more. One vial (1 mg) given over 10 min. If arrhythmia does not stop within 10 min after end of initial infusion, a second 1 mg/10-min infusion may be given.
Adults, Elderly weighing less than 60 kg. 0.01 mg/kg given over 10 min. If arrhythmia does not stop within 10 min after end of initial infusion, a second 0.01 mg/kg, 10-min infusion may be given.

SIDE EFFECTS/ADVERSE REACTIONS

Ibutilide is generally well tolerated.

Occasional
Ventricular extrasystoles (5.1%), ventricular tachycardia (4.9%), headache (3.6%), hypotension, orthostatic hypotension (2%)
Rare
Bundle-branch block, AV block, bradycardia, hypertension

PRECAUTIONS AND CONTRAINDICATIONS

None known

DRUG INTERACTIONS OF CONCERN TO DENTISTRY

• Potential for arrhythmia: drugs that prolong the QT interval, such as antidepressants

SERIOUS REACTIONS

❗ Sustained polymorphic ventricular tachycardia, occasionally with QT prolongation (torsades de pointes) occurs rarely.
❗ Overdose results in CNS toxicity, including CNS depression, rapid and gasping breathing, and seizures.
❗ Expect prolongation of repolarization may be exaggerated.
❗ Existing arrhythmias may worsen or new arrhythmias may develop.

DENTAL CONSIDERATIONS

General:
• Acute-use drug for use in hospitals, emergency rooms, or cardiac labs.
• Patients who have received this drug for arrhythmias may be at risk when it is combined with other drugs that prolong the QT interval.
Consultations:
• Medical consultation may be required to assess disease control and patient's ability to tolerate stress.
Teach Patient/Family to:
• Update health and medication history if physician makes any changes in evaluation or drug

regimens; include OTC, herbal, and nonherbal remedies in the update

idarubicin hydrochloride

eye-dah-roo´-bi-sin
high-droh-klor´-ide
(Idamycin PFS, Zavedos)
Do not confuse idarubicin with doxorubicin, or Idamycin with Adriamycin.

CATEGORY AND SCHEDULE
Pregnancy Risk Category: D

Drug Class: Anthracycline antibiotic; antineoplastic

MECHANISM OF ACTION
An anthracycline antibiotic that inhibits nucleic acid synthesis by interacting with the enzyme topoisomerase II, which promotes DNA strand supercoiling. *Therapeutic Effect:* Causes death of rapidly dividing cells.

USES
Treatment of acute myeloid leukemia (AML).

PHARMACOKINETICS
Widely distributed. Protein binding: 97%. Rapidly metabolized in the liver to active metabolite. Primarily eliminated by biliary excretion. Not removed by hemodialysis. *Half-life:* 4–46 hr; metabolite: 8–92 hr.

INDICATIONS AND DOSAGES
▸ **AML**
IV
Adults. 8–12 mg/m^2/day for 3 days in combination with Ara-C.
Children (solid tumor). 5 mg/m^2 once a day for 3 days.

Children (leukemia). 10–12 mg/m^2 once a day for 3 days.
▸ **Dosage in Hepatic or Renal Impairment**
Dosage is modified on the basis of serum creatinine or bilirubin level.

Serum Level	Dose Reduction
Serum creatinine 2 mg/dl or more	25%
Serum bilirubin greater than 2.5 mg/dl	50%
Serum bilirubin greater than 5 mg/dl	Do not give

SIDE EFFECTS/ADVERSE REACTIONS
Frequent
Nausea, vomiting, complete alopecia (scalp, axillary, pubic hair), abdominal cramping, diarrhea, mucositis
Occasional
Hyperpigmentation of nailbeds, phalangeal and dermal creases, fever, headache
Rare
Conjunctivitis, neuropathy

PRECAUTIONS AND CONTRAINDICATIONS
Preexisting arrhythmias, cardiomyopathy, myelosuppression, pregnancy, severe CHF

DRUG INTERACTIONS OF CONCERN TO DENTISTRY
Dental drug interactions have not been studied

SERIOUS REACTIONS
❗ Myelosuppression may cause hematologic toxicity (manifested principally as leukopenia and, to a lesser extent, anemia and thrombocytopenia), usually within

10–15 days of starting therapy. Blood counts typically return to normal levels by the third wk.
! Cardiotoxicity (either acute, manifested as transient ECG abnormalities, or chronic, manifested as CHF) may occur.

DENTAL CONSIDERATIONS

General:
• If additional analgesia is required for dental pain, consider alternative analgesics (NSAIDs) in patients taking narcotics for acute or chronic pain.
• Examine for oral manifestation of opportunistic infection.
• This drug may be used in the hospital or on an outpatient basis. Confirm the patient's disease and treatment status.
• Chlorhexidine mouth rinse prior to and during chemotherapy may reduce severity of mucositis.
• Patient on chronic drug therapy may rarely present with symptoms of blood dyscrasias, which can include infection, bleeding, and poor healing. If dyscrasia is present, caution patient to prevent oral tissue trauma when using oral hygiene aids.
• Palliative medication may be required for management of oral side effects.

Consultations:
• Consult physician; prophylactic or therapeutic antiinfectives may be indicated if surgery or periodontal treatment is required.
• Medical consultation may be required to assess immunologic status during cancer chemotherapy and determine safety risk, if any, posed by the required dental treatment.
• Medical consultation may be required to assess disease control and patient's ability to tolerate stress.

Teach Patient/Family to:
• Be aware of oral side effects
• Use effective oral hygiene to prevent soft tissue inflammation
• Report oral lesions, soreness, or bleeding to dentist
• Prevent trauma when using oral hygiene aids
• Update health and medication history if physician makes any changes in evaluation or drug regimens; include OTC, herbal, and nonherbal remedies in the update

idursulfase
eye-dur-sul´-face
(Elaprase)

CATEGORY AND SCHEDULE
Pregnancy Risk Category: C

Drug Class: Enzyme

MECHANISM OF ACTION
A recombinant form of iduronate-2-sulfatase that allows for catabolism of glycosaminoglycans. Hunter syndrome is a disease caused by insufficient levels of this lysosomal enzyme, iduronate-2-sulfate.
Therapeutic Effect: Replaces enzyme (iduronate-2-sulfatase).

USES
Treatment of Hunter syndrome

PHARMACOKENETICS
Half-life: 44–48 min.

INDICATIONS AND DOSAGES
▶ **Hunter Syndrome**
IV
Adults. 0.5 mg/kg once a wk.

Children (5 yr and older). 0.5 mg/kg once a wk.

SIDE EFFECTS/ADVERSE REACTIONS:

Frequent
Fever, headache, antibody development, arthralgia, limb pain, pruritus, hypertension, malaise, visual disturbance, wheezing, musculoskeletal pain, musculoskeletal dysfunction, chest wall, urticaria, abscess, pruritic rash, skin disorder, atrial abnormality, anxiety, irritability, dyspepsia, infusion-site edema, superficial injury

Rare
Angioedema, cardiac arrhythmia, cyanosis, hypotension, infection, pulmonary embolism, respiratory distress, respiratory failure, seizure

PRECAUTIONS AND CONTRAINDICATIONS

Hypersensitivity to idursulfase or its components

Caution
Impaired respiratory function, fever

DRUG INTERACTIONS OF CONCERN TO DENTISTRY

None reported

SERIOUS REACTIONS

! Anaphylactic reactions have been reported.

DENTAL CONSIDERATIONS

General
• Monitor vital signs at every appointment due to cardiovascular side effects.
• Consider semisupine chair position for patient comfort due to respiratory complications.
• Avoid aspirin and NSAIDs.

• Consider visual disturbances when presenting instructions to patients.

Consultations:
• Consult physician to determine disease control and ability of patient to tolerate dental procedures.

Teach Patient/Family to:
• Update medication/health history whenever symptoms of disease or medication regimen is changed
• Use effective, atraumatic oral hygiene measures to reduce soft-tissue inflammation
• Use home fluoride products for anticaries effect

ifosfamide
eye-fos´-fah-mide
(Holoxan[AUS], Ifex)

CATEGORY AND SCHEDULE
Pregnancy Risk Category: D

Drug Class: Alkylating agent; antineoplastic

MECHANISM OF ACTION

An alkylating agent that inhibits DNA and RNA protein synthesis by cross-linking with DNA and RNA strands, preventing cell growth. Cell cycle-phase nonspecific. ***Therapeutic Effect:*** Interferes with DNA and RNA function.

USES

Treatment of cancer of the testicles as well as some other kinds of cancer

PHARMACOKINETICS

Metabolized in the liver to active metabolite. Crosses the blood-brain barrier (to a limited extent). Primarily excreted in urine. Removed by hemodialysis. ***Half-life:*** 15 hr.

INDICATIONS AND DOSAGES
▶ **Germ Cell Testicular Carcinoma**
IV
Adults. 700–2000 mg/m²/day for 5 consecutive days. Repeat every 3 wk or after recovery from hematologic toxicity. Administer with mesna.
Children. 1200–1800 mg/m²/day for 5 days every 21–28 days.

SIDE EFFECTS/ADVERSE REACTIONS
Frequent
Alopecia, nausea, vomiting
Occasional
Confusion, somnolence, hallucinations, infection
Rare
Dizziness, seizures, disorientation, fever, malaise, stomatitis

PRECAUTIONS AND CONTRAINDICATIONS
Pregnancy, severe myelosuppression

DRUG INTERACTIONS OF CONCERN TO DENTISTRY
Dental drug interactions have not been studied

SERIOUS REACTIONS
! Hemorrhagic cystitis with hematuria and dysuria occurs frequently if a protective agent (mesna) is not used.
! Myelosuppression, characterized by leukopenia and, to a lesser extent, thrombocytopenia, occurs frequently.
! Pulmonary toxicity, hepatotoxicity, nephrotoxicity, cardiotoxicity, and CNS toxicity (manifested as confusion, hallucinations, somnolence, and coma) may require discontinuation of therapy.

DENTAL CONSIDERATIONS
General:
• Determine why patient is taking the drug.
• If additional analgesia is required for dental pain, consider alternative analgesics (NSAIDs) in patients taking narcotics for acute or chronic pain.
• Examine for oral manifestation of opportunistic infection.
• Avoid products that affect platelet function, such as aspirin and NSAIDs.
• This drug may be used in the hospital or on an outpatient basis. Confirm the patient's disease and treatment status.
• Chlorhexidine mouth rinse prior to and during chemotherapy may reduce severity of mucositis.
• Patient on chronic drug therapy may rarely present with symptoms of blood dyscrasias, which can include infection, bleeding, and poor healing. If dyscrasia is present, caution patient to prevent oral tissue trauma when using oral hygiene aids.
• Palliative medication may be required for management of oral side effects.
• Short appointments and a stress reduction protocol may be required for anxious patients.
• Patients may be at risk of bleeding; check for oral signs.
• Oral infections should be eliminated and/or treated aggressively.
Consultations:
• Medical consultation should include routine blood counts including platelet counts and bleeding time.
• Consult physician; prophylactic or therapeutic antiinfectives may be indicated if surgery or periodontal treatment is required.

- Medical consultation may be required to assess immunologic status during cancer chemotherapy and determine safety risk, if any, posed by the required dental treatment.
- Medical consultation may be required to assess disease control and patient's ability to tolerate stress.

Teach Patient/Family to:
- Be aware of oral side effects
- Use effective oral hygiene to prevent soft tissue inflammation
- Report oral lesions, soreness, or bleeding to dentist
- Prevent trauma when using oral hygiene aids
- Update health and medication history if physician makes any changes in evaluation or drug regimens; include OTC, herbal, and nonherbal remedies in the update

---

imatinib mesylate
im´-ah-tin-ib
(Gleevec, Glivec[AUS])

CATEGORY AND SCHEDULE
Pregnancy Risk Category: D

Drug Class: Antineoplastic

MECHANISM OF ACTION
Inhibits Bcr-Abl tyrosine kinase, an enzyme created by the Philadelphia chromosome abnormality found in patients with chronic myeloid leukemia (CML). *Therapeutic Effect:* Suppresses tumor growth during the three stages of CML; blast crisis, accelerated phase, and chronic phase.

USES
Treatment of CML in blast crisis, accelerated phase or chronic phase after failure of interferon-α therapy; GI stromal tumors

PHARMACOKINETICS
Well absorbed after PO administration. Binds to plasma proteins, particularly albumin. Metabolized in the liver. Eliminated mainly in the feces as metabolites. *Half-life:* 18 hr.

INDICATIONS AND DOSAGES
▶ **CML**
PO
Adults, Elderly. 400 mg/day for patients in chronic-phase CML; 600 mg/day for patients in accelerated phase or blast crisis. May increase dosage from 400 to 600 mg/day for patients in chronic phase or from 600 to 800 mg (given as 300–400 mg twice a day) for patients in accelerated phase or blast crisis in the absence of a severe drug reaction or severe neutropenia or thrombocytopenia in the following circumstances: progression of the disease, failure to achieve a satisfactory hematologic response after 3 mo or more of treatment, or loss of a previously achieved hematologic response.
Children: 260 mg/m^2 a day as a single daily dose or in 2 divided doses.

SIDE EFFECTS/ADVERSE REACTIONS
Frequent
Nausea, diarrhea, vomiting, headache, fluid retention (periorbital, lower extremities), rash, musculoskeletal pain, muscle cramps, arthralgia
Occasional
Abdominal pain, cough, myalgia, fatigue, fever, anorexia, dyspepsia, constipation, night sweats, pruritus

Rare
Nasopharyngitis, petechiae, asthenia, epistaxis

PRECAUTIONS AND CONTRAINDICATIONS
Known hypersensitivity to imatinib
Caution
Fluid retention, edema risk; neutropenia, thrombocytopenia, GI irritation, liver function abnormalities; safety in lactation or pediatric patients has not been studied

DRUG INTERACTIONS OF CONCERN TO DENTISTRY
• Increased plasma levels with CYP3A4 isoenzyme inhibitors: ketoconazole; possibly macrolide antibiotics, itraconazole, benzodiazepines
• Use acetaminophen with caution or avoid if hepatotoxicity is present
• Possible decrease in plasma concentrations: dexamethasone, carbamazepine, St. John's wort (herb)

SERIOUS REACTIONS
! Severe fluid retention (manifested as pleural effusion, pericardial effusion, pulmonary edema, and ascites) and hepatotoxicity occur rarely.
! Neutropenia and thrombocytopenia are expected responses to the drug.
! Respiratory toxicity, manifested as dyspnea and pneumonia, may occur.

DENTAL CONSIDERATIONS
General:
• Prophylactic or therapeutic antibiotics may be indicated to prevent or treat infection if surgery or periodontal debridement is required.
• Patients taking opioids for acute or chronic pain should be given alternative analgesics for dental pain.

• Short appointments and a stress reduction protocol may be required for anxious patients.
• Consider local hemostasis measures to control excessive bleeding.
• Patients on chronic drug therapy may rarely have symptoms of blood dyscrasias, which can include infection, bleeding, and poor healing.
• Consider semisupine chair position for patient comfort if GI side effects occur.
Consultations:
• In a patient with symptoms of blood dyscrasias, request a medical consultation for blood studies and postpone treatment until normal values are reestablished.
• Consultation with physician may be necessary if sedation or general anesthesia is required.
• Medical consultation should include routine blood counts, including platelet counts and bleeding time.
Teach Patient/Family to:
• Use effective oral hygiene to prevent soft tissue inflammation, infection
• Inform dentist of unusual bleeding episodes following dental treatment

imipramine
ih-mih´-prah-meen
(Apo-Imipramine[CAN], Melipramine[AUS], Tofranil, Tofranil-PM)
Do not confuse imipramine with desipramine.

CATEGORY AND SCHEDULE
Pregnancy Risk Category: D

Drug Class: Antidepressant (tricyclic)

MECHANISM OF ACTION

A tricyclic antidepressant, antibulimic, anticataplectic, antinarcoleptic, antineuralgic, antineuritic, and antipanic agent that blocks the reuptake of neurotransmitters, such as norepinephrine and serotonin, at presynaptic membranes, increasing their concentration at postsynaptic receptor sites. *Therapeutic Effect:* Relieves depression and controls nocturnal enuresis.

USES

Treatment of depression, enuresis in children

PHARMACOKINETICS

PO: Steady state 2–5 days. *Half-life:* 6–20 hr; metabolized by liver; excreted by kidneys, feces; crosses placenta; excreted in breast milk.

INDICATIONS AND DOSAGES

▸ **Depression**

PO

Adults. Initially, 75–100 mg/day. May gradually increase to 300 mg/day for hospitalized patients, or 200 mg/day for outpatients; then reduce dosage to effective maintenance level, 50–150 mg/day. *Elderly.* Initially, 10–25 mg/day at bedtime. May increase by 10–25 mg every 3–7 days. Range: 50–150 mg/day. *Children.* 1.5 mg/kg/day. May increase by 1 mg/kg every 3–4 days. Maximum: 5 mg/kg/day.

▸ **Enuresis**

PO

Children older than 6 yr. Initially, 10–25 mg at bedtime. May increase by 25 mg/day. Maximum: 50 mg for children older than 12 yr.

SIDE EFFECTS/ADVERSE REACTIONS

Frequent

Somnolence, fatigue, dry mouth, blurred vision, constipation, delayed micturition, orthostatic hypotension, diaphoresis, impaired concentration, increased appetite, urine retention, photosensitivity

Occasional

GI disturbances (nausea, metallic taste)

Rare

Paradoxical reactions, (agitation, restlessness, nightmares, insomnia), extrapyramidal symptoms (particularly fine hand tremors)

PRECAUTIONS AND CONTRAINDICATIONS

Acute recovery period after MI, use within 14 days of MAOIs.

Caution

Suicidal patients, severe depression, increased intraocular pressure, narrow-angle glaucoma, urinary retention, cardiac disease, hepatic disease, hyperthyroidism, electroshock therapy, elective surgery, elderly, MAOIs

DRUG INTERACTIONS OF CONCERN TO DENTISTRY

• Increased anticholinergic effects: muscarinic blockers, antihistamines, phenothiazines
• Increased effects of direct-acting sympathomimetics (epinephrine, levonordefrin)
• Potential risk of increased CNS depression: alcohol, barbiturates, benzodiazepines, other CNS depressants
• Decreased antihypertensive effects: clonidine, guanadrel, guanethidine
• Avoid concurrent use with St. John's wort (herb)

• Suspected increased tricyclic antidepressant effects: fluconazole, ketoconazole
• Increased serum levels of carbamazepine
• Caution in using drugs metabolized by CYP2D6: increased effects

SERIOUS REACTIONS

! Overdose may produce seizures; cardiovascular effects, such as severe orthostatic hypotension, dizziness, tachycardia, palpitations, and arrhythmias; and altered temperature regulation, including hyperpyrexia or hypothermia.
! Abrupt discontinuation after prolonged therapy may produce headache, malaise, nausea, vomiting, and vivid dreams.

DENTAL CONSIDERATIONS

General:
• Monitor vital signs at every appointment because of cardiovascular side effects.
• Assess salivary flow as a factor in caries, periodontal disease, and candidiasis.
• Patients on chronic drug therapy may rarely have symptoms of blood dyscrasias, which can include infection, bleeding, and poor healing.
• After supine positioning, have patient sit upright for at least 2 min to avoid orthostatic hypotension.
• Use vasoconstrictors with caution, in low doses, and with careful aspiration. Avoid use of gingival retraction cord with epinephrine.
• Place on frequent recall because of oral side effects.
Consultations:
• In a patient with symptoms of blood dyscrasias, request a medical consultation for blood studies and postpone dental treatment until normal values are reestablished.

• Medical consultation may be required to assess disease control.
• Physician should be informed if significant xerostomic side effects occur (e.g., increased caries, sore tongue, problems eating or swallowing, difficulty wearing prosthesis) so that a medication change can be considered.
Teach Patient/Family to:
• Use effective oral hygiene to prevent soft tissue inflammation
• Prevent injury when using oral hygiene aids
• When chronic dry mouth occurs, advise patient to:
  • Avoid mouth rinses with high alcohol content because of drying effects
  • Use sugarless gum, frequent sips of water, or saliva substitutes
  • Use daily home fluoride products for anticaries effect

imiquimod
im-ick´-wih-mod
(Aldara)

CATEGORY AND SCHEDULE
Pregnancy Risk Category: C

Drug Class: Immune response modifier

MECHANISM OF ACTION
An immune response modifier whose mechanism of action is unknown.
Therapeutic Effect: Reduces genital and perianal warts.

USES
Treatment of external genital and perianal warts, condylomata acuminata

PHARMACOKINETICS

Minimal absorption after topical administration. Minimal excretion in urine and feces.

INDICATIONS AND DOSAGES

▸ **Warts/Condyloma Acuminata**
Topical
Adults, Elderly, Children 12 yr and older. Apply 3 times a wk before normal sleeping hours; leave on skin 6–10 hr. Remove following treatment period. Continue therapy for maximum of 16 wk.

SIDE EFFECTS/ADVERSE REACTIONS

Frequent
Local skin reactions: erythema, itching, burning, erosion, excoriation/flaking, fungal infections (women)
Occasional
Pain, induration, ulceration, scabbing, soreness, headache, flu-like symptoms

PRECAUTIONS AND CONTRAINDICATIONS

History of hypersensitivity to imiquimod
Caution
Has not been evaluated in papilloma viral diseases, cream may weaken condoms and diaphragms, external use only, lactation, children younger 18 yr

DRUG INTERACTIONS OF CONCERN TO DENTISTRY

None reported

SERIOUS REACTIONS

None reported

DENTAL CONSIDERATIONS
General:
• Oral manifestations of the disease may occur in the oral mucosa.

• Patient may have history of other sexually transmitted diseases (STDs).
Consultations:
• Medical consultation may be required to assess disease control.
Teach Patient/Family to:
• Report oral lesions to the dentist
• Update health and drug history if physician makes any changes in evaluation or drug regimens

indapamide

in-dap´-ah-mide
(Dapa-tabs[AUS], Indahexal[AUS], Insig[AUS], Lozide[CAN], Lozol, Natrilix[AUS], Natrilix SR[AUS])
Do not confuse indapamide with iodamide or iopamidol.

CATEGORY AND SCHEDULE

Pregnancy Risk Category: B
(D if used in pregnancy-induced hypertension)

Drug Class: Diuretic, thiazide-like

MECHANISM OF ACTION

A thiazide-like diuretic that blocks reabsorption of water, sodium, and potassium at the cortical diluting segment of the distal tubule; also reduces plasma and extracellular fluid volume and peripheral vascular resistance by direct effect on blood vessels. *Therapeutic Effect:* Promotes diuresis and reduces B/P.

USES

Treatment of edema, hypertension

PHARMACOKINETICS

PO: Onset 1–2 hr, peak 2 hr, duration up to 36 hr. *Half-life:* 14–18 hr; excreted in urine, feces.

INDICATIONS AND DOSAGES
▸ **Edema**
PO
Adults. Initially, 2.5 mg/day, may increase to 5 mg/day after 1 wk.
▸ **Hypertension**
PO
Adults, Elderly. Initially, 1.25 mg, may increase to 2.5 mg/day after 4 wk or 5 mg/day after additional 4 wk.

SIDE EFFECTS/ADVERSE REACTIONS
Frequent
Fatigue, numbness of extremities, tension, irritability, agitation, headache, dizziness, light-headedness, insomnia, muscle cramps
Occasional
Tingling of extremities, urinary frequency, urticaria, rhinorrhea, flushing, weight loss, orthostatic hypotension, depression, blurred vision, nausea, vomiting, diarrhea or constipation, dry mouth, impotence, rash, pruritus

PRECAUTIONS AND CONTRAINDICATIONS
Hypersensitivity, anuria
Caution
Hypokalemia, dehydration, ascites, hepatic disease, severe renal disease

DRUG INTERACTIONS OF CONCERN TO DENTISTRY
• Decreased hypotensive response: NSAIDs, especially indomethacin

SERIOUS REACTIONS
! Vigorous diuresis may lead to profound water and electrolyte depletion, resulting in hypokalemia, hyponatremia, and dehydration.
! Acute hypotensive episodes may occur.
! Hyperglycemia may occur during prolonged therapy.
! Pancreatitis, blood dyscrasias, pulmonary edema, allergic pneumonitis, and dermatologic reactions occur rarely.
! Overdose can lead to lethargy and coma without changes in electrolytes or hydration.

DENTAL CONSIDERATIONS
General:
• Monitor vital signs at every appointment because of cardiovascular side effects.
• Patients on chronic drug therapy may rarely have symptoms of blood dyscrasias, which can include infection, bleeding, and poor healing.
• After supine positioning, have patient sit upright for at least 2 min before standing to avoid orthostatic hypotension.
• Assess salivary flow as a factor in caries, periodontal disease, and candidiasis.
• Limit use of sodium-containing products, such as saline IV fluids, for patients with a dietary salt restriction.
• Stress from dental procedures may compromise cardiovascular function; determine patient risk.
• Short appointments and a stress reduction protocol may be required for anxious patients.
• Patients on diuretic therapy should be monitored for serum K+ levels.
Consultations:
• In a patient with symptoms of blood dyscrasias, request a medical consultation for blood studies and postpone dental treatment until normal values are reestablished.
• Medical consultation may be required to assess disease control and patient's ability to tolerate stress.

Teach Patient/Family to:
• Use effective oral hygiene to prevent soft tissue inflammation
• Use caution to prevent injury when using oral hygiene aids
• When chronic dry mouth occurs, advise patient to:
  • Avoid mouth rinses with high alcohol content because of drying effects
  • Use sugarless gum, frequent sips of water, or saliva substitutes
  • Use daily home fluoride products for anticaries effect

indinavir
in-din′-ah-veer
(Crixivan)
Do not confuse indinavir with Denavir.

CATEGORY AND SCHEDULE
Pregnancy Risk Category: C

Drug Class: Antiviral

MECHANISM OF ACTION
A protease inhibitor that suppresses HIV protease, an enzyme necessary for splitting viral polyprotein precursors into mature and infectious viral particles. **Therapeutic Effect:** Interrupts HIV replication, slowing the progression of HIV infection.

USES
Treatment of HIV infection; prophylaxis after needle stick with AZT and lamivudine within 2 hr of needle stick

PHARMACOKINETICS
Rapidly absorbed after PO administration. Protein binding: 60%. Metabolized in the liver. Primarily excreted in urine. Unknown if removed by hemodialysis. **Half-life:** 1.8 hr (increased in impaired hepatic function).

INDICATIONS AND DOSAGES
▶ **HIV Infection (in combination with other antiretrovirals)**
PO
Adults. 800 mg (two 400-mg capsules) q8h.
▶ **HIV Infection in Patients with Hepatic Insufficiency**
PO
Adults. 600 mg q8h.

SIDE EFFECTS/ADVERSE REACTIONS
Frequent
Nausea, abdominal pain, headache, diarrhea
Occasional
Vomiting, asthenia, fatigue, insomnia, accumulation of fat in waist, abdomen, or back of neck
Rare
Abnormal taste sensation, heartburn, symptomatic urinary tract disease, transient renal dysfunction

PRECAUTIONS AND CONTRAINDICATIONS
Hypersensitivity to indinavir; nephrolithiasis
Caution
Nephrolithiasis (requires adequate hydration), hyperbilirubinemia, serum transaminase elevation, hepatic impairment, dose reduction of rifabutin required, lactation, children

DRUG INTERACTIONS OF CONCERN TO DENTISTRY
- Contraindicated with triazolam, midazolam
- Reduce dose when given with ketoconazole

SERIOUS REACTIONS
! Nephrolithiasis (flank pain with or without hematuria) occurs in 4% of patients.

DENTAL CONSIDERATIONS
General:
- Consider semisupine chair position when GI side effects occur.
- Assess salivary flow as a factor in caries, periodontal disease, and candidiasis.
- Monitor vital signs at every appointment because of cardiovascular side effects.
- Examine for oral manifestation of opportunistic infection.
- Patients with gastroesophageal reflux may have oral symptoms, including burning mouth, secondary candidiasis, and signs of tooth erosion.

Consultations:
- Medical consultation may be required to assess disease control.

Teach Patient/Family to:
- Use effective oral hygiene to prevent soft tissue inflammation
- Report oral lesions, soreness, or bleeding to dentist
- Update health history/drug record if physician makes any changes in evaluation or drug regimens
- When chronic dry mouth occurs, advise patient to:
  - Avoid mouth rinses with high alcohol content because of drying effects
  - Use daily home fluoride products for anticaries effect
  - Use sugarless gum, frequent sips of water, or saliva substitutes

indomethacin
in-doe-meth′-ah-sin
(Apo-Indomethacin[CAN], Arthrexin[AUS], Indocid[CAN], Indocin, Indocin-IV, Indocin-SR, Novomethacin[CAN])
Do not confuse Indocin with Imodium or Vicodin.

CATEGORY AND SCHEDULE
Pregnancy Risk Category: B
(D if used after 34 wk gestation, close to delivery, or for longer than 48 hr)

Drug Class: Nonsteroidal antiinflammatory

MECHANISM OF ACTION
An NSAID that produces analgesic and antiinflammatory effects by inhibiting prostaglandin synthesis. Also increases the sensitivity of the premature ductus to the dilating effects of prostaglandins.
Therapeutic Effect: Reduces the inflammatory response and intensity of pain. Closure of the patent ductus arteriosus.

USES
Treatment of rheumatoid arthritis, osteoarthritis, ankylosing rheumatoid spondylitis, acute gouty arthritis

PHARMACOKINETICS
PO: Onset 1–2 hr, peak 3 hr, duration 4–6 hr; 99% plasma-protein binding; metabolized in liver, kidneys; excreted in urine, bile, feces, breast milk; crosses placenta

INDICATIONS AND DOSAGES
▶ **Moderate-to-Severe Rheumatoid Arthritis, Osteoarthritis, Ankylosing Spondylitis**
PO
Adults, Elderly. Initially, 25 mg 2–3 times a day; increased by 25–50 mg/wk up to 150–200 mg/day. Or 75 mg/day (extended-release) up to 75 mg twice a day.
Children. 1–2 mg/kg/day. Maximum: 150–200 mg/day.
▶ **Acute Gouty Arthritis**
PO
Adults, Elderly. Initially, 100 mg, then 50 mg 3 times a day.
▶ **Acute Shoulder Pain**
PO
Adults, Elderly. 75–150 mg/day in 3–4 divided doses.
▶ **Usual Rectal Dosage**
Adults, Elderly. 50 mg 4 times a day.
Children. Initially, 1.5–2.5 mg/kg/day, increased up to 4 mg/kg/day. Maximum: 150–200 mg/day.
▶ **Patent Ductus Arteriosus**
IV
Neonates. Initially, 0.2 mg/kg. Subsequent doses are on the basis of age, as follows:
Neonates older than 7 days. 0.25 mg/kg for second and third doses.
Neonates 2–7 days. 0.2 mg/kg for second and third doses.
Neonates less than 48 hr. 0.1 mg/kg for second and third doses.

SIDE EFFECTS/ADVERSE REACTIONS
Frequent
Headache, nausea, vomiting, dyspepsia, dizziness
Occasional
Depression, tinnitus, diaphoresis, somnolence, constipation, diarrhea, bleeding disturbances in patent ductus arteriosus

Rare
Hypertension, confusion, urticaria, pruritus, rash, blurred vision

PRECAUTIONS AND CONTRAINDICATIONS
• Active GI bleeding or ulcerations; hypersensitivity to aspirin, indomethacin, or other NSAIDs; renal impairment, thrombocytopenia.
Caution
• Lactation, children, bleeding disorders, GI disorders, cardiac disorders, hypersensitivity to other antiinflammatory agents, depression

DRUG INTERACTIONS OF CONCERN TO DENTISTRY
• Increased GI bleeding, ulceration: corticosteroids, alcohol, aspirin, other NSAIDs
• Renal toxicity: acetaminophen (high doses, prolonged use)
• Possible risk of decreased renal function: cyclosporine
• When prescribed for dental pain:
  • Risk of increased effects: oral anticoagulants, oral antidiabetics, lithium, methotrexate
  • Decreased antihypertensive effects of diuretics, β-adrenergic blockers, ACE inhibitors
  • Increased toxicity of zidovudine
  • First-time users of SSRIs also taking NSAIDs may have a higher risk of GI side effects; until more data are available, it may be advisable to avoid use of NSAIDs in these patients (Br J Clin Pharmacol 55:591–595, 2003)

SERIOUS REACTIONS
! Paralytic ileus and ulceration of the esophagus, stomach, duodenum, or small intestine may occur.
! Patients with impaired renal function may develop hyperkalemia and worsening of renal impairment.

! Indomethacin use may aggravate epilepsy, parkinsonism, and depression or other psychiatric disturbances.

! Nephrotoxicity, including dysuria, hematuria, proteinuria, and nephrotic syndrome, occurs rarely.

! Metabolic acidosis or alkalosis, apnea, and bradycardia occur rarely in patients with patent ductus arteriosus.

DENTAL CONSIDERATIONS

General:

• Avoid prescribing aspirin-containing products.

• Patients on chronic drug therapy may rarely have symptoms of blood dyscrasias, which can include infection, bleeding, and poor healing.

• Assess salivary flow as a factor in caries, periodontal disease, and candidiasis.

• Consider semisupine chair position for patients with arthritic disease.

Consultations:

• In a patient with symptoms of blood dyscrasias, request a medical consultation for blood studies and postpone dental treatment until normal values are reestablished.

• Medical consultation may be required to assess disease control.

Teach Patient/Family to:

• Use effective oral hygiene to prevent soft tissue inflammation

• Use caution to prevent injury when using oral hygiene aids

• When chronic dry mouth occurs, advise patient to:

  • Avoid mouth rinses with high alcohol content because of drying effects

  • Use sugarless gum, frequent sips of water, or saliva substitutes

  • Use daily home fluoride products for anticaries effect

infliximab

in-flicks´-ih-mab
(Remicade)
Do not confuse Remicade with Reminyl.

CATEGORY AND SCHEDULE
Pregnancy Risk Category: C

Drug Class: Antiinflammatory

MECHANISM OF ACTION
A monoclonal antibody that binds to tumor necrosis factor (TNF), inhibiting functional activity of TNF. Reduces infiltration of inflammatory cells. *Therapeutic Effect:* Decreases inflamed areas of the intestine.

USES
Reduces signs and symptoms, progression of structural damage in rheumatoid arthritis in combination with methotrexate; improvement of physical function in moderate-to-severe rheumatoid arthritis in combination with methotrexate; reduction in signs and symptoms in patients with Crohn's disease with inadequate response to conventional therapy, long-term control of remission-level Crohn's disease; reduces and maintains fistulas in Crohn's disease

PHARMACOKINETICS

Route	Onset	Peak	Duration
IV (Crohn's disease)	1–2 wk	N/A	8–48 wk
IV (Rheumatoid arthritis)	3–7 days	N/A	6–12 wk

Absorbed into the GI tissue; primarily distributed in the vascular compartment. *Half-life:* 9.5 days.

INDICATIONS AND DOSAGES
▶ **Moderate-to-Severe Crohn's Disease**
IV Infusion
Adults, Elderly. 5 mg/kg as a single IV infusion.
▶ **Fistulizing Crohn's Disease**
IV Infusion
Adults, Elderly. Initially, 5 mg/kg followed by additional 5-mg/kg doses at 2 and 6 wk after first infusion.
▶ **Rheumatoid Arthritis**
IV Infusion
Adults, Elderly. 3 mg/kg; followed by additional doses at 2 and 6 wk after first infusion: Then q8wk.

SIDE EFFECTS/ADVERSE REACTIONS
Frequent
Headache, nausea, fatigue, fever
Occasional
Fever or chills during infusion, pharyngitis, vomiting, pain, dizziness, bronchitis, rash, rhinitis, cough, pruritus, sinusitis, myalgia, back pain
Rare
Hypotension or hypertension, paresthesia, anxiety, depression, insomnia, diarrhea, urinary tract infection

PRECAUTIONS AND CONTRAINDICATIONS
Sensitivity to infliximab or murine proteins, sepsis, serious active infection
Caution
Risk of serious infections, risk of autoimmunity, chronic use increases risk of lymphoma, do not give live vaccines to patients taking this drug, patients should be tested for tuberculosis before starting therapy, no data on lactation or pediatric use

DRUG INTERACTIONS OF CONCERN TO DENTISTRY
No drug interaction studies conducted

SERIOUS REACTIONS
! Hypersensitivity reaction, lupus-like syndrome, and severe hepatic reactions may occur.

DENTAL CONSIDERATIONS
General:
• Determine why patient is taking the drug.
• Question patient about other drugs being taken.
• Examine for oral manifestation of opportunistic infection.
• Report oral infections to patient's physician; treat infections aggressively.
Consultations:
• Medical consultation may be required to assess disease control and patient's ability to tolerate stress.
Teach Patient/Family to:
• Use effective oral hygiene to prevent soft tissue inflammation, infection
• Immediately report any signs or symptoms of oral infection

insulin
in´-su-lin
Rapid acting: Insulin Lispro (Humalog); Insulin Aspart (Novolog, NovoMix 30[AUS], Novorapid[AUS]); Regular Insulin (Actrapid[AUS], Humulin R, Novolin R, Regular Iletin II); Intermediate acting: NPH (Humulin N, Novolin N, NPH Iletin II); Lente: (Humulin L, Lente Iletin II, Monotard[aus], Novolin L); Long acting: Insulin Glargine (Lantus)

CATEGORY AND SCHEDULE
Pregnancy Risk Category: B

Drug Class: Hormone, antidiabetic

MECHANISM OF ACTION

An exogenous insulin that facilitates passage of glucose, potassium, and magnesium across the cellular membranes of skeletal and cardiac muscle and adipose tissue. Controls storage and metabolism of carbohydrates, protein, and fats. Promotes conversion of glucose to glycogen in the liver. *Therapeutic Effect:* Controls glucose levels in diabetic patients.

USES

Treatment of severe ketoacidosis, Type 1 (IDDM) and Type 2 (NIDDM; when diet, weight control, exercise, or oral hypoglycemics are not sufficient); hyperkalemia, hyperalimentation

PHARMACOKINETICS

Drug Form	Onset (hr)	Peak (hr)	Duration (hr)
Lispro	0.25	0.5–1.5	4–5
Insulin aspart	1/6	1–3	3–5
Regular	0.5–1	2–4	5–7
NPH	1–2	6–14	24+
Lente	1–3	6–14	24+
Insulin glargine	N/A	N/A	24

Long Acting: Lantus.

INDICATIONS AND DOSAGES

▶ **Treatment of Insulin-Dependent Type 1 Diabetes Mellitus and Non-Insulin-Dependent Type 2 Diabetes Mellitus When Diet or Weight Control Has Failed to Maintain Satisfactory Blood Glucose Levels or in Event of Fever, Infection, Pregnancy, Surgery, or Trauma, or Severe Endocrine, Hepatic or Renal Dysfunction; Emergency Treatment of Ketoacidosis (regular insulin); to Promote Passage of Glucose Across Cell Membrane in Hyperalimentation (regular insulin): to Facilitate Intracellular Shift of Potassium in Hyperkalemia (regular insulin)**

Subcutaneous
Adults, Elderly, Children.
0.5–1 unit/kg/day.
Adolescents (during growth spurt).
0.8–1.2 unit/kg/day.

SIDE EFFECTS/ADVERSE REACTIONS

Occasional
Localized redness, swelling, and itching caused by improper injection technique or allergy to cleansing solution or insulin

Infrequent
Somogyi effect, including rebound hyperglycemia with chronically excessive insulin dosages: systemic allergic reaction, marked by rash, angioedema, and anaphylaxis; lipodystrophy or depression at injection site due to breakdown of adipose tissue; lipohypertrophy or accumulation of subcutaneous tissue at injection site due to inadequate site rotation

Rare
Insulin resistance

PRECAUTIONS AND CONTRAINDICATIONS

Hypersensitivity or insulin resistance may require change of type or species source of insulin

DRUG INTERACTIONS OF CONCERN TO DENTISTRY

• Increased hypoglycemia: salicylates, NSAIDs (large doses and chronic use), alcohol
• Hyperglycemia: corticosteroids, epinephrine

SERIOUS REACTIONS

❗ Severe hypoglycemia caused by hyperinsulinism may occur with insulin overdose, decrease or delay of food intake, or excessive exercise and in those with brittle diabetes.

❗ Diabetic ketoacidosis may result from stress, illness, omission of insulin dose, or long-term poor insulin control.

DENTAL CONSIDERATIONS

General:
• Monitor vital signs at every appointment
• Potential for hypoglycemia.
• Place on frequent recall to evaluate healing response.
• Diabetics may be more susceptible to infection and have delayed wound healing.
• Assess salivary flow as a factor in caries, periodontal disease, and candidiasis.
• Prophylactic antibiotics may be indicated in uncontrolled diabetics to prevent infection if surgery or deep scaling is planned.
• Ensure that patient is following prescribed diet and regularly takes medication.
• Question patient about self-monitoring of drug's antidiabetic effect, including blood glucose values or finger-stick records.
• Keep a readily available source of sugar or fruit juice in case of insulin overdose.
Consultations:
• Medical consultation may be required to assess disease control and patient's ability to tolerate stress.
• Medical consultation may include data from patient's blood glucose monitoring, including glycosylated hemoglobin or HbA$_{1c}$ testing.

Teach Patient/Family to:
• Use effective oral hygiene to prevent soft tissue inflammation
• Use caution to prevent injury when using oral hygiene aids
• Avoid mouth rinses with high alcohol content because of drying effects

insulin glargine
in´-su-lin glare´-jeen
(Lantus)

CATEGORY AND SCHEDULE
Pregnancy Risk Category: C

Drug Class: Hormone, antidiabetic

MECHANISM OF ACTION
An exogenous insulin that facilitates passage of glucose, potassium, magnesium across cellular membranes of skeletal and cardiac muscle, adipose tissue; controls storage and metabolism of carbohydrates, protein, fats. Promotes conversion of glucose to glycogen in liver. *Therapeutic Effect:* Controls glucose levels in diabetic patients.

USES
Treatment of severe ketoacidosis, type 1 (IDDM) and type 2 (NIDDM; when diet, weight control, exercise, or oral hypoglycemics are not sufficient); hyperkalemia, hyperalimentation

PHARMACOKINETICS

Drug Form	Onset (hr)	Peak (hr)	Duration (hr)
Insulin glargine	N/A	N/A	24

Metabolized at the carboxyl terminus of the B chain in the subcutaneous depot to form two active metabolites. Unchanged drug and degradation products are present throughout circulation.

INDICATIONS AND DOSAGES
▶ **Treatment of Insulin-Dependent Type 1 Diabetes Mellitus, Non-Insulin-Dependent Type 2 Diabetes Mellitus When Diet or Weight Control Therapy Has Failed to Maintain Satisfactory Blood Glucose Levels or in Event of Fever, Infection, Pregnancy, Severe Endocrine, Liver or Renal Dysfunction, Surgery, or Trauma, Regular Insulin Used in Emergency Treatment of Ketoacidosis, to Promote Passage of Glucose Across Cell Membrane in Hyperalimentation, to Facilitate Intracellular Shift of Potassium in Hyperkalemia**
Subcutaneous
Adults, Elderly, Children. 10 units once daily, preferably at bedtime, adjusted according to patient response.

SIDE EFFECTS/ADVERSE REACTIONS
Frequent
Hypoglycemia
Occasional
Local redness, swelling, itching, caused by improper injection technique or allergy to cleansing solution or insulin
Infrequent
Systemic allergic reaction, marked by rash, angioedema, and anaphylaxis, lipodystrophy or depression at injection site due to breakdown of adipose tissue, lipohypertrophy or accumulation of subcutaneous tissue at injection site due to lack of adequate site rotation

Rare
Insulin resistance

PRECAUTIONS AND CONTRAINDICATIONS
Hypersensitivity or insulin resistance may require change of type or species source of insulin

DRUG INTERACTIONS OF CONCERN TO DENTISTRY
• Increased hypoglycemia: salicylates, NSAIDs (large doses and chronic use), alcohol
• Hyperglycemia: corticosteroids, epinephrine

SERIOUS REACTIONS
! Severe hypoglycemia caused by hyperinsulinism may occur in overdose of insulin, decrease or delay of food intake, excessive exercise, or those with brittle diabetes.
! Diabetic ketoacidosis may result from stress, illness, omission of insulin dose, or long-term poor insulin control.

DENTAL CONSIDERATIONS
General:
• Monitor vital signs at every appointment
• Potential for hypoglycemia.
• Place on frequent recall to evaluate healing response.
• Diabetics may be more susceptible to infection and have delayed wound healing.
• Assess salivary flow as a factor in caries, periodontal disease, and candidiasis.
• Prophylactic antibiotics may be indicated in uncontrolled diabetics to prevent infection if invasive procedures are planned.
• Ensure that patient is following prescribed diet and regularly takes medication.

• Question patient about self-monitoring of drug's antidiabetic effect, including blood glucose values or finger-stick records.
• Keep a readily available source of sugar or fruit juice in case of insulin overdose.

Consultations:
• Medical consultation may be required to assess disease control and patient's ability to tolerate stress.
• Medical consultation may include data from patient's blood glucose monitoring, including glycosylated hemoglobin or HbA_{1c} testing.

Teach Patient/Family to:
• Use effective oral hygiene to prevent soft tissue inflammation
• Use caution to prevent injury when using oral hygiene aids
• Avoid mouth rinses with high alcohol content because of drying effects

insulin glulisine
in´-su-lin gluh´-lih-seen
(Apidra)

CATEGORY AND SCHEDULE
Pregnancy Risk Category: C

Drug Class: Hormone, antidiabetic

MECHANISM OF ACTION
A recombinant, rapid-acting insulin analog that facilitates passage of glucose, potassium, magnesium across cellular membranes of skeletal and cardiac muscle, adipose tissue; controls storage and metabolism of carbohydrates, protein, fats. Promotes conversion of glucose to glycogen in liver. **Therapeutic Effect:** Controls glucose levels in diabetic patients.

USES
Treatment of severe ketoacidosis, type 1 (IDDM) and type 2 (NIDDM; when diet, weight control, exercise, or oral hypoglycemics are not sufficient); hyperkalemia, hyperalimentation

PHARMACOKINETICS

Drug Form	Onset (min)	Peak (min)	Duration (hr)
Insulin glulisine	20 min	55 min	5 hr

INDICATIONS AND DOSAGES
▸ **Diabetes Mellitus (Type 1 and Type 2)**
Subcutaneous, infusion pump
Adults, Elderly, Children.
Individualize per patient needs.

SIDE EFFECTS/ADVERSE REACTIONS
Occasional
Local redness, swelling, itching, caused by improper injection technique or allergy to cleansing solution or insulin
Infrequent
Somogyi effect, including rebound hyperglycemia with chronically excessive insulin doses. Systemic allergic reaction, marked by rash, angioedema, and anaphylaxis, lipodystrophy or depression at injection site due to breakdown of adipose tissue, lipohypertrophy or accumulation of subcutaneous tissue at injection site due to lack of adequate site rotation
Rare
Insulin resistance

PRECAUTIONS AND CONTRAINDICATIONS

Current hypoglycemic episode, hypersensitivity or insulin resistance may require change of type or species source of insulin

DRUG INTERACTIONS OF CONCERN TO DENTISTRY

• Increased hypoglycemia: salicylates, NSAIDs (large doses and chronic use), alcohol
• Hyperglycemia: corticosteroids, epinephrine

SERIOUS REACTIONS

! Severe hypoglycemia caused by hyperinsulinism may occur in overdose of insulin, decrease or delay of food intake, excessive exercise, or those with brittle diabetes.
! Diabetic ketoacidosis may result from stress, illness, omission of insulin dose, or long-term poor insulin control.

DENTAL CONSIDERATIONS
General:
• Monitor vital signs at every appointment
• Potential for hypoglycemia.
• Place on frequent recall to evaluate healing response.
• Diabetics may be more susceptible to infection and have delayed wound healing.
• Assess salivary flow as a factor in caries, periodontal disease, and candidiasis.
• Prophylactic antibiotics may be indicated in uncontrolled diabetics to prevent infection if surgery or deep scaling is planned.
• Ensure that patient is following prescribed diet and regularly takes medication.

• Question patient about self-monitoring of drug's antidiabetic effect, including blood glucose values or finger-stick records.
• Keep a readily available source of sugar or fruit juice in case of insulin overdose.
Consultations:
• Medical consultation may be required to assess disease control and patient's ability to tolerate stress.
• Medical consultation may include data from patient's blood glucose monitoring, including glycosylated hemoglobin or HbA_{1c} testing.
Teach Patient/Family to:
• Use effective oral hygiene to prevent soft tissue inflammation
• Use caution to prevent injury when using oral hygiene aids
• Avoid mouth rinses with high alcohol content because of drying effects

interferon alfa-2a
in-ter-fear´-on al´-fa
(Roferon-A)
Do not confuse interferon alfa-2a with interferon alfa-2b.

CATEGORY AND SCHEDULE
Pregnancy Risk Category: C

Drug Class: Biologic response modifier

MECHANISM OF ACTION
A biological response modifier that inhibits viral replication in virus-infected cells, suppresses cell proliferation, increases phagocytic action of macrophage, and augments specific lymphocytic cell toxicity.
Therapeutic Effect: Prevents rapid growth of malignant cells; inhibits hepatitis virus.

USES

Treatment of hairy-cell leukemia in patients older than 18 yr, AIDS-related Kaposi's sarcoma (KS), chronic hepatitis C, chronic myelogenous leukemia

PHARMACOKINETICS

Well absorbed after IM and subcutaneous administration. Undergoes proteolytic degradation during reabsorption in kidneys. *Half-life:* 2 hr (IM); 3 hr (subcutaneous).

INDICATIONS AND DOSAGES

▸ **Hairy Cell Leukemia**
IM, Subcutaneous
Adults. Initially, 3 million units/day for 16–24 wk. Maintenance: 3 million units 3 times a wk. Do not use 36-million-unit vial.
▸ **Chronic Myelocytic Leukemia**
IM, Subcutaneous
Adults. 9 million units/day.
▸ **Melanoma**
IM, Subcutaneous
Adults, Elderly. 12 million units/m^2 3 times a wk for 3 mo.
▸ **AIDS-Related KS**
IM, Subcutaneous
Adults. Initially, 36 million units/day for 10–12 wk, may give 3 million units on day 1, 9 million units on day 2, 18 million units on day 3, then 36 million units/day for remaining 10–12 wk. Maintenance: 36 million units/day 3 times a wk.
▸ **Chronic Hepatitis C**
IM, Subcutaneous
Adults, Elderly. 6 million units 3 times a wk for 3 mo, then 3 million units 3 times a wk for 9 mo.

SIDE EFFECTS/ADVERSE REACTIONS

Frequent
Flu-like symptoms, nausea, vomiting, cough, dyspnea, hypotension, edema, chest pain, dizziness, diarrhea, weight loss, altered taste, abdominal discomfort, confusion, paresthesia, depression, visual and sleep disturbances, diaphoresis, lethargy
Occasional
Alopecia (partial), rash, dry throat or skin, pruritus, flatulence, constipation, hypertension, palpitations, sinusitis
Rare
Hot flashes, hypermotility, Raynaud's syndrome, bronchospasm, earache, ecchymosis

PRECAUTIONS AND CONTRAINDICATIONS

Autoimmune hepatitis
Caution
Severe hypotension, dysrhythmia, tachycardia, lactation, children younger than 18 yr, severe renal or hepatic disease, convulsion disorder, thrombophlebitis, coagulation disorders, hemophilia, GI bleeding; closely monitor patients; severe, life-threatening neuropsychiatric, autoimmune, ischemic, or infectious disorders may cause or aggravate these conditions

DRUG INTERACTIONS OF CONCERN TO DENTISTRY

• Risk of hepatotoxicity in severe liver disease: acetaminophen

SERIOUS REACTIONS

❗ Arrhythmias, CVA, transient ischemic attacks, CHF, pulmonary edema, and MI occur rarely.

DENTAL CONSIDERATIONS

General:
• Determine why the patient is taking the drug.
• Monitor vital signs at every appointment because of cardiovascular side effects.

- Patients on chronic drug therapy may rarely have symptoms of blood dyscrasias, which can include infection, bleeding, and poor healing.
- Palliative medication may be required for oral side effects.
- Assess salivary flow as a factor in caries, periodontal disease, and candidiasis.
- Consider semisupine chair position for patient comfort if GI side effects occur.
- Avoid elective dental procedures if severe neutropenia (more than 500 cells/mm^3) or thrombocytopenia (more than 50,000 cell/mm^3) is present.
- Antibiotic prophylaxis is indicated in severely neutropenic patients.
- Patient history should include all medications and herbal or nonherbal remedies taken by the patient.
- Severe side effects may require deferring elective dental procedures until drug therapy is completed.
- Evaluate efficacy of oral hygiene home care; preventive appointments may be necessary.

Consultations:
- Medical consultation may be required to assess disease control.
- In a patient with symptoms of blood dyscrasias, request a medical consultation for blood studies and postpone treatment until normal values are reestablished.
- Liver function tests may be required to determine chronic liver disease.

Teach Patient/Family to:
- Use effective oral hygiene to prevent soft tissue inflammation
- Report oral lesions, soreness, or bleeding to dentist
- Update medical/drug records if physician makes any changes in evaluation or drug regimens

- When chronic dry mouth occurs, advise patient to:
  - Avoid mouth rinses with high alcohol content because of drying effects
  - Use sugarless gum, frequent sips of water, or saliva substitutes
  - Use daily home fluoride products for anticaries effect

interferon alfa-2a/2b
in-ter-fear´-on al´-fa
(Roferon-A)/(Intron-A)

CATEGORY AND SCHEDULE
Pregnancy Risk Category: C

Drug Class: Biologic response modifier

MECHANISM OF ACTION
A biologic response modifier that inhibits viral replication in virus-infected cells. ***Therapeutic Effect:*** Suppresses cell proliferation; increases phagocytic action of macrophages; augments specific lymphocytic cell toxicity.

USES
Treatment of hairy-cell leukemia, malignant melanoma, and AIDS-related Kaposi's sarcoma (KS). They are also used to treat laryngeal papillomatosis (growths in the respiratory tract) in children, genital warts, and some kinds of hepatitis.

PHARMACOKINETICS
Interferon alfa-2a
Well absorbed after IM, subcutaneous administration. Undergoes proteolytic degradation during reabsorption in kidney. *Half-life:* IM: 2 hr; Subcutaneous: 3 hr.

Interferon alfa-2b
Well absorbed after IM,
subcutaneous administration.
Undergoes proteolytic degradation
during reabsorption in kidney.
Half-life: 2–3 hr.

INDICATIONS AND DOSAGES
▶ **Hairy-Cell Leukemia**
Interferon alfa-2a
Subcutaneous/IM
Adults. Initially, 3 million units/day
for 16–24 wk. Maintenance:
3 million units 3 times a wk.
Do not use 36-million-unit vial.
Interferon alfa-2b
Subcutaneous/IM
Adults. 2 million units/m^2 3 times a
wk. If severe adverse reactions occur,
modify dose or temporarily
discontinue.
▶ **Chronic Myelocytic Leukemia (CML)**
Interferon alfa-2a
Subcutaneous/IM
Adults. 9 million units daily.
▶ **Condylomata Acuminate**
Interferon alfa-2b
Intralesional
Adults. 1 million units/lesion 3 times
a wk for 3 wk. Use only 10-million-
units vial, reconstitute with no more
than 1 ml diluent. Use tuberculin
(TB) syringe with 25- or 26-gauge
needle. Give in evening with
acetaminophen, which alleviates side
effects.
▶ **Melanoma**
Interferon alfa-2a
Subcutaneous/IM
Adults, Elderly. 12 million units/m^2
3 times a wk for 3 mo.
Interferon alfa-2b
IV
Adults. Initially, 20 million units/m^2
5 times a wk for 4 wk. Maintenance:
10 million units IM/Subcutaneous
for 48 wk.

▶ **AIDS-Related KS**
Interferon alfa-2a
Subcutaneous/IM
Adults. Initially, 36 million units/day
for 10–12 wk, may give 3 million
units on day 1; 9 million units on
day 2; 18 million units on day 3;
then begin 36 million units/day for
remainder of 10–12 wk.
Maintenance: 36 million units/day
3 times a wk.
Interferon alfa-2b
Subcutaneous/IM
Adults. 30 million units/m^2 3 times a
wk. Use only 50 million units vials.
If severe adverse reactions occur,
modify dose or temporarily
discontinue.
▶ **Chronic Hepatitis B**
Interferon alfa-2b
Subcutaneous/IM
Adults. 30–35 million units/wk,
5 million units/day or 10 million
units 3 times a wk.
▶ **Chronic Hepatitis C**
Interferon alfa-2a
Subcutaneous/IM
Adults. Initially, 6 million units once
a day for 3 wk, then 3 million units
3 times a wk for 6 mo.
Interferon alfa-2b
Subcutaneous/IM
Adults. 3 million units 3 times a wk
for up to 6 mo, for up to 18–24 mo
for chronic hepatitis C.

SIDE EFFECTS/ADVERSE REACTIONS
Frequent
Interferon alfa-2a: Flu-like
symptoms, including fever, fatigue,
headache, aches, pains, anorexia,
chills, nausea, vomiting, coughing,
dyspnea, hypotension, edema, chest
pain, dizziness, diarrhea, weight loss,
taste change, abdominal discomfort,
confusion, paresthesia, depression,

visual and sleep disturbances, diaphoresis, lethargy
Interferon alfa-2b: Flu-like symptoms, including fever, fatigue, headache, aches, pains, anorexia, and chills, rash with hairy cell leukemia (KS only)
KS: All previously mentioned side effects plus depression, dyspepsia, dry mouth or thirst, alopecia, rigors
Occasional
Interferon alfa-2a: Partial alopecia, rash, dry throat or skin, pruritus, flatulence, constipation, hypertension, palpitations, sinusitis
Interferon alfa-2b: Dizziness, pruritus, dry skin, dermatitis, alteration in taste
Rare
Interferon alfa-2a: Hot flashes, hypermotility, Raynaud's syndrome, bronchospasm, earache, ecchymosis
Interferon alfa-2b: Confusion, leg cramps, back pain, gingivitis, flushing, tremors, nervousness, eye pain

PRECAUTIONS AND CONTRAINDICATIONS

Hypersensitivity to any component of the formulations.
Caution
Preexisting psoriasis and sarcoidosis, do not use in patients with platelet counts less than 50,000/mm^3, preexisting CV disease, suicidal tendency, depression, preexisting psychiatric diseases, depressed bone marrow; safety and efficacy in lactation and children younger than 18 yr have not been established

DRUG INTERACTIONS OF CONCERN TO DENTISTRY

• Risk of hepatotoxicity in severe liver disease: acetaminophen

SERIOUS REACTIONS

! Arrhythmias, stroke, transient ischemic attacks, CHF, pulmonary edema, and MI occur rarely with interferon alfa-2a.
! Hypersensitivity reaction occurs rarely with interferon alfa-2b.
! Severe adverse reactions of flu-like symptoms appear dose related with interferon alfa-2b.

DENTAL CONSIDERATIONS

General:
• Determine why the patient is taking the drug.
• Monitor vital signs at every appointment because of cardiovascular side effects.
• After supine positioning, have patient sit upright for at least 2 min to avoid orthostatic hypotension.
• Palliative medication may be required for oral side effects.
• Assess salivary flow as a factor in caries, periodontal disease, and candidiasis.
• Patients on chronic drug therapy may rarely have symptoms of blood dyscrasias, which can include infection, bleeding, and poor healing.
• Consider semisupine chair position for patient comfort if GI side effects occur.
• Avoid elective dental procedures if severe neutropenia (fewer than 500 cells/mm^3) or thrombocytopenia (fewer than 50,000 cell/mm^3) is present.
• Antibiotic prophylaxis is indicated in severely neutropenic patients.
• Patient history should include all medications and herbal or nonherbal remedies taken by the patient.
• Severe side effects may require deferring elective dental procedures until drug therapy is completed.

• Evaluate efficacy of oral hygiene home care; preventive appointments may be necessary.
Consultations:
• Medical consultation may be required to assess disease control.
• In a patient with symptoms of blood dyscrasias, request a medical consultation for blood studies and postpone treatment until normal values are reestablished
• Liver function tests may be required to determine chronic liver disease.
Teach Patient/Family to:
• Use effective oral hygiene to prevent soft tissue inflammation
• Report oral lesions, soreness, or bleeding to dentist
• Update medical/drug records if physician makes any changes in evaluation or drug regimens
• When chronic dry mouth occurs, advise patient to:
  • Avoid mouth rinses with high alcohol content because of drying effects
  • Use sugarless gum, frequent sips of water, or saliva substitutes
  • Use daily home fluoride products for anticaries effect

interferon alfa-2b
in-ter-fear´-on al´-fa
(Intron-A)
Do not confuse interferon alfa-2b with interferon alfa-2a.

CATEGORY AND SCHEDULE
Pregnancy Risk Category: C

Drug Class: Biologic response modifier

MECHANISM OF ACTION
A biological response modifier that inhibits viral replication in virus-infected cells, suppresses cell proliferation, increases phagocytic action of macrophages, and augments specific cytotoxicity of lymphocytes for target cells.
Therapeutic Effect: Prevents rapid growth of malignant cells; inhibits hepatitis virus.

USES
Treatment of hairy-cell leukemia in patients older than 18 yr, malignant melanoma, chronic hepatitis B, follicular lymphoma, AIDS-related Kaposi's sarcoma (KS), chronic hepatitis C, condylomata acuminata

PHARMACOKINETICS
Well absorbed after IM and subcutaneous administration. Undergoes proteolytic degradation during reabsorption in kidneys.
Half-life: 2–3 hr.

INDICATIONS AND DOSAGES
▶ **Hairy-Cell Leukemia**
IM, Subcutaneous
Adults. 2 million units/m^2 3 times a wk. If severe adverse reactions occur, modify dose or temporarily discontinue drug.
▶ **Condyloma Acuminatum**
Intralesional
Adults. 1 million units/lesion 3 times a wk for 3 wk. Use only 10-million-unit vial, and reconstitute with no more than 1 ml diluent.
▶ **AIDS-Related KS**
IM, Subcutaneous
Adults. 30 million units/m^2 3 times a wk. Use only 50-million-unit vials. If severe adverse reactions occur, modify dose or temporarily discontinue drug.
▶ **Chronic Hepatitis C**
IM, Subcutaneous
Adults. 3 million units 3 times a wk for up to 6 mo. For patients who

tolerate therapy and whose
ALT(SGPT) level normalizes within
16 wk, therapy may be extended for
up to 18–24 mo.
▶ **Chronic Hepatitis B**
IM, Subcutaneous
Adults. 30–35 million units weekly,
either as 5 million units/day or
10 million units 3 times a wk.
▶ **Malignant Melanoma**
IV
Adults. Initially, 20 million units/m^2
5 times a wk for 4 wk. Maintenance:
10 million units IM or
subcutaneously 3 times a wk for
48 wk.
▶ **Follicular Lymphoma**
Subcutaneous
Adults. 5 million units 3 times a
wk for up to 18 mo.

SIDE EFFECTS/ADVERSE REACTIONS
Frequent
Flu-like symptoms, rash (only in
patients with hairy-cell leukemia KS)
Patients with KS: All previously
mentioned side effects and
depression, dyspepsia, dry mouth or
thirst, alopecia, rigors
Occasional
Dizziness, pruritus, dry skin,
dermatitis, altered taste
Rare
Confusion, leg cramps, back pain,
gingivitis, flushing, tremors,
nervousness, eye pain

PRECAUTIONS AND CONTRAINDICATIONS
Hypersensitivity

DRUG INTERACTIONS OF CONCERN TO DENTISTRY
• Risk of hepatotoxicity in severe
liver disease: acetaminophen

SERIOUS REACTIONS
! Hypersensitivity reactions occur
rarely.
! Severe flu-like symptoms may
occur at higher doses.

DENTAL CONSIDERATIONS
General:
• Determine why the patient is taking
the drug.
• Monitor vital signs at every
appointment because of
cardiovascular side effects.
• Palliative medication may be
required for oral side effects.
• Assess salivary flow as a factor in
caries, periodontal disease, and
candidiasis.
• Patients on chronic drug therapy
may rarely have symptoms of blood
dyscrasias, which can include
infection, bleeding, and poor healing.
• Consider semisupine chair position
for patient comfort if GI side effects
occur.
• Avoid elective dental procedures
if severe neutropenia (more than
500 cells/mm^3) or thrombocytopenia
(more than 50,000 cell/mm^3) is
present.
• Antibiotic prophylaxis is indicated
in severely neutropenic patients.
• Patient history should include all
medications and herbal or nonherbal
remedies taken by the patient.
• Severe side effects may require
deferring elective dental procedures
until drug therapy is completed.
• Evaluate efficacy of oral hygiene
home care; preventive appointments
may be necessary.
Consultations:
• Medical consultation may be
required to assess disease control.
• In a patient with symptoms of
blood dyscrasias, request a medical
consultation for blood studies and

postpone treatment until normal values are reestablished.
• Liver function tests may be required to determine chronic liver disease.

Teach Patient/Family to:
• Use effective oral hygiene to prevent soft tissue inflammation
• Report oral lesions, soreness, or bleeding to dentist
• Update medical/drug records if physician makes any changes in evaluation or drug regimens
• When chronic dry mouth occurs, advise patient to:
  • Avoid mouth rinses with high alcohol content because of drying effects
  • Use sugarless gum, frequent sips of water, or saliva substitutes
  • Use daily home fluoride products for anticaries effect

interferon alfa-n3
in-ter-fear´-on al´-fa
(Alferon N)

CATEGORY AND SCHEDULE
Pregnancy Risk Category: C

Drug Class: Biologic response modifier

MECHANISM OF ACTION
A biological response modifier that inhibits viral replication in virus-infected cells, suppresses cell proliferation, increases phagocytic action of macrophages, and augments specific cytotoxicity of lymphocytes for target cells.
Therapeutic Effect: Inhibits viral growth in condylomata acuminatum.

USES
Intralesional treatment of refractory or recurring external condylomata acuminata in patients 18 yr or older

PHARMACOKINETICS
Plasma levels below detectable limits.

INDICATIONS AND DOSAGES
▶ **Condyloma Acuminatum**
Intralesional
Adults, Children 18 yr and older.
0.05 ml (250,000 international units) per wart twice a wk up to 8 wk. Maximum dose/treatment session: 0.5 ml (2.5 million international units). Do not repeat for 3 mo after initial 8 wk course unless warts enlarge or new warts appear.

SIDE EFFECTS/ADVERSE REACTIONS
Frequent
Flu-like symptoms
Occasional
Dizziness, pruritus, dry skin, dermatitis, altered taste
Rare
Confusion, leg cramps, back pain, gingivitis, flushing, tremor, nervousness, eye pain

PRECAUTIONS AND CONTRAINDICATIONS
Previous history of anaphylactic reaction to egg protein, mouse immunoglobulin, or neomycin
Caution
CV disease, unstable angina, uncontrolled CHF, severe pulmonary disease, diabetes mellitus with ketoacidosis, coagulation disorders, severe myelosuppression, seizure disorders, risk of transmitting blood-borne infectious disease, lactation, use in children younger than 18 yr has not been established

DRUG INTERACTIONS OF CONCERN TO DENTISTRY
None reported

SERIOUS REACTIONS
! Hypersensitivity reaction occurs rarely.
! Severe flu-like symptoms may occur at higher doses.

DENTAL CONSIDERATIONS
General:
• Determine why the patient is taking the drug.
• Following injection, advise patient to take acetaminophen (if there are no contraindications for its use) in pm to ease flu-like symptoms.
• Advise patient if dental drugs prescribed have a potential for photosensitivity.
• Consider semisupine chair position for patient comfort if GI side effects occur.
Consultations:
• Medical consultation may be required to assess disease control.
Teach Patient/Family to:
• Update medical/drug records if physician makes any changes in evaluation or drug regimens

interferon gamma-1b
in-ter-fear´-on gamm´-ah
(Actimmune, Imukin[AUS])

CATEGORY AND SCHEDULE
Pregnancy Risk Category: C

Drug Class: Biologic response modifier

MECHANISM OF ACTION
A biological response modifier that induces activation of macrophages in blood monocytes to phagocytes, which is necessary in the body's cellular immune response to intracellular and extracellular pathogens. Enhances phagocytic function and antimicrobial activity of monocytes. *Therapeutic Effect:* Decreases signs and symptoms of serious infections in chronic granulomatous disease.

USES
Reduces the severity and frequency of infections associated with chronic granulomatous disease; delays disease progression in patients with severe, malignant osteoporosis

PHARMACOKINETICS
Slowly absorbed after subcutaneous administration.

INDICATIONS AND DOSAGES
▶ Chronic Granulomatous Disease; Severe, Malignant Osteopetrosis
Subcutaneous
Adults, Children older than 1 yr.
50 mcg/m^2 (1.5 million units/m^2) in patients with body surface area (BSA) greater than 0.5 m^2; 1.5 mcg/kg/dose in patients with BSA 0.5 m^2 or less. Give 3 times a wk.

SIDE EFFECTS/ADVERSE REACTIONS
Frequent
Fever, headache, rash, chills, fatigue, diarrhea
Occasional
Vomiting, nausea
Rare
Weight loss, myalgia, anorexia

PRECAUTIONS AND CONTRAINDICATIONS
Hypersensitivity to *E. coli*-derived products

Caution
Cardiac disease, seizure disorders, CNS disorders, myelosuppression, lactation, children younger than 1 yr; monitor hematologic values q3mo

DRUG INTERACTIONS OF CONCERN TO DENTISTRY
None reported

SERIOUS REACTIONS
! Interferon gamma-1b may exacerbate preexisting CNS disturbances, including decreased mental status, gait disturbance, and dizziness, as well as cardiac disorders.

DENTAL CONSIDERATIONS
General:
• Determine why the patient is taking the drug.
• Patients on chronic drug therapy may rarely have symptoms of blood dyscrasias, which can include infection, bleeding, and poor healing.
• Ask patient about side effects associated with drug use (abnormal hematologic values).
• Consider semisupine chair position for patient comfort if GI side effects occur.
• Place on frequent recall to evaluate healing response.
• Severe side effects may require deferring elective dental procedures until drug therapy is completed.
• Antibiotic prophylaxis is indicated in severely neutropenic patients.
• Avoid elective dental procedures if severe neutropenia (fewer than 500 cells/mm^3) or thrombocytopenia (fewer than 50,000 cell/mm^3) is present.
Consultations:
• In a patient with symptoms of blood dyscrasias, request a medical consultation for blood studies and

postpone dental treatment until normal values are reestablished.
• Medical consultation may be required to assess disease control and patient's ability to tolerate stress.
Teach Patient/Family to:
• Use effective oral hygiene to prevent soft tissue inflammation
• Use caution to prevent trauma when using oral hygiene aids
• Update medical history and drug records if physician makes any changes in evaluation or drug regimens

ipratropium bromide
eye-pra-troep´-ee-um broh´-mide
(Apo-Ipravent[CAN], Aproven[AUS], Atrovent, Atrovent Aerosol[AUS], Atrovent Nasal[AUS], Atrovent NPH, Novo-Ipramide[CAN], Nu-Ipratropium[CAN], PMS-Ipratropium[CAN])
Do not confuse Atrovent with Alupent.

CATEGORY AND SCHEDULE
Pregnancy Risk Category: B

Drug Class: Anticholinergic bronchodilator

MECHANISM OF ACTION
An anticholinergic that blocks the action of acetylcholine at parasympathetic sites in bronchial smooth muscle. *Therapeutic Effect:* Causes bronchodilation and inhibits nasal secretions.

USES
Treatment of bronchodilation during bronchospasm in those with COPD, bronchitis, emphysema, asthma; not for rapid bronchodilation, maintenance treatment only;

rhinorrhea, rhinorrhea associated with allergic and nonallergic perennial rhinitis in children age 6–11 yr, rhinorrhea associated with common cold

PHARMACOKINETICS

Route	Onset	Peak	Duration
Inhalation	1–3 min	1–2 hr	4–6 hr

Minimal systemic absorption after inhalation. Metabolized in the liver (systemic absorption). Primarily eliminated in feces. *Half-life:* 1.5–4 hr.

INDICATIONS AND DOSAGES
▶ **Bronchospasm, Acute Treatment**
Inhalation
Adults, Elderly, Children. 4–8 puffs as needed.
Nebulization
Adults, Elderly, Children 12 yr and older. 500 mcg q30min for 3 doses, then q2–4h as needed.
Children younger than 12 yr. 250 mcg q20min for 3 doses, then q2–4h as needed.
▶ **Bronchospasm, Maintenance Treatment**
Inhalation
Adults, Elderly, Children 12 yr and older. 2–3 puffs q6h.
Children younger than 12 yr. 1–2 puffs q6h.
Nebulization
Adults, Elderly, Children 12 yr and older.
500 mcg q6h.
Children younger than 12 yr. 250–500 mcg q6h.
▶ **Rhinorrhea**
Intranasal
Adults, Children older than 5 yr. 2 sprays of 0.06% solution 3–4 times a day.
Adults, Children older than 6 yr. 2 sprays of (0.03%) solution 2–3 times a day.

SIDE EFFECTS/ADVERSE REACTIONS
Frequent
Inhalation: Cough, dry mouth, headache, nausea
Nasal: Dry nose and mouth, headache, nasal irritation
Occasional
Inhalation: Dizziness, transient increased bronchospasm
Rare
Inhalation: Hypotension, insomnia, metallic or unpleasant taste, palpitations, urine retention
Nasal: Diarrhea or constipation, dry throat, abdominal pain, stuffy nose

PRECAUTIONS AND CONTRAINDICATIONS
History of hypersensitivity to atropine
Caution
Lactation, children younger than 12 yr, narrow-angle glaucoma, prostatic hypertrophy, bladder neck obstruction

DRUG INTERACTIONS OF CONCERN TO DENTISTRY
• Increased effects of anticholinergic drugs

SERIOUS REACTIONS
! Worsening of angle-closure glaucoma, acute eye pain, and hypotension occur rarely.

DENTAL CONSIDERATIONS
General:
• Monitor vital signs at every appointment because of cardiovascular and respiratory side effects.
• Assess salivary flow as a factor in caries, periodontal disease, and candidiasis.

- Acute asthmatic episodes may be precipitated in the dental office. Sympathomimetic inhalants should be available for emergency use.
- Consider semisupine chair position for patients with respiratory disease.
- Place on frequent recall because of oral side effects.

Consultations:
- Medical consultation may be required to assess disease control and patient's ability to tolerate stress.

Teach Patient/Family to:
- Rinse mouth with water after each inhaled dose to prevent dryness
- When chronic dry mouth occurs, advise patient to:
  - Avoid mouth rinses with high alcohol content because of drying effects
  - Use sugarless gum, frequent sips of water, or saliva substitutes
  - Use daily home fluoride products for anticaries effect

irbesartan
erb-ah-sar´-tan
(Avapro, Karvea[AUS])

CATEGORY AND SCHEDULE
Pregnancy Risk Category: C
(D if used in second or third trimester)

Drug Class: Angiotensin II receptor antagonist, antihypertensive

MECHANISM OF ACTION
An angiotensin II receptor, type AT1, antagonist that blocks the vasoconstrictor and aldosterone-secreting effects of angiotensin II, inhibiting the binding of angiotensin II to the AT1 receptors. ***Therapeutic Effect:*** Causes vasodilation, decreases peripheral resistance, and decreases B/P.

USES
Treatment of hypertension alone or in combination with other antihypertensive drugs; nephropathy in type 2 diabetes

PHARMACOKINETICS
Rapidly and completely absorbed after PO administration. Protein binding: 90%. Undergoes hepatic metabolism to inactive metabolite. Recovered primarily in feces and, to a lesser extent, in urine. Not removed by hemodialysis. ***Half-life:*** 11–15 hr.

INDICATIONS AND DOSAGES
▶ **Hypertension Alone or in Combination with Other Antihypertensives**
PO
Adults, Elderly, Children 13 yr and older. Initially, 75–150 mg/day. May increase to 300 mg/day.
Children 6–12 yr. Initially, 75 mg/day. May increase to 150 mg/day.
▶ **Nephropathy**
PO
Adults, Elderly. Target dose of 300 mg/day.

SIDE EFFECTS/ADVERSE REACTIONS
Occasional
Upper respiratory tract infection, fatigue, diarrhea, cough
Rare
Heartburn, dizziness, headache, nausea, rash

PRECAUTIONS AND CONTRAINDICATIONS
Bilateral renal artery stenosis, biliary cirrhosis or obstruction, primary hyperaldosteronism, severe hepatic insufficiency

Caution
Hypersensitivity to other angiotensin
II receptor antagonists, volume- or
salt-depleted patients, renal
impairment, lactation, children

DRUG INTERACTIONS OF CONCERN TO DENTISTRY
None reported

SERIOUS REACTIONS
! Overdosage may manifest as
hypotension and tachycardia.
Bradycardia occurs less often.

DENTAL CONSIDERATIONS
General:
• Monitor vital signs at every
appointment because of
cardiovascular side effects.
• Limit use of sodium-containing
products, such as saline IV fluids,
for those patients with a dietary salt
restriction.
• Stress from dental procedures may
compromise cardiovascular function;
determine patient risk.
• Short appointments and a stress-
reduction protocol may be required
for anxious patients.
• Use precaution if sedation or
general anesthesia is required; risk of
hypotensive episode.
• After supine positioning, have
patient sit upright for at least 2 min
before standing to avoid orthostatic
hypotension.
• Consider semisupine chair position
for patient comfort if GI side effects
occur.
Consultations:
• Consultation with physician may
be necessary if sedation or general
anesthesia is required.
• Medical consultation may be
required to assess disease control and
patient's ability to tolerate stress; risk
of hypotensive episode.

Teach Patient/Family to:
• Update health and drug history if
physician makes any changes in
evaluation or drug regimens

isocarboxazid
eye-soe-kar-box´-ah-zid
(Marplan)

CATEGORY AND SCHEDULE
Pregnancy Risk Category: C

Drug Class: Antidepressant–
monoamine oxidase inhibitor

MECHANISM OF ACTION
An antidepressant that inhibits the
MAO enzyme system at CNS storage
sites. The reduced MAO activity
causes an increased concentration in
epinephrine, norepinephrine,
serotonin, and dopamine at neuron
receptor sites. **Therapeutic Effect:**
Produces antidepressant effect.

USES
Treatment of depression

PHARMACOKINETICS
PO: Good absorption; maximum
MAO inhibition 5–10 days, duration
up to 2 wk; metabolized by liver;
excreted by kidneys.

INDICATIONS AND DOSAGES
▸ **Depression Refractory to
Other Antidepressants or
Electroconvulsive Therapy**
PO
Adults, Elderly. Initially,
10 mg 3 times a day. May increase
to 60 mg/day.

SIDE EFFECTS/ADVERSE REACTIONS
Frequent
Postural hypotension, drowsiness, decreased sexual ability, weakness, trembling, visual disturbances
Occasional
Tachycardia, peripheral edema, nervousness, chills, diarrhea, anorexia, constipation, xerostomia
Rare
Hepatitis, leukopenia, parkinsonian syndrome

PRECAUTIONS AND CONTRAINDICATIONS
Cardiovascular disease (CVD), cerebrovascular disease, liver impairment, pheochromocytoma, liver impairment
Caution
Suicidal patients, concurrent use with other antidepressants (patients must stop taking MAOI 14 days before initiating therapy with other antidepressants), general anesthesia, severe depression, schizophrenia, diabetes mellitus, lactation, children younger than 16 yr

DRUG INTERACTIONS OF CONCERN TO DENTISTRY
• Increased pressor effects: indirect-acting sympathomimetics (ephedrine)
• Hyperpyretic crisis, convulsions, hypertensive episode: meperidine, possibly other opioids, carbamazepine
• Increased anticholinergic effects: anticholinergics, antihistamines
• Increased effects of alcohol, barbiturates, benzodiazepines, CNS depressants, SSRIs, tricyclic antidepressants, cyclobenzaprine, bupropion, buspirone, dextromethorphan, antihypertensive

SERIOUS REACTIONS
! Hypertensive crisis, marked by severe hypertension, occipital headache radiating frontally, neck stiffness or soreness, nausea, vomiting, sweating, fever or chilliness, clammy skin, dilated pupils, palpitations, tachycardia or bradycardia, and constricting chest pain.

DENTAL CONSIDERATIONS
General:
• Monitor vital signs at every appointment because of cardiovascular side effects.
• After supine positioning, have patient sit upright for at least 2 min to avoid orthostatic hypotension.
• Patients on chronic drug therapy may rarely have symptoms of blood dyscrasias, which can include infection, bleeding, and poor healing.
• Consider semisupine chair position for patient comfort if GI side effects occur.
• Assess salivary flow as a factor in caries, periodontal disease, and candidiasis.
• Hypertensive episodes are possible even though there are no specific contraindications to vasoconstrictor use in local anesthetics.
• Short appointments and a stress-reduction protocol may be required for anxious patients.
Consultations:
• Medical consultation may be required to assess disease control and patient's ability to tolerate stress.
• In a patient with symptoms of blood dyscrasias, request a medical consultation for blood studies and postpone treatment until normal values are reestablished.
Teach Patient/Family:
• When chronic dry mouth occurs, advise patient to:

• To avoid mouth rinses with high alcohol content because of drying effects
• To use daily home fluoride products for anticaries effect
• To use sugarless gum, frequent sips of water, or saliva substitutes

isoetharine hydrochloride
eye-soe-eth´-ah-reen
high-droh-klor´-ide
(Beta-2, Bronkometer, Bronkosol, Dey-Lute)

CATEGORY AND SCHEDULE
Pregnancy Risk Category: C

Drug Class: Adrenergic β_2-agonist

MECHANISM OF ACTION
A sympathomimetic (adrenergic agonist) that stimulates β_2-adrenergic receptors in the lungs, resulting in relaxation of bronchial smooth muscle. **Therapeutic Effect:** Relieves bronchospasm, reduces airway resistance.

USES
Treatment of bronchospasm, asthma

PHARMACOKINETICS
Rapidly, well absorbed from the GI tract. Extensive metabolism in GI tract. Unknown extent metabolized in liver and lungs. Excreted in urine. **Half-life:** 4 hr.

INDICATIONS AND DOSAGES
▶ **Bronchospasm**
Hand-bulb Nebulizer
Adults, Elderly. 4 inhalations (range: 3–7 inhalations) undiluted. May be repeated up to 5 times a day.
Metered Dose Inhalation

Adults, Elderly. 1–2 inhalations q4h. Wait 1 min before administering second inhalation.
IPPB, Oxygen Aerolization
Adults, Elderly. 0.5–1 ml of a 0.5% or 0.5 ml of a 1% solution diluted 1:3.

SIDE EFFECTS/ADVERSE REACTIONS
Occasional
Tremor, nausea, nervousness, palpitations, tachycardia, peripheral vasodilation, dryness of mouth, throat, dizziness, vomiting, headache, increased B/P, insomnia

PRECAUTIONS AND CONTRAINDICATIONS
History of hypersensitivity to sympathomimetics
Caution
Cardiac disorders, hyperthyroidism, diabetes mellitus, prostatic hypertrophy

DRUG INTERACTIONS OF CONCERN TO DENTISTRY
• Increased effects of both drugs: other sympathomimetics
• Increased dysrhythmia: halogenated hydrocarbon anesthetics

SERIOUS REACTIONS
! Excessive sympathomimetic stimulation may produce palpitations, extrasystoles, tachycardia, chest pain, slight increase in B/P followed by a substantial decrease, chills, sweating, and blanching of skin.
! Too frequent or excessive use may lead to loss of bronchodilating effectiveness and severe and paradoxical bronchoconstriction.

DENTAL CONSIDERATIONS

General:
- Assess salivary flow as a factor in caries, periodontal disease, and candidiasis.
- Consider semisupine chair position for patients with respiratory disease.
- Acute asthmatic episodes may be precipitated in the dental office. Sympathomimetic inhalants should be available for emergency use.

Consultations:
- Medical consultation may be required to assess disease control and patient's ability to tolerate stress.

Teach Patient/Family to:
- Rinse mouth with water after each inhaled dose to prevent dryness
- When chronic dry mouth occurs, advise patient to:
  - Avoid mouth rinses with high alcohol content because of drying effects
  - Use sugarless gum, frequent sips of water, or saliva substitutes
  - Use daily home fluoride products for anticaries effect

isoniazid

eye-soe-nye´-ah-zid
(INH, Isotamine[CAN], Nydrazid, PMS Isoniazid[CAN])

CATEGORY AND SCHEDULE

Pregnancy Risk Category: C

Drug Class: Antitubercular

MECHANISM OF ACTION

An isonicotinic acid derivative that inhibits mycolic acid synthesis and causes disruption of the bacterial cell wall and loss of acid-fast properties in susceptible mycobacteria. Active only during bacterial cell division.

Therapeutic Effect: Bactericidal against actively growing intracellular and extracellular susceptible mycobacteria.

USES

Treatment and prevention of tuberculosis (TB)

PHARMACOKINETICS

Readily absorbed from the GI tract. Protein binding: 10%–15%. Widely distributed (including to CSF). Metabolized in the liver. Primarily excreted in urine. Removed by hemodialysis. ***Half-life:*** 0.5–5 hr.

INDICATIONS AND DOSAGES

▶ **TB (in combination with one or more antituberculars)**
PO, IM
Adults, Elderly. 5 mg/kg/day as a single dose. Maximum 300 mg/day.
Children. 10–15 mg/kg/day as a single dose. Maximum 300 mg/day.

▶ **Prevention of TB**
PO, IM
Adults, Elderly. 300 mg/day as a single dose.
Children. 10 mg/kg/day as a single dose. Maximum 300 mg/day.

SIDE EFFECTS/ADVERSE REACTIONS

Frequent
Nausea, vomiting, diarrhea, abdominal pain
Rare
Pain at injection site, hypersensitivity reaction

PRECAUTIONS AND CONTRAINDICATIONS

Acute hepatic disease, history of hypersensitivity reactions or hepatic injury with previous isoniazid therapy

Caution
Renal disease; diabetic retinopathy cataracts; ocular defects; hepatic disease; fatal hepatitis, especially in black women and Hispanic women; children younger than 13 yr, monitor liver function

DRUG INTERACTIONS OF CONCERN TO DENTISTRY
• Increased hepatotoxicity: alcohol, acetaminophen, carbamazepine
• Decreased effectiveness: glucocorticoids, especially prednisolone
• Increased plasma concentration: benzodiazepines, alfentanil
• Decreased effect of ketoconazole, miconazole

SERIOUS REACTIONS
! Rare reactions include neurotoxicity (as evidenced by ataxia and paraesthesia), optic neuritis, and hepatotoxicity.

DENTAL CONSIDERATIONS
General:
• Patients on chronic drug therapy may rarely have symptoms of blood dyscrasias, which can include infection, bleeding, and poor healing.
• Medical consultation may be required to assess disease control.
• Examine for evidence of oral signs of disease.
Consultations:
• In a patient with symptoms of blood dyscrasias, request a medical consultation for blood studies and postpone dental treatment until normal values are reestablished.
Teach Patient/Family to:
• Use caution to prevent injury when using oral hygiene aids

isoproterenol
eye-soe-proe-ter´-eh-nole
(Isuprel)

CATEGORY AND SCHEDULE
Pregnancy Risk Category: C

Drug Class: Adrenergic β_1- and β_2-agonist

MECHANISM OF ACTION
A sympathomimetic (adrenergic agonist) that stimulates β_1-adrenergic receptors. ***Therapeutic Effect:*** Increases myocardial contractility, stroke volume, cardiac output.

USES
Treatment of bronchospasm during anesthesia

PHARMACOKINETICS
Readily absorbed. Metabolized in liver. Primarily excreted in urine. ***Half-life:*** 2.5–5 min.

INDICATIONS AND DOSAGES
▶ **Arrhythmias**
IV Bolus
Adults, Elderly. Initially, 0.02–0.06 mg (1–3 ml of diluted solution). Subsequent dose range: 0.01–0.2 mg (0.5–10 ml of diluted solution).
IV Infusion
Adults, Elderly. Initially, 5 mcg/min (1.25 ml/min of diluted solution). Subsequent dose range: 2–20 mcg/min.
Children. 2.5 mcg/min or 0.1 mcg/kg per min.
▶ **Complete Heart Block Following Closure of Ventricular Septal Defects**
IV
Adults, Elderly. 0.04–0.06 mg (2–3 ml of diluted solution).
Infants. 0.01–0.03 (0.5–1.5 ml of diluted solution).

▶ **Shock**

IV Infusion

Adults, Elderly. Rate of 0.5–5 mcg/min (0.25–2.5 ml of 1:500,000 dilution); rate of infusion on the basis of clinical response (heart rate, central venous pressure, systemic B/P, urine flow measurements).

SIDE EFFECTS/ADVERSE REACTIONS

Frequent

Palpitations, tachycardia, restlessness, nervousness, tremors, insomnia, anxiety

Occasional

Increased sweating, headache, nausea, flushed skin, dizziness, coughing

PRECAUTIONS AND CONTRAINDICATIONS

Tachycardia due to digitalis toxicity, preexisting arrhythmias, angina, precordial distress, hypersensitivity to isoproterenol or any component of the formulation

Caution

Cardiac disorders, hyperthyroidism, diabetes mellitus, prostatic hypertrophy

DRUG INTERACTIONS OF CONCERN TO DENTISTRY

• Hypotension, tachycardia: haloperidol, loxapine, phenothiazines, thioxanthenes
• Increased dysrhythmia: halogenated-hydrocarbon anesthetics

SERIOUS REACTIONS

! Excessive sympathomimetic stimulation may cause palpitations, extrasystoles, tachycardia, chest pain, slight increase in B/P followed by a substantial decrease, chills, sweating, and blanching of skin.

! Ventricular arrhythmias may occur if heart rate is above 130 beats/min.

! Parotid gland swelling may occur with prolonged use.

DENTAL CONSIDERATIONS

General:

• This drug is used only in conjunction with general anesthesia procedures.

isosorbide

eye-soe-sor´-bide
isosorbide dinitrate
(Apo-ISDN[CAN], Cedocard[CAN], Dilatrate, Isogen[AUS], Isordil, Sorbidin[AUS]);
isosorbide mononitrate
(Duride[AUS], Imdur, Imtrate[AUS], ISMO, Monodur Durules[AUS], Monoket)
Do not confuse with Inderal, Isuprel, K-Dur, or Plendil.

CATEGORY AND SCHEDULE

Pregnancy Risk Category: C

Drug Class: Nitrate antianginal

MECHANISM OF ACTION

A nitrate that stimulates intracellular cyclic guanosine monophosphate (GMP). *Therapeutic Effect:* Relaxes vascular smooth muscle of both arterial and venous vasculature. Decreases preload and afterload.

USES

Treatment of chronic stable angina pectoris

PHARMACOKINETICS

Route	Onset	Peak	Duration
Sublingual	2–10 min	N/A	1–2 days
Chewable	3 min	N/A	0.5–2 hr
PO	45–60 min	N/A	4–6 hr
Sustained-release	30 min	N/A	6–12 hr

Mononitrate well absorbed after PO administration. Dinitrate poorly absorbed and metabolized in the liver to its activate metabolite isosorbide mononitrate. Excreted in urine and feces. *Half-life:* 1–4 hr, dinitrate; 4 hr, mononitrate.

INDICATIONS AND DOSAGES
▶ **Acute Angina, Prophylactic Management in Situations Likely to Provoke Attack**
Sublingual
Adults, Elderly. Initially, 2.5–5 mg. Repeat at 5–10 min intervals. No more than 3 doses in 15–30 min period.
▶ **Acute Prophylactic Management of Angina**
Sublingual
Adults, Elderly. 5–10 mg q2–3h.
▶ **Long-Term Prophylaxis of Angina**
PO
Adults, Elderly. Initially, 5–20 mg 3–4 times a day. Maintenance: 10–40 mg q6h. Consider 2–3 times a day, last dose no later than 7 pm to minimize intolerance.
PO (Mononitrate)
Adults, Elderly. 20 mg 2 times a day, 7 hr apart. First dose upon awakening in morning.
PO (Extended Release)
Adults, Elderly. Initially, 40 mg. Maintenance: 40–80 mg 2–3 times a day. Consider 1–2 times a day, last dose at 2 pm to minimize intolerance.

PO (Imdur)
Adults, Elderly. 60–120 mg/day as single dose.
▶ **CHF**
PO (Chewable)
Adults, Elderly. 5–10 mg every 2–3 hr.

SIDE EFFECTS/ADVERSE REACTIONS
Frequent
Burning and tingling at oral point of dissolution (sublingual), headache (may be severe) occurs mostly in early therapy, diminishes rapidly in intensity, usually disappears during continued treatment; transient flushing of face and neck, dizziness (especially if patient is standing immobile or is in a warm environment), weakness, postural hypotension, nausea, vomiting, restlessness
Occasional
GI upset, blurred vision, dry mouth

PRECAUTIONS AND CONTRAINDICATIONS
Closed-angle glaucoma, GI hypermotility or malabsorption (extended-release tablets), head trauma, hypersensitivity to nitrates, increased intracranial pressure, postural hypotension, severe anemia (extended-release tablets)
Caution
Postural hypotension, lactation, children

DRUG INTERACTIONS OF CONCERN TO DENTISTRY
• Increased effects: alcohol, other vasodilator-type drugs
• Severe hypotension: sildenafil, vardenafil, tadalafil

SERIOUS REACTIONS

! Blurred vision or dry mouth may occur (drug should be discontinued).
! Severe postural hypotension manifested by fainting, pulselessness, cold or clammy skin, and diaphoresis may occur.
! Tolerance may occur with repeated, prolonged therapy (minor tolerance with intermittent use of sublingual tablets). Tolerance may not occur with extended-release form.
! High dose tends to produce severe headache.

DENTAL CONSIDERATIONS

General:
• Monitor vital signs at every appointment because of cardiovascular side effects.
• After supine positioning, have patient sit upright for at least 2 min before standing to avoid orthostatic hypotension.
• Stress from dental procedures may compromise cardiovascular function; determine patient risk.
• Assess salivary flow as a factor in caries, periodontal disease, and candidiasis.
• Short appointments and a stress-reduction protocol may be required for anxious patients.
• Consider semisupine chair position for patients with respiratory distress.
• Use vasoconstrictors with caution, in low doses, and with careful aspiration. Avoid use of gingival retraction cord with epinephrine.
• Nitroglycerin should be available in case of an acute anginal episode.
Consultations:
• Medical consultation may be required to assess disease control and patient's ability to tolerate stress.
Teach Patient/Family:
• When chronic dry mouth occurs, advise patient to:

• Avoid mouth rinses with high alcohol content because of drying effects
• Use sugarless gum, frequent sips of water, or saliva substitutes
• Use daily home fluoride products for anticaries effect

isosorbide dinitrate/ isosorbide mononitrate

ahy-suh-sawr´-bayd
dahy-nahy´-treyt
isosorbide dinitrate (Apo-ISDN[CAN], Cedocard[CAN], Dilatrate, Isogen[AUS], Isordil, Sorbidin[AUS]); isosorbide mononitrate (Duride[AUS], Imdur, Imdur Durules[AUS], Imtrate[AUS], ISMO, Monodur Durules[AUS], Monoket)
Do not confuse Isordil with Isuprel or Plendil, or Imdur with Inderal or K-Dur.

CATEGORY AND SCHEDULE
Pregnancy Risk Category: C

Drug Class: Nitrate antianginal

MECHANISM OF ACTION
A nitrate that stimulates intracellular cyclic guanosine monophosphate. *Therapeutic Effect:* Relaxes vascular smooth muscle of both arterial and venous vasculature. Decreases preload and afterload.

USES
Treatment of chronic stable angina pectoris

PHARMACOKINETICS

Route	Onset	Peak	Duration
Dinitrate	2–5 min	N/A	1–2 hr
Sublingual oral (chewable)	2–5 min	N/A	1–2 hr
Oral	15–40 min	N/A	4–6 hr
Oral (sustained release)	30 min	N/A	12 hr
Mononitrate oral (extended release)	60 min	N/A	N/A

Dinitrate poorly absorbed and metabolized in the liver to its active metabolite isosorbide mononitrate. Mononitrate well absorbed after PO administration. Excreted in urine and feces. *Half-life:* Dinitrate, 1–4 hr; mononitrate, 4 hr.

INDICATIONS AND DOSAGES
▸ **Angina**
PO (isosorbide dinitrate)
Adults, Elderly. 5–40 mg 4 times a day. Sustained-release: 40 mg q8–12h.
PO (isosorbide mononitrate)
Adults, Elderly. 5–10 mg twice a day given 7 hr apart. Sustained-release: Initially, 30–60 mg/day in morning as a single dose. May increase dose at 3-day intervals. Maximum: 240 mg/day.

SIDE EFFECTS/ADVERSE REACTIONS
Frequent
Burning and tingling at oral point of dissolution (sublingual), headache (possibly severe) occurs mostly in early therapy, diminishes rapidly in intensity, and usually disappears during continued treatment, transient flushing of face and neck, dizziness (especially if patient is standing immobile or is in a warm environment), weakness, orthostatic hypotension, nausea, vomiting, restlessness
Occasional
GI upset, blurred vision, dry mouth

PRECAUTIONS AND CONTRAINDICATIONS
Closed-angle glaucoma, GI hypermotility or malabsorption (extended-release tablets), head trauma, hypersensitivity to nitrates, increased intracranial pressure, orthostatic hypotension, severe anemia (extended-release tablets)

DRUG INTERACTIONS OF CONCERN TO DENTISTRY
• Increased effects: alcohol and other drugs that can lower B/P
• Severe hypotension: sildenafil, vardenafil, tadalafil

SERIOUS REACTIONS
! Blurred vision or dry mouth may occur (drug should be discontinued).
! Isosorbide administration may cause severe orthostatic hypotension manifested by fainting, pulselessness, cold or clammy skin, and diaphoresis.
! Tolerance may occur with repeated, prolonged therapy, but may not occur with the extended-release form. Minor tolerance may be seen with intermittent use of sublingual tablets.
! High dosage tends to produce severe headache.

DENTAL CONSIDERATIONS
General:
• Monitor vital signs at every appointment because of cardiovascular side effects.
• After supine positioning, have patient sit upright for at least 2 min

before standing to avoid orthostatic hypotension.
- Assess salivary flow as a factor in caries, periodontal disease, and candidiasis.
- Stress from dental procedures may compromise cardiovascular function; determine patient risk.
- Use vasoconstrictors with caution, in low doses, and with careful aspiration. Avoid use of gingival retraction cord with epinephrine.
- Short appointments and a stress-reduction protocol may be required for anxious patients.
- Nitroglycerin should be available in case of acute anginal episode.

Consultations:
- Medical consultation may be required to assess disease control and patient's ability to tolerate stress.

Teach Patient/Family to:
- Use effective oral hygiene to prevent soft tissue inflammation
- When chronic dry mouth occurs, advise patient to:
  - Avoid mouth rinses with high alcohol content because of drying effects
  - Use sugarless gum, frequent sips of water, or saliva substitutes
  - Use daily home fluoride products for anticaries effect

isotretinoin
eye-soe-tret´-ih-noyn
(Accutane, Amnesteem, Claravis, Isotrex[CAN], Sotret)
Do not confuse Accutane with Accupril or Accurbron.

CATEGORY AND SCHEDULE
Pregnancy Risk Category: X

Drug Class: Retinoic acid isomer, vitamin A derivative

MECHANISM OF ACTION
Reduces the size of sebaceous glands and inhibits their activity. *Therapeutic Effect:* Decreases sebum production; produces antikeratinizing and antiinflammatory effects.

USES
Treatment of severe recalcitrant cystic acne; unapproved: severe rosacea

PHARMACOKINETICS
Metabolized in the liver; major metabolite active. Eliminated in urine and feces. *Half-life:* 21 hr; metabolite, 21–24 hr.

INDICATIONS AND DOSAGES
▶ **Recalcitrant Cystic Acne That Is Unresponsive to Conventional Acne Therapies**
PO
Adults. Initially, 0.5–2 mg/kg/day divided into 2 doses for 15–20 wk. May repeat after at least 2 mo off therapy.

SIDE EFFECTS/ADVERSE REACTIONS
Frequent
Cheilitis (inflammation of lips), dry skin and mucous membranes, skin fragility, pruritus, epistaxis, dry nose and mouth, conjunctivitis, hypertriglyceridemia, nausea, vomiting, abdominal pain
Occasional
Musculoskeletal symptoms (including bone pain, arthralgia, generalized myalgia), photosensitivity
Rare
Decreased night vision, depression

PRECAUTIONS AND CONTRAINDICATIONS

Hypersensitivity to isotretinoin or parabens (component of capsules)

Caution

Lactation, diabetes, photosensitivity, hepatic disease, depressive illness, children younger than 12 yr; potential musculoskeletal side effects (osteoporosis, osteopenia, bone fracture and delayed healing of bone fractures) have been spontaneously reported in Accutane users

DRUG INTERACTIONS OF CONCERN TO DENTISTRY

- Additive photosensitization: tetracycline
- Pseudotumor cerebri, intracranial hypertension: minocycline, doxycycline, tetracycline
- Increased tissue drying: alcohol
- Contraindicated with all tetracyclines (demeclocycline, doxycycline, minocycline, tetracycline)
- Avoid additional vitamin A supplements

SERIOUS REACTIONS

! Inflammatory bowel disease and pseudotumor cerebri (benign intracranial hypertension) have been associated with isotretinoin therapy.

DENTAL CONSIDERATIONS

General:
- Patients on chronic drug therapy may rarely have symptoms of blood dyscrasias, which can include infection, bleeding, and poor healing.
- Assess salivary flow as a factor in caries, periodontal disease, and candidiasis.
- Exaggerated healing response characterized by exuberant granulation tissue has been reported.

- Apply lubricant to dry lips for patient comfort before dental procedures.

Consultations:
- In a patient with symptoms of blood dyscrasias, request a medical consultation for blood studies and postpone dental treatment until normal values are reestablished.

Teach Patient/Family to:
- Use effective oral hygiene to prevent soft tissue inflammation
- When chronic dry mouth occurs, advise patient to:
  - Avoid mouth rinses with high alcohol content because of drying effects
  - Use sugarless gum, frequent sips of water, or saliva substitutes
  - Use daily home fluoride products for anticaries effect

isoxsuprine hydrochloride

eye-sox´-soo-preen
high-droh-klor´-ide
(Vasodilan)

CATEGORY AND SCHEDULE

Pregnancy Risk Category: C

Drug Class: Peripheral vasodilator

MECHANISM OF ACTION

The mechanism of action of isoxsuprine hydrochloride is not fully understood. Increases muscle blood flow. May have a direct action on vascular smooth muscle. β-adrenergic stimulation of the uterus. *Therapeutic Effect:* Relieves symptoms associated with cerebral vascular insufficiency. Inhibits preterm labor.

USES

Treatment of symptoms of
cerebrovascular insufficiency;
peripheral vascular disease, including
arteriosclerosis obliterans,
thromboangiitis obliterans,
Raynaud's disease

PHARMACOKINETICS

The pharmacokinetics of isoxsuprine
hydrochloride is not fully
understood. *Half-life:* Unknown.

INDICATIONS AND DOSAGES

▸ **Raynaud's Syndrome**
IV infusion
Adults, Elderly. 10–20 mg 3–4 times
a day.

SIDE EFFECTS/ADVERSE REACTIONS

Rare
Hypotension, tachyarrhythmia, rash,
abdominal discomfort, nausea,
dizziness

PRECAUTIONS AND CONTRAINDICATIONS

Arterial bleeding (recent),
immediately postpartum
Caution
Tachycardia

DRUG INTERACTIONS OF CONCERN TO DENTISTRY

• Increased effects: alcohol and
drugs that also lower B/P

SERIOUS REACTIONS

! Pulmonary edema occurs rarely.

DENTAL CONSIDERATIONS

General:
• Monitor vital signs at every
appointment because of
cardiovascular and respiratory side
effects.

• After supine positioning, have
patient sit upright for at least 2 min
before standing to avoid orthostatic
hypotension.
• Short appointments and a stress-
reduction protocol may be required
for anxious patients.
• Drugs used for conscious sedation
that lower B/P may potentiate the
hypotensive effects.
• Use vasoconstrictors with
caution, in low doses, and with
careful aspiration. Avoid use of
gingival retraction cord with
epinephrine.
Consultations:
• Medical consultation may be
required to assess disease
control and patient's ability to
tolerate stress.

---

isradipine

is-rad´-ih-peen
(DynaCirc, DynaCirc CR)
Do not confuse DynaCirc with
Dynabac or Dynacin.

CATEGORY AND SCHEDULE

Pregnancy Risk Category: C

Drug Class: Calcium channel
blocker

MECHANISM OF ACTION

An antihypertensive that inhibits
calcium movement across cardiac
and vascular smooth-muscle cell
membranes. Potent peripheral
vasodilator that does not depress SA
or AV nodes. *Therapeutic Effect:*
Produces relaxation of coronary
vascular smooth muscle and
coronary vasodilation. Increases
myocardial oxygen delivery to those
with vasospastic angina.

USES
Treatment of essential hypertension, alone or with a thiazide diuretic; unapproved: angina, Raynaud's disease

PHARMACOKINETICS

Route	Onset	Peak	Duration
PO	2–3 hr	2–4 wk (with multiple doses) 8–16 hr (with single dose)	N/A
PO (Controlled-release)	2 hr	8–10 hr	N/A

Well absorbed from the GI tract. Protein binding: 95%. Metabolized in the liver (undergoes first-pass effect). Primarily excreted in urine. Not removed by hemodialysis.
Half-life: 8 hr.

INDICATIONS AND DOSAGES
▶ **Hypertension**
PO
Adults, Elderly. Initially 2.5 mg twice a day. May increase by 2.5 mg at 2- to 4-wk intervals. Range: 5–20 mg/day

SIDE EFFECTS/ADVERSE REACTIONS
Frequent
Peripheral edema, palpitations (higher frequency in females)
Occasional
Facial flushing, cough
Rare
Angina, tachycardia, rash, pruritus

PRECAUTIONS AND CONTRAINDICATIONS
Cardiogenic shock, CHF, heart block, hypotension, sinus bradycardia, ventricular tachycardia
Caution
CHF, hypotension, hepatic disease, lactation, children, renal disease, elderly

DRUG INTERACTIONS OF CONCERN TO DENTISTRY
• Decreased effect: indomethacin, possibly other NSAIDs, phenobarbital
• Increased effect: parenteral and inhalational general anesthetics, other drugs with hypotensive actions, itraconazole
• Increased effects of carbamazepine

SERIOUS REACTIONS
! Overdose produces nausea, drowsiness, confusion, and slurred speech.
! CHF occurs rarely.

DENTAL CONSIDERATIONS
General:
• Monitor cardiac status; take vital signs at each appointment because of cardiovascular side effects. Consider a stress-reduction protocol to prevent stress-induced angina during the dental appointment.
• After supine positioning, have patient sit upright for at least 2 min before standing to avoid orthostatic hypotension.
• Place on frequent recall to monitor gingival condition.
• Limit use of sodium-containing products, such as saline IV fluids, for patients with a dietary salt restriction.
• Assess salivary flow as a factor in caries, periodontal disease, and candidiasis.

• Use vasoconstrictors with caution, in low doses, and with careful aspiration. Avoid use of gingival retraction cord with epinephrine.
• Patients on chronic drug therapy may rarely have symptoms of blood dyscrasias, which can include infection, bleeding, and poor healing.
Consultations:
• In a patient with symptoms of blood dyscrasias, request a medical consultation for blood studies and postpone dental treatment until normal values are reestablished.
• Medical consultation may be required to assess disease control and patient's ability to tolerate stress.
Teach Patient/Family to:
• Use effective oral hygiene to prevent soft tissue inflammation and minimize gingival enlargement
• Schedule frequent oral prophylaxis
• When chronic dry mouth occurs, advise patient to:
  • Avoid mouth rinses with high alcohol content because of drying effects
  • Use sugarless gum, frequent sips of water, or saliva substitutes
  • Use daily home fluoride products for anticaries effect

itraconazole
it-ra-con´-ah-zoll
(Sporanox)
Do not confuse Sporanox with Suprax.

CATEGORY AND SCHEDULE
Pregnancy Risk Category: C

Drug Class: Antifungal, systemic (triazole)

MECHANISM OF ACTION
A fungistatic antifungal that inhibits the synthesis of ergosterol, a vital component of fungal cell formation *Therapeutic Effect:* Damages the fungal cell membrane, altering its function.

USES
Treatment of Aspergillosis, blastomycosis, histoplasmosis (pulmonary and extrapulmonary); fungal infections of nails (onychomycosis); *Candida* infections of esophagus or mouth (oral sol only)

PHARMACOKINETICS
Moderately absorbed from the GI tract. Absorption is increased if the drug is taken with food. Protein binding: 99%. Widely distributed, primarily in the fatty tissue, liver, and kidneys. Metabolized in the liver to active metabolite. Primarily excreted in urine. Not removed by hemodialysis.
Half-life: 21 hr; metabolite, 12 hr.

INDICATIONS AND DOSAGES
▸ **Blastomycosis, Histoplasmosis**
PO
Adults, Elderly. Initially, 200 mg once a day. Maximum: 400 mg/day in 2 divided doses.
IV
Adults, Elderly. 200 mg twice a day for 4 doses, then 200 mg once a day.
▸ **Aspergillosis**
PO
Adults, Elderly. 600 mg/day in 3 divided doses for 3–4 days, then 200–400 mg/day in 2 divided doses.
IV
Adults, Elderly. 200 mg twice a day for 4 doses, then 200 mg once a day.
▸ **Esophageal Candidiasis**
PO
Adults, Elderly. Swish 10 ml in mouth for several seconds, then swallow. Maximum: 200 mg/day.

▶ **Oropharyngeal Candidiasis**
PO
Adults, Elderly. Vigorously swish
10 ml in mouth for several seconds
(20 ml total daily dose) once a day.

SIDE EFFECTS/ADVERSE REACTIONS
Frequent
Nausea, rash
Occasional
Vomiting, headache, diarrhea,
hypertension, peripheral edema,
fatigue, fever
Rare
Abdominal pain, dizziness, anorexia,
pruritus

PRECAUTIONS AND CONTRAINDICATIONS
Hypersensitivity to itraconazole,
fluconazole, ketoconazole, or
miconazole
Caution
Lactation, liver toxicity, oral
anticoagulants (monitor patient),
strong inhibitor of CYP 3A4
isoenzymes—note drug interactions

DRUG INTERACTIONS OF CONCERN TO DENTISTRY
• Increased risk of rhabdomyolysis:
lovastatin, simvastatin
• Increased risk of hypoglycemia:
oral antidiabetics
• Increased metabolism:
phenobarbital, carbamazepine
• May increase plasma levels of
cyclosporine
• Increased depression with
triazolam, midazolam
• Inhibits metabolism of certain
benzodiazepines: (e.g., midazolam,
triazolam), buspirone, allopurinol
(Zyloprim), felodipine
• Decreased effects: didanosine
• Increased plasma levels:
saquinavir, nisoldipine, haloperidol,
carbamazepine, erythromycin,
clarithromycin
• Avoid itraconazole use with
HMG-Co A reductase inhibitors
(statins) or lower their dose
• May inhibit warfarin metabolism
• Suspected increase in plasma
levels: cola beverages
• Decrease in plasma levels:
grapefruit juice
• Decreased effects: didanosine
(take 2 hr before didanosine tabs)
• May increase levels and side
effects of HMG-Co A reductase
inhibitors (statins)
• Increased plasma levels of
alfentanil, buspirone, carbamazepine,
corticosteroids, zolpidem
• Suspected decrease in oral
contractive effectiveness;
suggest alternative method of
contraception

SERIOUS REACTIONS
! Hepatitis (as evidenced by
anorexia, abdominal pain, unusual
fatigue or weakness, jaundiced
skin or sclera, and dark urine)
occurs rarely.

DENTAL CONSIDERATIONS
General:
• Monitor vital signs at every
appointment because of
cardiovascular side effects.
• Determine why the patient is taking
the drug.
• Consider semisupine chair position
for patient comfort because of
GI effects of drug.
Consultations:
• Medical consultation may be
required to assess patient's ability to
tolerate stress.

kanamycin sulfate
kan-ah-mye´-sin suhl´-feyt
(Kantrex)

CATEGORY AND SCHEDULE
Pregnancy Risk Category:
Unavailable for irrigating solution.

Drug Class: Aminoglycoside;
antibiotic

MECHANISM OF ACTION
An aminoglycoside antibiotic that
irreversibly binds to protein on bacterial
ribosomes. *Therapeutic Effect:*
Interferes with protein synthesis of
susceptible microorganisms.

USES
Treatment of wound, surgical site
irrigation

INDICATIONS AND DOSAGES
▶ **Wound and Surgical Site Irrigation**
Adults, Elderly. 0.25% solution to
irrigate pleural space, ventricular or
abscess cavities, wounds, or surgical
sites.

SIDE EFFECTS/ADVERSE REACTIONS
Occasional
Hypersensitivity reactions
(fever, pruritus, rash, urticaria)
Rare
Headache

PRECAUTIONS AND CONTRAINDICATIONS
Hypersensitivity to kanamycin, other
aminoglycosides (cross-sensitivity),
or their components

DRUG INTERACTIONS OF CONCERN TO DENTISTRY
• Increased risk of nephrotoxicity,
ototoxicity and neuromuscular
blockade: concurrent use with other
aminoglycosides
• Risk of inactivation: β-lactam
antiinfectives

SERIOUS REACTIONS
None known

DENTAL CONSIDERATIONS
General:
• For selected infections in
the hospital setting, provide
palliative emergency dental
treatment only.
• Examine for oral manifestation of
opportunistic infection.
• Determine why patient is taking
the drug.
• Caution regarding allergy to
medication.
Consultations:
• Medical consultation may be
required to assess disease control.
Teach Patient/Family to:
• Use effective oral hygiene to
prevent soft tissue inflammation
• Report oral lesions, soreness, or
bleeding to dentist
• Prevent trauma when using oral
hygiene aids

ketamine
key´-tah-meen
(Ketalar)

CATEGORY AND SCHEDULE
Pregnancy Risk Category: B

Drug Class: Anesthetic, general

MECHANISM OF ACTION
A rapidly acting general anesthetic
that selectively blocks afferent
impulses and interacts with CNS
transmitter systems. *Therapeutic
Effect:* Produces an anesthetic state

characterized by profound analgesia and normal pharyngeal-laryngeal reflexes.

USES
Production of loss of consciousness before and during surgery

PHARMACOKINETICS

Route	Onset	Peak	Duration
IM (anesthetic)	3–4 min	N/A	12–25 min
IM (analgesic)	30 min	N/A	15–30 min
IV (anesthetic)	30 sec	N/A	5–10 min
IV (analgesic)	10–15 min	N/A	N/A

Rapidly distributed. Metabolized in the liver. Primarily excreted in urine. *Half-life:* Distribution: 10–15 min, elimination: 2–3 hr.

INDICATIONS AND DOSAGES
▸ **Sole Anesthetic for Short Diagnostic and Surgical Procedures That Do Not Require Skeletal Muscle Relaxation, Induction of Anesthesia Before Administering Other General Anesthetics, Supplement to Low-Potency Agents**
IV
Adults, Elderly. 1–4.5 mg/kg.
Children. 0.5–2 mg/kg.
IM
Adults, Elderly. 3–8 mg/kg.
Children. 3–7 mg/kg.

SIDE EFFECTS/ADVERSE REACTIONS
Frequent
Increased B/P and pulse rate; emergence reaction (marked by dreamlike state, delirium, hallucinations, and vivid imagery and occasionally accompanied by confusion, excitement, and irrational behavior; lasts from a few hr to 24 hr after ketamine administration)
Occasional
Pain at injection site
Rare
Rash

PRECAUTIONS AND CONTRAINDICATIONS
Aneurysms, angina, CHF, elevated intracranial pressure, hypertension, psychotic disorders, thyrotoxicosis

DRUG INTERACTIONS OF CONCERN TO DENTISTRY
• Increased risk of hypotension and respiratory depression: all CNS depressants

SERIOUS REACTIONS
❗ Continuous or repeated intermittent infusion may result in extreme somnolence and circulatory or respiratory depression.
❗ Too-rapid IV administration of ketamine may produce severe hypotension, respiratory depression, and irregular muscle movements.
❗ Prolonged respiratory depression: nondepolarizing muscle relaxants

DENTAL CONSIDERATIONS
General
• Warning: Ketamine should be administered by persons trained in the administration of general anesthesia. Patients must be continually monitored, and facilities for maintenance of a patent airway, ventilatory support, oxygen supplementation, and circulatory resuscitation must be immediately available. Strict aseptic technique must be followed in handling ketamine.
• Monitor for increased B/P and pulse rate; emergence reactions including hallucinations, delirium,

dreamlike states, vivid imagery often accompanied by confusion, excitement, and irrational behavior.
● Responsible person must drive the patient home after recovery.
● Use safety measures: side rails, night light, and call bell within reach.
Consultations:
● Consultation with physician may be necessary if sedation or general anesthesia is required.
Teach Patient/Family:
● To avoid performing tasks that require mental alertness or motor skills for 24 hr after anesthesia has been discontinued

ketoconazole
kee-toe-kon´-ah-zole
(Apo-Ketocomazole[CAN], Nizoral, Nizoral AD, Sebizole[AUS])
Do not confuse Nizoral with Nasarel.

CATEGORY AND SCHEDULE
Pregnancy Risk Category: C
OTC (1% shampoo only)

Drug Class: Imidazole antifungal

MECHANISM OF ACTION
A fungistatic antifungal that inhibits the synthesis of ergosterol, a vital component of fungal cell formation. ***Therapeutic Effect:*** Damages the fungal cell membrane, altering its function.

USES
Treatment of systemic candidiasis, chronic mucocutaneous candidiasis, cutaneous candidiasis, candiduria, coccidioidomycosis, histoplasmosis, chromomycosis, para-coccidioidomycosis, severe recalcitrant cutaneous dermatophyte infections

PHARMACOKINETICS
PO: Peak 1–2 hr. *Half-life:* 2 hr, terminal 8 hr; highly protein bound; metabolized in liver; excreted in bile, feces; requires acid pH for absorption; distributed poorly to CSF.

INDICATIONS AND DOSAGES
▸ **Histoplasmosis, Blastomycosis, Systemic Candidiasis, Chronic Mucocutaneous Candidiasis, Coccidioidomycosis, Paracoccidioidomycosis, Chromomycosis, Seborrheic Dermatitis, Tinea Corporis, *Tinea capitis, Tinea manus, Tinea cruris, Tinea pedis, Tinea unguium* (onychomycosis), Oral Thrush, Candiduria**
PO
Adults, Elderly. 200–400 mg/day.
Children. 3.3–6.6 mg/kg/day.
Maximum: 800 mg/day in 2 divided doses.
Topical
Adults, Elderly. Apply to affected area 1–2 times a day for 2–4 wk.
Shampoo
Adults, Elderly. Use twice a wk for 4 wk, allowing at least 3 days between shampooing. Use intermittently to maintain control.

SIDE EFFECTS/ADVERSE REACTIONS
Occasional
Nausea, vomiting
Rare
Abdominal pain, diarrhea, headache, dizziness, photophobia, pruritus
Topical: itching, burning, irritation

PRECAUTIONS AND CONTRAINDICATIONS
Hypersensitivity, lactation, fungal meningitis, loratadine, triazolam, dofetilide

Caution
Renal disease, hepatic disease, drug-induced achlorhydria, potent inhibitor of CYP3A4 isoenzymes

DRUG INTERACTIONS OF CONCERN TO DENTISTRY
• Hepatotoxicity: alcohol, high-dose long-term use, acetaminophen, carbamazepine, sulfonamides
• Decreased absorption: antacids (take 2 hr after ketoconazole), proton pump inhibitors
• Leukocyte disorders: tacrolimus
• Contraindicated with triazolam, lovastatin, dofetilide
• Inhibits the metabolism of certain benzodiazepines (e.g., midazolam, triazolam)
• May inhibit metabolism of warfarin
• Decreased effects: didanosine (take 2 hr before didanosine tabs)
• May increase plasma levels and side effects of HMG-CoA reductase inhibitors (statins), cyclosporine
• Increased serum levels of indinavir, saquinavir, ritonavir, nisoldipine, haloperidol, carbamazepine, tricyclic antidepressants, buspirone, zolpidem, corticosteroids
• Suspected decrease in oral contraceptive effectiveness; may need to suggest additional contraception

SERIOUS REACTIONS
! Hematologic toxicity (as evidenced by thrombocytopenia, hemolytic anemia, and leukopenia) occurs occasionally.
! Hepatotoxicity may occur within 1 wk to several mo after starting therapy.
! Anaphylaxis occurs rarely.

DENTAL CONSIDERATIONS
General:
• To prevent reinoculation of *Candida* infection, dispose of tooth brush or other contaminated oral hygiene devices used during period of infection.
• Determine if medication controls disease.
• Place on frequent recall to evaluate healing response.
• Assess salivary flow as a factor in caries, periodontal disease, and candidiasis.
Teach Patient/Family to:
• Avoid mouth rinses with high alcohol content because of drying effects

ketoprofen
kee-toe-proe´-fen
(Apo-Keto[CAN], Novo-Keto-EC, Orudis[AUS], Orudis KT[CAN], Orudis SR[AUS], Oruvail, Oruvail SR[AUS], Rhodis[CAN])

CATEGORY AND SCHEDULE
Pregnancy Risk Category: B (D if used in third trimester or near delivery)
OTC (tablets)

Drug Class: Nonsteroidal antiinflammatory

MECHANISM OF ACTION
An NSAID that produces analgesic and antiinflammatory effects by inhibiting prostaglandin synthesis. *Therapeutic Effect:* Reduces the inflammatory response and intensity of pain.

USES

Treatment of osteoarthritis, rheumatoid arthritis, dysmenorrhea; OTC: minor aches and pains

PHARMACOKINETICS

PO: Peak 2 hr. *Half-life:* 3–3.5 hr; 99% plasma-protein binding; metabolized in liver; excreted in urine (metabolites), breast milk

INDICATIONS AND DOSAGES
▸ **Acute or Chronic Rheumatoid Arthritis and Osteoarthritis**
PO
Adults. Initially, 75 mg 3 times a day or 50 mg 4 times a day.
Elderly. Initially, 25–50 mg 3–4 times a day. Maintenance: 150–300 mg/day in 3–4 divided doses.
PO (Extended Release)
Adults, Elderly. 100–200 mg once a day.
▸ **Mild-to-Moderate Pain, Dysmenorrhea**
PO
Adults, Elderly. 25–50 mg q6–8h. Maximum: 300 mg/day.
▸ **OTC Dosage**
PO
Adults, Elderly. 12.5 mg q4–6h. Maximum: 6 tabs/day.
▸ **Dosage in Renal Impairment**
Mild. 150 mg/day maximum. Severe. 100 mg/day maximum.

SIDE EFFECTS/ADVERSE REACTIONS

Frequent
Dyspepsia
Occasional
Nausea, diarrhea or constipation, flatulence, abdominal cramps, headache
Rare
Anorexia, vomiting, visual disturbances, fluid retention

PRECAUTIONS AND CONTRAINDICATIONS

Active peptic ulcer disease, chronic inflammation of the GI tract, GI bleeding or ulceration, history of hypersensitivity to aspirin or NSAIDs.
Caution
Lactation, children, bleeding disorders, GI disorders, cardiac disorders, hypersensitivity to other antiinflammatory agents, elderly, children younger than 16 yr
Potential for increased adverse cardiovascular events in patients at risk for thromboembolism

DRUG INTERACTIONS OF CONCERN TO DENTISTRY

• GI ulceration, bleeding: aspirin, other NSAIDs, alcohol, corticosteroids
• Nephrotoxicity: acetaminophen (prolonged use)
• Possible risk of decreased renal function: cyclosporine
• Increased photosensitizing effect: tetracycline
• First-time users of SSRIs also taking NSAIDs may have a higher risk of GI side effects; until more data are available, it may be advisable to avoid use of NSAIDs in these patients (Br J Clin Pharmacol 55:591–595, 2003)
• When prescribed for dental pain:
  • Risk of increased effects: oral anticoagulants, oral antidiabetics, lithium, methotrexate
  • Decreased effects of diuretics

SERIOUS REACTIONS

! Rare reactions with long-term use include peptic ulcer disease, GI bleeding, gastritis, severe hepatic reactions (cholestasis, jaundice), nephrotoxicity (dysuria, hematuria, proteinuria, nephrotic syndrome), and severe hypersensitivity reaction (bronchospasm, angioedema).

DENTAL CONSIDERATIONS

General:
• Patients on chronic drug therapy may rarely have symptoms of blood dyscrasias, which can include infection, bleeding, and poor healing.
• Assess salivary flow as a factor in caries, periodontal disease, and candidiasis.
• Avoid prescribing for dental use in pregnancy.
• Avoid prescribing aspirin-containing products or giving to patient taking aspirin.
• Consider semisupine chair position for patients with arthritic disease.

Consultations:
• In a patient with symptoms of blood dyscrasias, request a medical consultation for blood studies and postpone dental treatment until normal values are reestablished.
• Medical consultation may be required to assess disease control.

Teach Patient/Family to:
• Use effective oral hygiene to prevent soft tissue inflammation
• Use caution to prevent injury when using oral hygiene aids
• When chronic dry mouth occurs, advise patient to:
  • Avoid mouth rinses with high alcohol content because of drying effects
  • Use sugarless gum, frequent sips of water, or saliva substitutes
  • Use daily home fluoride products for anticaries effect

ketorolac tromethamine
kee-tor´-oh-lak tro-meth´-ay-meen
(Acular, Acular LS, Acular PF, Toradol)
Do not confuse Acular with Acthar or Ocular.

CATEGORY AND SCHEDULE
Pregnancy Risk Category: C
(D if used in third trimester)

Drug Class: Nonsteroidal antiinflammatory

MECHANISM OF ACTION
An NSAID that inhibits prostaglandin synthesis and reduces prostaglandin levels in the aqueous humor. *Therapeutic Effect:* Relieves pain stimulus and reduces intraocular inflammation.

USES
Short-term treatment of acute mild-to-moderate pain

PHARMACOKINETICS

Route	Onset	Peak	Duration
PO	30–60 min	1.5–4 hr	4–6 hr
IV/IM	30 min	1–2 hr	4–6 hr

Readily absorbed from the GI tract, after IM administration. Protein binding: 99%. Largely metabolized in the liver. Primarily excreted in urine. Not removed by hemodialysis. *Half-life:* 3.8–6.3 hr (increased with impaired renal function and in the elderly).

INDICATIONS AND DOSAGES
▶ **Short-Term Relief of Mild-to-Moderate Pain (multiple doses)**
PO
Adults, Elderly. 10 mg q4–6h.
Maximum: 40 mg/24 hr.
IV, IM
Adults younger than 65 yr. 30 mg q6h. Maximum: 120 mg/24 hr.
Adults 65 yr and older, those with renal impairment, those weighing less than 50 kg. 15 mg q6h.
Maximum: 60 mg/24 hr.
Children 2–16 yr. 0.5 mg/kg q6h.
▶ **Short-Term Relief of Mild-to-Moderate Pain (single dose)**
IV
Adults younger than 65 yr, Children 17 yr and older weighing more than 50 kg. 30 mg.
Adults 65 yr and older, with renal impairment, weighing less than 50 kg. 15 mg.
Children 2–16 yr. 0.5 mg/kg.
Maximum: 15 mg.
IM
Adults younger than 65 yr, Children 17 yr and older, weighing more than 50 kg. 60 mg.
Adults 65 yr and older, with renal impairment, weighing less than 50 kg. 30 mg.
Children 2–16 yr. 1 mg/kg.
Maximum: 15 kg.
▶ **Allergic Conjunctivitis**
Ophthalmic
Adults, Elderly, Children 3 yr and older. 1 drop 4 times a day.
▶ **Cataract Extraction**
Ophthalmic
Adults, Elderly. 1 drop 4 times a day.
Begin 24 hr after surgery and continue for 2 wk.
▶ **Refractive Surgery**
Ophthalmic
Adults, Elderly. 1 drop 4 times a day for 3 days.

SIDE EFFECTS/ADVERSE REACTIONS
Frequent
Headache, nausea, abdominal cramps or pain, dyspepsia, oral lichenoid reaction
Occasional
Diarrhea
Ophthalmic: Transient stinging and burning
Rare
Constipation, vomiting, flatulence, stomatitis, dizziness
Ophthalmic: Ocular irritation, allergic reactions, superficial ocular infection, keratitis

PRECAUTIONS AND CONTRAINDICATIONS
Active peptic ulcer disease, chronic inflammation of GI tract, GI bleeding or ulceration, history of hypersensitivity to aspirin or NSAIDs.
Caution
Children, GI disorders, cardiac disorders, hypersensitivity to other antiinflammatory agents
Increased potential for adverse cardiovascular events in patients at risk for thromboembolism

DRUG INTERACTIONS OF CONCERN TO DENTISTRY
• GI ulceration, bleeding: aspirin, alcohol, corticosteroids
• Contraindicated with probenecid
• Possible risk of decreased renal function: cyclosporine
• First-time users of SSRIs also taking NSAIDs may have a higher risk of GI side effects; until more data are available, it may be advisable to avoid use of NSAIDs in these patients (Br J Clin Pharmacol 55:591–595, 2003)
• When prescribed for dental pain:
    • Risk of increased effects: oral anticoagulants, oral antidiabetics, lithium, methotrexate

- Decreased antihypertensive effects of diuretics, β-blockers, ACE inhibitors

DRUG INTERACTIONS OF CONCERN TO DENTISTRY
None reported

SERIOUS REACTIONS
! Rare reactions with long-term use include peptic ulcer disease, GI bleeding, gastritis, severe hepatic reactions (cholestasis, jaundice), nephrotoxicity (glomerular nephritis, interstitial nephritis, nephrotic syndrome), and an acute hypersensitivity reaction (including fever, chills, and joint pain).

DENTAL CONSIDERATIONS
General:
- Assess salivary flow as a factor in caries, periodontal disease, and candidiasis.
- Avoid prescribing for dental use in pregnancy.
- Avoid prescribing aspirin or other NSAIDs.
- Avoid long-term use for chronic pain syndromes; combined use of IV or IM and oral doses must not exceed 5 days.
Consultations:
- Medical consultation may be required to assess disease control.
Teach Patient/Family to:
- Avoid mouth rinses with high alcohol content because of drying effects

Ketorolac Tromethamine (Ocular)
General:
- Determine why patient is taking the drug.

- Avoid dental light in patient's eyes; offer dark glasses for patient comfort.

ketotifen fumarate
kee-toe-tye´-fen fyoo´-mah-rate
(Apo-Ketotifen[CAN], Novo-Ketotifen[CAN], Zaditen[CAN], Zaditor)

CATEGORY AND SCHEDULE
Pregnancy Risk Category: C

Drug Class: Antihistamine

MECHANISM OF ACTION
Selective histamine H_1-antagonist and mast cell stabilizer, suppresses release of mediators from cells involved in hypersensitivity reactions, and decreases chemotaxis and activation of eosinophils. *Therapeutic Effect:* Reduces symptoms of allergic conjunctivitis.

USES
Temporary prevention of itching of the eyes caused by allergic conjunctivitis

PHARMACOKINETICS
None reported

INDICATIONS AND DOSAGES
▶ Allergic Conjunctivitis
Ophthalmic
Adults, Elderly, Children 3 yr or older. 1 drop into affected eye q8–12h.

SIDE EFFECTS/ADVERSE REACTIONS
Frequent
Conjunctival infection, headache, rhinitis

Occasional
Allergic reaction, burning, stinging,
eyelid disorder, flu-like syndrome,
keratitis, mydriasis, ocular discharge
or pain, pharyngitis, photophobia,
rash

PRECAUTIONS AND CONTRAINDICATIONS

Hypersensitivity to ketotifen or any
component of the formulation
(the preservative is benzalkonium
chloride)

Caution
Prevent contamination of ophthalmic
solution by careful use, do not wear
contact lens if eyes are red, delay
inserting contacts up to 10 min after
drops are placed in eyes; lactation,
children younger than 3 yr

DRUG INTERACTIONS OF CONCERN TO DENTISTRY

None reported

SERIOUS REACTIONS

! No serious signs and symptoms
have been seen after ingestion up to
20 mg.

DENTAL CONSIDERATIONS

General:
• Avoid dental light in patient's eyes;
offer dark glasses for patient
comfort.

labetalol hydrochloride

la-bet´-ah-lole high-droh-klor´-ide
(Normodyne, Presolol[AUS], Trandate)
Do not confuse Trandate with tramadol or Trental.

CATEGORY AND SCHEDULE

Pregnancy Risk Category: C (D if used in second or third trimester)

Drug Class: Nonselective adrenergic β-blocker and selective α$_1$-blocker; antihypertensive

MECHANISM OF ACTION

An antihypertensive that blocks α$_1$-, β$_1$-, and β$_2$(large doses)-adrenergic receptor sites. Large doses increase airway resistance. *Therapeutic Effect:* Slows sinus heart rate; decreases peripheral vascular resistance, cardiac output, and B/P.

USES

Treatment of mild-to-severe hypertension

PHARMACOKINETICS

Route	Onset	Peak	Duration
PO	0.5–2 hr	2–4 hr	8–12 hr
IV	2–5 min	5–15 min	2–4 hr

Completely absorbed from the GI tract. Protein binding: 50%. Undergoes first-pass metabolism. Metabolized in the liver. Primarily excreted in urine. Not removed by hemodialysis. *Half-life:* PO, 6–8 hr; IV, 5.5 hr.

INDICATIONS AND DOSAGES

▶ **Hypertension**

PO

Adults. Initially, 100 mg twice a day adjusted in increments of 100 mg twice a day q2–3 days. Maintenance: 200–400 mg twice a day. Maximum: 2.4 g/day.

Elderly. Initially, 100 mg 1–2 times a day. May increase as needed.

▶ **Severe Hypertension, Hypertensive Emergency**

IV

Adults. Initially, 20 mg. Additional doses of 20–80 mg may be given at 10-min intervals, up to a total dose of 300 mg.

IV Infusion

Adults. Initially, 2 mg/min up to total dose of 300 mg.

PO (after IV therapy)

Adults. Initially, 200 mg; then, 200–400 mg in 6–12 hr. Increase dose at 1-day intervals to desired level.

SIDE EFFECTS/ADVERSE REACTIONS

Frequent

Drowsiness, difficulty sleeping, unusual fatigue or weakness, diminished sexual ability, transient scalp tingling

Occasional

Dizziness, dyspnea, peripheral edema, depression, anxiety, constipation, diarrhea, nasal congestion, nausea, vomiting, abdominal discomfort

Rare

Altered taste, dry eyes, increased urination, paresthesia

PRECAUTIONS AND CONTRAINDICATIONS

Bronchial asthma, cardiogenic shock, second- or third-degree heart block, severe bradycardia, uncontrolled CHF

Caution
Major surgery, lactation, diabetes mellitus, renal disease, thyroid disease, COPD, well-compensated heart failure, CAD, nonallergic bronchospasm

DRUG INTERACTIONS OF CONCERN TO DENTISTRY
- Decreased metabolism: lidocaine
- Decreased effect: sympathomimetics
- Decreased hypotensive effects: indomethacin and other NSAIDs
- Increased hypotension, myocardial depression: hydrocarbon-inhalation anesthetics
- Increased plasma levels: diphenhydramine

SERIOUS REACTIONS
! Labetolol administration may precipitate or aggravate CHF because of decreased myocardial stimulation.
! Abrupt withdrawal may precipitate ischemic heart disease, producing sweating, palpitations, headache, and tremors.
! May mask signs and symptoms of acute hypoglycemia (tachycardia, B/P changes) in patients with diabetes.

DENTAL CONSIDERATIONS
General:
- Monitor vital signs at every appointment because of cardiovascular side effects.
- Patients on chronic drug therapy may rarely have symptoms of blood dyscrasias, which can include infection, bleeding, and poor healing.
- Assess salivary flow as a factor in caries, periodontal disease, and candidiasis.
- After supine positioning, have patient sit upright for at least 2 min before standing to avoid orthostatic hypotension.

- Limit use of sodium-containing products, such as saline IV fluids, for patients with a dietary salt restriction.
- Stress from dental procedures may compromise cardiovascular function; determine patient risk.
- Short appointments and a stress-reduction protocol may be required for anxious patients.
Consultations:
- Medical consultation may be required to assess disease control and patient's ability to tolerate stress.
- In a patient with symptoms of blood dyscrasias, request a medical consultation for blood studies and postpone dental treatment until normal values are reestablished.
Teach Patient/Family:
- When chronic dry mouth occurs, advise patient to:
  - Avoid mouth rinses with high alcohol content because of drying effects
  - Use sugarless gum, frequent sips of water, or saliva substitutes
  - Use daily home fluoride products for anticaries effect

lamivudine
la-miv´-yoo-deen
(Epivir, Epivir-HBV, Heptovir[CAN], Zeffix[AUS])
Do not confuse lamivudine with lamotrigine.

CATEGORY AND SCHEDULE
Pregnancy Risk Category: C

Drug Class: Antiviral, nucleoside analog

MECHANISM OF ACTION
An antiviral that inhibits HIV reverse transcriptase by viral DNA chain

termination. Also inhibits RNA- and DNA-dependent DNA polymerase, an enzyme necessary for HIV replication. ***Therapeutic Effect:*** Interrupts HIV replication, slowing the progression of HIV infection.

USES
Used in combination with zidovudine for the treatment of HIV infection and to reduce disease progression and death in AIDS; HBV dose form: chronic hepatitis B associated with evidence of hepatitis B viral replication and liver inflammation

PHARMACOKINETICS
Rapidly and completely absorbed from the GI tract. Protein binding: less than 36%. Widely distributed (crosses the blood-brain barrier). Primarily excreted unchanged in urine. Not removed by hemodialysis or peritoneal dialysis. ***Half-life:*** 11–15 hr (intracellular), 2–11 hr (serum, adults), 1.7–2 hr (serum, children) (increased in impaired renal function).

INDICATIONS AND DOSAGES
▶ **HIV Infection (in combination with other antiretrovirals)**
PO
Adults, Children 12–16 yr, weighing 50 kg (100 lb) or more. 150 mg twice a day or 300 mg once a day.
Adults weighing less than 50 kg. 2 mg/kg twice a day.
Children 3 mo–11 yr. 4 mg/kg twice a day (up to 150 mg/dose).
▶ **Chronic Hepatitis B**
PO
Adults, Children 17 yr and older. 100 mg/day.
Children younger than 17 yr. 3 mg/kg/day. Maximum: 100 mg/day.

▶ **Dosage in Renal Impairment**
Dosage and frequency are modified on the basis of creatinine clearance.

Creatinine Clearance	Dosage
50 ml/min or higher	150 mg twice a day
30–59 ml/min	150 mg once a day
15–29 ml/min	150 mg first dose, then 100 mg once a day
5–14 ml/min	150 mg first dose, then 50 mg once a day
Less than 5 ml/min	50 mg first dose, then 25 mg once a day

SIDE EFFECTS/ADVERSE REACTIONS
Frequent
Headache, nausea, malaise and fatigue, nasal disturbances, diarrhea, cough, musculoskeletal pain, neuropathy, insomnia, anorexia, dizziness, fever or chills
Occasional
Depression, myalgia, abdominal cramps, dyspepsia, arthralgia

PRECAUTIONS AND CONTRAINDICATIONS
Hypersensitivity, history of pancreatitis as child
Caution
Reduce dose in renal disease, lactation

DRUG INTERACTIONS OF CONCERN TO DENTISTRY
None reported

SERIOUS REACTIONS
❗ Pancreatitis occurs in 13% of pediatric patients.

! Anemia, neutropenia, and thrombocytopenia occur rarely.

DENTAL CONSIDERATIONS

General:
- Patients on chronic drug therapy may rarely have symptoms of blood dyscrasias, which can include infection, bleeding, and poor healing.
- Examine for oral manifestation of opportunistic infections.

Consultations:
- In a patient with symptoms of blood dyscrasias, request a medical consultation for blood studies and postpone dental treatment until normal values are reestablished.
- Medical consultation may be required to assess disease control and patient's ability to tolerate stress.

Teach Patient/Family to:
- Use effective oral hygiene to prevent soft tissue inflammation
- Use caution to prevent trauma when using oral hygiene aids
- See dentist immediately if secondary oral infection occurs

lamotrigine

la-moe-trih´-jeen

(Apo-Lamotrigine[CAN], Lamictal, Lamictal CD)

Do not confuse lamotrigine with lamivudine.

CATEGORY AND SCHEDULE

Pregnancy Risk Category: C

Drug Class: Antiepileptic

MECHANISM OF ACTION

An anticonvulsant whose exact mechanism is unknown. May block voltage-gated sodium channels, thus stabilizing neuronal membranes and regulating presynaptic transmitter release of excitatory amino acids. *Therapeutic Effect:* Reduces seizure activity.

USES

Adjunctive treatment of refractory partial seizures in adults and adjunctive treatment for Lennox-Gastaut syndrome in pediatric and adult patients; long-term maintenance of bipolar 1 disorder

PHARMACOKINETICS

Rapidly absorbed from the GI tract. Protein binding: 55%. Metabolized primarily by glucuronic acid conjugation. Excreted in the urine. *Half-life:* 13–30 hr.

INDICATIONS AND DOSAGES

▸ **Seizure Control in Patients Receiving Enzyme-Inducing Antiepileptic Drug (EIAEDs), but Not Valproic Acid**

PO

Adults, Elderly, Children older than 12 yr. Recommended as add-on therapy: 50 mg once a day for 2 wk, followed by 100 mg/day in 2 divided doses for 2 wk. Maintenance: Dosage may be increased by 100 mg/day every wk, up to 300–500 mg/day in 2 divided doses.

Children 2–12 yr. 0.6 mg/kg/day in 2 divided doses for 2 wk, then 1.2 mg/kg/day in 2 divided doses for wk 3 and 4. Maintenance: 5–15 mg/kg/day. Maximum: 400 mg/day.

▸ **Seizure Control in Patients Receiving Combination Therapy of EIAEDs and Valproic Acid**

PO

Adults, Elderly, Children older than 12 yr. 25 mg every other day for 2 wk, followed by 25 mg once a day for 2 wk. Maintenance: Dosage may be increased by 25–50 mg/day q1–2wk, up to 150 mg/day in 2 divided doses.

Children 2–12 yr. 0.15 mg/kg/day in 2 divided doses for 2 wk, then 0.3 mg/kg/day in 2 divided doses for wk 3 and 4. Maintenance: 1–5 mg/kg/day in 2 divided doses. Maximum: 200 mg/day.

▸ **Conversion to Monotherapy for Patients Receiving EIAED**
PO
Adults, Elderly, Children 16 yr and older. 500 mg/day in 2 divided doses. Titrate to desired dose while maintaining EIAED at fixed level, then withdraw EIAED by 20% each wk over a 4-wk period.

▸ **Conversion to Monotherapy for Patients Receiving Valproic Acid**
PO
Adults, Elderly, Children 16 yr and older. Titrate lamotrigine to 200 mg/day, maintaining valproic acid dose. Maintain lamotrigine dose and decrease valproic acid to 500 mg/day, no greater than 500 mg/day/wk, then maintain 500 mg/day for 1 wk. Increase lamotrigine to 300 mg/day and decrease valproic acid to 250 mg/day. Maintain for 1 wk, then discontinue valproic acid and increase lamotrigine by 100 mg/day each wk until maintenance dose of 500 mg/day reached.

▸ **Bipolar Disorder in Patients Receiving EIAED**
PO
Adults, Elderly. 50 mg/day for 2 wk, then 100 mg/day for 2 wk, then 200 mg/day for 1 wk, then 300 mg/day for 1 wk, then up to usual maintenance dose 400 mg/day in divided doses.

▸ **Bipolar Disorder in Patients Receiving Valproic Acid**
PO
Adults, Elderly. 25 mg/day every other day for 2 wk, then 25 mg/day for 2 wk, then 50 mg/day for 1 wk, then 100 mg/day. Usual maintenance dose with valproic acid: 100 mg/day.

▸ **Discontinuation Therapy**
Adults, Children older than 12 yr.
A dosage reduction of approximately 50% per wk over at least 2 wk is recommended.

SIDE EFFECTS/ADVERSE REACTIONS
Frequent
Dizziness, diplopia, headache, ataxia, nausea, blurred vision, somnolence, rhinitis, dry mouth, halitosis
Occasional
Rash, pharyngitis, vomiting, cough, flu-like symptoms, diarrhea, dysmenorrhea, fever, insomnia, dyspepsia
Rare
Constipation, tremors, anxiety, pruritus, vaginitis, hypersensitivity reaction

PRECAUTIONS AND CONTRAINDICATIONS
Hypersensitivity.
Caution
Elderly, children younger than 16 yr, dose adjustment with other anticonvulsants, seizure risk with drug withdrawal, renal or hepatic impairment; can cause Stevens-Johnson syndrome, toxic epidermal necrolysis.

DRUG INTERACTIONS OF CONCERN TO DENTISTRY
• Increased excretion: chronic, high-dose acetaminophen (900 mg 3 times a day), but significance is unclear; carbamazepine
• Increased blood levels of carbamazepine

SERIOUS REACTIONS

! Abrupt withdrawal may increase seizure frequency.

! Serious rashes, including Stevens-Johnson syndrome, requiring hospitalization and discontinuation of treatment have been reported.

DENTAL CONSIDERATIONS

General:
• Early-morning appointments and a stress-reduction protocol may be required for anxious patients.
• Determine type of epilepsy, seizure frequency, and quality of seizure control.
• Evaluate respiration characteristics and rate.
• Assess salivary flow as factor in caries, periodontal disease, and candidiasis.
• Patients on chronic drug therapy may rarely have symptoms of blood dyscrasias, which can include infection, bleeding, and poor healing.
• Place on frequent recall because of oral side effects.
Consultations:
• Medical consultation may be required to assess disease control and the patient's ability to tolerate stress.
• In a patient with symptoms of blood dyscrasias, request a medical consultation for blood studies and postpone dental treatment until normal values are reestablished.
Teach Patient/Family to:
• Use effective oral hygiene to prevent soft tissue inflammation
• Use electric tooth brush if patient has difficulty holding conventional devices
• When chronic dry mouth occurs, advise patient to:
  • Avoid mouth rinses with high alcohol content because of drying effects

• Use daily home fluoride products for anticaries effect
• Use sugarless gum, frequent sips of water, or saliva substitutes

lansoprazole

lan-soe-pray´-zole
(Prevacid, Prevacid IV, Prevacid Solu-Tab, Zoton[AUS])
Do not confuse Prevacid with Pepcid, Pravachol, or Prevpac.

CATEGORY AND SCHEDULE

Pregnancy Risk Category: B

Drug Class: Antisecretory, proton pump inhibitor

MECHANISM OF ACTION

A proton pump inhibitor that selectively inhibits the parietal cell membrane enzyme system (hydrogen-potassium adenosine triphosphatase) or proton pump. ***Therapeutic Effect:*** Suppresses gastric acid secretion.

USES

Short-term treatment for healing and symptomatic relief of active duodenal ulcer and benign gastric ulcer, erosive esophagitis, and gastroesophageal reflux disease (GERD); maintenance of healing of duodenal ulcers; long-term treatment of pathologic hypersecretory syndromes; NSAID-associated gastric ulcers in patients who continue NSAID use; short-term treatment of symptomatic GERD

PHARMACOKINETICS

Route	Onset	Peak	Duration
PO (15 mg)	2–3 hr	N/A	8–24 hr
PO (30 mg)	1–2 hr	N/A	Longer than 24 hr

Rapid and complete absorption (food may decrease absorption) once drug has left stomach. Protein binding: 97%. Distributed primarily to gastric parietal cells and converted to two active metabolites. Extensively metabolized in the liver. Eliminated in bile and urine. Not removed by hemodialysis. *Half-life:* 1.5 hr (increased in the elderly and in those with hepatic impairment).

INDICATIONS AND DOSAGES
▶ **Duodenal Ulcer**
PO
Adults, Elderly. 15 mg/day, before eating, preferably in the morning, for up to 4 wk.
▶ **Erosive Esophagitis**
PO
Adults, Elderly. 30 mg/day, before eating, for up to 8 wk. If healing does not occur within 8 wk (in 5%–10% of cases), may give for additional 8 wk. Maintenance: 15 mg/day.
IV
Adults, Elderly. 30 mg once a day for up to 7 days. Switch to oral lansoprazole therapy as soon as patient can tolerate oral route.
▶ **Gastric Ulcer**
PO
Adults. 30 mg/day for up to 8 wk.
▶ **NSAID Gastric Ulcer**
PO
Adults, Elderly. (Healing): 30 mg/day for up to 8 wk. (Prevention): 15 mg/day for up to 12 wk.

▶ **Healed Duodenal Ulcer, GERD**
PO
Adults. 15 mg/day.
▶ **Usual Pediatric Dosage**
Children 3 mo–14 yr, weighing more than 20 kg. 30 mg once daily.
Children 3 mo–14 yr, weighing 10–20 kg. 15 mg once daily.
Children 3 mo–14 yr, weighing less than 10 kg. 7.5 mg once daily.
▶ **Helicobacter Pylori Infection**
PO
Adults. 30 mg twice a day for 10 days (with amoxicillin and clarithromycin).
▶ **Pathologic Hypersecretory Conditions (including Zollinger-Ellison syndrome)**
PO
Adults, Elderly. 60 mg/day. Individualize dosage according to patient needs and for as long as clinically indicated. Administer up to 120 mg/day in divided doses.

SIDE EFFECTS/ADVERSE REACTIONS
Occasional
Diarrhea, abdominal pain, rash, pruritus, altered appetite
Rare
Nausea, headache

PRECAUTIONS AND CONTRAINDICATIONS
Hypersensitivity
Caution
Children younger than 18 yr, elderly (limit doses to 30 mg/day), severe hepatic disease.

DRUG INTERACTIONS OF CONCERN TO DENTISTRY
• Drug interactions not established but potentially can interfere with absorption of amoxicillin, ketoconazole

SERIOUS REACTIONS
! Bilirubinemia, eosinophilia, and hyperlipemia occur rarely.

DENTAL CONSIDERATIONS
General:
• Consider semisupine chair position for patient comfort because of GI effects of disease.
• Question the patient about tolerance of NSAIDs or aspirin related to GI problem.
• Patients with GERD may have oral symptoms, including burning mouth, secondary candidiasis, and oral signs of dental erosion.
• Assess salivary flow as factor in caries, periodontal disease, and candidiasis.
Teach Patient/Family:
• When chronic dry mouth occurs, advise patient to:
  • Avoid mouth rinses with high alcohol content because of drying effects
  • Use daily home fluoride products for anticaries effect
  • Use sugarless gum, frequent sips of water, or saliva substitutes

lanthanum carbonate
lan-thah´-num kar´-boh-nate
(Fosrenol)

CATEGORY AND SCHEDULE
Pregnancy Risk Category: C

Drug Class: Phosphate binder

MECHANISM OF ACTION
A phosphate regulator that dissociates in the acidic environment of the upper GI tract to lanthanum ions, which bind to dietary phosphate released from food during digestion, forming highly insoluble lanthanum phosphate complexes. *Therapeutic Effect:* Reduces phosphate absorption.

USES
Treatment of end-stage renal disease

PHARMACOKINETICS
Phosphate complexes are eliminated in urine.

INDICATIONS AND DOSAGES
▶ **Reduce Serum Phosphate in End-Stage Renal Disease**
PO
Adults, Elderly. 750 mg–1500 mg in divided doses, taken with or immediately after a meal. Dosage may be titrated in 750-mg increments q2–3wk on the basis of serum phosphate levels.

SIDE EFFECTS/ADVERSE REACTIONS
Frequent
Nausea, vomiting, dialysis graft occlusion, abdominal pain

PRECAUTIONS AND CONTRAINDICATIONS
None known.

DRUG INTERACTIONS OF CONCERN TO DENTISTRY
None reported

SERIOUS REACTIONS
None known.

DENTAL CONSIDERATIONS
General:
• Question patient about renal dialysis history and use of other medications.
• Dental drugs known to interact with antacid products should not be taken within 2 hr of lanthanum carbonate.
• Dental procedures must be scheduled to appropriately sequence with dialysis regimen.

• Question patient about coexisting cardiovascular disease, related medications, and any bleeding problems.
• Avoid nephrotoxic drugs; dose adjustment may be required for renal-excreted drugs.
• Oral infections should be eliminated and/or treated aggressively.
• Patient may have AV shunt in place.
• Monitor and record vital signs.
• Consider semisupine chair position for patient comfort if GI side effects occur.
• Question patient about tolerance of NSAIDS or aspirin related to GI disease.
• After supine positioning, have patient sit upright for at least 2 min before taking to avoid orthostatic hypotension.
• Antiinfective prophylaxis may be indicated for patient on dialysis; consult physician.
Consultations:
• Consultation with physician may be necessary if sedation or general anesthesia is required.
• Medical consultation may be required to assess disease control and patient's ability to tolerate stress.
Teach Patient/Family to:
• Use effective oral hygiene to prevent soft tissue inflammation
• Prevent trauma when using oral hygiene aids
• Update health and medication history if physician makes any changes in evaluation/drug regimens; include OTC, herbal, and nonherbal drugs in the update

latanoprost
la-ta´-noe-prost
(Xalatan)
Do not confuse with Xanax.

CATEGORY AND SCHEDULE
Pregnancy Risk Category: C

Drug Class: Prostaglandin F_{2a} analogue

MECHANISM OF ACTION
An ophthalmic agent that is a prostanoid selective FP receptor agonist. *Therapeutic Effect:* Reduces intraocular pressure (IOP) by reducing aqueous humor production.

USES
Treatment of open-angle glaucoma and ocular hypertension in patients intolerant to other IOP-lowering drugs

PHARMACOKINETICS
Absorbed through the cornea where the isopropyl ester prodrug is hydrolyzed to acid form to become biologically active. Highly lipophilic. The acid of latanoprost can be measured in the aqueous humor during the first 4 hr and in the plasma only during the first hr after local administration. Cornea, latanoprost, is hydrolyzed to the biologically active acid. Metabolized in liver if it reaches systemic circulation. Metabolized to 1,2-dinor metabolite and 1,2,3,4-tetranor metabolite. Primarily eliminated by the kidneys. *Half-life:* 17 min.

INDICATIONS AND DOSAGES
▶ **Glaucoma, Ocular Hypertension**
Ophthalmic

Adults, Elderly. 1 drop (1.5 mcg) in affected eye(s) once daily, in the evening.

SIDE EFFECTS/ADVERSE REACTIONS
Frequent
Blurred vision
Occasional
Eyelash changes, eyelid skin darkening, iris pigmentation
Rare
Macular edema

PRECAUTIONS AND CONTRAINDICATIONS
Hypersensitivity to latanoprost or benzalkonium chloride, or any other component of the formulation
Caution
Gradual change in eye color, avoid contamination of sterile solution, renal or hepatic impairment, remove contact lens before using, administer at least 5 min apart if other ophthalmic drug is also used, nursing, pediatrics

DRUG INTERACTIONS OF CONCERN TO DENTISTRY
None reported at this time; avoid use of anticholinergic drugs, atropine-like drugs, propantheline, and diazepam (benzodiazepines) in patient with glaucoma

SERIOUS REACTIONS
❗ Pigmentation is expected to increase as long as latanoprost is administered but after discontinuation, pigmentation of the iris is likely to be permanent while pigmentation of the periorbital tissue and eyelash changes has been reported as reversible.
❗ Inflammation (iritis/uveitis) and macular edema, including cystoid macular edema have been reported.

DENTAL CONSIDERATIONS
General:
• Check compliance of patient with prescribed drug regimen for glaucoma.
• Avoid dental light in patient's eyes; offer dark glasses for patient comfort.
Consultations:
• Medical consultation may be required to assess disease control.

---

leflunomide
le-flu´-na-mide
(Arava)

CATEGORY AND SCHEDULE
Pregnancy Risk Category: X

Drug Class: Antiarthritic, immunosuppressive

MECHANISM OF ACTION
An immunomodulatory agent that inhibits dihydroorotate dehydrogenase, the enzyme involved in autoimmune process that leads to rheumatoid arthritis. *Therapeutic Effect:* Reduces signs and symptoms of rheumatoid arthritis and slows structural damage.

USES
Reduction of signs and symptoms and to retard structural damage in active rheumatoid arthritis as demonstrated by x-ray erosion and joint space narrowing

PHARMACOKINETICS
Well absorbed after PO administration. Protein binding: greater than 99%. Metabolized to

active metabolite in the GI wall and liver. Excreted through both renal and biliary systems. Not removed by hemodialysis. *Half-life:* 16 days.

INDICATIONS AND DOSAGES
▶ **Rheumatoid Arthritis**
PO
Adults, Elderly. Initially, 100 mg/day for 3 days, then 10–20 mg/day.

SIDE EFFECTS/ADVERSE REACTIONS
Frequent
Diarrhea, respiratory tract infection, alopecia, rash, nausea

PRECAUTIONS AND CONTRAINDICATIONS
Pregnancy or plans to become pregnant, chronic renal or hepatic insufficiency, rifampin
Caution
Chronic renal or hepatic insufficiency, rifampin, children younger than 18 yr

DRUG INTERACTIONS OF CONCERN TO DENTISTRY
None reported

SERIOUS REACTIONS
! Transient thrombocytopenia and leukopenia occur rarely.

DENTAL CONSIDERATIONS
General:
• Monitor vital signs at every appointment because of cardiovascular side effects.
• Consider semisupine chair position for patient comfort if GI side effects occur.
• Examine for oral manifestation of opportunistic infection.
• If acute oral infection occurs, inform physician.

• Assess salivary flow as a factor in caries, periodontal disease, and candidiasis.
Consultations:
• Consult the patient's family if needed.
Teach Patient/Family to:
• Use effective oral hygiene to prevent soft tissue inflammation
• Use electric tooth brush if patient has difficulty holding conventional devices
• When chronic dry mouth occurs, advise patient to:
  • Avoid mouth rinses with high alcohol content because of drying effects
  • Use daily home fluoride products for anticaries effect
  • Use sugarless gum, frequent sips of water, or saliva substitutes

lepirudin
leh-peer-oo´-din
(Refludan)

CATEGORY AND SCHEDULE
Pregnancy Risk Category: B

Drug Class: Anticoagulant; thrombin inhibitor, hirudin

MECHANISM OF ACTION
An anticoagulant that inhibits thrombogenic action of thrombin (independent of antithrombin II and not inhibited by platelet factor 4). One molecule of lepirudin binds to one molecule of thrombin.
Therapeutic Effect: Produces dose-dependent increases in aPTT.

USES
Treatment of heparin-induced thrombocytopenia and other thromboembolic conditions

PHARMACOKINETICS

Distributed primarily in extracellular fluid. Primarily eliminated by the kidneys. *Half-life:* 1.3 hr (increased in impaired renal function).

INDICATIONS AND DOSAGES
▸ **Heparin-Induced Thrombocytopenia and Associated Thromboembolic Disease to Prevent Further Thromboembolic Complications**
IV, IV Infusion
Adults, Elderly. 0.2–0.4 mg/kg, IV slowly over 15–20 sec, followed by IV infusion of 0.1–0.15 mg/kg/hr for 2–10 days or longer.
▸ **Dosage in Renal Impairment**
Initial dose is decreased to 0.2 mg/kg, with infusion rate adjusted on the basis of creatinine clearance.

Creatinine Clearance	% of Standard Infusion Rate	Infusion Rate (mg/kg/hr)
45–60	50	0.075
30–44	30	0.045
15–29	15	0.0225

SIDE EFFECTS/ADVERSE REACTIONS
Frequent
Bleeding from gums, puncture sites, or wounds, hematuria, fever, GI and rectal bleeding
Occasional
Epistaxis; allergic reaction, such as rash and pruritus; vaginal bleeding

PRECAUTIONS AND CONTRAINDICATIONS
None known

DRUG INTERACTIONS OF CONCERN TO DENTISTRY
● Increased risk of bleeding: drugs that interfere with coagulation and platelet function, such as NSAIDs, aspirin, ginkgo biloba (herb)

SERIOUS REACTIONS
! Overdose is characterized by excessively high aPTT.
! Intracranial bleeding occurs rarely.
! Abnormal hepatic function occurs in 6% of patients.

DENTAL CONSIDERATIONS
General:
● Patients are at risk of bleeding; check for oral signs.
● Provide palliative dental care for dental emergencies only.
● Determine why patient is taking the drug.
● Avoid products that affect platelet function, such as aspirin and NSAIDs.
● Consider local hemostasis measures to prevent excessive bleeding.
Consultations:
● Medical consultation should include partial prothrombin time, prothrombin time, and INR.
● Medical consultation may be required to assess disease control and patient's ability to tolerate stress.
Teach Patient/Family to:
● Use soft tooth brush to reduce risk of bleeding
● Use effective oral hygiene to prevent soft tissue inflammation
● Report oral lesions, soreness, or bleeding to dentist
● Prevent trauma when using oral hygiene aids
● Update health and medication history if physician makes any changes in evaluation or drug

regimens; include OTC, herbal, and nonherbal drugs in the update

letrozole
leh´-troe-zoll
(Femara)
Do not confuse Femara with Femhrt.

CATEGORY AND SCHEDULE
Pregnancy Risk Category: D

Drug Class: Antineoplastic

MECHANISM OF ACTION
Decreases the level of circulating estrogen by inhibiting aromatase, an enzyme that catalyzes the final step in estrogen production. *Therapeutic Effect:* Inhibits the growth of breast cancers that are stimulated by estrogens.

USES
Treatment of locally advanced or metastatic breast cancer in postmenopausal women either hormone receptor positive or hormone receptor unknown; advanced breast cancer in postmenopausal women with disease progression following antiestrogen therapy

PHARMACOKINETICS
Rapidly and completely absorbed. Metabolized in the liver. Primarily eliminated by the kidneys. Unknown if removed by hemodialysis. *Half-life:* Approximately 2 days.

INDICATIONS AND DOSAGES
▶ **Breast Cancer**
PO
Adults, Elderly. 2.5 mg/day. Continue until tumor progression is evident.

SIDE EFFECTS/ADVERSE REACTIONS
Frequent
Musculoskeletal pain (back, arm, leg), nausea, headache
Occasional
Constipation, arthralgia, fatigue, vomiting, hot flashes, diarrhea, abdominal pain, cough, rash, anorexia, hypertension, peripheral edema
Rare
Asthenia, somnolence, dyspepsia, weight gain, pruritus

PRECAUTIONS AND CONTRAINDICATIONS
Hypersensitivity
Caution
Lactation, children (no studies), for postmenopausal women only, thrombocytopenia and decreased lymphocyte counts, liver impairment

DRUG INTERACTIONS OF CONCERN TO DENTISTRY
None reported

SERIOUS REACTIONS
None known

DENTAL CONSIDERATIONS
General:
• Patients taking opioids for acute or chronic pain should be given alternative analgesics for dental pain.
• Patients on chronic drug therapy may rarely have symptoms of blood dyscrasias, which can include infection, bleeding, and poor healing.
• Palliative medication may be required for management of oral side effects.
• Examine for oral manifestation of opportunistic infection.
• Consider semisupine chair position for patient comfort if GI side effects occur.

• Monitor vital signs at every appointment because of cardiovascular and respiratory side effects.

Consultations:

• In a patient with symptoms of blood dyscrasias, request a medical consultation for blood studies and postpone treatment until normal values are reestablished.

Teach Patient/Family to:

• Use effective oral hygiene to prevent soft tissue inflammation

• Be aware of the possibility of secondary oral infection and the need to see dentist immediately if signs of infection occur

leucovorin calcium (folinic acid, citrovorum factor)

loo-koe-vor´-in kal´-see-um (Calcium Leucovorin[AUS], Wellcovorin)

Do not confuse Wellcovorin with Wellbutrin or Wellferon.

CATEGORY AND SCHEDULE

Pregnancy Risk Category: C

Drug Class: Folic acid antagonist antidote, antineoplastic adjunct

MECHANISM OF ACTION

An antidote to folic acid antagonists that may limit methotrexate action on normal cells by competing with methotrexate for the same transport processes into the cells. *Therapeutic Effect:* Reverses toxic effects of folic acid antagonists. Reverses folic acid deficiency.

USES

Treatment of megaloblastic or macrocytic anemia caused by folic acid deficiency, overdose of folic acid antagonist, methotrexate toxicity, toxicity caused by pyrimethamine or trimethoprim; used with fluorouracil in colorectal cancer

PHARMACOKINETICS

Readily absorbed from the GI tract. Widely distributed. Primarily concentrated in the liver. Metabolized in the liver and intestinal mucosa to active metabolite. Primarily excreted in urine. *Half-life:* 15 min; metabolite, 30–35 min.

INDICATIONS AND DOSAGES

▸ **Conventional Rescue Dosage in High-Dose Methotrexate Therapy**

PO, IV, IM

Adults, Elderly, Children. 10 mg/m^2 IM or IV one time, then PO q6h until serum methotrexate level is less than 10×8 M. If 24-hr serum creatinine level increases by 50% or greater over baseline or methotrexate level exceeds $5 \times 10 \times 6$ M or 48-hr level exceeds $9 \times 10 \times 7$ M, increase to 100 mg/m^2 IV q3h until methotrexate level is less than 10×8 M.

▸ **Folic Acid Antagonist Overdose**

PO

Adults, Elderly, Children. 2–15 mg/ day for 3 days or 5 mg every 3 days.

▸ **Megaloblastic Anemia**

IM

Adults, Elderly, Children. 3–6 mg/day.

▸ **Megaloblastic Anemia Secondary to Folate Deficiency**

IM

Adults, Elderly, Children. 1 mg/day.

▸ **Prevention of Hematologic Toxicity (for toxoplasmosis), with Sulfadiazine**

PO, IV

Adults, Elderly, Children. 5–10 mg/ day, repeat every 3 days.

▶ **Prevention of Hematologic Toxicity with Pyrimethamine, PCP**
PO, IV
Adults, Children. 25 mg once a wk.

SIDE EFFECTS/ADVERSE REACTIONS
Frequent
When combined with chemotherapeutic agents: Diarrhea, stomatitis, nausea, vomiting, lethargy or malaise or fatigue, alopecia, anorexia
Occasional
Urticaria, dermatitis

PRECAUTIONS AND CONTRAINDICATIONS
Pernicious anemia, other megaloblastic anemias secondary to vitamin B12 deficiency

DRUG INTERACTIONS OF CONCERN TO DENTISTRY
None reported

SERIOUS REACTIONS
! Excessive dosage may negate chemotherapeutic effects of folic acid antagonists.
! Anaphylaxis occurs rarely.
! Diarrhea may cause rapid clinical deterioration.

DENTAL CONSIDERATIONS
General:
• Signs of folate deficiency may appear in oral tissues.
• Determine why the patient is taking the drug.
• Patients with severe anemia or cancer or those receiving cancer chemotherapy may have oral complaints. Palliative therapy may be required.
Consultations:
• Medical consultation may be required to assess disease control.

Teach Patient/Family to:
• Use effective oral hygiene to prevent soft tissue inflammation
• Use caution to prevent trauma when using oral hygiene aids
• Report oral lesions, soreness, or bleeding to dentist
• See dentist immediately if secondary oral infection occurs
• Update medical/drug records if physician makes any changes in evaluation or drug regimens; include OTC, herbal, and nonherbal drugs in the update

leuprolide acetate
loo´-proe-lide ass´-eh-tayte
(Eligard, Lucrin[AUS], Lucrin Depot Inj[AUS], Lupron, Lupron Depot, Lupron Depot Ped, Viadur)
Do not confuse leuprolide or Lupron with Lopurin or Nuprin.

CATEGORY AND SCHEDULE
Pregnancy Risk Category: X

Drug Class: Antineoplastic hormone; gonadotropin-releasing hormone

MECHANISM OF ACTION
A gonadotropin-releasing hormone analog and antineoplastic agent that stimulates the release of luteinizing hormone (LH) and follicle-stimulating hormone (FSH) from the anterior pituitary gland. *Therapeutic Effect:* Produces pharmacologic castration and decreases the growth of abnormal prostate tissue in males; causes endometrial tissue to become inactive and atrophic in females; and decreases the rate of pubertal development in children with central precocious puberty.

USES
Treatment of metastatic prostate cancer, management of endometriosis, central precocious puberty

PHARMACOKINETICS
Rapidly and well absorbed after subcutaneous administration. Absorbed slowly after IM administration. Protein binding: 43%–49%. *Half-life:* 3–4 hr.

INDICATIONS AND DOSAGES
▸ **Advanced Prostatic Carcinoma**
IM (Lupron Depot)
Adults, Elderly. 7.5 mg every mo or 22.5 mg q3mo or 30 mg q4mo.
Subcutaneous (Eligard)
Adults, Elderly. 7.5 mg every mo or 22.5 mg q3mo or 30 mg q4mo.
Subcutaneous (Lupron)
Adults, Elderly. 1 mg/day.
Subcutaneous (Viadur)
Adults, Elderly. 65 mg implanted q12mo.
▸ **Endometriosis**
IM (Lupron Depot)
Adults, Elderly. 3.75 mg/mo for up to 6 mo or 11.25 mg q3mo for up to 2 doses.
▸ **Uterine Leiomyomata**
IM (with iron [Lupron Depot])
Adults, Elderly. 3.75 mg/mo for up to 3 mo or 11.25 mg as a single injection.
▸ **Precocious Puberty**
IM (Lupron Depot)
Children. 0.3 mg/kg/dose every 28 days. Minimum: 7.5 mg. If down-regulation is not achieved, titrate upward in 3.75-mg increments q4wk.
Subcutaneous (Lupron)
Children. 20–45 mcg/kg/day. Titrate upward by 10 mcg/kg/day if down-regulation is not achieved.

SIDE EFFECTS/ADVERSE REACTIONS
Frequent
Hot flashes (ranging from mild flushing to diaphoresis)
Females: Amenorrhea, spotting
Occasional
Arrhythmias; palpitations; blurred vision; dizziness; edema; headache; burning, itching, or swelling at injection site; nausea; insomnia; weight gain
Females: Deepening voice, hirsutism, decreased libido, increased breast tenderness, vaginitis, altered mood
Males: Constipation, decreased testicle size, gynecomastia, impotence, decreased appetite, angina
Rare
Males: Thrombophlebitis

PRECAUTIONS AND CONTRAINDICATIONS
Pernicious anemia, pregnancy

DRUG INTERACTIONS OF CONCERN TO DENTISTRY
None reported

SERIOUS REACTIONS
❗ Signs and symptoms of metastatic prostatic carcinoma (such as bone pain, dysuria or hematuria, and weakness or paresthesia of the lower extremities) occasionally worsen 1 to 2 wk after the initial dose but then subside with continued therapy.
❗ Pulmonary embolism and MI occur rarely.

DENTAL CONSIDERATIONS
General:
• If additional analgesia is required for dental pain, consider alternative analgesics (NSAIDs) in patients taking narcotics for acute or chronic pain.
• Monitor and record vital signs.

- Assess salivary flow as a factor in caries, periodontal disease, and candidiasis
- This drug may be used in the hospital or on an outpatient basis. Confirm the patient's disease and treatment status.
- Consider semisupine chair position for patient comfort if GI side effects occur.
- Question patient about tolerance of NSAIDS or aspirin related to GI disease.
- Patient on chronic drug therapy may rarely present with symptoms of blood dyscrasias, which can include infection, bleeding, and poor healing. If dyscrasia is present, caution patient to prevent oral tissue trauma when using oral hygiene aids.
- Examine for oral manifestation of opportunistic infection.

Consultations:
- Medical consultation may be required to assess immunologic status during cancer chemotherapy and determine safety risk, if any, posed by the required dental treatment.
- Consider consulting with physician before prescribing drugs that may cause constipation (narcotics).
- Medical consultation may be required to assess disease control and patient's ability to tolerate stress.
- In a patient with symptoms of blood dyscrasias, request a medical consultation for blood studies and postpone treatment until normal values are reestablished.

Teach Patient/Family:
- When chronic dry mouth occurs advise patient to:
  - Avoid mouth rinses with high alcohol content due to drying effects
  - Use daily home fluoride products for anticaries effect
  - Use sugarless gum, frequent sips of water, or saliva substitutes
- Prevent trauma when using oral hygiene aids
- Report oral lesions, soreness, or bleeding to dentist
- Update health and medication history if physician makes any changes in evaluation or drug regimens; include OTC, herbal, and nonherbal drugs in the update

levalbuterol
lee-val-byoot´-err-all
(Xopenex)
Do not confuse Xopenex with Xanax.

CATEGORY AND SCHEDULE
Pregnancy Risk Category: C

Drug Class: Bronchodilator

MECHANISM OF ACTION
A sympathomimetic that stimulates β_2-adrenergic receptors in the lungs resulting in relaxation of bronchial smooth muscle. **Therapeutic Effect:** Relieves bronchospasm and reduces airway resistance.

USES
Treatment or prevention of bronchospasm in adults and children older than 6 yr with reversible obstructive airway disease

PHARMACOKINETICS

Route	Onset	Peak	Duration
Inhalation	10–17 min	1.5 hr	5–6 hr

Metabolized in the liver to inactive metabolite. **Half-life:** 3.3–4 hr.

INDICATIONS AND DOSAGES
▶ **Treatment and Prevention of Bronchospasm**
Nebulization
Adults, Elderly, Children 12 yr and older. Initially, 0.63 mg 3 times a day 6–8 hr apart. May increase to 1.25 mg 3 times a day with dose monitoring.
Children 3–11 yr. Initially 0.31 mg 3 times a day. Maximum: 0.63 mg 3 times a day.

SIDE EFFECTS/ADVERSE REACTIONS
Frequent
Tremors, nervousness, headache, throat dryness and irritation
Occasional
Cough, bronchial irritation
Rare
Somnolence, diarrhea, dry mouth, flushing, diaphoresis, anorexia

PRECAUTIONS AND CONTRAINDICATIONS
History of hypersensitivity to sympathomimetics
Caution
Paradoxic bronchospasm, cardiovascular disorders, seizures, diabetes, hyperthyroidism, coronary insufficiency, cardiac arrhythmias, hypertension, not to exceed recommended dose, β-adrenergic blockers, MAOIs, tricyclic antidepressants, lactation, children younger than 12 yr

DRUG INTERACTIONS OF CONCERN TO DENTISTRY
• Significant reduction of effects: β-adrenergic blockers
• Potentiation of cardiovascular effects: MAOIs, tricyclic antidepressants, methylxanthines
• No specific dental drug interactions reported

SERIOUS REACTIONS
! Excessive sympathomimetic stimulation may produce palpitations, extrasystoles, tachycardia, chest pain, a slight increase in B/P followed by a substantial decrease, chills, diaphoresis, and blanching of skin.
! Too-frequent or excessive use may lead to decreased bronchodilating effectiveness and severe, paradoxical bronchoconstriction.

DENTAL CONSIDERATIONS
General:
• Monitor vital signs at every appointment because of cardiovascular side effects.
• Assess salivary flow as a factor in caries, periodontal disease, and candidiasis.
• Consider semisupine chair position for patients with respiratory disease.
• Short midday appointments and a stress-reduction protocol may be required for anxious patients.
• Be aware that aspirin or sulfite preservatives in vasoconstrictor-containing products can exacerbate asthma.
• Acute asthmatic episodes may be precipitated in the dental office. Rapid-acting sympathomimetic inhalants should be available for emergency use. A stress reduction protocol may be required.
Consultations:
• Medical consultation may be required to assess disease control and patient's ability to tolerate stress.
Teach Patient/Family to:
• Rinse mouth with water after each dose of inhalation dosage forms to prevent dryness

- When chronic dry mouth occurs, advise patient to:
  - Avoid mouth rinses with high alcohol content because of drying effects
  - Use daily home fluoride products for anticaries effect
  - Use sugarless gum, frequent sips of water, or saliva substitutes

levetiracetam
leva-tir-ass´-eh-tam
(Keppra)
Do not confuse Keppra with Kaletra.

CATEGORY AND SCHEDULE
Pregnancy Risk Category: C

Drug Class: Antiepileptic

MECHANISM OF ACTION
An anticonvulsant that inhibits burst firing without affecting normal neuronal excitability. *Therapeutic Effect:* Prevents seizure activity.

USES
Adjunctive therapy in adults with partial-onset seizures

PHARMACOKINETICS
PO: Bioavailability 100%, onset 1 hr, peak plasma levels 20 min–2 hr. *Half-life:* 6–8 hr, less than 10% plasma protein bound, limited hepatic metabolism, renal excretion (66%)

INDICATIONS AND DOSAGES
▸ **Partial-Onset Seizures**
PO
Adults, Elderly. Initially, 500 mg q12h. May increase by 1000 mg/day q2wk. Maximum: 3000 mg/day.
Children 4–16 yr. 10–20 mg/kg/day in 2 divided doses. May increase at

weekly intervals by 10–20 mg/kg. Maximum: 60 mg/kg.
▸ **Dosage in Renal Impairment**
Dosage is modified on the basis of creatinine clearance.

Creatinine Clearance (ml/min)	Dosage
Higher than 80 ml/min	500–1500 mg q12h
50–80 ml/min	500–1000 mg q12h
30–50 ml/min	250–750 mg q12h
Less than 30 ml/min	250–500 mg q12h
End-stage renal disease using dialysis	500–1000 mg q12h, after dialysis, a 250- to 500-mg supplemental dose is recommended.

SIDE EFFECTS/ADVERSE REACTIONS
Frequent
Somnolence, asthenia, headache, infection
Occasional
Dizziness, pharyngitis, pain, depression, nervousness, vertigo, rhinitis, anorexia
Rare
Amnesia, anxiety, emotional lability, cough, sinusitis, anorexia, diplopia

PRECAUTIONS AND CONTRAINDICATIONS
Hypersensitivity reaction
Caution
Lactation, children, blood dyscrasias

DRUG INTERACTIONS OF CONCERN TO DENTISTRY
None reported

SERIOUS REACTIONS
None known.

DENTAL CONSIDERATIONS
General:
• Short appointments and a stress-reduction protocol may be required for anxious patients.
• Ask patient about type of epilepsy, seizure frequency, and quality of seizure control.
Consultation:
• Medical consultation may be required to assess disease control and patient's ability to tolerate stress.
• In patients with symptoms of blood dyscrasias, request a medical consultation for blood studies and postpone treatment until normal values are reestablished.
Teach Patient/Family to:
• Update health and drug history if physician makes changes in evaluation or drug regimens; include OTC, herbal, and nonherbal drugs in the update

levobetaxolol hydrochloride
le-vo-bay-tax´-oh-lol
high-droh-klor´-ide
(Betaxon)
Do not confuse with levobunolol.

CATEGORY AND SCHEDULE
Pregnancy Risk Category: C

Drug Class: Antiglaucoma agent (ophthalmic)

MECHANISM OF ACTION
An antiglaucoma agent that blocks β_1-adrenergic receptors. Reduces aqueous humor production.
Therapeutic Effect: Reduces intraocular pressure (IOP).

USES
Treatment of certain types of glaucoma

PHARMACOKINETICS

Route	Onset	Peak	Duration
Eye drops	30 min	2 hr	12 hr

INDICATIONS AND DOSAGES
▶ **Glaucoma, Ocular Hypertension**
Ophthalmic
Adults, Elderly. Instill 1 drop 2 times a day.

SIDE EFFECTS/ADVERSE REACTIONS
Frequent
Ocular discomfort
Occasional
Blurred vision
Rare
Anxiety, dizziness, vertigo, headache

PRECAUTIONS AND CONTRAINDICATIONS
Sinus bradycardia, second- or third-degree atrioventricular (AV) block, cardiogenic shock, overt heart failure, hypersensitivity to betaxolol, levobetaxolol, or any component of levobetaxolol formulations

DRUG INTERACTIONS OF CONCERN TO DENTISTRY
None reported

SERIOUS REACTIONS
! Diabetes, hypothyroidism, bradycardia, tachycardia, hypertension, hypotension, heart block, alopecia, dermatitis, psoriasis, arthritis, tendonitis, dyspnea and other respiratory symptoms (e.g., bronchitis, pneumonia, rhinitis, sinusitis, pharyngitis) occur rarely.
! Ophthalmic overdosage may produce bradycardia, hypotension, bronchospasm, and acute cardiac failure.

DENTAL CONSIDERATIONS

General:
• Determine why patient is taking the drug.
• Avoid drugs with anticholinergic activity, such as antihistamines, opioids, benzodiazepines, propantheline, atropine, and scopolamine.
• Avoid dental light in patient's eyes; offer dark glasses for patient comfort.
• Question glaucoma patient about compliance with prescribed drug regimen.

Consultations:
• Medical consultation may be required to assess disease control.

Teach Patient/Family to:
• Update health and medication history if physician makes any changes in evaluation or drug regimens; include OTC, herbal, and nonherbal drugs in the update

levobunolol hydrochloride

lee-vo-byoo´-no-lol
high-droh-klor´-ide
(AK-Beta, Betagan,
Novo-Levobunolol[CAN],
Optho-Bunolol[CAN],
PMS-Levobunolol[CAN])
Do not confuse with levobetaxolol.

CATEGORY AND SCHEDULE

Pregnancy Risk Category: C

Drug Class: Antiglaucoma agent (ophthalmic)

MECHANISM OF ACTION

A nonselective β-blocker that blocks $β_1$- and $β_2$-adrenergic receptors. ***Therapeutic Effect:*** Reduces intraocular pressure (IOP). Decreases production of aqueous humor.

USES

Treatment of certain types of glaucoma

PHARMACOKINETICS

Well absorbed after administration. Metabolized in liver. Primarily excreted in urine. ***Half-life:*** 6.1 hr.

INDICATIONS AND DOSAGES

▸ **Glaucoma, Ocular Hypertension**
Ophthalmic
Adults, Elderly. Instill 1–2 drops in affected eye(s) once daily.

SIDE EFFECTS/ADVERSE REACTIONS

Frequent
Burning/stinging, eye irritation, visual disturbances
Occasional
Increased light sensitivity, watering of eye
Rare
Dry eye, conjunctivitis, eye pain, diarrhea, dyspepsia

PRECAUTIONS AND CONTRAINDICATIONS

Cardiogenic shock, overt cardiac failure, second- or third-degree heart block, sinus bradycardia, hypersensitivity to levobunolol or any component of the formulation.

DRUG INTERACTIONS OF CONCERN TO DENTISTRY

• Patient with glaucoma: avoid use of anticholinergic drugs, atropine-like drugs, propantheline, and diazepam (benzodiazepines)

SERIOUS REACTIONS

! Abrupt withdrawal may result in sweating, headache, and fatigue.
! Ophthalmic overdosage may produce bradycardia, hypotension, bronchospasm, and acute cardiac failure.

DENTAL CONSIDERATIONS

General:
• Check compliance of patient with prescribed drug regimen for glaucoma.
• Avoid dental light in patient's eyes; offer dark glasses for patient comfort.

Consultations:
• Consultation with physician may be necessary if sedation or anesthesia is required.

---

levocabastine
lev-oh-kab´-ah-steen
(Livostin)

CATEGORY AND SCHEDULE
Pregnancy Risk Category: C

Drug Class: Antihistamine, H_1- receptor antagonist

MECHANISM OF ACTION
An antiallergic agent that selectively antagonizes H_1 receptor. **Therapeutic Effect:** Blocks histamine-associated symptoms of seasonal allergic conjunctivitis.

USES
Temporary relief of seasonal allergic conjunctivitis

PHARMACOKINETICS
Duration of action is about 2 hr. Minimal systemic absorption.

INDICATIONS AND DOSAGES
▶ **Allergic Conjunctivitis**
Ophthalmic
Adults, Elderly, Children 12 yr or older. 1 drop 4 times a day, for up to 2 wk.

SIDE EFFECTS/ADVERSE REACTIONS
Frequent
Transient stinging, burning, discomfort, headache
Occasional
Dry mouth, fatigue, eye dryness, lacrimation and discharge, eyelid edema
Rare
Rash, erythema, nausea, dyspnea

PRECAUTIONS AND CONTRAINDICATIONS
Wearing of soft contact lenses (product contains benzalkonium chloride), hypersensitivity to levocabastine or any component of the formulation
Caution
Lactation, children younger than 12 yr

DRUG INTERACTIONS OF CONCERN TO DENTISTRY
None reported

SERIOUS REACTIONS
None reported

DENTAL CONSIDERATIONS
General:
• Question patient about history of allergy to avoid using other potential allergens.

- Avoid dental light in patient's eyes; offer dark glasses for patient comfort.
- Evaluate respiration characteristics and rate.
- Use for less than 2 wk should not present a problem with dry mouth.

Teach Patient/Family:
- When chronic dry mouth occurs, advise patient to:
  - Avoid mouth rinses with high alcohol content because of drying effects
  - Use daily home fluoride products for anticaries effect
  - Use sugarless gum, frequent sips of water, or saliva substitutes

levodopa
lev-oh-dope´-ah
(Dopar, Larodopa)

CATEGORY AND SCHEDULE
Pregnancy Risk Category: C

Drug Class: Antiparkinson agent

MECHANISM OF ACTION
A dopamine prodrug that is converted to dopamine in basal ganglia. Increases dopamine concentrations in the brain, inhibiting hyperactive cholinergic activity.
Therapeutic Effect: Decreases signs and symptoms of Parkinson's disease.

USES
Treatment of Parkinsonism of various causes

PHARMACOKINETICS
About 30% absorbed. May be reduced with high-protein meal. Protein binding: minimal. Crosses blood-brain barrier. Converted to dopamine. Eliminated primarily in urine and to a lesser amount in feces and expired air. Not removed by hemodialysis. **Half-life:** 0.75–1.5 hr.

INDICATIONS AND DOSAGES
▶ **Parkinsonism**
PO
Adults, Elderly. Initially, 0.5–1 g 2–4 times a day. May increase in increments not exceeding 0.75 g every 3–7 days, up to a maximum of 8 g/day.

SIDE EFFECTS/ADVERSE REACTIONS
Frequent
Uncontrolled body movements of the face, tongue, arms, and upper body; nausea and vomiting; anorexia
Occasional
Depression, anxiety, confusion, nervousness, difficulty urinating, irregular heartbeats, hiccoughs, dizziness, lightheadedness, decreased appetite, blurred vision, constipation, dry mouth, flushed skin, headache, insomnia, diarrhea, unusual tiredness, darkening of urine, discolored sweat
Rare
Hypertension, ulcer, hemolytic anemia, marked by tiredness or weakness.

PRECAUTIONS AND CONTRAINDICATIONS
Nonselective MAOI therapy, hypersensitivity to levodopa or any component of its formulation
Caution
Renal disease, cardiac disease, hepatic disease, respiratory disease, MI with dysrhythmia, convulsions, peptic ulcer, asthma, endocrine disease, affective disorders, psychosis, lactation, children younger than 12 yr

DRUG INTERACTIONS OF CONCERN TO DENTISTRY

• Decreased absorption: anticholinergics
• Decreased therapeutic effect: benzodiazepines, pyridoxine (vitamin B6), tricyclic antidepressants

SERIOUS REACTIONS

! High incidence of involuntary dystonic, and dyskinetic movements may be noted in patients on long-term therapy.
! Mental changes, such as paranoid ideation, psychotic episodes, and depression, may be noted.
! Numerous mild-to-severe CNS psychiatric disturbances may include reduced attention span, anxiety, nightmares, daytime somnolence, euphoria, fatigue, paranoia, and hallucinations.

DENTAL CONSIDERATIONS
General:
• Patients on chronic drug therapy may rarely have symptoms of blood dyscrasias, which can include infection, bleeding, and poor healing.
• Assess salivary flow as a factor in caries, periodontal disease, and candidiasis.
• After supine positioning, have patient sit upright for at least 2 min before standing to avoid orthostatic hypotension.
• Avoid dental light in patient's eyes; offer dark glasses for patient comfort.
Consultations:
• In a patient with symptoms of blood dyscrasias, request a medical consultation for blood studies and postpone dental treatment until normal values are reestablished.
• Take precautions if dental surgery is anticipated and anesthesia is required.

• Medical consultation may be required to assess disease control.
Teach Patient/Family to:
• Use electric tooth brush if patient has difficulty holding conventional devices
• When chronic dry mouth occurs, advise patient to:
  • Avoid mouth rinses with high alcohol content because of drying effects
  • Use sugarless gum, frequent sips of water, or saliva substitutes
  • Use daily home fluoride products for anticaries effect

levofloxacin
lev-oh-flox´-ah-sin
(Iquix, Levaquin, Quixin)

CATEGORY AND SCHEDULE
Pregnancy Risk Category: C

Drug Class: Fluoroquinolone antiinfective

MECHANISM OF ACTION
A fluoroquinolone that inhibits the enzyme DNA gyrase in susceptible microorganisms, interfering with bacterial cell replication and repair. *Therapeutic Effect:* Bactericidal.

USES
Treatment of acute infections caused by susceptible bacterial strains causing acute maxillary sinusitis, acute bacterial exacerbation of chronic bronchitis, community-acquired pneumonia, nosocomial pneumonia, complicated and uncomplicated skin and skin-structure infections, uncomplicated UTI, and acute pyelonephritis;

nosocomial pneumonia; chronic
bacterial prostatitis

PHARMACOKINETICS

Well absorbed after both PO and IV
administration. Protein binding:
24%–8%. Penetrates rapidly and
extensively into leukocytes, epithelial
cells, and macrophages. Lung
concentrations are 2–5 times higher
than those of plasma. Eliminated
unchanged in the urine. Partially
removed by hemodialysis.
Half-life: 8 hr.

INDICATIONS AND DOSAGES
▶ **Bronchitis**
PO, IV
Adults, Elderly. 500 mg q24h for
7 days.
▶ **Community-Acquired Pneumonia**
PO
Adults, Elderly. 750 mg/day for
5 days.
▶ **Pneumonia**
PO, IV
Adults, Elderly. 500 mg q24h for
7–14 days.
▶ **Acute Maxillary Sinusitis**
PO, IV
Adults, Elderly. 500 mg q24h for
10–14 days.
▶ **Skin and Skin-Structure Infections**
PO, IV
Adults, Elderly. 500 mg q24h for
7–10 days.
▶ **UTIs, Acute Pyelonephritis**
PO, IV
Adults, Elderly. 250 mg q24h for
10 days.
▶ **Bacterial Conjunctivitis**
Ophthalmic
*Adults, Elderly, Children 1 yr and
older.* 1–2 drops q2h for 2 days (up
to 8 times a day), then 1–2 drops q4h
for 5 days.
▶ **Corneal Ulcer**
Ophthalmic

*Adults, Elderly, Children older than
5 yr.* Days 1–3: Instill 1–2 drops
q30min to 2 hr while awake and
4–6 hr after retiring. Days 4 through
completion: 1–2 drops q1–4h while
awake.
▶ **Dosage in Renal Impairment**
For bronchitis, pneumonia, sinusitis,
and skin and skin-structure
infections, dosage and frequency are
modified on the basis of creatinine
clearance.

Creatinine Clearance	Dosage
50–80 ml/min	No change
20–49 ml/min	500 mg initially, then 250 mg q24h
10–19 ml/min	500 mg initially, then 250 mg q48h

Dialysis 500 mg initially, then
250 mg q48h
For UTIs and pyelonephritis, dosage
and frequency are modified on the
basis of creatinine clearance.

Creatinine Clearance	Dosage
20 ml/min	No change
10–19 ml/min	250 mg initially, then 250 mg q48h

SIDE EFFECTS/ADVERSE REACTIONS
Occasional
Diarrhea, nausea, abdominal pain,
dizziness, drowsiness, headache,
light-headedness
Ophthalmic: Local burning or
discomfort, margin crusting, crystals
or scales, foreign body sensation,
ocular itching, altered taste
Rare
Flatulence; altered taste; pain;
inflammation or swelling in calves,

hands, or shoulder; chest pain; difficulty breathing; palpitations; edema; tendon pain
Ophthalmic: Corneal staining, keratitis, allergic reaction, eyelid swelling, tearing, reduced visual acuity

PRECAUTIONS AND CONTRAINDICATIONS

Hypersensitivity to levofloxacin, other fluoroquinolones, or nalidixic acid
Caution
Children younger than 18 yr; seizure disorders, renal insufficiency, excessive exposure to sunlight, alterations in blood glucose (diabetes), lactation, drink fluids liberally; tendon rupture of shoulder, hand, and Achilles tendon, monitor blood glucose

DRUG INTERACTIONS OF CONCERN TO DENTISTRY

• Interference with absorption: solutions with multivalent cations (e.g., magnesium)
• Increased seizure risk: NSAIDs
• May increase effects of warfarin (monitor bleeding)

SERIOUS REACTIONS

! Antibiotic-associated colitis and other superinfections may occur from altered bacterial balance.
! Hypersensitivity reactions, including photosensitivity (as evidenced by rash, pruritus, blisters, edema, and burning skin), have occurred in patients receiving fluoroquinolones.

DENTAL CONSIDERATIONS
General:
• Determine why patient is taking the drug.

• If dental drugs prescribed, advise patient of potential for photosensitivity.
Consultations:
• Consult with patient's physician if an acute dental infection occurs and another antiinfective is required.
Teach Patient/Family to:
• Minimize exposure to sunlight and wear sunscreen if sun exposure is planned
• Discontinue treatment and inform dentist immediately if patient experiences pain or inflammation of a tendon, and to rest and refrain from exercise

levothyroxine
lev-oh-thye-rox´-een
(Droxine[AUS], Eltroxin[CAN], Eutroxsig[AUS], Levothroid, Levoxyl, Novothyrox[CAN], Oroxine[AUS], Synthroid, Unithroid)
Do not confuse levothyroxine with liothyronine.

CATEGORY AND SCHEDULE
Pregnancy Risk Category: A

Drug Class: Thyroid hormone

MECHANISM OF ACTION
A synthetic isomer of thyroxine involved in normal metabolism, growth, and development, especially of the CNS in infants. Possesses catabolic and anabolic effects.
Therapeutic Effect: Increases basal metabolic rate, enhances gluconeogenesis, and stimulates protein synthesis.

USES
Treatment of hypothyroidism, myxedema coma, thyroid hormone replacement, cretinism, chronic

thyroiditis, euthyroid goiters, management of thyroid cancer

PHARMACOKINETICS

Variable, incomplete absorption from the GI tract. Protein binding: greater than 99%. Widely distributed. Deiodinated in peripheral tissues, minimal metabolism in the liver. Eliminated by biliary excretion. *Half-life:* 6–7 days.

INDICATIONS AND DOSAGES
▸ **Hypothyroidism**
PO
Adults, Elderly. Initially, 12.5–50 mcg. May increase by 25–50 mcg/day q2–4wk. Maintenance: 100–200 mcg/day.
Children 13 yr and older. 150 mcg/day.
Children 6–12 yr. 100–125 mcg/day.
Children 1–5 yr. 75–100 mcg/day.
Children 7–11 mo. 50–75 mcg/day.
Children 3–6 mo. 25–50 mcg/day.
Children 3 mo and younger.
10–15 mcg/day.
▸ **Thyroid Suppression Therapy**
PO
Adults, Elderly. 2–6 mcg/kg/day for 7–10 days.
▸ **Thyroid Stimulating Hormone Suppression in Thyroid Cancer, Nodules, Euthyroid Goiters**
PO
Adults, Elderly. 2–6 mcg/kg/day for 7–10 days.
IV
Adults, Elderly, Children. Initial dosage approximately half the previously established oral dosage.

SIDE EFFECTS/ADVERSE REACTIONS
Occasional
Reversible hair loss at the start of therapy (in children)

Rare
Dry skin, GI intolerance, rash, hives, pseudotumor cerebri or severe headache in children

PRECAUTIONS AND CONTRAINDICATIONS
Hypersensitivity to tablet components, such as tartrazine; allergy to aspirin; lactose intolerance; MI and thyrotoxicosis uncomplicated by hypothyroidism; treatment of obesity
Caution
Elderly, angina pectoris, hypertension, ischemia, cardiac disease, lactation

DRUG INTERACTIONS OF CONCERN TO DENTISTRY
• Increased effects of sympathomimetics when thyroid doses are not carefully monitored or in patients with coronary artery disease

SERIOUS REACTIONS
! Excessive dosage produces signs and symptoms of hyperthyroidism, including weight loss, palpitations, increased appetite, tremors, nervousness, tachycardia, hypertension, headache, insomnia, and menstrual irregularities.
! Cardiac arrhythmias occur rarely.

DENTAL CONSIDERATIONS
General:
• Uncontrolled hypothyroid patients may be more responsive to CNS depressants.
• Increased nervousness, excitability, sweating, or tachycardia may indicate a patient with uncontrolled hyperthyroidism or a dose of medication that is too high.
• Uncontrolled patients should be referred for medical treatment.
• Observe appropriate limitations of vasoconstrictor doses.

• Monitor vital signs at every appointment because of CV side effects.
Consultations:
• Medical consultation may be required to assess disease control.

lidocaine hydrocloride
lye´-doe-kane high-droh-klor´-ide
(Lidoderm, Lignocaine Gel[AUS], Xylocaine, Xylocaine Aerosol[AUS], Xylocaine Ointment[AUS], Xylocaine Viscous Topical Solution[AUS], Xylocard[CAN], Zilactin-L[CAN])

CATEGORY AND SCHEDULE
Pregnancy Risk Category: B

Drug Class: Antidysrhythmic (class IB)

MECHANISM OF ACTION
An amide anesthetic that inhibits conduction of nerve impulses. *Therapeutic Effect:* Causes temporary loss of feeling and sensation. Also an antiarrhythmic that decreases depolarization, automaticity, excitability of the ventricle during diastole by direct action. *Therapeutic Effect:* Inhibits ventricular arrhythmias.

USES
Ventricular tachycardia, ventricular dysrhythmias during cardiac surgery, MI, digitalis toxicity, cardiac catheterization; for acute management only

PHARMACOKINETICS

Route	Onset	Peak	Duration
IV	30–90 sec	N/A	10–20 min
Local anesthetic	2.5 min	N/A	30–60 min

Completely absorbed after IM administration. Protein binding: 60%–80%. Widely distributed. Metabolized in the liver. Primarily excreted in urine. Minimally removed by hemodialysis.
Half-life: 1–2 hr.

INDICATIONS AND DOSAGES
▶ **Rapid Control of Acute Ventricular Arrhythmias after an MI, Cardiac Catheterization, Cardiac Surgery, or Digitalis-Induced Ventricular Arrhythmias**
IM
Adults, Elderly. 300 mg (or 4.3 mg/kg). May repeat in 60–90 min.
IV
Adults, Elderly. Initially, 50–100 mg (1 mg/kg) IV bolus at rate of 25–50 mg/min. May repeat in 5 min. Give no more than 200–300 mg in 1 hr. Maintenance: 20–50 mcg/kg/min (1–4 mg/min) as IV infusion.
Children, Infants. Initially, 0.5–1 mg/kg IV bolus; may repeat but total dose not to exceed 3–5 mg/kg. Maintenance: 10–50 mcg/kg/min as IV infusion.
▶ **Dental or Surgical Procedures, Childbirth**
Infiltration or nerve block
Adults. Local anesthetic dosage varies with procedure, degree of anesthesia, vascularity, duration. Maximum dose: 4.5 mg/kg. Do not repeat within 2 hr.
▶ **Local Skin Disorders (minor burns, insect bites, prickly heat, skin manifestations of**

chickenpox, abrasions), and **Mucous Membrane Disorders (local anesthesia of oral, nasal, and laryngeal mucous membranes; local anesthesia of respiratory, urinary tract; relief of discomfort of pruritus ani, hemorrhoids, pruritus vulvae)**
Topical
Adults, Elderly. Apply to affected areas as needed.
▶ **Treatment of Shingles-Related Skin Pain**
Topical (Dermal patch)
Adults, Elderly. Apply to intact skin over most painful area (up to 3 applications once for up to 12 hr in a 24-hr period).

SIDE EFFECTS/ADVERSE REACTIONS
CNS effects are generally dose related and of short duration
Occasional
IM: Pain at injection site
Topical: Burning, stinging, tenderness at application site
Rare
Generally with high dose: Drowsiness; dizziness; disorientation; light-headedness; tremors; apprehension; euphoria; sensation of heat, cold, or numbness; blurred or double vision; ringing or roaring in ears (tinnitus); nausea

PRECAUTIONS AND CONTRAINDICATIONS
Adams-Stokes syndrome, hypersensitivity to amide-type local anesthetics, septicemia (spinal anesthesia), supraventricular arrhythmias, Wolff-Parkinson-White syndrome
Caution
Lactation, children, renal disease, liver disease, CHF, respiratory depression, malignant hyperthermia

(questionable), elderly; need to monitor ECG

DRUG INTERACTIONS OF CONCERN TO DENTISTRY
Patch Form
None reported

SERIOUS REACTIONS
❗ Although serious adverse reactions to lidocaine are uncommon, high dosage by any route may produce cardiovascular depression, bradycardia, hypotension, arrhythmias, heart block, cardiovascular collapse, and cardiac arrest.
❗ Potential for malignant hyperthermia.
❗ CNS toxicity may occur, especially with regional anesthesia use, progressing rapidly from mild side effects to tremors, somnolence, seizures, vomiting, and respiratory depression.
❗ Methemoglobinemia (evidenced by cyanosis) has occurred following topical application of lidocaine for teething discomfort and laryngeal anesthetic spray.

DENTAL CONSIDERATIONS

Patch Form
General:
• Use no more than one patch per area, remove after 15 min to avoid toxicity.
Teach Patient/Family to:
• Prevent injury while numbness is present and to refrain from gum chewing and eating after dental treatment
• Report unresolved oral lesions to dentist

L

lidocaine transoral delivery system
lye´-doe-kane
(DentiPatch)

CATEGORY AND SCHEDULE
Pregnancy Risk Category: B

Drug Class: Amide local anesthetic

MECHANISM OF ACTION
Inhibits nerve impulses from sensory nerves, which produces anesthesia.

USES
Mild topical anesthesia of mucous membranes of the mouth before superficial dental procedures

PHARMACOKINETICS
Topical: Onset 2.5 min, duration of approximately 30 min after removal; blood levels less than 0.1 ng/ml limited absorption; hepatic metabolism, urinary excretion.

INDICATIONS AND DOSAGES
Topical
Adult. Apply one patch to area of application after drying with gauze; leave in place until local anesthesia is produced, but no longer than 15 min

SIDE EFFECTS/ADVERSE REACTIONS
Oral: Taste alteration, stomatitis, erythema, mucosa irritation
CNS: Headache, excitatory or depressor actions, dizziness, nervousness, confusion, tinnitus, twitching, tremors (associated with excessive systemic absorption)
CV: Bradycardia, hypotension, cardiovascular collapse (with excessive systemic absorption)
GI: Nausea

Misc: Allergic reactions to this agent or to other ingredients in the formulation (rare)

PRECAUTIONS AND CONTRAINDICATIONS
Hypersensitivity to amide-type local anesthetics
Caution
Local anesthetic toxicity, no pediatric (children younger than 12 yr) or geriatric studies have been made, liver dysfunction, onset longer for maxilla, lactation, contains phenylalanine (caution phenylketonurics)

DRUG INTERACTIONS OF CONCERN TO DENTISTRY
None reported

SERIOUS REACTIONS
! CNS excitation and depression, potential respiratory depression (at high blood levels).
! Bradycardia, hypotension, cardiovascular collapse, cardiac arrest (at high blood levels).
! Serious allergic reactions (rare).

DENTAL CONSIDERATIONS
General:
• Use no more than one patch per area, remove after 15 min to avoid toxicity.
Teach Patient/Family to:
• Prevent injury while numbness is present and to refrain from gum chewing and eating after dental treatment
• Report unresolved oral lesions to dentist

lincomycin HCL
lin-koe-my´-sin
(Bactramycin, Lincocin, Lincomycin)

CATEGORY AND SCHEDULE
Pregnancy Risk Category: B

Drug Class: Antibacterial

MECHANISM OF ACTION
A lincosamide antibiotic that specifically binds on the 50S subunit and affects the process of peptide chain initiation. *Therapeutic Effect:* Inhibits protein synthesis of the bacterial cell wall.

USES
Infections caused by group A β-hemolytic streptococci, pneumococci, staphylococci (respiratory tract, skin, soft tissue, UTIs; osteomyelitis; septicemia), and anaerobes

PHARMACOKINETICS
Rapidly absorbed from the GI tract. Protein binding: Unknown. Metabolized in liver. Primarily excreted in urine. Not removed by hemodialysis. *Half-life:* 5.4 hr (prolonged with renal or hepatic impairment).

INDICATIONS AND DOSAGES
▶ **Serious Infection Due to Susceptible Strains of Streptococci, Pneumococci, and Staphylococci**
PO
Adults. 500 mg 3 times a day (500 mg approximately q8h).
Children older than 1 mo. 30 mg/kg/day (15 mg/lb/day) divided into 3 or 4 equal doses.
▶ **More Severe Infection Due to Susceptible Strains of Streptococci, Pneumococci, and Staphylococci**
PO
Adults. 500 mg or more 4 times a day (500 mg or more approximately q6h).
Children older than 1 mo. 60 mg/kg/day (30 mg/lb/day) divided into 3 or 4 equal doses.

▶ **Serious Infection Due to Susceptible Strains of Streptococci, Pneumococci, and Staphylococci**
IM
Adults. 600 mg (2 ml) q24h.
Children older than 1 mo. One injection of 10 mg/kg (5 mg/lb) q24h.
▶ **More Severe Infection Due to Susceptible Strains of Streptococci, Pneumococci, and Staphylococci**
IM
Adults. 600 mg (2 ml) q12h or more often.
Children older than 1 mo. One injection of 10 mg/kg (5 mg/lb) q12h or more often.
▶ **Serious Infection Due to Susceptible Strains of Streptococci, Pneumococci, and Staphylococci**
IV
Adults. 600 mg (2 ml) to 1 g q8–12h
Children older than 1 mo. One injection of 10 mg/kg (5 mg/lb) q12h or more often. Depending on the severity of the infection, 10–20 mg/kg/day (5–10 mg/lb/day) can be infused in divided doses as described for adults.
▶ **More Severe Infection Due to Susceptible Strains of Streptococci, Pneumococci, and Staphylococci**
IV
Adults. 600 mg (2 ml) to 1 g q8–12h. Maximum: 8 g/day. Intravenous doses are given on the basis of 1 g lincomycin diluted in not less than 100 ml of appropriate solution and infused over a period of not less than 1 hr.
Subconjunctival Injection
Adults. Inject 0.25 ml (75 mg).
▶ **Dosage in Renal Impairment**
An appropriate dose is 25%–30% of that recommended for patients with normally functioning kidneys.

SIDE EFFECTS/ADVERSE REACTIONS
Frequent
Abdominal pain, nausea, vomiting, diarrhea
Occasional
Phlebitis, thrombophlebitis with IV administration, pain, induration at IM injection site, allergic reaction, urticaria, pruritus, tinnitus, vertigo
Rare
Dermatitis

PRECAUTIONS AND CONTRAINDICATIONS
History of hypersensitivity to clindamycin or lincomycin
Caution
Renal disease, liver disease, GI disease, elderly, lactation

DRUG INTERACTIONS OF CONCERN TO DENTISTRY
• Decreased action of erythromycin
• Oral contraceptives: advise patient of a potential risk for decreased contraceptive action, to maintain compliance with oral contraceptive use while using antibiotics, and to consider the use of additional nonhormonal contraception

SERIOUS REACTIONS
ALERT
❗ Antibiotic-associated colitis, as evidenced by severe abdominal pain and tenderness, fever, and watery and severe diarrhea, may occur during and several wk after lincomycin therapy.
❗ Cardiopulmonary arrest and hypotension have been reported.

DENTAL CONSIDERATIONS
General:
• Determine why the patient is taking the drug.

Consultations:
• Medical consultation may be required to assess disease control.
Teach Patient/Family to:
• Use effective oral hygiene to prevent soft tissue inflammation
• Use caution to prevent injury when using oral hygiene aids
• Notify dentist if diarrhea occurs
• When used for dental infection, advise patient to:
  • Report sore throat, oral burning sensation, fever, fatigue, any of which could indicate superinfection
  • Take at prescribed intervals and complete dosage regimen
  • Immediately notify the dentist if signs or symptoms of infection increase

linezolid
lin-ez´-oh-lid
(Zyvox, Zyvoxam)
Do not confuse Zyvox with Zoverax.

CATEGORY AND SCHEDULE
Pregnancy Risk Category: C

Drug Class: Antibiotic, oxazolidinone derivative

MECHANISM OF ACTION
An oxalodinone antiinfective that binds to a site on bacterial 23S ribosomal RNA, preventing the formation of a complex that is essential for bacterial translation.
Therapeutic Effect: Bacteriostatic against enterococci and staphylococci; bactericidal against streptococci.

USES
Treatment of vancomycin-resistant *E. faeceum* infections; nosocomial pneumonia caused by *S. aureus* (methicillin resistant and susceptible) and *S. pneumoniae* (penicillin susceptible); complicated skin and skin-structure infections caused by *S. aureus* (methicillin resistant and susceptible), *S. pyogenes*, or *S. agalactiae;* uncomplicated skin and skin-structure infections caused by *S. aureus* (methicillin susceptible); community-acquired pneumonia caused by *S. pneumoniae* (penicillin susceptible) or *S. aureus* (methicillin susceptible); and diabetic foot infections without osteomyelitis caused by gram-positive bacteria

PHARMACOKINETICS
Rapidly and extensively absorbed after PO administration. Protein binding: 31%. Metabolized in the liver by oxidation. Excreted in urine. *Half-life:* 4–5.4 hr.

INDICATIONS AND DOSAGES
▸ **Vancomycin-Resistant Infections**
PO, IV
Adults, Elderly, Children older than 11 yr. 600 mg q12h for 14–28 days.
▸ **Pneumonia, Complicated Skin, and Skin-Structure Infections**
PO, IV
Adults, Elderly, Children older than 11 yr. 600 mg q12h for 10–14 days.
▸ **Uncomplicated Skin and Skin-Structure Infections**
PO
Adults, Elderly. 400 mg q12h for 10–14 days.
Children older than 11 yr. 600 mg q12h for 10–14 days.
Children 5–11 yr. 10 mg/kg/dose q12h for 10–14 days.
▸ **Usual Neonate Dosage**
PO, IV
Neonates. 10 mg/kg/dose q8–12h.

SIDE EFFECTS/ADVERSE REACTIONS
Occasional
Diarrhea, nausea, headache
Rare
Altered taste, vaginal candidiasis, fungal infection, dizziness, tongue discoloration

PRECAUTIONS AND CONTRAINDICATIONS
Hypersensitivity
Caution
May promote overgrowth of nonsusceptible bacterial strains, monitor platelet counts in patients at risk for bleeding, lactation, pediatric doses not established, use longer than 28 days, selectively inhibits monoamine oxidase enzymes, potentiation of serotonergic drugs, hepatic disease, hemodialysis patients; risk of myelosuppression, monitor CBC counts, avoid tyramine-containing foods

DRUG INTERACTIONS OF CONCERN TO DENTISTRY
• Potential to increase pressor effects of indirect-action sympathomimetic drugs and vasopressors, such as dopaminergic drugs, phenylephrine, phenylpropanolamine, and pseudoephedrine
• Interactions with vasoconstrictors in local anesthetics has not been studied

SERIOUS REACTIONS
! Thrombocytopenia and myelosuppression occur rarely.
! Antibiotic-associated colitis and other superinfections may result from altered bacterial balance.

DENTAL CONSIDERATIONS
General:
• Determine why patient is taking the drug.

• Use vasoconstrictor with caution, in low doses, and with careful aspiration. Avoid using gingival retraction cord containing epinephrine.
• Patients on chronic drug therapy may rarely have symptoms of blood dyscrasias, which can include infection, bleeding, and poor healing.
• Examine for oral manifestation of opportunistic infection.
• Consider semisupine chair position for patient comfort if GI side effects occur.

Consultations:
• In a patient with symptoms of blood dyscrasias, request a medical consultation for blood studies and postpone treatment until normal values are reestablished.
• Medical consultation may be required to assess disease control and patient's ability to tolerate stress.
• Physician consultation is advised in the presence of an acute dental infection requiring another antibiotic.

Teach Patient/Family to:
• See dentist immediately if secondary oral infection occurs
• Report sore throat, oral burning sensation, fever, fatigue, any of which could indicate presence of a superinfection

liothyronine (T3)
lye-oh-thye′-roe-neen
(Cytomel, Tertroxin[AUS], Triostat)
Do not confuse liothyronine with levothyroxine.

CATEGORY AND SCHEDULE
Pregnancy Risk Category: A

Drug Class: Thyroid hormone

MECHANISM OF ACTION
A synthetic form of triiodothyronine (T3), a thyroid hormone involved in normal metabolism, growth, and development, especially of the CNS in infants. Possesses catabolic and anabolic effects. *Therapeutic Effect:* Increases basal metabolic rate, enhances gluconeogenesis, and stimulates protein synthesis.

USES
Treatment of hypothyroidism, myxedema coma, thyroid hormone replacement, cretinism, nontoxic goiter, T3 suppression test; thyroiditis, euthyroid goiter

PHARMACOKINETICS
PO: Peak 12–48 hr. *Half-life:* 0.6–1.4 days.

INDICATIONS AND DOSAGES
▶ **Hypothyroidism**
PO
Adults, Elderly. Initially, 25 mcg/day. May increase in increments of 12.5–25 mcg/day q1–2wk. Maximum 100 mcg/day.
Children. Initially, 5 mcg/day. May increase by 5 mcg/day q3–4wk. Maintenance: 100 mcg/day (children older than 3 yr); 50 mcg/day (children 1–3 yr); 20 mcg/day (infants).
▶ **Myxedema**
PO
Adults, Elderly. Initially, 5 mcg/day. Increase by 5–10 mcg q1–2wk (after 25 mcg/day has been reached, may increase in 12.5-mcg increments). Maintenance: 50–100 mcg/day.
▶ **Nontoxic Goiter**
PO
Adults, Elderly. Initially, 5 mcg/day. Increase by 5–10 mcg/day q1–2wk. When 25 mcg/day has been reached,

may increase by 12.5–25 mcg/day
q1–2wk. Maintenance: 75 mcg/day.
Children. 5 mcg/day. May increase
by 5 mcg q1–2wk. Maintenance:
15–20 mcg/day.
▸ **Congenital Hypothyroidism**
PO
Children. Initially, 5 mcg/day.
Increase by 5 mcg/day q3–4 days.
Maintenance: Full adult dosage
(children older than 3 yr); 50 mcg/day
(children 1–3 yr); 20 mcg/day
(infants).
▸ **T3 suppression Test**
PO
Adults, Elderly. 75–100 mcg/day for
7 days; then repeat I131 thyroid
uptake test.
▸ **Myxedema Coma, Precoma**
IV
Adults, Elderly. Initially, 25–50 mcg
(10–20 mcg in patients with
cardiovascular disease). Total dose at
least 65 mcg/day.

SIDE EFFECTS/ADVERSE REACTIONS
Occasional
Reversible hair loss at start of
therapy (in children)
Rare
Dry skin, GI intolerance, rash, hives,
pseudotumor cerebri or severe
headache in children

PRECAUTIONS AND CONTRAINDICATIONS
MI and thyrotoxicosis uncomplicated
by hypothyroidism; obesity
Caution
Elderly, angina pectoris,
hypertension, ischemia, cardiac
disease, lactation

DRUG INTERACTIONS OF CONCERN TO DENTISTRY
• Hypertension, tachycardia:
ketamine

• Increased effects of
sympathomimetics when thyroid doses
are not carefully monitored or in
patients with coronary artery disease

SERIOUS REACTIONS
! Excessive dosage produces signs
and symptoms of hyperthyroidism,
including weight loss, palpitations,
increased appetite, tremors, nervousness,
tachycardia, hypertension, headache,
insomnia, and menstrual irregularities.
! Cardiac arrhythmias occur rarely.

DENTAL CONSIDERATIONS
General:
• Patients with uncontrolled
hypothyroidism may be more
responsive to CNS depressants.
• Increased nervousness, excitability,
sweating, or tachycardia may indicate
a patient with uncontrolled
hyperthyroidism or a dose of
medication that is too high.
Uncontrolled patients should be
referred for medical treatment.
Consultations:
• Medical consultation may be
required to assess disease control.
• Observe appropriate limitations of
vasoconstrictor doses.

liotrix
lye´-oh-trix
(Thyrolar, Thyrolar-1, Thyrolar-1/2,
Thyrolar-1/4, Thyrolar-2,
Thyrolar-3)

CATEGORY AND SCHEDULE
Pregnancy Risk Category: A

Drug Class: Thyroid hormone

MECHANISM OF ACTION
A synthetic form of levothyroxine
(T4) and triiodothyronine (T3)

involved in normal metabolism, growth, and development, especially the CNS of infants. Possesses catabolic and anabolic effects. *Therapeutic Effect:* Increases basal metabolic rate, enhances gluconeogenesis, stimulates protein synthesis.

USES

Treatment of hypothyroidism, thyroid hormone replacement, thyroiditis, euthyroid goiter

PHARMACOKINETICS

T4 is partially absorbed from the GI tract. T3 is almost completely absorbed. Widely distributed. Deiodinated in peripheral tissues, minimal metabolism in the liver. *Half-life:* Unknown.

INDICATIONS AND DOSAGES
▶ **Hypothyroidism**
PO
Adults, Elderly. Initially, 50 mcg (0.05 mg) levothyroxine and 12.5 mcg (0.0125 mg) liothyronine per day, with increments of a like amount at monthly intervals until the desired result is obtained. Maintenance: 50–100 mcg (0.05–0.1 mg) levothyroxine and 12.5–25 mcg (0.0125–0.025 mg) liothyronine per day.
▶ **Congenital Hypothyroidism**
PO
Children older than 12 yr. More than 150 mcg of levothyroxine per day.
Children 6–12 yr. 100–150 mcg of levothyroxine per day.
Children 1–5 yr. 75–100 mcg of levothyroxine per day.
Children 6–12 mo. 50–75 mcg of levothyroxine per day.
Children 0–6 mo. 25–50 mcg of levothyroxine per day.

▶ **Myxedema**
PO
Adults, Elderly. Initially, 12.5 mcg (0.0125 mg) levothyroxine and 3.1 mcg (0.0031 mg) liothyronine per day, with increments of a like amount q2–3wk until the desired result is obtained. Maintenance: 50–100 mcg (0.05–0.1 mg) levothyroxine and 12.5–25 mcg (0.0125–0.025 mg) liothyronine per day.
▶ **Thyroid Cancer**
PO
Adults, Elderly. Larger amounts of thyroid hormone than those used for replacement therapy are required.
▶ **Thyroid Suppression Therapy**
PO
Adults, Elderly. Usual dosage of levothyroxine 2.6 mcg/kg/day for 7–10 days.

SIDE EFFECTS/ADVERSE REACTIONS
Occasional
Reversible hair loss at the start of therapy (in children)
Rare
Dry skin, GI intolerance, rash, hives, pseudotumor cerebri or severe headache in children

PRECAUTIONS AND CONTRAINDICATIONS
Uncorrected adrenal cortical insufficiency, untreated thyrotoxicosis, or hypersensitivity to any of active constituents
Caution
Elderly, angina pectoris, hypertension, ischemia, cardiac disease, lactation

DRUG INTERACTIONS OF CONCERN TO DENTISTRY
• Hypertension, tachycardia: ketamine
• Increased effects of sympathomimetics when thyroid doses are not carefully monitored or in patients with coronary artery disease

SERIOUS REACTIONS
! Excessive dosage produces signs and symptoms of hyperthyroidism, including weight loss, palpitations, increased appetite, tremors, nervousness, tachycardia, hypertension, headache, insomnia, menstrual irregularities.
! Cardiac arrhythmias occur rarely.

DENTAL CONSIDERATIONS
General:
• Patients with uncontrolled hypothyroidism may be more responsive to CNS depressants.
• Increased nervousness, excitability, sweating, or tachycardia may indicate a patient with uncontrolled hyperthyroidism or a dose of medication that is too high. Uncontrolled patients should be referred for medical treatment.
• Observe appropriate limitations of vasoconstrictor doses.
Consultations:
• Medical consultation may be required to assess disease control.
Teach Patient/Family to:
• Use effective oral hygiene to prevent soft tissue inflammation
• Avoid mouth rinses with high alcohol content because of drying effects

lisinopril
lye-sin´-oh-pril
(Apo-Lisinopril[CAN], Fibsol[AUS], Lisodur[AUS], Prinivil, Zestril)
Do not confuse lisinopril with fosinopril; Prinivil with Desyrel, Plendil, Proventil, or Restoril; Fibsol with Lioresal; or Zestril with Zostrix. Do not confuse lisinopril's combination form Zestoretic with Prilosec.

CATEGORY AND SCHEDULE
Pregnancy Risk Category: C (D if used in second or third trimester)

Drug Class: Angiotensin-converting enzyme (ACE) inhibitor

MECHANISM OF ACTION
This ACE inhibitor suppresses the renin-angiotensin-aldosterone system and prevents conversion of angiotensin I to angiotensin II, a potent vasoconstrictor; may also inhibit angiotensin II at local vascular and renal sites. Decreases plasma angiotensin II, increases plasma renin activity, and decreases aldosterone secretion. *Therapeutic Effect:* Reduces peripheral arterial resistance, B/P, afterload, pulmonary capillary wedge pressure (preload), and pulmonary vascular resistance. In those with heart failure, also decreases heart size, increases cardiac output, and exercise tolerance time.

USES
Treatment of mild-to-moderate hypertension, post-MI if hemodynamically stable, heart failure

PHARMACOKINETICS

Route	Onset	Peak	Duration
PO	1 hr	6 hr	24 hr

Incompletely absorbed from the GI tract. Protein binding: 25%. Primarily excreted unchanged in urine. Removed by hemodialysis. *Half-life:* 12 hr (half-life is prolonged in those with impaired renal function).

INDICATIONS AND DOSAGES
▶ **Hypertension (used alone)**
PO
Adults. Initially, 10 mg/day. May increase by 5–10 mcg/day at 1- to 2-wk intervals. Maximum: 40 mg/day.
Elderly. Initially, 2.5–5 mg/day. May increase by 2.5–5 mg/day at 1- to 2-wk intervals. Maximum: 40 mg/day.
▶ **Hypertension (used in combination with other antihypertensives)**
PO
Adults. Initially, 2.5–5 mg/day titrated to patient's needs.
▶ **Adjunctive Therapy for Management of Heart Failure**
PO
Adults, Elderly. Initially, 2.5–5 mg/day. May increase by no more than 10 mg/day at intervals of at least 2 wk. Maintenance: 5–40 mg/day.
▶ **Improve Survival in Patients after an MI**
PO
Adults, Elderly. Initially, 5 mg, then 5 mg after 24 hr, 10 mg after 48 hr, then 10 mg/day for 6 wk. For patients with low systolic B/P, give 2.5 mg/day for 3 days, then 2.5–5 mg/day.

▶ **Dosage in Renal Impairment**
Titrate to patient's needs after giving the following initial dose:

Creatinine Clearance	% Normal Dose
10–50 ml/min	50–75
Less than 10 ml/min	25–50

SIDE EFFECTS/ADVERSE REACTIONS
Frequent
Headache, dizziness, postural hypotension
Occasional
Chest discomfort, fatigue, rash, abdominal pain, nausea, diarrhea, upper respiratory infection
Rare
Palpitations, tachycardia, peripheral edema, insomnia, paresthesia, confusion, constipation, dry mouth, muscle cramps

PRECAUTIONS AND CONTRAINDICATIONS
History of angioedema from previous treatment with ACE inhibitors
Caution
Lactation, renal disease, hyperkalemia

DRUG INTERACTIONS OF CONCERN TO DENTISTRY
• Increased hypotension: alcohol, phenothiazines
• Decreased hypotensive effects: indomethacin and possibly other NSAIDs, sympathomimetics
• Suspected reduction in the antihypertensive and vasodilator effects by salicylates; monitor B/P if used concurrently

SERIOUS REACTIONS
! Excessive hypotension ("first-dose syncope") may occur in patients with

CHF and severe salt and volume depletion.

❗ Angioedema (swelling of face and lips) and hyperkalemia occurs rarely.

❗ Agranulocytosis and neutropenia may be noted in patients with collagen vascular disease, including scleroderma and systemic lupus erythematosus, and impaired renal function.

❗ Nephrotic syndrome may be noted in patients with history of renal disease.

DENTAL CONSIDERATIONS

General:
• Monitor vital signs at every appointment because of cardiovascular and respiratory side effects.
• After supine positioning, have patient sit upright for at least 2 min before standing to avoid orthostatic hypotension.
• Patients on chronic drug therapy may rarely have symptoms of blood dyscrasias, which can include infection, bleeding, and poor healing.
• Assess salivary flow as a factor in caries, periodontal disease, and candidiasis.
• Limit use of sodium-containing products, such as saline IV fluids, for patients with a dietary salt restriction.
• Use vasoconstrictors with caution, in low doses, and with careful aspiration.
• Short appointments and a stress-reduction protocol may be required for anxious patients.

Consultations:
• Medical consultation may be required to assess disease control and patient's ability to tolerate stress.
• In a patient with symptoms of blood dyscrasias, request a medical consultation for blood studies and

postpone dental treatment until normal values are reestablished.
• Take precautions if dental surgery is anticipated and sedation or general anesthesia is required; risk of hypotensive episode.

Teach Patient/Family to:
• Use effective oral hygiene to prevent soft tissue inflammation
• Use caution to prevent injury when using oral hygiene aids
• When chronic dry mouth occurs, advise patient to:
  • Avoid mouth rinses with high alcohol content because of drying effects
  • Use sugarless gum, frequent sips of water, or saliva substitutes
  • Use daily home fluoride products for anticaries effect

lithium carbonate/ lithium citrate

lith´-ee-um kahr´-buh-neyt/sit´-rayte lithium carbonate (Duralith[CAN], Eskalith, Lithi.carb[AUS], Lithobid, Quilonum SR[AUS]) lithium citrate (Cibalith-S)
Do not confuse Lithobid with Levbid, Lithostat, or Lithotabs.

CATEGORY AND SCHEDULE
Pregnancy Risk Category: D

Drug Class: Antimanic, inorganic salt

MECHANISM OF ACTION
A psychotherapeutic agent that affects the storage, release, and reuptake of neurotransmitters. Antimanic effect may result from increased norepinephrine reuptake

and serotonin receptor sensitivity. *Therapeutic Effect:* Produces antimanic and antidepressant effects.

USES
Treatment of manic-depressive illness (manic phase), prevention of bipolar manic depressive psychosis

PHARMACOKINETICS
Rapidly and completely absorbed from the GI tract. Primarily excreted unchanged in urine. Removed by hemodialysis. *Half-life:* 18–24 hr (increased in elderly).

INDICATIONS AND DOSAGES
ALERT
During acute phase, a therapeutic serum lithium concentration of 1–1.4 mEq/L is required. For long-term control, the desired level is 0.5–1.3 mEq/L. Monitor serum drug concentration and clinical response.
▸ **Prevention or Treatment of Acute Mania, Manic Phase of Bipolar Disorder (manic-depressive illness)**
PO
Adults. 300 mg 3–4 times a day or 450–900 mg slow-release form twice a day. Maximum: 2.4 g/day.
Elderly. 300 mg twice a day. May increase by 300 mg/day q1wk. Maintenance: 900–1200 mg/day.
Children 12 yr and older. 600–1800 mg/day in 3–4 divided doses (2 doses/day for slow-release).
Children younger than 12 yr. 15–60 mg/kg/day in 3–4 divided doses.

SIDE EFFECTS/ADVERSE REACTIONS
Occasional
Fine hand tremor, polydipsia, polyuria, mild nausea, dry mouth
Rare
Weight gain, bradycardia or tachycardia, acne, rash, muscle twitching, cold and cyanotic extremities, pseudotumor cerebri (eye pain, headache, tinnitus, vision disturbances)

PRECAUTIONS AND CONTRAINDICATIONS
Debilitated patients, severe cardiovascular disease, severe dehydration, severe renal disease, severe sodium depletion
Caution
Elderly, thyroid disease, seizure disorders, diabetes mellitus, systemic infection, urinary retention

DRUG INTERACTIONS OF CONCERN TO DENTISTRY
• Increased toxicity: aspirin, indomethacin, other NSAIDs, haloperidol, metronidazole, carbamazepine
• Increased effects of neuromuscular blocking agents

SERIOUS REACTIONS
❗ A lithium serum concentration of 1.5–2.0 mEq/L may produce vomiting, diarrhea, drowsiness, confusion, incoordination, coarse hand tremor, muscle twitching, and T-wave depression on ECG.
❗ A lithium serum concentration of 2.0–2.5 mEq/L may result in ataxia, giddiness, tinnitus, blurred vision, clonic movements, and severe hypotension.
❗ Acute toxicity may be characterized by seizures, oliguria, circulatory failure, coma, and death.

DENTAL CONSIDERATIONS
General:
• Assess salivary flow as a factor in caries, periodontal disease, and candidiasis.
• After supine positioning, have patient sit upright for at least 2 min

before standing to avoid orthostatic hypotension.
Consultations:
• Medical consultation may be required to assess disease control.
Teach Patient/Family to:
• Use effective oral hygiene to prevent soft tissue inflammation
• Use caution to prevent injury when using oral hygiene aids
• When chronic dry mouth occurs, advise patient to:
 • Avoid mouth rinses with high alcohol content because of drying effects
 • Use sugarless gum, frequent sips of water, or saliva substitutes
 • Use daily home fluoride products for anticaries effect

lodoxamide
loe-dox´-ah-mide
(Alomide)

CATEGORY AND SCHEDULE
Pregnancy Risk Category: B

Drug Class: Mast cell stabilizer

MECHANISM OF ACTION
A mast cell stabilizer that prevents increase in cutaneous vascular permeability, antigen-stimulated histamine release, and may prevent calcium influx into mast cells. *Therapeutic Effect:* Inhibits sensitivity reaction.

USES
Treatment of vernal keratoconjunctivitis, vernal conjunctivitis, keratitis

PHARMACOKINETICS
Non-detectable absorption.
Half-life: 8.5 hr.

INDICATIONS AND DOSAGES
▶ Treatment of Vernal Keratoconjunctivitis, Conjunctivitis, and Keratitis
Ophthalmic
Adults, Elderly, Children 2 yr or older. 1–2 drops 4 times a day, for up to 3 mo.

SIDE EFFECTS/ADVERSE REACTIONS
Frequent
Transient stinging, burning, instillation discomfort
Occasional
Ocular itching, blurred vision, dry eye, tearing/discharge/foreign body sensation, headache, dry mouth
Rare
Scales on lid/lash, ocular swelling, sticky sensation, dizziness, somnolence, nausea, sneezing, dry nose, rash

PRECAUTIONS AND CONTRAINDICATIONS
Wearing soft contact lenses (product contains benzalkonium chloride), hypersensitivity to lodoxamide tromethamine or any component of the formulation
Caution
Children younger than 2 yr, lactation

DRUG INTERACTIONS OF CONCERN TO DENTISTRY
None reported

SERIOUS REACTIONS
None reported

DENTAL CONSIDERATIONS
General:
• Question patient about history of allergy to avoid use of other potential allergens.

- Avoid dental light in patient's eyes; offer dark glasses for patient comfort.
- Use for less than 2 wk should not present a problem with dry mouth.

Teach Patient/Family:
- When chronic dry mouth occurs advise patient to:
  - Avoid mouth rinses with high alcohol content due to drying effects
  - Use daily home fluoride products for anticaries effect
  - Use sugarless gum, frequent sips of water, or saliva substitutes

lomefloxacin hydrochloride

low-meh-flocks´-ah-sin high-droh-klor´-ide (Maxaquin)

CATEGORY AND SCHEDULE

Pregnancy Risk Category: C

Drug Class: Fluoroquinolone antiinfective

MECHANISM OF ACTION

A quinolone that inhibits the enzyme DNA gyrase in susceptible microorganisms, interfering with bacterial cell replication and repair. **Therapeutic Effect:** Bactericidal.

USES

Treatment of lower respiratory tract infections (pneumonia, bronchitis); GU infections (prostatitis, UTIs); preoperatively to reduce UTIs in transurethral and transrectal surgical procedures caused by susceptible gram-negative organisms

PHARMACOKINETICS

Well absorbed from the GI tract. Protein binding: 10%. Widely distributed. Metabolized in the liver. Primarily excreted in urine. Not removed by hemodialysis. **Half-life:** 4–6 hr (increased with impaired renal function and in the elderly).

INDICATIONS AND DOSAGES
▸ **Complicated UTIs**
PO
Adults, Elderly. 400 mg/day for 10–14 days.
▸ **Uncomplicated UTIs**
PO
Adults (Females). 400 mg/day for 3 days.
▸ **Lower Respiratory Tract Infections**
PO
Adults, Elderly. 400 mg/day for 10 days.
▸ **Surgical Prophylaxis**
PO
Adults, Elderly. 400 mg 2–6 hr before surgery.
▸ **Dosage in Renal Impairment**
Dosage and frequency are modified on the basis of creatinine clearance.

Creatinine Clearance	Dosage
41 ml/min and higher	No change
10–40 ml/min	400 mg initially, then 200 mg/day for 10–14 days

SIDE EFFECTS/ADVERSE REACTIONS

Occasional
Nausea, headache, photosensitivity, dizziness
Rare
Diarrhea

PRECAUTIONS AND CONTRAINDICATIONS

Hypersensitivity to quinolones.

Caution
Lactation, children, elderly, renal disease, seizure disorders, excessive sunlight; tendon rupture in shoulder, hand, and Achilles tendons

DRUG INTERACTIONS OF CONCERN TO DENTISTRY
• Decreased effects: antacids
• Increased levels of cyclosporine, caffeine

SERIOUS REACTIONS
! Antibiotic-associated colitis and other superinfections may result from altered bacterial balance.
! Hypersensitivity reactions, including photosensitivity (as evidenced by rash, pruritus, blisters, edema, and burning skin), have occurred in patients receiving fluoroquinolones.
! Arthropathy may occur if the drug is given to children younger than 18 yr.

DENTAL CONSIDERATIONS
General:
• Because of drug interactions, do not use ingestible sodium bicarbonate products, such as the Prophy-Jet air polishing system, until 2 hr after drug use.
• Use caution in prescribing caffeine-containing analgesics.
• Determine why the patient is taking the drug.
• Avoid dental light in patient's eyes; offer dark glasses for patient comfort.
• Ruptures of the shoulder, hand, and Achilles tendons that required surgical repair or resulted in prolonged disability have been reported with this drug.
Consultations:
• Consult with patient's physician if an acute dental infection occurs and another antiinfective is required.

Teach Patient/Family to:
• Use caution to prevent injury when using oral hygiene aids
• Avoid mouth rinses with high alcohol content because of drying effects
• Minimize exposure to sunlight and wear sunscreen if sun exposure is planned
• Discontinue treatment and inform dentist immediately if patient experiences pain or inflammation of a tendon, and to rest and refrain from exercise

lomustine
low-meuw´-steen
(CeeNU)

CATEGORY AND SCHEDULE
Pregnancy Risk Category: D

L

Drug Class: Antineoplastic alkylating agent

MECHANISM OF ACTION
An alkylating agent and nitrosourea that inhibits DNA and RNA protein synthesis by cross-linking with DNA and RNA strands, preventing cell division. Cell cycle-phase nonspecific. *Therapeutic Effect:* Interferes with DNA and RNA function.

USES
Treatment of Hodgkin's disease; lymphomas; melanomas; multiple myeloma; brain, lung, bladder, kidney, colon cancer

PHARMACOKINETICS
PO: Well absorbed. *Half-life:* 16–48 hr; 50% protein bound; metabolized in liver; excreted in

urine; crosses blood-brain barrier; excreted in breast milk.

INDICATIONS AND DOSAGES
▶ **Disseminated Hodgkin's Disease, Primary and Metastatic Brain Tumors**
PO
Adults, Elderly. 100–130 mg/m^2 as single dose. Repeat dose at intervals of at least 6 wk but not until circulating blood elements have returned to acceptable levels. Adjust dose on the basis of hematologic response to previous dose.
Children. 75–150 mg/m^2 as a single dose every 6 wk.

SIDE EFFECTS/ADVERSE REACTIONS
Frequent
Nausea, vomiting (occurring 45 min–6 hr after dose and lasting 12–24 hr); anorexia (often follows for 2–3 days)
Occasional
Neurotoxicity (confusion, slurred speech), stomatitis, darkening of skin, diarrhea, rash, pruritus, alopecia

PRECAUTIONS AND CONTRAINDICATIONS
Pregnancy
Caution
Radiation therapy, geriatric patient, lactation

DRUG INTERACTIONS OF CONCERN TO DENTISTRY
• This drug depresses bone marrow function, which may increase risk of bleeding; avoid drugs that can increase bleeding, such as aspirin, NSAIDs

SERIOUS REACTIONS
! Myelosuppression may result in hematologic toxicity, manifested principally as leukopenia, mild anemia, and thrombocytopenia. Leukopenia occurs about 6 wk after a dose, thrombocytopenia about 4 wk after a dose; both persist for 1–2 wk.
! Refractory anemia and thrombocytopenia occur commonly if lomustine therapy continues for more than 1 yr.
! Hepatotoxicity occurs infrequently.
! Large cumulative doses of lomustine may result in renal damage.

DENTAL CONSIDERATIONS
General:
• Patients on chronic drug therapy may rarely have symptoms of blood dyscrasias, which can include infection, bleeding, and poor healing.
• Consider semisupine chair position for patient comfort if GI side effects occur.
• Palliative medication may be required for oral side effects.
• Consider local hemostasis measures to prevent excessive bleeding.
• Prophylactic antibiotics may be indicated to prevent infection if surgery or deep scaling is planned.
• Patients taking opioids for acute or chronic pain should be given alternative analgesics for dental pain.
• Avoid prescribing aspirin-containing products.
Consultations:
• In a patient with symptoms of blood dyscrasias, request a medical consultation for blood studies and postpone dental treatment until normal values are reestablished.
• Patients on cancer chemotherapy should have an adequate WBC count before completing dental procedures that may produce a wound. Consult to determine blood count before appointment.

Teach Patient/Family to:
• Use effective oral hygiene to prevent soft tissue inflammation
• Use caution to prevent trauma when using oral hygiene aids
• See dentist immediately if secondary oral infection occurs
• Report oral lesions, soreness, or bleeding to dentist
• Avoid mouth rinses with high alcohol content because of drying and irritating effects
• Update medical/drug records if physician makes any changes in evaluation or drug regimens; include OTC, herbal, and nonherbal drugs in the update

loperamide hydrochloride
loe-per´-ah-mide
high-droh-klor´-ide
(Apo-Loperamide[CAN], Gastro-Stop[AUS], Imodium, Imodium A-D, Loperacap[CAN], Novo-Loperamide[CAN])
Do not confuse Imodium with Indocin or Ionamin.

CATEGORY AND SCHEDULE
Pregnancy Risk Category: B
OTC liquid, tablets

Drug Class: Antidiarrheal (opioid)

MECHANISM OF ACTION
An antidiarrheal that directly affects the intestinal wall muscles.
Therapeutic Effect: Slows intestinal motility and prolongs transit time of intestinal contents by reducing fecal volume, diminishing loss of fluid and electrolytes, and increasing viscosity and bulk of stool.

USES
Treatment of diarrhea (cause undetermined), chronic diarrhea, ileostomy discharge

PHARMACOKINETICS
Poorly absorbed from the GI tract. Protein binding: 97%. Metabolized in the liver. Eliminated in feces and excreted in urine. Not removed by hemodialysis. **Half-life:** 9.1–14.4 hr.

INDICATIONS AND DOSAGES
▸ **Acute Diarrhea**
PO (capsules)
Adults, Elderly. Initially, 4 mg; then 2 mg after each unformed stool. Maximum: 16 mg/day.
Children 9–12 yr, weighing more than 30 kg. Initially, 2 mg 3 times a day for 24 hr.
Children 6–8 yr, weighing 20–30 kg. Initially, 2 mg twice a day for 24 hr.
Children 2–5 yr, weighing 13–20 kg. Initially, 1 mg 3 times a day for 24 hr. Maintenance: 1 mg/10 kg only after loose stool.
▸ **Chronic Diarrhea**
PO
Adults, Elderly. Initially, 4 mg; then 2 mg after each unformed stool until diarrhea is controlled.
Children. 0.08–0.24 mg/kg/day in 2–3 divided doses. Maximum: 2 mg/dose.
▸ **Traveler's Diarrhea**
PO
Adults, Elderly. Initially, 4 mg; then 2 mg after each loose bowel movement (LBM). Maximum: 8 mg/day for 2 days.
Children 9–11 yr. Initially, 2 mg; then 1 mg after each LBM. Maximum: 6 mg/day for 2 days.
Children 6–8 yr. Initially, 1 mg; then 1 mg after each LBM. Maximum: 4 mg/day for 2 days.

SIDE EFFECTS/ADVERSE REACTIONS
Frequent
Dry mouth
Rare
Somnolence, abdominal discomfort, allergic reaction (such as rash and itching)

PRECAUTIONS AND CONTRAINDICATIONS
Acute ulcerative colitis (may produce toxic megacolon), diarrhea associated with pseudomembranous enterocolitis due to broad-spectrum antibiotics or to organisms that invade intestinal mucosa (such as *Escherichia coli*, shigella, and salmonella), patients who must avoid constipation
Caution
Lactation, children younger than 2 yr, liver disease, dehydration, bacterial disease

DRUG INTERACTIONS OF CONCERN TO DENTISTRY
• Increased action: opioid analgesics

SERIOUS REACTIONS
! Toxicity results in constipation, GI irritation, including nausea and vomiting, and CNS depression. Activated charcoal is used to treat loperamide toxicity.

DENTAL CONSIDERATIONS
General:
• Assess salivary flow as a factor in caries, periodontal disease, and candidiasis.
• Evaluate respiration characteristics and rate.
• Consider semisupine chair position for patient comfort because of GI effects of drug.
• This drug product is normally used only for a few doses for acute problems; however, some patients may have to take it for longer time periods as dictated by contributing disease.
Teach Patient/Family:
• When chronic dry mouth occurs, advise patient to:
  • Avoid mouth rinses with high alcohol content because of drying effects
  • Use sugarless gum, frequent sips of water, or saliva substitutes
  • Use daily home fluoride products for anticaries effect

loracarbef
lor-ah-kar´-bef
(Lorabid)
Do not confuse loracarbef or Lorabid with Lortab.

CATEGORY AND SCHEDULE
Pregnancy Risk Category: B

Drug Class: Antibiotic, second-generation cephalosporin

MECHANISM OF ACTION
A second-generation cephalosporin that binds to bacterial cell membranes and inhibits cell wall synthesis. *Therapeutic Effect:* Bactericidal.

USES
Treatment of gram-negative organisms: *H. influenzae, E. coli, P. mirabilis*, Klebsiella; gram-positive organisms: *S. pneumoniae, S. pyogenes, S. aureus;* upper/lower respiratory tract infection, acute maxillary sinusitis, pharyngitis, tonsillitis; urinary tract and skin infections; otitis media; some in vitro activity against anaerobes

PHARMACOKINETICS
Peak 1 hr. *Half-life:* 1 hr; excreted in urine as unchanged drug

INDICATIONS AND DOSAGES
▶ **Bronchitis**
PO
Adults, Elderly, Children 12 yr and older. 200–400 mg q12h for 7 days.
▶ **Pharyngitis**
PO
Adults, Elderly, Children 12 yr and older. 200 mg q12h for 10 days.
Children 6 mo–11 yr. 7.5 mg/kg q12h for 10 days.
▶ **Pneumonia**
PO
Adults, Elderly, Children 12 yr and older. 400 mg q12h for 14 days.
▶ **Sinusitis**
PO
Adults, Elderly, Children 12 yr and older. 400 mg q12h for 10 days.
Children 6 mo–11 yr. 15 mg/kg q12h for 10 days.
▶ **Skin and Soft-Tissue Infections**
PO
Adults, Elderly, Children 12 yr and older. 200 mg q12h for 7 days.
Children 6 mo–11 yr. 7.5 mg/kg q12h for 7 days.
▶ **UTIs**
PO
Adults, Elderly, Children 6 mo–12 yr. 200–400 mg q12h for 7–14 days.
▶ **Otitis Media**
PO
Children 6 mo–12 yr. 15 mg/kg q12h for 10 days.

SIDE EFFECTS/ADVERSE REACTIONS
Frequent
Abdominal pain, anorexia, nausea, vomiting, diarrhea
Occasional
Rash, pruritus

Rare
Dizziness, headache, vaginitis

PRECAUTIONS AND CONTRAINDICATIONS
History of anaphylactic reaction to penicillins or hypersensitivity to cephalosporins
Caution
Lactation, children, renal disease

DRUG INTERACTIONS OF CONCERN TO DENTISTRY
• Decreased effects: tetracyclines, erythromycins, lincomycins
• When used for dental infection: potential low risk to reduce effect of oral contraceptives

SERIOUS REACTIONS
! Antibiotic-associated colitis and other superinfections may result from altered bacterial balance.
! Hypersensitivity reactions (ranging from rash, urticaria, and fever to anaphylaxis) occur in less than 5% of patients—most commonly in patients with a history of drug allergies, especially to penicillins.

DENTAL CONSIDERATIONS
General:
• Take precautions regarding allergy to medication.
• Determine why the patient is taking the drug.
• Examine for evidence of oral manifestations of blood dyscrasias (infection, bleeding, poor healing).
Consultations:
• Medical consultation may be required to assess disease control.
• Medical consultation for blood studies (CBC); leukopenic or thrombocytopenic side effects may result in infection, delayed healing, and excessive bleeding. Postpone

elective dental treatment until normal values are maintained.

Teach Patient/Family to:
• Use effective oral hygiene to prevent soft tissue inflammation

loratadine
lore-at´-ah-deen
(Alavert, Claratyne[AUS], Claritin, Claritin RediTab, Dimetapp, Tavist ND)

CATEGORY AND SCHEDULE
Pregnancy Risk Category: B

Drug Class: Antihistamine, H_1 histamine antagonist

MECHANISM OF ACTION
A long-acting antihistamine that competes with histamine for H_1 receptor sites on effector cells. *Therapeutic Effect:* Prevents allergic responses mediated by histamine, such as rhinitis, urticaria, and pruritus.

USES
Treatment of seasonal allergic rhinitis, idiopathic chronic urticaria

PHARMACOKINETICS

Route	Onset	Peak	Duration
PO	1–3 hr	8–12 hr	Longer than 24 hr

Rapidly and almost completely absorbed from the GI tract. Protein binding: 97%; metabolite, 73%–77%. Distributed mainly to the liver, lungs, GI tract, and bile. Metabolized in the liver to active metabolite; undergoes extensive first-pass metabolism. Eliminated in urine and feces. Not removed by hemodialysis.

Half-life: 8.4 hr; metabolite, 28 hr (increased in elderly and hepatic impairment).

INDICATIONS AND DOSAGES
▸ **Allergic Rhinitis, Urticaria**
PO
Adults, Elderly, Children 6 yr and older. 10 mg once a day.
Children 2–5 yr. 5 mg once a day.
▸ **Dosage in Hepatic Impairment**
For adults, elderly, and children 6 yr and older dosage is reduced to 10 mg every other day.

SIDE EFFECTS/ADVERSE REACTIONS
Frequent
Headache, fatigue, somnolence
Occasional
Dry mouth, nose, or throat
Rare
Photosensitivity

PRECAUTIONS AND CONTRAINDICATIONS
Hypersensitivity to loratadine or its ingredients
Caution
Increased intraocular pressure, bronchial asthma, patients at risk for syncope or drowsiness, reduce dose in renal impairment to every other day

DRUG INTERACTIONS OF CONCERN TO DENTISTRY
• Increased CNS depression: all CNS depressants, alcohol
• Increased anticholinergic effect: anticholinergics, antihistamines, antiparkinsonian drugs
• Increased plasma concentration: ketoconazole

SERIOUS REACTIONS
None known

DENTAL CONSIDERATIONS
General:
• Assess salivary flow as a factor in caries, periodontal disease, and candidiasis.
• Consider semisupine chair position for patients with respiratory disease.
• Conscious sedation drugs may produce synergistic, sedative action.
Teach Patient/Family to:
• Use effective oral hygiene to prevent soft tissue inflammation
• When chronic dry mouth occurs, advise patient to:
  • Avoid mouth rinses with high alcohol content because of drying effects
  • Use sugarless gum, frequent sips of water, or saliva substitutes
  • Use daily home fluoride products for anticaries effect

lorazepam
lor-ah´-zeh-pam
(Apo-Lorazepam[CAN], Ativan, Lorazepam Intensol, Novolorazepam[CAN])
Do not confuse lorazepam with Alprazolam.

CATEGORY AND SCHEDULE
Pregnancy Risk Category: D
Controlled Substance Schedule: IV

Drug Class: Benzodiazepine, antianxiety

MECHANISM OF ACTION
A benzodiazepine that enhances the action of the inhibitory neurotransmitter gamma-aminobutyric acid in the CNS, affecting memory, as well as motor, sensory, and cognitive function.
Therapeutic Effect: Produces anxiolytic, anticonvulsant, sedative,

muscle relaxant, and antiemetic effects.

USES
Treatment of anxiety, preoperatively in sedation, acute alcohol withdrawal symptoms, muscle spasm

PHARMACOKINETICS

Route	Onset	Peak	Duration
PO	60 min	N/A	8–12 hr
IV	15–30 min	N/A	8–12 hr
IM	30–60 min	N/A	8–12 hr

Well absorbed after PO and IM administration. Protein binding: 85%. Widely distributed. Metabolized in the liver. Primarily excreted in urine. Not removed by hemodialysis. *Half-life:* 10–20 hr.

INDICATIONS AND DOSAGES
▶ **Anxiety**
PO
Adults. 1–10 mg/day in 2–3 divided doses. Average: 2–6 mg/day.
Elderly. Initially, 0.5–1 mg/day. May increase gradually. Range: 0.5–4 mg.
IV
Adults, Elderly. 0.02–0.06 mg/kg q2–6h.
IV Infusion
Adults, Elderly. 0.01–0.1 mg/kg/h.
PO, IV
Children. 0.05 mg/kg/dose q4–8h. Range: 0.02–0.1 mg/kg. Maximum: 2 mg/dose.
▶ **Insomnia Due to Anxiety**
PO
Adults. 2–4 mg at bedtime.
Elderly. 0.5–1 mg at bedtime.
▶ **Preoperative Sedation**
IV
Adults, Elderly. 0.044 mg/kg 15–20 min before surgery. Maximum total dose: 2 mg.

IM
Adults, Elderly. 0.05 mg/kg 2 hr before procedure. Maximum total dose: 4 mg.

▸ **Status Epilepticus**
IV
Adults, Elderly. 4 mg over 2–5 min. May repeat in 10–15 min. Maximum: 8 mg in 12-hr period.
Children. 0.1 mg/kg over 2–5 min. May give second dose of 0.05 mg/kg in 15–20 min. Maximum: 4 mg.
Neonates. 0.05 mg/kg. May repeat in 10–15 min.

SIDE EFFECTS/ADVERSE REACTIONS
Frequent
Somnolence (initially in the morning), ataxia, confusion
Occasional
Blurred vision, slurred speech, hypotension, headache
Rare
Paradoxical CNS restlessness or excitement in elderly or debilitated

PRECAUTIONS AND CONTRAINDICATIONS
Angle-closure glaucoma; preexisting CNS depression; severe hypotension; severe uncontrolled pain
Caution
Elderly, debilitated, hepatic disease, renal disease, myasthenia gravis

DRUG INTERACTIONS OF CONCERN TO DENTISTRY
• Increased effects: alcohol, all CNS depressants, probenecid
• Increased sedation, hallucination: scopolamine
• Possible increase in CNS side effects of kava kava (herb)

SERIOUS REACTIONS
❗ Abrupt or too-rapid withdrawal may result in pronounced restlessness, irritability, insomnia, hand tremors, abdominal or muscle cramps, diaphoresis, vomiting, and seizures.
❗ Overdose results in somnolence, confusion, diminished reflexes, and coma.

DENTAL CONSIDERATIONS
General:
• After supine positioning, have patient sit upright for at least 2 min before standing to avoid orthostatic hypotension.
• Elderly persons are more prone to orthostatic hypotension and have increased sensitivity to anticholinergic and sedative effects; use lower dose.
• When administered with opioid analgesic, reduce dose of opioid by one third.
• Psychologic and physical dependence may occur with chronic administration.
• Have someone drive patient to and from dental office when drug used for conscious sedation.
Consultations:
• Medical consultation may be required to assess disease control.
Teach Patient/Family to:
• Use effective oral hygiene to prevent soft tissue inflammation
• Avoid mouth rinses with high alcohol content because of drying effects

losartan
lo-sar´-tan
(Cozaar)
Do not confuse Cozaar with Zocor.

CATEGORY AND SCHEDULE
Pregnancy Risk Category: C (D if used in second or third trimesters)

Drug Class: Angiotensin II receptor antagonist

MECHANISM OF ACTION

An angiotensin II receptor, type AT1, antagonist that blocks vasoconstrictor and aldosterone-secreting effects of angiotensin II, inhibiting the binding of angiotensin II to the AT1 receptors. *Therapeutic Effect:* Causes vasodilation, decreases peripheral resistance, and decreases B/P.

USES

Treatment of hypertension, as a single drug or in combination with other antihypertensives; for reduction of stroke risk in patients with hypertension and left ventricular hypertrophy; neuropathy in type 2 diabetes mellitus

PHARMACOKINETICS

Route	Onset	Peak	Duration
PO	N/A	6 hr	24 hr

Well absorbed after PO administration. Protein binding: 98%. Undergoes first-pass metabolism in the liver to active metabolites. Excreted in urine and via the biliary system. Not removed by hemodialysis. *Half-life:* 2 hr, metabolite: 6–9 hr.

INDICATIONS AND DOSAGES
▶ **Hypertension**
PO
Adults, Elderly. Initially, 50 mg once a day. Maximum: May be given once or twice a day, with total daily doses ranging from 25–100 mg.
▶ **Nephropathy**
PO
Adults, Elderly. Initially, 50 mg/day. May increase to 100 mg/day based on B/P response.
▶ **Stroke Reduction**
PO
Adults, Elderly. 50 mg/day. Maximum: 100 mg/day.

▶ **Hypertension in Patients with Impaired Hepatic Function**
PO
Adults, Elderly. Initially, 25 mg/day.

SIDE EFFECTS/ADVERSE REACTIONS
Frequent
Upper respiratory tract infection
Occasional
Dizziness, diarrhea, cough
Rare
Insomnia, dyspepsia, heartburn, back and leg pain, muscle cramps, myalgia, nasal congestion, sinusitis

PRECAUTIONS AND CONTRAINDICATIONS
Hypersensitivity, second or third trimester of pregnancy
Caution
Lactation, children, sodium-and volume-depleted patients, renal impairment.

DRUG INTERACTIONS OF CONCERN TO DENTISTRY
• Potential for increased hypotensive effects with other hypotensive drugs and sedatives
• Suspected increase in antihypertensive effects: fluconazole, ketoconazole; monitor B/P if used concurrently

SERIOUS REACTIONS
! Overdosage may manifest as hypotension and tachycardia. Bradycardia occurs less often.

DENTAL CONSIDERATIONS
General:
• Monitor vital signs at every appointment because of cardiovascular effects.
• Limit use of sodium-containing products, such as saline IV fluids, for

patients with a dietary salt restriction.
- Stress from dental procedures may compromise cardiovascular function; determine patient risk.
- Assess salivary flow as a factor in caries, periodontal disease, and candidiasis.
- Short appointments and a stress-reduction protocol may be required for anxious patients.
- Consider semisupine chair position for patient comfort because of respiratory side effects of drug.
- Use precaution if sedation or general anesthesia is required; risk of hypotensive episode.

Consultations:
- Medical consultation may be required to assess disease control and patient's ability to tolerate stress.

Teach Patient/Family to:
- Update health and drug history if physician makes any changes in evaluation or drug regimens; include OTC, herbal, and nonherbal drugs in the update
- When chronic dry mouth occurs, advise patient to:
  - Avoid mouth rinses with high alcohol content because of drying effects
  - Use daily home fluoride products for anticaries effect
  - Use sugarless gum, frequent sips of water, or saliva substitutes

loteprednol
loh-teh-pred´-nol
(Alrex, Lotemax)

CATEGORY AND SCHEDULE
Pregnancy Risk Category: C

Drug Class: Topical glucocorticoid

MECHANISM OF ACTION
A glucocorticoid that inhibits accumulation of inflammatory cells at inflammation sites, phagocytosis, lysosomal enzyme release and synthesis and/or release of mediators of inflammation. ***Therapeutic Effect:*** Prevents and suppresses cell and tissue immune reactions, inflammatory process.

USES
Treatment of steroid-responsive inflammation of the conjunctiva, cornea, and anterior segments of the globe associated with allergic conjunctivitis, acne rosacea, iritis, superficial punctate keratitis, and so on when topical steroid use is acceptable to reduce inflammation and edema, postoperative inflammation after ocular surgery (Lotemax 0.5%); temporary relief of symptoms of seasonal allergic conjunctivitis (Alrex 0.2%)

PHARMACOKINETICS
Metabolized by enzymes in the eye, minimizing systemic adverse effects.

INDICATIONS AND DOSAGES
▶ **Treatment of Seasonal Allergic Conjunctivitis, Giant Papillary Conjunctivitis, Ureitis**
Ophthalmic
Adults, Elderly. Instill 1 drop 4 times a day for 4–6 wk.

SIDE EFFECTS/ADVERSE REACTIONS
Frequent
Blurred vision
Occasional
Decreased vision, watering of eyes, eye pain, nausea, vomiting, burning, stinging, redness of eyes

PRECAUTIONS AND CONTRAINDICATIONS
Acute epithelial herpes simplex keratitis, fungal diseases of ocular

structures, vaccinia, varicella, ocular tuberculosis, hypersensitivity, after removal of corneal foreign body, mycobacterial eye infection, acute, purulent, untreated eye infection

Caution

Prolonged use may result in glaucoma, increased risk of secondary ocular infections, delayed healing after cataract surgery; avoid contamination of sterile container; lactation, safety in children not established

DRUG INTERACTIONS OF CONCERN TO DENTISTRY

None reported

SERIOUS REACTIONS

! Glaucoma with optic nerve damage, cataract formation, and secondary ocular infection occur rarely.

DENTAL CONSIDERATIONS

General:
• Avoid dental light in patient's eyes; offer dark glasses for patient comfort.
• Determine why patient is taking the drug.

loteprednol etabonate; tobramycin

loe-te-pred´-nol eh-tah-bone´-ayte; toe-bra-mye´-sin
(Zylet)

CATEGORY AND SCHEDULE

Pregnancy Risk Category: C

Drug Class: Corticosteroid, ophthalmic; antiinflammatory, steroidal, ophthalmic

MECHANISM OF ACTION

A combination ophthalmic product of an aminoglycoside and a glucocorticoid. Loteprednol is a glucocorticoid that inhibits accumulation of inflammatory cells at inflammation sites, phagocytosis, lysosomal enzyme release and synthesis, and/or release of mediators of inflammation. Tobramycin is an antibiotic that irreversibly binds to protein on bacterial ribosomes.

Therapeutic Effect: Prevents and suppresses cell and tissue immune reactions and inflammatory process. Interferes with protein synthesis of susceptible microorganisms.

USES

Treatment of inflammation of the eye, which may occur with certain eye problems or following eye surgery.

PHARMACOKINETICS

Limited systemic absorption.

INDICATIONS AND DOSAGES

▶ **Steroid-Responsive Inflammatory Ocular Conditions for Which a Corticosteroid Is Indicated and Where Superficial Bacterial Ocular Infection or a Risk of Bacterial Ocular Infection Exists**

Ophthalmic

Adults, Elderly. Apply 1 or 2 drops into the affected eye(s) q4–6h. During the initial 24–48 hr, the dosing may be increased to every 1–2 hr. Gradually decrease by improvement in clinical signs.

SIDE EFFECTS/ADVERSE REACTIONS

Frequent
Blurred vision
Occasional
Tearing, burning, itching, redness, swelling of eyelid, decreased vision, eye pain
Rare
Nausea, vomiting

PRECAUTIONS AND CONTRAINDICATIONS
Viral diseases of the cornea and conjunctiva including epithelial herpes simplex keratitis (dendritic keratitis), vaccinia, varicella, and mycobacterial infection of the eye and fungal diseases of ocular structures, hypersensitivity to any of loteprednol, tobramycin or any component of the formulation and to other corticosteroids

DRUG INTERACTIONS OF CONCERN TO DENTISTRY
None reported

SERIOUS REACTIONS
! Glaucoma with optic nerve damage, cataract formation, and secondary ocular infection occurs rarely.
! Secondary infection, especially fungal infections of the cornea, may occur after use of this medication. These infections are more frequent with long-term applications.

DENTAL CONSIDERATIONS
General:
• Avoid dental light in patient's eyes; offer dark glasses for patient comfort.
• Determine why patient is taking the drug.

lovastatin
lo´-va-sta-tin
(Altoprev, Lotrel, Mevacor)
Do not confuse lovastatin with Leustatin or Livostin, or Mevacor with Mivacron.

CATEGORY AND SCHEDULE
Pregnancy Risk Category: X

Drug Class: Cholesterol-lowering agent

MECHANISM OF ACTION
An antihyperlipidemic that inhibits HMG-CoA reductase, the enzyme that catalyzes the early step in cholesterol synthesis. **Therapeutic Effect:** Decreases low-density lipoproteins (LDL) cholesterol, very low-density lipoproteins (VLDL) cholesterol, plasma triglycerides; increases high-density lipoproteins (HDL) cholesterol.

USES
As an adjunct in homozygous familial hypercholesterolemia, mixed hyperlipidemia, elevated serum triglyceride levels, and type IV hyperproteinemia; also reduces total cholesterol LDL-C, apoB, and triglyceride levels; patient should first be placed on cholesterol-lowering diet; primary prevention of CHD and to slow CHD progression

PHARMACOKINETICS

Route	Onset	Peak	Duration
PO	3 days	4–6 wk	N/A

Incompletely absorbed from the GI tract (increased on empty stomach). Protein binding: 95%. Hydrolyzed in the liver to active metabolite. Primarily eliminated in feces. Not removed by hemodialysis. **Half-life:** 1.1–1.7 hr.

INDICATIONS AND DOSAGES
▶ **Hyperlipoproteinemia, Primary Prevention of Coronary Artery Disease**
PO
Adults, Elderly. Initially, 20–40 mg/day with evening meal. Increase at 4-wk intervals up to maximum of 80 mg/day. Maintenance: 20–80 mg/day in single or divided doses.
PO (Extended-Release)

Adults, Elderly. Initially, 20 mg/day. May increase at 4-wk intervals up to 60 mg/day.
Children 10–17 yr. 10–40 mg/day with evening meal.

▸ **Heterozygous Familial Hypercholesterolemia**
PO
Children 10–17 yr. Initially, 10 mg/day. May increase to 20 mg/day after 8 wk and 40 mg/day after 16 wk if needed.

SIDE EFFECTS/ADVERSE REACTIONS
Generally well tolerated. Side effects usually mild and transient.
Frequent
Headache, flatulence, diarrhea, abdominal pain or cramps, rash, and pruritus
Occasional
Nausea, vomiting, constipation, dyspepsia
Rare
Dizziness, heartburn, myalgia, blurred vision, eye irritation

PRECAUTIONS AND CONTRAINDICATIONS
Active liver disease, pregnancy, unexplained elevated liver function tests
Caution
Past liver disease, alcoholics, severe acute infections, trauma, hypotension, uncontrolled seizure disorders, severe metabolic disorders, electrolyte imbalances

DRUG INTERACTIONS OF CONCERN TO DENTISTRY
• Increased myalgia, rhabdomyolysis: erythromycin, cyclosporine
• Contraindicated with itraconazole, ketoconazole, erythromycin

SERIOUS REACTIONS
❗ There is a potential for cataract development.

DENTAL CONSIDERATIONS
General:
• Consider semisupine chair position for patient comfort because of GI side effects.
Teach Patient/Family to:
• Avoid mouth rinses with high alcohol content because of drying effects

loxapine
lox´-ah-peen
(Apo-Loxapine[CAN], Loxapac[CAN], Loxitane)

CATEGORY AND SCHEDULE
Pregnancy Risk Category: C

Drug Class: Antipsychotic

MECHANISM OF ACTION
A dibenzodiazepine derivative that interferes with the binding of dopamine at postsynaptic receptor sites in brain. Strong anticholinergic effects. ***Therapeutic Effect:*** Suppresses locomotor activity, produces tranquilization.

USES
Treatment of psychotic disorders

PHARMACOKINETICS
Onset of action occurs within 1 hr. Metabolized to active metabolites 8-hydroxyloxapine, 7-hydroxyloxapine, and 8-hydroxyamoxapine. Excreted in urine. ***Half-life:*** 4 hr.

INDICATIONS AND DOSAGES
▸ **Psychotic Disorders**
PO
Adults. 10 mg 2 times a day. Increase dosage rapidly during first wk to 50 mg, if needed. Usual therapeutic, maintenance range: 60–100 mg daily

in 2–4 divided doses. Maximum: 250 mg/day.

SIDE EFFECTS/ADVERSE REACTIONS
Frequent
Blurred vision, confusion, drowsiness, dry mouth, dizziness, lightheadedness
Occasional
Allergic reaction (rash, itching), decreased urination, constipation, decreased sexual ability, enlarged breasts, headache, photosensitivity, nausea, vomiting, insomnia, weight gain

PRECAUTIONS AND CONTRAINDICATIONS
Severe CNS depression, comatose states, hypersensitivity to loxapine or any component of the formulation
Caution
Lactation, seizure disorders, hepatic disease, cardiac disease, prostatic hypertrophy, cardiac conditions, children younger than 16 yr

DRUG INTERACTIONS OF CONCERN TO DENTISTRY
• Increased effects of both drugs: anticholinergics
• Increased CNS depression: alcohol, all CNS depressants
• Decreased effects of sympathomimetics, carbamazepine

SERIOUS REACTIONS
! Extrapyramidal symptoms frequently noted are akathisia (motor restlessness, anxiety). Less frequently noted are akinesia (rigidity, tremors, salivation, mask-like facial expression, reduced voluntary movements). Infrequently noted dystonias: torticollis (neck muscle spasm), opisthotonos (rigidity of back muscles), and oculogyric crisis (rolling back of eyes). Tardive dyskinesia (protrusion of tongue, puffing of cheeks, chewing/puckering of mouth) occurs rarely but may be irreversible. Risk is greater in female elderly patients.

DENTAL CONSIDERATIONS
General:
• Patients on chronic drug therapy may rarely have symptoms of blood dyscrasias, which can include infection, bleeding, and poor healing.
• Assess salivary flow as a factor in caries, periodontal disease, and candidiasis.
• Assess for presence of extrapyramidal motor symptoms, such as tardive dyskinesia and akathisia. Extrapyramidal motor activity may complicate dental treatment.
• After supine positioning, have patient sit upright for at least 2 min before standing to avoid orthostatic hypotension.
Consultations:
• In a patient with symptoms of blood dyscrasias, request a medical consultation for blood studies and postpone dental treatment until normal values are reestablished.
• If signs of tardive dyskinesia or akathisia are present, refer to physician.
• Physician should be informed if significant xerostomic side effects occur (e.g., increased caries, sore tongue, problems eating or swallowing, difficulty wearing prosthesis) so that a medication change can be considered.

Teach Patient/Family to:
• Use effective oral hygiene
to prevent soft tissue
inflammation
• Use caution to prevent
injury when using oral
hygiene aids
• Use electric tooth brush if patient
has difficulty holding conventional
devices

• When chronic dry mouth occurs,
advise patient to:
  • Avoid mouth rinses with high
  alcohol content because of drying
  effects
  • Use sugarless gum, frequent sips
  of water, or saliva substitutes
  • Use daily home fluoride products
  for anticaries effect

mafenide
ma´-fe-nide
(Sulfamylon)

CATEGORY AND SCHEDULE
Pregnancy Risk Category: C

Drug Class: Antibacterial, topical; antifungal, topical

MECHANISM OF ACTION
A topical antiinfective that decreases the number of bacteria in avascular tissue of second- and third-degree burns. **Therapeutic Effect:** Bacteriostatic. Promotes spontaneous healing of deep partial-thickness burns.

USES
Prevention and treatment of bacterial or fungal infections

PHARMACOKINETICS
Absorbed through devascularzied areas into systemic circulation following topical administration. Excreted in the form of its metabolite rho-carboxyben-zen esulfonamide.

INDICATIONS AND DOSAGES
▶ Burns
Topical
Adults, Elderly, Children. Apply 1–2 times a day.

SIDE EFFECTS/ADVERSE REACTIONS
Difficult to distinguish side effects and effects of severe burn
Frequent
Pain, burning upon application
Occasional
Allergic reaction (usually 10–14 days after initiation): itching, rash, facial edema, swelling; unexplained syndrome of marked hyperventilation with respiratory alkalosis
Rare
Delay in eschar separation, excoriation of new skin

PRECAUTIONS AND CONTRAINDICATIONS
Hypersensitivity to mafenide or sulfite or any other component of the formulation

DRUG INTERACTIONS OF CONCERN TO DENTISTRY
None reported

SERIOUS REACTIONS
❗ Hemolytic anemia, porphyria, bone marrow depression, superinfections (especially with fungi), metabolic acidosis occurs rarely.

DENTAL CONSIDERATIONS
General:
• Dental management depends on extent and severity of burns and patient's ability to cooperate; above all use aseptic techniques.
• Provide palliative dental care for dental emergencies only.
• Monitor and record vital signs.
Consultations:
• Medical consultation may be required to assess disease control and patient's ability to tolerate stress.
• Consult patient's physician if an acute dental infection occurs and another antiinfective is required.
Teach Patient/Family to:
• Use effective oral hygiene to prevent soft tissue inflammation
• Prevent trauma when using oral hygiene aids

magaldrate
mag´-ahl-drate (Iosopan Plus,
Lowsium Plus, Riopan Plus)

CATEGORY AND SCHEDULE
Pregnancy Risk Category: C

Drug Class: Antacid/aluminum/
magnesium hydroxide

MECHANISM OF ACTION
An antacid that causes fewer hydrogen
ions to be available for diffusion
through the GI mucosa. *Therapeutic
Effect:* Reduces and neutralizes
gastric acid.

USES
An antacid for hyperacidity

PHARMACOKINETICS
Onset 10–15 min, duration longer
than 3 hr.

INDICATIONS AND DOSAGES
▶ **Hyperacidity and Gas**
PO
Adults, Elderly. 540–1080 mg
between meals and at bedtime.

SIDE EFFECTS/ADVERSE REACTIONS
Rare

Constipation, diarrhea, fluid
retention, dizziness or
lightheadedness, continuing
discomfort, irregular heartbeat, loss
of appetite, mood or mental changes,
muscle weakness, unusual tiredness
or weakness, weight loss, chalky
taste

PRECAUTIONS AND CONTRAINDICATIONS
Hypersensitivity to magaldrate,
colostomy or ileostomy, appendicitis,
ulcerative colitis, diverticulits

Caution
Elderly, fluid restriction, decreased
GI motility, GI obstruction,
dehydration, renal disease, sodium-
restricted diets, colitis, gastric outlet
obstruction syndrome, colostomy

DRUG INTERACTIONS OF CONCERN TO DENTISTRY
• Decreased absorption of
anticholinergics, corticosteroids,
sodium fluoride, tetracycline,
ketoconazole, chlordiazepoxide,
ciprofloxacin, metronidazole

SERIOUS REACTIONS
None known.

DENTAL CONSIDERATIONS
General:
• If prescribing oral form of a drug
for which risk of decreased
absorption is reported, advise taking
doses at least 2 hr after or before
antacid use.
• Avoid drugs that could exacerbate
upper GI distress (aspirin and
NSAIDs).
• Consider semisupine chair position
for patient comfort because of GI
effects of disease.

maprotiline
mah-pro´-tih-leen
(Ludiomil)

CATEGORY AND SCHEDULE
Pregnancy Risk Category: B

Drug Class: Tetracyclic
antidepressant

MECHANISM OF ACTION
A tetracyclic compound that blocks
reuptake norepinephrine by CNS
presynaptic neuronal membranes,
increasing availability at postsynaptic

neuronal receptor sites, and enhances synaptic activity. ***Therapeutic Effect:*** Produces antidepressant effect, with prominent sedative effects and low anticholinergic activity.

USES
Treatment of depression, depression with anxiety, manic depression

PHARMACOKINETICS
Slowly and completely absorbed after PO administration. Protein binding: 88%. Metabolized in liver by hydroxylation and oxidative modification. Excreted in urine. Unknown if removed by hemodialysis. ***Half-life:*** 27–58 hr.

INDICATIONS AND DOSAGES
▶ **Mild to Moderate Depression**
PO
Adults. 75 mg/day to start, in 1–4 divided doses.
Elderly. 50–75 mg/day.
In 2 wk, increase dosage gradually in 25 mg increments until therapeutic response is achieved. Reduce to lowest effective maintenance level.
▶ **Severe Depression**
PO
Adults. 100–150 mg/day in 1–4 divided doses. May increase gradually to maximum 225 mg/day.
▶ **Usual Elderly Dosage**
PO
Initially, 25 mg at bedtime. May increase by 25 mg q3–7 days. Maintenance: 50–75 mg/day.

SIDE EFFECTS/ADVERSE REACTIONS
Frequent
Drowsiness, fatigue, dry mouth, blurred vision, constipation, delayed micturition, postural hypotension, excessive sweating, disturbed concentration, increased appetite, urinary retention
Occasional
GI disturbances (nausea, GI distress, metallic taste sensation), photosensitivity
Rare
Paradoxical reaction (agitation, restlessness, nightmares, insomnia), extrapyramidal symptoms (particularly fine hand tremors)

PRECAUTIONS AND CONTRAINDICATIONS
Acute recovery period following MI, Within 14 days of MAOI ingestion, known or suspected seizure disorder, hypersensitivity to maprotiline or any component of the formulation
Caution
Suicidal patients, severe depression, increased intraocular pressure, narrow-angle glaucoma, urinary retention, cardiac disease, hepatic or renal disease, hypothyroidism, hyperthyroidism, electroshock therapy, elective surgery, elderly, lactation, prostate hypertrophy, schizophrenia, MAOIs

DRUG INTERACTIONS OF CONCERN TO DENTISTRY
• Increased effects of direct-acting sympathomimetics (epinephrine)
• Potential risk of increased CNS depression: alcohol, and all CNS depressants
• Decreased antihypertensive effect: clonidine, guanadrel, guanethidine

SERIOUS REACTIONS
! Higher incidence of seizures than with tricyclic antidepressants, especially in those with no previous history of seizures.
! High dosage may produce cardiovascular effects, such as severe postural hypotension, dizziness,

tachycardia, palpitations, and arrhythmias.

! May also result in altered temperature regulation (hyperpyrexia or hypothermia).

! Abrupt withdrawal from prolonged therapy may produce headache, malaise, nausea, vomiting, and vivid dreams.

DENTAL CONSIDERATIONS

General:

• Monitor vital signs at every appointment because of cardiovascular side effects.

• Patients on chronic drug therapy may rarely have symptoms of blood dyscrasias, which can include infection, bleeding, and poor healing.

• Assess salivary flow as a factor in caries, periodontal disease, and candidiasis.

• After supine positioning, have patient sit upright for at least 2 min before standing to avoid orthostatic hypotension.

• Use of epinephrine in gingival retraction cord is contraindicated. Use vasoconstrictors with caution, in low doses, and with careful aspiration.

Consultations:

• In a patient with symptoms of blood dyscrasias, request a medical consultation for blood studies and postpone dental treatment until normal values are reestablished.

• Take precautions if dental surgery is anticipated and anesthesia is required.

• Medical consultation may be required to assess disease control.

• Physician should be informed if significant xerostomic side effects occur (e.g., increased caries, sore tongue, problems eating or swallowing, difficulty wearing

prosthesis) so that a medication change can be considered.

Teach Patient/Family to:

• Use effective oral hygiene to prevent soft tissue inflammation

• Use caution to prevent injury when using oral hygiene aids

• When chronic dry mouth occurs, advise patient to:

  • Avoid mouth rinses with high alcohol content because of drying effects

  • Use sugarless gum, frequent sips of water, or saliva substitutes

  • Use daily home fluoride products for anticaries effect

mebendazole
meh-ben´-dah-zole
(Vermox)

CATEGORY AND SCHEDULE
Pregnancy Risk Category: C

Drug Class: Anthelmintic; carbamate

MECHANISM OF ACTION
A synthetic benzimidazole derivative that degrades parasite cytoplasmic microtubules and irreversibly blocks glucose uptake in helminthes and larvae. Vermicidal. *Therapeutic Effect:* Depletes glycogen, decreases ATP, causes helminth death.

USES
Treatment of pinworms, roundworms, hookworms, whipworms, thread-worms, pork tapeworms, dwarf tapeworms, beef tapeworms, hydatid cyst

PHARMACOKINETICS
Poorly absorbed from GI tract (absorption increases with food).

Metabolized in liver. Primarily eliminated in feces. *Half-life:* 2.5–9 hr (half-life increased with impaired renal function).

INDICATIONS AND DOSAGES
▶ **Trichuriasis, Ascariasis, Hookworm**
PO
Adults, Elderly, Children older than 2 yr. 1 tablet in morning and at bedtime for 3 days.
▶ **Enterobiasis**
PO
Adults, Elderly, Children older than 2 yr. 1 tablet one time.

SIDE EFFECTS/ADVERSE REACTIONS
Occasional
Nausea, vomiting, headache, dizziness, transient abdominal pain, diarrhea with massive infection and expulsion of helminths
Rare
Fever

PRECAUTIONS AND CONTRAINDICATIONS
Hypersensitivity to mebendazole or any component of the formulation

DRUG INTERACTIONS OF CONCERN TO DENTISTRY
• Decreased plasma levels: carbamazepine

SERIOUS REACTIONS
! High dosage may produce reversible myelosuppression (granulocytopenia, leukopenia, neutropenia).

DENTAL CONSIDERATIONS
General:
• Determine why patient is taking the drug.

• Patient on chronic drug therapy may rarely present with symptoms of blood dyscrasias, which can include infection, bleeding, and poor healing. If dyscrasia is present, caution patient to prevent oral tissue trauma when using oral hygiene aids.
• Question patient about other drugs he or she is taking.
Consultations:
• In a patient with symptoms of blood dyscrasias, request a medical consultation for blood studies and postpone treatment until normal values are reestablished.

mecasermin
mek-ah-sir´-men
(Increlex)

CATEGORY AND SCHEDULE
Pregnancy Risk Category: C

Drug Class: Growth hormone

MECHANISM OF ACTION
An insulin-like growth factor-1 (IGF-1) that stimulates the uptake of glucose, fatty acids, and amino acids so that metabolism supports growing tissues. *Therapeutic Effect:* Promotes effects of growth hormone.

USES
Treatment for growth failure in children with severe primary IGF-1 deficiency

PHARMACOKINETICS
Absorption has not been determined. Protein binding: greater than 80% bound to IGFBP-3 and acid-labile subunit. Metabolized in liver and kidney. *Half-life:* 5.8 hr.

INDICATIONS AND DOSAGES
▶ **Primary IGF-1 deficiency (severe)**
SC
Children. Initially, 0.04–0.08 mg/kg
twice a day. Maintenance: May
increase by 0.04 mg/kg per dose.
Maximum: 0.12 mg/kg twice a day.
The drug should be given shortly
before or after (20 min) a meal or
snack—do not administer when the
meal or snack is omitted.
Intravenous administration is
contraindicated.

SIDE EFFECTS/ADVERSE REACTIONS:
Occasional
Hyper/hypoglycemia, headache,
snoring, tonsillar hypertrophy, heart
murmur, convulsion, dizziness,
vomiting, arthralgia, bone pain,
extremity pain, muscular atrophy,
injection site reactions, papilledema,
ear pain, hypoacusis, middle ear
fluid, otitis media, serous otitis
media, tympanometry abnormal,
hematuria, lymphadenopathy, iron-
deficiency anemia, ovarian cysts,
thymus hypertrophy, thyromegaly,
increased liver enzymes
Rare
Hypoglycemic seizure, loss of
consciousness secondary to
hypoglycemia, intracranial hypertension

PRECAUTIONS AND CONTRAINDICATIONS
Hypersensitivity to mecasermin or its
components
Caution
Avoid in patients with closed epiphyses,
active or suspected neoplasia, driving
or operating machinery due to
hypoglycemic effects

DRUG INTERACTIONS OF CONCERN TO DENTISTRY
None reported

SERIOUS REACTIONS
! Lymphoid tissue (e.g., tonsillar)
hypertrophy associated with
complications, such as snoring, sleep
apnea, and chronic middle-ear
effusions have been reported.
! Intracranial hypertension with
papilledema, visual changes,
headache, nausea and/or vomiting
have been reported.
! Local or systemic allergic reactions
may occur.

DENTAL CONSIDERATIONS
General:
• Potential acute hypoglycemia

meclizine
mek´-lih-zeen
(Antivert, Bonamine[CAN], Bonine)
Do not confuse Antivert with Axert.

CATEGORY AND SCHEDULE
Pregnancy Risk Category: B

Drug Class: Antihistamine

MECHANISM OF ACTION
An anticholinergic that reduces
labyrinthine excitability and
diminishes vestibular stimulation of
the labyrinth, affecting the
chemoreceptor trigger zone.
Therapeutic Effect: Reduces nausea,
vomiting, and vertigo.

USES
Treatment of vertigo, motion sickness

PHARMACOKINETICS

Route	Onset	Peak	Duration
PO	30–60 min	N/A	12–24 hr

Well absorbed from the GI tract.
Widely distributed. Metabolized in

the liver. Primarily excreted in urine.
Half-life: 6 hr.

INDICATIONS AND DOSAGES
▶ **Motion Sickness**
PO
Adults, Elderly, Children 12 yr and older. 12.5–25 mg 1 hr before travel. May repeat q12–24h. May require a dose of 50 mg.
▶ **Vertigo**
PO
Adults, Elderly, Children 12 yr and older. 25–100 mg/day in divided doses, as needed.

SIDE EFFECTS/ADVERSE REACTIONS
Frequent
Drowsiness
Occasional
Blurred vision; dry mouth, nose, or throat

PRECAUTIONS AND CONTRAINDICATIONS
Hypersensitivity to cyclizines
Caution
Children, narrow-angle glaucoma, urinary retention, lactation, prostatic hypertrophy, elderly, asthma, hypersensitivity to cyclizines.

DRUG INTERACTIONS OF CONCERN TO DENTISTRY
● Increased effect of alcohol, other CNS depressants, anticholinergics

SERIOUS REACTIONS
❗ A hypersensitivity reaction, marked by eczema, pruritus, rash, cardiac disturbances, and photosensitivity, may occur.
❗ Overdose may produce CNS depression (manifested as sedation, apnea, cardiovascular collapse, or death) or severe paradoxical

reactions (such as hallucinations, tremor, and seizures).
❗ Children may experience paradoxical reactions, including restlessness, insomnia, euphoria, nervousness, and tremors.
❗ Overdose in children may result in hallucinations, seizures, and death.

DENTAL CONSIDERATIONS
General:
● Assess salivary flow as a factor in caries, periodontal disease, and candidiasis.
Teach Patient/Family:
● When chronic dry mouth occurs, advise patient to:
  ● Avoid mouth rinses with high alcohol content because of drying effects
  ● Use daily home fluoride products for anticaries effect
  ● Use sugarless gum, frequent sips of water, or saliva substitutes

meclofenamate sodium
me-kloe-fen´-a-mate soe´-dee-um
(Meclomen[CAN])
Do not confuse with meclizine.

CATEGORY AND SCHEDULE
Pregnancy Risk Category: B (D if used in third trimester or near delivery)

Drug Class: Nonsteroidal antiinflammatory

MECHANISM OF ACTION
A nonsteroidal antiinflammatory drug that inhibits prostaglandin synthesis by decreasing activity of the enzyme, cyclooxygenase, which results in decreased formation of prostaglandin precursors.

Therapeutic Effect: Reduces inflammatory response and intensity of pain stimulus reaching sensory nerve endings.

USES
Treatment of mild-to-moderate pain, osteoarthritis, rheumatoid arthritis, dysmenorrhea

PHARMACOKINETICS
PO route, onset 15 min, peak 0.5–1.5 hr, duration 2–4 hr. Completely absorbed from the GI tract. Widely distributed. Protein binding: greater than 99%. Metabolized in liver. Primarily excreted in urine and feces as metabolites. Not removed by hemodialysis. *Half-life:* 2–3.3 hr.

INDICATIONS AND DOSAGES
▶ **Mild-to-Moderate Pain**
PO
Adults, Elderly. 50 mg q4–6h as needed.
▶ **Excessive Menstrual Blood Loss and Primary Dysmenorrhea**
PO
Adults, Elderly. 100 mg 3 times a day for 6 days, starting at the onset of menstrual flow.
▶ **Rheumatoid Arthritis, Osteoarthritis**
PO
Adults, Elderly. 200–400 mg 3–4 times a day.

SIDE EFFECTS/ADVERSE REACTIONS
Frequent
Diarrhea, nausea, abdominal cramping/pain, dyspepsia (heartburn, indigestion, epigastric pain), oral lichenoid reaction
Occasional
Flatulence, rash, dizziness
Rare
Constipation, anorexia, stomatitis, headache, ringing in the ears, rash

PRECAUTIONS AND CONTRAINDICATIONS
Active peptic ulcer disease, chronic inflammation of GI tract, GI bleeding disorders, GI ulceration, history of hypersensitivity to aspirin or NSAIDs
Caution
Lactation, children younger than 14 yr, bleeding disorders, upper GI disorders, cardiac disorders, hypersensitivity to other antiinflammatory agents

DRUG INTERACTIONS OF CONCERN TO DENTISTRY
• GI ulceration, bleeding: aspirin, alcohol, corticosteroids, biphosphonates
• Nephrotoxicity: acetaminophen (prolonged use)
• Possible risk of decreased renal function: cyclosporine
• First-time users of SSRIs also taking NSAIDs may have a higher risk of GI side effects; until more data are available, it may be advisable to avoid use of NSAIDs in these patients (Br J Clin Pharmacol 55:591–595, 2003)
• When prescribed for dental pain:
  • Risk of increased effects: oral anticoagulants, oral antidiabetics, lithium, methotrexate
  • Decreased effects of diuretics, β-adrenergic blockers

SERIOUS REACTIONS
❗ Overdosage may result in headache, seizure, vomiting, and cerebral edema.
❗ Peptic ulcer disease, GI bleeding, gastritis, severe hepatic reactions, such as jaundice, nephrotoxicity, marked by hematuria, dysuria, proteinuria, and severe hypersensitivity reaction, including

bronchospasm, and facial edema occur rarely.

DENTAL CONSIDERATIONS

General:
- Increased potential for adverse cardiovascular events in patients at risk for thromboembolism
- Patients on chronic drug therapy may rarely have symptoms of blood dyscrasias, which can include infection, bleeding, and poor healing.
- Assess salivary flow as a factor in caries, periodontal disease, and candidiasis.
- Avoid prescribing for dental use in last trimester of pregnancy.
- Avoid prescribing aspirin-containing products.
- Consider semisupine chair position for patients with rheumatic disease.

Consultations:
- In a patient with symptoms of blood dyscrasias, request a medical consultation for blood studies and postpone dental treatment until normal values are reestablished.
- Medical consultation may be required to assess disease control.

Teach Patient/Family to:
- Use effective oral hygiene to prevent soft tissue inflammation
- Use caution to prevent injury when using oral hygiene aids
- When chronic dry mouth occurs, advise patient to:
    - Avoid mouth rinses with high alcohol content because of drying effects
    - Use sugarless gum, frequent sips of water, or saliva substitutes
    - Use daily home fluoride products for anticaries effect

medroxyprogesterone acetate

me-drox´-ee-proe-jess´-te-rone ass´-ih-tate
(Depo-Provera, Depo-Provera Contraceptive, Novo-Medrone[CAN], Provera, Ralovera[AUS])
Do not confuse medroxyprogesterone with hydroxyprogesterone, methylprednisolone, or methyltestosterone.

CATEGORY AND SCHEDULE
Pregnancy Risk Category: X

Drug Class: Progestogen

MECHANISM OF ACTION
A hormone that transforms endometrium from proliferative to secretory in an estrogen-primed endometrium. Inhibits secretion of pituitary gonadotropins. *Therapeutic Effect:* Prevents follicular maturation and ovulation. Stimulates growth of mammary alveolar tissue and relaxes uterine smooth muscle. Corrects hormonal imbalance.

USES
Treatment of uterine bleeding (abnormal), secondary amenorrhea, endometrial cancer, metastatic renal cancer, contraceptive; with estrogens to reduce incidence of endometrial hyperplasia, cancer

PHARMACOKINETICS
Slowly absorbed after IM administration. Protein binding: 90%. Metabolized in the liver. Primarily excreted in urine. *Half-life:* 30 days.

INDICATIONS AND DOSAGES
▸ **Endometrial Hyperplasia**
PO
Adults. 2.5–10 mg/day for 14 days.
▸ **Secondary Amenorrhea**
PO
Adults. 5–10 mg/day for 5–10 days, beginning at any time during menstrual cycle or 2.5 mg/day.
▸ **Abnormal Uterine Bleeding**
PO
Adults. 5–10 mg/day for 5–10 days, beginning on calculated day 16 or day 21 of menstrual cycle.
▸ **Endometrial, Renal Carcinoma**
IM
Adults, Elderly. Initially, 400–1000 mg; repeat at 1-wk intervals. If improvement occurs and disease is stabilized, begin maintenance with as little as 400 mg/mo.
▸ **Prevention of Pregnancy**
IM
Adults. 150 mg q3mo.

SIDE EFFECTS/ADVERSE REACTIONS
Frequent
Transient menstrual abnormalities (including spotting, change in menstrual flow or cervical secretions, and amenorrhea) at initiation of therapy
Occasional
Edema, weight change, breast tenderness, nervousness, insomnia, fatigue, dizziness
Rare
Alopecia, depression, dermatologic changes, headache, fever, nausea

PRECAUTIONS AND CONTRAINDICATIONS
Carcinoma of breast; estrogen-dependent neoplasm; history of or active thrombotic disorders, such as cerebral apoplexy, thrombophlebitis, or thromboembolic disorders; hypersensitivity to progestins; known or suspected pregnancy; missed abortion; severe hepatic dysfunction; undiagnosed abnormal genital bleeding; use as pregnancy test
Caution
Lactation, hypertension, asthma, blood dyscrasias, gallbladder disease, CHF, diabetes mellitus, bone disease, depression, migraine headache, convulsive disorders, hepatic disease, renal disease, family history of cancer of breast or reproductive tract

SERIOUS REACTIONS
❗ Thrombophlebitis, pulmonary or cerebral embolism, and retinal thrombosis occur rarely.

DENTAL CONSIDERATIONS
General:
• Place on frequent recall to evaluate inflammatory and healing response.
Teach Patient/Family to:
• Use effective oral hygiene to prevent soft tissue inflammation

medrysone
meh´-dri-sone
(HMS Liquifilm)

CATEGORY AND SCHEDULE
Pregnancy Risk Category: C

Drug Class: Antiinflammatory, steroidal, ophthalmic; corticosteroid, ophthalmic

MECHANISM OF ACTION
A topical synthetic corticosteroid that inhibits accumulation of inflammatory cells at inflammation sites.

Therapeutic Effect: Inhibits inflammatory process.

USES
Prevention of permanent damage to the eye, which may occur with certain eye problems. Also provides relief from redness, irritation, and other discomfort.

PHARMACOKINETICS
Absorbed through aqueous humor. Metabolized in liver if absorbed. Excreted in urine and feces.

INDICATIONS AND DOSAGES
▶ **Ophthalmic Disorders**
Ophthalmic
Adults, Elderly, Children 3 yr and older. Instill 1 drop up to every 4 hr.

SIDE EFFECTS/ADVERSE REACTIONS
Frequent
Blurred vision
Occasional
Decreased vision, watering of eyes, eye pain, burning, stinging, redness of eyes, nausea, vomiting

PRECAUTIONS AND CONTRAINDICATIONS
Active superficial herpes simplex, conjunctival or corneal viral disease, fungal diseases of the eye, ocular tuberculosis, hypersensitivity to medrysone or any component of the formulation

DRUG INTERACTIONS OF CONCERN TO DENTISTRY
None reported

SERIOUS REACTIONS
! Systemic absorption may occur with topical application.
! Cataracts, corneal thinning, corneal ulcers, delayed wound healing, optic nerve damage, and glaucoma have been reported.

DENTAL CONSIDERATIONS

GENERAL:
• Determine why patient is taking the drug.
• Avoid dental light in patient's eyes; offer dark glasses for patient comfort.

mefenamic acid
meh-feh-nam´-ik
(Apo-Mefenamic[CAN], Nu-Mefenamic[CAN], PMS-Mefenamic Acid[CAN], Ponstan[CAN], Ponstel)

CATEGORY AND SCHEDULE
Pregnancy Risk Category: C (D if used in third trimester or near delivery)

Drug Class: Nonsteroidal antiinflammatory

MECHANISM OF ACTION
A nonsteroidal antiinflammatory that produces analgesic and antiinflammatory effect by inhibiting prostaglandin synthesis. *Therapeutic Effect:* Reduces inflammatory response and intensity of pain stimulus reaching sensory nerve endings.

USES
Treatment of mild-to-moderate pain, dysmenorrhea, inflammatory disease

PHARMACOKINETICS
Rapidly absorbed from the GI tract. Protein binding: high. Metabolized in liver. Partially excreted in urine

and partially in the feces. Not removed by hemodialysis. *Half-life:* 3.5 hr.

INDICATIONS AND DOSAGES

▶ **Mild-to-Moderate Pain, Lower Back Pain, Dysmenorrhea**

PO

Adults, Elderly, Children 14 yr and older. Initially, 500 mg to start, then 250 mg q4h as needed. Maximum: 1 wk of therapy.

SIDE EFFECTS/ADVERSE REACTIONS

Occasional

Dyspepsia, including heartburn, indigestion, flatulence, abdominal cramping, constipation, nausea, diarrhea, epigastric pain, vomiting, headache, nervousness, dizziness, bleeding, elevated liver function tests, tinnitus, oral lichenoid reaction

Rare

Fluid retention, arrhythmias, tachycardia, confusion, drowsiness, rash, dry eyes, blurred vision, hot flashes

PRECAUTIONS AND CONTRAINDICATIONS

History of hypersensitivity to aspirin or NSAIDs, pregnancy

Caution

Lactation, children, bleeding disorders, GI disorders, cardiac disorders, hypersensitivity to other antiinflammatory agents

DRUG INTERACTIONS OF CONCERN TO DENTISTRY

• GI bleeding, ulceration: aspirin, alcohol, corticosteroids
• Nephrotoxicity: acetaminophen (prolonged use and high doses)
• Possible risk of decreased renal function: cyclosporine
• First-time users of SSRIs also taking NSAIDs may have a higher risk of GI side effects; until more data are available, it may be

advisable to avoid use of NSAIDs in these patients (Br J Clin Pharmacol 55:591–595, 2003)
• When prescribed for dental pain:
  • Risk of increased effects of oral anticoagulants, oral antidiabetics, lithium, methotrexate
  • Decreased effects of diuretics

SERIOUS REACTIONS

! Peptic ulcer, GI bleeding, gastritis, and severe hepatic reaction, such as cholestasis and jaundice, occur rarely.
! Nephrotoxicity, including dysuria, hematuria, proteinuria, and nephrotic syndrome and severe hypersensitivity reaction, marked by bronchospasm, and angioedema occur rarely.

DENTAL CONSIDERATIONS

General:
• Avoid prescribing for dental use in last trimester of pregnancy.
• Avoid prescribing aspirin-containing products.
• Potential for increased adverse cardiovascular events in patients at risk for thromboembolism.

Consultations:
• Medical consultation may be required to assess disease control.

mefloquine

meh´-flow-quine
(Lariam)
Do not confuse with Librium.

CATEGORY AND SCHEDULE

Pregnancy Risk Category: C

Drug Class: Antimalarial

MECHANISM OF ACTION

A quinolone-methanol compound structurally similar to quinine that destroys the asexual blood forms of malarial pathogens, *Plasmodium falciparum, P. vivax, P. malariae, P. ovale.* **Therapeutic Effect:** Inhibits parasite growth.

USES
Prevention or treatment of malaria, a red blood cell infection transmitted by the bite of a mosquito

PHARMACOKINETICS
Well absorbed from the GI tract. Protein binding: 98%. Widely distributed, including CSF. Metabolized in liver. Primarily excreted in urine. *Half-life:* 21–22 days.

INDICATIONS AND DOSAGES
▶ **Suppression of Malaria**
PO
Adults. 250 mg base weekly starting 1 wk before travel, continuing weekly during travel and for 4 wk after leaving endemic area.
Children more than 45 kg. 250 mg weekly starting 1 wk before travel, continuing weekly during travel and for 4 wk after leaving endemic area.
Children 45–31 kg. 187.5 mg ($^3/_4$ tablet) weekly starting 1 wk before travel, continuing weekly during travel and for 4 wk after leaving endemic area.
Children 30–20 kg. 125 mg ($^1/_2$ tablet) weekly starting 1 wk before travel, continuing weekly during travel and for 4 wk after leaving endemic area.
Children 19–15 kg. 62.5 mg ($^1/_4$ tablet) weekly starting 1 wk before travel, continuing weekly during travel and for 4 wk after leaving endemic area.
▶ **Treatment of Malaria**
PO
Adults. 1250 mg as a single dose.

Children. 15–25 mg/kg in a single dose. Maximum: 1250 mg.

SIDE EFFECTS/ADVERSE REACTIONS
Occasional
Mild transient headache, difficulty concentrating, insomnia, light headedness, vertigo, diarrhea, nausea, vomiting, visual disturbances, tinnitus
Rare
Aggressive behavior, anxiety, bradycardia, depression, hallucinations, hypotension, panic attacks, paranoia, psychosis, syncope, tremors

PRECAUTIONS AND CONTRAINDICATIONS
Cardiac abnormalities, severe psychiatric disorders, epilepsy, history of hypersensitivity to mefloquine

DRUG INTERACTIONS OF CONCERN TO DENTISTRY
None reported

SERIOUS REACTIONS
! Prolonged therapy may result in peripheral neuritis, neuromyopathy, hypotension, ECG changes, agranulocytosis, aplastic anemia, thrombocytopenia, seizures, and psychosis.
! Overdosage may result in headache, vomiting, visual disturbance, drowsiness, and seizures.

DENTAL CONSIDERATIONS
General:
• Consider semisupine chair position for patient comfort if GI side effects occur.
• Question patient about tolerance of NSAIDs or aspirin related to GI disease.

- Determine why patient is taking the drug.
- Be aware of patient's disease, its severity and frequence of NSAIDS or aspirin related to GI disease.
- TGB.
- Monitor and record vital signs.
Consultations:
- Medical consultation may be required to assess disease control and patient's ability to tolerate stress.
Teach Patient/Family to:
- Prevent trauma when using oral hygiene aids
- Avoid performing tasks that require mental alertness

megestrol acetate
meh-jess´-trole ass´-eh-tayte
(Apo-Megestrol[CAN], Megace, Megostat[AUS])

CATEGORY AND SCHEDULE
Pregnancy Risk Category: X (for suspension), D (for tablets)

Drug Class: Progestin

MECHANISM OF ACTION
A hormone and antineoplastic agent that suppresses the release of luteinizing hormone from the anterior pituitary gland by inhibiting pituitary function. *Therapeutic Effect:* Shrinks tumors. Also increases appetite by an unknown mechanism.

USES
Treatment of breast, endometrial cancer, renal cell cancer; AIDS wasting syndrome

PHARMACOKINETICS
Well absorbed from the GI tract. Metabolized in the liver; excreted in urine.

INDICATIONS AND DOSAGES
▶ **Palliative Treatment of Advanced Breast Cancer**
PO
Adults, Elderly. 160 mg/day in 4 equally divided doses.
▶ **Palliative Treatment of Advanced Endometrial Carcinoma**
PO
Adults, Elderly. 40–320 mg/day in divided doses. Maximum: 800 mg/day in 1–4 divided doses.
▶ **Anorexia, Cachexia, Weight Loss**
PO
Adults, Elderly. 800 mg (20 ml)/day.

SIDE EFFECTS/ADVERSE REACTIONS
Frequent
Weight gain secondary to increased appetite
Occasional
Nausea, breakthrough bleeding, backache, headache, breast tenderness, carpal tunnel syndrome
Rare
Feelings of coldness

PRECAUTIONS AND CONTRAINDICATIONS
Hypersensitivity

SERIOUS REACTIONS
❗ Thrombophlebitis and pulmonary embolism occur rarely.

DENTAL CONSIDERATIONS
General:
- Place on frequent recall to evaluate inflammatory and healing response.
- Patients receiving chemotherapy may require palliative treatment for stomatitis.
Teach Patient/Family to:
- Use effective oral hygiene to prevent soft tissue inflammation

M

meloxicam
mel-oks´-ih-kam
(Mobic)

CATEGORY AND SCHEDULE
Pregnancy Risk Category: C
(D if used in third trimester or near delivery)

Drug Class: Nonsteroidal antiinflammatory

MECHANISM OF ACTION
An NSAID that produces analgesic and antiinflammatory effects by inhibiting prostaglandin synthesis. **Therapeutic Effect:** Reduces the inflammatory response and intensity of pain.

USES
Relief of signs and symptoms of osteoarthritis

PHARMACOKINETICS

Route	Onset	Peak	Duration
PO (analgesic)	30 min	4–5 hr	N/A

Well absorbed after PO administration. Protein binding: 99%. Metabolized in the liver. Eliminated in urine and feces. Not removed by hemodialysis. **Half-life:** 15–20 hr.

INDICATIONS AND DOSAGES
▶ **Osteoarthritis, Rheumatoid Arthritis**
PO
Adults. Initially, 7.5 mg/day. Maximum: 15 mg/day.

SIDE EFFECTS/ADVERSE REACTIONS
Frequent
Dyspepsia, headache, diarrhea, nausea
Occasional
Dizziness, insomnia, rash, pruritus, flatulence, constipation, vomiting
Rare
Somnolence, urticaria, photosensitivity, tinnitus

PRECAUTIONS AND CONTRAINDICATIONS
Aspirin-induced nasal polyps associated with bronchospasm
Caution
Preexisting asthma, anaphylactic reactions to NSAIDs, serious GI side effects may occur, GI ulcer or GI bleeding; avoid in late pregnancy, liver dysfunction, dehydration, long-term use, edema, heart failure, hypertension, ACE inhibitors, lactation, elderly

DRUG INTERACTIONS OF CONCERN TO DENTISTRY
• Increased risk of GI side effects: long-duration NSAIDs, aspirin (except low-dose form), oral glucocorticoids, alcoholism, smoking, older age, and generally poor health
• Increased blood levels: lithium
• Reduced natriuretic effect: furosemide and other loop diuretics
• First-time users of SSRIs also taking NSAIDs may have a higher risk of GI side effects; until more data are available, it may be advisable to avoid use of NSAIDs in these patients (Br J Clin Pharmacol 55:591–595, 2003)

SERIOUS REACTIONS
! Rare reactions with long-term use include peptic ulcer disease, GI

bleeding, gastritis, severe hepatic
reaction (jaundice), nephrotoxicity
(hematuria, dysuria, proteinuria), and
a severe hypersensitivity reaction
(bronchospasm, angioedema).

DENTAL CONSIDERATIONS

General:
- Potential for increased adverse
cardiovascular events in patients at
risk for thromboembolism
- Assess salivary flow as a factor in
caries, periodontal disease, and
candidiasis.
- Patients on chronic drug therapy
may rarely have symptoms of blood
dyscrasias, which can include
infection, bleeding, and poor healing.
- Consider semisupine chair position
for patient comfort if GI side effects
occur.

Consultations:
- In a patient with symptoms of
blood dyscrasias, request a medical
consultation for blood studies and
postpone treatment until normal
values are reestablished.

Teach Patient/Family to:
- Use electric tooth brush if patient
has difficulty holding conventional
devices
- Update health and drug history if
physician makes any changes in
evaluation or drug regimens; include
OTC, herbal, and nonherbal drugs in
the update
- Use effective oral hygiene to
prevent soft tissue inflammation
- Prevent trauma when using oral
hygiene aids
- When chronic dry mouth occurs,
advise patient to:
  - Avoid mouth rinses with high
  alcohol content because of drying
  effects
  - Use daily home fluoride products
  for anticaries effect
  - Use sugarless gum, frequent sips
  of water, or saliva substitutes

melphalan
mel´-fah-lan
(Alkeran)
Do not confuse Alkeran with
Leukeran, or melphalan with
Mephyton or Myleran.

CATEGORY AND SCHEDULE
Pregnancy Risk Category: D

Drug Class: Antineoplastic

MECHANISM OF ACTION
An alkylating agent that inhibits
protein synthesis primarily by cross-
linking with strands of DNA
and RNA, producing cell death.
Cell cycle-phase nonspecific.
Therapeutic Effect: Disrupts nucleic
acid function.

USES
Palliative treatment of multiple
myeloma and nonresectable
epithelial carcinoma of the ovary

PHARMACOKINETICS
Half-life: 1.5 hr; first-pass hepatic
metabolism; plasma levels vary;
metabolites excreted in urine

INDICATIONS AND DOSAGES
▶ **Ovarian Carcinoma**
PO
Adults, Elderly. 0.2 mg/kg/day for
5 successive days. Repeat at 4- to
6-wk intervals.
▶ **Multiple Myeloma**
PO
Adults. Initially, 6 mg once a day,
adjusted as indicated; or 0.15 mg/kg/
day for 7 days or 0.25 mg/kg/day for
4 days. Repeat at 4- to 6-wk intervals.
IV
Adults. 16 mg/m²/dose every 2 wk
for 4 doses, then repeated monthly
according to protocol.

▶ **Dosage in Renal Impairment**

PO, IV

BUN level greater than 30 mg/dl.
Decrease melphalan dosage by 50%.
*Serum creatinine level greater than
1.5 mg/dl.* Decrease the melphalan
dosage by 50%.

SIDE EFFECTS/ADVERSE REACTIONS

Frequent
Nausea, vomiting (may be severe
with large dose)
Occasional
Diarrhea, stomatitis, rash, pruritus,
alopecia

PRECAUTIONS AND CONTRAINDICATIONS

Pregnancy, severe
myelosuppression
Caution
Severe bone marrow depression risk,
renal impairment.

DRUG INTERACTIONS OF CONCERN TO DENTISTRY

• Increased toxicity: antineoplastics,
radiation

SERIOUS REACTIONS

! Myelosuppression may cause
hematologic toxicity, manifested
principally as leukopenia and
thrombocytopenia and, to lesser
extent, anemia, pancytopenia, and
agranulocytosis. Leukopenia may
occur as early as 5 days after drug
initiation.

! WBC and platelet counts return to
normal levels during the fifth wk of
therapy, but leukopenia and
thrombocytopenia may last more
than 6 wk after the drug is
discontinued.

! Hyperuricemia, marked by
hematuria, crystalluria, and flank
pain, may occur.

DENTAL CONSIDERATIONS

General:
• Patients receiving chemotherapy
may be taking chronic opioids for
pain. Consider NSAIDs for dental
pain management.
• Patients receiving chemotherapy
may require palliative therapy for
stomatitis.
• Patients on chronic drug therapy
may rarely have symptoms of blood
dyscrasias, which can include
infection, bleeding, and poor
healing.
Consultations:
• Medical consultation may be
required to assess disease control.
• In a patient with symptoms of
blood dyscrasias, request a medical
consultation for blood studies and
postpone dental treatment until
normal values are reestablished.
Teach Patient/Family to:
• See dentist immediately if
secondary oral infection occurs
• When chronic dry mouth occurs,
advise patient to:
  • Avoid mouth rinses with high
  alcohol content because of drying
  effects
  • Use sugarless gum, frequent sips
  of water, or saliva substitutes
  • Use daily home fluoride products
  for anticaries effect

memantine hydrochloride

meh-man´-teen high-droh-klor´-ide
(Ebixa[AUS], Namenda)

CATEGORY AND SCHEDULE

Pregnancy Risk Category: B

Drug Class: NMDA receptor
antagonist

MECHANISM OF ACTION

A neurotransmitter inhibitor that decreases the effects of glutamate, the principle excitatory neurotransmitter in the brain. Persistent CNS excitation by glutamate is thought to cause the symptoms of Alzheimer's disease. *Therapeutic Effect:* May reduce clinical deterioration in moderate to severe Alzheimer's disease.

USES

Treatment of moderate-to-severe dementia of Alzheimer's disease

PHARMACOKINETICS

Rapidly and completely absorbed after PO administration. Protein binding: 45%. Undergoes little metabolism; most of the dose is excreted unchanged in urine. *Half-life:* 60–80 hr.

INDICATIONS AND DOSAGES
▸ **Alzheimer's Disease**
PO
Adults, Elderly. Initially, 5 mg once a day. May increase dosage at intervals of at least 1 wk in 5-mg increments to 10 mg/day (5 mg twice a day), then 15 mg/day (5 mg and 10 mg as separate doses), and finally 20 mg/day (10 mg twice a day). Target dose: 20 mg/day.

SIDE EFFECTS/ADVERSE REACTIONS
Occasional
Dizziness, headache, confusion, constipation, hypertension, cough
Rare
Back pain, nausea, fatigue, anxiety, peripheral edema, arthralgia, insomnia

PRECAUTIONS AND CONTRAINDICATIONS
Severe renal impairment
Caution
Moderate to severe renal impairment, alkaline urine pH, safety and efficacy in nursing mothers and pediatric patients have not been established

DRUG INTERACTIONS OF CONCERN TO DENTISTRY
None reported

SERIOUS REACTIONS
None known

DENTAL CONSIDERATIONS
• Monitor vital signs at every appointment because of cardiovascular side effects.
General:
• Patients with Alzheimer's disease may be taking other drugs; get a complete drug history.
• Drug may be used late in disease process; ensure caregiver or responsible person understands informed consent.
• Place on frequent recall to evaluate oral health.
Consultations:
• Consultation with physician may be necessary if sedation or general anesthesia is required.
Teach Patient/Family to:
• Use electric tooth brush if patient has difficulty holding conventional devices
• Use effective oral hygiene to prevent soft tissue inflammation/infection
• Prevent trauma when using oral hygiene aids
• Update health and drug history and reporting changes in health status, drug regimen, or disease/treatment status; include OTC, herbal, and nonherbal drugs in the update

meperidine hydrochloride
me-per´-ih-deen
high-droh-klor´-ide
(Demerol, Pethidine Injection[AUS])
Do not confuse with Demulen or Dymelor.

CATEGORY AND SCHEDULE
Pregnancy Risk Category: B
(D if used for prolonged periods or at high dosages at term)
Controlled Substance: Schedule II

Drug Class: Synthetic narcotic analgesic

MECHANISM OF ACTION
An opioid agonist that binds to opioid receptors in the CNS. **Therapeutic Effect:** Alters the perception of and emotional response to pain.

USES
Treatment of moderate-to-severe pain, preoperatively in sedation techniques

PHARMACOKINETICS

Route	Onset	Peak	Duration
PO	15 min	60 min	2–4 hr
IV	Less than 5 min	5–7 min	2–3 hr
IM	10–15 min	30–50 min	2–4 hr
Subcutaneous	10–15 min	30–50 min	2–4 hr

Variably absorbed from the GI tract; well absorbed after IM administration. Protein binding: 60%–80%. Widely distributed. Metabolized in the liver to active metabolite. Primarily excreted in urine. Not removed by hemodialysis.

Half-life: 2.4–4 hr; metabolite 8–16 hr (increased in hepatic impairment and disease).

INDICATIONS AND DOSAGES
▶ **Analgesia**
PO, IM, Subcutaneous
Adults, Elderly. 50–150 mg q3–4h.
Children. 1.1–1.5 mg/kg q3–4h.
Don't exceed single dose of 100 mg.
▶ **Patient-Controlled Analgesia**
IV
Adults. Loading dose: 50–100 mg.
Intermittent bolus: 5–30 mg.
Lockout interval: 10–20 min.
Continuous infusion: 5–40 mg/hr.
Maximum (4-hr): 200–300 mg.
▶ **Dosage in Renal Impairment**
Dosage is based on creatinine clearance.

Creatinine Clearance	Dosage
10–50 ml/min	75% of usual dose
Less than 10 ml/min	50% of usual dose

SIDE EFFECTS/ADVERSE REACTIONS
Frequent
Sedation, hypotension (including orthostatic hypotension), diaphoresis, facial flushing, dizziness, nausea, vomiting, constipation
Occasional
Confusion, arrhythmias, tremors, urine retention, abdominal pain, dry mouth, headache, irritation at injection site, euphoria, dysphoria
Rare
Allergic reaction (rash, pruritus), insomnia

PRECAUTIONS AND CONTRAINDICATIONS
Delivery of premature infant, diarrhea due to poisoning, use within 14 days of MAOIs

. **Caution**
Addictive personality, lactation,
increased intracranial pressure, MI
(acute), severe heart disease,
respiratory depression, hepatic
disease, renal disease, children
younger than 18 yr

DRUG INTERACTIONS OF CONCERN TO DENTISTRY
• Increased effects with all CNS
depressants, neuromuscular blocking
agents
• Contraindication: MAOIs,
sibutramine
• Increased effects of
anticholinergics
• Suspected increase in
normeperidine levels: ritonavir
• Increased risk of hypotension:
antihypertensive drugs

SERIOUS REACTIONS
! Overdose results in respiratory
depression, skeletal muscle
flaccidity, cold or clammy skin,
cyanosis, and extreme somnolence
progressing to seizures, stupor, and
coma. The antidote is 0.4 mg
naloxone.
! The patient who uses meperidine
repeatedly may develop a tolerance
to the drug's analgesic effect and
physical dependence.

DENTAL CONSIDERATIONS
General:
• After supine positioning, have
patient sit upright for at least 2 min
before standing to avoid orthostatic
hypotension.
• Psychologic and physical
dependence may occur with chronic
administration.
Teach Patient/Family to:
• Avoid mouth rinses with high
alcohol content because of drying
effects

mephentermine sulfate
meh-fen´-ter-meen sull´-fate
(Wyamine Sulfate)

CATEGORY AND SCHEDULE
Pregnancy Risk Category: C

Drug Class: Sympathomimetic

MECHANISM OF ACTION
A sympathomimetic amine that acts
indirectly by releasing
norepinephrine and directly by
exerting a slight effect on α and
β_1 receptors and a moderate effect on
β_2 receptors mediating vasodilation.
Therapeutic Effect: Produces
cardiac stimulation.

USES
Treatment of hypotension due to
anesthesia, ganglionic blockade, or
hemorrhage

PHARMACOKINETICS
Onset of action occurs immediately
and persists 15–30 min. Metabolized
in liver. Excreted in urine.
Half-life: 17–18 hr.

INDICATIONS AND DOSAGES
▶ **Hypotension (secondary to spinal anesthesia)**
IM/IV
Adults. 30–45 mg as a single
injection.
▶ **Prophylaxis of hypotension in spinal anesthesia**
IM/IV
Adults. 30–45 mg 10–20 min before
anesthesia.

SIDE EFFECTS/ADVERSE REACTIONS
Occasional
Anxiety, nervousness, cardiac
arrhythmias, increased B/P

M

PRECAUTIONS AND CONTRAINDICATIONS

Concurrent use or within 14 days of discontinuation of MAOI therapy, hypotension induced by chlorpromazine, hypersensitivity to mephentermine or sympathomimetic amines

DRUG INTERACTIONS OF CONCERN TO DENTISTRY

• Increased risk of arrhythmia: halogenated hydrocarbon anesthetics

SERIOUS REACTIONS

! Mephentermine may produce arrhythmias, including transient extrasystoles, AV block, and hypertension.
! CNS effects, including hyperexcitability, prolonged wakefulness, weeping, incoherence, convulsions, flushing, tremors, and hallucinations, may occur with large doses of mephentermine.

DENTAL CONSIDERATIONS

General:
• For use in hospitals or emergency rooms for selected hypotensive episodes.

mephobarbital
me´-foe-bar´-bi-tal
(Mebaral)

CATEGORY AND SCHEDULE

Pregnancy Risk Category: D
Controlled substance: Schedule IV

Drug Class: Barbiturate anticonvulsant

MECHANISM OF ACTION

A barbiturate that increases seizure threshold in the motor cortex. *Therapeutic Effect:* Depresses monosynaptic and polysynaptic transmission in the CNS.

USES

Treatment of generalized tonic-clonic (grand mal) or absence (petit mal) seizures, sedation

PHARMACOKINETICS

PO route onset 20–60 min, peak N/A, duration 6–8 hr. Well absorbed after PO administration. Widely distributed. Metabolized in liver to active metabolite, a form of phenobarbital. Minimally excreted in urine. Removed by hemodialysis. *Half-life:* 34 hr.

INDICATIONS AND DOSAGES
▸ **Epilepsy**
PO
Adults, Elderly. 400–600 mg/day in divided doses or at bedtime.
Children older than 5 yr. 32–64 mg 3 or 4 times a day.
Children younger than 5 yr. 16–32 mg 3 or 4 times a day.
▸ **Sedation**
PO
Adults, Elderly. 32–100 mg/day in 3–4 divided doses.
Children. 16–32 mg in 3–4 divided doses.

SIDE EFFECTS/ADVERSE REACTIONS
Frequent
Dizziness, lightheadedness, somnolence
Occasional
Confusion, headache, insomnia, mental depression, nervousness, nightmares, unusual excitement
Rare
Rash, paradoxical CNS hyperactivity or nervousness in children, excitement or restlessness in elderly, generally noted during first 2 wk of therapy, particularly noted in presence of uncontrolled pain

PRECAUTIONS AND CONTRAINDICATIONS

Porphyria, history of hypersensitivity to mephobarbital or other barbiturates.

Caution
Hepatic disease, renal disease, lactation, alcoholism, drug abuse, hyperthyroidism

DRUG INTERACTIONS OF CONCERN TO DENTISTRY
• Increased effects: alcohol, all CNS depressants
• Decreased effects of corticosteroids, doxycycline, carbamazepine

SERIOUS REACTIONS
! Abrupt withdrawal after prolonged therapy may produce effects including markedly increased dreaming, nightmares or insomnia, tremors, sweating, vomiting, to hallucinations, delirium, seizures, and status epilepticus.
! Skin eruptions appear as hypersensitivity reaction.
! Blood dyscrasias, liver disease, and hypocalcemia occur rarely.
! Overdosage produces cold or clammy skin, hypothermia, severe CNS depression, cyanosis, rapid pulse, and Cheyne-Stokes respirations.
! Toxicity may result in severe renal impairment.

DENTAL CONSIDERATIONS
General:
• Determine type of epilepsy, seizure frequency, and quality of seizure control. A stress reduction protocol may be required.
• Monitor vital signs at every appointment because of cardiovascular and respiratory side effects.
• Patients on chronic drug therapy may rarely have symptoms of blood dyscrasias, which can include infection, bleeding, and poor healing.
• Barbiturates induce liver microsomal enzymes, which alters the metabolism of other drugs.
• Avoid drugs that may lower seizure threshold (phenothiazines).

• Be sure patient is regularly taking medication.
Consultations:
• In a patient with symptoms of blood dyscrasias, request a medical consultation for blood studies and postpone dental treatment until normal values are reestablished.
• Medical consultation may be required to assess disease control and patient's ability to tolerate stress.
Teach Patient/Family to:
• Use effective oral hygiene to prevent soft tissue inflammation
• Use caution to prevent injury when using oral hygiene aids
• Avoid mouth rinses with high alcohol content because of drying effects

mepivacaine HCl (local)

M

me-piv´-ah-kane high-droh-klor´-ide
(Carbocaine Caudal 1.5%[AUS], Carbocaine HCl, Polocaine, Polocaine-MPF)

CATEGORY AND SCHEDULE
Pregnancy Risk Category: C

Drug Class: Amide local anesthetic

MECHANISM OF ACTION
An amide anesthetic that inhibits conduction of nerve impulses. *Therapeutic Effect:* Causes temporary loss of feeling and sensation.

USES
Local dental anesthesia, nerve block, caudal anesthesia, epidural, pain relief, paracervical block, transvaginal block or infiltration

PHARMACOKINETICS

Onset	Peak	Duration
3–20 min	N/A	2–2.5 hr

Protein binding: 75%. Rapidly metabolized in liver. Small amount is excreted in urine. *Half-life:* 1.9–3.2 hr; 8.7–9 hr (neonates).

INDICATIONS AND DOSAGES

Recommended Concentrations and Doses of Mepivacaine

Concentration	Total Dose		Comments
	ml	mg	
Cervical, Brachial Intercostal, Pudendal Nerve Block			
1%	5–40	50–400	Pudendal block; half of total dose injected each side
2%	5–20	100–400	
Transvaginal Block (Paracervical and Pudendal)			
1%	Up to 30 (both sides)	Up to 300 both sides)	Half of total dose injected each side
Paracervical Block			
1%	Up to 20 (both sides)	Up to 200 (both sides)	Half of total dose injected each side. This is maximum recommended dose per 90-min period in obstetrical patients. Inject slowly, 5 min. between sides.
Caudal and Epidural Block			
1%	15–30	150–300	Use only single-dose vials that do not contain a preservative.
1.5%	10–25	150–375	
2%	10–20	200–400	
Infiltration			
1%	Up to 30	Up to 300	An equivalent amount of a 0.5% solution (prepared by diluting the 1% solution with sodium chloride) injection can be used for large areas.
Therapeutic Block (Pain Management)			
1%	1–5	10–50	
2%	1–5	20–100	

▸ **Regional Anesthesia**
Children younger than 3 yr or weighing less than 30 lb. Maximum dose of mepivacaine should not exceed 4.4 mg/kg. Concentrations greater than 1.5% should be avoided.

SIDE EFFECTS/ADVERSE REACTIONS

CNS and cardiovascular effects are generally dose related and of short duration

Occasional
Burning, stinging, tenderness

Rare
Generally with high dose:
Drowsiness, dizziness, disorientation, light-headedness, tremors, apprehension, euphoria, blurred or double vision, ringing or roaring in ears (tinnitus), nausea, sensation of heat, cold, numbness

PRECAUTIONS AND CONTRAINDICATIONS

Hypersensitivity to any local anesthetic agent of the amide-type or to other components of solutions of mepivacaine

Caution
Elderly, severe drug allergies.

DRUG INTERACTIONS OF CONCERN TO DENTISTRY

• CNS depressants: may see increased risk of CNS depression with all CNS depressants, especially in children and when larger doses are used
• Avoid placing dental cartridges in disinfectant solutions with heavy metals or surface-active agents; may see release of metal ions into local anesthetic solutions with tissue irritation following injection
• Avoid excessive exposure of dental cartridges to light or heat, which hastens deterioration of vasoconstrictor; observe for color change in local anesthetic solution
• Risk of cardiovascular side effects: rapid intravascular administration of local anesthetic containing vasoconstrictor, either alone or in patients taking tricyclic antidepressants, MAOIs, digitalis drugs, cocaine, phenothiazines, β-blockers, and in the presence of halogenated-hydrocarbon general anesthetics; use lowest effective vasoconstrictor dose and careful aspiration techniques
• Avoid use of vasoconstrictors in patients with uncontrolled hyperthyroidism, diabetes, angina, or hypertension; refer these patients for medical treatment before elective dental procedures

SERIOUS REACTIONS

! CNS toxicity may occur, especially with regional anesthesia use, progressing rapidly from mild side effects to tremors, somnolence, seizures, vomiting, and respiratory depression.
! Allergic reactions, bradyarrhythmia, cardiac arrest, fetal bradycardia, heart block, hypotension, seizure, and ventricular arrhythmia have been reported.
! Allergic reactions occur rarely.

DENTAL CONSIDERATIONS

General:
• Drug is often used with a vasoconstrictor for increased duration of action.
• Monitor vital signs at every appointment because of cardiovascular and respiratory side effects.
• Lubricate dry lips before injection.

Teach Patient/Family to:
• Use care to prevent injury while numbness exists and to refrain from

M

chewing gum and eating following dental anesthesia
- Report any signs of infection, muscle pain, or fever to dentist when feeling returns
- Report any unusual soft tissue reactions

meprobamate
meh-proe-ba´-mate
(Miltown, Novo-Mepro[CAN])

CATEGORY AND SCHEDULE
Pregnancy Risk Category: D
Schedule IV

Drug Class: Sedative-hypnotic, anxiolytic

MECHANISM OF ACTION
A carbamate derivative that affects the thalamus and limbic system. Appears to inhibit multi-neuronal spinal reflexes. ***Therapeutic Effect:*** Relieves pain or muscle spasms.

USES
Treatment of anxiety disorders

PHARMACOKINETICS
Slowly absorbed from the GI tract. Protein binding: 0%–30%. Metabolized in liver. Excreted in urine and feces. Moderately dialyzable. ***Half-life:*** 10 hr.

INDICATIONS AND DOSAGES
▸ Anxiety Disorders
PO
Adults, Children 12 yr and older. 400 mg 3–4 times. Maximum: 2400 mg/day.
Children 6–12 yr. 100–200 mg 2–3 times a day.
Elderly. Use lowest effective dose. 200 mg 2–3 times a day

▸ Dosage in Renal Impairment

Creatinine Clearance	Dosage Interval
10–50 ml/min	Every 9–12 hr
Less than 10 ml/min	Every 12–18 hr

SIDE EFFECTS/ADVERSE REACTIONS
Frequent
Drowsiness, dizziness

Occasional
Tachycardia, palpitations, headache, lightheadedness, dermatitis, diarrhea, nausea, vomiting, dyspnea, rash, weakness, blurred vision, wheezing

PRECAUTIONS AND CONTRAINDICATIONS
Acute intermittent porphyria, hypersensitivity to meprobamate or related compounds

Caution
Suicidal patients, severe depression, renal disease, hepatic disease, elderly

DRUG INTERACTIONS OF CONCERN TO DENTISTRY
- Increased effects: CNS depressants, alcohol

SERIOUS REACTIONS
▮ Agranulocytosis, aplastic anemia, leucopenia, anaphylaxis, cardiac arrhythmias, hypotensive crisis, syncope, Stevens-Johnson syndrome and bullous dermatitis have been reported.
▮ Overdose may cause CNS depression, ataxia, coma, shock, hypotension, and death.

DENTAL CONSIDERATIONS
General:
- Monitor vital signs at every appointment because of cardiovascular side effects.
- Patients on chronic drug therapy may rarely have symptoms of blood

dyscrasias, which can include infection, bleeding, and poor healing.
* Assess salivary flow as a factor in caries, periodontal disease, and candidiasis.
* Avoid dental light in patient's eyes; offer dark glasses for patient comfort.
* Determine why the patient is taking the drug.
* Psychologic and physical dependence may occur with chronic administration.
Consultations:
* In a patient with symptoms of blood dyscrasias, request a medical consultation for blood studies and postpone dental treatment until normal values are reestablished.
* Medical consultation may be required to assess disease control.
Teach Patient/Family to:
* Use effective oral hygiene to prevent soft tissue inflammation
* Use caution to prevent injury when using oral hygiene aids
* When chronic dry mouth occurs, advise patient to:
  * Avoid mouth rinses with high alcohol content because of drying effects
  * Use sugarless gum, frequent sips of water, or saliva substitutes
  * Use daily home fluoride products for anticaries effect

mercaptopurine (6-MP)
mur-cap-tow-pure´-een
(Purinethol)

CATEGORY AND SCHEDULE
Pregnancy Risk Category: D

Drug Class:
Antineoplastic-antimetabolite

MECHANISM OF ACTION
An antimetabolite that is incorporated into RNA and DNA, blocks purine synthesis, and inhibits DNA and RNA synthesis.
Therapeutic Effect: Causes death of cancer cells.

USES
Treatment of acute lymphatic leukemia (ALL), acute myelogenous leukemia (AML)

PHARMACOKINETICS
Incompletely absorbed when taken orally; metabolized in liver; excreted in urine.

INDICATIONS AND DOSAGES
▶ **ALL**
PO
Adults, Elderly, Children. 2.5–5 mg/kg once a day as induction dose.
Maintenance: 1.5–2.5 mg/kg/day.
▶ **Dosage in Renal Impairment:**
Creatinine clearance less than 50 ml/min. Administer usual dose q48h.

SIDE EFFECTS/ADVERSE REACTIONS
Frequent
Myelosuppression (leading to leukopenia, thrombocytopenia, anemia), intrahepatic cholestasis, hepatic necrosis
Occasional
Drug fever, hyperpigmentation, rash, hyperuricemia, nausea, vomiting, diarrhea, stomatitis, anorexia, abdominal pain, mucositis

PRECAUTIONS AND CONTRAINDICATIONS
Pregnancy, severe myelosuppression or hepatic disease
Caution
Renal disease

M

DRUG INTERACTIONS OF CONCERN TO DENTISTRY

• Increased risk of hepatotoxicity: hepatotoxic drugs

SERIOUS REACTIONS

! Myelosuppression, hepatic necrosis, and gastroenteritis may occur.

DENTAL CONSIDERATIONS

General:

• Patients on chronic drug therapy may rarely have symptoms of blood dyscrasias, which can include infection, bleeding, and poor healing.
• Avoid prescribing aspirin-containing products.
• Prophylactic antibiotics may be indicated to prevent infection if surgery or deep scaling is planned.
• Patients receiving chemotherapy may require palliative treatment for stomatitis.

Consultations:

• In a patient with symptoms of blood dyscrasias, request a medical consultation for blood studies and postpone dental treatment until normal values are reestablished.

Teach Patient/Family to:

• Use effective oral hygiene to prevent soft tissue inflammation
• Use caution to prevent injury when using oral hygiene aids
• Avoid mouth rinses with high alcohol content

---

meropenem

mare-oh-peh´-nem
(Merrem IV)

CATEGORY AND SCHEDULE

Pregnancy Risk Category: B

Drug Class: Antiinfective, miscellaneous; carbapenem

MECHANISM OF ACTION

A carbapenem that binds to penicillin-binding proteins and inhibits bacterial cell wall synthesis. ***Therapeutic Effect:*** Produces bacterial cell death.

USES

Treatment of infections caused by bacteria

PHARMACOKINETICS

After IV administration, widely distributed into tissues and body fluids, including CSF. Protein binding: 2%. Primarily excreted unchanged in urine. Removed by hemodialysis. ***Half-life:*** 1 hr.

INDICATIONS AND DOSAGES

▸ **Mild-to-Moderate Infections**
IV
Adults, Elderly. 0.5–1 g q8h.
Children 3 mo and older. 20 mg/kg/ dose q8h.
Children younger than 3 mo. 20 mg/kg/dose q8–12h.

▸ **Meningitis**
IV
Adults, Elderly, Children weighing 50 kg or more. 2 g q8h.
Children 3 mo and older weighing less than 50 kg. 40 mg/kg q8h. Maximum: 2 g/dose.

▸ **Dosage in Renal Impairment**
Dosage and frequency are modified on the basis of creatinine clearance.

Creatinine Clearance	Dosage	Interval
26–49 ml/min	Recommended dose (1000 mg)	q12h
10–25 ml/min	$\frac{1}{2}$ of recommended dose	q12h
Less than 10 ml/min	$\frac{1}{2}$ of recommended dose	q24h

SIDE EFFECTS/ADVERSE REACTIONS
Frequent
Diarrhea, nausea, vomiting, headache, inflammation at injection site
Occasional
Oral candidiasis, rash, pruritus
Rare
Constipation, glossitis

PRECAUTIONS AND CONTRAINDICATIONS
None known

DRUG INTERACTIONS OF CONCERN TO DENTISTRY
• Increased or prolonged plasma levels: probenecid

SERIOUS REACTIONS
❗ Antibiotic-associated colitis and other superinfections may occur.
❗ Anaphylactic reactions have been reported.
❗ Seizures may occur in those with CNS disorders (including brain lesions and a history of seizures), bacterial meningitis, or impaired renal function.

DENTAL CONSIDERATIONS
General:
• For selected infections in the hospital setting: provide emergency dental treatment only.
• Examine for oral manifestation of opportunistic infection.
• Determine why patient is taking the drug.
• Caution regarding allergy to medication.
Consultations:
• Consult patient's physician if an acute dental infection occurs and another antiinfective is required.
• Medical consultation may be required to assess disease control.

Teach Patient/Family to:
• Use effective oral hygiene to prevent soft tissue inflammation
• Report oral lesions, soreness, or bleeding to dentist
• Prevent trauma when using oral hygiene aids

---

mesalamine/ 5 aminosalicylic acid(5-ASA)
mez-al´-a-meen
ah-mee-no-sal-i-sill´-ik
(Asacol, Fiv-Canasa, Mesasal[CAN], Pentasa, Rowasa, Salofalk[CAN])
Do not confuse Asacol with Os-Cal.

CATEGORY AND SCHEDULE
Pregnancy Risk Category: B

Drug Class: Antiinflammatory

MECHANISM OF ACTION
A salicylic acid derivative that locally inhibits arachidonic acid metabolite production, which is increased in patients with chronic inflammatory bowel disease. *Therapeutic Effect:* Blocks prostaglandin production and diminishes inflammation in the colon.

USES
Treatment of inflammatory bowel disease, ulcerative colitis, maintenance for remission of ulcerative colitis

PHARMACOKINETICS
Poorly absorbed from the colon. Moderately absorbed from the GI tract. Metabolized in the liver to active metabolite. Unabsorbed portion eliminated in feces; absorbed portion excreted in urine. Unknown if removed by hemodialysis.

Half-life: 0.5–1.5 hr; metabolite, 5–10 hr.

INDICATIONS AND DOSAGES
▸ **Ulcerative Colitis, Proctosigmoiditis, Proctitis**
PO (Asacol)
Adults, Elderly. 800 mg 3 times a day for 6 wk.
Children. 50 mg/kg/day q8–12h.
PO (Pentasa)
Adults, Elderly. 1 g 4 times a day for 8 wk.
Children. 50 mg/kg/day q6–12h.
Rectal (retention enema)
Adults, Elderly. 60 ml (4 g) at bedtime; retain overnight (about 8 hr) for 3–6 wk.
Rectal (suppositories)
Adults, Elderly. 1 suppository (500 mg) twice a day, retain 1–3 hr for 3–6 wk.
▸ **To Maintain Remission in Ulcerative Colitis**
PO (Asacol)
Adults, Elderly. 1.6 g/day in divided doses.
PO (Pentasa)
Adults, Elderly. 1 g 4 times a day

SIDE EFFECTS/ADVERSE REACTIONS
Mesalamine is generally well tolerated, with only mild and transient effects
Frequent
PO: Abdominal cramps or pain, diarrhea, dizziness, headache, nausea, vomiting, rhinitis, unusual fatigue
Rectal: Abdominal or stomach cramps, flatulence, headache, nausea
Occasional
PO: Hair loss, decreased appetite, back or joint pain, flatulence, acne
Rectal: Hair loss
Rare
Rectal: Anal irritation

PRECAUTIONS AND CONTRAINDICATIONS
Hypersensitivity, renal disease, lactation, children, sulfite sensitivity
Caution
Renal disease, lactation, children, sulfite sensitivity

SERIOUS REACTIONS
! Sulfite sensitivity may occur in susceptible patients, manifested by cramping, headache, diarrhea, fever, rash, hives, itching, and wheezing. Discontinue drug immediately.
! Hepatitis, pancreatitis, and pericarditis occur rarely with oral forms.

DENTAL CONSIDERATIONS
General:
• Consider semisupine chair position for patient comfort because of GI effects of disease.
Consultations
• To reduce any potential risk of antibiotic-associated pseudomembranous colitis, a consultation is recommended before selecting an antibiotic for a dental infection.

mesna
mez´-na
(Mesnex, Uromitexan[CAN])

CATEGORY AND SCHEDULE
Pregnancy Risk Category: B

Drug Class: Cytoprotective agent; antineoplastic adjunct, antidote

MECHANISM OF ACTION
An antineoplastic adjunct and cytoprotective agent that binds with

and detoxifies urotoxic metabolites of ifosfamide and cyclophosphamide. ***Therapeutic Effect:*** Inhibits ifosfamide- and cyclophosphamide-induced hemorrhagic cystitis.

USES
Detoxifying agent used as a protectant against hemorrhagic cystitis induced by ifosamide, cyclophosphamide

PHARMACOKINETICS
Rapidly metabolized after IV administration to mesna disulfide, which is reduced to mesna in kidney. Excreted in urine. ***Half-life:*** 24 min.

INDICATIONS AND DOSAGES
▸ **Prevention of Hemorrhagic Cystitis in Patients Receiving Ifosfamide**
IV
Adults, Elderly. 20% of ifosfamide dose at time of ifosfamide administration and 4 and 8 hr after each dose of ifosfamide. Total dose: 60% of ifosfamide dosage. Range: 60%–160% of the daily ifosfamide dose.
▸ **Prevention of Hemorrhagic Cystitis in Patients Receiving Cyclophosphamide**
PO
Adults, Elderly. 40% of cyclophosphamide dose q4h for 3 doses.
IV
Adults, Elderly. 20% of cyclophosphamide dose at time of cyclophosphamide administration and q3h for 3–4 doses.

SIDE EFFECTS/ADVERSE REACTIONS
Frequent
Bad taste, soft stools
Large doses: Diarrhea, myalgia, headache, fatigue, nausea, hypotension, allergic reaction

PRECAUTIONS AND CONTRAINDICATIONS
None known

DRUG INTERACTIONS OF CONCERN TO DENTISTRY
None reported

SERIOUS REACTIONS
❗ Hematuria occurs rarely.

DENTAL CONSIDERATIONS
General:
• Patient will be taking ifosfamide or cyclophosphamide; determine use and disease.
• Question patient about other diseases and medications taken.
• Note side effects and precautions associated with chemotherapeutic drugs.

Consultations:
• Medical consultation should include routine blood counts including platelet counts and bleeding time.
• Consult physician; prophylactic or therapeutic antiinfectives may be indicated if surgery or periodontal treatment is required.
• Medical consultation may be required to assess immunologic status during cancer chemotherapy and determine safety risk, if any, posed by the required dental treatment.
• Medical consultation may be required to assess disease control and patient's ability to tolerate stress.

Teach Patient/Family to:
• Use effective oral hygiene to prevent soft tissue inflammation
• Prevent trauma when using oral hygiene aids
• Report oral lesions, soreness, or bleeding to dentist
• Update health and medication history if physician makes any

changes in evaluation or drug regimens; include OTC, herbal, and nonherbal drugs in the update

mesoridazine besylate

mez-oh-rid´-ah-zeen bes-il´-ayte (Serentil)

Do not confuse Serentil with Proventil, Serevent, or sertraline.

CATEGORY AND SCHEDULE

Pregnancy Risk Category: C

Drug Class: Phenothiazine antipsychotic

MECHANISM OF ACTION

A phenothiazine that blocks dopamine at postsynaptic receptor sites in the brain. *Therapeutic Effect:* Diminishes schizophrenic behavior. Also has anticholinergic and sedative effects.

USES

Treatment of psychotic disorders, schizophrenia when inadequate response with other antipsychotic drugs

PHARMACOKINETICS

PO: Onset erratic, peak 2 hr, duration 4-6 hr.

IM: Onset 15–30 min, peak 30 min, duration 6–8 hr. Metabolized by liver, excreted in urine, crosses placenta, excreted in breast milk.

INDICATIONS AND DOSAGES

▶ **Schizophrenia**
PO
Adults, Elderly. 25–50 mg 3 times a day. Maximum: 400 mg/day.
IM

Adults, Elderly. Initially, 25 mg. May repeat in 30–60 min. Range: 25–200 mg.

▶ **Severe Behavioral Problems (combativeness or explosive, hyperexcitable behavior) Associated with Neurologic Diseases**
PO
Elderly. Initially, 10 mg once or twice a day. May increase at 4–7 day intervals. Maximum: 250 mg.
IM
Adults, Elderly. Initially, 25 mg. May repeat in 30–60 min. Range: 25–200 mg.

SIDE EFFECTS/ADVERSE REACTIONS

Frequent
Orthostatic hypotension, dizziness, syncope (occur frequently after first injection, occasionally after subsequent injections, and rarely with oral form)

Occasional
Somnolence (during early therapy), dry mouth, blurred vision, lethargy, constipation or diarrhea, nasal congestion, peripheral edema, urine retention

Rare
Ocular changes, altered skin pigmentation (in those taking high doses for prolonged periods), darkening of urine

PRECAUTIONS AND CONTRAINDICATIONS

Coma, myelosuppression, severe cardiovascular disease, severe CNS depression, subcortical brain damage

Caution
Lactation, seizure disorders, hypertension, hepatic disease, cardiac disease, prostatic hypertrophy, intestinal obstruction,

respiratory conditions, dose-related prolongation of QTc interval

DRUG INTERACTIONS OF CONCERN TO DENTISTRY

• Increased sedation: other CNS depressants, alcohol, barbiturate anesthetics, opioid analgesics
• Hypotension, tachycardia: epinephrine
• Increased extrapyramidal effects: phenothiazines and related drugs (haloperidol, droperidol), metoclopramide
• Additive photosensitization: tetracyclines
• Increased anticholinergic effects: anticholinergics

SERIOUS REACTIONS

! Abrupt withdrawal after long-term therapy may precipitate nausea, vomiting, gastritis, dizziness, and tremors.
! Blood dyscrasias, particularly agranulocytosis and mild leukopenia, may occur.
! Mesoridazine use may lower the seizure threshold.

DENTAL CONSIDERATIONS

General:
• Monitor vital signs at every appointment because of cardiovascular side effects.
• Patients on chronic drug therapy may rarely have symptoms of blood dyscrasias, which can include infection, bleeding, and poor healing.
• After supine positioning, have patient sit upright for at least 2 min before standing to avoid orthostatic hypotension.
• Assess salivary flow as a factor in caries, periodontal disease, and candidiasis.
• Avoid dental light in patient's eyes; offer dark glasses for patient comfort.

• Assess for presence of extrapyramidal motor symptoms, such as tardive dyskinesia and akathisia. Extrapyramidal motor activity may complicate dental treatment.
• Geriatric patients are more susceptible to drug effects; use lower dose.
• Use vasoconstrictors with caution, in low doses, and with careful aspiration. Avoid use of gingival retraction cord with epinephrine.
Consultations:
• In a patient with symptoms of blood dyscrasias, request a medical consultation for blood studies and postpone dental treatment until normal values are reestablished.
• Take precautions if dental surgery is anticipated and anesthesia is required.
• Refer to physician if signs of tardive dyskinesia or akathisia are present.
• Physician should be informed if significant xerostomic side effects occur (e.g., increased caries, sore tongue, problems eating or swallowing, difficulty wearing prosthesis) so that a medication change can be considered.
Teach Patient/Family to:
• Use effective oral hygiene to prevent soft tissue inflammation
• Use caution to prevent injury when using oral hygiene aids
• Use electric tooth brush if patient has difficulty holding conventional devices
• When chronic dry mouth occurs, advise patient to:
  • Avoid mouth rinses with high alcohol content because of drying effects
  • Use sugarless gum, frequent sips of water, or saliva substitutes
  • Use daily home fluoride products for anticaries effect

metaproterenol sulfate

met-ah-proe-ter´-eh-nole suhl´-feyt
(Alupent)
Do not confuse metaproterenol with metipranolol or metoprolol, or Alupent with Atrovent.

CATEGORY AND SCHEDULE
Pregnancy Risk Category: C

Drug Class: Selective β_2-agonist

MECHANISM OF ACTION
A sympathomimetic that stimulates β_2-adrenergic receptors, resulting in relaxation of bronchial smooth muscle. ***Therapeutic Effect:*** Relieves bronchospasm and reduces airway resistance.

USES
Treatment of bronchial asthma, bronchospasm

PHARMACOKINETICS
3% absorbed through lungs after inhalation. Primarily metabolized in the GI tract. Duration 1–5 hr following a single dose (reduced to 1–2.5 hr after repetitive dosing).

INDICATIONS AND DOSAGES
▶ **Treatment of Bronchospasm**
PO
Adults, Children 10 yr and older. 20 mg 3–4 times a day.
Elderly. 10 mg 3–4 times a day. May increase to 20 mg/dose.
Children 6–9 yr. 10 mg 3–4 times a day.
Children 2–5 yr. 1.3–2.6 mg/kg/day in 3–4 divided doses.
Children younger than 2 yr. 0.4 mg/kg 3–4 times a day.
Inhalation
Adults, Elderly, Children 12 yr and older. 2–3 inhalations q3–4h.
Maximum: 12 inhalations/24 hr.

Nebulization
Adults, Elderly, Children 12 yr and older. 10–15 mg (0.2–0.3 ml) of 5% q4–6h.
Children younger than 12 yr, Infants. 0.5–1 mg/kg (0.01–0.02 ml/kg) of 5% q4–6h.

SIDE EFFECTS/ADVERSE REACTIONS
Frequent

Rigors, tremors, anxiety, nausea, dry mouth
Occasional

Dizziness, vertigo, asthenia, headache, GI distress, vomiting, cough, dry throat
Rare

Somnolence, diarrhea, altered taste

PRECAUTIONS AND CONTRAINDICATIONS
Angle-closure glaucoma, preexisting arrhythmias associated with tachycardia
Caution

Cardiac disorders, hyperthyroidism, diabetes mellitus, prostatic hypertrophy.

DRUG INTERACTIONS OF CONCERN TO DENTISTRY
* Increased effects of both drugs: other sympathomimetics, CNS stimulants
* Increased dysrhythmias: halogenated hydrocarbon anesthetics

SERIOUS REACTIONS
! Excessive sympathomimetic stimulation may cause palpitations, extrasystoles, tachycardia, chest pain, a slight increase in B/P followed by a substantial decrease, chills, diaphoresis, and blanching of skin.
! Too-frequent or excessive use may lead to decreased drug effectiveness and severe, paradoxical bronchoconstriction.

DENTAL CONSIDERATIONS

General:
- Assess salivary flow as a factor in caries, periodontal disease, and candidiasis.
- Consider semisupine chair position for patients with respiratory disease.
- Short appointments and a stress reduction protocol may be required for anxious patients.
- Be aware that aspirin or sulfite preservatives in vasoconstrictor-containing products can exacerbate asthma.
- Acute asthmatic episodes may be precipitated in the dental office. Sympathomimetic inhalants should be available for emergency use.

Consultations:
- Medical consultation may be required to assess disease control and patient's ability to tolerate stress.

Teach Patient/Family to:
- Rinse mouth with water after each inhaled dose to prevent dryness
- When chronic dry mouth occurs, advise patient to:
  - Avoid mouth rinses with high alcohol content because of drying effects
  - Use sugarless gum, frequent sips of water, or saliva substitutes
  - Use daily home fluoride products for anticaries effect

metaraminol
met-ar-am´-eh-nol
(Aramine)

CATEGORY AND SCHEDULE
Pregnancy Risk Category: D

Drug Class: Adrenergic agonists

MECHANISM OF ACTION
An α-adrenergic receptor agonist that causes vasoconstriction, reflex bradycardia, inhibits GI smooth muscle and vascular smooth muscle supplying skeletal muscle and increases heart rate and force of heart muscle contraction.
Therapeutic Effect: Increases both systolic and diastolic pressure.

USES
Treatment and prevention of hypotension due to hemorrhage, spinal anesthesia, and shock associated with brain damage

PHARMACOKINETICS

Route	Onset	Peak	Duration
IM (Pressor Effect)	10 min	N/A	20–60 min
IV	1–2 min	N/A	
SC	5–20 min	N/A	

Metabolized in the liver. Excreted in the urine and the bile.

INDICATIONS AND DOSAGES
▶ **Prevention of Hypotension**
IM/Subcutaneous
Adults, Elderly. 2–10 mg as a single dose.
Children. 0.01 mg/kg as a single dose.
▶ **Adjunctive Treatment of Hypotension**
IV
Adults, Elderly. 15–100 mg IV infusion, administered at a rate to maintain the desired B/P.
▶ **Severe Shock**
IV
Adults, Elderly. 0.5–5 mg direct IV injection followed by 15–100 mg IV infusion in 250–500 ml fluid for control of B/P.

SIDE EFFECTS/ADVERSE REACTIONS

Occasional
Tachycardia, hypertension, cardiac arrhythmias, flushing, palpitations, hypotension, angina, tremors, nervousness, headache, dizziness, weakness, sloughing of skin, nausea, abscess formation, diaphoresis

PRECAUTIONS AND CONTRAINDICATIONS

Cyclopropane or halothane anesthesia, use of MAOIs, pregnancy, hypersensitivity to metaraminol

DRUG INTERACTIONS OF CONCERN TO DENTISTRY

• Increased risk of arrhythmia: halogenated hydrocarbon anesthetics

SERIOUS REACTIONS

! Overdosage produces hypertension, cerebral hemorrhage, cardiac arrest, and seizures.

DENTAL CONSIDERATIONS

General:
• Acute-use drug for use in hospitals or emergency rooms for selected hypotensive episodes.

metaxalone
me-tax´-ah-lone
(Skelaxin)

CATEGORY AND SCHEDULE
Pregnancy Risk Category: C

Drug Class: Muscle relaxant

MECHANISM OF ACTION
A central depressant whose exact mechanism is unknown. Many effects due to its central depressant

actions. *Therapeutic Effect:* Relieves pain or muscle spasms.

USES
Adjunct to rest, physical therapy, and other measures for relief of discomfort associated with acute, painful musculoskeletal conditions

PHARMACOKINETICS
PO route onset 1 hr, peak 3 hr, duration 4–6 hr. Well absorbed from the GI tract. Metabolized in liver. Primarily excreted in urine. *Half-life:* 9 hr.

INDICATIONS AND DOSAGES
▶ Muscle Relaxant
PO
Adults, Elderly, Children older than 12 yr. 800 mg 3–4 times a day.

SIDE EFFECTS/ADVERSE REACTIONS

Occasional
Drowsiness, headache, lightheadedness, dermatitis, nausea, vomiting, stomach cramps, dyspnea

PRECAUTIONS AND CONTRAINDICATIONS

Impaired renal or hepatic function, history of drug-induced hemolytic anemias or other anemias, history of hypersensitivity to metaxalone
Caution
Preexisting hepatic impairment, lactation, children younger than 12 yr, alcohol use

DRUG INTERACTIONS OF CONCERN TO DENTISTRY

• No data reported; however, this drug does cause a nonspecific CNS depression: monitor patients if other CNS depressants are used

SERIOUS REACTIONS
! Overdose may cause CNS depression, coma, shock, and respiratory depression.

DENTAL CONSIDERATIONS
General:
• Determine why patient is taking the drug.
• Patients on chronic drug therapy may rarely have symptoms of blood dyscrasias, which can include infection, bleeding, and poor healing.
• Consider semisupine chair position for patient comfort if GI side effects occur.
Consultations:
• In a patient with symptoms of blood dyscrasias, request a medical consultation for blood studies and postpone treatment until normal values are reestablished.
Teach Patient/Family to:
• Update health and drug history if physician makes any changes in evaluation or drug regimens; include OTC, herbal, and nonherbal drugs in the update

metformin hydrochloride
met-for´-min high-droh-klor´-ide
(Diabex[AUS], Diaformin[AUS], Fortamet, Glucohexal[AUS], Glucomet[AUS], Glucophage, Glucophage XL, Glycon[CAN], Novo-Metformin[CAN], Riomet)

CATEGORY AND SCHEDULE
Pregnancy Risk Category: B

Drug Class: Oral hypoglycemic, biguanide derivative

MECHANISM OF ACTION
An antihyperglycemic that decreases hepatic production of glucose. Decreases absorption of glucose and improves insulin sensitivity.
Therapeutic Effect: Improves glycemic control, stabilizes or decreases body weight, and improves lipid profile.

USES
Treatment of Type 2 diabetes mellitus

PHARMACOKINETICS
Slowly, incompletely absorbed after oral administration. Food delays or decreases the extent of absorption. Protein binding: Negligible. Primarily distributed to intestinal mucosa and salivary glands. Primarily excreted unchanged in urine. Removed by hemodialysis.
Half-life: 3–6 hr.

INDICATIONS AND DOSAGES
▸ **Diabetes Mellitus**
PO (500-mg, 1000-mg tablet)
Adults, Elderly. Initially, 500 mg twice a day, with morning and evening meals. May increase in 500-mg increments every wk, in divided doses. May give twice a day up to 2000 mg/day (e.g., 1000 mg twice a day [with morning and evening meals]). If 2500 mg/day are required, give 3 times a day with meals. Maximum: 2500 mg/day.
Children 10–16 yr. Initially, 500 mg twice a day. May increase by 500 mg/day at weekly intervals. Maximum: 2000 mg/day.
PO (850-mg tablet)
Adults, Elderly. Initially, 850-mg/day, with morning meal. May increase dosage in 850-mg increments every other wk, in divided doses. Maintenance: 850 mg twice a day, with morning and evening meals. Maximum: 2550 mg/day (850 mg 3 times a day).
PO (Extended-Release tablets)
Adults, Elderly. Initially, 500 mg once a day. May increase by 500 mg/day at weekly intervals. Maximum: 2000 mg once a day.

▶ **Adjunct to Insulin Therapy**
PO
Adults, Elderly. Initially, 500 mg/day.
May increase by 500 mg at 7-day
intervals. Maximum: 2500 mg/day
(2000 mg/day for extended-release
form).

SIDE EFFECTS/ADVERSE REACTIONS
Occasional
GI disturbances (including diarrhea,
nausea, vomiting, abdominal
bloating, flatulence, and anorexia)
that are transient and resolve
spontaneously during therapy
Rare
Unpleasant or metallic taste that
resolves spontaneously during
therapy

PRECAUTIONS AND CONTRAINDICATIONS
Acute CHF, MI, cardiovascular
collapse, renal disease or
dysfunction, respiratory failure,
septicemia.
Caution
Elderly, lactation, children, interferes
with vitamin B_{12} absorption; avoid
alcohol use

DRUG INTERACTIONS OF CONCERN TO DENTISTRY
None reported

SERIOUS REACTIONS
! Lactic acidosis occurs rarely but is
a fatal complication in 50% of cases.
Lactic acidosis is characterized by an
increase in blood lactate levels
(higher than 5 mmol/L), a decrease
in blood pH, and electrolyte
disturbances. Signs and symptoms of
lactic acidosis include unexplained
hyperventilation, myalgia, malaise,
and somnolence, which may advance
to cardiovascular collapse (shock),

acute CHF, acute MI, and prerenal
azotemia.

DENTAL CONSIDERATIONS
General:
• Short appointments and a stress
reduction protocol may be required
for anxious patients.
• Consider semisupine chair position
for patient comfort if GI side effects
occur.
• Question patient about self-
monitoring of drug's antidiabetic
effect, including blood glucose
values or finger-stick records.
• Ensure that patient is following
prescribed diet and regularly takes
medication.
• Diabetics may be more susceptible
to infection and have delayed wound
healing.
• Place on frequent recall to evaluate
healing response.
Consultations:
• Medical consultation may be
required to assess disease control and
patient's ability to tolerate stress.
• Notify physician immediately if
symptoms of lactic acidosis are
observed (myalgia, respiratory
distress, weakness, diarrhea, malaise,
muscle cramps, somnolence).
• Medical consultation may include
data from patient's blood glucose
monitoring, including glycosylated
hemoglobin or HbA1c testing.
• Oral and maxillofacial surgical
procedures associated with
significantly restricted food intake
require a medical consultation and
temporary cessation of metformin
use.
Teach Patient/Family to:
• Use effective oral hygiene to
prevent soft-tissue inflammation
• Understand that alteration of taste
may be due to drug side effects

methadone hydrochloride

meth´-ah-done high-droh-klor´-ide
(Dolophine, Metadol[CAN],
Methadone Intensol, Methadose,
Physeptone[AUS])

CATEGORY AND SCHEDULE
Pregnancy Risk Category: B
(D if used for prolonged periods or
at high dosages at term)
Controlled Substance: Schedule II

Drug Class: Synthetic narcotic
analgesic

MECHANISM OF ACTION
An opioid agonist that binds with
opioid receptors in the CNS.
Therapeutic Effect: Alters the
perception of and emotional response
to pain; reduces withdrawal
symptoms from other opioid drugs.

USES
Treatment of severe pain, opioid
withdrawal program

PHARMACOKINETICS

Route	Onset	Peak	Duration
Oral	0.5–1 hr	1.5–2 hr	6–8 hr
IM	10–20 min	N/A	4–5 hr
IV	N/A	15–30 min	3–4 hr

Well absorbed after IM injection.
Protein binding: 80%–85%.
Metabolized in the liver. Primarily
excreted in urine. Not removed by
hemodialysis. *Half-life:* 15–25 hr.

INDICATIONS AND DOSAGES
▶ **Analgesia**
PO
Adults, Elderly. Initially, 5–10 mg
q3–4h.

Children. 0.1–0.2 mg/kg q6h as
needed. Maximum: 10 mg/dose.
IV, IM, Subcutaneous
Adults, Elderly. Initially, 2.5–10 mg
q3–4h.
▶ **Narcotic Addiction**
IM, PO
Adults, Elderly. 15–40 mg once daily
or as needed. Reduce dose at 1–2 day
intervals based on patient response.
Maintenance: Individualized.

SIDE EFFECTS/ADVERSE REACTIONS
Frequent

Sedation, decreased B/P (including
orthostatic hypotension), diaphoresis,
facial flushing, constipation,
dizziness, nausea, vomiting
Occasional

Confusion, urine retention,
palpitations, abdominal cramps,
visual changes, dry mouth, headache,
decreased appetite, anxiety, insomnia
Rare

Allergic reaction (rash, pruritus)

PRECAUTIONS AND CONTRAINDICATIONS
Delivery of premature infant,
diarrhea due to poisoning,
hypersensitivity to narcotics, labor
Caution

Addictive personality, lactation,
increased intracranial pressure, MI
(acute), severe heart disease,
respiratory depression, hepatic
disease, renal disease, children
younger than 18 yr

DRUG INTERACTIONS OF CONCERN TO DENTISTRY
* Increased CNS depression: alcohol,
narcotics, sedative-hypnotics,
skeletal muscle relaxants,
benzodiazepines, and other CNS
depressants

M

• Increased effects of anticholinergics

SERIOUS REACTIONS

! Overdose results in respiratory depression, skeletal muscle flaccidity, cold or clammy skin, cyanosis, and extreme somnolence progressing to seizures, stupor, and coma. The antidote is 0.4 mg naloxone.

! The patient who uses methadone long-term may develop a tolerance to the drug's analgesic effect and physical dependence.

DENTAL CONSIDERATIONS

General:
• Assess salivary flow as a factor in caries, periodontal disease, and candidiasis.
• Psychologic and physical dependence may occur with chronic administration.
• Determine why the patient is taking the drug.
• Be aware of the needs of patients who are in recovery from substance abuse.
• In an opioid-dependent patient, NSAIDs are the drugs of choice for posttreatment pain control.

Consultations:
• Patients in the methadone maintenance program should not receive additional opioids or other controlled substances without a consultation.

Teach Patient/Family:
• When chronic dry mouth occurs, advise patient to:
  • Avoid mouth rinses with high alcohol content because of drying effects
  • Use sugarless gum, frequent sips of water, or saliva substitutes
  • Use daily home fluoride products for anticaries effect

methamphetamine
meth-am-fet´-ah-meen
(Desoxyn, Gradumet)
Do not confuse with Dextran, dextromethorphan, or Excedrin.

CATEGORY AND SCHEDULE
Pregnancy Risk Category: C
Controlled substance: Schedule II

Drug Class: Amphetamine

MECHANISM OF ACTION
A sympathomimetic amine related to amphetamine and ephedrine that enhances CNS stimulant activity. Peripheral actions include elevation of systolic and diastolic B/P and weak bronchodilator and respiratory stimulant action. *Therapeutic Effect:* Increases motor activity, mental alertness; decreases drowsiness, fatigue.

USES
Treatment of exogenous obesity, minimal brain dysfunction, attention deficit hyperactivity disorder (ADHD)

PHARMACOKINETICS
Rapidly absorbed from the GI tract. Metabolized in liver. Primarily excreted in the urine. Unknown if removed by hemodialysis.
Half-life: 4–5 hr.

INDICATIONS AND DOSAGES
▶ ADHD
PO
Adults, Children 6 yr and older.
Initially, 2.5–5 mg 1–2 times a day. Increase by 5 mg/day at weekly intervals until therapeutic response achieved.

▶ **Appetite Suppressant**
PO
Adults, Children 12 yr and older.
5 mg daily, given 30 min before
meals. Extended-release 10–15 mg
in the morning.

SIDE EFFECTS/ADVERSE REACTIONS
Frequent
Irregular pulse, increased motor
activity, talkativeness, nervousness,
mild euphoria, insomnia
Occasional
Headache, chills, dry mouth, GI
distress, worsening depression in
patients who are clinically depressed,
tachycardia, palpitations, chest pain

PRECAUTIONS AND CONTRAINDICATIONS
Advanced arteriosclerosis, agitated
states, glaucoma, history of drug
abuse, history of hypersensitivity to
sympathomimetic amines,
hyperthyroidism, moderate to severe
hypertension, symptomatic
cardiovascular disease, within
14 days following discontinuation of
an MAOI
Caution
Gilles de la Tourette's syndrome,
lactation, children younger than 6 yr

DRUG INTERACTIONS OF CONCERN TO DENTISTRY
• Increased effect of
methamphetamine: CNS stimulants,
sympathomimetics
• Decreased effects of both drugs:
haloperidol, sedative-hypnotics
• Ventricular dysrhythmia: inhalation
anesthetics

SERIOUS REACTIONS
❗ Overdose may produce skin pallor,
flushing, arrhythmias, and psychosis.

❗ Abrupt withdrawal following
prolonged administration of high
dosage may produce lethargy which
may last for weeks.
❗ Prolonged administration to
children with ADHD may produce a
temporary suppression of normal
weight and height patterns.

DENTAL CONSIDERATIONS
General:
• Assess salivary flow as a factor in
caries, periodontal disease, and
candidiasis.
Consultations:
• Physician should be informed if
significant xerostomic side effects
occur (e.g., increased caries, sore
tongue, problems eating or
swallowing, difficulty wearing
prosthesis) so that a medication
change can be considered.
Teach Patient/Family:
• When chronic dry mouth occurs,
advise patient to:
  • Avoid mouth rinses with high
  alcohol content because of drying
  effects
  • Use sugarless gum, frequent sips
  of water, or saliva substitutes
  • Use daily home fluoride products
  for anticaries effect

methazolamide
meth-ah-zole´-ah-mide
(Apo-Methazolamide[CAN],
Glauctabs, Neptazane)
Do not confuse with nefazodone.

CATEGORY AND SCHEDULE
Pregnancy Risk Category: C

Drug Class: Carbonic anhydrase
inhibitor

MECHANISM OF ACTION

A noncompetitive inhibitor of carbonic anhydrase that inhibits the enzyme at the luminal border of cells of the proximal tubule. Increases urine volume and changes to an alkaline pH with subsequent decreases in the excretion of titratable acid and ammonia. *Therapeutic Effect:* Produces a diuretic and antiglaucoma effect.

USES

Treatment of open-angle glaucoma or preoperatively in narrow-angle glaucoma; can be used with miotic, osmotic agents

PHARMACOKINETICS

PO route onset 2–4 hr, peak 6–8 hr, duration 10–18 hr. Well absorbed slowly from the GI tract. Protein binding: 55%. Distributed into the tissues (including CSF). Metabolized slowly from the GI tract. Partially excreted in urine. Not removed by hemodialysis. *Half-life:* 14 hr.

INDICATIONS AND DOSAGES
▶ **Glaucoma**
PO
Adults, Elderly. 50–100 mg/day 2–3 times a day.

SIDE EFFECTS/ADVERSE REACTIONS
Occasional

Paresthesias, hearing dysfunction or tinnitus, fatigue, malaise, loss of appetite, taste alteration, nausea, vomiting, diarrhea, polyuria, drowsiness, confusion, hypokalemia
Rare

Metabolic acidosis, electrolyte imbalance, transient myopia, urticaria, melena, hematuria, glycosuria, hepatic insufficiency, flaccid paralysis, photosensitivity, convulsions, and rarely, crystalluria, renal calculi

PRECAUTIONS AND CONTRAINDICATIONS

Kidney or liver dysfunction, severe pulmonary obstruction, hypersensitivity to methazolamide or any component of the formulation
Caution

Hypercalciuria, lactation, children

DRUG INTERACTIONS OF CONCERN TO DENTISTRY
Methazolamide (neptazane, gluctabs)

• Toxicity: salicylates (high doses)
• Hypokalemia: corticosteroids (systemic use)

SERIOUS REACTIONS

• Malaise and complaints of tiredness and myalgia are signs of excessive dosing and acidosis in the elderly.
• Stevens-Johnson syndrome, toxic epidermal necrolysis, fulminant hepatic necrosis, agranulocytosis, aplastic anemia, and other blood dyscrasias have been reported and have caused fatalities.

DENTAL CONSIDERATIONS

Neptazane, Gluctabs
General:

• Avoid dental light in patient's eyes; offer dark glasses for patient comfort.
• Avoid prescribing aspirin-containing products.
• Consider semisupine chair position for patient comfort if GI side effects occur.
• Question patient about tolerance of NSAIDs or aspirin related to GI disease.

• Patient on chronic drug therapy may rarely present with symptoms of blood dyscrasias, which can include infection, bleeding, and poor healing.

• Caution patient to prevent oral tissue trauma when using oral hygiene aids.

Consultations:

• In a patient with symptoms of blood dyscrasias, request a medical consultation for blood studies and postpone treatment until normal values are reestablished.

Teach Patient/Family to:

• Use effective oral hygiene to prevent soft tissue inflammation

• Prevent trauma when using oral hygiene aids

• Update health and medication history if physician makes any changes in evaluation or drug regimens; include OTC, herbal, and nonherbal drugs in the update

methenamine
meh-theh´-nah-meen
(Dehydral[CAN], Hiprex,
Hip-Rex[CAN], Mandelamine,
Urasal[CAN], Urex)

CATEGORY AND SCHEDULE
Pregnancy Risk Category: C

Drug Class: Urinary
antiinfective

MECHANISM OF ACTION
A hippuric acid salt that hydrolyzes to formaldehyde and ammonia in acidic urine. *Therapeutic Effect:* Formaldehyde has antibacterial action. Bactericidal.

USES
Prophylaxis and treatment of uncomplicated UTIs

PHARMACOKINETICS
Readily absorbed from the GI tract. Partially metabolized by hydrolysis (unless protected by enteric coating) and partially by the liver. Primarily excreted in urine. *Half-life:* 3–6 hr.

INDICATIONS AND DOSAGES
▶ UTI
PO
Adults, Elderly. 1 g 2 times/day (as hippurate). 1 g 4 times/day (as mandelate).
Children 6–12 yr. 25–50 mg/kg/day q12h (as hippurate). 50–75 mg/kg/day q6h (as mandelate).

SIDE EFFECTS/ADVERSE REACTIONS
Occasional
Rash, nausea, dyspepsia, difficulty urinating
Rare
Bladder irritation, increased liver enzymes

PRECAUTIONS AND CONTRAINDICATIONS
Moderate to severe renal impairment, hepatic impairment (hippurate salt), tartrazine sensitivity (Hiprex contains tartrazine), hypersensitivity to methenamine or any of its components
Caution
Renal disease, lactation

DRUG INTERACTIONS OF CONCERN TO DENTISTRY
None reported

SERIOUS REACTIONS
! Crystalluria can occur when methenamine is given in large doses.

M

DENTAL CONSIDERATIONS

General:
- Determine why the patient is taking the drug.
- Antibiotics for dental infections are not contraindicated, but a physician notification may be advisable.
- Palliative treatment may be required for oral side effects.
- Consider semisupine chair position for patient comfort because of GI effects of drug.

methimazole
meth-im´-ah-zole
(Tapazole)

CATEGORY AND SCHEDULE
Pregnancy Risk Category: D

Drug Class: Thyroid hormone antagonist

MECHANISM OF ACTION
A thiomidazole derivative that inhibits synthesis of thyroid hormone by interfering with the incorporation of iodine into tyrosyl residues.
Therapeutic Effect: Effectively treats hyperthyroidism by decreasing thyroid hormone levels.

USES
Treatment of hyperthyroidism

PHARMACOKINETICS
PO: Onset 30–40 min, duration 2–4 hr. *Half-life:* 1–2 hr; excreted in urine, bile, breast milk; crosses placenta.

INDICATIONS AND DOSAGES
▶ **Hyperthyroidism**
PO
Adults, Elderly. Initially, 15–60 mg/day in 3 divided doses. Maintenance: 5–15 mg/day.

Children. Initially, 0.4 mg/kg/day in 3 divided doses. Maintenance: $^1/_2$ the initial dose.

SIDE EFFECTS/ADVERSE REACTIONS
Frequent
Fever, rash, pruritus
Occasional
Dizziness, loss of taste, nausea, vomiting, stomach pain, peripheral neuropathy or numbness in fingers, toes, face
Rare
Swollen lymph nodes or salivary glands

PRECAUTIONS AND CONTRAINDICATIONS
Hypersensitivity, infection, bone marrow depression, hepatic disease, pregnancy (first or second trimester)
Caution
Infection, bone marrow depression, hepatic disease

DRUG INTERACTIONS OF CONCERN TO DENTISTRY
- Increased cardiovascular side effects in uncontrolled patients: anticholinergics and sympathomimetics
- Patients with uncontrolled hyperthyroidism are at risk when vasoconstrictors are used
- Patients with uncontrolled hypothyroidism may be more responsive to CNS depressants

SERIOUS REACTIONS
❗ Agranulocytosis as long as 4 mo after therapy, pancytopenia, and hepatitis have occurred.

DENTAL CONSIDERATIONS
General:
- Monitor vital signs at every appointment because of cardiovascular effects of disease.

- Patients on chronic drug therapy may rarely have symptoms of blood dyscrasias; examine for evidence of oral manifestations of blood dyscrasias (infection, bleeding, poor healing).
- Evaluate for clotting ability during periodontal instrumentation.
- Evaluate for control of hyperthyroidism. Patients with uncontrolled condition should not be treated in the dental office until thyroid values are normalized.
- Patients with uncontrolled condition should be referred for medical evaluation and treatment.

Consultations:
- Medical consultation may be required to assess disease control.
- Medical consultation for blood studies (CBC); leukopenic or thrombocytopenic side effects may result in infection, delayed healing, and excessive bleeding. Postpone elective dental treatment until normal values are maintained.

Teach Patient/Family to:
- Use effective oral hygiene to prevent soft tissue inflammation
- Use caution in use of oral hygiene aids to prevent injury

methocarbamol
meth-oh-kar´-ba-mole
(Carbacot, Robaxin)

CATEGORY AND SCHEDULE
Pregnancy Risk Category: C

Drug Class: Skeletal muscle relaxant

MECHANISM OF ACTION
A carbamate derivative of guaifenesin that causes skeletal muscle relaxation by general CNS depression.

Therapeutic Effect: Relieves muscle spasticity.

USES
Adjunct for relief in painful musculoskeletal conditions

PHARMACOKINETICS
Rapidly and almost completely absorbed from the GI tract. Protein binding: 46%–50%. Metabolized in liver by dealkylation and hydroxylation. Primarily excreted in urine as metabolites. *Half-life:* 1–2 hr.

INDICATIONS AND DOSAGES
▶ **Musculoskeletal Spasm**
IM/IV
Adults, Children 16 yr and older. 1 g q8h for no more than 3 consecutive days. May repeat course of therapy after a drug-free interval of 48 hr.
PO
Adults, Children 16 yr and older. 1.5 g 4 times a day for 2–3 days (up to 8 g/day may be given in severe conditions). Decrease to 4–4.5 g/day in 3–6 divided doses.
Elderly. Initially, 500 mg 4 times a day. May gradually increase dosage.
▶ **Tetanus Spasm**
IV
Adults. 1–3 g q6h until oral dosing is possible. Injection should be used no more than 3 consecutive days.
Children. 15 mg/kg/dose or 500 mg/m^2/dose q6h as needed. Maximum: 1.8 g/m^2/day for 3 days only.

SIDE EFFECTS/ADVERSE REACTIONS
Frequent
Transient drowsiness, weakness, dizziness, lightheadedness, nausea, vomiting
Occasional
Headache, constipation, anorexia, hypotension, confusion, blurred vision, vertigo, facial flushing, rash

Rare
Paradoxical CNS excitement and restlessness, slurred speech, tremors, dry mouth, diarrhea, nocturia, impotence, bradycardia, hypotension, syncope

PRECAUTIONS AND CONTRAINDICATIONS
Hypersensitivity to methocarbamol or any component of the formulation, renal impairment (injection formulation)
Caution
Renal disease, hepatic disease, addictive personalities, myasthenia gravis, epilepsy

DRUG INTERACTIONS OF CONCERN TO DENTISTRY
• Increased CNS depression: alcohol, narcotics, sedative-hypnotics

SERIOUS REACTIONS
! Anaphylactoid reactions, leukopenia, and seizures (intravenous form) have been reported.
! Methocarbamol overdosage results in cardiac arrhythmias, nausea, vomiting, drowsiness, and coma.

DENTAL CONSIDERATIONS
General:
• Determine why the patient is taking the drug.
• Consider semisupine chair position for patient comfort if back is involved.
Teach Patient/Family to:
• Use effective oral hygiene to prevent soft tissue inflammation
• Use caution to prevent injury when using oral hygiene aids
• Avoid mouth rinses with high alcohol content because of drying effects

methotrexate sodium
meth-oh-trex´-ate soe´-dee-um
(Apo-Methotrexate[CAN], Ledertrexate[AUS], Methoblastin[AUS], Rheumatrex, Trexall)
Do not confuse Trexall with Trexan.

CATEGORY AND SCHEDULE
Pregnancy Risk Category: D (X for patients with psoriasis or rheumatoid arthritis)

Drug Class: Folic acid antagonist, antineoplastic

MECHANISM OF ACTION
An antimetabolite that competes with enzymes necessary to reduce folic acid to tetrahydrofolic acid, a component essential to DNA, RNA, and protein synthesis. This action inhibits DNA, RNA, and protein synthesis. **Therapeutic Effect:** Causes death of cancer cells.

USES
Treatment of acute lymphocytic leukemia (ALL), non-Hodgkins lymphoma; in combination with other drugs for breast, lung, head, neck cancer; lymphosarcoma; psoriasis; gestational choriocarcinoma; hydatidiform mole; rheumatoid arthritis

PHARMACOKINETICS
Variably absorbed from the GI tract. Completely absorbed after IM administration. Protein binding: 50%–60%. Widely distributed. Metabolized intracellularly in the liver. Primarily excreted in urine. Removed by hemodialysis but not by peritoneal dialysis. **Half-life:** 8–12 hr (large doses, 8–15 hr).

INDICATIONS AND DOSAGES

▶ **Trophoblastic Neoplasms**

PO, IM

Adults, Elderly. 15–30 mg/day for 5 days; repeat in 7 days for 3–5 courses.

▶ **Head and Neck Cancer**

PO, IV, IM

Adults, Elderly. 25–50 mg/m² once weekly.

▶ **Choriocarcinoma, Chorioadenoma Destruens, Hydatidiform Mole**

PO, IM

Adults, Elderly. 15–30 mg/day for 5 days; repeat 3–5 times with 1–2 wk between courses.

▶ **Breast Cancer**

IV

Adults, Elderly. 30–60 mg/m² days 1 and 8 q3–4wk.

▶ **ALL**

PO, IV, IM

Adults, Elderly. Induction: 3.3 mg/m²/day in combination with other chemotherapeutic agents. Maintenance: 30 mg/m²/wk PO or IM in divided doses or 2.5 mg/kg IV every 14 days.

▶ **Burkitt's Lymphoma**

PO

Adults. 10–25 mg/day for 4–8 days; repeat with 7- to 10-day rest between courses.

▶ **Lymphosarcoma**

PO

Adults, Elderly.
0.625–2.5 mg/kg/day.

▶ **Mycosis Fungoides**

PO

Adults, Elderly. 2.5–10 mg/day.

IM

Adults, Elderly. 50 mg/wk or 25 mg twice a wk.

▶ **Rheumatoid Arthritis**

PO

Adults, Elderly. 7.5 mg once a wk or 2.5 mg q12h for 3 doses once a wk. Maximum: 20 mg/wk.

▶ **Juvenile Rheumatoid Arthritis**

PO, IM, Subcutaneous

Children. 5–15 mg/m²/wk as a single dose or in 3 divided doses given q12h.

▶ **Psoriasis**

PO

Adults, Elderly. 10–25 mg once a wk or 2.5–5 mg q12h for 3 doses once a wk.

IM

Adults, Elderly. 10–25 mg once a wk.

▶ **Antineoplastic Dosage for Children**

PO, IM

Children. 7.5–30 mg/m²/wk or q2wk.

IV

Children. 10–33,000 mg/m² bolus or continuous infusion over 6–42 hr.

▶ **Dosage in Renal Impairment**

Creatinine clearance 61–80 ml/min. Reduce dose by 25%.

Creatinine clearance 51–60 ml/min. Reduce dose by 33%.

Creatinine clearance 10–50 ml/min. Reduce dose by 50%–70%.

SIDE EFFECTS/ADVERSE REACTIONS

Frequent

Nausea, vomiting, stomatitis; burning and erythema at psoriatic site (in patients with psoriasis)

Occasional

Diarrhea, rash, dermatitis, pruritus, alopecia, dizziness, anorexia, malaise, headache, drowsiness, blurred vision

PRECAUTIONS AND CONTRAINDICATIONS

Preexisting myelosuppression, severe hepatic or renal impairment

Caution

Renal disease, lactation, drugs with potential for hepatotoxicity, monitor for hepatic toxicity, methotrexate-induced lung disease

DRUG INTERACTIONS OF CONCERN TO DENTISTRY
- Increased toxicity: aspirin, alcohol, NSAIDs
- Possible fatal interactions: NSAIDs, high-dose IV methotrexate
- Suspected increase in methotrexate toxicity: amoxicillin, tetracycline, doxycycline

SERIOUS REACTIONS
❗ GI toxicity may produce gingivitis, glossitis, pharyngitis, stomatitis, enteritis, and hematemesis.
❗ Hepatotoxicity is more likely to occur with frequent small doses than with large intermittent doses.
❗ Pulmonary toxicity may be characterized by interstitial pneumonitis.
❗ Hematologic toxicity, which may develop rapidly from marked myelosuppression, may be manifested as leukopenia, thrombocytopenia, anemia, and hemorrhage.
❗ Dermatologic toxicity may produce a rash, pruritus, urticaria, pigmentation, photosensitivity, petechiae, ecchymosis, and pustules.
❗ Severe nephrotoxicity may produce azotemia, hematuria, and renal failure.

DENTAL CONSIDERATIONS
General:
- Patients on chronic drug therapy may rarely have symptoms of blood dyscrasias, which can include infection, bleeding, and poor healing.
- Avoid prescribing aspirin- or NSAID-containing products.
- Place on frequent recall because of increased risk for infection and to evaluate healing response.
- Determine why the patient is taking the drug.

- Palliative treatment may be necessary if stomatitis or oral desquamative lesions occur.
Consultations:
- In a patient with symptoms of blood dyscrasias, request a medical consultation for blood studies and postpone dental treatment until normal values are reestablished.
- Medical consultation may be required to assess disease control.
Teach Patient/Family to:
- Use effective oral hygiene to prevent soft tissue inflammation
- Use caution to prevent injury when using oral hygiene aids
- Use palliative therapy for sore mouth
- Avoid mouth rinses with high alcohol content because of drying effects

methsuximide
meth-sux´-ih-mide
(Celontin)
Do not confuse with methoxsalen.

CATEGORY AND SCHEDULE
Pregnancy Risk Category: C

Drug Class: Anticonvulsant

MECHANISM OF ACTION
An anticonvulsant agent that increases the seizure threshold, suppresses paroxysmal spike-and-wave pattern in absence seizures and depresses nerve transmission in the motor cortex. *Therapeutic Effect:* Controls absence (petit mal) seizures.

USES
Treatment of refractory absence seizures (petit mal)

PHARMACOKINETICS
Rapidly metabolized in liver to active metabolite, *N*-desmethylmeth-suximide. Primarily excreted in urine. Unknown if removed by hemodialysis.
Half-life: 1.4 hr.

INDICATIONS AND DOSAGES
▶ **Absence Seizures**
PO
Adults, Elderly. Initially, 300 mg/day for the first wk. Increase dosage by 300 mg/day at weekly intervals until response is attained. Maintenance: 1200 mg/day at 2–4 times a day. Do not exceed 1000 mg/day in children 12–15 yr, 1200 mg/day in patients older than 15 yr.
Children. Initially, 10–15 mg/kg/day 3–4 times a day. Increase at weekly intervals. Maximum: 30 mg/kg/day.

SIDE EFFECTS/ADVERSE REACTIONS
Frequent
Drowsiness, dizziness, nausea, vomiting
Occasional
Visual abnormalities, such as spots before eyes, difficulty focusing, blurred vision, dry mouth or pharynx, tongue irritation, nervousness, insomnia, headache, constipation or diarrhea, rash, weight loss, proteinuria, edema

PRECAUTIONS AND CONTRAINDICATIONS
Hypersensitivity to succinimides or any component of the formulation
Caution
Hepatic disease, renal disease, lactation

DRUG INTERACTIONS OF CONCERN TO DENTISTRY
• Enhanced CNS depression: alcohol, CNS depressants

• Decreased effects: phenothiazines, thioxanthenes, barbiturates
• Changes in seizure pattern, frequency: haloperidol

SERIOUS REACTIONS
❗ Toxic reactions appear as blood dyscrasias, including aplastic anemia, agranulocytosis, thrombocytopenia, leukopenia, leukocytosis, eosinophilia, cardiovascular disturbances, such as CHF, hypotension or hypertension, thrombophlebitis, arrhythmias, and dermatologic effects, such as rash, urticaria, pruritus, photosensitivity.
❗ Abrupt withdrawal may precipitate status epilepticus.

DENTAL CONSIDERATIONS
General:
• Patients on chronic drug therapy may rarely have symptoms of blood dyscrasias, which can include infection, bleeding, and poor healing.
• Avoid dental light in patient's eyes; offer dark glasses for patient comfort.
• Determine type of epilepsy, seizure frequency, and quality of seizure control. A stress reduction protocol may be required.
• Place on frequent recall to monitor gingival condition.
Consultations:
• In a patient with symptoms of blood dyscrasias, request a medical consultation for blood studies and postpone dental treatment until normal values are reestablished.
• Take precautions if dental surgery is anticipated and anesthesia is required.
• Medical consultation may be required to assess disease control.
Teach Patient/Family to:
• Use effective oral hygiene to prevent soft tissue inflammation

- Use caution to prevent injury when using oral hygiene aids
- Avoid mouth rinses with high alcohol content if oral side effects occur

methyldopa/ methyldopate

meth-ill-doe´-pa/meth-ill-doe´-payte
(Aldomet, Apo-Methyldopa[CAN], Hydopa[AUS], Novomedopa[CAN], Nudopa[AUS])
Do not confuse Aldomet with Anzemet.

CATEGORY AND SCHEDULE
Pregnancy Risk Category: B

Drug Class: Centrally acting antihypertensive

MECHANISM OF ACTION
An antihypertensive agent that stimulates central inhibitory alpha-adrenergic receptors, lowers arterial pressure, and reduces plasma renin activity. ***Therapeutic Effect:*** Reduces B/P.

USES
Treatment of hypertension

PHARMACOKINETICS
PO: Peak 4–6 hr, duration 12–24 hr
IV: Peak 2 hr, duration 10–16 hr
Metabolized by liver, excreted in urine.

INDICATIONS AND DOSAGES
▸ **Moderate to Severe Hypertension**
PO
Adults. Initially, 250 mg 2–3 times a day for 2 days. Adjust dosage at intervals of 2 days (minimum).
Elderly. Initially, 125 mg 1–2 times a day. May increase by 125 mg

q2–3 days. Maintenance:
500 mg–2 g/day in 2–4 divided doses.
Children. Initially, 10 mg/kg/day in 2–4 divided doses. Adjust dosage at intervals of 2 days (minimum). Maximum: 65 mg/kg/day or 3 g/day, whichever is less.
IV
Adults. 250–1000 mg q6–8h. Maximum: 4 g/day.
Children. Initially, 2–4 mg/kg/dose. May increase to 5–10 mg/kg/dose in 4–6 hr if no response. Maximum: 65 mg/kg/day or 3 g/day, whichever is less.

SIDE EFFECTS/ADVERSE REACTIONS

Frequent
Peripheral edema, somnolence, headache, dry mouth

Occasional
Mental changes (such as anxiety, depression), decreased sexual function or libido, diarrhea, swelling of breasts, nausea, vomiting, light-headedness, paraesthesia, rhinitis

PRECAUTIONS AND CONTRAINDICATIONS
Hepatic disease, pheochromocytoma

Caution
Liver disease, eclampsia, severe cardiac disease

DRUG INTERACTIONS OF CONCERN TO DENTISTRY
- Decreased effects: indomethacin and other NSAIDs
- Increased pressor response: epinephrine and other sympathomimetics
- Increased sedation: haloperidol, alcohol, CNS depressants
- Increased hypotensive action of general anesthetics

SERIOUS REACTIONS

! Hepatotoxicity (abnormal liver function test results, jaundice, hepatitis), hemolytic anemia, unexplained fever and flu-like symptoms may occur. If these conditions appear, discontinue the medication and contact the physician.

DENTAL CONSIDERATIONS

General:
• Monitor vital signs at every appointment because of cardiovascular side effects.
• Patients on chronic drug therapy may rarely have symptoms of blood dyscrasias, which can include infection, bleeding, and poor healing.
• Assess salivary flow as a factor in caries, periodontal disease, and candidiasis.
• Limit use of sodium-containing products, such as saline IV fluids, for patients with a dietary salt restriction.
• After supine positioning, have patient sit upright for at least 2 min before standing to avoid orthostatic hypotension.
• Stress from dental procedures may compromise cardiovascular function; determine patient risk and consider use of stress-reduction protocol.
Consultations:
• In a patient with symptoms of blood dyscrasias, request a medical consultation for blood studies and postpone dental treatment until normal values are reestablished.
• Medical consultation may be required to assess disease control and patient's ability to tolerate stress.
Teach Patient/Family to:
• Use effective oral hygiene to prevent soft tissue inflammation
• Use caution to prevent injury when using oral hygiene aids

• When chronic dry mouth occurs, advise patient to:
  • Avoid mouth rinses with high alcohol content because of drying effects
  • Use sugarless gum, frequent sips of water, or saliva substitutes
  • Use daily home fluoride products for anticaries effect

methylergonovine
meth-ill-er-gon´-oh-veen
(Methergine)

CATEGORY AND SCHEDULE
Pregnancy Risk Category: C

Drug Class: Oxytocic

MECHANISM OF ACTION
An ergot alkaloid that stimulates α-adrenergic and serotonin receptors, producing arterial vasoconstriction. Causes vasospasm of coronary arteries and directly stimulates uterine muscle. *Therapeutic Effect:* Increases strength and frequency of uterine contractions. Decreases uterine bleeding.

USES
Treatment of hemorrhage postpartum or postabortion, uterine contractions

PHARMACOKINETICS

Route	Onset	Peak	Duration
PO	5–10 min	N/A	N/A
IV	Immediate	N/A	3 hr
IM	2–5 min	N/A	N/A

Rapidly absorbed from the GI tract after IM administration. Distributed rapidly to plasma, extracellular fluid, and tissues. Metabolized in the liver

and undergoes first-pass effect. Primarily excreted in urine.
Half-life: IV (alpha phase), 2–3 min or less; IV (beta phase), 20–30 min or longer.

INDICATIONS AND DOSAGES
▶ **Prevention and Treatment of Postpartum and Postabortion Hemorrhage Caused by Atony or Involution**
PO
Adults. 0.2 mg 3–4 times a day. Continue for up to 7 days.
IV, IM
Adults. Initially, 0.2 mg. May repeat q2–4h for no more than a total of 5 doses.

SIDE EFFECTS/ADVERSE REACTIONS
Frequent
Nausea, uterine cramping, vomiting
Occasional
Abdominal pain, diarrhea, dizziness, diaphoresis, tinnitus, bradycardia, chest pain
Rare
Allergic reaction, such as rash and itching; dyspnea; severe or sudden hypertension

PRECAUTIONS AND CONTRAINDICATIONS
Hypertension, pregnancy, toxemia, untreated hypocalcemia

DRUG INTERACTIONS OF CONCERN TO DENTISTRY
• Increased effects: sympathomimetics

SERIOUS REACTIONS
❗ Severe hypertensive episodes may result in CVA, serious arrhythmias, and seizures. Hypertensive effects are more frequent with patient susceptibility, rapid IV

administration, and concurrent use of regional anesthesia or vasoconstrictors.
❗ Peripheral ischemia may lead to gangrene.

DENTAL CONSIDERATIONS
General:
• Acute-use drug normally given in the hospital; provide palliative dental care for dental emergencies only.
Teach Patient/Family to:
• Follow up with definitive dental care at an opportune date

methylphenidate hydrochloride
meth-ill-fen´-ih-date
high-droh-klor´-ide
(Attenta[AUS], Concerta, Metadate CD, Metadate ER, Methylin, Methylin ER, PMS-Methylphenidate[CAN], Riphenidate[CAN], Ritalin, Ritalin LA, Ritalin SR)
Do not confuse Ritalin with Rifadin.

CATEGORY AND SCHEDULE
Pregnancy Risk Category: C
Controlled Substance: Schedule II

Drug Class: CNS stimulant, related to amphetamines

MECHANISM OF ACTION
A CNS stimulant that blocks the reuptake of norepinephrine and dopamine into presynaptic neurons.
Therapeutic Effect: Decreases motor restlessness and fatigue; increases motor activity, attention span, and mental alertness; produces mild euphoria.

USES

Treatment of attention deficit hyperactivity disorder (ADHD), narcolepsy

PHARMACOKINETICS

Onset	Peak	Duration
Immediate release	2 hr	3–5 hr
Sustained release	4–7 hr	3–8 hr
Extended release	N/A	8–12 hr

Slowly and incompletely absorbed from the GI tract. Protein binding: 15%. Metabolized in the liver. Eliminated in urine and in feces by biliary system. Unknown if removed by hemodialysis. *Half-life:* 2–4 hr.

INDICATIONS AND DOSAGES
▶ **ADHD**
PO
Children 6 yr and older. Immediate release: Initially, 2.5–5 mg before breakfast and lunch. May increase by 5–10 mg/day at weekly intervals. Maximum: 60 mg/day.
PO (Concerta)
Children 6 yr and older. Initially, 18 mg once a day; may increase by 18 mg/day at weekly intervals. Maximum: 72 mg/day.
PO (Metadate CD)
Children 6 yr and older. Initially, 20 mg/day. May increase by 20 mg/day at weekly intervals. Maximum: 60 mg/day.
PO (Ritalin LA)
Children 6 yr and older. Initially, 20 mg/day. May increase by 10 mg/day at weekly intervals. Maximum: 60 mg/day.
PO (Metadate ER, Methylin ER, Ritalin SR)
Children 6 yr and older. May replace regular tablets after daily dose is titrated and 8-hr dosage corresponds to sustained-release or extended-release tablet size.
▶ **Narcolepsy**
PO
Adults, Elderly. 10 mg 2–3 times a day. Range: 10–60 mg/day.

SIDE EFFECTS/ADVERSE REACTIONS
Frequent
Anxiety, insomnia, anorexia
Occasional
Dizziness, drowsiness, headache, nausea, abdominal pain, fever, rash, arthralgia, vomiting
Rare
Blurred vision, Tourette syndrome (marked by uncontrolled vocal outbursts, repetitive body movements, and tics), palpitations

PRECAUTIONS AND CONTRAINDICATIONS
Avoid use within 14 days of MAOIs
Caution
Hypertension, depression, seizures, lactation, drug abuse

DRUG INTERACTIONS OF CONCERN TO DENTISTRY
• Increased effects of CNS stimulants, tricyclic antidepressants, SSRIs, sympathomimetics

SERIOUS REACTIONS
! Prolonged administration to children with ADHD may delay growth.
! Overdose may produce tachycardia, palpitations, arrhythmias, chest pain, psychotic episode, seizures, and coma.
! Hypersensitivity reactions and blood dyscrasias occur rarely.

M

DENTAL CONSIDERATIONS

General:
- Monitor vital signs often because of cardiovascular side effects.
- Patients on chronic drug therapy may rarely have symptoms of blood dyscrasias, which can include infection, bleeding, and poor healing.
- Assess salivary flow as a factor in caries, periodontal disease, and candidiasis.
- Use vasoconstrictors with caution, in low doses, and with careful aspiration.
- Determine why the patient is taking the drug.

Consultations:
- In a patient with symptoms of blood dyscrasias, request a medical consultation for blood studies and postpone dental treatment until normal values are reestablished.
- Medical consultation may be required to assess disease control.

Teach Patient/Family to:
- Use effective oral hygiene to prevent soft tissue inflammation
- Use caution to prevent injury when using oral hygiene aids
- When chronic dry mouth occurs, advise patient to:
  - Avoid mouth rinses with high alcohol content because of drying effects
  - Use sugarless gum, frequent sips of water, or saliva substitutes
  - Use daily home fluoride products for anticaries effect

methylprednisolone

meth-il-pred-niss´-oh-lone
methylprednisolone (Medrol)
methylprednisolone acetate (Depo-Medrol, Depo-Nisolone[AUS])
methylprednisolone sodium succinate (A-Methapred, Solu-Medrol)
Do not confuse methylprednisolone with medroxyprogesterone or Medrol with Mebaral.

CATEGORY AND SCHEDULE
Pregnancy Risk Category: C

Drug Class: Glucocorticoid, immediate acting

MECHANISM OF ACTION
An adrenocortical steroid that suppresses migration of polymorphonuclear leukocytes and reverses increased capillary permeability. *Therapeutic Effect:* Decreases inflammation.

USES
Treatment of severe inflammation, shock, adrenal insufficiency, collagen disorders

PHARMACOKINETICS

Route	Onset	Peak	Duration
PO	N/A	1–2 hr	30–36 hr
IM	N/A	4–8 days	1–4 wk

Well absorbed from the GI tract after IM administration. Widely distributed. Metabolized in the liver. Excreted in urine. Removed by hemodialysis. *Half-life:* 3.5 hr.

INDICATIONS AND DOSAGES

▶ **Substitution Therapy for Deficiency States: Acute or Chronic Adrenal Insufficiency, Adrenal Insufficiency Secondary to Pituitary Insufficiency, and Congenital Adrenal Hyperplasia; Nonendocrine Disorders: Allergic, Collagen, Hepatic, Intestinal Tract, Ocular, Renal, and Skin Diseases; Arthritis; Bronchial Asthma; Cerebral Edema; Malignancies; and Rheumatic Carditis**

PO
Adults, Elderly.
Initially, 4–48 mg/day.
IV (methylprednisolone sodium succinate)
Adults, Elderly. 40–250 mg q4–6h.
High dosage: 30 mg/kg over at least 30 min. Repeat q4–6h for 48–72 hr.

▶ **Spinal Cord Injury**
IV Bolus
Adults, Elderly. 30 mg/kg over 15 min. Maintenance dose: 5.4 mg/kg/h over 23 hr, to be given within 45 min of bolus dose.
IM (methylprednisolone acetate)
Adults, Elderly. 10–80 mg/day.
Intra-articular, Intralesional
Adults, Elderly. 4–40 mg, up to 80 mg q1–5wk.

▶ **Antiinflammatory/ Immunosuppressant**
PO/IM/IV
Pediatric. 0.5–1.7 mg/kg/day or 5–25 mg/m²/day in 2–4 divided doses.

SIDE EFFECTS/ADVERSE REACTIONS

Frequent
Insomnia, heartburn, anxiety, abdominal distention, diaphoresis, acne, mood swings, increased appetite, facial flushing, GI distress, delayed wound healing, increased susceptibility to infection, diarrhea or constipation

Occasional
Headache, edema, tachycardia, change in skin color, frequent urination, depression

Rare
Psychosis, increased blood coagulability, hallucinations

PRECAUTIONS AND CONTRAINDICATIONS

Administration of live virus vaccines, systemic fungal infection

Caution
Diabetes mellitus, glaucoma, osteoporosis, seizure disorders, ulcerative colitis, CHF, myasthenia gravis, renal disease, esophagitis, peptic ulcer, rifampin

DRUG INTERACTIONS OF CONCERN TO DENTISTRY

● Decreased action: barbiturates, rifampin, rifabutin
● Increased GI side effects: alcohol, salicylates, NSAIDs
● Increased action: ketoconazole, macrolide antibiotics
● Hepatotoxicity: acetaminophen (chronic, high doses)

SERIOUS REACTIONS

❗ Long-term therapy may cause hypocalcemia, hypokalemia, muscle wasting (especially in arms and legs), osteoporosis, spontaneous fractures, amenorrhea, cataracts, glaucoma, peptic ulcer disease, and CHF.

❗ Abruptly withdrawing the drug after long-term therapy may cause anorexia, nausea, fever, headache, sudden severe myalgia, rebound inflammation, fatigue, weakness, lethargy, dizziness, and orthostatic hypotension.

M

M

DENTAL CONSIDERATIONS
General:
• Patients on chronic drug therapy may rarely have symptoms of blood dyscrasias, which can include infection, bleeding, and poor healing.
• Assess salivary flow as a factor in caries, periodontal disease, and candidiasis.
• Symptoms of oral infections may be masked.
• Place on frequent recall to evaluate healing response.
• Prophylactic antibiotics may be indicated to prevent infection if surgery or deep scaling is planned.
• Avoid prescribing aspirin-containing products.
• Determine dose and duration of steroid therapy for each patient to assess risk for stress tolerance and immunosuppression.
• Patients who have been or are currently on chronic steroid therapy (longer than 2 wk) may require supplemental steroids for dental treatment.
Consultations:
• In a patient with symptoms of blood dyscrasias, request a medical consultation for blood studies and postpone dental treatment until normal values are reestablished.
• Medical consultation may be required to assess disease control.
• Consultation may be required to confirm steroid dose and duration of use.
Teach Patient/Family to:
• Use effective oral hygiene to prevent soft tissue inflammation
• Use caution to prevent injury when using oral hygiene aids because of reduced healing response
• When chronic dry mouth occurs, advise patient to:

• Avoid mouth rinses with high alcohol content because of drying effects
• Use sugarless gum, frequent sips of water, or saliva substitutes
• Use daily home fluoride products for anticaries effect

methyltestosterone
meth-il-tes-tos-´te-rone
(Android, Android-10, Android-25, Oreton Methyl, Testred, Virilon)
Do not confuse with methylprednisolone.

CATEGORY AND SCHEDULE
Pregnancy Risk Category: X
Controlled substance: Schedule III

Drug Class: Androgens, hormones/hormone modifiers

MECHANISM OF ACTION
A synthetic testosterone derivative with androgen activity that promotes growth and development of male sex organs and maintains secondary sex characteristics in androgen-deficient males. **Therapeutic Effect:** Treats hypogonadism and delayed puberty in males.

USES
Replacement of the hormone when the body is unable to produce enough on its own; to stimulate the beginning of puberty in certain boys who are late starting puberty naturally; to treat certain types of breast cancer in females.

PHARMACOKINETICS
Well absorbed from the GI tract. Protein binding: 98%. Metabolized in liver. Primarily excreted in urine.

Unknown if removed by hemodialysis. *Half-life:* 10–100 min.

INDICATIONS AND DOSAGES
▶ **Breast Cancer**
PO
Adults, Elderly. 50–200 mg/day.
▶ **Delayed Puberty**
PO
Adults. 10–50 mg/day.
Adults, Elderly. 50–200 mg/day.
▶ **Hypogonadism**
PO
Adults. 10–50 mg/day.

SIDE EFFECTS/ADVERSE REACTIONS
Frequent
Gynecomastia, acne, amenorrhea or other menstrual irregularities
Females: Hirsutism, deepening of voice, clitoral enlargement that may not be reversible when drug is discontinued
Occasional
Edema, nausea, insomnia, oligospermia, priapism, male pattern of baldness, bladder irritability, hypercalcemia in immobilized patients or those with breast cancer, hypercholesterolemia
Rare
Polycythemia

PRECAUTIONS AND CONTRAINDICATIONS
Pregnancy, prostatic or breast cancer in males, hypersensitivity to methyltestosterone or any other component of its formulation

DRUG INTERACTIONS OF CONCERN TO DENTISTRY
Edema: ACTH, corticosteroids

SERIOUS REACTIONS
! Cholestatic jaundice, hepatocellular neoplasms, peliosis hepatitis, edema

with or without CHF and suppression of clotting factors II, V, VII, and X have been reported.

DENTAL CONSIDERATIONS
General:
• Determine why patient is taking the drug.
• Short appointments and a stress reduction protocol may be required for anxious patients.
• Possible risk of bleeding when used concurrently with oral anticoagulants and aspirin.
Consultations:
• Medical consultation may be required to assess disease control.
Teach Patient/Family to:
• Use effective oral hygiene to prevent soft tissue inflammation
• Update health and medication history if physician makes any changes in evaluation or drug regimens; include OTC, herbal, and nonherbal drugs in the update

M

metipranolol hydrochloride
met-ee-pran´-oh-lol
high-droh-klor´-ide
(OptiPranolol)
Do not confuse with metoprolol or propranolol.

CATEGORY AND SCHEDULE
Pregnancy Risk Category: C

Drug Class: Antiglaucoma agent (ophthalmic)

MECHANISM OF ACTION
An antiglaucoma agent that non-selectively blocks β-adrenergic receptors. Reduces aqueous humor production. *Therapeutic Effect:* Reduces intraocular pressure (IOP).

USES
Treatment of certain types of glaucoma

PHARMACOKINETICS

Route	Onset	Peak	Duration
Eye drops	0.5–3 hr	2–7 hr	24 hr or more

Systemic absorption may occur.

INDICATIONS AND DOSAGES
▸ **Glaucoma, Ocular Hypertension**
Ophthalmic
Adults, Elderly. Instill 1 drop 2 times a day.

SIDE EFFECTS/ADVERSE REACTIONS
Frequent
Eye burning/stinging, hyperemia, blurred vision, headache, fatigue
Occasional
Sensitivity to light, dizziness, hypotension
Rare
Dry eye, conjunctivitis, eye pain, rash, muscle pain

PRECAUTIONS AND CONTRAINDICATIONS
Bronchial asthma or chronic obstructive pulmonary disease, cardiogenic shock, overt cardiac failure, second- or third- degree heart AV block, severe sinus bradycardia, hypersensitivity to metipranolol or any component of the formulation

DRUG INTERACTIONS OF CONCERN TO DENTISTRY
- Avoid or use with caution: drugs with anticholinergic effects

SERIOUS REACTIONS
❗ Ophthalmic overdosage may produce bradycardia, hypotension, bronchospasm, and acute cardiac failure.
❗ Arrhythmias and myocardial infarction have been reported.

DENTAL CONSIDERATIONS
General:
- Determine why patient is taking the drug.
- Avoid drugs with anticholinergic activity, such as antihistamines, opioids, benzodiazepines, propantheline, atropine, and scopolamine.
- Avoid dental light in patient's eyes; offer dark glasses for patient comfort.
- Protect patient's eyes from accidental spatter during dental treatment.
- Question glaucoma patient about compliance with prescribed drug regimen.
Consultations:
- Medical consultation may be required to assess disease control.
Teach Patient/Family to:
- Update health and medication history if physician makes any changes in evaluation or drug regimens; include OTC, herbal, and nonherbal drugs in the update

metoclopramide
met-oh-kloe-pra´-mide
(Apo-Metoclop[CAN], Maxolon[AUS], Pramin[AUS], Reglan)
Do not confuse Reglan with Renagel.

CATEGORY AND SCHEDULE
Pregnancy Risk Category: B

Drug Class: Central dopamine receptor antagonist

MECHANISM OF ACTION
A dopamine receptor antagonist that stimulates motility of the upper GI tract and decreases reflux into the esophagus. Also raises the threshold of activity in the chemoreceptor trigger zone. *Therapeutic Effect:* Accelerates intestinal transit and gastric emptying; relieves nausea and vomiting.

USES
Prevention of nausea, vomiting induced by chemotherapy, radiation, delayed gastric emptying, gastroesophageal reflux, diabetic gastroparesis

PHARMACOKINETICS

Route	Onset	Peak	Duration
PO	30–60 min	N/A	N/A
IV	1–3 min	N/A	N/A
IM	10–15 min	N/A	N/A

Well absorbed from the GI tract. Metabolized in the liver. Protein binding: 30%. Primarily excreted in urine. Not removed by hemodialysis. *Half-life:* 4–6 hr.

INDICATIONS AND DOSAGES
▶ **Prevention of Chemotherapy-Induced Nausea and Vomiting**
IV
Adults, Elderly, Children. 1–2 mg/kg 30 min before chemotherapy; repeat q2h for 2 doses, then q3h as needed.
▶ **Postoperative Nausea and Vomiting**
IV
Adults, Elderly, Children 15 yr and older. 10 mg; repeat q6–8h as needed.
Children 14 yr and younger. 0.1–0.2 mg/kg/dose; repeat q6–8h as needed.

▶ **Diabetic Gastroparesis**
PO, IV
Adults. 10 mg 30 min before meals and at bedtime for 2–8 wk.
PO
Elderly. Initially, 5 mg 30 min before meals and at bedtime. May increase to 10 mg.
IV
Elderly. 5 mg over 1–2 min. May increase to 10 mg.
▶ **Symptomatic Gastroesophageal Reflux**
PO
Adults. 10–15 mg up to 4 times a day, or single doses up to 20 mg as needed.
Elderly. Initially, 5 mg 4 times a day. May increase to 10 mg.
Children. 0.4–0.8 mg/kg/day in 4 divided doses.
▶ **To Facilitate Small Bowel Intubation (single dose)**
IV Adults, Elderly. 10 mg as a single dose.
Children 6–14 yr. 2.5–5 mg as a single dose.
Children younger than 6 yr. 0.1 mg/kg as a single dose.
▶ **Dosage in Renal Impairment**
Dosage is modified on the basis of creatinine clearance.

Creatinine Clearance	% of normal dose
40–50 ml/min	75%
10–40 ml/min	50%
Less than 10 ml/min	25%–50%

SIDE EFFECTS/ADVERSE REACTIONS
Frequent
Somnolence, restlessness, fatigue, lethargy
Occasional
Dizziness, anxiety, headache, insomnia, breast tenderness, altered

menstruation, constipation, rash, dry mouth, galactorrhea, gynecomastia
Rare
Hypotension or hypertension, tachycardia

PRECAUTIONS AND CONTRAINDICATIONS

Concurrent use of medications likely to produce extrapyramidal reactions, GI hemorrhage, GI obstruction or perforation, history of seizure disorders, pheochromocytoma
Caution
Lactation, GI hemorrhage, CHF, asthma, hypertension, renal failure; extrapyramidal diseases, depression, concurrently with or within 14 days of discontinuing MAOIs

DRUG INTERACTIONS OF CONCERN TO DENTISTRY

• Decreased GI action: anticholinergics, opioids
• Increased sedation: alcohol, other CNS depressants
• Increased effects of succinylcholine

SERIOUS REACTIONS

! Extrapyramidal reactions occur most commonly in children and young adults (18–30 yr) receiving large doses (2 mg/kg) during chemotherapy and are usually limited to akathisia (involuntary limb movement and facial grimacing).

DENTAL CONSIDERATIONS

General:
• Assess salivary flow as a factor in caries, periodontal disease, and candidiasis.
• Assess for presence of extrapyramidal motor symptoms, such as tardive dyskinesia and akathisia. Extrapyramidal motor activity may complicate dental treatment.

• Determine why the patient is taking the drug.
• Consider semisupine chair position for patient comfort because of GI effects of disease.
Teach Patient/Family:
• When chronic dry mouth occurs, advise patient to:
  • Avoid mouth rinses with high alcohol content because of drying effects
  • Use sugarless gum, frequent sips of water, or saliva substitutes
  • Use daily home fluoride products for anticaries effect

metolazone

met-tole´-ah-zone
(Mykrox, Zaroxolyn)
Do not confuse metolazone with methazolamide or metoprolol, or Zaroxolyn with Zarontin.

CATEGORY AND SCHEDULE

Pregnancy Risk Category: B
(D if used in pregnancy-induced hypertension)

Drug Class: Diuretic with thiazide-like effects

MECHANISM OF ACTION

A thiazide-like diuretic and antihypertensive. As a diuretic, blocks reabsorption of sodium, potassium, and chloride at the distal convoluted tubule, increasing renal excretion of sodium and water. As an antihypertensive, reduces plasma and extracellular fluid volume and peripheral vascular resistance.
Therapeutic Effect: Promotes diuresis and reduces B/P.

USES

Treatment of edema, hypertension, CHF

PHARMACOKINETICS

Route	Onset	Peak	Duration
PO (diuretic)	1 hr	2 hr	12–24 hr

Incompletely absorbed from the GI tract. Protein binding: 95%. Primarily excreted unchanged in urine. Not removed by hemodialysis. *Half-life:* 14 hr.

INDICATIONS AND DOSAGES

▶ **Edema**

PO (Zaroxolyn)

Adults, Elderly. 5–10 mg/day.
May increase to 20 mg/day in edema associated with renal disease or heart failure.

Children. 0.2–0.4 mg/kg/day in 1–2 divided doses.

▶ **Hypertension**

PO (Zaroxolyn)

Adults, Elderly. 2.5–5 mg/day.

PO (Mydrox)

Adults, Elderly. Initially, 0.5 mg/day. May increase up to 1 mg/day.

SIDE EFFECTS/ADVERSE REACTIONS

Expected

Increase in urinary frequency and urine volume

Frequent

Dizziness, light-headedness, headache

Occasional

Muscle cramps and spasm, fatigue, lethargy

Rare

Asthenia, palpitations, depression, nausea, vomiting, abdominal bloating, constipation, diarrhea, urticaria

PRECAUTIONS AND CONTRAINDICATIONS

Anuria, hepatic coma or precoma, history of hypersensitivity to sulfonamides or thiazide diuretics, renal decompensation

Caution

Hypokalemia, renal disease, hepatic disease, gout, COPD, lupus erythematosus, diabetes mellitus

DRUG INTERACTIONS OF CONCERN TO DENTISTRY

• Increased photosensitization: tetracycline
• Decreased hypotensive response: indomethacin and other NSAIDs

SERIOUS REACTIONS

! Vigorous diuresis may lead to profound water and electrolyte depletion, resulting in hypokalemia, hyponatremia, and dehydration.
! Acute hypotensive episodes may occur.
! Hyperglycemia may occur during prolonged therapy.
! Pancreatitis, paresthesia, blood dyscrasias, pulmonary edema, allergic pneumonitis, and dermatologic reactions occur rarely.
! Overdose can lead to lethargy and coma without changes in electrolytes or hydration.

DENTAL CONSIDERATIONS

General:

• Patients on chronic drug therapy may rarely have symptoms of blood dyscrasias, which can include infection, bleeding, and poor healing.
• Assess salivary flow as a factor in caries, periodontal disease, and candidiasis.
• After supine positioning, have patient sit upright for at least 2 min before standing to avoid orthostatic hypotension.
• Short appointments and a stress-reduction protocol may be required for anxious patients.
• Limit use of sodium-containing products, such as saline IV fluids, for

patients with a dietary salt restriction.
- Stress from dental procedures may compromise cardiovascular function; determine patient risk.

Consultations:
- In a patient with symptoms of blood dyscrasias, request a medical consultation for blood studies and postpone dental treatment until normal values are reestablished.
- Medical consultation may be required to assess disease control and patient's ability to tolerate stress.

Teach Patient/Family to:
- Use effective oral hygiene to prevent soft tissue inflammation
- Use caution to prevent injury when using oral hygiene aids
- When chronic dry mouth occurs, advise patient to:
  - Avoid mouth rinses with high alcohol content because of drying effects
  - Use sugarless gum, frequent sips of water, or saliva substitutes
  - Use daily home fluoride products for anticaries effect

metoprolol tartrate

me-toe´-pro-lole tahr´-treyt
(Apo-Metoprolol[CAN],
Betaloc[CAN], Lopresor[AUS],
Lopressor, Metohexal[AUS],
Metolol[AUS], Minax[AUS], Nu-
Metop[CAN], PMS-Metoprolol[CAN],
Toprol XL)
Do not confuse metoprolol with
metaproterenol or metolazone.

CATEGORY AND SCHEDULE
Pregnancy Risk Category: C (D if used in second or third trimester)

Drug Class: Antihypertensive, selective β_1-blocker

MECHANISM OF ACTION
An antianginal, antihypertensive, and MI adjunct that selectively blocks β_1-adrenergic receptors; high dosages may block β_2-adrenergic receptors. Decreases oxygen requirements. Large doses increase airway resistance. *Therapeutic Effect:* Slows sinus node heart rate, decreases cardiac output, and reduces B/P. Also decreases myocardial ischemia severity.

USES
Treatment of mild-to-moderate hypertension, acute MI to reduce risk of cardiovascular mortality, angina pectoris, CHF

PHARMACOKINETICS

Route	Onset	Peak	Duration
PO	10–15 min	N/A	6 hr
PO (extended release)	N/A	6–12 hr	5–8 hr
IV	Immediate	20 min	5–8 hr

Well absorbed from the GI tract. Protein binding: 12%. Widely distributed. Metabolized in the liver (undergoes significant first-pass metabolism). Primarily excreted in urine. Removed by hemodialysis. *Half-life:* 3–7 hr.

INDICATIONS AND DOSAGES
▶ **Mild-to-Moderate Hypertension**
PO
Adults. Initially, 100 mg/day as single or divided dose. Increase at weekly (or longer) intervals. Maintenance: 100–450 mg/day.
Elderly. Initially, 25 mg/day. Range: 25–300 mg/day.
PO (Extended-Release)
Adults. 50–100 mg/day as single dose. May increase at least at weekly

intervals until optimum B/P attained.
Maximum: 200 mg/day.
Elderly. Initially, 25–50 mg/day as a
single dose. May increase at
1- to 2-wk intervals.
▸ **Chronic, Stable Angina Pectoris**
PO
Adults. Initially, 100 mg/day as
single or divided dose. Increase at
weekly (or longer) intervals.
Maintenance: 100–450 mg/day.
PO (Extended-Release)
Adults. Initially, 100 mg/day as
single dose. May increase at least at
weekly intervals until optimum
clinical response achieved.
Maximum: 200 mg/day.
▸ **CHF**
PO (Extended-Release)
Adults. Initially, 25 mg/day. May
double dose q2wk. Maximum:
200 mg/day.
▸ **Early Treatment of MI**
IV
Adults. 5 mg q2min for 3 doses,
followed by 50 mg orally q6h for
48 hr. Begin oral dose 15 min after
last IV dose. Or, in patients who do
not tolerate full IV dose, give 25–50 mg
orally q6h, 15 min after last IV dose.
▸ **Late Treatment and Maintenance
after an MI**
PO
Adults. 100 mg twice a day for at
least 3 mo.

SIDE EFFECTS/ADVERSE REACTIONS
Metoprolol is generally well
tolerated, with transient and mild
side effects
Frequent
Diminished sexual function,
drowsiness, insomnia, unusual
fatigue or weakness
Occasional
Anxiety, nervousness, diarrhea,
constipation, nausea, vomiting, nasal
congestion, abdominal discomfort,
dizziness, difficulty breathing, cold
hands or feet
Rare
Altered taste, dry eyes, nightmares,
paraesthesia, allergic reaction
(rash, pruritus)

PRECAUTIONS AND CONTRAINDICATIONS
Cardiogenic shock, MI with a heart
rate less than 45 beats/min or systolic
B/P less than 100 mm Hg, overt
heart failure, second- or third-degree
heart block, sinus bradycardia
Caution
Major surgery, lactation, diabetes
mellitus, renal disease, thyroid
disease, COPD, heart failure, CAD,
nonallergic bronchospasm, hepatic
disease

DRUG INTERACTIONS OF CONCERN TO DENTISTRY
• Increased hypotension,
bradycardia: fentanyl derivatives,
inhalation anesthetics
• Decreased antihypertensive effects:
indomethacin and possibly other
NSAIDs, sympathomimetics
• May slow metabolism of lidocaine
• Decreased β-blocking effects
(or decreased β-adrenergic effects) of
epinephrine, levonordefrin,
isoproterenol, and other
sympathomimetics
• Increased plasma concentrations:
diphenhydramine
• Decreased effects: didanosine
(take 2 hr before didanosine tabs)

SERIOUS REACTIONS
❗ Overdose may produce profound
bradycardia, hypotension, and
bronchospasm.
❗ Abrupt withdrawal of metoprolol
may result in diaphoresis,
palpitations, headache,

tremulousness, exacerbation of angina, MI, and ventricular arrhythmias.

! Metoprolol administration may precipitate CHF and MI in patients with heart disease; thyroid storm in those with thyrotoxicosis; and peripheral ischemia in those with existing peripheral vascular disease.

! Hypoglycemia may occur in patients with previously controlled diabetes mellitus.

DENTAL CONSIDERATIONS

General:
• Monitor vital signs at every appointment because of cardiovascular and respiratory side effects.
• After supine positioning, have patient sit upright for at least 2 min before standing to avoid orthostatic hypotension.
• Patients on chronic drug therapy may rarely have symptoms of blood dyscrasias, which can include infection, bleeding, and poor healing.
• Assess salivary flow as a factor in caries, periodontal disease, and candidiasis.
• Stress from dental procedures may compromise cardiovascular function; determine patient risk.
• Short appointments and a stress-reduction protocol may be required for anxious patients.
• Use vasoconstrictors with caution, in low doses, and with careful aspiration. Avoid use of gingival retraction cord with epinephrine.
• Determine why patient is taking the drug.
Consultations:
• In a patient with symptoms of blood dyscrasias, request a medical consultation for blood studies and postpone dental treatment until normal values are reestablished.

• Medical consultation may be required to assess disease control and patient's ability to tolerate stress.
• Take precautions if general anesthesia is required for dental surgery.
Teach Patient/Family to:
• Use effective oral hygiene to prevent soft tissue inflammation
• Use caution to prevent injury when using oral hygiene aids
• When chronic dry mouth occurs, advise patient to:
  • Avoid mouth rinses with high alcohol content because of drying effects
  • Use sugarless gum, frequent sips of water, or saliva substitutes
  • Use daily home fluoride products for anticaries effect

metronidazole hydrochloride
me-troe-ni´-da-zole high-droh-klor´-ide
(Apo-Metronidazole[CAN], Flagyl, Flagyl ER, MetroCream, MetroGel, Metrogyl[AUS], MetroLotion, Metronidazole IV[AUS], Metronide[AUS], NidaGel[CAN], Noritate, Novonidazol[CAN], Rozex[AUS])

CATEGORY AND SCHEDULE
Pregnancy Risk Category: B

Drug Class: Trichomonacide, amebicide, antiinfective

MECHANISM OF ACTION
A nitroimidazole derivative that disrupts bacterial and protozoal DNA, inhibiting nucleic acid synthesis.
Therapeutic Effect: Produces bactericidal, antiprotozoal, amebicidal, and trichomonacidal effects.

Produces antiinflammatory and immunosuppressive effects when applied topically.

USES

Treatment of intestinal amebiasis, amebic abscess, trichomoniasis, refractory trichomoniasis, bacterial anaerobic infections, giardiasis

PHARMACOKINETICS

Well absorbed from the GI tract; minimally absorbed after topical application. Protein binding: less than 20%. Widely distributed; crosses blood-brain barrier. Metabolized in the liver to active metabolite. Primarily excreted in urine; partially eliminated in feces. Removed by hemodialysis. *Half-life:* 8 hr (increased in alcoholic hepatic disease and in neonates).

INDICATIONS AND DOSAGES
▶ **Amebiasis**
PO
Adults, Elderly. 500–750 mg q8h.
Children. 35–50 mg/kg/day in divided doses q8h.
▶ **Trichomoniasis**
PO
Adults, Elderly. 250 mg q8h or 2 g as a single dose.
Children. 15–30 mg/kg/day in divided doses q8h.
▶ **Anaerobic Skin and Skin-Structure, CNS, Lower Respiratory Tract, Bone, Joint, Intraabdominal, and Gynecologic Infections; Endocarditis; Septicemia**
PO, IV
Adults, Elderly, Children. 30 mg/kg/day in divided doses q6h.
Maximum: 4 g/day.
▶ **Antibiotic-Associated Pseudomembranous Colitis**
PO
Adults, Elderly. 250–500 mg 3–4 times a day for 10–14 days.

Children. 30 mg/kg/day in divided doses q6h for 7–10 days.
▶ *Helicobacter Pylori* **Infections**
PO
Adults, Elderly. 250–500 mg 3 times a day (in combination).
Children. 15–20 mg/kg/day in 2 divided doses.
▶ **Bacterial Vaginosis**
PO
Adults. 750 mg at bedtime for 7 days.
Intravaginal
Adults. One applicatorful twice a day or once a day at bedtime for 5 days.
▶ **Rosacea**
Topical
Adults. Apply thin layer of lotion to affected area twice a day or cream once a day.

SIDE EFFECTS/ADVERSE REACTIONS
Frequent
Systemic: Anorexia, nausea, dry mouth, metallic taste
Vaginal: Symptomatic cervicitis and vaginitis, abdominal cramps, uterine pain
Occasional
Systemic: Diarrhea or constipation, vomiting, dizziness, erythematous rash, urticaria, reddish brown urine
Topical: Transient erythema, mild dryness, burning, irritation, stinging, tearing when applied too close to eyes
Vaginal: Vaginal, perineal, or vulvar itching; vulvar swelling
Rare
Mild, transient leukopenia; thrombophlebitis with IV therapy

PRECAUTIONS AND CONTRAINDICATIONS
Hypersensitivity to metronidazole or other nitroimidazole derivatives (also parabens with topical application)
Caution
Candida infections; avoid unnecessary use because shown to be carcinogenic in rodents

M

DRUG INTERACTIONS OF CONCERN TO DENTISTRY
* Antabuse-like reaction: alcohol, alcohol-containing products
* Decreased action: phenobarbital
* Possible increase in blood levels of tacrolimus
* Enhanced effects of warfarin, carbamazepine

SERIOUS REACTIONS
! Oral therapy may result in furry tongue, glossitis, cystitis, dysuria, pancreatitis, and flattening of T waves on ECG readings.
! Peripheral neuropathy, manifested as numbness and tingling in hands or feet, is usually reversible if treatment is stopped immediately after neurologic symptoms appear.
! Seizures occur occasionally.

DENTAL CONSIDERATIONS
General:
* Patients on chronic drug therapy may rarely have symptoms of blood dyscrasias, which can include infection, bleeding, and poor healing.
* Assess salivary flow as a factor in caries, periodontal disease, and candidiasis.
* Determine why the patient is taking the drug.
Consultations:
* In a patient with symptoms of blood dyscrasias, request a medical consultation for blood studies and postpone dental treatment until normal values are reestablished.
* Medical consultation may be required to assess disease control.
Teach Patient/Family to:
* Avoid alcoholic beverages
* Report taste alterations
* Use effective oral hygiene to prevent soft tissue inflammation
* Use caution to prevent injury when using oral hygiene aids

* When chronic dry mouth occurs, advise patient to:
  * Avoid mouth rinses with high alcohol content because of drying effects
  * Use sugarless gum, frequent sips of water, or saliva substitutes
  * Use daily home fluoride products for anticaries effect

metyrosine
me-tye´-roe-seen
(Demser)

CATEGORY AND SCHEDULE
Pregnancy Risk Category: C

Drug Class: Antihypertensives

MECHANISM OF ACTION
A tyrosine hydroxylase inhibitor that blocks conversion of tyrosine to dihydroxyphenylalanine, the rate-limiting step in the biosynthetic pathway of catecholamines.
Therapeutic Effect: Reduces levels of endogenous catecholamines.

USES
Treatment of high B/P (hypertension) caused by a disease called pheochromocytoma (a noncancerous tumor of the adrenal gland)

PHARMACOKINETICS
Well absorbed from the GI tract. Metabolized in the liver. Excreted primarily in the urine. **Half-life:** 7.2 hr.

INDICATIONS AND DOSAGES
▶ **Pheochromocytoma (preoperative)**
PO
Adults, Elderly. Initially, 250 mg 4 times a day. Increase by 250–500 mg/day up to 4 g/day.

Maintenance: 2–4 g/day in 4 divided
doses for 5–7 days.

SIDE EFFECTS/ADVERSE REACTIONS
Frequent
Drowsiness, extrapyramidal
symptoms, diarrhea
Occasional
Galactorrhea, edema of the breasts,
nausea, vomiting, dry mouth,
impotence, nasal congestion
Rare
Lower extremity edema, urinary
problems, urticaria, anemia,
depression, disorientation

PRECAUTIONS AND CONTRAINDICATIONS
Hypertension of unknown etiology,
hypersensitivity to metyrosine or any
component of the formulation

DRUG INTERACTIONS OF CONCERN TO DENTISTRY
• Increased CNS depression with
CNS depressants

SERIOUS REACTIONS
! Serious or life-threatening allergic
reaction characterized by
hallucinations, hematuria,
hyperstimulation after withdrawal,
severe lower extremity edema, and
parkinsonism.

DENTAL CONSIDERATIONS
General:
• Medication may be used in
anticipation of surgery to remove the
adrenal tumor.
• Hypertension may preclude all
dental care except for palliative
emergency treatment.
• Question patient about compliance
with drug therapy.
• Risk of increased CNS depression
when other CNS depressants are used.

• Use stress-reduction protocol
• Trismus may be a symptom of
excessive doses of this drug.
• Determine why patient is taking
the drug.
• Monitor and record vital signs.
• Use vasoconstrictor with caution,
in low doses, and with careful
aspiration. Avoid using gingival
retraction cord containing
epinephrine.
• Assess for presence of
extrapyramidal motor symptoms,
such as tardive dyskinesia and
akathisia; extrapyramidal motor
activity may complicate dental
treatment. Advise seeing physician if
tardive dyskinesia or akathisia is
present.
Consultations:
• Medical consultation may be
required to assess disease control and
patient's ability to tolerate stress.
Teach Patient/Family to:
• Use effective oral hygiene to
prevent soft tissue inflammation
• Not drive or perform other tasks
requiring mental alertness

mexiletine hydrochloride
mex-il´-eh-teen high-droh-klor´-ide
(Mexitil)

CATEGORY AND SCHEDULE
Pregnancy Risk Category: C

Drug Class: Antidysrhythmic
(class IB, lidocaine analog)

MECHANISM OF ACTION
An antiarrhythmic that shortens
duration of action potential and
decreases effective refractory period
in the His-Purkinje system of the
myocardium by blocking sodium
transport across myocardial

cell membranes. ***Therapeutic Effect:*** Suppresses ventricular arrhythmias.

USES
Treatment of documented life-threatening ventricular dysrhythmias

PHARMACOKINETICS
PO: Peak 2–3 hr. ***Half-life:*** 12 hr; metabolized by liver; excreted unchanged by kidneys (10%); excreted in breast milk.

INDICATIONS AND DOSAGES
▸ **Arrhythmia**
PO
Adults, Elderly. Initially, 200 mg q8h. Adjust dosage by 50–100 mg at 2- to 3-day intervals. Maximum: 1200 mg/day.

SIDE EFFECTS/ADVERSE REACTIONS
Frequent
GI distress, including nausea, vomiting, and heartburn; dizziness; light-headedness; tremors
Occasional
Nervousness, change in sleep habits, headache, visual disturbances, paresthesia, diarrhea or constipation, palpitations, chest pain, rash, respiratory difficulty, edema

PRECAUTIONS AND CONTRAINDICATIONS
Cardiogenic shock, preexisting second- or third-degree AV block, right bundle-branch block without presence of pacemaker
Caution
Lactation, children, renal disease, liver disease, CHF, respiratory depression, myasthenia gravis

DRUG INTERACTIONS OF CONCERN TO DENTISTRY
• No specific interactions are reported with dental drugs; however, any drug that could affect the cardiac action of mexiletine should be used

in the least effective dose, such as other local anesthetics, vasoconstrictors, and anticholinergics

SERIOUS REACTIONS
❗ Mexiletine has the ability to worsen existing arrhythmias or produce new ones.
❗ CHF may occur, and existing CHF may worsen.

DENTAL CONSIDERATIONS
General:
• Monitor vital signs at every appointment because of cardiovascular side effects.
• Patients on chronic drug therapy may rarely have symptoms of blood dyscrasias, which can include infection, bleeding, and poor healing.
• Assess salivary flow as a factor in caries, periodontal disease, and candidiasis.
• Stress from dental procedures may compromise cardiovascular function; determine patient risk and use stress-reduction protocols.
Consultations:
• In a patient with symptoms of blood dyscrasias, request a medical consultation for blood studies and postpone dental treatment until normal values are reestablished.
• Medical consultation should be made to assess disease control.
• Medical consultation may be required to assess patient's ability to tolerate stress.
Teach Patient/Family to:
• Use effective oral hygiene to prevent soft tissue inflammation
• Use caution to prevent injury when using oral hygiene aids
• When chronic dry mouth occurs, advise patient to:
  • Avoid mouth rinses with high alcohol content because of drying effects
  • Use sugarless gum, frequent sips of water, or saliva substitutes

• Use daily home fluoride products for anticaries effect

miconazole
mih-kon´-ah-zole
(Femizol-M, Micatin, Micozole[CAN], Monistat[CAN], Monistat-3, Monistat-7, Monistat-Derm)

CATEGORY AND SCHEDULE
Pregnancy Risk Category: C

Drug Class: Antifungal

MECHANISM OF ACTION
An imidazole derivative that inhibits synthesis of ergosterol (vital component of fungal cell formation), damaging cell membrane.
Therapeutic Effect: Fungistatic; may be fungicidal, depending on concentration.

USES
Treatment of tinea pedis, tinea cruris, tinea corporis, tinea versicolor, vaginal or vulval *Candida albicans*

PHARMACOKINETICS
Parenteral: Widely distributed in tissues. Metabolized in liver. Primarily excreted in urine.
Half-life: 24 hr. Topical: No systemic absorption following application to intact skin. Intravaginally: Small amount absorbed systemically.

INDICATIONS AND DOSAGES
▶ **Coccidioidomycosis**
IV
Adults, Elderly. 1.8–3.6 g/day for 3–20 wk or longer.
▶ **Cryptococcosis**
IV
Adults, Elderly. 1.2–2.4 g/day for 3–12 wk or longer.

▶ **Petriellidiosis**
IV
Adults, Elderly. 0.6–3.0 g/day for 5–20 wk or longer.
▶ **Candidiasis**
IV
Adults, Elderly. 0.6–1.8 g/day for 1–20 wk or longer.
▶ **Paracoccidioidomycosis**
IV
Adults, Elderly. 0.2–1.2 g/day for 2–16 wk or longer.
▶ **Usual Dosage for Children**
IV
20–40 mg/kg/day in 3 divided doses. (Do not exceed 15 mg/kg for any 1 infusion.)
▶ **Vulvovaginal Candidiasis**
Intravaginally
Adults, Elderly. One 200 mg suppository at bedtime for 3 days; one 100 mg suppository or one applicatorful at bedtime for 7 days.
▶ **Topical Fungal Infections, Cutaneous Candidiasis**
Topical
Adults, Elderly, Children 2 yr and older. Apply liberally 2 times a day, morning and evening.

SIDE EFFECTS/ADVERSE REACTIONS
Frequent
Phlebitis, fever, chills, rash, itching, nausea, vomiting
Occasional
Dizziness, drowsiness, headache, flushed face, abdominal pain, constipation, diarrhea, decreased appetite
Topical: Itching, burning, stinging, erythema, urticaria
Vaginal: Vulvovaginal burning, itching, irritation, headache, skin rash

PRECAUTIONS AND CONTRAINDICATIONS
Children younger than 1 yr old, hypersensitivity to miconazole or any component of the formulation

Topically: Children younger than
2 yr old
Caution
Lactation

DRUG INTERACTIONS OF CONCERN TO DENTISTRY
• Warfarin anticoagulants: potential
for increased bleeding
• Drugs metabolized by CYP hepatic
isoenzyme system: potential
increased blood levels of metabolized
drugs (e.g., benzodiazepines,
phenytoin, anesthetics)

SERIOUS REACTIONS
! Anemia, thrombocytopenia, and
liver toxicity occur rarely

DENTAL CONSIDERATIONS
General:
• Examine oral mucous membranes
for signs of fungal infection.
• Broad-spectrum antibiotics may
evoke vaginal yeast infections.
Teach Patient/Family to:
• Prevent reinoculation of *Candida*
infection by disposing of toothbrush
or other contaminated oral hygiene
devices used during period of infection

midazolam hydrochloride
mid-az´-zoe-lam
high-droh-klor´-ide
(Apo-Midazolam[CAN],
Hypnovel[AUS], Versed)
Do not confuse Versed with
VePesid.

CATEGORY AND SCHEDULE
Pregnancy Risk Category: D
Controlled substance: Schedule IV

Drug Class: Benzodiazepine,
sedative, anesthesia adjunct

MECHANISM OF ACTION
A benzodiazepine that enhances the
action of gamma-aminobutyric acid,
one of the major inhibitory
neurotransmitters in the brain.
Therapeutic Effect: Produces
anxiolytic, hypnotic, anticonvulsant,
muscle relaxant, and amnestic
effects.

USES
Conscious sedation, general
anesthesia induction, sedation for
diagnostic endoscopic procedures,
intubation, preoperative sedation,
amnesia

PHARMACOKINETICS

Route	Onset	Peak	Duration
PO	10–20 min	N/A	N/A
IV	1–5 min	5–7 min	20–30 min
IM	5–15 min	15–60 min	2–6 hr

Well absorbed after IM
administration. Protein binding:
97%. Metabolized in the liver to
active metabolite. Primarily excreted
in urine. Not removed by
hemodialysis. ***Half-life:*** 1–5 hr.

INDICATIONS AND DOSAGES
▶ **Preoperative Sedation**
PO
Children. 0.25–0.5 mg/kg.
Maximum: 20 mg.
IV
Children 6–12 yr. 0.025–0.05 mg/kg.
Children 6 mo–5 yr. 0.05–0.1 mg/kg.
IM
Adults, Elderly. 0.07–0.08 mg/kg
30–60 min before surgery.
Children. 0.1–0.15 mg/kg 30–60 min
before surgery. Maximum: 10 mg.

▶ **Conscious Sedation for Diagnostic, Therapeutic, and Endoscopic Procedures**
IV
Adults, Elderly. 1–2.5 mg over 2 min. Titrate as needed. Maximum total dose: 2.5–5 mg.

▶ **Conscious Sedation During Mechanical Ventilation**
IV
Adults, Elderly. 0.01–0.05 mg/kg; may repeat q10–15min until adequately sedated. Then continuous infusion at initial rate of 0.02–0.1 mg/kg/hr (1–7 mg/hr).
Children older than 32 wk. Initially, 1 mcg/kg/min as continuous infusion.
Children 32 wk and younger. Initially, 0.5 mcg/kg/min as continuous infusion.

▶ **Status Epilepticus**
IV
Children older than 2 mo. Loading dose of 0.15 mg/kg followed by continuous infusion of 1 mcg/kg/min. Titrate as needed. Range: 1–18 mcg/kg/min.

SIDE EFFECTS/ADVERSE REACTIONS
Frequent
Decreased respiratory rate, tenderness at IM or IV injection site, pain during injection, oxygen desaturation, hiccups
Occasional
Hypotension, paradoxical CNS reaction
Rare
Nausea, vomiting, headache, coughing

PRECAUTIONS AND CONTRAINDICATIONS
Acute alcohol intoxication, acute angle-closure glaucoma, coma, shock

Caution
COPD, CHF, chronic renal failure, chills, elderly, debilitated, children younger than 18 yr; to be used only by health care professionals skilled in airway maintenance and ventilation and resuscitation techniques

DRUG INTERACTIONS OF CONCERN TO DENTISTRY
• Prolonged respiratory depression: all CNS depressants, including alcohol, barbiturates, narcotics. All doses of midazolam must be reduced when used in combination with any CNS depressant. Serious respiratory and cardiovascular depression, including death, has occurred when midazolam is used in combination with other CNS depressants or given too rapidly. Medically compromised and elderly patients are at greater risk.
• Increased serum levels and prolonged effect of benzodiazepines: erythromycin, clarithromycin, ketoconazole, itraconazole, fluconazole, miconazole (systemic), diltiazem, fluvoxamine
• Contraindicated with nelfinavir, ritonavir, indinavir, saquinavir
• Possible increase in CNS side effects: kava kava (herb)
• Suspected increase in midazolam effects when used in general anesthesia: atorvastatin (Anesthesia 58:899–904, 2003)

SERIOUS REACTIONS
! Inadequate or excessive dosage or improper administration may result in cerebral hypoxia, agitation, involuntary movements, hyperactivity, and combativeness.
! A too-rapid IV rate, excessive doses, or a single large dose

M

increases the risk of respiratory depression or arrest.

! Respiratory depression or apnea may produce hypoxia and cardiac arrest.

DENTAL CONSIDERATIONS
General:
• Monitor vital signs every 5 min during general anesthesia because of cardiovascular and respiratory side effects. Monitor vital signs at regular intervals during recovery.
• Degree of CNS depression is dose dependent; titrate all doses.
• Drug produces amnesia, especially in the elderly patient.
• Longer recovery period could be observed in an obese patient because half-life may be extended.
• Assist patient with ambulation until drowsy period has passed.
Teach Patient/Family to:
• Avoid driving or potentially hazardous activities until drowsiness or weakness subsides
• Be aware amnesia occurs; events may not be remembered
• Treat overdose: O$_2$, vasopressors, flumazenil, resuscitation measures as required

---

midodrine
mid´-oh-drin
(Amatine, ProAmatine)
Do not confuse Amatine or ProAmatine with amantadine or protamine.

CATEGORY AND SCHEDULE
Pregnancy Risk Category: C

Drug Class: Vasopressor; orthostatic hypotension adjunct

MECHANISM OF ACTION
A vasopressor that forms the active metabolite desglymidodrine, an α_1-agonist, activating alpha receptors of the arteriolar and venous vasculature. **Therapeutic Effect:** Increases vascular tone and B/P.

USES
Treatment of symptomatic orthostatic; hypotension

PHARMACOKINETICS
Peak 1–2 hr. **Half-life:** 3–4 hr, bioavailability 90%.

INDICATIONS AND DOSAGES
▶ **Orthostatic Hypotension**
PO
Adults, Elderly. 10 mg 3 times a day. Give during the day when patient is upright, such as upon arising, midday, and late afternoon. Do not give later than 6 pm.
▶ **Dosage in Renal Impairment**
For adults and elderly patients, give 2.5 mg 3 times a day; increase gradually, as tolerated.

SIDE EFFECTS/ADVERSE REACTIONS
Frequent
Paresthesia, piloerection, pruritus, dysuria, supine hypertension
Occasional
Pain, rash, chills, headache, facial flushing, confusion, dry mouth, anxiety

PRECAUTIONS AND CONTRAINDICATIONS
Acute renal function impairment, persistent hypertension, pheochromocytoma, severe cardiac disease, thyrotoxicosis, urine retention

DRUG INTERACTIONS OF CONCERN TO DENTISTRY
• Risk of increased pressor effects: α-adrenergic agonists

SERIOUS REACTIONS
None known

General:
• Carefully review patient's medical and drug history.
• Supine hypotension is a serious side effect; a more upright chair position is highly desirable.
• Determine why patient is taking the drug.
• Monitor and record vital signs.
• Use vasoconstrictor with caution, in low doses, and with careful aspiration. Avoid using gingival retraction cord containing epinephrine.
• Examine for oral manifestation of opportunistic infection.
• Assess salivary flow as a factor in caries, periodontal disease, and candidiasis.
• Be aware of patient's disease, its severity, and frequency when known.
• Short appointments and a stress-reduction protocol may be required for anxious patients.
• Precaution if dental surgery is anticipated or general anesthesia is required.
Consultations:
• Medical consultation may be required to assess disease control and patient's ability to tolerate stress.
Teach Patient/Family to:
• Use OTC medications, such as cough, cold, and diet preparations, cautiously because that may affect B/P
• When chronic dry mouth occurs advise patient to:

• Avoid mouth rinses with high alcohol content due to drying effects
• Use daily home fluoride products for anticaries effect
• Use sugarless gum, frequent sips of water, or saliva substitutes

miglitol
mig-lee´-tall
(Glyset)

CATEGORY AND SCHEDULE
Pregnancy Risk Category: B

Drug Class: Oligosaccharide, glucosidase enzyme inhibitor

MECHANISM OF ACTION
An α-glucosidase inhibitor that delays the digestion of ingested carbohydrates into simple sugars such as glucose. ***Therapeutic Effect:*** Produces smaller rise in blood glucose concentration after meals.

USES
Treatment of type 2 diabetes when diet control is ineffective in controlling blood glucose levels, used as single agent or in combination with other oral hypoglycemics

PHARMACOKINETICS
PO: Peak plasma levels 2–3 hr; negligible plasma protein binding, not metabolized, urinary excretion.

INDICATIONS AND DOSAGES
▸ **Diabetes Mellitus**
PO
Adults, Elderly. Initially, 25 mg 3 times a day with first bite of each main meal. Maintenance: 50 mg

3 times a day. Maximum: 100 mg
3 times a day.

SIDE EFFECTS/ADVERSE REACTIONS
Frequent

Flatulence, loose stools, diarrhea,
abdominal pain
Occasional

Rash

PRECAUTIONS AND CONTRAINDICATIONS

Colonic ulceration, diabetic
ketoacidosis, hypersensitivity to
miglitol, inflammatory bowel
disease, partial intestinal
obstruction
Caution

Renal impairment, hypoglycemia,
lactation, children

DRUG INTERACTIONS OF CONCERN TO DENTISTRY

None reported

DENTAL CONSIDERATIONS
General:

• Ensure that patient is following
prescribed diet and regularly takes
medication.
• Type 2 patients may also be using
insulin. Should symptomatic
hypoglycemia occur while taking this
drug, use glucose rather than sucrose
because of interference with sucrose
metabolism.
• Place on frequent recall to evaluate
healing response.
• Short appointments and a stress-
reduction protocol may be required
for anxious patients.
• Diabetics may be more susceptible
to infection and have delayed wound
healing.
• Consider semisupine chair position
for patient comfort if GI side effects
occur.

• Question patient about self-
monitoring of drug's antidiabetic
effect, including blood glucose
values or finger-stick records.
• Examine for oral manifestation of
opportunistic infection.
Consultations:

• Medical consultation may be
required to assess disease control
and patient's ability to tolerate
stress.
• Medical consultation may
include data from patient's blood
glucose monitoring, including
glycosylated hemoglobin or HbA$_{1c}$
testing.
Teach Patient/Family to:

• Update health and drug history if
physician makes any changes in
evaluation or drug regimens; include
OTC, herbal, and nonherbal drugs
in update
• Use effective oral hygiene to
prevent soft tissue inflammation

miglustat
mig´-lew-stat
(Zavesca)

CATEGORY AND SCHEDULE
Pregnancy Risk Category: X

Drug Class: Enzyme inhibitor

MECHANISM OF ACTION

A Gaucher disease agent that inhibits
the enzyme, glucosylceramide
synthase, reducing the rate of
synthesis of most glycosphingolipids.
Allows the residual activity of the
deficient enzyme,
glucocerebrosidase, to be more
effective in degrading lysosomal
storage within tissues. *Therapeutic
Effect:* Minimizes conditions

associated with Gaucher's disease, such as anemia and bone disease.

USES
Treatment of adult patients with mild to moderate type 1 Gaucher disease for whom enzyme replacement therapy is not an option

PHARMACOKINETICS
PO: Maximum plasma levels 2–2.5 hr. *Half-life:* about 6–7 hr; oral bioavailability 97%, no plasma protein binding, excreted unchanged in urine.

INDICATIONS AND DOSAGES
▶ **Gaucher's Disease**
PO
Adults, Elderly. One 100-mg capsule 3 times a day at regular intervals.
▶ **Dosage in Renal Impairment**
Patients with creatinine clearance of 50–70 ml/min. Dosage is reduced to 100 mg twice a day.
Patients with creatinine clearance of 30–49 ml/min. Dosage is 100 mg once a day.

SIDE EFFECTS/ADVERSE REACTIONS
Expected
Diarrhea, weight loss, dry mouth
Frequent
Hand tremors, flatulence, headache, abdominal pain, nausea
Occasional
Paresthesia, anorexia, dyspepsia, leg cramps, vomiting

PRECAUTIONS AND CONTRAINDICATIONS
Women who are or may become pregnant
Caution
Efficacy and safety not evaluated in patients younger than 18 yr or older than 65 yr, renal impairment, women

of reproductive age, provide pretreatment neurologic evaluation, lactation

DRUG INTERACTIONS OF CONCERN TO DENTISTRY
None reported

SERIOUS REACTIONS
! Thrombocytopenia occurs in 7% of patients.
! Overdose produces dizziness and neutropenia.

DENTAL CONSIDERATIONS
General:
• Ask patient about disease control.
• Question patient about nosebleeds or other bleeding events.
• Short appointments and a stress-reduction protocol may be required for anxious patients.
• Avoid products that affect platelet function, such as aspirin and NSAIDs.
• Patients on chronic drug therapy may rarely have symptoms of blood dyscrasias, which can include infection, bleeding, and poor healing.
• Assess salivary flow as a factor in caries, periodontal disease, and candidiasis.
• Consider semisupine chair position for patient comfort as needed.
• Place on frequent recall to evaluate healing response.
Consultations:
• Medical consultation may be required to assess disease control and patient's ability to tolerate stress.
• Medical consultation should include routine blood counts, including platelet counts and bleeding time.
• In a patient with symptoms of blood dyscrasias, request a medical consultation for blood studies and

postpone treatment until normal values are reestablished.
Teach Patient/Family to:
• Inform dentist of unusual bleeding episodes following dental treatment
• Use effective oral hygiene to prevent soft tissue inflammation/infection
• Use electric tooth brush if patient has difficulty holding conventional devices

minocycline hydrochloride
mi-noe-sye´-kleen
high-droh-klor´-ide
(Akamin[AUS], Dynacin, Minocin, Minomycin[AUS], Myrac, Novo Minocycline[CAN])
Do not confuse Dynacin with Dynabac or Minocin with Mithracin or niacin.

CATEGORY AND SCHEDULE
Pregnancy Risk Category: D

Drug Class: Tetracycline antiinfective

MECHANISM OF ACTION
A tetracycline antibiotic that inhibits bacterial protein synthesis by binding to ribosomes. **Therapeutic Effect:** Bacteriostatic.

USES
Treatment of syphilis, *C. trachomatis* infection, gonorrhea, lymphogranuloma venereum, rickettsial infections, inflammatory acne, *M. marinum*, *Neisseria* meningitis carriers, actinomycosis, anthrax, ANUG, AA-induced periodontitis, and other susceptible infections; dental product is an adjunct to scaling and root planing in adult periodontitis

PHARMACOKINETICS
PO: Peak 2–3 hr. **Half-life:** 11–17 hr; 55%–88% protein bound; excreted in urine, feces, breast milk; crosses placenta.

INDICATIONS AND DOSAGES
▸ **Mild, Moderate, or Severe Prostate, Urinary Tract, and CNS Infections (excluding meningitis); Uncomplicated Gonorrhea; Inflammatory Acne; Brucellosis; Skin Granulomas; Cholera; Trachoma; Nocardiasis; Yaws; and Syphilis When Penicillins Are Contraindicated**
PO
Adults, Elderly. Initially, 100–200 mg, then 100 mg q12h or 50 mg q6h.
IV
Adults, Elderly. Initially, 200 mg, then 100 mg q12h up to 400 mg/day.
PO, IV
Children older than 8 yr. Initially, 4 mg/kg, then 2 mg/kg q12h.

SIDE EFFECTS/ADVERSE REACTIONS
Frequent
Dizziness, light-headedness, diarrhea, nausea, vomiting, abdominal cramps, possibly severe photosensitivity, drowsiness, vertigo
Occasional
Altered pigmentation of skin or mucous membranes, rectal or genital pruritus, stomatitis

PRECAUTIONS AND CONTRAINDICATIONS
Children younger than 8 yr, hypersensitivity to tetracyclines, last half of pregnancy
Caution
Hepatic disease, lactation

DRUG INTERACTIONS OF CONCERN TO DENTISTRY

• Decreased effect: antacids, milk, or other calcium- and aluminum-containing products
• Decreased effect of penicillins
• Oral contraceptives: advise patient of a potential risk for decreased contraceptive action, to maintain compliance with oral contraceptive use while using antibiotics, and to consider the use of additional nonhormonal contraception
• Contraindicated with isotretinoin (Accutane)
• Drug interactions of concern to dentistry minocycline HCl (microspheres)

SERIOUS REACTIONS

! Superinfection (especially fungal), anaphylaxis, and benign intracranial hypertension may occur.
! Bulging fontanelles occur rarely in infants.

DENTAL CONSIDERATIONS

General:
• This drug is reported to cause intrinsic staining in erupted permanent teeth not associated with the calcification stage.
• The drug readily distributes to gingival crevicular fluid.
• Do not prescribe drug during pregnancy or in patients younger than 8 yr because of tooth discoloration.
• Caution patients about driving or performing other tasks requiring alertness.
• Advise patient if dental drugs prescribed have a potential for photosensitivity.
• Do not use ingestible sodium bicarbonate products, such as the Prophy-Jet air polishing system, at the same time dose is taken; take minocycline 2 hr later.
• Determine why the patient is taking the drug.

Consultations:
• Medical consultation may be required to assess disease control.

Teach Patient/Family to:
• Use effective oral hygiene to prevent soft tissue inflammation
• Use caution to prevent injury when using oral hygiene aids
• Avoid mouth rinses with high alcohol content because of drying effects
• When used for dental infection, advise patient to:
  • Report sore throat, oral burning sensation, fever, fatigue, any of which could indicate superinfection
  • Take at prescribed intervals and complete dosage regimen
  • Immediately notify the dentist if signs or symptoms of infection increase

Microspheres
General:
• Follow all general precautions when using tetracyclines.

Teach Patient/Family to:
• Avoid eating hard, crunchy foods for 1 wk
• Postpone tooth brushing for 12 hr
• Postpone use of interproximal cleaning devices for 10 days
• Notify dentist immediately if pain, swelling, or other unexpected symptoms occur

M

minoxidil
mih-nox´-ih-dill
(Apo-Gain[CAN], Loniten,
Milnox[CAN], Regaine[AUS],
Rogaine, Rogaine Extra Strength)
Do not confuse Loniten with
Lotensin.

CATEGORY AND SCHEDULE
Pregnancy Risk Category: C
OTC (topical solution)

Drug Class: Antihypertensive

MECHANISM OF ACTION
An antihypertensive and hair growth
stimulant that has direct action on
vascular smooth muscle, producing
vasodilation of arterioles.
Therapeutic Effect: Decreases
peripheral vascular resistance and
B/P; increases cutaneous blood flow;
stimulates hair follicle epithelium
and hair follicle growth.

USES
Treatment of severe hypertension not
responsive to other therapy (used
with a diuretic and α-adrenergic
antagonist); topically to treat
androgenic alopecia

PHARMACOKINETICS

Route	Onset	Peak	Duration
PO	0.5 hr	2–8 hr	2–5 days

Well absorbed from the GI tract;
minimal absorption after topical
application. Protein binding: None.
Widely distributed. Metabolized in
the liver to active metabolite.
Primarily excreted in urine. Removed
by hemodialysis. *Half-life:* 4.2 hr.

INDICATIONS AND DOSAGES
▶ **Severe Symptomatic Hypertension,
Hypertension Associated with Organ
Damage, Hypertension That Has
Failed to Respond to Maximal
Therapeutic Dosages of a Diuretic or
Two Other Antihypertensives**
PO
Adults. Initially, 5 mg/day. Increase
with at least 3-day intervals to
10 mg, then 20 mg, then up to
40 mg/day in 1–2 doses.
Elderly. Initially, 2.5 mg/day.
May increase gradually.
Maintenance: 10–40 mg/day.
Maximum: 100 mg/day.
Children. Initially, 0.1–0.2 mg/kg
(5 mg maximum) daily. Gradually
increase at a minimum of 3-day
intervals. Maintenance:
0.25–1 mg/kg/day in 1–2 doses.
Maximum: 50 mg/day.
▶ **Hair Regrowth**
Topical
Adults. 1 ml to affected areas of
scalp 2 times a day. Total daily dose
not to exceed 2 ml.

SIDE EFFECTS/ADVERSE REACTIONS
Frequent
PO: Edema with concurrent weight
gain, hypertrichosis (elongation,
thickening, increased pigmentation
of fine body hair; develops in 80% of
patients within 3–6 wk after
beginning therapy)
Occasional
PO: T-wave changes (usually revert
to pretreatment state with continued
therapy or drug withdrawal)
Topical: Pruritus, rash, dry or flaking
skin, erythema
Rare
PO: Breast tenderness, headache,
photosensitivity reaction
Topical: Allergic reaction, alopecia,
burning sensation at scalp, soreness

at hair root, headache, visual
disturbances

PRECAUTIONS AND CONTRAINDICATIONS
Pheochromocytoma
Caution
Lactation, children, renal disease,
CAD, CHF

DRUG INTERACTIONS OF CONCERN TO DENTISTRY
• Decreased effects: NSAIDs,
indomethacin, sympathomimetics
• Increased hypotension: CNS
depressant drug used in conscious
sedation technique may also lower
B/P

SERIOUS REACTIONS
! Tachycardia and angina pectoris
may occur because of increased
oxygen demands associated with
increased heart rate and cardiac
output.
! Fluid and electrolyte imbalance
and CHF may occur, especially if a
diuretic is not given concurrently
with minoxidil.
! Too rapid reduction in B/P may
result in syncope, CVA, MI, and
ocular or vestibular ischemia.
! Pericardial effusion and tamponade
may be seen in patients with
impaired renal function who are not
on dialysis.

DENTAL CONSIDERATIONS
General:
• Monitor vital signs at every
appointment because of
cardiovascular side effects.
• Patients on chronic drug therapy
may rarely have symptoms of blood
dyscrasias, which can include
infection, bleeding, and poor healing.
• Limit use of sodium-containing
products, such as saline IV fluids, for
patients with a dietary salt
restriction.
• Short appointments and a stress-
reduction protocol may be required
for anxious patients.
• After supine positioning, have
patient sit upright for at least 2 min
before standing to avoid orthostatic
hypotension.
Consultations:
• In a patient with symptoms of
blood dyscrasias, request a medical
consultation for blood studies and
postpone dental treatment until
normal values are reestablished.
• Medical consultation may be
required to assess disease control and
patient's ability to tolerate stress.

mirtazapine
mir-taz´-ah-peen
(Avanza[AUS], Mirtazon[AUS],
Remeron, Remeron Soltab)
Do not confuse Remeron with
Premarin.

CATEGORY AND SCHEDULE
Pregnancy Risk Category: C

Drug Class: Tetracyclic
antidepressant

MECHANISM OF ACTION
A tetracyclic compound that acts as
an antagonist at presynaptic
α_2-adrenergic receptors, increasing
both norepinephrine and serotonin
neurotransmission. Has low
anticholinergic activity. *Therapeutic
Effect:* Relieves depression and
produces sedative effects.

USES
Treatment of depression

PHARMACOKINETICS
Rapidly and completely absorbed
after PO administration; absorption
not affected by food. Protein binding:
85%. Metabolized in the liver.
Primarily excreted in urine.
Unknown if removed by
hemodialysis. *Half-life:* 20–40 hr
(longer in males [37 hr] than females
[26 hr]).

INDICATIONS AND DOSAGES
▸ **Depression**
PO
Adults. Initially, 15 mg at bedtime.
May increase by 15 mg/day q1–2wk.
Maximum: 45 mg/day.
Elderly. Initially, 7.5 mg at bedtime.
May increase by 7.5–15 mg/day
q1–2wk. Maximum: 45 mg/day.

SIDE EFFECTS/ADVERSE REACTIONS
Frequent
Somnolence, dry mouth,
increased appetite, constipation,
weight gain
Occasional
Asthenia, dizziness, flu-like
symptoms, abnormal dreams
Rare
Abdominal discomfort, vasodilation,
paresthesia, acne, dry skin, thirst,
arthralgia

PRECAUTIONS AND CONTRAINDICATIONS
Use within 14 days of MAOIs
Caution
Hepatic impairment, renal
impairment, elderly, nursing,
pediatric, suicidal ideation,
cardiovascular or cerebrovascular
disease aggravated by
hypotension, avoid
alcohol use

DRUG INTERACTIONS OF CONCERN TO DENTISTRY
• Impairment of cognitive and motor
performance with diazepam or other
drugs used in conscious sedation
• Use opioid analgesics with caution
because of impairment of cognitive
or motor performance; NSAIDs may
be a more appropriate choice

SERIOUS REACTIONS
❗ Mirtazapine poses a higher risk of
seizures than tricyclic
antidepressants, especially in those
with no previous history of seizures.
❗ Overdose may produce
cardiovascular effects, such as severe
orthostatic hypotension, dizziness,
tachycardia, palpitations, and
arrhythmias.
❗ Abrupt discontinuation after
prolonged therapy may produce
headache, malaise, nausea, vomiting,
and vivid dreams.
❗ Agranulocytosis occurs rarely.

DENTAL CONSIDERATIONS
General:
• Patients on chronic drug therapy
may rarely have symptoms of blood
dyscrasias, which can include
infection, bleeding, and poor healing.
• Assess salivary flow as a factor in
caries, periodontal disease, and
candidiasis.
• Monitor vital signs at every
appointment because of
cardiovascular side effects.
• Consider semisupine chair position
for patient comfort of GI or MS side
effects occur.
• Place on frequent recall if oral side
effects are a problem.
Consultations:
• In a patient with symptoms of
blood dyscrasias, request a medical
consultation for blood studies and

postpone dental treatment until normal values are reestablished.
• Take precaution if dental surgery is anticipated and sedation or general anesthesia is required; risk of hypotensive episode.
• Medical consultation may be required to assess disease control.
• Physician should be informed if significant xerostomic side effects occur (e.g., increased caries, sore tongue, problems eating or swallowing, difficulty wearing prosthesis) so that a medication change can be considered.
Teach Patient/Family to:
• Use effective oral hygiene to prevent soft tissue inflammation
• Use caution to prevent soft tissue trauma when using oral hygiene aids
• Update health history/drug record if physician makes any changes in evaluation or drug regimens; include OTC, herbal, and nonherbal drugs in update
• Not drive or perform other tasks requiring alertness
• When chronic dry mouth occurs, advise patient to:
  • Avoid mouth rinses with high alcohol content because of drying effects
  • Use daily home fluoride products for anticaries effect
  • Use sugarless gum, frequent sips of water, or saliva substitutes

misoprostol
mis-oh-pros´-toll
(Cytotec)
Do not confuse with Cytomel.

CATEGORY AND SCHEDULE
Pregnancy Risk Category: X

Drug Class: Gastric mucosa protectant

MECHANISM OF ACTION
A prostaglandin that inhibits basal, nocturnal gastric acid secretion via direct action on parietal cells.
Therapeutic Effect: Increases production of protective gastric mucus.

USES
Prevention of NSAID-induced gastric ulcers

PHARMACOKINETICS
Rapidly absorbed from GI tract. Rapidly converted to active metabolite. Primarily excreted in urine. **Half-life:** 20–40 min.

INDICATIONS AND DOSAGES
▶ **Prevention of NSAID-Induced Gastric Ulcer**
PO
Adults. 200 mcg 4 times a day with food (last dose at bedtime). Continue for duration of NSAID therapy. May reduce dosage to 100 mcg if 200 mcg dose is not tolerable.
Elderly: 100–200 mcg 4 times a day with food.

SIDE EFFECTS/ADVERSE REACTIONS
Frequent
Abdominal pain, diarrhea
Occasional
Nausea, flatulence, dyspepsia, headache
Rare
Vomiting, constipation

PRECAUTIONS AND CONTRAINDICATIONS
Pregnancy (produces uterine contractions), hypersensitivity to misoprostol or any component of the formulation

Caution
Lactation, children, elderly, renal disease

SERIOUS REACTIONS

! Overdosage may produce sedation, tremors, convulsions, dyspnea, palpitations, hypotension, and bradycardia.

DENTAL CONSIDERATIONS

General:
• Avoid NSAIDs and salicylates in patients with upper active GI disease; acetaminophen/opioids are more appropriate for pain control in these patients.
Consultations:
• Medical consultation may be required to assess disease control.

mitotane
my´-tow-tane
(Lysodren)

CATEGORY AND SCHEDULE
Pregnancy Risk Category: C

Drug Class: Antineoplastic

MECHANISM OF ACTION
A hormonal agent that inhibits activity of the adrenal cortex.
Therapeutic Effect: Suppresses functional and nonfunctional adrenocortical neoplasms by direct cytoxic effect.

USES
Treatment of adrenocortical carcinoma

PHARMACOKINETICS
Adequately absorbed orally (40%).
Half-life: 18–159 days; hepatic metabolism; excreted in urine, bile.

INDICATIONS AND DOSAGES
▸ **Adrenocortical Carcinomas**
PO
Adults, Elderly. Initially, 2–6 g/day in 3–4 divided doses. Increase by 2–4 g/day every 3–7 days up to 9–10 g/day. Range: 2–16 g/day.

SIDE EFFECTS/ADVERSE REACTIONS
Frequent
Anorexia, nausea, vomiting, diarrhea, lethargy, somnolence, adrenocortical insufficiency, dizziness, vertigo, maculopapular rash, hypouricemia
Occasional
Blurred or double vision, retinopathy, hearing loss, excessive salivation, urine abnormalities (hematuria, cystitis, albuminuria), hypertension, orthostatic hypotension, flushing, wheezing, dyspnea, generalized aching, fever

PRECAUTIONS AND CONTRAINDICATIONS
Known hypersensitivity to mitotane
Caution
Lactation, hepatic disease, infection; caution: avoid use or discontinue if adrenal cortical suppression occurs

DRUG INTERACTIONS OF CONCERN TO DENTISTRY
• Increased CNS depression: all CNS depressants
• Decreased effects of corticosteroids; if glucocorticoid replacement is necessary, use hydrocortisone

SERIOUS REACTIONS
! Brain damage and functional impairment may occur with long-term, high-dosage therapy.

DENTAL CONSIDERATIONS

General:
- Evaluate respiration characteristics and rate.
- Drug may cause adrenal hypofunction, especially under conditions of stress such as surgery, trauma, or acute illness. Patients should be carefully monitored and given hydrocortisone or mineralocorticoid as needed.
- Consider semisupine chair position for patient comfort if GI side effects occur.
- Patients taking opioids for acute or chronic pain should be given alternative analgesics for dental pain.

Consultations:
- Medical consultation may be required to assess disease control and patient's ability to tolerate stress.

Teach Patient/Family to:
- See dentist immediately if secondary oral infection occurs
- Report oral lesions, soreness, or bleeding to dentist
- Update medical/drug records if physician makes any changes in evaluation or drug regimens; include OTC, herbal, and nonherbal drugs in update

mitoxantrone

my-toe-zan´-trone
(Novantrone, Onkotrone[AUS])

CATEGORY AND SCHEDULE
Pregnancy Risk Category: D

Drug Class: Antineoplastic, antiinfective, immunomodulator; synthetic anthraquinone

MECHANISM OF ACTION

An anthracenedione that inhibits B-cell, T-cell, and macrophage proliferation and DNA and RNA synthesis. Active throughout the entire cell cycle. ***Therapeutic Effect:*** Causes cell death.

PHARMACOKINETICS

Protein binding: 78%. Widely distributed. Metabolized in the liver. Primarily eliminated in feces by the biliary system. Not removed by hemodialysis. ***Half-life:*** 2.3–13 days.

USES

Treatment of some kinds of cancer. It is also used to treat some forms of multiple sclerosis.

PHARMACOKINETICS

Highly bound to plasma proteins, metabolized in liver, excreted via renal, hepatobiliary systems. ***Half-life:*** 24–72 hr.

INDICATIONS AND DOSAGES
▸ **Leukemias**
IV
Adults, Elderly, Children 2 yr and older. 12 mg/m² once a day for 2–3 days.
Children younger than 2 yr. 0.4 mg/kg once a day for 3–5 days.
▸ **Acute Leukemia in Relapse**
IV
Adults, Elderly, Children older than 2 yr. 8–12 mg/m² once a day for 4–5 days.
▸ **Acute Nonlymphocytic Leukemia**
IV
Adults, Elderly, Children older than 2 yr. 10 mg/m² once a day for 3–5 days.
▸ **Solid Tumors**
IV
Adults, Elderly. 12–14 mg/m² once q3–4wk.
Children. 18–20 mg/m² once q3–4wk.

M

▶ **Prostate Cancer**
IV
Adults, Elderly. 12–14 mg/m^2 every 21 days.
▶ **Multiple Sclerosis**
IV
Adults, Elderly. 12 mg/m^2/dose q3mo.

SIDE EFFECTS/ADVERSE REACTIONS
Frequent
Nausea, vomiting, diarrhea, cough, headache, stomatitis, abdominal discomfort, fever, alopecia
Occasional
Ecchymosis, fungal infection, conjunctivitis, UTI
Rare
Arrhythmias

PRECAUTIONS AND CONTRAINDICATIONS
Baseline left ventricular ejection fraction less than 50%, cumulative lifetime mitoxantrone dose of 140 mg/m^2 or more, multiple sclerosis with hepatic impairment

DRUG INTERACTIONS OF CONCERN TO DENTISTRY
None reported

SERIOUS REACTIONS
❗ Myelosuppression may be severe, resulting in GI bleeding, hematologic toxicity, sepsis, and pneumonia.
❗ Renal failure, seizures, jaundice, and CHF may occur.
❗ Cardiotoxicity has been reported during therapy.

DENTAL CONSIDERATIONS
General:
• Monitor and record vital signs.
• If additional analgesia is required for dental pain, consider alternative analgesics (NSAIDs) in patients taking narcotics for acute or chronic pain.
• Examine for oral manifestation of opportunistic infection.
• Avoid products that affect platelet function, such as aspirin and NSAIDs.
• This drug may be used in the hospital or on an outpatient basis. Confirm the patient's disease and treatment status.
• Chlorhexidine mouth rinse prior to and during chemotherapy may reduce severity of mucositis.
• Patient on chronic drug therapy may rarely present with symptoms of blood dyscrasias, which can include infection, bleeding, and poor healing. If dyscrasia is present, caution patient to prevent oral tissue trauma when using oral hygiene aids.
• Palliative medication may be required for management of oral side effects.
• Short appointments and a stress-reduction protocol may be required for anxious patients.
• Provide emergency dental care only during drug use.
• Patients may be at risk of bleeding, check for oral signs.
• Oral infections should be eliminated and treated aggressively.
• Patients may have received other chemotherapy or radiation, confirm medical and drug history.
• Place on frequent recall due to oral side effects
Consultations:
• Medical consultation should include routine blood counts including platelet counts and bleeding time.
• Consult physician; prophylactic or therapeutic antiinfectives may be indicated if surgery or periodontal treatment is required.

• Medical consultation may be required to assess immunologic status during cancer chemotherapy and determine safety risk, if any, posed by the required dental treatment.

• Medical consultation may be required to assess disease control and patient's ability to tolerate stress.

Teach Patient/Family to:

• See dentist immediately if secondary oral infection occurs

• Be aware of oral side effects

• Use effective oral hygiene to prevent soft tissue inflammation

• Report oral lesions, soreness, or bleeding to dentist

• Prevent trauma when using oral hygiene aids

• Update health and medication history if physician makes any changes in evaluation or drug regimens; include OTC, herbal, and nonherbal drugs in the update

modafinil
mode-ah-feen´-awl
(Alertec[CAN], Modavigil[AUS], Provigil)

CATEGORY AND SCHEDULE
Pregnancy Risk Category: C

Drug Class: CNS stimulant

MECHANISM OF ACTION
An α_1-agonist that may bind to dopamine reuptake carrier sites, increasing α activity and decreasing θ, and β brain wave activity.
Therapeutic Effect: Reduces the number of sleep episodes and total daytime sleep.

USES
Improvement of wakefulness in narcolepsy, obstructive sleep apnea, shift work sleep disorder

PHARMACOKINETICS
Well absorbed. Protein binding: 60%. Widely distributed. Metabolized in the liver. Excreted by the kidneys. Unknown if removed by hemodialysis. *Half-life:* 8–10 hr.

INDICATIONS AND DOSAGES
▶ **Narcolepsy, Other Sleep Disorders**
PO
Adults, Elderly. 200–400 mg/day.

SIDE EFFECTS/ADVERSE REACTIONS
Frequent
Anxiety, insomnia, nausea
Occasional
Anorexia, diarrhea, dizziness, dry mouth or skin, muscle stiffness, polydipsia, rhinitis, paraesthesia, tremor, headache, vomiting

PRECAUTIONS AND CONTRAINDICATIONS
Hypersensitivity
Caution
Ischemic heart disease, left ventricular hypertrophy, mitral valve prolapse, recent MI, unstable angina, renal impairment, hepatic impairment, lactation, children younger than 16 yr, drug abuse

DRUG INTERACTIONS OF CONCERN TO DENTISTRY
• No documented dental drug interactions reported; however, because it induces cytochrome P-450 isoenzymes, other P-450 isoenzyme inducers or inhibitors (antifungal agents, erythromycin) could result in a drug interaction

M

SERIOUS REACTIONS

❗ Agitation, excitation, hypertension, and insomnia may occur.

DENTAL CONSIDERATIONS

General:
• Monitor vital signs at every appointment because of cardiovascular side effects.
• Assess salivary flow as a factor in caries, periodontal disease, and candidiasis.
• Consider semisupine chair position for patient comfort because of GI side effects of drug.
• Short appointments and a stress reduction protocol may be required for anxious patients.

Teach Patient/Family to:
• Prevent trauma when using oral hygiene aids
• When chronic dry mouth occurs, advise patient to:
   • Avoid mouth rinses with high alcohol content because of drying effects
   • Use daily home fluoride products for anticaries effect
   • Use sugarless gum, frequent sips of water, or saliva substitutes

---

moexipril hydrochloride

moe-ex´-ah-pril
high-droh-klor´-ide
(Univasc)

CATEGORY AND SCHEDULE

Pregnancy Risk Category: C (D if used in second or third trimesters)

Drug Class: Angiotensin-converting enzyme (ACE) inhibitor

MECHANISM OF ACTION

An ACE inhibitor that suppresses the renin-angiotensin-aldosterone system and prevents conversion of angiotensin I to angiotensin II, a potent vasoconstrictor; may also inhibit angiotensin II at local vascular and renal sites.
Therapeutic Effect: Reduces peripheral arterial resistance and lowers B/P.

USES

Treatment of hypertension as a single drug or in combination with a thiazide diuretic

PHARMACOKINETICS

Route	Onset	Peak	Duration
PO	1 hr	3–6 hr	24 hr

Incompletely absorbed from the GI tract. Food decreases drug absorption. Rapidly converted to active metabolite. Protein binding: 50%. Primarily recovered in feces, partially excreted in urine. Unknown if removed by dialysis. ***Half-life:*** 1 hr, metabolite 2–9 hr.

INDICATIONS AND DOSAGES

▸ **Hypertension**
PO
Adults, Elderly. For patients not receiving diuretics, initial dose is 7.5 mg once a day 1 hr before meals. Adjust according to B/P effect. Maintenance: 7.5–30 mg a day in 1–2 divided doses 1 hr before meals.

▸ **Hypertension in Patients with Impaired Renal Function**
PO
Adults, Elderly. 3.75 mg once a day in patients with creatinine clearance of 40 ml/min. Maximum: May titrate up to 15 mg/day.

SIDE EFFECTS/ADVERSE REACTIONS
Occasional
Cough, headache, dizziness, fatigue
Rare
Flushing, rash, myalgia, nausea, vomiting

PRECAUTIONS AND CONTRAINDICATIONS
History of angioedema from previous treatment with ACE inhibitors
Caution
Food retards absorption, renal or hepatic impairment, CHF, SLE, scleroderma, renal artery stenosis, lactation, children

DRUG INTERACTIONS OF CONCERN TO DENTISTRY
• IV fluids containing potassium: risk of hyperkalemia
• Increased hypotension: other hypotensive drugs, alcohol, phenothiazines
• Decreased hypotensive effects: indomethacin, possibly other NSAIDs, sympathomimetics
• Suspected reduction in the antihypertensive and vasodilator effects by salicylates; monitor B/P if used concurrently

SERIOUS REACTIONS
! Excessive hypotension ("first-dose syncope") may occur in patients with CHF and in those who are severely salt or volume depleted.
! Angioedema (swelling of face and lips) and hyperkalemia occur rarely.
! Agranulocytosis and neutropenia may be noted in those with collagen vascular disease, including scleroderma and systemic lupus erythematosus, and impaired renal function.

! Nephrotic syndrome may be noted in those with history of renal disease.

DENTAL CONSIDERATIONS
General:
• Monitor vital signs at every appointment because of cardiovascular side effects.
• After supine positioning, have patient sit upright for at least 2 min before standing to avoid orthostatic hypotension.
• Take precautions if dental surgery is anticipated and general anesthesia is required.
• Patients on chronic drug therapy may rarely have symptoms of blood dyscrasias, which can include infection, bleeding, and poor healing.
• Stress from dental procedures may compromise cardiovascular function; determine patient risk.
• Assess salivary flow as a factor in caries, periodontal disease, and candidiasis.
• Short appointments and a stress-reduction protocol may be required for anxious patients.
Consultations:
• Medical consultation may be required to assess disease control and patient's ability to tolerate stress.
• In a patient with symptoms of blood dyscrasias, request a medical consultation for blood studies and postpone dental treatment until normal values are reestablished.
Teach Patient/Family to:
• Use effective oral hygiene to prevent soft tissue inflammation
• Use caution to prevent trauma when using oral hygiene aids
• Report oral lesions, soreness, or bleeding to dentist

- When chronic dry mouth occurs, advise patient to:
  - Avoid mouth rinses with high alcohol content because of drying effects
  - Use daily home fluoride products for anticaries effect
  - Use sugarless gum, frequent sips of water, or saliva substitutes

molindone
moe-lin´-done
(Moban)
Do not confuse with Mobic.

CATEGORY AND SCHEDULE
Pregnancy Risk Category: C

Drug Class: Antipsychotic

MECHANISM OF ACTION
An indole derivative of dihydroindole compounds that reduces spontaneous locomotion and aggressiveness. *Therapeutic Effect:* Suppresses behavioral response in psychosis.

USES
Treatment of psychotic disorders

PHARMACOKINETICS
Rapidly absorbed from the GI tract. Metabolized in liver. Excreted in feces, and a small amount excreted via lungs as carbon dioxide. Not removed by dialysis.
Half-life: unknown.

INDICATIONS AND DOSAGES
▶ Schizophrenia
PO
Adults, Children 12 yr and older. Initially, 50–75 mg/day, increased to 100 mg/day in 3–4 days. Maintenance: 5–15 mg 3–4 times a day (mild psychosis). Maintenance:

10–25 mg 3–4 times a day (moderate psychosis). Maintenance: 225 mg/day maximum in divided doses (severe psychosis).
Elderly. Start at a lower dose.

SIDE EFFECTS/ADVERSE REACTIONS
Frequent
Blurred vision, constipation, drowsiness, headache, extrapyramidal symptoms
Occasional
Mental depression
Rare
Skin rash, hot and dry skin, inability to sweat, muscle weakness, confusion, jaundice, convulsions

PRECAUTIONS AND CONTRAINDICATIONS
Severe CNS depression, hypersensitivity to molindone or any component of the formulation
Caution
Lactation, hypertension, hepatic disease, cardiac disease, Parkinson's disease, brain tumor, glaucoma, urinary retention, diabetes mellitus, respiratory disease, prostatic hypertrophy

DRUG INTERACTIONS OF CONCERN TO DENTISTRY
- Increased sedation: alcohol, other CNS depressants
- Increased anticholinergic effect: anticholinergics, antihistamines

SERIOUS REACTIONS
! Neuroleptic malignant syndrome or tardive dyskinesia has been reported.

DENTAL CONSIDERATIONS
General:
- Patients on chronic drug therapy may rarely have symptoms of blood dyscrasias, which can include infection, bleeding, and poor healing.

- Assess salivary flow as a factor in caries, periodontal disease, and candidiasis.
- After supine positioning, have patient sit upright for at least 2 min before standing to avoid orthostatic hypotension.
- Assess for presence of extrapyramidal motor symptoms, such as tardive dyskinesia and akathisia. Extrapyramidal motor activity may complicate dental treatment.
- Use vasoconstrictors with caution, in low doses, and with careful aspiration.

Consultations:
- In a patient with symptoms of blood dyscrasias, request a medical consultation for blood studies and postpone dental treatment until normal values are reestablished.
- Medical consultation may be required to assess disease control.

Teach Patient/Family to:
- Use effective oral hygiene to prevent soft tissue inflammation
- Use caution to prevent injury when using oral hygiene aids
- When chronic dry mouth occurs, advise patient to:
  - Avoid mouth rinses with high alcohol content because of drying effects
  - Use sugarless gum, frequent sips of water, or saliva substitutes
  - Use daily home fluoride products for anticaries effect

mometasone furoate monohydrate
mo-met´-ah-sone
(Allermax Aqueous[AUS], Asmanex Twisthaler, Elocon Cream[AUS], Elocon Ointment[AUS], Nasonex, Nasonex Nasal Spray[AUS], Novasone Cream[AUS], Novasone Lotion[AUS], Novasone Ointment[AUS])

CATEGORY AND SCHEDULE
Pregnancy Risk Category: C

Drug Class: Synthetic corticosteroid

MECHANISM OF ACTION
An adrenocorticosteroid that inhibits the release of inflammatory cells into nasal tissue, preventing early activation of the allergic reaction. *Therapeutic Effect:* Decreases response to seasonal and perennial rhinitis.

USES
Treatment of nasal symptoms of seasonal and perennial allergic rhinitis; prophylaxis of nasal symptoms of seasonal allergic rhinitis

PHARMACOKINETICS
Undetectable in plasma. Protein binding: 98%–99%. The swallowed portion undergoes extensive metabolism. Excreted primarily through bile and, to a lesser extent, urine. *Half-life:* 5.8 hr (nasal).

INDICATIONS AND DOSAGES
▶ **Allergic Rhinitis**
Nasal Spray
Adults, Elderly, Children 12 yr and older. 2 sprays in each nostril once a day.

Children 2–11 yr. 1 spray in each nostril once a day.

▶ **Asthma**
Inhalation
Adults, Elderly, Children 12 yr and older. Initially, inhale 220 mcg (1 puff) once a day. Maximum: 880 mcg once a day.

▶ **Skin Disease**
Topical
Adults, Elderly, Children 12 yr and older. Apply cream, lotion, or ointment to affected area once a day.

▶ **Nasal Polyp**
Nasal spray
Adults, Elderly. 2 sprays in each nostril twice a day.

SIDE EFFECTS/ADVERSE REACTIONS

Occasional
Inhalation: Headache, allergic rhinitis, upper respiratory infection, muscle pain, fatigue
Nasal: Nasal irritation, stinging
Topical: Burning
Rare
Inhalation: Abdominal pain, dyspepsia, nausea
Nasal: Nasal or pharyngeal candidiasis
Topical: Pruritus

PRECAUTIONS AND CONTRAINDICATIONS

Hypersensitivity to any corticosteroid, persistently positive sputum cultures for *Candida albicans*, status asthmaticus (inhalation), systemic fungal infections, untreated localized infection involving nasal mucosa
Caution
Caution in transferring patient from systemic to inhalation steroids; active or quiescent tuberculosis, untreated fungal, bacterial, or viral infections, lactation, safety and efficacy in

children younger than 12 yr not established

DRUG INTERACTIONS OF CONCERN TO DENTISTRY
None reported

SERIOUS REACTIONS
! An acute hypersensitivity reaction, including urticaria, angioedema, and severe bronchospasm, occurs rarely.
! Transfer from systemic to local steroid therapy may unmask previously suppressed bronchial asthma condition.

DENTAL CONSIDERATIONS
General:
• Allergic rhinitis may be a factor in mouth breathing and drying of oral tissues.
• Examine for oral manifestation of opportunistic infection.
Teach Patient/Family to:
• Gargle, rinse mouth with water, and expectorate after each aerosol dose

montelukast
mon-te´-loo-kast
(Singulair)

CATEGORY AND SCHEDULE
Pregnancy Risk Category: B

Drug Class: Selective leukotriene receptor antagonist

MECHANISM OF ACTION
An antiasthmatic that binds to cysteinyl leukotriene receptors, inhibiting the effects of leukotrienes on bronchial smooth muscle.
Therapeutic Effect: Decreases bronchoconstriction, vascular

permeability, mucosal edema, and mucus production.

USES

Prophylaxis and chronic treatment of asthma, seasonal allergic rhinitis

PHARMACOKINETICS

Route	Onset	Peak	Duration
PO	N/A	N/A	24 hr
PO (chewable)	N/A	N/A	24 hr

Rapidly absorbed from the GI tract. Protein binding: 99%. Extensively metabolized in the liver. Excreted almost exclusively in feces.
Half-life: 2.7–5.5 hr (slightly longer in the elderly).

INDICATIONS AND DOSAGES
▶ **Bronchial Asthma**
PO
Adults, Elderly, Adolescents older than 14 yr. One 10-mg tablet a day, taken in the evening.
Children 6–14 yr. One 5-mg chewable tablet a day, taken in the evening.
Children 1–5 yr. One 4-mg chewable tablet a day, taken in the evening.

SIDE EFFECTS/ADVERSE REACTIONS

Adults, Adolescents 15 yr and older
Frequent
Headache
Occasional
Influenza
Rare
Abdominal pain, cough, dyspepsia, dizziness, fatigue, dental pain

Children 6–14 yr
Rare
Diarrhea, laryngitis, pharyngitis, nausea, otitis media, sinusitis, viral infection

PRECAUTIONS AND CONTRAINDICATIONS
Hypersensitivity
Caution

Not for acute asthma attacks, not for treatment of exercise-induced bronchospasm or ASA-induced bronchospasm, chewable tablets contain aspartame, lactation; monitor patients when potent CYP3A4 isoenzyme inducers are used

DRUG INTERACTIONS OF CONCERN TO DENTISTRY
• None reported; however, monitor patients when inhibitors of CYP3A4 or CYP2C9 are prescribed

SERIOUS REACTIONS
None known

DENTAL CONSIDERATIONS
General:
• Midday appointments and a stress-reduction protocol may be required for anxious patients.
• Avoid prescribing aspirin-containing products.
• Acute asthmatic episodes may be precipitated in the dental office. Rapid-acting sympathomimetic inhalants should be available for emergency use.
• Be aware that aspirin or sulfite preservatives in vasoconstrictor-containing products can exacerbate asthma.
• Consider semisupine chair position for patients with respiratory disease or if GI side effects occur.
Consultations:
• Medical consultation may be required to assess disease control.
Teach Patient/Family to:
• Update health and drug history if physician makes any changes in evaluation or drug

M

regimens; include OTC, herbal, and nonherbal drugs in the update

moricizine hydrochloride

mor-iss´-ih-zeen
high-droh-klor´-ide
(Ethmozine)

CATEGORY AND SCHEDULE
Pregnancy Risk Category: B

Drug Class: Antidysrhythmic, type I

MECHANISM OF ACTION
An antiarrhythmic that prevents sodium current across myocardial cell membranes. Has potent local anesthetic activity and membrane stabilizing effects. Slows AV and His-Purkinje conduction and decreases action potential duration and effective refractory period. *Therapeutic Effect:* Suppresses ventricular arrhythmias.

USES
Treatment of documented life-threatening dysrhythmias

PHARMACOKINETICS
Peak 0.5–2.2 hr. *Half-life:* 1.5–3.5 hr; protein binding greater than 90%; metabolized by the liver; metabolites excreted in feces, urine.

INDICATIONS AND DOSAGES
▸ **Arrhythmias**
PO
Adults, Elderly. 200–300 mg q8h. May increase by 150 mg/day at no less than 3-day intervals.

SIDE EFFECTS/ADVERSE REACTIONS
Frequent
Dizziness, nausea, headache, fatigue, dyspnea
Occasional
Nervousness, paraesthesia, sleep disturbances, dyspepsia, vomiting, diarrhea, dry mouth

PRECAUTIONS AND CONTRAINDICATIONS
Cardiogenic shock, preexisting second- or third-degree AV block or right bundle-branch block without pacemaker
Caution
CHF, hypokalemia, hyperkalemia, sick sinus syndrome, lactation, children, impaired hepatic and renal function, cardiac dysfunction

DRUG INTERACTIONS OF CONCERN TO DENTISTRY
• No specific interactions are reported with dental drugs; however, any drug that could affect the cardiac action of moricizine (e.g., other local anesthetics, vasoconstrictors, anticholinergics) should be used in the lowest effective dose

SERIOUS REACTIONS
! Moricizine may worsen existing arrhythmias or produce new ones.
! Jaundice with hepatitis occurs rarely.
! Overdosage produces vomiting, lethargy, syncope, hypotension, conduction disturbances, exacerbation of CHF, MI, and sinus arrest.

DENTAL CONSIDERATIONS
General:
• Monitor vital signs at every appointment because of cardiovascular side effects.

• Assess salivary flow as a factor in caries, periodontal disease, and candidiasis.
• Stress from dental procedures may compromise cardiovascular function; determine patient risk.
Consultations:
• Medical consultation should be made to assess disease control and patient's ability to tolerate stress.
Teach Patient/Family to:
• Use effective oral hygiene to prevent soft tissue inflammation
• Use caution to prevent injury when using oral hygiene aids
• When chronic dry mouth occurs, advise patient to:
  • Avoid mouth rinses with high alcohol content because of drying effects
  • Use sugarless gum, frequent sips of water, or saliva substitutes
  • Use daily home fluoride products for anticaries effect

morphine sulfate

mor´-feen sull´-fate
(Anamorph[AUS], Astramorph, Avinza, DepoDur, Duramorph, Infumorph, Kadian, Kapanol[AUS], M-Eslon, Morphine Mixtures[AUS], MS Contin, MSIR, MS Mono[AUS], Oramorph SR, RMS, Roxanol, Statex[CAN])
Do not confuse morphine with hydromorphone, or Roxanol with Roxicet.

CATEGORY AND SCHEDULE

Pregnancy Risk Category: C
(D if used for prolonged periods or at high dosages at term)
Controlled Substance: Schedule II

Drug Class: Narcotic analgesic

MECHANISM OF ACTION

An opioid agonist that binds with opioid receptors in the CNS. *Therapeutic Effect:* Alters the perception of and emotional response to pain; produces generalized CNS depression.

USES

Treatment of severe pain

PHARMACOKINETICS

Route	Onset	Peak	Duration
Oral solution	N/A	1 hr	3–5 hr
Tablets	N/A	1 hr	3–5 hr
Tablets (ER)	N/A	3–4 hr	8–12 hr
IV	Rapid	0.3 hr	3–5 hr
IM	5–30 min	0.5–1 hr	3–5 hr
Epidural	N/A	1 hr	12–20 hr
Subcutaneous	N/A	1.1–5 hr	3–5 hr
Rectal	N/A	0.5–1 hr	3–7 hr

Variably absorbed from the GI tract. Readily absorbed after IM or subcutaneous administration. Protein binding: 20%–35%. Widely distributed. Metabolized in the liver. Primarily excreted in urine. Removed by hemodialysis. *Half-life:* 2–3 hr. (increased in patients with hepatic disease).

INDICATIONS AND DOSAGES
Alert
Dosage should be titrated to desired effect.
▶ **Analgesia**
PO (Prompt Release)
Adults, Elderly. 10–30 mg q3–4h as needed.
Children. 0.2–0.5 mg/kg q3–4h as needed.

Alert
For the Avinza dosage below, be aware that this drug is to be administered once a day only.

Alert
For the Kadian dosage information below, be aware that this drug is to be administered q12h or once a day only.

Alert
Be aware that pediatric dosages of extended-release preparations Kadian and Avinza have not been established.

Alert
For the MSContin and Oramorph SR dosage information below, be aware that the daily dosage is divided and given q8h or q12h.

PO (Extended-Release [Avinza])
Adults, Elderly. Dosage requirement should be established using prompt-release formulations and is based on total daily dose. Avinza is given once a day only.

PO (Extended-Release [Kadian])
Adults, Elderly. Dosage requirement should be established using prompt-release formulations and is based on total daily dose. Dose is given once a day or divided and given q12h.

PO (Extended-Release [MSContin, Oramorph SR])
Adults, Elderly. Dosage requirement should be established using prompt-release formulations and is based on total daily dose. Daily dose is divided and given q8h or q12h.
Children. 0.3–0.6 mg/kg/dose q12h.

IV
Adults, Elderly. 2.5–5 mg q3–4h as needed. Note: Repeated doses (e.g., 1–2 mg) may be given more frequently (e.g., every hr) if needed.
Children. 0.05–0.1 mg/kg q3–4h as needed.

IV Continuous Infusion

Adults, Elderly. 0.8–10 mg/h. Range: Up to 80 mg/h.
Children. 10–30 mcg/kg/hr.

IM
Adults, Elderly. 5–10 mg q3–4h as needed.
Children. 0.1 mg/kg q3–4h as needed.

Epidural
Adults, Elderly. Initially, 1–6 mg bolus, infusion rate: 0.1–1 mg/h. Maximum: 10 mg/24 h.

Intrathecal
Adults, Elderly. One tenth of the epidural dose: 0.2–1 mg/dose.

▶ **PCA**
IV
Adults, Elderly. Loading dose: 5–10 mg. Intermittent bolus: 0.5–3 mg. Lockout interval: 5–12 min. Continuous infusion: 1–10 mg/hr. 4-hr limit: 20–30 mg.

SIDE EFFECTS/ADVERSE REACTIONS
Frequent
Sedation, decreased B/P (including orthostatic hypotension), diaphoresis, facial flushing, constipation, dizziness, somnolence, nausea, vomiting

Occasional
Allergic reaction (rash, pruritus), dyspnea, confusion, palpitations, tremors, urine retention, abdominal cramps, vision changes, dry mouth, headache, decreased appetite, pain or burning at injection site

Rare
Paralytic ileus

PRECAUTIONS AND CONTRAINDICATIONS
Acute or severe asthma, GI obstruction, severe hepatic or renal impairment, severe respiratory depression, asthma, severe liver or renal impairment

Caution
Addictive personality, lactation, MI (acute), severe heart disease, elderly, respiratory depression, hepatic disease, renal disease, children younger than 18 yr

DRUG INTERACTIONS OF CONCERN TO DENTISTRY

• Increased CNS depression: alcohol, all CNS depressants
• Contraindication: MAOIs
• Increased effects of anticholinergics

SERIOUS REACTIONS

! Overdose results in respiratory depression, skeletal muscle flaccidity, cold or clammy skin, cyanosis, and extreme somnolence progressing to seizures, stupor, and coma.
! The patient who uses morphine repeatedly may develop a tolerance to the drug's analgesic effect and physical dependence.
! The drug may have a prolonged duration of action and cumulative effect in those with hepatic and renal impairment.

DENTAL CONSIDERATIONS

General:
• Monitor vital signs at every appointment because of cardiovascular and respiratory side effects.
• Assess salivary flow as a factor in caries, periodontal disease, and candidiasis.
• After supine positioning, have patient sit upright for at least 2 min before standing to avoid orthostatic hypotension.
• Psychologic and physical dependence may occur with chronic administration.

• Determine why the patient is taking the drug.
• Consider the use of NSAIDs when additional analgesia is required.
Teach Patient/Family:
• When chronic dry mouth occurs, advise patient to:
  • Use daily home fluoride products for anticaries effect
  • Avoid mouth rinses with high alcohol content because of drying effects
  • Use sugarless gum, frequent sips of water, or saliva substitutes

moxifloxacin hydrochloride

moks-ih-floks´-ah-sin high-dro-klor´-ide
(Avelox, Avelox IV, Vigamox)
Do not confuse Avelox with Avonex.

CATEGORY AND SCHEDULE
Pregnancy Risk Category: C

Drug Class: Fluoroquinolone antiinfective

MECHANISM OF ACTION
A fluoroquinolone that inhibits two enzymes, topoisomerase II and IV, in susceptible microorganisms.
Therapeutic Effect: Interferes with bacterial DNA replication. Prevents or delays emergence of resistant organisms. Bactericidal.

USES
Treatment of acute bacterial sinusitis (*S. pneumoniae, H. influenzae,* or *M. catarrhalis*); acute bacterial exacerbation of chronic bronchitis (*S. pneumoniae, H. influenzae, H. parainfluenzae, K. pneumoniae, M. catarrhalis,* or *S. aureus*); community-acquired pneumonia

(*S. pneumoniae, H. influenzae, M. catarrhalis, M. pneumoniae,* or *C. pneumoniae*); bacterial conjunctivitis caused by susceptible bacterial strains including selected aerobic gram-positive species, selected aerobic gram-negative species, and *C. trachomatis*

PHARMACOKINETICS

Well absorbed from the GI tract after PO administration. Protein binding: 50%. Widely distributed throughout body with tissue concentration often exceeding plasma concentration. Metabolized in liver. Primarily excreted in urine with a lesser amount in feces. *Half-life:* 10.7–13.3 hr.

INDICATIONS AND DOSAGES

▶ **Acute Bacterial Sinusitis, Community-Acquired Pneumonia**
PO, IV
Adults, Elderly. 400 mg q24h for 10 days.
▶ **Acute Bacterial Exacerbation of Chronic Bronchitis**
PO, IV
Adults, Elderly. 400 mg q24h for 5 days.
▶ **Skin and Skin-Structure Infection**
PO, IV
Adults, Elderly. 400 mg once a day for 7 days.
▶ **Topical Treatment of Bacterial Conjunctivitis Caused by Susceptible Strains of Bacteria**
Ophthalmic
Adults, Elderly, Children older than 1 yr. 1 drop 3 times a day for 7 days.

SIDE EFFECTS/ADVERSE REACTIONS

Frequent
Nausea, diarrhea
Occasional
Dizziness, headache, abdominal pain, vomiting

Ophthalmic: conjunctival irritation, reduced visual acuity, dry eye, keratitis, eye pain, ocular itching, swelling of tissue around cornea, eye discharge, fever, cough, pharyngitis, rash, rhinitis
Rare
Change in sense of taste, dyspepsia (heartburn, indigestion), photosensitivity

PRECAUTIONS AND CONTRAINDICATIONS

Hypersensitivity to quinolones
Caution
Divalent cations, retard absorption, not for use with class 1A and III antiarrhythmics, use in children not studied, cross resistance with other fluoroquinolones, may prolong QT interval in some patients, seizures, use with NSAIDs, children younger than 18 yr, lactation

DRUG INTERACTIONS OF CONCERN TO DENTISTRY

• Increased risk of CNS stimulation and seizures: NSAIDs
• Decreased absorption: divalent and trivalent antacids, iron and zinc salts
• Caution when using erythromycin, tricyclic antidepressants (no data, risk of QT interval)
• Increased risk of life-threatening arrhythmias: procainamide

DRUG INTERACTIONS OF CONCERN TO DENTISTRY

None reported

SERIOUS REACTIONS

! Pseudomembranous colitis as evidenced by fever, severe abdominal cramps or pain, and severe watery diarrhea may occur.
! Superinfection manifested as anal or genital pruritus, moderate to severe diarrhea, and stomatitis may occur.

DENTAL CONSIDERATIONS

General:
• Determine why patient is taking the drug.
• Examine for oral manifestation of opportunistic infection.
• Advise patient if dental drugs prescribed have a potential for photosensitivity.
• Ruptures of the shoulder, hand, and Achilles tendons that required surgical repair or resulted in prolonged disability have been reported with the use of fluoroquinolones. Question patient about history of side effects associated with fluoroquinolone use.
• Monitor vital signs at every appointment because of cardiovascular side effects.
• Patients on chronic drug therapy may rarely have symptoms of blood dyscrasias, which can include infection, bleeding, and poor healing.
• Consider semisupine chair position for patient comfort if GI side effects occur.

Consultations:
• In a patient with symptoms of blood dyscrasias, request a medical consultation for blood studies and postpone treatment until normal values are reestablished.
• Physician consultation is advised in the presence of an acute dental infection requiring another antibiotic.

Teach Patient/Family:
• If used for dental infection to:
  • Minimize exposure to sunlight and wear sunscreen if sun exposure is planned
  • Discontinue treatment and inform dentist immediately if patient experiences pain or inflammation of a tendon, and to rest and refrain from exercise

Moxifloxacin HCl (Vigamox)
General:
• Avoid dental light in patient's eyes.

mupirocin
mew-peer´-oh-sin
(Bactroban)
Do not confuse with Bactrim or Bacitracin

CATEGORY AND SCHEDULE
Pregnancy Risk Category: B

Drug Class: Topical antiinfective, pseudomonic acid A

MECHANISM OF ACTION
An antibacterial agent that inhibits bacterial protein, RNA synthesis. Less effective on DNA synthesis. Nasal: Eradicates nasal colonization of MRSA. **Therapeutic Effect:** Prevents bacterial growth and replication. Bacteriostatic.

USES
Treatment of Impetigo caused by *S. aureus*, β-hemolytic streptococci, *S. pyogenes;* nasal membranes: *S. aureus*

PHARMACOKINETICS
Metabolized in skin to inactive metabolite. Transported to skin surface; removed by normal skin desquamation.

INDICATIONS AND DOSAGES
▶ **Impetigo, Infected Traumatic Skin Lesions**
Topical
Adults, Elderly, Children. Apply 3 times a day (may cover with gauze).

▶ **Nasal colonization of resistant Staphylococcus aureus**
Intranasal
Adults, Elderly, Children 12 yr and older. Apply 2 times a day for 5 days.

SIDE EFFECTS/ADVERSE REACTIONS

Frequent
Nasal: Headache, rhinitis, upper respiratory congestion, pharyngitis, altered taste
Occasional
Nasal: Burning, stinging, cough
Topical: Pain, burning, stinging, itching
Rare
Nasal: Pruritis, diarrhea, dry mouth, epistaxis, nausea, rash
Topical: Rash, nausea, dry skin, contact dermatitis

PRECAUTIONS AND CONTRAINDICATIONS

Hypersensitivity to mupirocin or any component of the formulation
Caution
Lactation

DRUG INTERACTIONS OF CONCERN TO DENTISTRY

SERIOUS REACTIONS

! Superinfection may result in bacterial or fungal infections, especially with prolonged or repeated therapy.

DENTAL CONSIDERATIONS

General:
• The dentist may choose to postpone elective dental treatment if the infected site may be affected by dental treatment.

mycophenolate mofetil
my-co-fen´-oh-late
(CellCept)

CATEGORY AND SCHEDULE
Pregnancy Risk Category: C

Drug Class: Immunosuppressant

MECHANISM OF ACTION
An immunologic agent that suppresses the immunologically mediated inflammatory response by inhibiting inosine monophosphate dehydrogenase, an enzyme that deprives lymphocytes of nucleotides necessary for DNA and RNA synthesis, thus inhibiting the proliferation of T and B lymphocytes. ***Therapeutic Effect:*** Prevents transplant rejection.

USES
Prophylaxis of organ rejection in patients receiving allogenic renal or hepatic transplants, cardiac transplants (in combination with cyclosporine and corticosteroids)

PHARMACOKINETICS
Rapidly and extensively absorbed after PO administration (food decreases drug plasma concentration but doesn't affect absorption). Protein binding: 97%. Completely hydrolyzed to active metabolite mycophenolic acid. Primarily excreted in urine. Not removed by hemodialysis. ***Half-life:*** 17.9 hr.

INDICATIONS AND DOSAGES
▶ **Prevention of Renal Transplant Rejection**
PO, IV
Adults, Elderly. 1 g twice a day.

▶ **Prevention of Heart Transplant Rejection**
PO, IV
Adults, Elderly. 1.5 g twice a day.
▶ **Prevention of Liver Transplant Rejection**
PO
Adults, Elderly. 1.5 g twice a day.
IV
Adults, Elderly. 1 g twice a day.
▶ **Usual Pediatric Dosage**
PO
Children. 600 mg/m^2/dose twice a day. Maximum: 2 g/day.

SIDE EFFECTS/ADVERSE REACTIONS
Frequent
UTI, hypertension, peripheral edema, diarrhea, constipation, fever, headache, nausea
Occasional
Dyspepsia; dyspnea; cough; hematuria; asthenia; vomiting; edema; tremors; abdominal, chest, or back pain; oral candidiasis; acne
Rare
Insomnia, respiratory tract infection, rash, dizziness

PRECAUTIONS AND CONTRAINDICATIONS
Hypersensitivity to mycophenolic acid
Caution
Active GI diseases, lactation, reduce dose in severe chronic renal impairment, increased risk of development of lymphomas or other malignancies and susceptibility to infection

DRUG INTERACTIONS OF CONCERN TO DENTISTRY
• Increased plasma concentration: acyclovir, ganciclovir
• Decreased availability of MPA: drugs that alter the GI flora

SERIOUS REACTIONS
❗ Significant anemia, leukopenia, thrombocytopenia, neutropenia, and leukocytosis may occur, particularly in those undergoing renal transplant rejection.
❗ Sepsis and infection occur occasionally.
❗ GI tract hemorrhage occurs rarely.
❗ Patients receiving mycophenolate have an increased risk of developing neoplasms.

DENTAL CONSIDERATIONS
General:
• Determine why the patient is taking the drug.
• Short appointments and a stress-reduction protocol may be required for anxious patients.
• Patients who have been or are currently on chronic steroid therapy (longer than 2 wk) may require supplemental steroids for dental treatment.
• Patients on chronic drug therapy may rarely have symptoms of blood dyscrasias, which can include infection, bleeding, and poor healing.
• Place on frequent recall because of oral side effects.
• Determine dose and duration of steroid for patient to assess risk for stress tolerance and immunosuppression.
• Examine for oral manifestation of opportunistic infections.
• Monitor vital signs at every appointment because of cardiovascular and respiratory side effects.
• Consider semisupine chair position for patient comfort if GI side effects occur.
• Antibiotic prophylaxis is usually recommended in patients with organ transplants and immunosuppression.

M

• Monitor time since organ/tissue transplant; note duration of transplant and status of renal function.
• Place on frequent recall because of possible blood dyscrasias and oral side effects.

Consultations:
• Medical consultation may be required to assess disease control and patient's ability to tolerate stress.
• In a patient with symptoms of blood dyscrasias, request a medical consultation for blood studies and postpone dental treatment until normal values are reestablished.

• Request baseline B/P in renal transplant patients for patient evaluation before dental treatment.

Teach Patient/Family to:
• See dentist immediately if secondary oral infection occurs
• Use effective oral hygiene to prevent soft tissue inflammation
• Return to dentist frequently because of possible blood dyscrasias and oral side effects
• Report oral lesions, soreness, or bleeding to dentist

M

nabumetone

na-byu´-meh-tone
(Apo-Nabumetone, Relafen)

CATEGORY AND SCHEDULE

Pregnancy Risk Category: C
(D if used in third trimester or near
delivery)

Drug Class: Nonsteroidal
antiinflammatory

MECHANISM OF ACTION

An NSAID that produces analgesic
and antiinflammatory effects by
inhibiting prostaglandin synthesis.
Therapeutic Effect: Reduces the
inflammatory response and intensity
of pain.

USES

Treatment of osteoarthritis,
rheumatoid arthritis, acute or chronic
treatment

PHARMACOKINETICS

Readily absorbed from the GI tract.
Protein binding: 99%. Widely
distributed. Metabolized in the liver
to active metabolite. Primarily
excreted in urine. Not removed by
hemodialysis. **Half-life:** 22–30 hr.

INDICATIONS AND DOSAGES

▸ **Acute or Chronic Rheumatoid
Arthritis and Osteoarthritis**
PO
Adults, Elderly. Initially, 1000 mg as
a single dose or in 2 divided doses.
May increase up to 2000 mg/day as a
single or in 2 divided doses.

SIDE EFFECTS/ADVERSE
REACTIONS

Frequent
Diarrhea, abdominal cramps or pain,
dyspepsia, oral lichenoid reaction

Occasional
Nausea, constipation, flatulence,
dizziness, headache
Rare
Vomiting, stomatitis, confusion

PRECAUTIONS AND
CONTRAINDICATIONS

Active peptic ulcer disease, chronic
inflammation of GI tract, GI bleeding
or ulceration, history of
hypersensitivity to aspirin or NSAIDs,
history of significant renal impairment
Caution
Lactation, children, bleeding
disorders, GI disorders, cardiac
disorders, renal disorders, hepatic
dysfunction, elderly

DRUG INTERACTIONS OF
CONCERN TO DENTISTRY

• GI ulceration, bleeding: aspirin,
alcohol, corticosteroids
• May decrease effects of
nabumetone: salicylates
• Nephrotoxicity: acetaminophen
(prolonged use and high doses)
• Possible risk of decreased renal
function: cyclosporine
• First-time users of SSRIs also
taking NSAIDs may have a higher
risk of GI side effects; until more
data are available, it may be
advisable to avoid use of NSAIDs in
these patients (Br J Clin Pharmacol
55:591–595, 2003)

SERIOUS REACTIONS

! Overdose may result in acute
hypotension and tachycardia.
! Rare reactions with long-term use
include peptic ulcer disease,
GI bleeding, gastritis, nephrotoxicity
(dysuria, cystitis, hematuria,
proteinuria, nephrotic syndrome),
severe hepatic reactions (cholestasis,
jaundice), and severe hypersensitivity
reactions (bronchospasm,
angioedema).

N

DENTAL CONSIDERATIONS

General:
• Potential increase of adverse cardiovascular events in patients at risk for thromboembolism.
• Patients on chronic drug therapy may rarely have symptoms of blood dyscrasias, which can include infection, bleeding, and poor healing.
• Assess salivary flow as a factor in caries, periodontal disease, and candidiasis.
• Avoid prescribing for dental use in pregnancy.
• Avoid prescribing aspirin-containing products.
• Consider semisupine chair position for patients with arthritic disease.

Consultations:
• In patients with symptoms of blood dyscrasias, request a medical consultation for blood studies and postpone dental treatment until normal values are reestablished.
• Medical consultation may be required to assess disease control.

Teach Patient/Family to:
• Use effective oral hygiene to prevent soft tissue inflammation
• Use caution to prevent injury when using oral hygiene aids
• When chronic dry mouth occurs, advise patient to:
    • Avoid mouth rinses with high alcohol content because of drying effects
    • Use daily home fluoride products for anticaries effect
    • Use sugarless gum, frequent sips of water, or saliva substitutes

nadolol
nay´-doe-lole
(Apo-Nadol[CAN], Corgard, Novo-Nadolol[CAN])

CATEGORY AND SCHEDULE
Pregnancy Risk Category: C (D if used in second or third trimester)

Drug Class: Nonselective β-adrenergic blocker

MECHANISM OF ACTION
A nonselective β-blocker that blocks β_1- and β_2-adrenergenic receptors. Large doses increase airway resistance. ***Therapeutic Effect:*** Slows sinus heart rate, decreases cardiac output and B/P. Decreases myocardial ischemia severity by decreasing oxygen requirements.

USES
Treatment of chronic stable angina pectoris, mild-to-moderate hypertension; unapproved: dysrhythmias, MI prophylaxis, vascular headache

PHARMACOKINETICS
PO: Onset variable, peak 3–4 hr, duration 17–24 hr. ***Half-life:*** 16–20 hr; not metabolized; excreted in urine (unchanged), bile, breast milk

INDICATIONS AND DOSAGES
▸ **Mild-to-Moderate Hypertension, Angina**
PO
Adults. Initially, 40 mg/day. May increase by 40–80 mg at 3–7-day intervals.
Maximum: 240–360 mg/day.
Elderly. Initially, 20 mg/day. May increase gradually. Range: 20–240 mg/day.

▶ **Dosage in Renal Impairment**

Dosage is modified on the basis of creatinine clearance.

Creatinine Clearance	% of Usual Dosage
10–50 ml/min	50
Less than 10 ml/min	25

SIDE EFFECTS/ADVERSE REACTIONS

Nadolol is generally well tolerated, with transient and mild side effects

Frequent

Diminished sexual ability, drowsiness, unusual fatigue, or weakness

Occasional

Bradycardia, difficulty breathing, depression, cold hands or feet, diarrhea, constipation, anxiety, nasal congestion, nausea, vomiting

Rare

Altered taste, dry eyes, itching

PRECAUTIONS AND CONTRAINDICATIONS

Bronchial asthma, cardiogenic shock, CHF secondary to tachyarrhythmias, COPD, patients receiving MAOI therapy, second- or third-degree heart block, sinus bradycardia, uncontrolled cardiac failure

Caution

Diabetes mellitus, renal disease, lactation, hyperthyroidism, peripheral vascular disease, myasthenia gravis

DRUG INTERACTIONS OF CONCERN TO DENTISTRY

• Decreased effects: sympathomimetics (epinephrine, norepinephrine, isoproterenol)
• Slows metabolism of nadolol: lidocaine
• Increased hypotension, myocardial depression: fentanyl derivatives, hydrocarbon inhalation anesthetics
• Decreased hypotensive effect: indomethacin and other NSAIDs

SERIOUS REACTIONS

! Overdose may produce profound bradycardia and hypotension.
! Abrupt withdrawal of nadolol may result in diaphoresis, palpitations, headache, tremors, exacerbation of angina, MI, and ventricular arrhythmias.
! Nadolol administration may precipitate CHF and MI in patients with cardiac disease; thyroid storm in those with thyrotoxicosis; and peripheral ischemia in those with existing peripheral vascular disease.
! Hypoglycemia may occur in patients with previously controlled diabetes.

DENTAL CONSIDERATIONS

General:

• Monitor vital signs at every appointment because of cardiovascular side effects.
• Patients on chronic drug therapy may rarely have symptoms of blood dyscrasias, which can include infection, bleeding, and poor healing.
• After supine positioning, have patient sit upright for at least 2 min before standing to avoid orthostatic hypotension.
• Limit use of sodium-containing products, such as saline IV fluids, for patients with a dietary salt restriction.
• Assess salivary flow as a factor in caries, periodontal disease, and candidiasis.
• Stress from dental procedures may compromise cardiovascular function; determine patient risk.
• Short appointments and a stress-reduction protocol may be required for anxious patients.
• Consider semisupine chair position for patients with respiratory distress.

N

Consultations:
• In patients with symptoms of blood dyscrasias, request a medical consultation for blood studies and postpone dental treatment until normal values are reestablished.
• Take precautions if dental surgery is anticipated and anesthesia is required.
• Medical consultation may be required to assess disease control and patient's ability to tolerate stress.

Teach Patient/Family to:
• Use effective oral hygiene to prevent soft tissue inflammation
• Use caution to prevent injury when using oral hygiene aids
• When chronic dry mouth occurs, advise patient to:
  • Avoid mouth rinses with high alcohol content because of drying effects
  • Use daily home fluoride products for anticaries effect
  • Use sugarless gum, frequent sips of water, or saliva substitutes

nafarelin
naf-ah´-rell-in
(Synarel)

CATEGORY AND SCHEDULE
Pregnancy Risk Category: X

Drug Class: Gonadotropin; analog of gonadotropin-releasing hormone

MECHANISM OF ACTION
A gonadotropin inhibitor that initially stimulates the release of the pituitary gonadotropins, luteinizing hormone and follicle-stimulating hormone, then decreases secretion of gonadal steroids. *Therapeutic*

Effect: Temporarily increases ovarian steroidogenesis, abolishes the stimulatory effect on the pituitary gland, decreases secretion of gonadal steroids.

USES
Treatment of endometriosis, gonadotropin-dependent precocious puberty

PHARMACOKINETICS
Rapidly absorbed after nasal administration. Protein binding: 78%–84%, binds primarily to albumin. Metabolism: unknown. Excreted in urine. *Half-life:* 3 hr.

INDICATIONS AND DOSAGES
▸ **Endometriosis**
Intranasal
Adults. 400 mcg/day: 200 mcg (1 spray) into 1 nostril in morning, 1 spray into other nostril in evening. For patients with persistent regular menstruation after months of treatment, increase dose to 800 mcg/day (1 spray into each nostril in morning and evening).
▸ **Central Precocious Puberty**
Intranasal
Children. 1600 mcg/day: 400 mcg (2 sprays into each nostril in morning and evening; total 8 sprays).

SIDE EFFECTS/ADVERSE REACTIONS
Frequent
Hot flashes. muscle pain, decreased breast size, myalgia
Occasional
Nasal irritation, decreased libido, vaginal dryness, headache, emotional lability, acne
Rare
Insomnia, edema, weight gain, seborrhea, depression

PRECAUTIONS AND CONTRAINDICATIONS

Pregnancy, other agonist analogues, undiagnosed abnormal vaginal bleeding, hypersensitivity to nafarelin or any component of the formulation

DRUG INTERACTIONS OF CONCERN TO DENTISTRY

None reported

SERIOUS REACTIONS

None reported

DENTAL CONSIDERATIONS

General:
• Determine why patient is taking the drug.

naftifine

naf´-ti-feen
(Naftin)
Do not confuse with nafcillin or nafarelin.

CATEGORY AND SCHEDULE

Pregnancy Risk Category: B

Drug Class: Topical antifungal

MECHANISM OF ACTION

An antifungal that selectively inhibits the enzyme squalene epoxidase in a dose-dependent manner, which results in the primary sterol, ergosterol, within the fungal membrane not being synthesized. *Therapeutic Effect:* Results in fungal cell death. Fungistatic and fungicidal.

USES

Treatment of tinea cruris, tinea corporis, tinea pedis

PHARMACOKINETICS

Minimal systemic absorption. Metabolized in the liver. Excreted in the urine, as well as the feces and bile. *Half-life:* 48–72 hr.

INDICATIONS AND DOSAGES
▶ **Tinea Pedis, Tinea Cruris, Tinea Corporis**
Topical
Adults, Elderly, Children 12 yr and older. Apply cream 1 time a day for 4 wk or until signs and symptoms significantly improve. Apply gel 2 times a day for 4 wk or until signs and symptoms significantly improve.

SIDE EFFECTS/ADVERSE REACTIONS

Frequent
Burning, stinging
Occasional
Erythema, itching, dryness, irritation

PRECAUTIONS AND CONTRAINDICATIONS

Hypersensitivity to naftifine or any of its components
Caution
Lactation, children

DRUG INTERACTIONS OF CONCERN TO DENTISTRY

None reported

SERIOUS REACTIONS

! Excessive irritation may indicate hypersensitivity reaction.

nalbuphine hydrochloride

nal-byoo´-feen high-droh-klor´-ide
(Nubain)
Do not confuse Nubain with
Navane.

CATEGORY AND SCHEDULE

Pregnancy Risk Category: B
(D if used for prolonged periods or
at high dosages at term)

Drug Class: Narcotic agonist,
antagonist; opioid analgesic

MECHANISM OF ACTION

A narcotic agonist-antagonist that
binds with opioid receptors in the
CNS. May displace opioid agonists
and competitively inhibit their
action; may precipitate withdrawal
symptoms. **Therapeutic Effect:**
Alters the perception of and
emotional response to pain.

USES

Relief of moderate-to-severe pain,
preoperative sedation, obstetric
analgesia, adjunct to anesthesia

PHARMACOKINETICS

Route	Onset	Peak	Duration
IV	2–3 min	30 min	3–6 hr
IM	Less than 15 min	60 min	3–6 hr
Subcuta-neous	Less than 15 min	N/A	3–6 hr

Well absorbed after IM or
subcutaneous administration. Protein
binding: 50%. Metabolized in the
liver. Primarily eliminated in feces
by biliary secretion. **Half-life:**
3.5–5 hr.

INDICATIONS AND DOSAGES

▶ **Analgesia**
IV, IM, Subcutaneous
Adults, Elderly. 10 mg q3–6h as
needed. Don't exceed maximum
single dose of 20 mg or daily dose of
160 mg. For patients receiving
long-term narcotic analgesics of
similar duration of action, give
25% of usual dose.
Children. 0.1–0.15 mg/kg q3–6h as
needed.
▶ **Supplement to Anesthesia**
IV
Adults, Elderly. Induction: 0.3–3 mg/
kg over 10–15 min. Maintenance:
0.25–0.5 mg/kg as needed.

SIDE EFFECTS/ADVERSE REACTIONS

Frequent
Sedation
Occasional
Diaphoresis, cold and clammy skin,
nausea, vomiting, dizziness, vertigo,
dry mouth, headache
Rare
Restlessness, emotional lability,
paresthesia, flushing, paradoxical
reaction

PRECAUTIONS AND CONTRAINDICATIONS

Respiratory rate less than
12 breaths/min

DRUG INTERACTIONS OF CONCERN TO DENTISTRY

• Increased CNS and respiratory
depression: all CNS depressants
• Contraindicated with MAOIs
• Avoid use in narcotic-dependent
persons; risk of withdrawal reactions
• Increased risk of constipation:
anticholinergics
• Increased risk of orthostatic
hypotension: antihypertensive
medications

SERIOUS REACTIONS

! Abrupt withdrawal after prolonged use may produce symptoms of narcotic withdrawal, such as abdominal cramping, rhinorrhea, lacrimation, anxiety, fever, and piloerection (goosebumps).
! Overdose results in severe respiratory depression, skeletal muscle flaccidity, cyanosis, and extreme somnolence progressing to seizures, stupor, and coma.
! Repeated use may result in drug tolerance and physical dependence.

DENTAL CONSIDERATIONS

General:
• Avoid use in an opioid-dependent patient.
• Acute-use drug, question patient about use for pain.
• If additional analgesia is required for dental pain, consider alternative analgesics (NSAIDs) in patients taking narcotics for acute or chronic pain.
• Monitor and record vital signs.
• Assess salivary flow as a factor in caries, periodontal disease, and candidiasis.
Consultations:
• Medical consultation may be required to assess disease control.
Teach Patient/Family to:
• Use effective oral hygiene to prevent soft tissue inflammation
• Prevent trauma when using oral hygiene aids
• Avoid driving or other activities requiring mental alertness
• Avoid alcohol ingestion or CNS depressants; serious CNS depression may result
• Avoid OTC preparations that contain CNS depressants (antihistamines, cold remedies)

• When chronic dry mouth occurs advise patient to:
  • Avoid mouth rinses with high alcohol content due to drying effects
  • Use daily home fluoride products for anticaries effect
  • Use sugarless gum, frequent sips of water, or saliva substitutes

nalmefene hydrochloride
nal´-meh-feen
(Revex)

CATEGORY AND SCHEDULE
Pregnancy Risk Category: B

Drug Class: Opioid antagonist

MECHANISM OF ACTION
Reverses the effects of opioids by competitive antagonism of opioid receptors.

USES
Management of opioid overdose and complete or partial reversal of opioid drug effects, including respiratory depression

PHARMACOKINETICS
IV: Onset 2 min, peak plasma concentration 1.1–2.3 hr; can also be given IM or subcutaneously; hepatic metabolism; excreted in urine.

INDICATIONS AND DOSAGES
▶ **Reversal of Opioid Depression:**
IV
Adult. (100 mcg/ml strength) initial dose 0.25 mcg/kg followed by 0.25 mcg/kg, incremental dose at 2–5 min intervals; cumulative doses over 1.0 mcg/kg do not provide

additional therapeutic effect; titrate all doses

Body weight (kg)	ml of 100 mcg/ml solution
50	0.125
60	0.150
70	0.175
80	0.200
90	0.225
100	0.250

▸ **Known or Suspected Opioid Overdose**

IV

Adult. (1 mg/ml strength) initial 0.5 mg/70 kg; if needed, a second dose of 1.0 mg/70 kg, 2–5 min later; doses over 1.5 mg/70 kg are unlikely to be beneficial

SIDE EFFECTS/ADVERSE REACTIONS

Oral: Dry mouth
CNS: Dizziness, headache, dysphoria, perception of pain, nervousness
CV: Tachycardia, hypertension, dysrhythmia, hypotension
GI: Nausea, abdominal cramps, vomiting, diarrhea
Resp: Pharyngitis, pulmonary edema
GU: Urinary retention
Integ: Pruritus
MS: Myalgia, joint pain
Misc: Chills

PRECAUTIONS AND CONTRAINDICATIONS

Hypersensitivity
Caution
Nursing mothers, children, withdrawal symptoms in opioid addicts, renal impairment

DRUG INTERACTIONS OF CONCERN TO DENTISTRY

None reported

SERIOUS REACTIONS

❗ Precipitation of acute withdrawal syndrome in opioid-dependent individuals.
❗ Tachycardia, hypertension.

DENTAL CONSIDERATIONS

General:
• This drug is intended for acute use only, but listed side effects can sometimes be seen.
• There is a risk of seizures reported in animal studies; be aware of this potential.
• Serious cardiovascular events have been associated with opioid reversal in postoperative patients; doses should be carefully titrated to reduce these events.
• Buprenorphine depression may not be completely reversed.
• In all cases, the establishment of a patent airway, ventilatory assistance, oxygen administration, and circulatory access should complement or precede opioid antagonist use.
• Significant opioid depression occurring in the dental office may require relocation of the patient to a medical facility for comprehensive management.
• Patients discharged from the office or emergency facility should be carefully observed for the return of opioid-induced depression.

naloxone hydrochloride
nal-oks´-one high-droh-klor´-ide
(Narcan)
Do not confuse naltrexone or Narcan with Norcuron.

CATEGORY AND SCHEDULE
Pregnancy Risk Category: B

Drug Class: Narcotic antagonist

MECHANISM OF ACTION

A narcotic antagonist that displaces opioids at opioid-occupied receptor sites in the CNS. *Therapeutic Effect:* Reverses opioid-induced sleep or sedation, increases respiratory rate, raises B/P to normal range.

USES

Treatment of respiratory depression induced by narcotics, to reverse postoperative opioid depression

PHARMACOKINETICS

Route	Onset	Peak	Duration
IV	1–2 min	N/A	20–60 min
IM	2–5 min	N/A	20–60 min
Subcutaneous	2–5 min	N/A	20–60 min

Well absorbed after IM or subcutaneous administration. Metabolized in the liver. Primarily excreted in urine. *Half-life:* 1–1.7hr.

INDICATIONS AND DOSAGES
▶ **Opioid toxicity**
IV, IM, Subcutaneous
Adults, Elderly. 0.4–2 mg q2–3min as needed. May repeat q20–60min.
Children 5 yr and older and weighing 22 kg or more. 2 mg/dose; if no response, may repeat q2–3min. May need to repeat q20–60min.
Children younger than 5 yr and weighing less than 22 kg. 0.1 mg/kg; if no response, repeat q2–3min. May need to repeat q20–60min.
▶ **Postanesthesia Narcotic Reversal**
IV
Children. 0.01 mg/kg; may repeat q2–3min.
Neonatal Opioid-Induced Depression
IV
Neonates. May repeat q2–3min as needed. May need to repeat q1–2h.

SIDE EFFECTS/ADVERSE REACTIONS

None known; little or no pharmacologic effect in absence of narcotics

PRECAUTIONS AND CONTRAINDICATIONS

Respiratory depression due to nonopioid drugs
Caution
Opioid dependence

DRUG INTERACTIONS OF CONCERN TO DENTISTRY

• Antagonizes effects of opioid agonists
and mixed agonists/antagonists

SERIOUS REACTIONS

! Too-rapid reversal of narcotic-induced respiratory depression may result in nausea, vomiting, tremors, increased B/P, and tachycardia.
! Excessive dosage in postoperative patients may produce significant excitement, tremors, and reversal of analgesia.
! Patients with cardiovascular disease may experience hypotension or hypertension, ventricular tachycardia and fibrillation, and pulmonary edema.

DENTAL CONSIDERATIONS
General:
• This drug is intended for acute use only, but listed side effects can sometimes be seen.
• Risk of seizures reported in animal studies; be aware of this potential.
• Serious cardiovascular events have been associated with opioid reversal in postoperative patients; doses should be carefully titrated to reduce these events.
• Buprenorphine depression may not be completely reversed.

• In all cases, the establishment of a patent airway, ventilatory assistance, oxygen administration, and circulatory access should complement or precede opioid antagonist use.

• Significant opioid depression occurring in the dental office may require relocation of the patient to a medical facility for comprehensive management.

• Patients discharged from the office/emergency facility should be carefully observed for the return of opioid-induced depression.

naltrexone hydrochloride

nal-trex´-one high-droh-klor´-ide
(Revia)

CATEGORY AND SCHEDULE
Pregnancy Risk Category: C

Drug Class: Narcotic antagonist

MECHANISM OF ACTION
A narcotic antagonist that displaces opioids at opioid-occupied receptor sites in the CNS. ***Therapeutic Effect:*** Blocks physical effects of opioid analgesics; decreases craving for alcohol and relapse rate in alcoholism.

USES
Treatment of opioid addiction following detoxification, alcoholism

PHARMACOKINETICS
PO: Onset 15–30 min, peak 1–2 hr, duration is dose dependent. ***Half-life:*** 4 hr; extensive first-pass metabolism; metabolized by liver; excreted by kidneys; crosses placenta; excreted in breast milk.

INDICATIONS AND DOSAGES
▸ **Naloxone Challenge Test to Determine if Patient Is Opioid Dependent**
Alert
Expect to perform the naloxone challenge test if there is any question that the patient is opioid dependent. Don't administer naltrexone until the naloxone challenge test is negative.
IV
Adults, Elderly. Draw 2 ml (0.8 mg) of naloxone into syringe. Inject 0.5 ml (0.2 mg); while needle is still in vein, observe patient for 30 sec for withdrawal signs or symptoms. If no evidence of withdrawal, inject remaining 1.5 ml (0.6 mg); observe patient for additional 20 min for withdrawal signs or symptoms.
Subcutaneous
Adults, Elderly. Inject 2 ml (0.8 mg) of naloxone; observe patient for 45 min for withdrawal signs or symptoms.
▸ **Treatment of Opioid Dependence in Patients Who Have Been Opioid Free for at Least 7–10 Days**
PO
Adults, Elderly. Initially, 25 mg. Observe patient for 1 hr. If no withdrawal signs or symptoms appear, give another 25 mg. May be given as 100 mg every other day or 150 mg every 3 days.
▸ **Adjunctive Treatment of Alcohol Dependence**
PO
Adults, Elderly. 50 mg once a day.

SIDE EFFECTS/ADVERSE REACTIONS
Frequent
Alcoholism: Nausea, headache, depression
Narcotic addiction: Insomnia, anxiety, nervousness, headache, low energy, abdominal cramps, nausea, vomiting, arthralgia, myalgia

Occasional

Alcoholism: Dizziness, nervousness, fatigue, insomnia, vomiting, anxiety, suicidal ideation

Narcotic addiction: Irritability, increased energy, dizziness, anorexia, diarrhea or constipation, rash, chills, increased thirst

PRECAUTIONS AND CONTRAINDICATIONS

Acute hepatitis, acute opioid withdrawal, failed naloxone challenge test, hepatic failure, history of hypersensitivity to naltrexone, opioid dependence, positive urine screen for opioids

DRUG INTERACTIONS OF CONCERN TO DENTISTRY

• Decreased effects of opioid narcotics

SERIOUS REACTIONS

! Signs and symptoms of opioid withdrawal include stuffy or runny nose, tearing, yawning, diaphoresis, tremors, vomiting, piloerection, feeling of temperature change, bone pain, arthralgia, myalgia, abdominal cramps, and feeling of skin crawling.

! Accidental naltrexone overdose produces withdrawal symptoms within 5 min of ingestion that may last for up to 48 hr. Symptoms include confusion, visual hallucinations, somnolence, and significant vomiting and diarrhea.

! Hepatocellular injury may occur with large doses.

DENTAL CONSIDERATIONS

General:

• Monitor vital signs at every appointment because of cardiovascular and respiratory side effects.

• Patients on chronic drug therapy may rarely have symptoms of blood dyscrasias, which can include infection, bleeding, and poor healing.

• Patients should not be given opioid analgesics for dental pain management. Substitute with NSAID and long-acting local anesthetics.

• The dental professional must be aware of the patient's disease, and the patient must be active in treatment for chemical dependency.

Consultations:

• In patients with symptoms of blood dyscrasias, request a medical consultation for blood studies and postpone dental treatment until normal values are reestablished.

• Medical consultation may be required to assess disease control.

• Inform aftercare provider or counselor if sedative medications are required for proper management.

Teach Patient/Family to:

• Use effective oral hygiene to prevent soft tissue inflammation

• Use caution to prevent injury when using oral hygiene aids

naphazoline

naf-az´-oh-leen

(AK-Con, Albalon Liquifilm[AUS], Clear Eyes[AUS], Naphcon, Naphcon Forte[AUS], Privine, Vasocon)

CATEGORY AND SCHEDULE

Pregnancy Risk Category: C

Drug Class: Ophthalmic vasoconstrictor

MECHANISM OF ACTION

A sympathomimetic that directly acts on alpha-adrenergic receptors in conjunctival arterioles and nasal blood vessels. *Therapeutic Effect:* Causes vasoconstriction, resulting in decreased congestion.

USES

Relief of hyperemia, irritation in superficial corneal vascularity

PHARMACOKINETICS

Instillation: Duration 2–3 hr.

INDICATIONS AND DOSAGES

▶ **Nasal Congestion Due to Acute or Chronic Rhinitis, Common Cold, Hay Fever, or other Allergies**
Intranasal
Adults, Elderly, Children older than 12 yr. 1–2 drops or sprays in each nostril q3–6h.
Children 6–12 yr. 1 spray or drop in each nostril q6h as needed.
▶ **Control of Hyperemia in Patients with Superficial Corneal Vascularity; Relief of Congestion and Inflammation; for Use During Ocular Diagnostic Procedures**
Ophthalmic
Adults, Elderly, Children older than 6 yr. 1–2 drops in affected eye q3–4h for 3–4 days.

SIDE EFFECTS/ADVERSE REACTIONS

Occasional
Nasal: Burning, stinging, or drying of nasal mucosa; sneezing; rebound congestion
Ophthalmic: Blurred vision, dilated pupils, increased eye irritation

PRECAUTIONS AND CONTRAINDICATIONS

Angle-closure glaucoma, before peripheral iridectomy, patients with a narrow angle who do not have glaucoma
Caution
Hypertension, hyperthyroidism, elderly, severe arteriosclerosis, cardiac disease

DRUG INTERACTIONS OF CONCERN TO DENTISTRY

• Increased pressor effects: tricyclic antidepressants

SERIOUS REACTIONS

❗ If naphazoline is systemically absorbed, the patient may experience tachycardia, palpitations, headache, insomnia, light-headedness, nausea, nervousness, and tremors.
❗ Large doses may produce tachycardia, palpitations, light headedness, nausea, and vomiting.
❗ Overdose in patients older than 60 yr may produce hallucinations, CNS depression, and seizures.

DENTAL CONSIDERATIONS

General:
• Monitor vital signs at every appointment because of cardiovascular side effects.
• Avoid dental light in patient's eyes; offer dark glasses for patient comfort.

naproxen/naproxen sodium

na-prox´-en soe´-dee-um
naproxen:
(Crysanal[AUS], EC-Naprosyn,
Inza[AUS], Naprelan, Naprosyn)
naproxen sodium:
(Aleve, Anaprox, Anaprox DS,
Apo-Naprosyn[CAN],
Naprogesic[AUS], Novo-Naprox[CAN],
Nu-Naprox[CAN], Pamprin)
Do not confuse Aleve with Allese
or Anaprox with Anaspaz.

CATEGORY AND SCHEDULE

Pregnancy Risk Category: B
(D if used in third trimester or near
delivery)
OTC (220 mg gelcaps, 220 mg
tablets)

Drug Class: Nonsteroidal
antiinflammatory

MECHANISM OF ACTION

An NSAID that produces analgesic
and antiinflammatory effects by
inhibiting prostaglandin synthesis.
Therapeutic Effect: Reduces the
inflammatory response and intensity
of pain.

USES

Treatment of mild-to-moderate pain,
osteoarthritis, rheumatoid, juvenile,
gouty arthritis, ankylosing
spondylitis, primary dysmenorrhea;
unapproved: migraine, PMS, fever

PHARMACOKINETICS

Route	Onset	Peak	Duration
PO (analgesic)	Less than 1 hr	N/A	7 hr or less
PO (antirheu- matic)	Less than 14 days	2–4 wk	N/A

Completely absorbed from the GI
tract. Protein binding: 99%.
Metabolized in the liver. Primarily
excreted in urine. Not removed by
hemodialysis. *Half-life:* 13 hr.

INDICATIONS AND DOSAGES

▶ **Rheumatoid Arthritis,
Osteoarthritis, Ankylosing
Spondylitis**
PO
Adults, Elderly. 250–500 mg naproxen
(275–550 mg naproxen sodium) twice
a day or 250 mg naproxen (275 mg
naproxen sodium) in morning and
500 mg naproxen (550 mg naproxen
sodium) in evening. Naprelan:
750–1000 mg once a day.
▶ **Acute Gouty Arthritis**
PO
Adults, Elderly. Initially, 750 mg
naproxen (825 mg naproxen sodium),
then 250 mg naproxen (275 mg
naproxen sodium) q8h until attack
subsides. Naprelan: Initially,
1000–1500 mg, then 1000 mg
once a day until attack subsides.
▶ **Mild-to-Moderate Pain,
Dysmenorrhea, Bursitis, Tendinitis**
PO
Adults, Elderly. Initially, 500 mg
naproxen (550 mg naproxen sodium),
then 250 mg naparoxen (275 mg
naproxen sodium) q6–8h as needed.
Maximum: 1.25 g/day naproxen
(1.375 g/day naproxen sodium).
Naprelan: 1000 mg once a day.

N

▶ **Juvenile Rheumatoid Arthritis**
PO (naproxen only)
Children. 10–15 mg/kg/day in
2 divided doses. Maximum:
1000 mg/day.

SIDE EFFECTS/ADVERSE REACTIONS
Frequent
Nausea, constipation, abdominal
cramps or pain, heartburn, dizziness,
headache, somnolence, oral lichenoid
reaction
Occasional
Stomatitis, diarrhea, indigestion
Rare
Vomiting, confusion

PRECAUTIONS AND CONTRAINDICATIONS
Hypersensitivity to aspirin, naproxen,
or other NSAIDs
Caution
Lactation, children, bleeding
disorders, GI disorders, cardiac
disorders, hypersensitivity to other
antiinflammatory agents, elderly,
more than 2 alcohol drinks daily

DRUG INTERACTIONS OF CONCERN TO DENTISTRY
• GI ulceration, bleeding: aspirin,
alcohol, corticosteroids
• Nephrotoxicity: acetaminophen
(chronic use and high doses)
• Possible risk of decreased renal
function: cyclosporine
• Increased photosensitization:
tetracycline
• Increased plasma levels:
probenecid
• First-time users of SSRIs also
taking NSAIDs may have a higher
risk of GI side effects; until more
data are available, it may be
advisable to avoid use of NSAIDs in
these patients (Br J Clin Pharmacol
55:591–595, 2003)

• When prescribed for dental pain:
  • Risk of increased effects: oral
  anticoagulants, oral antidiabetics,
  thium, methotrexate
  • Decreased antihypertensive
  effects of diuretics, β-adrenergic
  blockers, and ACE inhibitors

SERIOUS REACTIONS
❗ Rare reactions with long-term use
include peptic ulcer disease,
GI bleeding, gastritis, severe hepatic
reactions (cholestasis, jaundice),
nephrotoxicity (dysuria, hematuria,
proteinuria, nephrotic syndrome),
and a severe hypersensitivity reaction
(fever, chills, bronchospasm).

DENTAL CONSIDERATIONS
General:
• Possible increased adverse
cardiovascular events in patients at
risk for thromboembolism
• Patients on chronic drug therapy
may rarely have symptoms of blood
dyscrasias, which can include
infection, bleeding, and poor healing.
• Assess salivary flow as a factor in
caries, periodontal disease, and
candidiasis.
• Avoid prescribing for dental use in
last trimester of pregnancy.
• Avoid prescribing aspirin-
containing products.
• Consider semisupine chair
position for patients with arthritic
disease.
Consultations:
• Inpatient swith symptoms of blood
dyscrasias, request a medical
consultation for blood studies and
postpone dental treatment until
normal values are reestablished.
• Medical consultation may be
required to assess disease control.
Teach Patient/Family to:
• Use effective oral hygiene to
prevent soft tissue inflammation

- Use caution to prevent injury when using oral hygiene aids
- When chronic dry mouth occurs, advise patient to:
  - Avoid mouth rinses with high alcohol content because of drying effects
  - Use daily home fluoride products for anticaries effect
  - Use sugarless gum, frequent sips of water, or saliva substitutes

naratriptan
nare-ah-trip´-tan
(Amerge, Naramig[AUS])
Do not confuse Amerge with Amaryl.

CATEGORY AND SCHEDULE
Pregnancy Risk Category: C

Drug Class: Serotonin agonist

MECHANISM OF ACTION
A serotonin receptor agonist that binds selectively to vascular receptors, producing a vasoconstrictive effect on cranial blood vessels. *Therapeutic Effect:* Relieves migraine headache.

USES
Acute treatment of migraine attacks with or without aura in adults

PHARMACOKINETICS
Well absorbed after PO administration. Protein binding: 28%–31%. Metabolized by the liver to inactive metabolite. Eliminated primarily in urine and, to a lesser extent, in feces. *Half-life:* 6 hr (increased in hepatic or renal impairment).

INDICATIONS AND DOSAGES
▸ **Acute Migraine Attack**
PO
Adults. 1 mg or 2.5 mg. If headache improves but then returns, dose may be repeated after 4 hr. Maximum: 5 mg/24 hr.
▸ **Dosage in Mild-to-Moderate Hepatic or Renal Impairment**
A lower starting dose is recommended. Do not exceed 2.5 mg/24 hr.

SIDE EFFECTS/ADVERSE REACTIONS
Occasional
Nausea
Rare
Paresthesia; dizziness; fatigue; somnolence; jaw, neck, or throat pressure

PRECAUTIONS AND CONTRAINDICATIONS
Basilar or hemiplegic migraine, cerebrovascular or peripheral vascular disease, coronary artery disease, ischemic heart disease (including angina pectoris, history of MI, silent ischemia, and Prinzmetal's angina), severe hepatic impairment (Child-Pugh grade C), severe renal impairment (serum creatinine less than 15 ml/min), uncontrolled hypertension, use within 24 hr of ergotamine-containing preparations or another serotonin receptor agonist, use within 14 days of MAOIs
Caution
Risk of serious cardiovascular events, including ischemia and MI; renal/hepatic dysfunction, SSRI antidepressants, lactation, use in children not established, not recommended in elderly

DRUG INTERACTIONS OF CONCERN TO DENTISTRY
- No specific interactions with dental drugs reported

• Should not be used within 24 hr of another 5-HT1 agonist

SERIOUS REACTIONS

❗ Corneal opacities and other ocular defects may occur.
❗ Cardiac reactions (including ischemia, coronary artery vasospasm, and MI) and noncardiac vasospasm-related reactions (such as hemorrhage and CVA), occur rarely, particularly in patients with hypertension, diabetes, or a strong family history of coronary artery disease; obese patients; smokers; males older than 40 yr; and postmenopausal women.

DENTAL CONSIDERATIONS

General:
• This is an acute-use drug; it is doubtful that patients will come to the office if acute migraine is present.
• Be aware of patient's disease, its severity, and its frequency when known.
Consultations:
• If treating chronic orofacial pain, consult with physician of record.
• Medical consultation may be required to assess disease control and patient's ability to tolerate stress.
Teach Patient/Family to:
• Update health and drug history if physician makes any changes in evaluation or drug regimens; include OTC, herbal, and nonherbal drugs in update
• Avoid mouth rinses with high alcohol content because of additional drying effects.

nateglinide
na-teg′-lin-ide
(Starlix)

CATEGORY AND SCHEDULE
Pregnancy Risk Category: C

Drug Class: Oral antidiabetic, meglitinide class

MECHANISM OF ACTION
An antihyperglycemic that stimulates release of insulin from β cells of the pancreas by depolarizing β cells, leading to an opening of calcium channels. Resulting calcium influx induces insulin secretion.
Therapeutic Effect: Lowers blood glucose concentration.

USES
Treatment of Type 2 diabetes mellitus when hyperglycemia cannot be controlled by diet and exercise, can be used in combination with metformin, not for patients who have been chronically treated with other antidiabetic drugs

PHARMACOKINETICS
PO: Rapid absorption, peak plasma levels 1 hr, bioavailability 73%, plasma protein binding 98%, hepatic metabolism (CYP450 2C9 isoenzyme [70%] and CYP450 3A4 isoenzyme [30%]); excretion renal (83%), feces (10%).

INDICATIONS AND DOSAGES
▸ **Diabetes Mellitus**
PO
Adult, Elderly. 120 mg 3 times a day before meals. Initially, 60 mg may be given.

SIDE EFFECTS/ADVERSE REACTIONS

Frequent

Upper respiratory tract infection

Occasional

Back pain, flu symptoms, dizziness, arthropathy, diarrhea

Rare

Bronchitis, cough

PRECAUTIONS AND CONTRAINDICATIONS

Diabetic ketoacidosis, type 1 diabetes mellitus

Caution

Hypoglycemia (geriatric, malnourished, adrenal insufficiency or pituitary insufficiency more susceptible to hypoglycemia), β-blocker may mask hypoglycemia, administer before meals, infection, hepatic dysfunction, lactation, children

DRUG INTERACTIONS OF CONCERN TO DENTISTRY

• Most drug interactions not clearly identified; may act as an inhibitor of CYP450 2C9 enzymes but not CYP450 3A4. Does not appear to interact with highly protein-bound drugs

• Potential potentiation of hypoglycemic effects: NSAIDs, salicylates, nonselective β-blockers

SERIOUS REACTIONS

! Hypoglycemia occurs in less than 2% of patients.

DENTAL CONSIDERATIONS

General:

• If dentist prescribes any of the drugs listed in the drug interaction section, monitor patient's blood sugar levels.

• Consider semisupine chair position for patient comfort if GI side effects occur.

• Ensure that patient is following prescribed diet and regularly takes medication.

• Place on frequent recall to evaluate healing response.

• Short appointments and a stress-reduction protocol may be required.

• Diabetics may be more susceptible to infection and have delayed wound healing.

Consultations:

• Medical consultation may include data from patient's blood glucose monitoring, including glycosylated hemoglobin or HbA_{1c} testing.

• Medical consultation may be required to assess disease control and patient's ability to tolerate stress.

Teach Patient/Family to:

• Prevent trauma when using oral hygiene aids

• Update health and drug history if physician makes any changes in evaluation or drug regimens

nedocromil sodium

ned-oh-crow´-mil soe´-dee-um
(Alocril, Mireze[CAN], Tilade, Tilade CFC Free[AUS])

CATEGORY AND SCHEDULE

Pregnancy Risk Category: B

Drug Class: Antiasthmatic, mast cell stabilizer

MECHANISM OF ACTION

A mast cell stabilizer that prevents the activation and release of inflammatory mediators, such as histamine, leukotrienes, mast cells, eosinophils, and monocytes.

Therapeutic Effect: Prevents both early and late asthmatic responses.

USES
Maintenance therapy in mild-to-moderate asthma; ophthalmic solution for allergic conjunctivitis

PHARMACOKINETICS
Inhalation: Peak 15 min, duration 4–6 hr. *Half-life:* 80 min; excreted unchanged in feces.

INDICATIONS AND DOSAGES
▶ **Mild-to-Moderate Asthma**
Oral Inhalation
Adults, Elderly, Children 6 yr and older. 2 inhalations 4 times a day. May decrease to 3 times a day then twice a day as asthma becomes controlled.
▶ **Allergic Conjunctivitis**
Ophthalmic
Adults, Elderly, Children 3 yr and older. 1–2 drops in each eye twice a day.

SIDE EFFECTS/ADVERSE REACTIONS
Frequent
Cough, pharyngitis, bronchospasm, headache, altered taste
Occasional
Rhinitis, upper respiratory tract infection, abdominal pain, fatigue
Rare
Diarrhea, dizziness

PRECAUTIONS AND CONTRAINDICATIONS
Hypersensitivity to this drug or lactose, status asthmaticus
Caution
Lactation, renal disease, hepatic disease, safety and efficacy of inhalation in children younger than 6 yr or ophthalmic solution in children younger than 3 yr not established

DRUG INTERACTIONS OF CONCERN TO DENTISTRY
None reported

SERIOUS REACTIONS
None known

DENTAL CONSIDERATIONS

Nedocromil Sodium (Alocril)
General:
• Determine why patient is taking the drug.
• Avoid dental light in patient's eyes; offer dark glasses for patient comfort.
• Users may report unpleasant taste while using this product.

Nedocromil Sodium
General:
• Assess salivary flow as a factor in caries, periodontal disease, and candidiasis.
• Consider semisupine chair position for patients with respiratory disease.
• Short appointments and a stress reduction protocol may be required for anxious patients.
• Be aware that aspirin or sulfite preservatives in vasoconstrictor-containing products can exacerbate asthma.
Consultations:
• Medical consultation may be required to assess disease control.
Teach Patient/Family to:
• Avoid mouth rinses with high alcohol content because of drying effects
• Rinse mouth with water after each inhaled dose to prevent dryness

nefazodone hydrochloride
neh-faz´-oh-doan
high-droh-klor´-ide

CATEGORY AND SCHEDULE
Pregnancy Risk Category: C

Drug Class: Antidepressant

MECHANISM OF ACTION
Exact mechanism is unknown. Appears to inhibit neuronal uptake of serotonin and norepinephrine and to antagonize α_1-adrenergic receptors. *Therapeutic Effect:* Relieves depression.

USES
Treatment of major depressive disorders

PHARMACOKINETICS
Rapidly and completely absorbed from the GI tract; food delays absorption. Protein binding: 99%. Widely distributed in body tissues, including CNS. Extensively metabolized to active metabolites. Excreted in urine and eliminated in feces. Unknown if removed by hemodialysis. *Half-life:* 2–4 hr.

INDICATIONS AND DOSAGES
▶ **Depression, Prevention of Relapse of Acute Depressive Episode**
PO
Adults. Initially, 200 mg/day in 2 divided doses. Gradually increase by 100–200 mg/day at intervals of at least 1 wk. Range: 300–600 mg/day.
Elderly. Initially, 100 mg/day in 2 divided doses. Subsequent dosage titration based on clinical response. Range: 200–400 mg/day.

Children. 300–400 mg/day.

SIDE EFFECTS/ADVERSE REACTIONS
Frequent
Headache, dry mouth, somnolence, nausea, dizziness, constipation, insomnia, asthenia, light-headedness
Occasional
Dyspepsia, blurred vision, diarrhea, infection, confusion, abnormal vision, pharyngitis, increased appetite, orthostatic hypotension, flushing, feeling of warmth, peripheral edema, cough, flulike symptoms

PRECAUTIONS AND CONTRAINDICATIONS
Use within 14 days of MAOIs.
Caution
Mania, hypomania, suicidal tendencies, seizures, history of MI or unstable heart conditions, hepatic impairment, lactation, children younger than 18 yr, elderly (requires dose adjustment), priapism history, alcohol use; risk in operating auto or hazardous machinery

DRUG INTERACTIONS OF CONCERN TO DENTISTRY
• Must not be used concurrently with or within 14 days of discontinuing MAOI
• Risk of significant adverse drug interaction with triazolam, alprazolam, alcohol-containing products
• Increased sedation: St. John's wort (herb)
• Acts as an inhibitor of CYP3A4 isoenzymes: risk of interaction with drugs metabolized by CYP3A4

SERIOUS REACTIONS

! Serious reactions, such as hyperthermia, rigidity, myoclonus, extreme agitation, delirium, and coma, will occur if the patient takes an MAOI concurrently or fails to let enough time elapse when switching from an MAOI to nefazodone or vice versa.

DENTAL CONSIDERATIONS

General:
• Assess salivary flow as a factor in caries, periodontal disease, and candidiasis.
• Take vital signs at every appointment because of cardiovascular side effects.
• After supine positioning, have patient sit upright for at least 2 min before standing to avoid postural hypotension.
• There is no information concerning the use of vasoconstrictors in patients taking this drug.
• Advise patient if dental drugs prescribed have a potential for photosensitivity.
Consultations:
• Medical consultation may be required to assess disease control.
• Physician should be informed if significant xerostomic side effects occur (e.g., increased caries, sore tongue, problems eating or swallowing, difficulty wearing prosthesis) so that a medication change can be considered.
• Because there is no experience with the use of conscious sedation or general anesthesia in patients taking this drug, a medical consultation is recommended for risk evaluation.
• Patients showing anorexia, jaundice, GI complaints, or malaise

should be referred for medical evaluation before treatment.
Teach Patient/Family:
• When chronic dry mouth occurs, advise patient to:
  • Avoid mouth rinses with high alcohol content because of drying effects
  • Use daily home fluoride products for anticaries effect
  • Use sugarless gum, frequent sips of water, or saliva substitutes

nelarabine

nel-ay′-reh-been
(Arranon)

CATEGORY AND SCHEDULE

Pregnancy Risk Category: D

Drug Class: Antineoplastic

MECHANISM OF ACTION

A prodrug of deoxyguanosine analogue 9-β-D-arabinofuranosylguanine (ara-G) that disrupts DNA synthesis. *Therapeutic Effect:* Induces cellular apoptosis.

USES

Treatment of relapsed or refractory T-cell acute lymphoblastic leukemia (ALL) and T-cell lymphoblastic lymphoma

PHARMACOKINETICS

Protein binding: less than 25%. Metabolized in liver to ara-G (active); also hydrolyzed to methylguanine. Excreted in urine. *Half-life:* 30 min (nelarabine); 3 hr (ara-G).

INDICATIONS AND DOSAGES

▶ **T-cell ALL (relapsed or refractory)**
IV
Adults. 1,500 mg/m² delivered as a
2-hr infusion on days 1, 3, and 5 of a
21-day treatment cycle. Treatment
cycles should be repeated until
evidence of disease progression is
observed.
Children. 650 mg/m² delivered as a
1-hr infusion daily for days 1–5 of a
21-day treatment cycle. Treatment
cycles should be repeated until
evidence of disease progression is
observed.

▶ **T-cell lymphoblastic lymphoma
(relapsed or refractory)**
IV
Adults. 1500 mg/m² delivered as a
2-hr infusion on days 1, 3, and 5 of a
21-day treatment cycle. Treatment
cycles should be repeated until
evidence of disease progression is
observed.
Children. 650 mg/m² delivered as a
1-hr infusion daily for days 1–5 of a
21-day treatment cycle. Treatment
cycles should be repeated until
evidence of disease progression is
observed.

SIDE EFFECTS/ADVERSE REACTIONS:

Frequent
Anemia, neutropenia,
thrombocytopenia, fatigue, nausea,
leukopenia, cough, fever, diarrhea,
vomiting, somnolence, dizziness,
constipation, peripheral neuropathy,
dyspnea, headache, hypoesthesia,
weakness, peripheral edema, febrile
neutropenia, hypokalemia, petechiae,
edema, pain, albumin decreased,
bilirubin increased, pleural effusion

Occasional
Abdominal pain, anorexia,
arthralgia, infection, ataxia, back
pain, muscle weakness, rigors,
stomatitis, hypotension, tachycardia,
hypocalcemia, confusion, epistaxis,
pneumonia, sinusitis, insomnia,
dehydration, limb pain, abnormal
gait, depressed level of
consciousness, hypomagnesemia,
depression, seizure,
hyper-/hypoglycemia, abdominal
distension, AST increased,
creatinine increased, noncardiac
chest pain, wheezing, chest pain,
tremor, blurred vision, motor
dysfunction, taste perversion,
amnesia, balance disorder, nerve
paralysis, sensory loss

Rare
Aphasia, cerebral hemorrhage, coma,
encephalopathy, hemiparesis,
hydrocephalus, lethargy,
leukoencephalopathy, loss of
consciousness, mental impairment,
neuropathic pain, nerve palsy,
nystagmus, paralysis, sciatica,
sensory disturbance, speech disorder,
demyelination, ascending peripheral
neuropathy, dysarthria, hyporeflexia,
hypertonia, incoordination, sinus
headache (1%)

PRECAUTIONS AND CONTRAINDICATIONS

Hypersensitivity to nelarabine or its
components
Caution
Do not breast-feed, compromised
bone marrow reserve, chickenpox,
herpes zoster, history of gout,
infection

N

DRUG INTERACTIONS OF CONCERN TO DENTISTRY
None reported

SERIOUS REACTIONS
❗ Severe neurologic events have been reported with the use of nelarabine including altered mental states, severe somnolence, convulsions, peripheral neuropathy ranging from numbness and paresthesias to motor weakness and paralysis.
❗ Demyelination and ascending peripheral neuropathies similar in appearance to Guillain-Barré syndrome have been reported.
❗ Leukopenia, anemia, neutropenia, and thrombocytopenia have been associated with nelarabine therapy.

DENTAL CONSIDERATIONS
General
● Monitor vital signs at every appointment because of cardiovascular and respiratory adverse effects
● Avoid aspirin and NSAIDs to prevent gastrointestinal irritation and excessive bleeding
● Examine patient carefully for oral manifestations of opportunistic infections, blood dyscrasias, and stomatitis and mucositis
● Confirm patient's disease status and treatment regimen
● Chlorhexidine mouthrinse prior to and during chemotherapy may reduce severity of mucositis
● Palliative medication may be required for management of oral adverse effects of drug
● Patient may be taking prophylactic antiinfective drug
● Place patient on frequent recall due to adverse oral effects of drug

Consultations:
● Consult physician to determine control of disease and ability of patient to tolerate dental procedures
● Consult physician to determine need for prophylactic or therapeutic antiinfective medications if oral surgery or periodontal treatment is required
● Consult physician to determine assess patient's immunologic and coagulation status and determine safety risk, if any, posed by the required dental treatment
Teach Patient/Family to:
● Be aware of oral adverse effects of drug
● Use atraumatic, effective oral hygiene measures to prevent or minimize soft tissue inflammation
● Report oral lesions, soreness, or bleeding to dentist
● Update health and medication history if physician makes any changes in evaluation or drug regimen; include OTC, herbal, and nonherbal drug in update

nelfinavir
nel-fin´-eh-veer
(Viracept)

CATEGORY AND SCHEDULE
Pregnancy Risk Category: B

Drug Class: Antiviral

MECHANISM OF ACTION
Inhibits the activity of HIV-1 protease, the enzyme necessary for the formation of infectious HIV.
Therapeutic Effect: Formation of immature noninfectious viral particles rather than HIV replication.

USES
Treatment of HIV infection when indicated by surrogate marker changes in patients receiving nelfinavir in combination with nucleoside analogues or alone for up to 24 wk

PHARMACOKINETICS
Well absorbed after PO administration (absorption increased with food). Protein binding: 98%. Metabolized in the liver. Highly bound to plasma proteins. Eliminated primarily in feces. Unknown if removed by hemodialysis.
Half-life: 3.5–5 hr.

INDICATIONS AND DOSAGES
▸ **HIV Infection**
PO
Adults. 750 mg (three 250-mg tablets) 3 times a day or 1250 mg twice a day in combination with nucleoside analogs (enhances antiviral activity).
Children 2–13 yr. 0–30 mg/kg/dose 3 times a day. Maximum: 750 mg q8h.

SIDE EFFECTS/ADVERSE REACTIONS
Frequent
Diarrhea
Occasional
Nausea, rash
Rare
Flatulence, asthenia

PRECAUTIONS AND CONTRAINDICATIONS
Concurrent administration with midazolam, rifampin, or triazolam
Caution
Pediatric use, phenylketonuria (powder contains phenylalanine), diabetes mellitus, hyperglycemia, hepatic impairment, development of resistance, hemophilia, lactation, children younger than 2 yr, an inhibitor of CYP3A4 isoenzymes; use with caution with drugs that are inducers of CYP3A4 or CYP2C19 isoenzymes

DRUG INTERACTIONS OF CONCERN TO DENTISTRY
• Contraindicated with triazolam, midazolam, and other drugs dependent on CYP3A4 for metabolism
• Increased plasma levels: azithromycin, ketoconazole
• Increased plasma concentrations of fentanyl

SERIOUS REACTIONS
None known

DENTAL CONSIDERATIONS
General:
• Examine for oral manifestation of opportunistic infection.
• Patients on chronic drug therapy may rarely have symptoms of blood dyscrasias, which can include infection, bleeding, and poor healing.
• Palliative medication may be required for management of oral side effects.
Consultations:
• In a patient with symptoms of blood dyscrasias, request a medical consultation for blood studies and postpone treatment until normal values are reestablished.
• Medical consultation may be required to assess disease control.
Teach Patient/Family to:
• Use effective oral hygiene to prevent soft tissue inflammation
• Use caution to prevent trauma when using oral hygiene aids
• Update health and drug history if physician makes any changes in evaluation or drug regimens; include

N

OTC, herbal, and nonherbal drugs in the update
• See dentist immediately if secondary oral infection occurs

neostigmine
nee-oh-stig´-meen
(Prostigmin)
Do not confuse neostigmine with physostigmine.

CATEGORY AND SCHEDULE
Pregnancy Risk Category: C

Drug Class: Cholinesterase inhibitor

MECHANISM OF ACTION
A cholinergic that prevents destruction of acetylcholine by inhibiting the enzyme acetylcholinesterase, thus enhancing impulse transmission across the myoneural junction. *Therapeutic Effect:* Improves intestinal and skeletal muscle tone; stimulates salivary and sweat gland secretions.

USES
Myasthenia gravis, nondepolarizing neuromuscular blocker, antagonist, bladder distention, postoperative ileus

PHARMACOKINETICS
PO: Onset 45–75 min, duration 2.5–4 hr.
IM/Subcutaneous: Onset 10–30 min, duration 2.5–4 hr.
IV: Onset 4–8 min, duration 2–4 hr Metabolized in liver, excreted in urine.

INDICATIONS AND DOSAGES
▶ **Myasthenia Gravis**
PO
Adults, Elderly. Initially, 15–30 mg 3–4 times a day. Increase as necessary. Maintenance: 150 mg/day (range of 15–375 mg).
Children. 2 mg/kg/day or 60 mg/m^2/day divided q3–4h.
IV, IM, Subcutaneous
Adults. 0.5–2.5 mg as needed.
Children. 0.01–0.04 mg/kg q2–4h.
▶ **Diagnosis of Myasthenia Gravis**
IM
Adults, Elderly. 0.022 mg/kg.
If cholinergic reaction occurs, discontinue tests and administer 0.4–0.6 mg or more atropine sulfate IV.
Children. 0.025–0.04 mg/kg preceded by atropine sulfate 0.011 mg/kg subcutaneously.
▶ **Prevention of Postoperative Urinary Retention**
IM, Subcutaneous
Adults, Elderly. 0.25 mg q4–6h for 2–3 days.
▶ **Postoperative Abdomonial Distention and Urine Retention**
IM, Subcutaneous
Adults, Elderly. 0.5–1 mg. Catheterize patient if voiding does not occur within 1 hr. After voiding, administer 0.5 mg q3h for 5 injections.
▶ **Reversal of Neuromuscular Blockade**
IV
Adults, Elderly. 0.5–2.5 mg given slowly.
Children. 0.025–0.08 mg/kg/dose.
Infants. 0.025–0.1 mg/kg/dose.

SIDE EFFECTS/ADVERSE REACTIONS
Frequent
Muscarinic effects (diarrhea, diaphoresis, increased salivation,

nausea, vomiting, abdominal cramps or pain)
Occasional
Muscarinic effects (urinary urgency or frequency, increased bronchial secretions, miosis, lacrimation)

PRECAUTIONS AND CONTRAINDICATIONS

GI or GU obstruction, peritonitis
Caution
Bradycardia, hypotension, seizure disorders, bronchial asthma, coronary occlusion, hyperthyroidism, dysrhythmias, peptic ulcer, megacolon, poor GI motility, lactation, children

DRUG INTERACTIONS OF CONCERN TO DENTISTRY

• Decreased action: hydrocarbon inhalation anesthetics, corticosteroids
• Decreased action of anticholinergics (may be contraindicated)
• Increased action of succinylcholine
• Increased toxicity of ester-type local anesthetics

SERIOUS REACTIONS

! Overdose produces a cholinergic crisis manifested as abdominal discomfort or cramps, nausea, vomiting, diarrhea, flushing, facial warmth, excessive salivation, diaphoresis, lacrimation, pallor, bradycardia or tachycardia, hypotension, bronchospasm, urinary urgency, blurred vision, miosis, and fasciculation (involuntary muscular contractions visible under the skin).

DENTAL CONSIDERATIONS

General:
• Monitor vital signs at every appointment because of cardiovascular and respiratory side effects.

• Early-morning and brief appointments are preferred because of effects of disease on oral musculature.
Consultations:
• Take precautions if dental surgery is anticipated and anesthesia is required.
• Medical consultation may be required to assess disease control and patient's tolerance for stress.

nesiritide

neh-sir´-ih-tide
(Natrecor)

CATEGORY AND SCHEDULE
Pregnancy Risk Category: C

Drug Class: Brain natriuretic peptide; endogenous hormone

MECHANISM OF ACTION

A brain natriuretic peptide that facilitates cardiovascular homeostasis and fluid status through counter regulation of the renin-angiotensin-aldosterone system, stimulating cyclic guanosine monophosphate, thereby leading to smooth-muscle cell relaxation. ***Therapeutic Effect:*** Promotes vasodilation, natriuresis, and diuresis, correcting CHF.

USES

Treatment of acutely decompensated CHF in patients who have dyspnea at rest or with minimal activity

PHARMACOKINETICS

Route	Onset	Peak	Duration
IV	15–30 min	1–2 hr	4 hr

N

Excreted primarily in the heart by the left ventricle. Metabolized by the natriuretic neutral endopeptidase enzymes on the vascular luminal surface. *Half-life:* 18–23 min.

INDICATIONS AND DOSAGES
▶ **Treatment of Acutely Decompensated CHF in Patients with Dyspnea at Rest or with Minimal Activity**
IV Bolus
Adults, Elderly. 2 mcg/kg followed by a continuous IV infusion of 0.01 mcg/kg/min. May be incrementally increased q3h to a maximum of 0.03 mcg/kg/min.

SIDE EFFECTS/ADVERSE REACTIONS
Frequent
Hypotension
Occasional
Headache, nausea, bradycardia
Rare
Confusion, paresthesia, somnolence, tremors

PRECAUTIONS AND CONTRAINDICATIONS
Cardiogenic shock, systolic B/P less than 90 mm Hg

DRUG INTERACTIONS OF CONCERN TO DENTISTRY
None reported

SERIOUS REACTIONS
! Ventricular arrhythmias, including ventricular tachycardia, atrial fibrillation, AV node conduction abnormalities, and angina pectoris occur rarely.

DENTAL CONSIDERATIONS
General:
• Acute-use drug for use in hospitals or emergency rooms.

• Review patient's medical and drug history.
• Only palliative dental care may be possible.
Consultations:
• Medical consultation may be required to assess disease control and patient's ability to tolerate stress.

---

nevirapine
neh-veer´-ah-peen
(Viramune)

CATEGORY AND SCHEDULE
Pregnancy Risk Category: C

Drug Class: Antiviral

MECHANISM OF ACTION
A nonnucleoside reverse transcriptase inhibitor that binds directly to HIV-1 reverse transcriptase, thus changing the shape of this enzyme and blocking RNA- and DNA-dependent polymerase activity.
Therapeutic Effect: Interferes with HIV replication, slowing the progression of HIV infection.

USES
Treatment in combination with nucleoside analogs for HIV-1 infection in adults who have demonstrated clinical or immunologic deterioration

PHARMACOKINETICS
Readily absorbed after PO administration. Protein binding: 60%. Widely distributed. Extensively metabolized in the liver. Excreted primarily in urine. *Half-life:* 45 hr (single dose), 25–30 hr (multiple doses).

INDICATIONS AND DOSAGES
▶ **HIV Infection**
PO
Adults. 200 mg once a day for
14 days (to reduce the risk of rash).
Maintenance: 200 mg twice a day in
combination with nucleoside
analogs.
Children older than 8 yr. 4 mg/kg
once a day for 14 days; then 4 mg/kg
twice a day. Maximum: 400 mg/day.
Children 2 mo–8 yr. 4 mg/kg once a
day for 14 days; then 7 mg/kg twice
a day.

SIDE EFFECTS/ADVERSE REACTIONS
Frequent
Rash, fever, headache, nausea,
granulocytopenia (more common in
children)
Occasional
Stomatitis (burning, erythema, or
ulceration of the oral mucosa;
dysphagia)
Rare
Paresthesia, myalgia, abdominal pain

PRECAUTIONS AND CONTRAINDICATIONS
Hypersensitivity, protease inhibitors
Caution
Severe life-threatening skin reactions
(Stevens-Johnson syndrome), fatal
hepatotoxicity has occurred, renal
dysfunction, lactation, children

DRUG INTERACTIONS OF CONCERN TO DENTISTRY
• Should not be given with
ketoconazole; monitor patients when
other CYP3A4 isoenzyme inhibitors
are used

SERIOUS REACTIONS
! Hepatitis and rash may become
severe and life threatening.

DENTAL CONSIDERATIONS
General:
• Determine why patient is taking
the drug.
• Examine for oral manifestation of
opportunistic infection.
Consultations:
• Medical consultation may be
required to assess disease control.
Teach Patient/Family to:
• Use effective oral hygiene to
prevent soft tissue inflammation
• Report oral lesions, soreness, or
bleeding to dentist
• Update health history/drug record
if physician makes any changes in
evaluation or drug regimens; include
OTC, herbal, and nonherbal drugs in
the update
• See dentist immediately if
secondary oral infection occurs

niacin, nicotinic acid
nye´-ah-sin, nih-koh´-tin-ik ass´-id
(Niacor, Niaspan, Nicotinex,
Slo-Niacin)
Do not confuse niacin, niacor, or
niaspan with minocin or nitro-bid.

CATEGORY AND SCHEDULE
Pregnancy Risk Category:
A (C if used at dosages above the
recommended daily allowance)
OTC

Drug Class: Vitamin B$_3$

MECHANISM OF ACTION
An antihyperlipidemic, water-soluble
vitamin that is a component of 2
coenzymes needed for tissue
respiration, lipid metabolism, and
glycogenolysis. Inhibits synthesis of
very low-density lipoproteins
(VLDLs). *Therapeutic Effect:*
Reduces total, low-density

lipoproteins (LDL), and VLDL
cholesterol levels and triglyceride
levels; increases high-density
lipoprotein (HDL) cholesterol
concentration.

USES

Treatment of pellagra,
hyperlipidemias (niacin), peripheral
vascular disease (niacin)

PHARMACOKINETICS

Readily absorbed from the GI tract.
Widely distributed. Metabolized in
the liver. Primarily excreted in urine.
Half-life: 45 min.

INDICATIONS AND DOSAGES

▶ **Hyperlipidemia**
PO (Immediate-Release)
Adults, Elderly. Initially, 50–100 mg
twice a day for 7 days. Increase
gradually by doubling dose every wk
up to 1–1.5 g/day in 2–3 doses.
Maximum: 3 g/day.
Children. Initially, 100–250 mg/day
(maximum: 10 mg/kg/day) in 3
divided doses. May increase by
100 mg/wk or 250 mg q2–3wk.
Maximum: 2250 mg/day.
PO (Timed-Release)
Adults, Elderly. Initially, 500 mg/day
in 2 divided doses for 1 wk; then
increase to 500 mg twice a day.
Maintenance: 2 g/day.

▶ **Nutritional Supplement**
PO
Adults, Elderly. 10–20 mg/day.
Maximum: 100 mg/day.

▶ **Pellegra**
PO
Adults, Elderly. 50–100 mg
3–4 times a day. Maximum:
500 mg/day.
Children. 50–100 mg 3 times a day.

SIDE EFFECTS/ADVERSE REACTIONS

Frequent
Flushing (especially of the face and
neck) occurring within 20 min of
drug administration and lasting for
30–60 min, GI upset, pruritus
Occasional
Dizziness, hypotension, headache,
blurred vision, burning or tingling of
skin, flatulence, nausea, vomiting,
diarrhea
Rare
Hyperglycemia, glycosuria, rash,
hyperpigmentation, dry skin

PRECAUTIONS AND CONTRAINDICATIONS

Active peptic ulcer disease, arterial
hemorrhaging, hepatic dysfunction,
hypersensitivity to niacin or
tartrazine (frequently seen in patients
sensitive to aspirin), severe
hypotension.
Caution
Glaucoma, cardiovascular disease,
CAD, diabetes mellitus, gout,
schizophrenia

DRUG INTERACTIONS OF CONCERN TO DENTISTRY

None reported

SERIOUS REACTIONS

! Arrhythmias occur rarely.

DENTAL CONSIDERATIONS

General:
• Take vital signs at every
appointment because of
cardiovascular side effects.
• After supine positioning, have
patient sit upright for at least 2 min
before standing to avoid postural
hypotension.
• Assess salivary flow as a factor in
caries, periodontal disease, and
candidiasis.

Teach Patient/Family:
• When chronic dry mouth occurs, advise patient to:
  • Avoid mouth rinses with high alcohol content because of drying effects
  • Use daily home fluoride products for anticaries effect
  • Use sugarless gum, frequent sips of water, or saliva substitutes

nicardipine hydrochloride

nye-card´-ih-peen
high-droh-klor´-ide
(Cardene, Cardene IV, Cardene SR)
Do not confuse nicardipine with nifedipine, cardene with codeine, or cardene SR with cardizem SR or codeine.

CATEGORY AND SCHEDULE
Pregnancy Risk Category: C

Drug Class: Calcium channel blocker

MECHANISM OF ACTION
An antianginal and antihypertensive agent that inhibits calcium ion movement across cell membranes, depressing contraction of cardiac and vascular smooth muscle.
Therapeutic Effect: Increases heart rate and cardiac output. Decreases systemic vascular resistance and B/P.

USES
Treatment of chronic stable angina pectoris, hypertension

PHARMACOKINETICS

Route	Onset	Peak	Duration
PO	N/A	1–2 hr	8 hr

Rapidly, completely absorbed from the GI tract. Protein binding: 95%. Undergoes first-pass metabolism in the liver. Primarily excreted in urine. Not removed by hemodialysis.
Half-life: 2–4 hr.

INDICATIONS AND DOSAGES
▶ **Chronic Stable (Effort-Associated) Angina**
PO
Adults, Elderly. Initially, 20 mg 3 times a day. Range: 20–40 mg 3 times a day.
▶ **Essential Hypertension**
PO
Adults, Elderly. Initially, 20 mg 3 times a day. Range: 20–40 mg 3 times a day.
PO (Sustained-Release)
Adults, Elderly. Initially, 30 mg twice a day. Range: 30–60 mg twice a day.
▶ **Short-term Treatment of Hypertension When Oral Therapy Is not Feasible or Desirable (substitute for oral nicardipine)**
IV
Adults, Elderly. 0.5 mg/hr (for patient receiving 20 mg PO q8h); 1.2 mg/hr (for patient receiving 30 mg PO q8h); 2.2 mg/hr (for patient receiving 40 mg PO q8h).
▶ **Patients not Already Receiving Nicardipine**
IV
Adults, Elderly (gradual B/P decrease). Initially, 5 mg/hr. May increase by 2.5 mg/hr q15min. After B/P goal is achieved, decrease rate to 3 mg/hr.
Adults, Elderly (rapid B/P decrease). Initially, 5 mg/hr. May increase by 2.5 mg/hr q5min. Maximum: 15 mg/hr until desired B/P attained. After B/P goal achieved, decrease rate to 3 mg/hr.
Changing from IV to Oral Antihypertensive Therapy

Adults, Elderly. Begin antihypertensives other than nicardipine when IV has been discontinued; for nicardipine, give first dose 1 hr before discontinuing IV.

▸ **Dosage in Hepatic Impairment**

For adults and elderly patients, initially give 20 mg twice a day; then titrate.

▸ **Dosage in Renal Impairment**

For adults and elderly patients, initially give 20 mg q8h (30 mg twice a day [sustained-release capsules]); then titrate.

SIDE EFFECTS/ADVERSE REACTIONS

Frequent

Headache, facial flushing, peripheral edema, light-headedness, dizziness

Occasional

Asthenia (loss of strength, energy), palpitations, angina, tachycardia

Rare

Nausea, abdominal cramps, dyspepsia, dry mouth, rash

PRECAUTIONS AND CONTRAINDICATIONS

Atrial fibrillation or flutter associated with accessory conduction pathways, cardiogenic shock, CHF, second- or third-degree heart block, severe hypotension, sinus bradycardia, ventricular tachycardia, within several hr of IV β-blocker therapy

Caution

CHF, hypotension, hepatic injury, lactation, children, renal disease, elderly

DRUG INTERACTIONS OF CONCERN TO DENTISTRY

• Decreased effect: indomethacin, possibly other NSAIDs, phenobarbital, St. John's wort (herb)

• Increased effect: parenteral and inhalational general anesthetics or other drugs with hypotensive actions

• Possible risk of increased plasma level, monitor patient: erythromycin, ketoconazole, other CYP3A4 inhibitors

• Increased effects of nondepolarizing muscle relaxants

• Increased effects of carbamazepine

SERIOUS REACTIONS

! Overdose produces confusion, slurred speech, somnolence, marked hypotension, and bradycardia.

DENTAL CONSIDERATIONS

General:

• Monitor cardiac status; take vital signs at each appointment because of CV side effects. Consider a stress reduction protocol to prevent stress-induced angina during the dental appointment.

• After supine positioning, have patient sit upright for at least 2 min before standing to avoid orthostatic hypotension.

• Place on frequent recall to monitor gingival condition.

• Limit use of sodium-containing products, such as saline IV fluids, for patients with a dietary salt restriction.

• Assess salivary flow as a factor in caries, periodontal disease, and candidiasis.

• Use vasoconstrictors with caution, in low doses, and with careful aspiration. Avoid use of gingival retraction cord with epinephrine.

Consultations:

• Medical consultation may be required to assess disease control and tolerance for stress.

Teach Patient/Family to:

• Use effective oral hygiene to prevent soft tissue inflammation and minimize gingival overgrowth

• Schedule frequent oral prophylaxis if hyperplasia occurs
• When chronic dry mouth occurs, advise patient to:
  • Avoid mouth rinses with high alcohol content because of drying effects
  • Use daily home fluoride products for anticaries effect
  • Use sugarless gum, frequent sips of water, or saliva substitutes

nicotine

nik´-oh-teen
(Commit, Habitrol[CAN], Nicabate[AUS], Nicabate CQ Clear[AUS], Nicabate CQ Lozenges[AUS], NicoDerm[CAN], NicoDerm CQ, Nicorette, Nicorette Plus[CAN], Nicotinell[AUS], Nicotrol, Nicotrol NS, Nicotrol Patch[CAN])
Do not confuse Nicoderm with Nitroderm.

CATEGORY AND SCHEDULE

Pregnancy Risk Category: D (transdermal)
OTC (Nicoderm transdermal patch, Nicotrol transdermal patch, Nicorette chewing gum)

Drug Class: Smoking deterrent

MECHANISM OF ACTION

A cholinergic-receptor agonist binds to acetylcholine receptors, producing both stimulating and depressant effects on the peripheral and central nervous systems. **Therapeutic Effect:** Provides a source of nicotine during nicotine withdrawal and reduces withdrawal symptoms.

USES

Cigarette smoking cessation program

PHARMACOKINETICS

Absorbed slowly after transdermal administration. Protein binding: 5%. Metabolized in the liver. Excreted primarily in urine. **Half-life:** 4 hr.

INDICATIONS AND DOSAGES

▶ **Smoking Cessation Aid to Relieve Nicotine Withdrawal Symptoms**
PO (Chewing gum)
Adults, Elderly. Usually, 10–12 pieces/day. Maximum: 30 pieces/day.
PO (Lozenge)
Adults, Elderly. One 4-mg or 2-mg lozenge q1–2h for the first 6 wk; 1 lozenge q2–4h for wk 7–9; and 1 lozenge q4–8h for wk 10–12. Maximum: 1 lozenge at a time, 5 lozenges/6 hr, 20 lozenges/day.
Transdermal
Adults, Elderly who smoke 10 cigarettes or more per day. Follow the guidelines below.
Step 1: 21 mg/day for 4–6 wk.
Step 2: 14 mg/day for 2 wk.
Step 3: 7 mg/day for 2 wk.
Adults, Elderly who smoke fewer than 10 cigarettes per day. Follow the guidelines below.
Step 1: 14 mg/day for 6 wk.
Step 2: 7 mg/day for 2 wk. Patients weighing less than 100 lb, patients with a history of cardiovascular disease. Initially, 14 mg/day for 4–6 wk, then 7 mg/day for 2–4 wk.
Transdermal (Nicotrol)
Adults, Elderly. 1 patch a day for 6 wk.
Nasal
Adults, Elderly. 1–2 doses/hr (1 dose = 2 sprays [1 in each nostril] = 1 mg). Maximum: 5 doses (5 mg)/hr; 40 doses (40 mg) /day.
Inhaler (Nicotrol)
Adults, Elderly. Puff on nicotine cartridge mouthpiece for about 20 min as needed.

N

SIDE EFFECTS/ADVERSE REACTIONS

Frequent
All forms: Hiccups, nausea
Gum: Mouth or throat soreness, nausea, hiccups
Transdermal: Erythema, pruritus, or burning at application site

Occasional
All forms: Eructation, GI upset, dry mouth, insomnia, diaphoresis, irritability
Gum: Hiccups, hoarseness
Inhaler: Mouth or throat irritation, cough

Rare
All forms: Dizziness, myalgia, arthralgia

PRECAUTIONS AND CONTRAINDICATIONS

Immediate post-MI period, life-threatening arrhythmias, severe or worsening angina

Caution
Skin disease, angina pectoris, MI, renal or hepatic insufficiency, peptic ulcer, serious cardiac dysrhythmias, hyperthyroidism, pheochromocytoma, insulin-dependent diabetes, elderly

DRUG INTERACTIONS OF CONCERN TO DENTISTRY

- Decreased dose at cessation of smoking: acetaminophen, caffeine, oxazepam, pentazocine
- Decreased metabolism of propoxyphene

DRUG INTERACTIONS OF CONCERN TO DENTISTRY NICOTINE POLACRILEX

- Increased blood levels with cessation of smoking: propoxyphene

SERIOUS REACTIONS

! Overdose produces palpitations, tachyarrhythmias, seizures, depression, confusion, diaphoresis, hypotension, rapid or weak pulse, and dyspnea. Lethal dose for adults is 40–60 mg. Death results from respiratory paralysis.

DENTAL CONSIDERATIONS

General:
- Assess salivary flow as a factor in caries, periodontal disease, and candidiasis.

Teach Patient/Family:
- When chronic dry mouth occurs, advise patient to:
  - Avoid mouth rinses with high alcohol content because of drying effects
  - Use daily home fluoride products to prevent caries
  - Use sugarless gum, frequent sips of water, or saliva substitutes
- When used in conjunction with a smoking cessation program in the dental office, teach:
  - All aspects of product drug; give package insert to patient and explain:
    - That patch is to be used only to deter smoking
    - Not to use during pregnancy; birth defects may occur
    - To keep used and unused system out of reach of children and pets; potentially toxic if chewed or swallowed
    - To apply once per day to a nonhairy, clean, dry area of skin on upper body or upper outer arm
    - To stop smoking immediately when beginning treatment with patch

- To apply promptly after removing from protective covering; system may lose strength

Nicotine Polacrilex
General:
- Take vital signs at every appointment because of cardiovascular side effects.
- Temporomandibular joint (TMJ) disorder may be aggravated by chewing because of heavier viscosity of gum.

Teach Patient/Family to:
- Use effective oral hygiene to prevent periodontal inflammation
- When chronic dry mouth occurs, advise patient to:
  - Avoid mouth rinses with high alcohol content because of drying effects
  - Use daily home fluoride products for anticaries effect
  - Use sugarless gum, frequent sips of water, or saliva substitutes
- When used in conjunction with a smoking cessation program in the dental office, teach:
  - All aspects of product use; give package insert to patient and explain:
    - That gum is to be used only to deter smoking
    - To avoid use in pregnancy; birth defects may occur
    - To stop smoking when beginning treatment with gum
    - To dispose of gum carefully because nicotine will still be present; to protect from children

nifedipine
nye-fed´-ih-peen
(Adalat 5[AUS], Adalat 10[AUS], Adalat 20[aus], Adalat CC, Adalat Oros[AUS], Apo-Nifed[CAN], Nifecard[AUS], Nifedicol XL, Nifehexal[AUS], Novo-Nifedin[CAN], Nyefax[AUS], Procardia, Procardia XL)
Do not confuse nifedipine with nicardipine or nimodipine.

CATEGORY AND SCHEDULE
Pregnancy Risk Category: C

Drug Class: Calcium channel blocker

MECHANISM OF ACTION
An antianginal and antihypertensive agent that inhibits calcium ion movement across cell membranes, depressing contraction of cardiac and vascular smooth muscle.
Therapeutic Effect: Increases heart rate and cardiac output. Decreases systemic vascular resistance and B/P.

USES
Treatment of chronic stable angina pectoris, vasospastic angina, hypertension (sustained release only)

PHARMACOKINETICS

Route	Onset	Peak	Duration
Sublingual	1–5 min	N/A	N/A
PO	20–30 min	N/A	4–8 hr
PO (extended release)	2 hr	N/A	24 hr

Rapidly, completely absorbed from the GI tract. Protein binding: 92%–98%. Undergoes first-pass metabolism in the liver. Primarily excreted in urine. Not removed by hemodialysis. *Half-life:* 2–5 hr.

INDICATIONS AND DOSAGES

▶ **Prinzmetal's Variant Angina, Chronic Stable (Effort-Associated) Angina**
PO
Adults, Elderly. Initially, 10 mg 3 times a day. Increase at 7- to 14-day intervals. Maintenance: 10 mg 3 times a day up to 30 mg 4 times a day.
PO (Extended-Release)
Adults, Elderly. Initially, 30–60 mg/day. Maintenance: Up to 120 mg/day.

▶ **Essential Hypertension**
PO (Extended-Release)
Adults, Elderly. Initially, 30–60 mg/day. Maintenance: Up to 120 mg/day.

SIDE EFFECTS/ADVERSE REACTIONS

Frequent
Peripheral edema, headache, flushed skin, dizziness
Occasional
Nausea, shakiness, muscle cramps and pain, somnolence, palpitations, nasal congestion, cough, dyspnea, wheezing, oral gingival enlargement
Rare
Hypotension, rash, pruritus, urticaria, constipation, abdominal discomfort, flatulence, sexual difficulties

PRECAUTIONS AND CONTRAINDICATIONS

Advanced aortic stenosis, severe hypotension
Caution
CHF, hypotension, sick sinus syndrome, second- or third-degree heart block, hypotension less than 90 mm Hg systolic, hepatic injury, lactation, children, renal disease.

DRUG INTERACTIONS OF CONCERN TO DENTISTRY

• Decreased effect: indomethacin, possibly other NSAIDs, phenobarbital
• Increased effect: parenteral and inhalational general anesthetics or other drugs with hypotensive actions
• Possible increase in effects, monitor patients: inhibitors of CYP3A4 isoenzyme
• Increased effects of nondepolarizing muscle relaxants
• Increased effects of carbamazepine

SERIOUS REACTIONS

! Nifedipine may precipitate CHF and MI in patients with cardiac disease and peripheral ischemia.
! Overdose produces nausea, somnolence, confusion, and slurred speech.

DENTAL CONSIDERATIONS

General:
• Monitor cardiac status; take vital signs at each appointment because of cardiovascular side effects. Consider a stress-reduction protocol to prevent stress-induced angina during the dental appointment.
• After supine positioning, have patient sit upright for at least 2 min before standing to avoid orthostatic hypotension at dismissal.
• Place on frequent recall to monitor gingival condition.
• Limit use of sodium-containing products, such as saline IV fluids, for patients with a dietary salt restriction.
• Assess salivary flow as a factor in caries, periodontal disease, and candidiasis.
• Use vasoconstrictors with caution, in low doses, and with careful aspiration. Avoid use of gingival retraction cord with epinephrine.
Consultations:
• Medical consultation may be required to assess disease control and stress tolerance.

Teach Patient/Family to:
• Use effective oral hygiene to prevent soft tissue inflammation and minimize gingival overgrowth
• Schedule frequent oral prophylaxis if hyperplasia occurs
• When chronic dry mouth occurs, advise patient to:
  • Avoid mouth rinses with high alcohol content because of drying effects
  • Use daily home fluoride products for anticaries effect
  • Use sugarless gum, frequent sips of water, or saliva substitutes

nilutamide
nih-lute´-ah-myd
(Anandron[CAN], Nilandron)

CATEGORY AND SCHEDULE
Pregnancy Risk Category: C

Drug Class: Hormone; antineoplastic

MECHANISM OF ACTION
An antiandrogen hormone and antineoplastic agent that competitively inhibits androgen action by binding to androgen receptors in target tissue.
Therapeutic Effect: Decreases growth of abnormal prostate tissue.

USES
Treatment of cancer of the prostate gland

PHARMACOKINETICS
Rapidly and completed absorbed; excreted in urine and feces as metabolites

INDICATIONS AND DOSAGES
▶ **Prostatic Carcinoma**
PO
Adults, Elderly. 300 mg once a day for 30 days, then 150 mg once a day. Begin on day of, or day after, surgical castration.

SIDE EFFECTS/ADVERSE REACTIONS
Frequent
Hot flashes, delay in recovering vision after bright illumination (such as sun, television, bright lights), decreased libido, diminished sexual function, mild nausea, gynecomastia, alcohol intolerance
Occasional
Constipation, hypertension, dizziness, dyspnea, UTIs

PRECAUTIONS AND CONTRAINDICATIONS
Severe hepatic impairment, severe respiratory insufficiency

DRUG INTERACTIONS OF CONCERN TO DENTISTRY
• Avoid drugs that may aggravate urinary retention when symptoms are present
• This is an inhibitor of CYP3A4 isoenzymes; no specific studies have been done, but use caution when prescribing drugs metabolized by this enzyme

SERIOUS REACTIONS
! Interstitial pneumonitis occurs rarely.

DENTAL CONSIDERATIONS
General:
• Monitor and record vital signs.
• If additional analgesia is required for dental pain, consider alternative analgesics (NSAIDs) in patients

N

taking narcotics for acute or chronic pain.
• Avoid dental light in patient's eyes; offer dark glasses for patient comfort.
• This drug may be used in the hospital or on an outpatient basis. Confirm the patient's disease and treatment status.
• Short appointments and a stress-reduction protocol may be required for anxious patients.

Consultations:
• Medical consultation may be required to assess immunologic status during cancer chemotherapy and determine safety risk, if any, posed by the required dental treatment.
• Medical consultation may be required to assess disease control and patient's ability to tolerate stress.

Teach Patient/Family to:
• Use effective oral hygiene to prevent soft tissue inflammation
• Prevent trauma when using oral hygiene aids
• Report oral lesions, soreness, or bleeding to dentist
• Update health and medication history if physician makes any changes in evaluation or drug regimens; include OTC, herbal, and nonherbal in the update

nimodipine
nye-mode´-ih-peen
(Nimotop)
Do not confuse nimodipine with nifedipine.

CATEGORY AND SCHEDULE
Pregnancy Risk Category: C

Drug Class: Calcium channel blockers

MECHANISM OF ACTION
A cerebral vasospasm agent that inhibits movement of calcium ions across vascular smooth-muscle cell membranes. ***Therapeutic Effect:*** Produces favorable effect on severity of neurologic deficits due to cerebral vasospasm. Exerts greatest effect on cerebral arteries; may prevent cerebral spasm.

USES
Relief of and control of angina pectoris (chest pain)

PHARMACOKINETICS
Rapidly absorbed from the GI tract. Protein binding: 95%. Metabolized in the liver. Excreted in urine; eliminated in feces. Not removed by hemodialysis. ***Half-life:*** terminal, 3 hr.

INDICATIONS AND DOSAGES
▶ **Improvement in Neurologic Deficits after Subarachnoid Hemorrhage from Ruptured Congenital Aneurysms**
PO
Adults, Elderly. 60 mg q4h for 21 days. Begin within 96 hr of subarachnoid hemorrhage.

SIDE EFFECTS/ADVERSE REACTIONS
Occasional
Hypotension, peripheral edema, diarrhea, headache
Rare
Allergic reaction (rash, hives), tachycardia, flushing of skin

PRECAUTIONS AND CONTRAINDICATIONS
Atrial fibrillation or flutter, cardiogenic shock, CHF, heart block, sinus bradycardia, ventricular

tachycardia, within several hr of IV β-blocker therapy

DRUG INTERACTIONS OF CONCERN TO DENTISTRY
• Hypotension: anesthetics, other antihypertensive medications
• Antagonism of antihypertensive effect: indomethacin and possibly other NSAIDs
• Possible reduction in antihypertensive effects: sympathomimetics

SERIOUS REACTIONS
! Overdose produces nausea, weakness, dizziness, somnolence, confusion, and slurred speech.

DENTAL CONSIDERATIONS
General:
• Patients may have significant neurologic deficit; dental care may not be practical.
• Caution: potential for interactions with drugs used in dentistry.
• Determine why patient is taking the drug.
• Monitor and record vital signs.
• After supine positioning, have patient sit upright for at least 2 min before standing to avoid orthostatic hypotension.
Consultations:
• This drug may be used in the hospital or on an outpatient basis. Confirm the patient's disease and treatment status.
• Medical consultation may be required to assess disease control and patient's ability to tolerate stress.
Teach Patient/Family to:
• Use effective oral hygiene to prevent soft tissue inflammation
• Use electric toothbrush if patient has difficulty holding conventional devices

• Update health and medication history if physician makes any changes in evaluation or drug regimens; include OTC, herbal, and nonherbal drugs in the update

nisoldipine
nye-soul´-dih-peen
(Sular)
Do not confuse with nicardipine.

CATEGORY AND SCHEDULE
Pregnancy Risk Category: C

Drug Class: Calcium channel antagonist (dihydropyridine group)

MECHANISM OF ACTION
A calcium channel blocker that inhibits calcium ion movement across cell membrane, depressing contraction of cardiac and vascular smooth muscle. *Therapeutic Effect:* Increases heart rate and cardiac output. Decreases systemic vascular resistance and B/P.

USES
Hypertension as a single agent or in combination with other antihypertensive medications

PHARMACOKINETICS
Poor absorption from the GI tract. Food increases bioavailability. Protein binding: more than 99%. Metabolism occurs in the gut wall. Primarily excreted in urine. Not removed by hemodialysis. *Half-life:* 7–12 hr.

INDICATIONS AND DOSAGES
▶ **Hypertension**
PO
Adults. Initially, 20 mg once daily, then increase by 10 mg/wk, or longer intervals until therapeutic BP response is attained.
Elderly. Initially, 10 mg once daily. Increase by 10 mg/wk to therapeutic response. Maintenance: 20–40 mg once daily. Maximum: 60 mg once daily.

SIDE EFFECTS/ADVERSE REACTIONS
Frequent
Giddiness, dizziness, lightheadedness, peripheral edema, headache, flushing, weakness, nausea, oral gingival enlargement
Occasional
Transient hypotension, heartburn, muscle cramps, nasal congestion, cough, wheezing, sore throat, palpitations, nervousness, mood changes
Rare
Increase in frequency, intensity, duration of anginal attack during initial therapy

PRECAUTIONS AND CONTRAINDICATIONS
Sick-sinus syndrome or second- or third-degree AV block (except in presence of pacemaker), hypersensitivity to nisoldipine or any component of the formulation
Caution
Avoid high-fat meals, severe coronary artery disease, monitor BP, CHF, severe hepatic impairment, do not break or crush tablets, lactation, geriatric patients

SERIOUS REACTIONS
! May precipitate CHF and MI in patients with cardiac disease and peripheral ischemia.

! Overdose produces nausea, drowsiness, confusion, and slurred speech.

DENTAL CONSIDERATIONS
General:
• Stress from dental procedures may compromise cardiovascular function; determine patient risk.
• Monitor vital signs at every appointment because of cardiovascular side effects.
• Short appointments and a stress reduction protocol may be required for anxious patients.
• Grapefruit juice may increase plasma levels.
• Limit use of sodium-containing products, such as saline IV fluids, for patients with a dietary salt restriction.
• After supine positioning, have patient sit upright for at least 2 min before standing to avoid orthostatic hypotension.
• Assess salivary flow as a factor in caries, periodontal disease, and candidiasis.
Consultations:
• Medical consultation may be required to assess disease control and patient's ability to tolerate stress.
Teach Patient/Family to:
• Schedule frequent oral prophylaxis if gingival enlargement occurs
• When chronic dry mouth occurs, advise patient to:
    • Avoid mouth rinses with high alcohol content because of drying effects
    • Use daily home fluoride products for anticaries effect
    • Use sugarless gum, frequent sips of water, or saliva substitutes

nitazoxanide
nigh-taz-oks´-ah-nide
(Alinia)

CATEGORY AND SCHEDULE
Pregnancy Risk Category: B

Drug Class: Antiprotozoals

MECHANISM OF ACTION
An antiparasitic that interferes with
the body's reaction to pyruvate
ferredoxin oxidoreductase, an
enzyme essential for anaerobic
energy metabolism. *Therapeutic
Effect:* Produces antiprotozoal
activity, reducing or terminating
diarrheal episodes.

USES
Treatment of diarrhea that is caused
by certain types of protozoa (tiny,
1-celled animals)

PHARMACOKINETICS
Rapidly hydrolyzed to an active
metabolite. Protein binding: 99%.
Excreted in the urine, bile, and feces.
Half-life: 2–4 hr.

INDICATIONS AND DOSAGES
▶ **Diarrhea**
PO
Children 12 yr and older. 200 mg
q12h.
Children 4–11 yr. 200 mg (10 ml)
q12h for 3 days.
Children 12–47 mo. 100 mg (5 ml)
q12h for 3 days.

SIDE EFFECTS/ADVERSE REACTIONS
Occasional
Abdominal pain
Rare
Diarrhea, vomiting, headache

PRECAUTIONS AND CONTRAINDICATIONS
History of sensitivity to aspirin and
salicylates

DRUG INTERACTIONS OF CONCERN TO DENTISTRY
None reported

SERIOUS REACTIONS
None known

DENTAL CONSIDERATIONS
General:
• This is an acute-use drug; patients
highly unlikely to present for
dental care.
• Ensure patients are well hydrated
and electrolytes reestablished
following recovery if they present for
dental treatment.
Consultations:
• Medical consultation may be
required to assess disease control.
Teach Patient/Family to:
• Maintain or reestablish oral
hygiene care

nitrofurantoin sodium
nye-troe-fyoor´-an-toyn
soe´-dee-um
(Apo-Nitrofurantoin[CAN],
Furadantin, Macrobid, Macrodantin,
Novo-Furan[CAN], Ralodantin[AUS])

CATEGORY AND SCHEDULE
Pregnancy Risk Category: B

Drug Class: Urinary tract
antiinfective

MECHANISM OF ACTION
An antibacterial UTI agent that
inhibits the synthesis of bacterial

DNA, RNA, proteins, and cell walls by altering or inactivating ribosomal proteins. ***Therapeutic Effect***: Bacteriostatic (bactericidal at high concentrations).

USES

Treatment of UTIs caused by *E. coli*, Klebsiella, Pseudomonas, *P. vulgaris, P. morganii*, Serratia, Citro-bacter, *S. aureus*

PHARMACOKINETICS

Microcrystalline form rapidly and completely absorbed; macrocrystalline form more slowly absorbed. Food increases absorption. Protein binding: 40%. Primarily concentrated in urine and kidneys. Metabolized in most body tissues. Primarily excreted in urine. Removed by hemodialysis. *Half-life:* 20–60 min.

INDICATIONS AND DOSAGES

▶ **UTIs**
PO (Furadantin, Macrodantin)
Adults, Elderly. 50–100 mg q6h. Maximum: 400 mg/day.
Children. 5–7 mg/kg/day in divided doses q6h. Maximum: 400 mg/day.
PO (Macrobid)
Adults, Elderly. 100 mg twice a day. Maximum: 400 mg/day.
▶ **Long-Term Prevention of UTIs**
PO
Adults, Elderly. 50–100 mg at bedtime.
Children. 1–2 mg/kg/day as a single dose. Maximum: 100 mg/day.

SIDE EFFECTS/ADVERSE REACTIONS

Frequent
Anorexia, nausea, vomiting, dark urine

Occasional
Abdominal pain, diarrhea, rash, pruritus, urticaria, hypertension, headache, dizziness, drowsiness
Rare
Photosensitivity, transient alopecia, asthmatic exacerbation in those with history of asthma

PRECAUTIONS AND CONTRAINDICATIONS

Anuria, oliguria, substantial renal impairment (creatinine clearance less than 40 ml/min); infants younger than 1 mo old because of the risk of hemolytic anemia
Caution
Lactation

DRUG INTERACTIONS OF CONCERN TO DENTISTRY

• Increased effects: anticholinergic drugs

SERIOUS REACTIONS

❗ Superinfection, hepatotoxicity, peripheral neuropathy (may be irreversible), Stevens-Johnson syndrome, permanent pulmonary function impairment, and anaphylaxis occur rarely.

DENTAL CONSIDERATIONS

General:
• Determine why the patient is taking the drug.
Consultations:
• Medical consultation may be required to assess disease control and to select an antiinfective if a dental infection is diagnosed.

nitrofurazone
nye-troe-fyoor´-ah-zone
(Furacin)
Do not confuse with nitrofurantoin.

CATEGORY AND SCHEDULE
Pregnancy Risk Category: C
OTC (ointment)

Drug Class: Coronary
vasodilator, antianginal; nitrate

MECHANISM OF ACTION
A synthetic nitrofuran that inhibits
bacterial enzymes involved in
carbohydrate metabolism.
Therapeutic Effect: Inhibits a variety
of enzymes. Bactericidal.

USES
Treatment of chronic stable angina
pectoris, prophylaxis of angina pain,
CHF associated with acute MI,
controlled hypotension in surgical
procedures

PHARMACOKINETICS
Not known

INDICATIONS AND DOSAGES
▶ Burns, Catheter-Related UTI,
Skin Grafts
Topical
Adults. Apply directly on lesion with
spatula or place on a piece of gauze
first. Use of a bandage is optional.
Preparation should remain on lesion
for at least 24 hr. Dressing may be
changed several times daily or left on
the lesion for a longer period.

SIDE EFFECTS/ADVERSE
REACTIONS
Occasional
Itching, rash, swelling

PRECAUTIONS AND
CONTRAINDICATIONS
Hypersensitivity to nitrofurazone or
any of its components

DRUG INTERACTIONS OF
CONCERN TO DENTISTRY
None reported

SERIOUS REACTIONS
❗ Use of nitrofurazone may
result in bacterial or fungal
overgrowth of nonsusceptible
pathogens, which may lead to
secondary infection.

DENTAL CONSIDERATIONS
General:
• Dental management depends on
extent and severity of burns and
patients ability to cooperate; use
aseptic techniques.
• Provide palliative dental care for
dental emergencies only.
• Monitor and record vital
signs.
Consultations:
• Medical consultation may be
required to assess disease
control and patient's ability to
tolerate stress.
• Consult patient's physician
if an acute dental infection
occurs and another antiinfective is
required.
Teach Patient/Family to:
• Use effective oral
hygiene to prevent soft tissue
inflammation
• Prevent trauma when using oral
hygiene aids

nitroglycerin

nye-troe-gli´-ser-in

(Anginine[AUS], Minitran,
Nitradisc[AUS], Nitrek, Nitro-Bid,
Nitro-Dur, Nitrogard,
Nitroject[CAN], Nitrolingual,
Nitrolingual Spray[AUS],
Nitrong-SR, NitroQuick, Nitrostat,
Nitro-Tab, Rectogesic[AUS],
Transiderm Nitro[AUS],
Trinipatch[CAN])
Do not confuse nitroglycerin with
nitroprusside; Nitro-Bid with
Nicobid; Nitro-Dur with Nicoderm;
Nitrostat with Hyperstat, Nilstat, or
Nystatin; or Nitrong-SR with
Nizoral.

CATEGORY AND SCHEDULE

Pregnancy Risk Category: B

Drug Class: Inorganic nitrate,
vasodilator

MECHANISM OF ACTION

A nitrate that decreases myocardial
oxygen demand. Reduces left
ventricular preload and afterload.
Therapeutic Effect: Dilates coronary
arteries and improves collateral
blood flow to ischemic areas within
myocardium. IV form produces
peripheral vasodilation.

USES

Treatment of chronic stable angina
pectoris, prophylaxis of angina pain,
CHF associated with acute MI,
controlled hypotension in surgical
procedures

PHARMACOKINETICS

Route	Onset	Peak	Duration
Sublingual	1–3 min	4–8 min	30–60 min
Translingual spray	2 min	4–10 min	30–60 min
Buccal tablet	2–5 min	4–10 min	2 hr
PO (extended release)	20–45 min	45–120 min	4–8 hr
Topical	15–60 min	30–120 min	2–12 hr
Transdermal patch	40–60 min	60–180 min	18–24 hr
IV	1–2 min	Immediate	3–5 min

Well absorbed after PO, sublingual,
and topical administration.
Undergoes extensive first-pass
metabolism. Metabolized in the liver
and by enzymes in the bloodstream.
Primarily excreted in urine.
Not removed by hemodialysis.
Half-life: 1–4 min.

INDICATIONS AND DOSAGES

▸ **Acute Relief of Angina Pectoris,
Acute Prophylaxis**
Lingual Spray
Adults, Elderly. 1 spray onto or under
tongue q3–5min until relief is noted
(no more than 3 sprays in 15-min
period).
Sublingual
Adults, Elderly. 0.4 mg q5min until
relief is noted (no more than 3 doses
in 15-min period). Use
prophylactically 5–10 min before
activities that may cause an acute
attack.
▸ **Long-Term Prophylaxis of Angina**
PO (Extended-Release)
Adults, Elderly. 2.5–9 mg q8–12h.
Topical
Adults, Elderly. Initially, ¹/₂ inch q8h.
Increase by ¹/₂ inch with each

application. Range: 1–2 inches q8h up to 4–5 inches q4h.
Transdermal Patch
Adults, Elderly. Initially, 0.2–0.4 mg/hr. Maintenance: 0.4–0.8 mg/hr. Consider patch on for 12–14 hr, patch off for 10–12 hr (prevents tolerance).

▶ CHF Associated with Acute MI
IV
Adults, Elderly. Initially, 5 mcg/min via infusion pump. Increase in 5-mcg/min increments at 3- to 5-min intervals until B/P response is noted or until dosage reaches 20 mcg/min; then increase as needed by 10 mcg/min. Dosage may be further titrated according to clinical, therapeutic response up to 200 mcg/min.
Children. Initially, 0.25–0.5 mcg/kg/min; titrate by 0.5–1 mcg/kg/min up to 20 mcg/kg/min.

SIDE EFFECTS/ADVERSE REACTIONS
Frequent
Headache (possibly severe; occurs mostly in early therapy, diminishes rapidly in intensity, and usually disappears during continued treatment), transient flushing of face and neck, dizziness (especially if patient is standing immobile or is in a warm environment), weakness, orthostatic hypotension
Sublingual: Burning, tingling sensation at oral point of dissolution
Ointment: Erythema, pruritus
Occasional
GI upset
Transdermal: Contact dermatitis

PRECAUTIONS AND CONTRAINDICATIONS
Allergy to adhesives (transdermal), closed-angle glaucoma, constrictive pericarditis (IV), early MI (sublingual), GI hypermotility or malabsorption (extended-release), head trauma, hypotension (IV), inadequate cerebral circulation (IV), increased intracranial pressure, nitrates, orthostatic hypotension, pericardial tamponade (IV), severe anemia, uncorrected hypovolemia (IV)
Caution
Postural hypotension, lactation

DRUG INTERACTIONS OF CONCERN TO DENTISTRY
• Increased hypotensive effects: alcohol, opioids, benzodiazepines, phenothiazines, and other drugs used in conscious sedation techniques

SERIOUS REACTIONS
❗ Nitroglycerin should be discontinued if blurred vision or dry mouth occurs.
❗ Severe orthostatic hypotension may occur, manifested by fainting, pulselessness, cold or clammy skin, and diaphoresis.
❗ Tolerance may occur with repeated, prolonged therapy; minor tolerance may occur with intermittent use of sublingual tablets.
❗ High doses of nitroglycerin tend to produce severe headache.

DENTAL CONSIDERATIONS
General:
• Take vital signs at every appointment because of cardiovascular side effects.
• After supine positioning, have patient sit upright for at least 2 min before standing to avoid orthostatic hypotension.
• Assess salivary flow as a factor in caries, periodontal disease, and candidiasis.
• Ensure that patient's drug is easily available if angina occurs.

- A benzodiazepine or nitrous oxide/oxygen may be prescribed to allay anxiety.
- Check expiration date on prescription to ensure drug activity. If bottle has been opened, the shelf life is 3 mo.
- Stress from dental procedures may compromise cardiovascular function; determine patient risk.
- Talk with patient about disease control (frequency of angina episodes).
- Use vasoconstrictors with caution, in low doses, and with careful aspiration. Avoid gingival retraction cord with epinephrine.
- Short appointments and a stress-reduction protocol may be required for anxious patients.
- Consider semisupine chair position for patients with cardiovascular disease.

Consultations:
- Medical consultation may be required to assess disease control and patient's ability to tolerate stress.

Teach Patient/Family to:
- Use effective oral hygiene to prevent soft tissue inflammation
- Use caution to prevent injury when using oral hygiene aids
- When chronic dry mouth occurs, advise patient to:
  - Avoid mouth rinses with high alcohol content because of drying effects
  - Use daily home fluoride products for anticaries effect
  - Use sugarless gum, frequent sips of water, or saliva substitutes

nizatidine
ni-za´-ti-deen
(Apo-Nizatidine[CAN], Axid, Axid AR, Tazac[AUS])
Do not confuse Axid with Ansaid.

CATEGORY AND SCHEDULE
Pregnancy Risk Category: B
OTC (75 mg capsules)

Drug Class: Histamine
H_2-receptor antagonist

MECHANISM OF ACTION
An antiulcer agent and gastric acid secretion inhibitor that inhibits histamine action at histamine 2 receptors of parietal cells.
Therapeutic Effect: Inhibits basal and nocturnal gastric acid secretion.

USES
Treatment of duodenal ulcer, Zollinger-Ellison syndrome, gastric ulcers, hypersecretory conditions, gastroesophageal reflux disease (GERD), stress ulcers; unapproved: GI symptoms associated with NSAID use in rheumatoid arthritis

PHARMACOKINETICS
Rapidly well absorbed from the GI tract. Protein binding: 35%. Metabolized in the liver. Primarily excreted in urine. Not removed by hemodialysis. *Half-life:* 1–2 hr (increased with impaired renal function).

INDICATIONS AND DOSAGES
▶ **Active Duodenal Ulcer**
PO
Adults, Elderly. 300 mg at bedtime or 150 mg twice a day.

▶ **Prevention of Duodenal Ulcer Recurrence**
PO
Adults, Elderly. 150 mg at bedtime.
▶ **GERD**
PO
Adults, Elderly. 150 mg twice a day.
▶ **Active Benign Gastric Ulcer**
PO
Adults, Elderly. 150 mg twice a day or 300 mg at bedtime.
PO, oral solution
Children 12 yr and older. 2 tsp twice a day.
▶ **Dyspepsia**
PO
Adults, Elderly. 75 mg 30–60 min before meals; no more than 2 tablets a day.
▶ **Dosage in Renal Impairment**
Dosage adjustment is based on creatinine clearance.

Creatinine Clearance	Active Ulcer	Maintenance Therapy
20–50 ml/min	150 mg every bedtime	150 mg every other day
Less than 20 ml/min	150 mg every other day	150 mg q3days

SIDE EFFECTS/ADVERSE REACTIONS
Occasional
Somnolence, fatigue
Rare
Diaphoresis, rash

PRECAUTIONS AND CONTRAINDICATIONS
Hypersensitivity to other H$_2$-antagonists

Caution
Hepatic disease, renal disease, lactation, children younger than 16 yr

DRUG INTERACTIONS OF CONCERN TO DENTISTRY
• Increased serum salicylate when administered with high doses of aspirin
• Decreased absorption of ketoconazole (take doses 2 hr apart)

SERIOUS REACTIONS
! Asymptomatic ventricular tachycardia, hyperuricemia not associated with gout, and nephrolithiasis occur rarely.

DENTAL CONSIDERATIONS
General:
• Avoid prescribing aspirin-containing products in patients with active GI disease.
Teach Patient/Family to:
• Avoid mouth rinses with high alcohol content because of drying effects

norepinephrine bitartrate
nor-ep-ih-nef´-rin bye-tar´-trate
(Levophed)
Do not confuse Levophed with Levid, or norepinephrine with epinephrine.

CATEGORY AND SCHEDULE
Pregnancy Risk Category: C

Drug Class: Adrenergic; catecholamine

MECHANISM OF ACTION
A sympathomimetic that stimulates
β_1-adrenergic receptors and
α-adrenergic receptors, increasing
peripheral resistance. Enhances
contractile myocardial force, increases
cardiac output. Constricts resistance
and capacitance vessels. *Therapeutic
Effect:* Increases systemic B/P and
coronary blood flow.

USES
Treatment of acute hypotension, shock

PHARMACOKINETICS

Route	Onset	Peak	Duration
IV	Rapid	1–2 min	N/A

Localized in sympathetic tissue.
Metabolized in the liver. Primarily
excreted in urine.

INDICATIONS AND DOSAGES
▸ **Acute Hypotension Unresponsive
to Fluid Volume Replacement**
IV
Adults, Elderly. Initially, administer
at 0.5–1 mcg/min. Adjust rate of flow
to establish and maintain desired B/P
(40 mm Hg below preexisting
systolic pressure). Average
maintenance dose: 8–12 mcg/min.
Children. Initially, 0.05–0.1 mcg/kg/
min; titrate to desired effect.
Maximum: 1–2 mcg/kg/min. Range:
0.5–3 mcg/min.

SIDE EFFECTS/ADVERSE REACTIONS
Norepinephrine produces less
pronounced and less frequent side
effects than epinephrine
Occasional
Anxiety, bradycardia, palpitations
Rare
Nausea, anginal pain, shortness of
breath, fever

PRECAUTIONS AND CONTRAINDICATIONS
Hypovolemic states (unless as an
emergency measure), mesenteric or
peripheral vascular thrombosis,
profound hypoxia

DRUG INTERACTIONS OF CONCERN TO DENTISTRY
• Risk of arrhythmia: halogenated
hydrocarbon anesthetics
• Risk of severe hypertension:
tricyclic antidepressants, MAOIs,
oxytocin, guanethidine

SERIOUS REACTIONS
! Extravasation may produce tissue
necrosis and sloughing.
! Overdose is manifested as severe
hypertension with violent headache
(which may be the first clinical sign of
overdose), arrhythmias, photophobia,
retrosternal or pharyngeal pain, pallor,
excessive sweating, and vomiting.
! Prolonged therapy may result in
plasma volume depletion.
Hypotension may recur if plasma
volume is not restored.

DENTAL CONSIDERATIONS
General:
• Acute-use drug for use in hospitals
or emergency rooms for selected
hypotensive episodes.

norethindrone
nor-eth´-in-drone
(Aygestin, Camila, Errin, Jolivette,
Micronor, Nora-BE, Nor-QD,
Norlutate[CAN])

CATEGORY AND SCHEDULE
Pregnancy Risk Category: X

Drug Class: Progesterone
derivative

MECHANISM OF ACTION
A synthetic progestin that is used as a single agent or in combination with estrogens for the treatment of gynecological disorders. It inhibits secretion of pituitary gonadotropin (LH) which prevents follicular maturation and ovulation.
Therapeutic Effect: Transforms endometrium from proliferative to secretory in an estrogen-primed endometrium, promotes mammary gland development, relaxes uterine smooth muscle.

USES
Treatment of uterine bleeding (abnormal), amenorrhea, endometriosis

PHARMACOKINETICS
Rapidly absorbed from the GI tract. Widely distributed. Protein binding: 61%. Metabolized in liver. Excreted in urine and feces. ***Half-life:*** 4–13 hr.

INDICATIONS AND DOSAGES
▸ **Contraception**
PO
Adults. 1 tablet/day.
▸ **Amenorrhea and Abnormal Uterine Bleeding**
PO
Adults. 5–20 mg/day cyclically (21 days on; 7 days off or continuously) or for acetate salt formulation, 2.5–10 mg cyclically.
▸ **Endometriosis**
PO
Adults. 10 mg/day for 2 wk increase at increments of 5 mg/day every 2 wk until 30 mg/day; continue for 6–9 mo or until breakthrough bleeding demands temporary termination. For acetate salt formulation, 5 mg/day for 14 days increase at increments of 2.5 mg/day every 2 wk up to 15 mg/day; continue for 6–9 mo or until breakthrough bleeding demands temporary termination.

SIDE EFFECTS/ADVERSE REACTIONS
Occasional
Breast tenderness, dizziness, headache, breakthrough bleeding, amenorrhea, menstrual irregularity, nausea, weakness
Rare
Mental depression, fever, insomnia, rash, acne, increased breast tenderness, weight gain/loss, changes in cervical erosion and secretions, cholestatic jaundice

PRECAUTIONS AND CONTRAINDICATIONS
Acute liver disease, benign or malignant liver tumors, hypersensitivity to norethindrone and any component of the formulation, known or suspected carcinoma of the breast, known or suspected pregnancy, undiagnosed abnormal genital bleeding
Caution
Lactation, hypertension, asthma, blood dyscrasias, gallbladder disease, CHF, diabetes mellitus, bone disease, depression, migraine headache, convulsive disorders, hepatic disease, renal disease, family history of breast or reproductive tract cancer

DRUG INTERACTIONS OF CONCERN TO DENTISTRY
• Decreased effectiveness of oral contraceptives (low risk), antibiotics, barbiturates

SERIOUS REACTIONS
❗ Thrombophlebitis, cerebrovascular disorders, retinal thrombosis, cholestatic jaundice, and pulmonary embolism occur rarely.

General:
- Place on frequent recall to evaluate gingival inflammation, if present.
- Increased incidence of dry socket has been reported after extraction.
- Monitor vital signs at each appointment.

Teach Patient/Family to:
- Use effective oral hygiene to prevent periodontal inflammation
- Use additional method of birth control while undergoing antibiotic therapy

norfloxacin

nor-flox´-ah-sin
(Apo-Norflox[CAN], Insensye[AUS], Norfloxacine[CAN], Noroxin, Novo-Norfloxacin[CAN], PMS-Norfloxacin[CAN], Roxin[AUS])

CATEGORY AND SCHEDULE
Pregnancy Risk Category: C

Drug Class: Fluoroquinolone antiinfective

MECHANISM OF ACTION
A quinolone that inhibits DNA gyrase in susceptible microorganisms, interfering with bacterial cell replication and repair. **Therapeutic Effect:** Bactericidal.

USES
Treatment of adult UTIs (including complicated) caused by *E. coli, E. cloacae, P. mirabilis, K. pneumoniae,* group D strep, indole-positive Proteus, *C. freundii, S. aureus;* sexually transmitted disease caused by *N. gonorrhoeae;* prostatitis caused by *E. coli*

PHARMACOKINETICS
PO: Peak 1 hr, steady state 2 days, half-life 3–4 hr; excreted in urine as active drug, metabolites

INDICATIONS AND DOSAGES
▶ **UTIs**
PO
Adults, Elderly. 400 mg twice a day for 7–21 days.
▶ **Prostatitis**
PO
Adults. 400 mg twice a day for 28 days.
▶ **Uncomplicated Gonococcal Infections**
PO
Adults. 800 mg as a single dose.
▶ **Dosage in Renal Impairment**
Dosage and frequency are modified on the basis of creatinine clearance.

Creatinine Clearance	Dosage
30 ml/min or higher	400 mg twice a day
Less than 30 ml/min	400 mg once a day

SIDE EFFECTS/ADVERSE REACTIONS
Frequent
Nausea, headache, dizziness
Rare
Vomiting, diarrhea, dry mouth, bitter taste, nervousness, drowsiness, insomnia, photosensitivity, tinnitus, crystalluria, rash, fever, seizures

PRECAUTIONS AND CONTRAINDICATIONS
Children younger than 18 yr because of risk of arthropathy; hypersensitivity to norfloxacin, other quinolones, or their components

Caution
Children, renal disease, seizure disorders, tendon rupture in shoulder, hand, and Achilles tendons

DRUG INTERACTIONS OF CONCERN TO DENTISTRY
• Decreased absorption: sodium bicarbonate

SERIOUS REACTIONS
! Superinfection, anaphylaxis, Stevens-Johnson syndrome, and arthropathy occur rarely.
! Hypersensitivity reactions, including photosensitivity (as evidenced by rash, pruritus, blisters, edema, and burning skin), have occurred in patients receiving fluoroquinolones.

DENTAL CONSIDERATIONS
General:
• Assess salivary flow as a factor in caries, periodontal disease, and candidiasis.
• Determine why the patient is taking the drug.
• Because of drug interaction, do not use ingestible sodium bicarbonate products, such as the Prophy-Jet air polishing system, until 2 hr after drug use.
• Avoid dental light in patient's eyes; offer dark glasses for patient comfort.
• Ruptures of the shoulder, hand, and Achilles tendons that required surgical repair or resulted in prolonged disability have been reported with this drug.
Consultations:
• Consult with patient's physician if an acute dental infection occurs and another antiinfective is required.
Teach Patient/Family to:
• Avoid mouth rinses with high alcohol content because of drying effects

• Discontinue treatment and inform dentist immediately if patient experiences pain or inflammation of a tendon, and to rest and refrain from exercise

norgestrel
nor-jes´-trel
(Ovrette)

CATEGORY AND SCHEDULE
Pregnancy Risk Category: X

Drug Class: Progesterone derivative

MECHANISM OF ACTION
A progestin that inhibits secretion of pituitary gonadotropin (LH), which prevents follicular maturation and ovulation. ***Therapeutic Effect:*** Transforms endometrium from proliferative to secretory in an estrogen-primed endometrium, promotes mammary gland development, relaxes uterine smooth muscle.

USES
Oral contraception

PHARMACOKINETICS
Well absorbed from the GI tract. Widely distributed. Protein binding: 97%. Metabolized in liver via reduction and conjugation. Primarily excreted in urine. ***Half-life:*** 20 hr.

INDICATIONS AND DOSAGES
▶ **Contraception, Female**
PO
Adults. 0.075 mg/day.

SIDE EFFECTS/ADVERSE REACTIONS
Frequent
Breakthrough bleeding or spotting at beginning of therapy, amenorrhea,

change in menstrual flow, breast tenderness
Occasional
Edema, weight gain or loss, rash, pruritus, photosensitivity, skin pigmentation
Rare
Pain or swelling at injection site, acne, mental depression, alopecia, hirsutism

PRECAUTIONS AND CONTRAINDICATIONS
Hypersensitivity to norgestrel or any component of the formulation, hypersensitivity to tartrazine, thromboembolic disorders, severe hepatic disease; breast cancer; undiagnosed vaginal bleeding, pregnancy
Caution
Lactation, hypertension, asthma, blood dyscrasias, gallbladder disease, CHF, diabetes mellitus, bone disease, depression, migraine headache, convulsive disorders, hepatic disease, renal disease, family history of breast or reproductive tract cancer

DRUG INTERACTIONS OF CONCERN TO DENTISTRY
• Decreased effectiveness of oral contraceptives: antibiotics, barbiturates

SERIOUS REACTIONS
! Thrombophlebitis, cerebrovascular disorders, retinal thrombosis, and pulmonary embolism occur rarely.

DENTAL CONSIDERATIONS
General:
• Place on frequent recall to evaluate gingival inflammation, if present.
• Increased incidence of dry socket has been reported after extraction.
• Monitor vital signs at each appointment.

Teach Patient/Family to:
• Use effective oral hygiene to prevent periodontal inflammation
• Quit smoking because it decreases risk of serious and adverse cardiovascular side effects
• Use an additional method of birth control while undergoing antibiotic therapy

nortriptyline hydrochloride
nor-trip´-ti-leen high-droh-klor´-ide (Allegron[AUS], Apo-Nortriptyline[CAN], Aventyl, Norventyl, Novo-Nortriptyline [CAN], Pamelor)
Do not confuse nortriptyline with amitriptyline, or aventyl with ambenyl or bentyl.

CATEGORY AND SCHEDULE
Pregnancy Risk Category: D

Drug Class:
Antidepressant–tricyclic

MECHANISM OF ACTION
A tricyclic antidepressant that blocks reuptake of the neurotransmitters norepinephrine and serotonin at neuronal presynaptic membranes, increasing their availability at postsynaptic receptor sites.
Therapeutic Effect: Relieves depression.

USES
Treatment of major depression

PHARMACOKINETICS
Well absorbed from the GI tract. Protein binding: 86%–95%. Metabolized in the liver. Primarily excreted in urine. *Half-life:* 17.6 hr.

INDICATIONS AND DOSAGES
▸ **Depression**
PO
Adults. 75–100 mg/day in
1–4 divided doses until therapeutic
response is achieved. Reduce dosage
gradually to effective maintenance
level.
Elderly. Initially, 10–25 mg at
bedtime. May increase by 25 mg
every 3–7 days. Maximum:
150 mg/day.
Children 12 yr and older.
30–50 mg/day in 3–4 divided doses.
Maximum: 150 mg/day.
Children 6–11 yr. 10–20 mg/day in
3–4 divided doses.
▸ **Enuresis**
PO
Children 12 yr and older.
25–35 mg/day.
Children 8–11 yr. 10–20 mg/day.
Children 6–7 yr. 10 mg/day.

SIDE EFFECTS/ADVERSE REACTIONS
Frequent
Somnolence, fatigue, dry mouth,
blurred vision, constipation, delayed
micturition, orthostatic hypotension,
diaphoresis, impaired concentration,
increased appetite, urine retention
Occasional
GI disturbances (nausea, GI distress,
metallic taste), photosensitivity
Rare
Paradoxic reactions (agitation,
restlessness, nightmares, insomnia),
extrapyramidal symptoms
(particularly fine hand tremors)

PRECAUTIONS AND CONTRAINDICATIONS
Acute recovery period after MI, use
within 14 days of MAOIs
Caution
Suicidal patients, severe depression,
increased intraocular pressure,
narrow-angle glaucoma, urinary
retention, cardiac disease, hepatic
disease, hyperthyroidism,
electroshock therapy, elective
surgery, MAOIs

DRUG INTERACTIONS OF CONCERN TO DENTISTRY
• Increased anticholinergic effects:
muscarinic blockers, antihistamines,
phenothiazines
• Increased effects of direct-acting
sympathomimetics (epinephrine,
levonordefrin)
• Potential risk of increased CNS
depression: alcohol, barbiturates,
benzodiazepines, and other CNS
depressants
• Decreased antihypertensive effect:
clonidine, guanadrel, guanethidine
• Avoid concurrent use with
St. John's wort (herb)

SERIOUS REACTIONS
! Overdose may produce seizures;
cardiovascular effects, such as severe
orthostatic hypotension, dizziness,
tachycardia, palpitations, and
arrhythmias; and altered temperature
regulation, such as hyperpyrexia or
hypothermia.
! Abrupt discontinuation after
prolonged therapy may produce
headache, malaise, nausea, vomiting,
and vivid dreams.

DENTAL CONSIDERATIONS
General:
• Take vital signs at every
appointment because of
cardiovascular side effects.
• Assess salivary flow as a factor in
caries, periodontal disease, and
candidiasis.
• Patients on chronic drug therapy
may rarely have symptoms of blood
dyscrasias, which can include
infection, bleeding, and poor healing.

• After supine positioning, have patient sit upright for at least 2 min before standing to avoid orthostatic hypotension.
• Use vasoconstrictors with caution, in low doses, and with careful aspiration. Avoid use of gingival retraction cord with epinephrine.
• Place on frequent recall because of oral side effects.

Consultations:
• In patients with symptoms of blood dyscrasias, request a medical consultation for blood studies and postpone dental treatment until normal values are reestablished.
• Medical consultation may be required to assess disease control.
• Physician should be informed if significant xerostomic side effects occur (e.g., increased caries, sore tongue, problems eating or swallowing, difficulty wearing prosthesis) so that a medication change can be considered.

Teach Patient/Family to:
• Use effective oral hygiene to prevent soft tissue inflammation
• Use caution to prevent injury when using oral hygiene aids
• When chronic dry mouth occurs, advise patient to:
  • Avoid mouth rinses with high alcohol content because of drying effects
  • Use daily home fluoride products for anticaries effect
  • Use sugarless gum, frequent sips of water, or saliva substitutes

nystatin
nye-stat´-in
(Mycostatin, Nilstat[CAN], Nyaderm, Nystop)
Do not confuse nystatin or mycostatin with nitrostat.

CATEGORY AND SCHEDULE
Pregnancy Risk Category: C

Drug Class: Antifungal

MECHANISM OF ACTION
A fungistatic antifungal that binds to sterols in the fungal cell membrane. ***Therapeutic Effect:*** Increases fungal cell-membrane permeability, allowing loss of potassium and other cellular components.

USES
Treatment of *Candida* species causing oral, vaginal, intestinal infections

PHARMACOKINETICS
PO: Poorly absorbed from the GI tract. Eliminated unchanged in feces. Topical: Not absorbed systemically from intact skin.

INDICATIONS AND DOSAGES
▸ **Intestinal Infections**
PO
Adults, Elderly. 500,000–1,000,000 units q8h.
▸ **Oral Candidiasis**
PO
Adults, Elderly, Children. 400,000–600,000 units 4 times a day.
Infants. 200,000 units 4 times a day.
▸ **Vaginal Infections**
Vaginal
Adults, Elderly, Adolescents. 1 tablet/day at bedtime for 14 days.

▸ **Cutaneous Candidal Infections**
Topical
Adults, Elderly, Children. Apply
2–4 times a day.

SIDE EFFECTS/ADVERSE REACTIONS
Occasional
PO: None known
Topical: Skin irritation
Vaginal: Vaginal irritation

PRECAUTIONS AND CONTRAINDICATIONS
Hypersensitivity

SERIOUS REACTIONS
! High dosages of oral form may produce nausea, vomiting, diarrhea, and GI distress.

DENTAL CONSIDERATIONS
General:
• Determine why the patient is taking the drug.
• Broad-spectrum antibiotic may contribute to oral Candida infections.
Teach Patient/Family to:
• Complete entire course of medication
• Not use commercial mouthwashes for mouth infection unless prescribed by dentist
• Soak full or partial dentures in a suitable antifungal solution nightly
• Prevent reinoculation of *Candida* infection by disposing of toothbrush or other contaminated oral hygiene devices used during period of infection

N

octreotide acetate

ok-tree´-oh-tide ass´-ih-tate
(Sandostatin, Sandostatin LAR)
Do not confuse octreotide with
OctreoScan, or Sandostatin with
Sandimmune or Sandoglobulin.

CATEGORY AND SCHEDULE

Pregnancy Risk Category: B

Drug Class: Secretory inhibitor,
growth hormone suppressant

MECHANISM OF ACTION

An antidiarrheal and growth
hormone suppressant that suppresses
the secretion of serotonin and
gastroenteropancreatic peptides and
enhances fluid and electrolyte
absorption from the GI tract.
Therapeutic Effect: Prolongs
intestinal transit time.

USES

Treatment of severe diarrhea and
other symptoms that occur with
certain intestinal tumors

PHARMACOKINETICS

Route	Onset	Peak	Duration
Subcutaneous	N/A	N/A	Up to 12 hr

Rapidly and completely absorbed
from injection site. Excreted in urine.
Removed by hemodialysis.
Half-life: 1.5 hr.

INDICATIONS AND DOSAGES

▸ **Diarrhea**
IV (Sandostatin)
Adults, Elderly. Initially, 50–100 mcg
q8h. May increase by 100 mcg/dose
q48h. Maximum: 500 mcg q8h.
Subcutaneous (Sandostatin)
Adults, Elderly. 50 mcg 1–2 times
a day.

IV, Subcutaneous (Sandostatin)
Children. 1–10 mcg/kg q12h.
▸ **Carcinoid Tumors**
IV, Subcutaneous (Sandostatin)
Adults, Elderly. 100–600 mcg/day in
2–4 divided doses.
IM (Sandostatin LAR)
Adults, Elderly. 20 mg q4wk.
▸ **Vipomas**
IV, Subcutaneous (Sandostatin)
Adults, Elderly. 200–300 mcg/day in
2–4 divided doses.
IM (Sandostatin LAR)
Adults, Elderly. 20 mg q4wk.
▸ **Esophageal Varices**
IV (Sandostatin)
Adults, Elderly. Bolus of 25–50 mcg
followed by IV infusion of
25–50 mcg/hr.
▸ **Acromegaly**
IV, Subcutaneous (Sandostatin)
Adults, Elderly. 50 mcg 3 times a
day. Increase as needed. Maximum:
500 mcg 3 times a day.
▸ **Acromegaly**
IM (Sandostatin LAR)
Adults, Elderly. 20 mg q4wk for
3 mo. Maximum: 40 mg q4wk.

SIDE EFFECTS/ADVERSE REACTIONS

Frequent
Diarrhea, nausea, abdominal
discomfort, headache, injection
site pain
Occasional
Vomiting, flatulence, constipation,
alopecia, facial flushing, pruritus,
dizziness, fatigue, arrhythmias,
ecchymosis, blurred vision
Rare
Depression, diminished libido,
vertigo, palpitations, dyspnea

PRECAUTIONS AND CONTRAINDICATIONS

None known

DRUG INTERACTIONS OF CONCERN TO DENTISTRY
• May cause decrease in vitamin B$_{12}$ levels

SERIOUS REACTIONS
! Patients using octreotide may develop cholelithiasis or, with prolonged high dosages, hypothyroidism.
! GI bleeding, hepatitis, and seizures occur rarely.

DENTAL CONSIDERATIONS
General:
• This drug is administered in several disease states; determine patient's medical and drug history and exact use to accurately plan patient management.
• Monitor and record vital signs.
• Consider semisupine chair position for patient comfort if GI side effects occur.
• Question patient about tolerance of NSAIDs or aspirin related to GI disease.
• This drug may be used in the hospital or on an outpatient basis. Confirm the patient's disease and treatment status.
• Patient may need assistance in getting into and out of dental chair. Adjust chair position for patient comfort.
• Examine for oral manifestation of opportunistic infection.
Consultations:
• Medical consultation may be required to assess disease control and patient's ability to tolerate stress.
Teach Patient/Family to:
• Use effective oral hygiene to prevent soft tissue inflammation
• Prevent trauma when using oral hygiene aids

• Use electric tooth brush if patient has difficulty holding conventional devices
• Update health and medication history if physician makes any changes in evaluation or drug regimens; include OTC, herbal, and nonherbal drugs in the update

ofloxacin
o-flox´-ah-sin
(Apo-Oflox[CAN], Floxin, Floxin Otic, Ocuflox)
Do not confuse Floxin with Flexeril or Flexon, or Ocuflox with Ocufen.

CATEGORY AND SCHEDULE
Pregnancy Risk Category: C

Drug Class: Fluoroquinolone antiinfective

MECHANISM OF ACTION
A fluoroquinolone antibiotic that inhibits DNA gyrase in susceptible microorganisms, interfering with bacterial cell replication and repair. **Therapeutic Effect:** Bactericidal.

USES
Treatment of lower respiratory tract infections (pneumonia, bronchitis), genitourinary infections (prostatitis, UTIs) caused by E. coli, K. pneumoniae, C. trachomatis, N. gonorrhoeae; skin and skin-structure infections

PHARMACOKINETICS
Rapidly and well absorbed from the GI tract. Protein binding: 20%–25%. Widely distributed (including to CSF). Metabolized in the liver. Primarily excreted in urine. Removed by hemodialysis. **Half-life:** 4.7–7 hr (increased in impaired renal function, cirrhosis, and the elderly).

INDICATIONS AND DOSAGES

▶ **UTIs**

PO, IV

Adults. 200 mg q12h.

▶ **Pelvic Inflammatory Disease (PID)**

PO

Adults. 400 mg q12h for 10–14 days.

▶ **Lower Respiratory Tract, Skin and Skin-Structure Infections**

PO, IV

Adults. 400 mg q12h for 10 days.

▶ **Prostatitis, Sexually Transmitted Diseases (Cervicitis, Urethritis)**

PO

Adults. 300 mg q12h.

▶ **Prostatitis**

IV

Adults. 300 mg q12h.

▶ **Sexually Transmitted Diseases**

IV

Adults. 400 mg as a single dose.

▶ **Acute, Uncomplicated Gonorrhea**

PO

Adults. 400 mg 1 time.

▶ **Usual Elderly Dosage**

PO

Elderly. 200–400 mg q12–24h for 7 days up to 6 wk.

▶ **Bacterial Conjunctivitis**

Ophthalmic

Adults, Elderly. 1–2 drops q2–4h for 2 days, then 4 times a day for 5 days.

▶ **Corneal Ulcers**

Ophthalmic

Adults. 1–2 drops q30min while awake for 2 days, then q60min while awake for 5–7 days, then 4 times a day.

▶ **Acute Otitis Media**

Otic

Children 1–12 yr. 5 drops into the affected ear 2 times a day for 10 days.

▶ **Otitis Externa**

Otic

Adults, Elderly, Children 12 yr and older. 10 drops into the affected ear once a day for 7 days.

Children 6 mo–11 yr. 5 drops into the affected ear once a day for 7 days.

▶ **Dosage in Renal Impairment**

After a normal initial dose, dosage and frequency are based on creatinine clearance.

Creatinine Clearance	Adjusted Dose	Dosage Interval
Greater than 50 ml/min	None	q12h
10–50 ml/min	None	q24h
Less than 10 ml/min	½	q24h

SIDE EFFECTS/ADVERSE REACTIONS

Frequent

Nausea, headache, insomnia

Occasional

Abdominal pain, diarrhea, vomiting, dry mouth, flatulence, dizziness, fatigue, drowsiness, rash, pruritus, fever

Rare

Constipation, paraesthesia

PRECAUTIONS AND CONTRAINDICATIONS

Hypersensitivity to any quinolones

Caution

Lactation, children younger than 18 yr, elderly, renal disease, seizure disorders, excessive sunlight, tendon rupture in shoulder, hand, and Achilles tendons

DRUG INTERACTIONS OF CONCERN TO DENTISTRY

• Decreased effects: antacids
• Possible increased risk of life-threatening arrhythmias: procainamide

SERIOUS REACTIONS

! Antibiotic-associated colitis and other superinfections may occur from altered bacterial balance.

! Hypersensitivity reactions, including photosensitivity (as evidenced by rash, pruritus, blisters, edema, and burning skin), have occurred in patients receiving fluoroquinolones.

! Arthropathy (swelling, pain, and clubbing of fingers and toes, degeneration of stress-bearing portion of a joint) may occur if the drug is given to children.

DENTAL CONSIDERATIONS

General:

• Because of drug interaction, do not use ingestible sodium bicarbonate products, such as the Prophy-Jet air polishing system, until 2 hr after drug use.

• Examine for oral manifestation of opportunistic infections.

• Avoid dental light in patient's eyes; offer dark glasses for patient comfort.

• Minimize exposure to sunlight and wear sunscreen if sun exposure is planned.

• Ruptures of the shoulder, hand, and Achilles tendons that required surgical repair or resulted in prolonged disability have been reported with this drug.

Consultations:

• Consult with patient's physician if an acute dental infection occurs and another antiinfective is required.

Teach Patient/Family to:

• Use effective oral hygiene to prevent soft tissue inflammation

• Avoid mouth rinses with high alcohol content because of drying effects

• Discontinue treatment and inform dentist immediately if patient experiences pain or inflammation of a tendon, and to rest and refrain from exercise

Ofloxacin (Optic)

General:

• Avoid dental light in patient's eyes; offer dark glasses for patient comfort and safety protection during dental treatment.

Ofloxacin Otic Solution

General:

• Determine why the patient is taking the drug.

• Severity or discomfort of infection may require postponement of elective dental treatment.

Consultations:

• Consult with patient's physician if an acute dental infection occurs and another antiinfective is required.

• Medical consultation may be required to assess disease control in the patient.

Teach Patient/Family:

• When chronic dry mouth occurs, advise patient to:

  • Avoid mouth rinses with high alcohol content because of drying effects

  • Use daily home fluoride products for anticaries effect

  • Use sugarless gum, frequent sips of water, or saliva substitutes

olanzapine

oh-lan´-za-peen
(Zyprexa, Zyprexa Intramuscular, Zyprexa Zydis)
Do not confuse olanzapine with olsalazine, or Zyprexa with Zyrtec.

CATEGORY AND SCHEDULE

Pregnancy Risk Category: C

Drug Class: Antipsychotic

MECHANISM OF ACTION

A dibenzepine derivative that antagonizes α_1-adrenergic, dopamine, histamine, muscarinic, and serotonin receptors. Produces anticholinergic, histaminic, and CNS depressant effects. *Therapeutic Effect:* Diminishes manifestations of psychotic symptoms.

USES

Treatment of psychotic disorders, schizophrenia, bipolar disorder; acute manic episode in bipolar 1 disorder in combination with lithium or valproate

PHARMACOKINETICS

Well absorbed after PO administration. Protein binding: 93%. Extensively distributed throughout the body. Undergoes extensive first-pass metabolism in the liver. Excreted primarily in urine and, to a lesser extent, in feces. Not removed by dialysis. *Half-life:* 21–54 hr.

INDICATIONS AND DOSAGES

▶ **Schizophrenia**

PO

Adults. Initially, 5–10 mg once daily. May increase by 10 mg/day at 5–7 day intervals. If further adjustments are indicated, may increase by 5–10 mg/day at 7-day intervals. Range: 10–30 mg/day.
Elderly. Initially, 2.5 mg/day. May increase as indicated. Range: 2.5–10 mg/day.
Children. Initially, 2.5 mg/day. Titrate as needed up to 20 mg/day.

▶ **Bipolar Mania**

PO

Adults. Initially, 10–15 mg/day. May increase by 5 mg/day at intervals of at least 24 hr. Maximum: 20 mg/day.

Children. Initially, 2.5 mg/day. Titrate as needed up to 20 mg/day.

▶ **Dosage for Elderly or Debilitated Patients and Those Predisposed to Hypotensive Reactions**

The initial dosage for these patients is 5 mg/day.

▶ **Control Agitation in Schizophrenic or Bipolar Patients**

IM

Adults, Elderly. 2.5–10 mg. May repeat 2 hr after first dose and 4 hr after second dose. Maximum: 30 mg/day.

SIDE EFFECTS/ADVERSE REACTIONS

Frequent
Somnolence, agitation, insomnia, headache, nervousness, hostility, dizziness, rhinitis
Occasional
Anxiety, constipation, nonaggressive atypical behavior, dry mouth, weight gain, orthostatic hypotension, fever, arthralgia, restlessness, cough, pharyngitis, visual changes (dim vision)
Rare
Tachycardia; back, chest, abdominal, or extremity pain; tremors

PRECAUTIONS AND CONTRAINDICATIONS

Hypersensitivity
Caution
Lactation, paralytic ileus, elderly; combination of age, smoking, and gender (female) may increase clearance rate; neuroleptic malignant syndrome, cardiovascular disease, cerebrovascular disease, seizures, orthostatic hypotension, Alzheimer's dementia, prostate hypertrophy, glaucoma; patients should be monitored for signs and symptoms of diabetes mellitus

DRUG INTERACTIONS OF CONCERN TO DENTISTRY
• Potentiation of orthostatic hypotension: diazepam, alcohol, other CNS depressants
• Increased anticholinergic effects: anticholinergic drugs
• Suspected reduction of plasma levels: carbamazepine

SERIOUS REACTIONS
❗ Rare reactions include seizures and neuroleptic malignant syndrome, a potentially fatal syndrome characterized by hyperpyrexia, muscle rigidity, irregular pulse or B/P, tachycardia, diaphoresis, and cardiac arrhythmias.
❗ Extrapyramidal symptoms and dysphagia may also occur.
❗ Overdose (300 mg) produces drowsiness and slurred speech.

DENTAL CONSIDERATIONS
General:
• Consider semisupine chair position for patient comfort because of GI effects of drug.
• Assess salivary flow as factor in caries, periodontal disease, and candidiasis.
• Monitor vital signs at every appointment because of cardiovascular side effects.
• After supine positioning, have patient sit upright for at least 2 min before standing to avoid orthostatic hypotension.
• Patients on chronic drug therapy may rarely have symptoms of blood dyscrasias, which can include infection, bleeding, and poor healing.
• Assess for presence of extrapyramidal motor symptoms, such as tardive dyskinesia and akathisia. Extrapyramidal motor activity may complicate dental treatment.

Consultations:
• In a patient with symptoms of blood dyscrasias, request a medical consultation for blood studies and postpone dental treatment until normal values are reestablished.
• Medical consultation may be required to assess disease control.
• Physician should be informed if significant xerostomic side effects occur (e.g., increased caries, sore tongue, problems eating or swallowing, difficulty wearing prosthesis) so that a medication change can be considered.
Teach Patient/Family to:
• Use effective oral hygiene to prevent soft tissue inflammation
• Use electric tooth brush if patient has difficulty holding conventional devices
• Use caution when driving or performing other tasks requiring alertness
• When chronic dry mouth occurs, advise patient to:
  • Avoid mouth rinses with high alcohol content because of drying effects
  • Use daily home fluoride products for anticaries effect
  • Use sugarless gum, frequent sips of water, or saliva substitutes

olmesartan medoxomil
ol-mess´-er-tan
(Benicar)

CATEGORY AND SCHEDULE
Pregnancy Risk Category: C (D if used in second or third trimester)

Drug Class: Angiotensin II (AT1) receptor antagonist

MECHANISM OF ACTION

An angiotensin II receptor, type AT1, antagonist that blocks the vasoconstrictor and aldosterone-secreting effects of angiotensin II, inhibiting the binding of angiotensin II to the AT1 receptors. *Therapeutic Effect:* Causes vasodilation, decreases peripheral resistance, and decreases B/P.

USES

Treatment of hypertension, as a single drug or in combination with other antihypertensives

PHARMACOKINETICS

Rapidly and completely absorbed after PO administration. Metabolized in the liver. Recovered primarily in feces and, to a lesser extent, in urine. Not removed by hemodialysis. *Half-life:* 13 hr.

INDICATIONS AND DOSAGES

▸ **Hypertension**

PO

Adults, Elderly, Patients with mildly impaired hepatic or renal function. 20 mg once a day in patients who are not volume depleted. After 2 wk of therapy, if further reduction in B/P is necessary, may increase dosage to 40 mg/day.

SIDE EFFECTS/ADVERSE REACTIONS

Occasional
Dizziness
Rare
Headache, diarrhea, upper respiratory tract infection

PRECAUTIONS AND CONTRAINDICATIONS

Bilateral renal artery stenosis
Caution
Discontinue drug if pregnancy occurs, use in volume- or salt-depleted patients, or in nursing mothers or pediatric patients has not been established, impaired renal function, CHF, renal artery stenosis

DRUG INTERACTIONS OF CONCERN TO DENTISTRY

No significant drug interactions have been reported, but increased hypotensive effects always are possible when used with other antihypertensives or sedatives

SERIOUS REACTIONS

! Overdosage may manifest as hypotension and tachycardia. Bradycardia occurs less often.

DENTAL CONSIDERATIONS

General:
• Monitor vital signs at every appointment because of cardiovascular side effects.
• Consider semisupine chair position for patient comfort if GI side effects occur.
• Limit use of sodium-containing products, such as saline IV fluids, for patients with a dietary salt restriction.
• Stress from dental procedures may compromise cardiovascular function; determine patient risk.
• Patients with hypertensive disease may be taking more than one drug to control B/P; although not specifically noted for this drug, postural hypotension is always a possibility.
• After supine positioning, have patient sit upright for at least 2 min before standing to avoid orthostatic hypotension.
• Short appointments and a stress-reduction protocol may be required for anxious patients.
• Use precaution if sedation or general anesthesia is required; risk of hypotensive episode.
Consultations:
• Medical consultation may be required to assess disease control and patient's ability to tolerate stress.

Teach Patient/Family to:
• Update health and drug history if physician makes any changes in evaluation or drug regimens; include OTC, herbal, and nonherbal drugs in the update

olopatadine
oh-loe-pa-ta´-deen
(Patanol)

CATEGORY AND SCHEDULE
Pregnancy Risk Category: C

Drug Class: antihistamine; mast cell stabilizer

MECHANISM OF ACTION
An antihistamine that inhibits histamine release from the mast cell. *Therapeutic Effect:* Inhibits symptoms associated with allergic conjunctivitis.

USES
Allergic conjunctivitis

PHARMACOKINETICS
The time to peak concentration is less than 2 hr and duration of action is 8 hr. Minimal absorption after topical administration. Metabolized to inactive metabolites. Primarily excreted in urine. *Half-life:* 3 hr.

INDICATIONS AND DOSAGES
▶ **Allergic Conjunctivitis**
Ophthalmic
Adults, Elderly, Children 3 yr and older. 1–2 drops in affected eye(s) twice daily q6–8h.

SIDE EFFECTS/ADVERSE REACTIONS
Occasional
Headache, weakness, cold syndrome, taste perversion, burning, stinging,

dry eyes, foreign body sensation, hyperemia, keratitis, eyelid edema, itching, pharyngitis, rhinitis, sinusitis

PRECAUTIONS AND CONTRAINDICATIONS
Hypersensitivity to olopatadine hydrochloride or any other component of the formulation
Caution
Topical use only, do not use while wearing contact lenses, lactation, children younger than 3 yr

DRUG INTERACTIONS OF CONCERN TO DENTISTRY
None reported

SERIOUS REACTIONS
None reported

DENTAL CONSIDERATIONS
General:
• Protect patient's eyes from accidental spatter during dental treatment.

O

olsalazine sodium
ohl-sal´-ah-zeen soe´-dee-um
(Dipentum)
Do not confuse olsalazine with olanzapine.

CATEGORY AND SCHEDULE
Pregnancy Risk Category: C

Drug Class: Antiinflammatory, salicylate derivative

MECHANISM OF ACTION
A salicylic acid derivative that is converted to mesalamine in the colon by bacterial action.

Blocks prostaglandin production in bowel mucosa. ***Therapeutic Effect:*** Reduces colonic inflammation in inflammatory bowel disease.

USES
Maintenance of remission of ulcerative colitis in patients intolerant to sulfasalazine

PHARMACOKINETICS
PO: Partially absorbed, peak 1.5 hr. *Half-life:* 5–10 hr; excreted in urine as 5-aminosalicylic acid and metabolites; crosses placenta.

INDICATIONS AND DOSAGES
▸ **Maintenance of Controlled Ulcerative Colitis**
PO
Adults, Elderly. 1 g/day in 2 divided doses, preferably q12h.

SIDE EFFECTS/ADVERSE REACTIONS
Frequent
Headache, diarrhea, abdominal pain or cramps, nausea
Occasional
Depression, fatigue, dyspepsia, upper respiratory tract infection, decreased appetite, rash, itching, arthralgia
Rare
Dizziness, vomiting, stomatitis

PRECAUTIONS AND CONTRAINDICATIONS
History of hypersensitivity to salicylates
Caution
Lactation, impaired hepatic function, severe allergy, bronchial asthma, renal disease

SERIOUS REACTIONS
❗ Sulfite sensitivity may occur in susceptible patients, manifested by cramping, headache, diarrhea, fever, rash, hives, itching, and wheezing. Discontinue drug immediately.
❗ Excessive diarrhea associated with extreme fatigue is noted rarely.

DENTAL CONSIDERATIONS
General:
• Consider semisupine chair position for patient comfort because of GI effects of disease.
Consultations:
• Avoid drugs that could aggravate an inflammatory colon disease; consultation is recommended before selection of an antibiotic.
Teach Patient/Family to:
• Use effective oral hygiene to prevent soft tissue inflammation
• Use caution to prevent injury when using oral hygiene aids
• Avoid mouth rinses with high alcohol content because of drying effects

omalizumab
oh-mah-liz´-uw-mab
(Xolair)

CATEGORY AND SCHEDULE
Pregnancy Risk Category: B

Drug Class: Anti-Ig E monoclonal antibody

MECHANISM OF ACTION
A monoclonal antibody that selectively binds to human immunoglobulin E (IgE), preventing it from binding to the surface of mast cells and basophils. ***Therapeutic Effect:*** Prevents or reduces the number of asthmatic attacks.

USES
Reduction of asthma exacerbation in patients with moderate to severe asthma who have a positive skin test or in vitro reactivity to a perennial aeroallergen not adequately controlled by inhaled glucocorticoids

PHARMACOKINETICS
Absorbed slowly after subcutaneous administration, with peak concentration in 7–8 days. Excreted in the liver, reticuloendothelial system, and endothelial cells. *Half-life:* 26 days.

INDICATIONS AND DOSAGES
▸ **Moderate to Severe Persistent Asthma in Patients Who Are Reactive to a Perennial Allergen and Whose Asthma Symptoms Have Been Inadequately Controlled with Inhaled Corticosteroids**
Subcutaneous
Adults, Elderly, Children 12 yr and older. 150–375 mg every 2 or 4 wk; dose and dosing frequency are individualized on the basis of weight and pretreatment immunoglobulin E (IgE) level (as shown below).
▸ **4-wk Dosing Table**

Pretreatment Serum IgE Levels (units/ml)	Weight 30–60 kg	Weight 61–70 kg	Weight 71–90 kg	Weight 91–150 kg
30 to 100	150 mg	150 mg	150 mg	300 mg
101–200	300 mg	300 mg	300 mg	See next table
201–300	300 mg	See next table	See next table	See next table

▸ **2-week Dosing Table**

Pretreatment Serum IgE Levels (units/ml)	Weight 30–60 kg	Weight 61–70 kg	Weight 71–90 kg	Weight 91–150 kg
101–200	See preceding table	See preceding table	See preceding table	225 mg
201–300	See preceding table	225 mg	225 mg	300 mg
301–400	225 mg	225 mg	300 mg	Do not dose
401–500	300 mg	300 mg	375 mg	Do not dose
501–600	300 mg	375 mg	Do not dose	Do not dose
601–700	375 mg	Do not dose	Do not dose	Do not dose

SIDE EFFECTS/ADVERSE REACTIONS
Frequent
Injection site ecchymosis, redness, warmth, stinging, and urticaria; viral infections; sinusitis; headache; pharyngitis
Occasional
Arthralgia, leg pain, fatigue, dizziness
Rare
Arm pain, earache, dermatitis, pruritus

PRECAUTIONS AND CONTRAINDICATIONS
Hypersensitivity
Caution
Possible risk of malignancy, anaphylactic reactions, not for acute asthma or status asthmaticus, do not abruptly discontinue glucocorticoid therapy, use in nursing mothers or children younger than 12 yr has not been established

O

DRUG INTERACTIONS OF CONCERN TO DENTISTRY
None reported

SERIOUS REACTIONS
! Anaphylaxis occurs within 2 hr of the first dose or subsequent doses in 0.1% of patients.
! Malignant neoplasms occur in 0.5% of patients.

DENTAL CONSIDERATIONS
General:
• Determine why patient is taking the drug.
• Be aware of patient's disease, its severity, and its frequency, when known.
• Question patient about other medications used for asthma or to prevent bronchoconstriction.
• Avoid drugs that may aggravate asthma.
• Short appointments and a stress reduction protocol may be required for anxious patients.
• Have patient bring personal short-acting bronchodilator to appointment for use in emergency.
• Acute asthmatic episodes may be precipitated in the dental office. Rapid-acting sympathomimetic inhalants should be available for emergency use. A stress-reduction protocol may be required.
Consultations:
• Consultation with physician may be necessary if sedation or general anesthesia is required.
• Medical consultation may be required to assess disease control and patient's ability to tolerate stress.
Teach Patient/Family to:
• Use effective oral hygiene to prevent soft tissue inflammation/infection
• Update health and drug history and report changes in health status,

drug regimen, or disease/treatment status

omeprazole
oh-mep´-rah-zole
(Losec[CAN], Maxor[AUS], Prilosec, Prilosec OTC, Probitor[AUS], Zegerid)
Do not confuse Prilosec with prilocaine, Prinivil, or Prozac.

CATEGORY AND SCHEDULE
Pregnancy Risk Category: C

Drug Class: Antisecretory, proton pump inhibitor

MECHANISM OF ACTION
A benzimidazole that is converted to active metabolites that irreversibly bind to and inhibit hydrogen-potassium adenosine triphosphatase, an enzyme on the surface of gastric parietal cells. Inhibits hydrogen ion transport into gastric lumen.
Therapeutic Effect: Increases gastric pH, reduces gastric acid production.

USES
Treatment of gastroesophageal reflux disease (GERD), severe erosive esophagitis, poorly responsive systemic GERD, pathologic hypersecretory conditions (Zollinger-Ellison syndrome, systemic mastocytosis, multiple endocrine adenomas), with clarithromycin, short-term treatment of gastric ulcers; not approved for long-term ulcer maintenance therapy

PHARMACOKINETICS

Route	Onset	Peak	Duration
PO	1 hr	2 hr	72 hr

Rapidly absorbed from the GI tract. Protein binding: 99%. Primarily distributed into gastric parietal cells. Metabolized extensively in the liver. Primarily excreted in urine. Unknown if removed by hemodialysis. *Half-life:* 0.5–1 hr (increased in patients with hepatic impairment).

INDICATIONS AND DOSAGES
▶ **Erosive Esophagitis, Poorly Responsive GERD, Active Duodenal Ulcer, Prevention and Treatment of NSAID-Induced Ulcers**
PO
Adults, Elderly. 20 mg/day.
▶ **To Maintain Healing of Erosive Esophagitis**
PO
Adults, Elderly. 20 mg/day.
▶ **Pathologic Hypersecretory Conditions**
PO
Adults, Elderly. Initially, 60 mg/day up to 120 mg 3 times a day.
▶ **Duodenal Ulcer Caused by *H. Pylori***
PO
Adults, Elderly. 20 mg twice a day for 10 days.
▶ **Active Benign Gastric Ulcer**
PO
Adults, Elderly. 40 mg/day for 4–8 wk.
▶ **Usual Pediatric Dosage**
Children older than 2 yr, weighing 20 kg and more. 20 mg/day.
Children older than 2 yr, weighing less than 20 kg. 10 mg/day.

SIDE EFFECTS/ADVERSE REACTIONS
Frequent
Headache
Occasional
Diarrhea, abdominal pain, nausea

Rare
Dizziness, asthenia or loss of strength, vomiting, constipation, upper respiratory tract infection, back pain, rash, cough

PRECAUTIONS AND CONTRAINDICATIONS
Hypersensitivity
Caution
Lactation, children

DRUG INTERACTIONS OF CONCERN TO DENTISTRY
• Increased serum levels: diazepam

SERIOUS REACTIONS
None known

DENTAL CONSIDERATIONS
General:
• Question the patient about tolerance of NSAIDs or aspirin related to GI problem.
• Consider semisupine chair position for patient comfort because of GI effects of disease.
• Assess salivary flow as a factor in caries, periodontal disease, and candidiasis.
Teach Patient/Family to:
• Use caution to prevent injury when using oral hygiene aids
• When chronic dry mouth occurs, advise patient to:
   • Avoid mouth rinses with high alcohol content because of drying effects
   • Use daily home fluoride products to prevent caries
   • Use sugarless gum, frequent sips of water, or saliva substitutes

O

oprelvekin (interleukin-2, IL-2)

oh-prel´-vee-kinn
(Neumega)
Do not confuse Neumega with Neupogen.

CATEGORY AND SCHEDULE

Schedule IV
Pregnancy Risk Category: C

Drug Class: Hematopoietic; platelet growth factor

MECHANISM OF ACTION

A hematopoietic that stimulates production of blood platelets, essential to the blood-clotting process. *Therapeutic Effect:* Increases platelet production.

USES

Prevention of low platelet counts caused by treatment with some cancer medicines

PHARMACOKINETICS

Peak 3.2 hr following single subcutaneous dose. *Half-life:* 6.9 hr. Rapidly excreted by the kidneys.

INDICATIONS AND DOSAGES

▶ **Prevention of Thrombocytopenia**
Subcutaneous
Adults. 50 mcg/kg once a day.
Children. 75–100 mcg/kg once a day.
Continue for 14–28 days or until platelet count reaches 50,000 cells/mcl after its nadir.

SIDE EFFECTS/ADVERSE REACTIONS

Frequent
Nausea or vomiting, fluid retention, neutropenic fever, diarrhea, rhinitis, headache, dizziness, fever, insomnia,
cough, rash, pharyngitis, tachycardia, vasodilation

PRECAUTIONS AND CONTRAINDICATIONS

None known.

DRUG INTERACTIONS OF CONCERN TO DENTISTRY

No data available

SERIOUS REACTIONS

❗ Transient atrial fibrillation or flutter occurs in 10% of patients and may be caused by increased plasma volume; oprelvekin is not directly arrhythmogenic. Arrhythmias are usually brief in duration and convert spontaneously to normal sinus rhythm.
❗ Papilledema may occur in children.

DENTAL CONSIDERATIONS

General:
• If bleeding problem has not been diagnosed; refer for evaluation prior to any dental treatment.
• Question patient about medical and drug history in relationship to bleeding problems.
• Provide dental treatment in conjunction with hematologist.
• Patients may present with localized gingival bleeding with incomplete clotting.
• Avoid elective dental procedures if severe neutropenia (more than 500 cells/mm³) or thrombocytopenia (fewer than 50,000 cells/mm³) is present.
• Avoid products that affect platelet function, such as aspirin and NSAIDs.
• Monitor and record vital signs.
• Consider local hemostasis measures to prevent excessive bleeding.

- Short appointments and a stress-reduction protocol may be required for anxious patients.
- Place on frequent recall to evaluate healing response

Consultations:
- Consultation with hematologist or physician of record required.
- Medical consultation should include routine blood counts, including platelet counts and bleeding time.
- Consultation with physician may be necessary if sedation or general anesthesia is required.
- In a patient with symptoms of blood dyscrasias, request a medical consultation for blood studies and postpone treatment until normal values are reestablished.
- Medical consultation should include PPT, PT, or INR.

Teach Patient/Family to:
- Use soft tooth brush to prevent trauma to oral tissues and risk of bleeding
- Use effective oral hygiene to prevent soft tissue inflammation
- Report oral lesions, soreness, or bleeding to dentist
- Update health and medication history if physician makes any changes in evaluation or drug regimens; include OTC, herbal, and nonherbal drugs in the update
- Prevent trauma when using oral hygiene aids

orlistat
ohr´-lih-stat
(Xenical)
Do not confuse Xenical with Xeloda.

CATEGORY AND SCHEDULE
Pregnancy Risk Category: B

Drug Class: Antiobesity

MECHANISM OF ACTION
A gastric and pancreatic lipase inhibitor that inhibits absorption of dietary fats by inactivating gastric and pancreatic enzymes. *Therapeutic Effect:* Resulting caloric deficit may positively affect weight control.

USES
Obesity management, including weight loss and maintenance in conjunction with a reduced-calorie diet; used in patients with a defined body mass index with other risk factors for cardiovascular disease

PHARMACOKINETICS
Minimal absorption after administration. Protein binding: 99%. Primarily eliminated unchanged in feces. Unknown if removed by hemodialysis. *Half-life:* 1–2 hr.

INDICATIONS AND DOSAGES
▶ Weight Reduction
PO
Adults, Elderly, Children 12–16 yr.
120 mg 3 times a day.

SIDE EFFECTS/ADVERSE REACTIONS
Frequent
Headache, abdominal discomfort, flatulence, fecal urgency, fatty or oily stool
Occasional
Back pain, menstrual irregularity, nausea, fatigue, diarrhea, dizziness
Rare
Anxiety, rash, myalgia, dry skin, vomiting

PRECAUTIONS AND CONTRAINDICATIONS
Cholestasis, chronic malabsorption syndrome
Caution
Adherence to dietary guidelines, supplemental fat-soluble vitamins

may be required along with betacarotene, nephrolithiasis, use in children not established

DRUG INTERACTIONS OF CONCERN TO DENTISTRY
None reported

SERIOUS REACTIONS
None known

General:
• Although no dental drug interactions are reported, observe expected outcomes of systemically administered drugs.
• Severely obese patients may have Type 2 diabetes or cardiovascular diseases.
• Consider semisupine chair position for patient comfort if GI side effects occur.
• Ensure that patient is following prescribed diet and regularly takes medication.

Consultations:
• Medical consultation may be required to assess disease control.

Teach Patient/Family to:
• Update health and drug history if physician makes any changes in evaluation or drug regimens; include OTC, herbal, and nonherbal drugs in the update

orphenadrine
or-fen´-ah-dreen
(Norflex, Orphenace[CAN], Rhoxal-orphenadrine[CAN])

CATEGORY AND SCHEDULE
Pregnancy Risk Category: C

Drug Class: Skeletal muscle relaxant

MECHANISM OF ACTION
A skeletal muscle relaxant that is structurally related to diphenhydramine and is thought to indirectly affect skeletal muscle by central atropine-like effects.
Therapeutic Effect: Relieves musculoskeletal pain.

USES
Treatment of pain in musculoskeletal conditions

PHARMACOKINETICS
Well absorbed after PO and IM absorption. Protein binding: low. Metabolized in liver. Primarily excreted in urine and feces.
Half-life: 14 hr.

INDICATIONS AND DOSAGES
▶ **Musculoskeletal Pain**
IM/IV
Adults, Elderly. 60 mg 2 times a day. Switch to oral form for maintenance.
PO
Adults, Elderly. 100 mg 2 times a day.

SIDE EFFECTS/ADVERSE REACTIONS
Frequent
Drowsiness, dizziness, muscular weakness, hypotension, dry mouth, nose, throat, and lips, urinary retention, thickening of bronchial secretions
Elderly: Sedation, dizziness, hypotension
Occasional
Elderly: Flushing, visual or hearing disturbances, paresthesia, diaphoresis, chill

PRECAUTIONS AND CONTRAINDICATIONS
Angle-closure glaucoma, myasthenia gravis, pyloric or duodenal

obstruction, stenosing peptic ulcer, prostatic hypertrophy, obstruction of the bladder neck, achalasia, cardiospasm (megaesophagus), hypersensitivity to orphenadrine or any component of the formulation
Caution
Children, cardiac disease, tachycardia, caution in lactation

DRUG INTERACTIONS OF CONCERN TO DENTISTRY

- Increased CNS effects: propoxyphene, CNS depressants, alcohol
- Increased anticholinergic effect: other anticholinergics

SERIOUS REACTIONS

❗ Hypersensitivity reaction, such as eczema, pruritus, rash, cardiac disturbances, and photosensitivity, may occur.
❗ Overdosage may vary from CNS depression, including sedation, apnea, hypotension, cardiovascular collapse, or death, to severe paradoxical reaction, such as hallucinations, tremors, and seizures.

DENTAL CONSIDERATIONS

General:
- Consider semisupine chair position for patients with back pain.
- Patients on chronic drug therapy may rarely have symptoms of blood dyscrasias, which can include infection, bleeding, and poor healing.
- Assess salivary flow as a factor in caries, periodontal disease, and candidiasis.

Consultations:
- In a patient with symptoms of blood dyscrasias, request a medical consultation for blood studies and postpone dental treatment until normal values are reestablished.

- Medical consultation may be required to assess disease control.

Teach Patient/Family to:
- Use effective oral hygiene to prevent soft tissue inflammation
- Use caution to prevent injury when using oral hygiene aids
- Use caution when driving or operating equipment because of risk of dizziness
- When chronic dry mouth occurs, advise patient to:
  - Avoid mouth rinses with high alcohol content because of drying effects
  - Use daily home fluoride products to prevent caries
  - Use sugarless gum, frequent sips of water, or saliva substitutes

oseltamivir
ah-suhl-tahm´-ah-veer
(Tamiflu)

CATEGORY AND SCHEDULE
Pregnancy Risk Category: C

Drug Class: Antiviral

MECHANISM OF ACTION
A selective inhibitor of influenza virus neuraminidase, an enzyme essential for viral replication. Acts against both influenza A and B viruses. *Therapeutic Effect:* Suppresses the spread of infection within the respiratory system and reduces the duration of clinical symptoms.

USES
Treatment of uncomplicated acute illness caused by influenza infection in adults who have been symptomatic for no more than 2 days; more effective against influenza type A virus;

prophylaxis for adults and children older than 13 yr

PHARMACOKINETICS

Readily absorbed. Protein binding: 3%. Extensively converted to active drug in the liver. Primarily excreted in urine. *Half-life:* 6–10 hr.

INDICATIONS AND DOSAGES

▶ **Influenza**
PO
Adults, Elderly. 75 mg 2 times a day for 5 days.
Children weighing more than 40 kg. 75 mg twice a day.
Children weighing 24–40 kg. 60 mg twice a day.
Children weighing 15–23 kg. 45 mg twice a day.
Children weighing less than 15 kg. 30 mg twice a day.
▶ **Prevention of Influenza**
PO
Adults, Elderly. 75 mg once a day.
▶ **Dosage in Renal Impairment**
PO
Adults, Elderly. Dosage is decreased to 75 mg once a day for at least 7 days and possibly up to 6 wk.

SIDE EFFECTS/ADVERSE REACTIONS

Frequent
Nausea, vomiting, diarrhea
Occasional
Abdominal pain, bronchitis, dizziness, headache, cough, insomnia, fatigue, vertigo

PRECAUTIONS AND CONTRAINDICATIONS

Hypersensitivity
Caution
Renal impairment, lactation

DRUG INTERACTIONS OF CONCERN TO DENTISTRY

None reported

SERIOUS REACTIONS

! Colitis, pneumonia, and pyrexia occur rarely.

DENTAL CONSIDERATIONS

General:
• Acute influenza patients are unlikely to be seen in the dental office except for dental emergencies.
• Consider semisupine chair position for patient comfort because of respiratory effects of disease.

oxacillin
ox-ah-sill´-in

CATEGORY AND SCHEDULE
Pregnancy Risk Category: B

Drug Class: Broad-spectrum antiinfective; penicillinase-resistant penicillin

MECHANISM OF ACTION
A penicillin that binds to bacterial membranes. *Therapeutic Effect:* Bactericidal.

USES
Treatment of infections caused by bacteria

PHARMACOKINETICS:
PO/IM: Peak 30–60 min, duration 4–6 hr **IV:** Peak 5 min, duration 4–6 hr. *Half-life:* 30–60 min. Metabolized in the liver; excreted in urine, bile, breast milk, crosses placenta.

INDICATIONS AND DOSAGES

▶ **Upper Respiratory Tract, Skin, and Skin-Structure Infections**

IV, IM

Adults, Elderly, Children weighing 40 kg or more. 250–500 mg q4–6h.
Children weighing less than 40 kg. 50 mg/kg/day in divided doses q6h. Maximum: 12 g/day.

▶ **Lower Respiratory Tract and Other Serious Infections**

IV, IM

Adults, Elderly, Children weighing 40 kg or more. 1 g q4–6h. Maximum: 12 g/day.
Children weighing less than 40 kg. 100 mg/kg/day in divided doses q4–6h.

SIDE EFFECTS/ADVERSE REACTIONS

Frequent

Mild hypersensitivity reaction (fever, rash, pruritus), GI effects (nausea, vomiting, diarrhea)

Occasional

Phlebitis, thrombophlebitis (more common in elderly), hepatotoxicity (with high IV dosage)

PRECAUTIONS AND CONTRAINDICATIONS

Hypersensitivity to any penicillin

DRUG INTERACTIONS OF CONCERN TO DENTISTRY

• Increased or prolonged plasma levels: probenecid
• Aminoglycosides: injections must be separated by 1 hr
• Possible decrease in antimicrobial effectiveness: tetracyclines, erythromycins, lincomycins
• Suspected increase in methotrexate toxicity
• When used for dental infection:
  • Oral contraceptives: advise patient of a potential risk for decreased contraceptive action, to maintain compliance with oral contraceptive while using antibiotics, and to consider the use of nonhormonal contraception

SERIOUS REACTIONS

! Antibiotic-associated colitis and other superinfections may result from altered bacterial balance.
! A mild to severe hypersensitivity reaction may occur in those allergic to penicillins.

DENTAL CONSIDERATIONS

General:
• Determine why patient is taking the drug.
• Caution regarding allergy to medication.

Consultations:
• Consult patient's physician if an acute dental infection occurs and another antiinfective is required.
• Medical consultation may be required to assess disease control.

Teach Patient/Family to:
• Use effective oral hygiene to prevent soft tissue inflammation
• Prevent trauma when using oral hygiene aids
• When antibiotics are used for dental infection:
  • Oral contraceptives: advise patient of a low potential risk for decreased contraceptive action, to maintain compliance with oral contraceptive use while using antibiotics, and to consider the use of additional nonhormonal contraception
  • Report sore throat, oral burning sensation, fever, or fatigue, any of which could indicate presence of a superinfection

O

oxaliplatin
ahks-al-eh-plah´-tin
(Eloxatin)

CATEGORY AND SCHEDULE
Pregnancy Risk Category: D

Drug Class: Antineoplastic;
platinum coordination complex

MECHANISM OF ACTION
A platinum-containing complex that
cross-links with DNA strands,
preventing cell division. Cell
cycle-phase nonspecific.
Therapeutic Effect: Inhibits DNA
replication.

USES
Treatment of metastatic carcinoma of
the colon or rectum in combination
with 5-FU/leucovorin

PHARMACOKINETICS
Rapidly distributed. Protein binding:
90%. Undergoes rapid, extensive
nonenzymatic biotransformation.
Excreted in urine. ***Half-life:*** 70 hr.

INDICATIONS AND DOSAGES
▶ **Metastatic Colon or Rectal Cancer
in Patients Whose Disease Has
Recurred or Progressed During or
Within 6 Mo of Completing First-Line
Therapy with Bolus 5-Fluorouracil
(5-FU), Leucovorin, and Irinotecan**
IV
Adults. Day 1: Oxaliplatin 85 mg/m^2
in 250–500 ml D5W and leucovorin
200 mg/m^2, both given
simultaneously over more than 2 hr
in separate bags using a Y-line,
followed by 5-FU 400 mg/m^2 IV
bolus given over 2–4 min, followed
by 5-FU 600 mg/m^2 in 500 ml D5W
as a 22-hr continuous IV infusion.
Day 2: Leucovorin 200 mg/m^2

IV infusion given over more than 2 hr,
followed by 5-FU 400 mg/m^2 IV
bolus given over 2–4 min, followed
by 5-FU 600 mg/m^2 in 500 ml D5W
as a 22-hr continuous IV infusion.
▶ **Ovarian Cancer**
IV
Adults. Cisplatin 100 mg/m^2 and
oxaliplatin 130 mg/m^2 every 3 wk.

SIDE EFFECTS/ADVERSE REACTIONS
Frequent
Peripheral or sensory neuropathy
(usually occurs in hands, feet,
perioral area, and throat but may
present as jaw spasm, abnormal
tongue sensation, eye pain, chest
pressure, or difficulty walking,
swallowing, or writing), nausea,
fatigue, diarrhea, vomiting,
constipation, abdominal pain, fever,
anorexia
Occasional
Stomatitis, earache, insomnia, cough,
difficulty breathing, backache, edema
Rare
Dyspepsia, dizziness, rhinitis,
flushing, alopecia

PRECAUTIONS AND CONTRAINDICATIONS
History of allergy to platinum
compounds

DRUG INTERACTIONS OF CONCERN TO DENTISTRY
None reported

SERIOUS REACTIONS
! Peripheral or sensory neuropathy
can occur, sometimes precipitated or
exacerbated by drinking or holding a
glass of cold liquid during the
IV infusion.
! Pulmonary fibrosis, characterized
by a nonproductive cough, dyspnea,
crackles, and radiologic pulmonary

infiltrates, may require drug discontinuation.

! Hypersensitivity reaction (rash, urticaria, pruritus) occurs rarely.

DENTAL CONSIDERATIONS

General:

• If additional analgesia is required for dental pain, consider alternative analgesics (NSAIDs) in patients taking narcotics for acute or chronic pain.

• Examine for oral manifestation of opportunistic infection.

• Avoid products that affect platelet function, such as aspirin and NSAIDs.

• This drug may be used in the hospital or on an outpatient basis. Confirm the patient's disease and treatment status.

• Chlorhexidine mouth rinse prior to and during chemotherapy may reduce severity of mucositis.

• Patient on chronic drug therapy may rarely present with symptoms of blood dyscrasias, which can include infection, bleeding, and poor healing. If dyscrasia is present, caution patient to prevent oral tissue trauma when using oral hygiene aids.

• Palliative medication may be required for management of oral side effects.

• Short appointments and a stress-reduction protocol may be required for anxious patients.

• Provide palliative emergency dental care during drug use.

• Patients may be at risk of bleeding; check for oral signs.

• Oral infections should be eliminated and treated aggressively.

• Monitor vital signs.

Consultations:

• Medical consultation should include routine blood counts,

including platelet counts and bleeding time.

• Consult physician; prophylactic or therapeutic antiinfectives may be indicated if surgery or periodontal treatment is required.

• Medical consultation may be required to assess immunologic status during cancer chemotherapy and determine safety risk, if any, posed by the required dental treatment.

• Medical consultation may be required to assess disease control and patient's ability to tolerate stress.

Teach Patient/Family to:

• See dentist immediately if secondary oral infection occurs

• Be aware of oral side effects

• Use effective oral hygiene to prevent soft tissue inflammation

• Report oral lesions, soreness, or bleeding to dentist

• Prevent trauma when using oral hygiene aids

• Update health and medication history if physician makes any changes in evaluation or drug regimens; include OTC, herbal, and nonherbal drugs in the update

• Avoid ice water rinses and exposure to cold to prevent exacerbation of neuropathy symptoms

oxandrolone

ox-an´-droe-lone
(Lonavar[AUS], Oxandrin)
Do not confuse with testolactone.

CATEGORY AND SCHEDULE

Pregnancy Risk Category: X
Controlled substance: Schedule III

Drug Class: Androgenic anabolic steroid

MECHANISM OF ACTION

A synthetic testosterone derivative that promotes growth and development of male sex organs, maintains secondary sex characteristics in androgen-deficient males. *Therapeutic Effect:* Androgenic and anabolic actions.

USES

Promotion of weight gain in catabolic or tissue wasting processes, such as extensive surgery, burns, infection, or trauma; HIV wasting syndrome; Turner's syndrome

PHARMACOKINETICS

Well absorbed from the GI tract. Protein binding: 94%–97%. Metabolized in liver. Primarily excreted in urine. Unknown if removed by hemodialysis. *Half-life:* 5–13 hr.

INDICATIONS AND DOSAGES
▶ **Weight Gain**

Adults, Elderly. 2.5–20 mg in divided doses 2–4 times a day usually for 2–4 wk. Course of therapy is based on individual response. Repeat intermittently as needed.
Children. Total daily dose is 0.1 mg/kg. Repeat intermittently as needed.

SIDE EFFECTS/ADVERSE REACTIONS
Frequent

Gynecomastia, acne, amenorrhea, other menstrual irregularities
Females: Hirsutism, deepening of voice, clitoral enlargement that may not be reversible when drug is discontinued
Occasional

Edema, nausea, insomnia, oligospermia, priapism, male pattern of baldness, bladder irritability, hypercalcemia in immobilized

patients or those with breast cancer, hypercholesterolemia
Rare
Polycythemia with high dosage

PRECAUTIONS AND CONTRAINDICATIONS

Nephrosis, carcinoma of breast or prostate hypercalcemia, pregnancy, hypersensitivity to oxandrolone or any component of the formulation
Caution
Diabetes mellitus, cardiovascular disease, MI, increased risk of prostatic hypertrophy, prostatic carcinoma, virilization (women), increased PT

DRUG INTERACTIONS OF CONCERN TO DENTISTRY
• Increased risk of bleeding: aspirin
• Edema: adrenocorticotropic hormone (ACTH), adrenal steroids

SERIOUS REACTIONS

! Peliotic hepatitis of the liver, spleen replaced with blood-filled cysts, hepatic neoplasms and hepatocellular carcinoma have been associated with prolonged high-dosage, anaphylactic reactions.

DENTAL CONSIDERATIONS
General:
• Monitor vital signs at every appointment because of cardiovascular side effects.
• Determine why the patient is taking the drug.
• Consider local hemostasis measures to prevent excessive bleeding.
• Short appointments and a stress-reduction protocol may be required for anxious patients.
• Avoid prescribing aspirin-containing products.

Consultations:
• If signs of anemia are observed in oral tissues, physician consultation may be required.
• Medical consultation may be required to assess disease control and patient's ability to tolerate stress.
• Medical consultation should include PPT or PT.

Teach Patient/Family to:
• Use effective oral hygiene to prevent soft tissue inflammation
• See dentist immediately if secondary oral infection occurs

oxaprozin
ox-ah-pro´-zin
(Daypro)
Do not confuse oxaprozin with oxazepam.

CATEGORY AND SCHEDULE
Pregnancy Risk Category: C
(D if used in third trimester or near delivery)

Drug Class: Nonsteroidal antiinflammatory

MECHANISM OF ACTION
An NSAID that produces analgesic and antiinflammatory effects by inhibiting prostaglandin synthesis. ***Therapeutic Effect:*** Reduces the inflammatory response and intensity of pain.

USES
Treatment of rheumatoid arthritis, osteoarthritis, and ankylosing spondylitis

PHARMACOKINETICS
Well absorbed from the GI tract. Protein binding: 99%. Widely distributed. Metabolized in the liver.

Primarily excreted in urine; partially eliminated in feces. Not removed by hemodialysis. ***Half-life:*** 42–50 hr.

INDICATIONS AND DOSAGES
▸ **Osteoarthritis**
PO
Adults, Elderly. 1200 mg once a day (600 mg in patients with low body weight or mild disease). Maximum: 1800 mg/day.
▸ **Rheumatoid Arthritis**
PO
Adults, Elderly. 1200 mg once a day. Range: 600–1800 mg/day.
▸ **Juvenile Rheumatoid Arthritis**
Children weighing more than 54 kg. 1200 mg/day.
Children weighing 32–54 kg. 900 mg/day.
Children weighing 22–31 kg. 600 mg/day.
▸ **Dosage in Renal Impairment**
For adults and elderly patients with renal impairment, the recommended initial dose is 600 mg/day; may be increased up to 1200 mg/day.

SIDE EFFECTS/ADVERSE REACTIONS
Occasional
Nausea, diarrhea, constipation, dyspepsia, edema
Rare
Vomiting, abdominal cramps or pain, flatulence, anorexia, confusion, tinnitus, insomnia, somnolence

PRECAUTIONS AND CONTRAINDICATIONS
Active peptic ulcer disease, chronic inflammation of GI tract, GI bleeding or ulceration, history of hypersensitivity to aspirin or NSAIDs
Caution
Lactation, children, bleeding disorders, GI disorders, cardiac

disorders, hypersensitivity to other antiinflammatory agents, diabetes

DRUG INTERACTIONS OF CONCERN TO DENTISTRY
- GI ulceration, bleeding: aspirin, alcohol, corticosteroids
- Decreased action: salicylates
- Nephrotoxicity: acetaminophen (prolonged use and high doses)
- Possible risk of decreased renal function: cyclosporine
- First-time users of SSRIs also taking NSAIDs may have a higher risk of GI side effects; until more data are available, it may be advisable to avoid use of NSAIDs in these patients (Br J Clin Pharmacol 55:591–595, 2003)
- When prescribed for dental pain:
  - Risk of increased effects: oral anticoagulants, oral antidiabetics, lithium, methotrexate
  - Decreased antihypertensive effects of diuretics, β-adrenergic blockers, and ACE inhibitors

SERIOUS REACTIONS
! Hypertension, acute renal failure, respiratory depression, GI bleeding, and coma occur rarely.

DENTAL CONSIDERATIONS
General:
- Patients on chronic drug therapy may rarely have symptoms of blood dyscrasias, which can include infection, bleeding, and poor healing.
- Assess salivary flow as a factor in caries, periodontal disease, and candidiasis.
- Avoid prescribing for dental use in pregnancy.
- Consider semisupine chair position for patients with arthritic disease.
Consultations:
- Medical consultation may be required to assess disease control.

- In a patient with symptoms of blood dyscrasias, request a medical consultation for blood studies and postpone dental treatment until normal values are reestablished.
Teach Patient/Family to:
- Use effective oral hygiene to prevent soft tissue inflammation
- Use caution to prevent injury when using oral hygiene aids
- When chronic dry mouth occurs, advise patient to:
  - Avoid mouth rinses with high alcohol content because of drying effects
  - Use daily home fluoride products to prevent caries
  - Use sugarless gum, frequent sips of water, or saliva substitutes

---

oxazepam
ox-a′-ze-pam
(Alepam[AUS], Apo-Oxazepam[CAN], Murelax[AUS], Serax, Serepax[AUS])
Do not confuse oxazepam with oxaprozin, or Serax with Eurax or Xerac.

CATEGORY AND SCHEDULE
Pregnancy Risk Category: D
Controlled Substance Schedule IV

Drug Class: Benzodiazepine

MECHANISM OF ACTION
A benzodiazepine that potentiates the effects of gamma-aminobutyric acid and other inhibitory neurotransmitters by binding to specific receptors in the CNS.
Therapeutic Effect: Produces anxiolytic effect and skeletal muscle relaxation.

USES
Treatment of anxiety, alcohol withdrawal

PHARMACOKINETICS
Well absorbed from the GI tract. Protein binding: 97%. Metabolized in the liver. Primarily excreted in urine. Not removed by hemodialysis. *Half-life:* 5–20 hr.

INDICATIONS AND DOSAGES
▶ **Mild-to-Moderate Anxiety**
PO
Adults. 10–15 mg 3–4 times a day.
▶ **Severe Anxiety**
PO
Adults. 15–30 mg 3–4 times a day.
▶ **Alcohol Withdrawal**
PO
Adults. 15–30 mg 3–4 times a day.
Elderly. Initially, 10–20 mg 3 times a day. May gradually increase up to 30–45 mg/day.

SIDE EFFECTS/ADVERSE REACTIONS
Frequent
Mild, transient somnolence at beginning of therapy
Occasional
Dizziness, headache
Rare
Paradoxic CNS reactions, such as hyperactivity or nervousness in children and excitement or restlessness in the elderly or debilitated (generally noted during the first 2 wk of therapy)

PRECAUTIONS AND CONTRAINDICATIONS
Angle-closure glaucoma; preexisting CNS depression; severe, uncontrolled pain
Caution
Elderly, debilitated, hepatic disease, renal disease

DRUG INTERACTIONS OF CONCERN TO DENTISTRY
• Increased effects: CNS depressants, alcohol, and anticonvulsant medications
• Possible increase in CNS side effects of kava kava (herb)

SERIOUS REACTIONS
! Abrupt or too-rapid withdrawal may result in pronounced restlessness, irritability, insomnia, hand tremors, abdominal or muscle cramps, diaphoresis, vomiting, and seizures.
! Overdose results in somnolence, confusion, diminished reflexes, and coma.

DENTAL CONSIDERATIONS
General:
• Monitor vital signs at every appointment because of cardiovascular side effects.
• Psychologic and physical dependence may occur with chronic administration.
• Geriatric patients are more susceptible to drug effects; use lower dose.
• Assess salivary flow as a factor in caries, periodontal disease, and candidiasis.
Consultations:
• Medical consultation may be required to assess disease control.
Teach Patient/Family to:
• Avoid mouth rinses with high alcohol content because of drying effects

oxcarbazepine
oks-kar-bays´-uh-peen
(Trileptal)

CATEGORY AND SCHEDULE
Pregnancy Risk Category: C

Drug Class: Anticonvulsant

MECHANISM OF ACTION

An anticonvulsant that blocks sodium channels, resulting in stabilization of hyperexcited neural membranes, inhibition of repetitive neuronal firing, and diminishing synaptic impulses. ***Therapeutic Effect:*** Prevents seizures.

USES

Monotherapy or adjunctive therapy of partial seizures in adults with epilepsy; monotherapy or adjunctive therapy for partial seizures in children (4–16 yr) with epilepsy

PHARMACOKINETICS

Completely absorbed from GI tract and extensively metabolized in the liver to active metabolite. Protein binding: 40%. Primarily excreted in urine. ***Half-life:*** 2 hr; metabolite, 6–10 hr.

INDICATIONS AND DOSAGES

▸ **Adjunctive Treatment of Seizures**
PO
Adults, Elderly. Initially, 600 mg/day in 2 divided doses. May increase by up to 600 mg/day at weekly intervals. Maximum: 2400 mg/day.
Children 4–16 yr. 8–10 mg/kg. Maximum: 600 mg/day. Maintenance (based on weight): 1800 mg/day for children weighing more than 39 kg; 1200 mg/day for children weighing 29.1–39 kg; and 900 mg/day for children weighing 20–29 kg.
▸ **Conversion to Monotherapy**
PO
Adults, Elderly. 600 mg/day in 2 divided doses (while decreasing concomitant anticonvulsant over 3–6 wk). May increase by 600 mg/day at weekly intervals up to 2400 mg/day.
Children. Initially, 8–10 mg/kg/day in 2 divided doses with simultaneous initial reduction of dose of concomitant antiepileptic.
▸ **Initiation of Monotherapy**
PO
Adults, Elderly. 600 mg/day in 2 divided doses. May increase by 300 mg/day every 3 days up to 1200 mg/day.
Children. Initially, 8–10 mg/kg/day in 2 divided doses. Increase at 3 day intervals by 5 mg/kg/day to achieve maintenance dose by weight;
(70 kg): 1500–2100 mg/day;
(60–69 kg): 1200–2100 mg/day;
(50–59 kg): 1200–1800 mg/day;
(41–49 kg): 1200–1500 mg/day;
(35–40 kg): 900–1500 mg/day;
(25–34 kg): 900–1200 mg/day;
(20–24 kg): 600–900 mg/day.
▸ **Dosage in Renal Impairment**
For patients with creatinine clearance less than 30 ml/min, give 50% of normal starting dose, then titrate slowly to desired dose.

SIDE EFFECTS/ADVERSE REACTIONS

Frequent
Dizziness, nausea, headache
Occasional
Vomiting, diarrhea, ataxia, nervousness, heartburn, indigestion, epigastric pain, constipation
Rare
Tremors, rash, back pain, epistaxis, sinusitis, diplopia

PRECAUTIONS AND CONTRAINDICATIONS

Hypersensitivity to this drug or carbamazepine
Caution
Development of hyponatremia, withdraw drug slowly to avoid seizures, cognitive CNS adverse effects, decreases effect of oral contraceptives, caution when used

with other anticonvulsants, renal impairment, lactation

DRUG INTERACTIONS OF CONCERN TO DENTISTRY
• No dental drug interactions reported; CYP450 3A4/5 enzyme inducers may decrease plasma levels
• Possible increase in CNS depression: all CNS depressants, alcohol

SERIOUS REACTIONS
! Clinically significant hyponatremia may occur.

DENTAL CONSIDERATIONS
General:
• Monitor vital signs at every appointment because of cardiovascular side effects.
• Patients on chronic drug therapy may rarely have symptoms of blood dyscrasias, which can include infection, bleeding, and poor healing.
• Assess salivary flow as a factor in caries, periodontal disease, and candidiasis
• Consider semisupine chair position for patient comfort if GI side effects occur.
• Short appointments and a stress reduction protocol may be required for anxious patients.
• Determine type of epilepsy, seizure frequency, and quality of seizure control.
Consultations:
• In a patient with symptoms of blood dyscrasias, request a medical consultation for blood studies and postpone treatment until normal values are reestablished.
• Medical consultation may be required to assess disease control and patient's ability to tolerate stress.
Teach Patient/Family to:
• Use effective oral hygiene to prevent soft tissue inflammation

• Prevent trauma when using oral hygiene aids
• When chronic dry mouth occurs, advise patient to:
  • Avoid mouth rinses with high alcohol content because of drying effects
  • Use daily home fluoride products for anticaries effect
  • Use sugarless gum, frequent sips of water, or saliva substitutes

oxiconazole
ox-i-con´-a-zole
(Oxistat, Oxizole[CAN])
Do not confuse with Nitrostat.

CATEGORY AND SCHEDULE
Pregnancy Risk Category: B

Drug Class: Antifungals, topical, dermatologics

MECHANISM OF ACTION
An antifungal agent that inhibits ergosterol synthesis. *Therapeutic Effect:* Destroys cytoplasmic membrane integrity of fungi. Fungicidal.

USES
Treatment of infections caused by a fungus

PHARMACOKINETICS
Low systemic absorption. Absorbed and distributed in each layer of the dermis. Excreted in the urine.

INDICATIONS AND DOSAGES
▶ *Tinea Pedis*
Topical
Adults, Elderly, Children 12 yr and older. Apply 1–2 times a day for 1 mo or until signs and symptoms significantly improve.

916 Oxidized Cellulose

▶ *Tinea cruris, Tinea corporis*
Topical
Adults, Elderly, Children 12 yr and older. Apply 1–2 times a day for 2 wk or until signs and symptoms significantly improve.

SIDE EFFECTS/ADVERSE REACTIONS
Occasional
Itching, local irritation, stinging, dryness

PRECAUTIONS AND CONTRAINDICATIONS
Not for ophthalmic use, hypersensitivity to oxiconazole or any other azole fungals

DRUG INTERACTIONS OF CONCERN TO DENTISTRY
None reported

SERIOUS REACTIONS
! Hypersensitivity reactions characterized by rash, swelling, pruritus, maceration, and a sensation of warmth may occur.

DENTAL CONSIDERATIONS
General:
• Determine why the patient is using this medication.

oxidized cellulose
oks´-ih-dye-zed cell´-you-lose
(Interceed, Surgicel)

CATEGORY AND SCHEDULE
Pregnancy Risk Category: Not reported

Drug Class: Cellulose hemostatic

MECHANISM OF ACTION
Oxidized cellulose is saturated with blood at the bleeding site and swells into a brownish or black gelatinous mass that aids in clot formation. When used in small amounts, it is absorbed from the sites of implantation with minimal tissue reaction. *Therapeutic Effect:* Reduces bleeding. Weak bactericidal action.

USES
Hemostasis in surgery, oral surgery, exodontia

PHARMACOKINETICS
Absorption occurs in 7–14 days. *Half-life:* Unknown.

INDICATIONS AND DOSAGES
▶ **Surgical Procedures to Assist in the Control of Capillary, Venous, and Small Arterial Hemorrhage When Ligation or Other Conventional Methods of Control Are Impractical or Ineffective**
Topical
Adults. Minimal amounts of an appropriate size are laid on the bleeding site or held firmly against the tissues until hemostasis is obtained.

SIDE EFFECTS/ADVERSE REACTIONS
Frequency Not Defined
Headache, nasal burning or stinging, sneezing, encapsulation of fluid

PRECAUTIONS AND CONTRAINDICATIONS
Use for packing or implantation in fractures or laminectomies, hemorrhage from large arteries, and nonhemorrhagic oozing surfaces; use as a wrap; use around the optic nerve and chiasm; applied as wadding or packing as a hemostatic agent;

hypersensitivity to oxidized cellulose or any component of the formulation
Caution
Do not autoclave; inactivation of topical thrombin

SERIOUS REACTIONS
! Pain, numbness, and paralysis have been reported.

DENTAL CONSIDERATIONS

General:
• Apply dry; use only amount needed to control bleeding.
• Place loosely and avoid packing; remove excess before closure in surgery; irrigate first, then remove using sterile technique.
• Ensure therapeutic response: decreased bleeding in surgery.
• Can be left in situ when necessary but should be removed once bleeding is controlled.
• Application of topical thrombin solution to the cellulose gauze will inactivate thrombin because of acidity.

---

oxybutynin
ox-ih-byoo´-ti-nin
(Ditropan, Ditropan XL, Oxytrol)
Do not confuse oxybutynin with Oxycontin, or Ditropan with diazepam.

CATEGORY AND SCHEDULE
Pregnancy Risk Category: B

Drug Class: Antispasmodic

MECHANISM OF ACTION
An anticholinergic that exerts antispasmodic (papaverine-like) and antimuscarinic (atropine-like) action on the detrusor smooth muscle of the bladder. *Therapeutic Effect:* Increases bladder capacity and delays desire to void.

USES
Antispasmodic for neurogenic bladder, overactive bladder

PHARMACOKINETICS

Route	Onset	Peak	Duration
PO	0.5–1 hr	3–6 hr	6–10 hr

Rapidly absorbed from the GI tract. Metabolized in the liver. Primarily excreted in urine. Unknown if removed by hemodialysis.
Half-life: 1–2.3 hr.

INDICATIONS AND DOSAGES
▶ **Neurogenic Bladder**
PO
Adults. 5 mg 2–3 times a day up to 5 mg 4 times a day.
Elderly. 2.5–5 mg twice a day. May increase by 2.5 mg/day every 1–2 days.
Children 5 yr and older. 5 mg twice a day up to 5 mg 4 times a day.
Children 1–4 yr. 0.2 mg/kg/dose 2–4 times a day.
PO (Extended-Release)
Adults.
5–10 mg/day up to 30 mg/day.
Transdermal
Adults. 3.9 mg applied twice a week. Apply every 3–4 days.

SIDE EFFECTS/ADVERSE REACTIONS
Frequent
Constipation, dry mouth, somnolence, decreased perspiration
Occasional
Decreased lacrimation or salivation, impotence, urinary hesitancy and retention, suppressed lactation, blurred vision, mydriasis, nausea or vomiting, insomnia

O

PRECAUTIONS AND CONTRAINDICATIONS

GI or GU obstruction, glaucoma, myasthenia gravis, toxic megacolon, ulcerative colitis

Caution

Lactation, suspected glaucoma, children younger than 12 yr, hiatal hernia, esophageal reflux, coronary heart disease, CHF, hypertension

DRUG INTERACTIONS OF CONCERN TO DENTISTRY

- Increased anticholinergic effect: anticholinergic drugs
- Increased depressant effect of both drugs: CNS depressants, alcohol

SERIOUS REACTIONS

! Overdose produces CNS excitation (including nervousness, restlessness, hallucinations, and irritability), hypotension or hypertension, confusion, tachycardia, facial flushing, and respiratory depression.

DENTAL CONSIDERATIONS

General:
- Assess salivary flow as a factor in caries, periodontal disease, and candidiasis.
- Monitor vital signs at every appointment because of cardiovascular side effects.
- Avoid dental light in patient's eyes; offer dark glasses for patient comfort.
- Consider semisupine chair position for patient comfort if GI side effects occur.

Consultations:
- Physician should be informed if significant xerostomic side effects occur (e.g., increased caries, sore tongue, problems eating or swallowing, difficulty wearing prosthesis) so that a medication change can be considered.

Teach Patient/Family to:
- Use effective oral hygiene to prevent soft tissue inflammation
- When chronic dry mouth occurs, advise patient to:
  - Avoid mouth rinses with high alcohol content because of drying effects
  - Use daily home fluoride products to prevent caries
  - Use sugarless gum, frequent sips of water, or saliva substitutes

oxycodone

ox-ee-koe´-done
(Endone[AUS], OxyContin, Oxydose, OxyFast, OxyIR, Oxynorm[AUS], Roxicodone, Roxicodone Intensol)
Do not confuse oxycodone with oxybutynin.

CATEGORY AND SCHEDULE

Pregnancy Risk Category: B
(D if used for prolonged periods or at high dosages at term)
Controlled Substance: Schedule II

Drug Class: Synthetic opioid analgesic

MECHANISM OF ACTION

An opioid analgesic that binds with opioid receptors in the CNS.
Therapeutic Effect: Alters the perception of and emotional response to pain.

USES

Treatment of moderate-to-severe pain, normally used in combination with aspirin or acetaminophen; combination products

PHARMACOKINETICS

Route	Onset	Peak	Duration
PO, immediate release	N/A	N/A	4–5 hr
PO, controlled release	N/A	N/A	12 hr

Moderately absorbed from the GI tract. Protein binding: 38%–45%. Widely distributed. Metabolized in the liver. Excreted in urine. Unknown if removed by hemodialysis.
Half-life: 2–3 hr (3.2 hr controlled-release).

INDICATIONS AND DOSAGES
▸ **Analgesia**
PO (Controlled-Release)
Adults, Elderly. Initially, 10 mg q12h. May increase every 1–2 days by 25%–50%. Usual: 40 mg/day (100 mg/day for cancer pain).
PO (Immediate-Release)
Adults, Elderly. Initially, 5 mg q6h as needed. May increase up to 30 mg q4h. Usual: 10–30 mg q4h as needed.
Children. 0.05–0.15 mg/kg/dose q4–6h.

SIDE EFFECTS/ADVERSE REACTIONS
Frequent
Somnolence, dizziness, hypotension (including orthostatic hypotension), anorexia
Occasional
Confusion, diaphoresis, facial flushing, urine retention, constipation, dry mouth, nausea, vomiting, headache
Rare
Allergic reaction, depression, paradoxic CNS hyperactivity or nervousness in children, paradoxic excitement and restlessness in elderly or debilitated patients

PRECAUTIONS AND CONTRAINDICATIONS
Hypersensitivity, addiction (narcotic)
Caution
Addictive personality, lactation, increased intracranial pressure, MI (acute), severe heart disease, respiratory depression, hepatic disease, renal disease, children younger than 18 yr, physical dependence

DRUG INTERACTIONS OF CONCERN TO DENTISTRY
• Increased effects with other CNS depressants: alcohol, other narcotics, sedative-hypnotics, skeletal muscle relaxants, phenothiazines, benzodiazepines
• Contraindication: MAOIs
• Increased effects of anticholinergics

SERIOUS REACTIONS
❗ Overdose results in respiratory depression, skeletal muscle flaccidity, cold or clammy skin, cyanosis, and extreme somnolence progressing to seizures, stupor, and coma.
❗ Hepatotoxicity may occur with overdose of the acetaminophen component of fixed-combination products.
❗ The patient who uses oxycodone repeatedly may develop a tolerance to the drug's analgesic effect and physical dependence.

DENTAL CONSIDERATIONS
General:
• Monitor vital signs at every appointment because of cardiovascular and respiratory side effects.
• Assess salivary flow as a factor in caries, periodontal disease, and candidiasis.

- Psychologic and physical dependence may occur with chronic administration.
- Determine why the patient is taking the drug.

Teach Patient/Family to:
- Avoid mouth rinses with high alcohol content because of drying effects

---

oxymetazoline
ox-ee-met-az´-oh-leen
(Afrin, Afrin 12-Hour, Afrin Children's Strength Nose Drops, Ocuclear, Sinex 12 Hour Long-Acting)

CATEGORY AND SCHEDULE
Pregnancy Risk Category: C
OTC

Drug Class: Nasal decongestant, sympathomimetic amine

MECHANISM OF ACTION
A direct-acting sympathomimetic amine that acts on alpha-adrenergic receptors in arterioles of the nasal mucosa to produce constriction.
Therapeutic Effect: Causes vasoconstriction resulting in decreased blood flow and decreased nasal congestion.

USES
Treatment of nasal congestion

PHARMACOKINETICS
Onset of action is about 10 min, and a duration of action is 7 hr or more. Absorption occurs from the nasal mucosa and can produce systemic effects, primarily following overdose or excessive use. Excreted mostly in the urine, as well as the feces.
Half-life: 5–8 hr.

INDICATIONS AND DOSAGES
▸ **Rhinitis**
Intranasal
Adults, Elderly, Children older than 6 yr. 2–3 drops/sprays (0.05% nasal solution) in each nostril q12h.
Children 2–5 yr. 2–4 drops or sprays (0.025% nasal solution) in each nostril q12h for up to 3 days.
▸ **Conjunctivitis**
Ophthalmic
Adults, Elderly, Children older than 6 yr. 1–2 drops (0.025% ophthalmic solution) q6h for 3–4 days.

SIDE EFFECTS/ADVERSE REACTIONS
Occasional
Burning, stinging, drying nasal mucosa, sneezing, rebound congestion, insomnia, nervousness

PRECAUTIONS AND CONTRAINDICATIONS
Narrow-angle glaucoma or hypersensitivity to oxymetazoline or other adrenergic agents
Caution
Children younger than 6 yr, elderly, diabetes, cardiovascular disease, hypertension, hyperthyroidism, increased intracranial pressure, prostatic hypertrophy, glaucoma

DRUG INTERACTIONS OF CONCERN TO DENTISTRY
- Increased risk of hypertension: tricyclic antidepressants, but it requires adequate systemic absorption of oxymetazoline

SERIOUS REACTIONS
! Large doses may produce tachycardia, hypertension, arrhythmias, palpitations, lightheadedness, nausea, and vomiting.

DENTAL CONSIDERATIONS

General:

• Excessive use can lead to rebound congestion and cardiovascular side effects; follow recommended dosing intervals.

• Extensive nasal swelling and congestion may interfere with optimal use of nitrous oxide/oxygen sedation.

oxymetholone

ox-ee-meth´-oh-lone
(Anadrol, Anapolon[CAN])
Do not confuse with oxycodone.

CATEGORY AND SCHEDULE

Pregnancy Risk Category: X
Controlled substance: Schedule III

Drug Class: Androgenic anabolic steroid

MECHANISM OF ACTION

An androgenic-anabolic steroid that is a synthetic derivative of testosterone synthesized to accentuate anabolic as opposed to androgenic effects. *Therapeutic Effect:* Improves nitrogen balance in conditions of unfavorable protein metabolism with adequate caloric and protein intake, stimulates erythropoiesis, suppresses gonadotropic functions of pituitary, and may exert a direct effect upon the testes.

USES

Anemia associated with bone marrow failure and red cell production deficiencies; aplastic anemia, myelofibrosis, and anemia caused by myelotoxic drugs

PHARMACOKINETICS

The pharmacokinetics of oxymetholone has been studied. Metabolized in the liver via reduction and oxidation. Unchanged oxymetholone and its metabolites are excreted in urine. *Half-life:* Unknown.

INDICATIONS AND DOSAGES

▶ **Anemia, Chronic Renal Failure, Acqured Aplastic Anemia, Chemotherapy-Induced Myelosuppresion, Fanconi's Anemia, Red Cell Aplasia**
PO
Adults, Elderly, Children. 1–5 mg/kg/day. Response is not immediate, and a minimum of 3–6 mo should be given.

SIDE EFFECTS/ADVERSE REACTIONS

Frequent
Gynecomastia, acne, amenorrhea, menstrual irregularities
Females: Hirsutism, deepening of voice, clitoral enlargement that may not be reversible when drug is discontinued
Occasional
Edema, nausea, insomnia, oligospermia, priapism, male pattern of baldness, bladder irritability, hypercalcemia in immobilized patients or those with breast cancer, hypercholesterolemia, inflammation and pain at IM injection site
Transdermal: Itching, erythema, skin irritation
Rare
Liver damage, hypersensitivity

PRECAUTIONS AND CONTRAINDICATIONS

Cardiac impairment, hypercalcemia, pregnancy/lactation, prostatic or breast cancer in males, metastatic

O

breast cancer in women with active hypercalcemia, nephrosis or nephritic phase nephritis, severe liver disease, hypersensitivity to oxymetholone or any of its components

Caution

Diabetes mellitus, cardiovascular disease, MI, increased risk of prostatic hypertrophy, prostatic carcinoma, virilization (women), increased PT

DRUG INTERACTIONS OF CONCERN TO DENTISTRY

- Increased risk of bleeding: aspirin
- Edema: ACTH, adrenal steroids

SERIOUS REACTIONS

! Cholestatic jaundice, hepatic necrosis and death occur rarely but have been reported in association with long-term androgenic-anabolic steroid use.

DENTAL CONSIDERATIONS

General:

- Monitor vital signs at every appointment because of cardiovascular side effects.

- Determine why the patient is taking the drug.
- Consider local hemostasis measures to prevent excessive bleeding.
- Short appointments and a stress-reduction protocol may be required for anxious patients.
- Avoid prescribing aspirin-containing products.

Consultations:

- Physician consultation may be required if signs of anemia are observed in oral tissues.
- Medical consultation may be required to assess disease control and patient's ability to tolerate stress.
- Medical consultation should include PPT or PT.

Teach Patient/Family to:

- Use effective oral hygiene to prevent soft tissue inflammation
- See dentist immediately if secondary oral infection occurs

paclitaxel

pak-leh-tax´-ell

(Abraxane, Anzatax[AUS], Onxol, Taxol)

Do not confuse paclitaxel with Paxil, or Taxol with Taxotere.

CATEGORY AND SCHEDULE

Pregnancy Risk Category: D

Drug Class: Antineoplastic

MECHANISM OF ACTION

An antimitotic agent in the taxoid family that disrupts the microtubular cell network, which is essential for cellular function. Blocks cells in the late G2 phase and M phase of the cell cycle. *Therapeutic Effect:* Inhibits cellular mitosis and replication.

USES

Treatment of metastatic ovarian cancer, non–small-cell lung cancer; second-line treatment for AIDS-related Kaposi's sarcoma (KS); adjuvant treatment of node-positive breast cancer sequential to a course of standard doxorubicin-containing combination chemotherapy

PHARMACOKINETICS

Does not readily cross the blood-brain barrier. Protein binding: 89%–98%. Metabolized in the liver to active metabolites; eliminated by bile. Not removed by hemodialysis. *Half-life:* 1.3–8.6 hr.

INDICATIONS AND DOSAGES
▶ **Ovarian Cancer**

IV

Adults. 135–175 mg/m²/dose over 1–24 hr q3wk.

▶ **Breast Carcinoma**

IV (Onxol, Taxol)

Adults, Elderly. 175 mg/m² over 3 hr q3wk.

PO (Abraxane)

Adults, Elderly. 260 mg/m² over 30 min q3wk.

▶ **Non–Small-Cell Lung Carcinoma**

IV

Adults, Elderly. 135 mg/m² over 24 hr, followed by cisplatin 75 mg/m² q3wk.

▶ **KS**

IV

Adults, Elderly. 135 mg/m²/dose over 3 hr q3wk or 100 mg/m²/dose over 3 hr q2wk.

▶ **Dosage in Hepatic Impairment**

Total Bilirubin	Total Dose
More than 3 mg/dl	Less than 50 mg/m²
1.6–3 mg/dl	Less than 75 mg/m²
1.5 mg/dl or less	Less than 135 mg/m²

SIDE EFFECTS/ADVERSE REACTIONS

Expected

Diarrhea, alopecia, nausea, vomiting

Frequent

Myalgia or arthralgia, peripheral neuropathy

Occasional

Mucositis, hypotension during infusion, pain or redness at injection site

Rare

Bradycardia

PRECAUTIONS AND CONTRAINDICATIONS

Baseline neutropenia (neutrophil count 1500 cells/mm³), hypersensitivity to drugs developed with Cremophor EL (polyoxyethylated castor oil).

P

Caution
Bone marrow depression, AV block, hepatic impairment, lactation, children, recent MI, angina pectoris, CHF history, current use of drug with effect on cardiac conduction system

DRUG INTERACTIONS OF CONCERN TO DENTISTRY
• Possible (not demonstrated) increase in action by strong inhibitors of CYP2C8 and CYP3A4 isoenzymes: diazepam, ketoconazole, midazolam (monitor patient if prescribed)

SERIOUS REACTIONS
! Neutropenic nadir occurs at approximately day 11 of paclitaxel therapy.
! Anemia and leukopenia are common reactions.
! Thrombocytopenia occurs occasionally.
! A severe hypersensitivity reaction, including dyspnea, severe hypotension, angioedema, and generalized urticaria, occurs rarely.

DENTAL CONSIDERATIONS
General:
• Consider semisupine chair position for patient comfort if GI side effects occur.
• Patients receiving chemotherapy may require palliative therapy for stomatitis.
• Patients on chronic drug therapy may rarely have symptoms of blood dyscrasias, which can include infection, bleeding, and poor healing.
Consultations:
• Medical consultation may be required to assess disease control.
Teach Patient/Family to:
• Use effective oral hygiene to prevent soft tissue inflammation

• Use caution to prevent trauma when using oral hygiene aids

palonosetron hydrochloride
pal-oh-noe´-seh-tron high-droh-klor´-ide
(Aloxi)

CATEGORY AND SCHEDULE
Pregnancy Risk Category: B

Drug Class: Antiemetics/ antivertigo, serotonin receptor antagonists

MECHANISM OF ACTION
A 5-HT$_3$ receptor antagonist that acts centrally in the chemoreceptor trigger zone and peripherally at the vagal nerve terminals.

USES
Prevention of nausea and vomiting associated with chemotherapy.

PHARMACOKINETICS
Protein binding: 52%. Eliminated in urine. *Half-life:* 40 hr.

INDICATIONS AND DOSAGES
▶ **Chemotherapy-Induced Nausea and Vomiting**
IV
Adults, Elderly. 0.25 mg as a single dose 30 min before starting chemotherapy.

SIDE EFFECTS/ADVERSE REACTIONS
Occasional
Headache, constipation
Rare
Diarrhea, dizziness, fatigue, abdominal pain, insomnia

PRECAUTIONS AND CONTRAINDICATIONS
None known

DRUG INTERACTIONS OF CONCERN TO DENTISTRY
None reported

SERIOUS REACTIONS
! Overdose may produce a combination of CNS stimulant and depressant effects.

DENTAL CONSIDERATIONS
General:
• For acute use in hospitals or cancer treatment centers.
Teach Patient/Family to:
• Be aware of possible oral side effects from concurrent chemotherapy

pamidronate disodium
pam-id´-row-nate die-soe´-dee-um
(Aredia, Pamisol[AUS])
Do not confuse Aredia with Adriamcyin.

CATEGORY AND SCHEDULE
Pregnancy Risk Category: D

Drug Class: Bone-resorption inhibitor, electrolyte modifier

MECHANISM OF ACTION
A bisphosphate that binds to bone and inhibits osteoclast-mediated calcium resorption. *Therapeutic Effect:* Lowers serum calcium concentrations.

USES
Treatment of moderate-to-severe Paget's disease, mild-to-moderate hypercalcemia associated with malignancy with or without bone metastases, osteolytic bone metastases in breast cancer, multiple myeloma patients

PHARMACOKINETICS

Route	Onset	Peak	Duration
IV	24–48 hr	5–7 days	N/A

After IV administration, rapidly absorbed by bone. Slowly excreted unchanged in urine. Unknown if removed by hemodialysis. *Half-life:* bone, 300 days; unmetabolized, 2.5 hr.

INDICATIONS AND DOSAGES
▸ **Hypercalcemia**
IV Infusion
Adults, Elderly. Moderate hypercalcemia (corrected serum calcium level 12–13.5 mg/dl): 60–90 mg. Severe hypercalcemia (corrected serum calcium level greater than 13.5 mg/dl): 90 mg.
▸ **Paget's Disease**
IV Infusion
Adults, Elderly. 30 mg/day for 3 days.
▸ **Osteolytic Bone Lesion**
90 mg over 4 hr once monthly.

SIDE EFFECTS/ADVERSE REACTIONS
Frequent
Temperature elevation (at least 1°C) 24–48 hr after administration; redness, swelling, induration, pain at catheter site in patients receiving 90 mg; anorexia, nausea, fatigue
Occasional
Constipation, rhinitis

PRECAUTIONS AND CONTRAINDICATIONS
Hypersensitivity to other bisphosphonates, such as etidronate, tiludronate, risedronate, and alendronate. Dental implants are

P

contraindicated for patients taking this drug.

DRUG INTERACTIONS OF CONCERN TO DENTISTRY

None reported

SERIOUS REACTIONS

! Hypophosphatemia, hypokalemia, hypomagnesemia, and hypocalcemia occur more frequently with higher dosages.

! Anemia, hypertension, tachycardia, atrial fibrillation, and somnolence occur more frequently with 90-mg doses.

! GI hemorrhage occurs rarely.

DENTAL CONSIDERATIONS

General:

• Increased risk for osteochemonecrosis; avoid invasive procedures and emphasize preventative care.

• Determine why patient is taking the drug.

• This drug may be used in the hospital or on an outpatient basis. Confirm the patient's disease and treatment status.

• Examine for oral manifestation of opportunistic infection.

• Monitor and record vital signs.

• Consider semisupine chair position for patient comfort if GI side effects occur.

• Question patient about tolerance of NSAIDs or aspirin related to GI disease.

• Be aware of the oral manifestations of Paget's disease (macrognathia, alveolar pain).

• Patients may have received other chemotherapy or radiation; confirm medical and drug history.

• Recent reports indicate osteonecrosis of the jaw may occur with the use of this drug.

Consultations:

• Medical consultation may be required to assess disease control and patient's ability to tolerate stress.

Teach Patient/Family to:

• Avoid drugs containing calcium, vitamin D, and antacids; possible antagonism of pamidronate

pancreatin/ pancrelipase

pan-kree-ah´-tin/pan-kree-lie´-pace (pancreatin: Ku-Zyme, Pancreatin; pancrelipase: Cotazym-S[AUS], Cotazym-S Forte[AUS], Creon, Pancrease[CAN], Pancrease MT, Ultrase, Viokase)

CATEGORY AND SCHEDULE

Pregnancy Risk Category: C

Drug Class: Digestant

MECHANISM OF ACTION

Digestive enzymes that replace endogenous pancreatic enzymes. *Therapeutic Effect:* Assist in digestion of protein, starch, and fats.

USES

Treatment of exocrine pancreatic secretion insufficiency, cystic fibrosis (digestive aid), steatorrhea, pancreatic enzyme deficiency, chronic pancreatitis

PHARMACOKINETICS

Not studied

INDICATIONS AND DOSAGES

▶ **Pancreatic Enzyme Replacement or Supplement when Enzymes Are Absent or Deficient, Such as with Chronic Pancreatitis, Cystic Fibrosis,**

or Ductal Obstruction from Cancer of the Pancreas or Common Bile Duct; to Reduce Malabsorption; Treatment of Steatorrhea Associated with Bowel Resection or Postgastrectomy Syndrome
PO
Adults, Elderly. 1–3 capsules or tablets before or with meals or snacks. May increase to 8 tablets/dose.
Children. 1–2 tablets with meals or snacks.

SIDE EFFECTS/ADVERSE REACTIONS
Rare
Allergic reaction, mouth irritation, shortness of breath, wheezing

PRECAUTIONS AND CONTRAINDICATIONS
Acute pancreatitis, exacerbation of chronic pancreatitis, hypersensitivity to pork protein

SERIOUS REACTIONS
! Excessive dosage may produce nausea, cramping, and diarrhea.
! Hyperuricosuria and hyperuricemia have occurred with extremely high dosages.

DENTAL CONSIDERATIONS
General:
• Consider semisupine chair position for patient comfort because of GI effects of disease.
• To avoid oral irritation, mouth should be rinsed or drug taken with liquid.

panitumumab
pan-ih-tu-mue´-mab
(Vectibix)

CATEGORY AND SCHEDULE
Pregnancy Risk Category: C

Drug Class: Antineoplastic

MECHANISM OF ACTION
An antineoplastic agent that binds specifically to epidermal growth factor (EGFR) on normal and tumor cells, and competively inhibits the binding of ligands for EGFR. Blocks phosphorylation and activation of intracellular tyrosine kinases, resulting in inhibition of cell survival, growth, proliferation and transformation. *Therapeutic Effect:* Inhibits growth and survival of selected human tumor cell lines expressing EGFR.

USES
Treatment of EGFR-positive metastatic colorectal cancer

PHARMACOKINETICS
Half-life: 4–11 days. Other pharmacokinetic parameters have not been clearly established.

INDICATIONS AND DOSAGES
▸ **EGFR-Positive Metastatic Colorectal Cancer**
IV infusion
Adults. 6 mg/kg administered over 60 min every 14 days. Doses higher than 1000 mg should be administered over 90 min.
▸ **Dosing Adjustments**
Infusion reactions
Infusion reactions, mild-to-moderate (grade 1 or 2). Reduce the infusion rate by 50% for the duration of infusion.

Infusion reactions, severe (grade 3 or 4). Immediately and permanently discontinue.

▶ **Dermatologic Toxicity**

Dermatologic toxicity (grade 3 or 4). Withhold panitumumab if skin toxicity does not improve to grade 2 or lower within 1 mo, permanently discontinue.

Dermatologic toxicity (grade 2 or lower), and the patient is symptomatically improved after withholding no more than 2 doses of panitumumab. Treatment may be resumed at 50% of the original dose. If toxicities recur, permanently discontinue drug. If toxicities do not recur, subsequent doses may be increased in increments of 25% of the original dose until the recommended dose of 6 mg/kg is obtained.

Safety and efficacy have not been established in children.

SIDE EFFECTS/ADVERSE REACTIONS:

Frequent

Dermatologic toxicity, erythema, acneiform rash, pruritus, hypomagnesemia, fatigue, exfoliation, abdominal pain, paronychia, nausea, rash, diarrhea, constipation, fissures, vomiting, cough, acne, peripheral edema, dry skin

Occasional

Nail disorder, stomatitis, mucositis, eyelash growth, conjunctivitis, ocular hyperemia, lacrimation increased

Rare

Infusion reactions, eye/eyelid irritation

PRECAUTIONS AND CONTRAINDICATIONS

Hypersensitivity to panitumumab or its components; sunlight may exacerbate skin reactions

DRUG INTERACTIONS OF CONCERN TO DENTISTRY

None reported

SERIOUS REACTIONS

❗ Dermatologic toxicities have been reported.

❗ Severe infusion-related reactions have been reported.

❗ Pulmonary fibrosis has been reported.

DENTAL CONSIDERATIONS

General:

• Examine patient for signs of adverse drug effects, including stomatitis and mucositis

• Be prepared to manage nausea and vomiting related to drug use

• Avoid aspirin and NSAIDs to reduce GI irritation

Consultations:

• Consult physician to determine degree of disease control and ability of patient to tolerate dental procedures

Teach Patient/Family to:

• Be aware of oral side effects of drug

• Report oral lesions, soreness or bleeding to dentist

• Use effective, atraumatic oral hygiene to minimize soft tissue inflammation

• Update health and medication history if physician makes any changes in evaluation or drug regimen; include OTC, herbal, and nonherbal drugs in the update

pantoprazole
pan-toe´-pra-zole
(Protonix, Pantoloc, Somac[AUS])
Do not confuse Protonix with
Lotronex.

CATEGORY AND SCHEDULE
Pregnancy Risk Category: B

Drug Class: Gastrointestinal,
proton pump inhibitor

MECHANISM OF ACTION
A benzimidazole that is converted
to active metabolites that irreversibly
bind to and inhibit hydrogen-
potassium adenosine triphophate,
an enzyme on the surface of gastric
parietal cells. Inhibits hydrogen
ion transport into gastric lumen.
Therapeutic Effect: Increases gastric
pH and reduces gastric acid production.

USES
Short-term treatment of esophageal
erosion and ulceration associated with
gastroesophageal reflux disease (GERD)

PHARMACOKINETICS

Route	Onset	Peak	Duration
PO	N/A	N/A	24 hr

Rapidly absorbed from the GI tract.
Protein binding: 98%. Primarily
distributed into gastric parietal cells.
Metabolized extensively in the liver.
Primarily excreted in urine.
Not removed by hemodialysis.
Half-life: 1 hr.

INDICATIONS AND DOSAGES
▶ **Erosive Esophagitis**
PO
Adults, Elderly. 40 mg/day for up to
8 wk. If not healed after 8 wk, may
continue an additional 8 wk.

IV
Adults, Elderly. 40 mg/day for
7-10 days
▶ **Hypersecretory Conditions**
PO
Adults, Elderly. Initially, 40 mg twice
a day. May increase to 240 mg/day.
IV
Adults, Elderly. 80 mg twice a day.
May increase to 80 mg q8hr.

SIDE EFFECTS/ADVERSE REACTIONS
Rare
Diarrhea, headache, dizziness,
pruritus, rash

PRECAUTIONS AND CONTRAINDICATIONS
Caution is warranted with a chronic
or current hepatic disease. It is
unknown if pantoprazole crosses the
placenta or is distributed in breast
milk. Safety and efficacy of
pantoprazole have not been
established in children. No age-
related precautions have been noted
in the elderly. Serum chemistry
laboratory values, including serum
creatinine and cholesterol levels,
should be obtained before therapy.

DRUG INTERACTIONS OF CONCERN TO DENTISTRY
• None reported.

SERIOUS REACTIONS
None known.

DENTAL CONSIDERATIONS
General:
• Avoid aspirin and NSAIDs for pain
control if GI disease requires
• Consider semisupine chair position
for patient comfort because of possible
regurgitation of stomach contents
• Patients with gastroesophageal
reflux may have oral symptoms,

including burning mouth, secondary
candidiasis and dental erosion
Consultations:
• Consultation is only required if GI
disease is severe or associated with
other systemic conditions
Teach Patient/Family to:
• Report symptoms of oral adverse
effects of GI disease

papaverine hydrochloride
pa-pav´-er-een
(Papacon, Para-Time SR, Pavabid
Plateau, Pavacot, Pavagen)

CATEGORY AND SCHEDULE
Pregnancy Risk Category: C

Drug Class: Peripheral
vasodilator

MECHANISM OF ACTION
A vasodilating agent that acts
directly on the heart muscle to
depress conduction and prolong the
refractory period. **Therapeutic
Effect:** Relaxes smooth muscle.

USES
Treatment of arterial spasm resulting
in cerebral and peripheral ischemia;
myocardial ischemia associated with
vascular spasm or dysrhythmias;
angina pectoris; peripheral
pulmonary embolism; visceral spasm
as in ureteral, biliary, and GI colic
PVD; unapproved: with
phentolamine or alprostadil for
intracavernous injection for
impotence

PHARMACOKINETICS
Protein binding: 90%. Primarily
excreted in urine as inactive
metabolites. **Half-life:** Unknown.

INDICATIONS AND DOSAGES
▸ **Vascular Spasm**
IV/IM
Adults, Elderly. Inject 1–4 ml slowly
and repeat q3h as indicated.
▸ **Vascular Spasm**
PO
Adults, Elderly. One capsule q12h.
In difficult cases, administration may
be increased to one capsule q8h or
2 capsules q12h.

SIDE EFFECTS/ADVERSE REACTIONS
Frequency Not Defined
Capsules: Nausea, abdominal
distress, anorexia, constipation,
malaise, drowsiness, vertigo,
perspiration, headache, diarrhea,
skin rash
Injection: General discomfort,
nausea, abdominal discomfort,
anorexia, constipation, diarrhea,
skin rash, malaise, vertigo, headache,
intensive flushing of the face,
perspiration, increased depth of
respiration, increased heart rate,
slight rise in B/P, excessive sedation

PRECAUTIONS AND CONTRAINDICATIONS
Complete atrioventricular heart
block, impotence by intracorporeal
injection, hypersensitivity to
papaverine or any component of
the formulation
Caution
Cardiac dysrhythmias, glaucoma,
pregnancy category C, lactation,
drug dependency, children, hepatic
hypersensitivity, Parkinson's disease

DRUG INTERACTIONS OF CONCERN TO DENTISTRY
• Increased hypotension:
alcohol, other drugs that may
also lower B/P

SERIOUS REACTIONS

❗ Hepatotoxicity has been reported.
❗ Priapism has been reported.

DENTAL CONSIDERATIONS

General:
• Monitor vital signs at every appointment because of cardiovascular and respiratory side effects.
• Short appointments and a stress reduction protocol may be required for anxious patients.
Consultations:
• Stress from dental procedures may compromise cardiovascular function; determine patient risk.
• Medical consultation may be required to assess disease control.
Teach Patient/Family to:
• Avoid mouth rinses with high alcohol content
• Use effective oral hygiene to prevent soft tissue inflammation

paregoric
par-eh-gor´-ik
Do not confuse with opium tincture.

CATEGORY AND SCHEDULE
Pregnancy Risk Category: B (D if used for prolonged periods, high dosages at term)
Controlled substance: Schedule III

Drug Class: Antidiarrheal

MECHANISM OF ACTION
An opioid agonist that contains many narcotic alkaloids, including morphine. It inhibits gastric motility due to its morphine content.
Therapeutic Effect: Decreases digestive secretions, increases GI muscle tone, and reduces GI propulsion.

USES
Treatment of diarrhea

PHARMACOKINETICS
Variably absorbed from the GI tract. Protein binding: low. Metabolized in liver. Primarily excreted in urine primarily as morphine glucuronide conjugates and unchanged drug—morphine, codeine, papaverine, etc. Unknown if removed by hemodialysis. *Half-life:* 2–3 hr.

INDICATIONS AND DOSAGES
▸ **Antidiarrheal**
PO
Adults, Elderly. 5–10 ml 1–4 times a day.
Children. 0.25–0.5 ml/kg/dose 1–4 times a day.

SIDE EFFECTS/ADVERSE REACTIONS
Frequent
Constipation, drowsiness, nausea, vomiting
Occasional
Paradoxic excitement, confusion, pounding heartbeat, facial flushing, decreased urination, blurred vision, dizziness, dry mouth, headache, hypotension, decreased appetite, redness, burning, pain at injection site
Rare
Hallucinations, depression, stomach pain, insomnia

PRECAUTIONS AND CONTRAINDICATIONS
Diarrhea caused by poisoning until the toxic material is removed, hypersensitivity to morphine sulfate or any component of the formulation, pregnancy (prolonged use or high dosages near term)
Caution
Liver disease, addiction-prone individuals, prostatic

hypertrophy (severe), caution in lactation, safety and efficacy in pediatric patients not established

DRUG INTERACTIONS OF CONCERN TO DENTISTRY
• Increased action of both drugs: alcohol, all other CNS depressants
• Decreased peristalsis: anticholinergic drugs

SERIOUS REACTIONS
! Overdosage results in cold or clammy skin, confusion, convulsions, decreased B/P, restlessness, pinpoint pupils, bradycardia, respiratory depression, decreased level of consciousness, and severe weakness.
! Tolerance to analgesic effect and physical dependence may occur with repeated use.

DENTAL CONSIDERATIONS
General:
• Psychologic and physical dependence may occur with chronic administration.
• Determine why the patient is taking the drug.
Teach Patient/Family to:
• Avoid mouth rinses with high alcohol content because of drying effects

paromomycin
par-oh-moe-mye´-sin
(Humatin)
Do not confuse with Humira.

CATEGORY AND SCHEDULE
Pregnancy Risk Category: C

Drug Class: Amebicide

MECHANISM OF ACTION
An antibacterial agent that acts directly on amoebas and against normal and pathogenic organisms in the GI tract. Interferes with bacterial protein synthesis by binding to 30S ribosomal subunits. ***Therapeutic Effect:*** Produces amoebicidal effects.

USES
Treatment of intestinal amebiasis, adjunct in hepatic coma

PHARMACOKINETICS
Poorly absorbed from the GI tract and most of the dose is eliminated unchanged in feces.

INDICATIONS AND DOSAGES
▸ **Intestinal Amebiasis**
PO
Adults, Elderly, Children. 25–35 mg/kg/day q8h for 5–10 days.
▸ **Hepatic Coma**
PO
Adults, Elderly. 4 g/day q6–12h for 5–6 days.

SIDE EFFECTS/ADVERSE REACTIONS
Occasional
Diarrhea, abdominal cramps, nausea, vomiting, heartburn
Rare
Rash, pruritus, vertigo

PRECAUTIONS AND CONTRAINDICATIONS
Intestinal obstruction, renal failure, hypersensitivity to paromomycin or any of its components

DRUG INTERACTIONS OF CONCERN TO DENTISTRY
• Possible degradation by penicillins and cephalosporins

SERIOUS REACTIONS

! Overdosage may result in nausea, vomiting, and diarrhea.

DENTAL CONSIDERATIONS

General:
• Determine why patient is taking the drug.
• Consider semisupine chair position for patient comfort due to GI effects of disease.
• Question patient about tolerance of NSAIDs or aspirin related to GI disease.
• Postpone elective dental treatment until symptoms are controlled.

Consultations:
• Medical consultation may be required to assess disease control.

Teach Patient/Family to:
• Update health and medication history if physician makes any changes in evaluation or drug regimens; include OTC, herbal, and nonherbal drugs in the update
• Report sore throat, oral burning sensation, fever, or fatigue, any of which could indicate presence of a superinfection

paroxetine hydrochloride

par-ox´-eh-teen high-droh-klor´-ide
(Aropax 20[AUS], Paxeva, Paxil, Paxil CR, Paxtine[AUS])
Do not confuse paroxetine with pyridoxine, or Paxil with Doxil or Taxol.

CATEGORY AND SCHEDULE

Pregnancy Risk Category: C

Drug Class: Antidepressant

MECHANISM OF ACTION

An antidepressant, anxiolytic, and antiobsessional agent that selectively blocks uptake of the neurotransmitter serotonin at neuronal presynaptic membranes, thereby increasing its availability at postsynaptic receptor sites. *Therapeutic Effect:* Relieves depression, reduces obsessive-compulsive behavior, decreases anxiety.

USES

Treatment of depression, panic disorder, obsessive-compulsive disorder, social anxiety disorder; generalized anxiety disorder, posttraumatic stress disorder; premenstrual dysphoric disorder

PHARMACOKINETICS

Well absorbed from the GI tract. Protein binding: 95%. Widely distributed. Metabolized in the liver. Excreted in urine. Not removed by hemodialysis. *Half-life:* 24 hr.

INDICATIONS AND DOSAGES

▸ **Depression**
PO
Adults. Initially, 20 mg/day. May increase by 10 mg/day at intervals of more than 1 wk. Maximum: 50 mg/day.
PO (Controlled-Release)
Adults. Initially, 25 mg/day. May increase by 12.5 mg/day at intervals of more than 1 wk. Maximum: 62.5 mg/day.
▸ **Generalized Anxiety Disorder**
PO
Adults. Initially, 20 mg/day. May increase by 10 mg/day at intervals of more than 1 wk. Range: 20–50 mg/day.
▸ **Obsessive-Compulsive Disorder**
PO
Adults. Initially, 20 mg/day. May increase by 10 mg/day at intervals of more than 1 wk. Range: 20–60 mg/day.

▶ **Panic Disorder**
PO
Adults. Initially, 10–20 mg/day.
May increase by 10 mg/day at
intervals of more than 1 wk.
Range: 10–60 mg/day.
▶ **Social Anxiety Disorder**
PO
Adults. Initially 20 mg/day.
Range: 20–60 mg/day.
▶ **Posttraumatic Stress Disorder**
PO
Adults. Initially, 20 mg/day. May
increase by 10 mg/day at intervals of
more than 1 wk. Range:
20–50 mg/day.
▶ **Premenstrual Dysphoric Disorder**
PO (Paxil CR)
Adults. Initially, 12.5 mg/day. May
increase by 12.5 mg at weekly
intervals to a maximum of 25 mg/day.
▶ **Usual Elderly Dosage**
PO
Initially, 10 mg/day. May increase
by 10 mg/day at intervals of
more than 1 wk. Maximum:
40 mg/day.
PO (Controlled-Release)
Initially, 12.5 mg/day. May increase
by 12.5 mg/day at intervals of
more than 1 wk. Maximum:
50 mg/day.

SIDE EFFECTS/ADVERSE REACTIONS
Frequent
Nausea, somnolence, headache, dry
mouth, asthenia, constipation,
dizziness, insomnia, diarrhea,
diaphoresis, tremor
Occasional
Decreased appetite, respiratory
disturbance (such as increased
cough), anxiety, nervousness,
flatulence, paresthesia, yawning,
decreased libido, sexual dysfunction,
abdominal discomfort

Rare
Palpitations, vomiting, blurred
vision, altered taste, confusion

PRECAUTIONS AND CONTRAINDICATIONS
Use within 14 days of MAOIs
Caution
Lactation, elderly, oral
anticoagulants, renal or hepatic
impairment, children with suspected
higher risk of suicide ideation, other
serotonergic drugs

DRUG INTERACTIONS OF CONCERN TO DENTISTRY
• Possible increased side effects:
highly protein-bound drugs (aspirin),
other antidepressants, alcohol
• Possible inhibition of fluoxetine
metabolism: erythromycin,
clarithromycin
• Increased half-life of diazepam
• First-time users of SSRIs also
taking NSAIDs may have a higher
risk of GI side effects; until more
data are available, it may be
advisable to avoid use of NSAIDs in
these patients (Br J Clin Pharmacol
55:591–595, 2003)

SERIOUS REACTIONS
! Abnormal bleeding, hyponatremia,
seizures, hypomania, and suicidal
thoughts have been reported.

DENTAL CONSIDERATIONS
General:
• After supine positioning, have
patient sit upright for at least 2 min
before standing to avoid orthostatic
hypotension.
• Assess salivary flow as a factor
in caries, periodontal disease, and
candidiasis.
• Avoid dental light in patient's eyes;
offer dark glasses for patient
comfort.

Consultations:
• Medical consultation may be required to assess disease control and patient's ability to tolerate stress.
• Physician should be informed if significant xerostomic side effects occur (e.g., increased caries, sore tongue, problems eating or swallowing, difficulty wearing prosthesis) so that a medication change can be considered.

Teach Patient/Family:
• When chronic dry mouth occurs, advise patient to:
  • Avoid mouth rinses with high alcohol content because of drying effects
  • Use daily home fluoride products to prevent caries
  • Use sugarless gum, frequent sips of water, or saliva substitutes

pegfilgrastim
peg-fil-gras´-tim
(Neulasta)
Do not confuse Neulasta with Neumega.

CATEGORY AND SCHEDULE
Pregnancy Risk Category: C

Drug Class: Hematopoietic agent

MECHANISM OF ACTION
A colony-stimulating factor that regulates production of neutrophils within bone marrow. Also a glycoprotein that primarily affects neutrophil progenitor proliferation, differentiation, and selected end-cell functional activation. **Therapeutic Effect:** Increases phagocytic ability and antibody-dependent destruction; decreases incidence of infection.

USES
To decrease infection in patients receiving antineoplastics that are myelosuppressive; to increase WBC in patients with drug-induced neutropenia

PHARMACOKINETICS
Readily absorbed after subcutaneous administration. **Half-life:** 15–80 hr.

INDICATIONS AND DOSAGES
▶ **Myelosuppression**
Subcutaneous
Adults, Elderly. Give as a single 6-mg injection once per chemotherapy cycle.

SIDE EFFECTS/ADVERSE REACTIONS
Frequent
Bone pain, nausea, fatigue, alopecia, diarrhea, vomiting, constipation, anorexia, abdominal pain, arthralgia, generalized weakness, peripheral edema, dizziness, stomatitis, mucositis, neutropenic fever

PRECAUTIONS AND CONTRAINDICATIONS
Hypersensitivity to *Escherichia coli*–derived proteins, within 14 days before and 24 hr after cytotoxic chemotherapy

DRUG INTERACTIONS OF CONCERN TO DENTISTRY
None reported

SERIOUS REACTIONS
❗ Allergic reactions, such as anaphylaxis, rash, and urticaria, occur rarely.
❗ Cytopenia resulting from an antibody response to growth factors occurs rarely.

P

! Splenomegaly occurs rarely; assess for left upper abdominal or shoulder pain.
! Adult respiratory distress syndrome (ARDS) may occur in patients with sepsis.

DENTAL CONSIDERATIONS

General:
• Patients may have a history of chemotherapy or radiation; confirm medical and drug history.
• Determine type of chemotherapeutic agents used and related oral side effects.
• Monitor and record vital signs.
• Examine for oral manifestation of opportunistic infection.
Consultations:
• Medical consultation may be required to assess disease control and patient's ability to tolerate stress.
Teach Patient/Family to:
• Use effective oral hygiene to prevent soft tissue inflammation
• Prevent trauma when using oral hygiene aids
• Report oral lesions, soreness, or bleeding to dentist

peginterferon alfa-2a

peg-inn-ter-fear´-on al´-fah
(Pegasys)

CATEGORY AND SCHEDULE
Pregnancy Risk Category: C

Drug Class: Biologic response modifier

MECHANISM OF ACTION
An immunomodulator that binds to specific membrane receptors on the cell surface, inhibiting viral replication in virus-infected cells, suppressing cell proliferation, and producing reversible decreases in leukocyte and platelet counts. *Therapeutic Effect:* Inhibits hepatitis C virus.

USES
Treatment of adults with chronic hepatitis C with compensated liver disease who have not been previously treated with interferon-alfa.

PHARMACOKINETICS
Subcutaneous: Peak serum levels 72–96 hr; cleared from the body at 94 ml/hr; no data in children
Readily absorbed after subcutaneous administration. Excreted by the kidneys. *Half-life:* 80 hr.

INDICATIONS AND DOSAGES
▸ **Hepatitis C**
Subcutaneous
Adults 18 yr and older, Elderly.
180 mcg (1 ml) injected in abdomen or thigh once weekly for 48 wk.
▸ **Dosage in Renal Impairment**
For patients who require hemodialysis, dosage is 135 mg injected in abdomen or thigh once weekly for 48 wk.
▸ **Dosage in Hepatic Impairment**
For patients with progressive ALT (SGPT) increases above baseline values, dosage is 90 mcg injected in abdomen or thigh once weekly for 48 wk.

SIDE EFFECTS/ADVERSE REACTIONS
Frequent
Headache
Occasional
Alopecia, nausea, insomnia, anorexia, dizziness, diarrhea,

abdominal pain, flu-like symptoms, psychiatric reactions (depression, irritability, anxiety), injection site reaction, impaired concentration, diaphoresis, dry mouth, nausea, vomiting

PRECAUTIONS AND CONTRAINDICATIONS

Autoimmune hepatitis, decompensated hepatic disease, infants, neonates

Caution

Preexisting cardiac disease, may aggravate hypothyroidism, hyperthyroidism, hyperglycemia, hypoglycemia, diabetes, ophthalmologic disorders, lactation, children; closely monitor patients, severe
life-threatening neuropsychiatric, autoimmune, ischemic, or infectious disorders may cause or aggravate these conditions

DRUG INTERACTIONS OF CONCERN TO DENTISTRY

• Risk of hepatotoxicity in severe liver disease: acetaminophen

SERIOUS REACTIONS

! Serious, acute hypersensitivity reactions, such as urticaria, angioedema, bronchoconstriction, and anaphylaxis, may occur. Other rare reactions include pancreatitis, colitis, endocrine disorders (e.g., diabetes mellitus), hyperthyroidism or hypothyroidism, ophthalmologic disorders, and pulmonary disorders.

DENTAL CONSIDERATIONS

General:

• Determine why patient is taking the drug.

• Assess salivary flow as a factor in caries, periodontal disease, and candidiasis.

• Consider semisupine chair position for patient comfort if GI side effects occur.

• Question patient about tolerance of NSAIDs or aspirin related to GI disease.

• Patients on chronic drug therapy may rarely have symptoms of blood dyscrasias, which can include infection, bleeding, and poor healing.

• Avoid elective dental procedures if severe neutropenia (fewer than 500 cells/mm^3) or thrombocytopenia (fewer than 50,000 cell/mm^3) is present.

• Severe side effects may require postponing elective dental procedures until drug therapy is completed.

Consultations:

• Medical consultation may be required to assess disease control in the patient.

• In a patient with symptoms of blood dyscrasias, request a medical consultation for blood studies and postpone treatment until normal values are reestablished

• Liver function tests may be required to determine chronic liver disease.

Teach Patient/Family to:

• Use effective oral hygiene to prevent soft tissue inflammation/infection

• Evaluate efficacy of oral hygiene home care; preventive appointments may be necessary

• Prevent trauma when using oral hygiene aids

• When chronic dry mouth occurs, advise patient to:
  • Avoid mouth rinses with high alcohol content because of drying effects
  • Use daily home fluoride products for anticaries effect
  • Use sugarless gum, frequent sips of water, or saliva substitutes

peginterferon alfa-2b

peg-inn-ter-fear´-on al´-fah
(PEG-Intron)

CATEGORY AND SCHEDULE
Pregnancy Risk Category: C

Drug Class: Biologic response
modifier

MECHANISM OF ACTION
An immunomodulator that inhibits
viral replication in virus-infected
cells, suppresses cell proliferation,
increases phagocytic action of
macrophages, and augments specific
cytotoxicity of lymphocytes for
target cells. *Therapeutic Effect:*
Inhibits hepatitis C virus.

USES
Treatment of adults with chronic
hepatitis C with compensated liver
disease who have not been previously
treated with interferon-alfa;
peginterferon alfa-2b can be used
with ribavirin

PHARMACOKINETICS
Subcutaneous: Peak serum levels
72–96 hr; cleared from the body at
94 ml/hr; no data in children,
pharmacokinetic data are limited

INDICATIONS AND DOSAGES
▶ **Chronic Hepatitis C, Monotherapy**
Subcutaneous
Adults 18 yr and older, Elderly.
Administer appropriate dosage (see
chart below) once weekly for 1 yr on
the same day each wk.

Vial Strength	Weight (kg)	mcg*	ml*
100 mcg/ml	37–45	40	0.4
	46–56	50	0.5
160 mcg/ml	57–72	64	0.4
	73–88	80	0.5
240 mcg/ml	89–106	96	0.4
	107–136	120	0.5
300 mcg/ml	137–160	150	0.5

*Of peginterferon alpha-2b to administer

▶ **Chronic Hepatitis C**
Subcutaneous combination therapy
with ribavirin (400 mg twice a day).
Initially, 1.5 mcg/kg/wk.

SIDE EFFECTS/ADVERSE REACTIONS
Frequent
Flu-like symptoms; inflammation,
bruising, pruritus, and irritation at
injection site
Occasional
Psychiatric reactions (depression,
anxiety, emotional lability,
irritability), insomnia, alopecia,
diarrhea
Rare
Rash, diaphoresis, dry skin,
dizziness, flushing, vomiting,
dyspepsia

PRECAUTIONS AND CONTRAINDICATIONS
Autoimmune hepatitis,
decompensated hepatic disease,
history of psychiatric disorders
Caution
Preexisting cardiac disease,
may aggravate hypothyroidism,
hyperthyroidism, hyperglycemia,
hypoglycemia, diabetes,
ophthalmologic disorders,
lactation, children; closely monitor
patients, severe life-threatening
neuropsychiatric, autoimmune,
ischemic, or infectious disorders

may cause or aggravate these conditions

DRUG INTERACTIONS OF CONCERN TO DENTISTRY

• Risk of hepatotoxicity in severe liver disease: acetaminophen

SERIOUS REACTIONS

❗ Serious, acute hypersensitivity reactions (such as urticaria, angioedema, bronchoconstriction, and anaphylaxis), pulmonary disorders, endocrine disorders (e.g., diabetes mellitus), hypothyroidism, hyperthyroidism, and pancreatitis occur rarely.

❗ Ulcerative colitis may occur within 12 wk of starting treatment.

DENTAL CONSIDERATIONS

General:

• Determine why patient is taking the drug.

• Assess salivary flow as a factor in caries, periodontal disease, and candidiasis.

• Consider semisupine chair position for patient comfort if GI side effects occur.

• Question patient about tolerance of NSAIDs or aspirin related to GI disease.

• Patients on chronic drug therapy may rarely have symptoms of blood dyscrasias, which can include infection, bleeding, and poor healing.

• Avoid elective dental procedures if severe neutropenia (fewer than 500 cells/mm^3) or thrombocytopenia (fewer than 50,000 cell/mm^3) is present.

• Severe side effects may require postponing elective dental procedures until drug therapy is completed.

Consultations:

• Medical consultation may be required to assess disease control in the patient.

• In a patient with symptoms of blood dyscrasias, request a medical consultation for blood studies and postpone treatment until normal values are reestablished.

• Liver function tests may be required to determine chronic liver disease.

Teach Patient/Family to:

• Use effective oral hygiene to prevent soft tissue inflammation/infection

• Evaluate efficacy of oral hygiene home care; preventive appointments may be necessary

• Prevent trauma when using oral hygiene aids

• When chronic dry mouth occurs, advise patient to:

  • Avoid mouth rinses with high alcohol content because of drying effects

  • Use daily home fluoride products for anticaries effect

  • Use sugarless gum, frequent sips of water, or saliva substitutes

P

pegvisomant

peg-vis´-oh-mant
(Somavert)
Do not confuse Somavert with somatrem or somatropin.

CATEGORY AND SCHEDULE

Pregnancy Risk Category: B

Drug Class: Acroegaly agent

MECHANISM OF ACTION

A protein that selectively binds to growth hormone (GH) receptors on cell surfaces, blocking the binding of endogenous GHs and interfering with GH signal transduction. *Therapeutic Effect:* Decreases serum concentrations of insulin-like growth factor 1 (IGF-1) and other GH-responsive serum proteins.

USES

Treatment of acromegaly in those patients who have an inadequate response to other treatment

PHARMACOKINETICS

Not distributed extensively into tissues after subcutaneous administration. Less than 1% excreted in urine. *Half-life:* 6 days.

INDICATIONS AND DOSAGES
▸ **Acromegaly**
Subcutaneous
Adults, Elderly. Initially, 40 mg as a loading dose, then 10 mg daily. After 4–6 wk, adjust dosage in 5-mg increments if serum IGF-1 level is still elevated, or in 5-mg decrements if IGF-1 level has decreased below the normal range. Maximum: 30 mg daily.

SIDE EFFECTS/ADVERSE REACTIONS
Frequent
Infection (cold symptoms, upper respiratory tract infection, blister, ear infection)
Occasional
Back pain, dizziness, injection site reaction, peripheral edema, sinusitis, nausea
Rare
Diarrhea, paresthesia

PRECAUTIONS AND CONTRAINDICATIONS
Latex allergy (stopper on vial contains latex)

DRUG INTERACTIONS OF CONCERN TO DENTISTRY
• Opioids: decreased serum levels

SERIOUS REACTIONS
❗ Pegvisomant use may markedly elevate liver function test results, including serum transaminase levels.
❗ Substantial weight gain occurs rarely.

DENTAL CONSIDERATIONS
General:
• Confirm history of previous medical, surgical, or radiation treatment for this disease.
• Monitor vital signs.
• Patient may complain of temporomandibular dysfunction (TMD) due to disease.
• Place on frequent recall to evaluate healing response
Consultations:
• Physician consultation should include liver function tests.
Teach Patient/Family to:
• Use effective oral hygiene to prevent soft tissue inflammation
• Prevent trauma when using oral hygiene aids
• Update health and medication history if physician makes any changes in evaluation or drug regimens; include OTC, herbal, and nonherbal drugs in the update

pemirolast potassium
peh-meer´-oh-last poe-tass´-ee-um
(Alamast)

CATEGORY AND SCHEDULE
Pregnancy Risk Category: C

Drug Class:
Ophthalmic

MECHANISM OF ACTION

An antiallergic agent that prevents activation and release of mediators of inflammation (e.g., mast cells). *Therapeutic Effect:* Reduces symptoms of allergic conjunctivitis.

USES

Relief of allergic conjunctivitis

PHARMACOKINETICS

Detected in plasma. Excreted in urine. *Half-life:* 4.5 hr.

INDICATIONS AND DOSAGES
▶ Allergic Conjunctivitis
Ophthalmic
Adults, Elderly, Children 3 yr and older. 1–2 drops in affected eye(s) 4 times a day.

SIDE EFFECTS/ADVERSE REACTIONS

Frequent
Headache, rhinitis, cold and flu symptoms
Occasional
Transient ocular stinging, burning, itching, dry eye, foreign body sensation, tearing
Rare
Sinusitis, sneezing/nasal congestion

PRECAUTIONS AND CONTRAINDICATIONS

Hypersensitivity to pemirolast potassium or any other component of the formulation
Caution
Lactation, children, do not wear contact lens if eyes are red, may affect soft contact lens, if no red eyes wait 10 min after using to place soft contacts

DRUG INTERACTIONS OF CONCERN TO DENTISTRY

None reported

SERIOUS REACTIONS

None reported

DENTAL CONSIDERATIONS
General:
• Question patient about history of allergies to avoid using other potential allergens.
• Avoid dental light in patient's eyes; offer dark glasses for patient comfort.

---

pemoline
pem´-oh-leen
(Cylert, PemADD, PemADD CT)

CATEGORY AND SCHEDULE
Pregnancy Risk Category: B
Controlled Substance: Schedule IV

Drug Class: CNS stimulant

MECHANISM OF ACTION

A CNS stimulant that blocks the reuptake mechanism present in dopaminergic neurons in the cerebral cortex and subcortical structures. *Therapeutic Effect:* Reduces motor restlessness and fatigue, increases alertness, elevates mood.

USES

Treatment of attention deficit hyperactivity disorder (ADHD)

PHARMACOKINETICS

PO: Peak 2–4 hr, duration 8 hr. *Half-life:* 12 hr; metabolized (50%) by liver; excreted (40%) by kidneys.

INDICATIONS AND DOSAGES
▶ ADHD
PO
Children 6 yr and older. Initially, 37.5 mg/day as a single dose in morning. May increase by 18.75 mg

P

at weekly intervals until therapeutic response is achieved. Range: 56.25–75 mg/day. Maximum: 112.5 mg/day.

SIDE EFFECTS/ADVERSE REACTIONS
Frequent
Anorexia, insomnia
Occasional
Nausea, abdominal discomfort, diarrhea, headache, dizziness, somnolence

PRECAUTIONS AND CONTRAINDICATIONS
Family history of Tourette syndrome, hepatic impairment, motor tics
Caution
Renal disease, lactation, drug abuse, children younger than 6 yr; liver function monitoring recommended

DRUG INTERACTIONS OF CONCERN TO DENTISTRY
• Increased irritability, stimulation: caffeine-containing products and food

SERIOUS REACTIONS
! Visual disturbances, rash, and dyskinetic movements of the tongue, lips, face, and extremities have occurred.
! Large doses of pemoline may produce extreme nervousness and tachycardia.
! Hepatic effects, such as hepatitis and jaundice, appear to be reversible when the drug is discontinued.
! Prolonged administration to children with ADHD may temporarily delay growth.

DENTAL CONSIDERATIONS
General:
• Keep dental appointments short because of effects of disease.

Teach Patient/Family to:
• Use electric tooth brush for effective plaque control

penbutolol
pen-beaut´-oh-lol
(Levatol)
Do not confuse with pindolol.

CATEGORY AND SCHEDULE
Pregnancy Risk Category: C
(D if used in the second or third trimester)

Drug Class: Nonselective β-adrenergic blocker

MECHANISM OF ACTION
An antihypertensive that possesses nonselective beta-blocking. Has moderate intrinsic sympathomimetic activity. ***Therapeutic Effect:*** Reduces cardiac output, decreases B/P, increases airway resistance, and decreases myocardial ischemia severity.

USES
Treatment of hypertension alone or with other antihypertensive drugs

PHARMACOKINETICS
Rapidly and extensively absorbed from the GI tract. Protein binding: 80%–90%. Metabolized in liver. Excreted primarily via urine. ***Half-life:*** 17–26 hr.

INDICATIONS AND DOSAGES
▶ **Hypertension**
PO
Adults. Initially, 20 mg/day as a single dose. May increase to 40–80 mg/day.
Elderly. Initially, 10 mg/day.

SIDE EFFECTS/ADVERSE REACTIONS

Frequent

Decreased sexual ability, drowsiness, trouble sleeping, unusual tiredness/weakness

Occasional

Diarrhea, bradycardia, depression, cold hands/feet, constipation, anxiety, nasal congestion, nausea, vomiting

Rare

Altered taste, dry eyes, itching, numbness of fingers, toes, scalp

PRECAUTIONS AND CONTRAINDICATIONS

Bronchial asthma or related bronchospastic conditions, cardiogenic shock, pulmonary edema, second- or third-degree AV block, severe bradycardia, overt cardiac failure, hypersensitivity to penbutolol or any component of the formulation

Caution

Diabetes mellitus, renal disease, lactation, hyperthyroidism, COPD, hepatic disease, children, myasthenia gravis, peripheral vascular disease, hypotension

DRUG INTERACTIONS OF CONCERN TO DENTISTRY

• Decreased hypotensive effect: indomethacin, NSAIDs
• Increased hypotension, myocardial depression: hydrocarbon inhalation anesthetics
• Hypertension, bradycardia: sympathomimetics (epinephrine, ephedrine)
• Slow metabolism of lidocaine

SERIOUS REACTIONS

! Abrupt withdrawal may result in sweating, palpitations, headache, and tremulousness.

! Hypoglycemia may occur in patients with previously controlled diabetes.

DENTAL CONSIDERATIONS

General:

• Monitor vital signs at every appointment because of cardiovascular side effects.
• Patients on chronic drug therapy may rarely have symptoms of blood dyscrasias, which can include infection, bleeding, and poor healing.
• Limit use of sodium-containing products, such as saline IV fluids, for patients with a dietary salt restriction.
• Assess salivary flow as a factor in caries, periodontal disease, and candidiasis.
• After supine positioning, have patient sit upright for at least 2 min before standing to avoid orthostatic hypotension.
• Stress from dental procedures may compromise cardiovascular function; determine patient risk.
• Short appointments and a stress-reduction protocol may be required for anxious patients.
• Use vasoconstrictor with caution, in low doses, and with careful aspiration.
• Avoid using gingival retraction cord containing epinephrine.

Consultations:

• In a patient with symptoms of blood dyscrasias, request a medical consultation for blood studies and postpone dental treatment until normal values are reestablished.
• Medical consultation may be required to assess disease control and patient's ability to tolerate stress.

Teach Patient/Family to:

• Use caution to prevent injury when using oral hygiene aids

P

- Use effective oral hygiene to prevent soft tissue inflammation
- If taste alterations occur, consider drug as potential cause
- When chronic dry mouth occurs, advise patient to:
  - Avoid mouth rinses with high alcohol content because of drying effects
  - Use daily home fluoride products to prevent caries
  - Use sugarless gum, frequent sips of water, or saliva substitutes

---

penciclovir
pen-sye´-kloe-veer
(Denavir, Vectavir[South Africa, Costa Rica, Dominican Republic, El Salvador, Germany, Guatemala, Honduras, Israel, Nicaragua, Panama])
Do not confuse with acyclovir.

CATEGORY AND SCHEDULE
Pregnancy Risk Category: B

Drug Class: Antiviral

MECHANISM OF ACTION
Penciclovir triphosphate inhibits HSV polymerase competitively with deoxyguanosine triphosphate. Consequently, herpes viral DNA synthesis and, therefore, replication are selectively inhibited. *Therapeutic Effect:* An antiviral compound that has inhibitory activity against human herpes virus types 1 (HHV-1) and 2 (HHV-2).

USES
Treatment of recurrent herpes labialis (cold sores)

PHARMACOKINETICS
Measurable penciclovir concentrations were not detected in plasma or urine. The systemic absorption of penciclovir following topical administration has not been evaluated.

INDICATIONS AND DOSAGES
▶ **Herpes Labialis (cold sores)**
Topical
Adolescents, Adults. Penciclovir should be applied every 2 hr during waking hr for a period of 4 days. Treatment should be started as early as possible (i.e., during the prodrome or when lesions appear).

SIDE EFFECTS/ADVERSE REACTIONS
Frequent
Headache
Occasional
Change in sense of taste; decreased sensitivity of skin, particularly to touch; redness of the skin; skin rash (maculopapular, erythematous), local edema, skin discoloration; pruritus; hypoesthesia; parathesias; parosmia; urticaria; oral/pharyngeal edema
Rare
Mild pain, burning, or stinging

PRECAUTIONS AND CONTRAINDICATIONS
Hypersensitivity to penciclovir or any of its components
Caution
Acyclovir-resistant herpes viruses, patients younger than 18 yr, use on mucous membranes not recommended, avoid applications near the eye, lactation

DRUG INTERACTIONS OF CONCERN TO DENTISTRY
- None reported.

SERIOUS REACTIONS
- None reported.

DENTAL CONSIDERATIONS
General:
- Use in immunocompromised patients not established.

• Postpone dental treatment when oral herpetic lesions are present.
Teach Patient/Family to:
• Dispose of toothbrush or other contaminated oral hygiene devices used during period of infection to prevent reinoculation of herpetic infection
• Apply with a finger cot or latex glove to prevent herpes infection on fingers

penicillin
pen-ih-sil´-in
(Amoxicillin, Ampicillin, Bacampicillin, Carbenicillin, Cloxacillin, Dicloxacillin, Flucloxacillin, Methicillin, Mezlocillin, Nafcillin, Oxacillin, Penicillin G benzathine, Penicillin G potassium, Penicillin V potassium, Piperacillin, Pivampicillin, Pivmecillinam, Ticarcillin; Penicillin and beta-lactamase inhibitors; Amoxicillin/Clavulanate Potassium, Ampicillin/Sulbactam Sodium, Piperacillin Sodium/Tazobactam Sodium, Ticarcillin Disodium/Clavulanate Potassium)

CATEGORY AND SCHEDULE
Pregnancy Risk Category: B

Drug Class: Antibiotics

MECHANISM OF ACTION
Penicillins bind to bacterial cell wall, inhibiting bacterial cell wall synthesis. *Therapeutic Effect:* Inhibits bacterial cell wall synthesis. β-lactamase inhibitors: inhibit the action of bacterial β-lactamase. *Therapeutic Effect:* Protects the penicillin from enzymatic degradation.

USES
Treatment of sepsis, meningitis, pericarditis, endocarditis, pneumonia, UTIs, septicemia, meningitis, intraabdominal infections, gonorrhea, syphilis, and bone and joint infections

PHARMACOKINETICS
Penicillins are generally well absorbed from the GI tract after oral administration. Widely distributed to most tissues and body fluids. Protein binding: 20%. Partially metabolized in liver. Primarily excreted in urine. *Half-life:* Varies (half-life increased in reduced renal function).

INDICATIONS AND DOSAGES
Penicillins may be used to treat a large number of infections, including pneumonia and other respiratory diseases, urinary tract infections, septicemia, meningitis, intraabdominal infections, gonorrhea, syphilis, and bone and joint infections. Doses vary depending on the drug used. In general, penicillins should be taken on an empty stomach. Patients with impaired renal function may require dose adjustment.

SIDE EFFECTS/ADVERSE REACTIONS
Frequent
GI disturbances (mild diarrhea, nausea, or vomiting), headache, oral or vaginal candidiasis
Occasional
Generalized rash, urticaria

PRECAUTIONS AND CONTRAINDICATIONS
Hypersensitivity to any penicillin, infectious mononucleosis

P

DRUG INTERACTIONS OF CONCERN TO DENTISTRY
- Decreased antimicrobial effect of penicillin: tetracyclines, erythromycins, lincomycins
- Increased penicillin concentrations: aspirin, probenecid
- Suspected increased risk of methotrexate toxicity
- Oral contraceptives: advise patient of a potential risk for decreased contraceptive action, to maintain compliance with oral contraceptive use while using antibiotics, and to consider the use of additional nonhormonal contraception

DRUG INTERACTIONS OF CONCERN TO DENTISTRY
Penicillin G Potassium, Aqueous (Pfizerpen), Penicillin V Potassium/ Penicillin V
- Increased or prolonged plasma levels: probenecid
- Possible decrease in antimicrobial effectiveness: tetracyclines, erythromycins, lincomycins
- When used for dental infection:
  - Oral contraceptives: advise patient of a potential low risk for decreased contraceptive action, to maintain compliance with oral contraceptive while using antibiotics, and to consider the use of additional nonhormonal contraception

SERIOUS REACTIONS
! Altered bacterial balance may result in potentially fatal superinfections and antibiotic-associated colitis as evidenced by abdominal cramps, watery or severe diarrhea, and fever.
! Severe hypersensitivity reactions, including anaphylaxis and acute interstitial nephritis occur rarely.

Penicillin G Benzathine
Penicillin G Potassium, Aqueous (Pfizerpen)
General:
- Take precautions regarding allergy to medication.
- Determine why the patient is taking the drug.
- Place on frequent recall to evaluate healing response.

Consultations:
- Medical consultation may be required to assess disease control.

Teach Patient/Family to:
- When used for dental infection, advise patient to:
  - Report sore throat, oral burning sensation, fever, fatigue, any of which could indicate superinfection
  - Take at prescribed intervals and complete dosage regimen
  - Immediately notify the dentist if signs or symptoms of infection increase
- Use with caution in patients with a history of antibiotic-associated colitis.
- Use effective oral hygiene to prevent soft tissue inflammation
- Prevent trauma when using oral hygiene aids
- Report sore throat, oral burning sensation, fever, or fatigue, any of which could indicate presence of a superinfection

penicillin G benzathine

pen-ih-sil´-lin G benz´-ah-thene
(Bicillin LA, Permapen)
Do not confuse penicillin G
benzathine with penicillin G
potassium or penicillin G procaine.

CATEGORY AND SCHEDULE
Pregnancy Risk Category: B

Drug Class: Benzathine salt
of natural penicillin G

MECHANISM OF ACTION
A penicillin that inhibits bacterial
cell wall synthesis by binding to one
or more of the penicillin-binding
proteins of bacteria. *Therapeutic
Effect:* Bactericidal.

USES
Treatment of respiratory infections,
scarlet fever, erysipelas, otitis media,
pneumonia, skin and soft tissue
infections, bejel, pinta, yaws;
effective for gram-positive cocci
(*Staphylococcus, S. pyogenes,
S. viridans, S. faecalis, S. bovis,
S. pneumoniae*), gram-negative cocci
(*N. gonorrhoeae*), gram-positive
bacilli (*B. anthracis, C. perfringens,
C. tetani, C. diphtheriae,
L. monocytogenes*), gram-negative
bacilli (*E. coli, P. mirabilis,
Salmonella, Shigella, Enterobacter,
S. moniliformis*), spirochetes
(*T. pallidum*), Actinomyces

PHARMACOKINETICS
IM: Very slow absorption,
hydrolyzed to penicillin G, duration
21–28 days. *Half-life:* 30–60 min;
excreted in urine, breast milk;
crosses placenta.

INDICATIONS AND DOSAGES
▶ **Group A Streptococcal Infections**
IM
Adults, Elderly. 1.2 million units as a
single dose.
Children. 25,000–50,000 units/kg as
a single dose.
▶ **Prevention of Rheumatic Fever**
IM
Adults, Elderly. 1.2 million units
every 3–4 wk or 600,000 units twice
monthly.
Children. 25,000–50,000 units/kg
every 3–4 wk.
▶ **Early Syphilis**
IM
Adults, Elderly. 2.4 million units
divided and administered in 2
separate injection sites.
▶ **Congenital Syphilis**
IM
Children. 50,000 units/kg weekly for
3 wk.
▶ **Syphilis of More Than 1 Year's
Duration**
IM
Adults, Elderly. 2.4 million units
divided and administered in 2
separate injection sites weekly for
3 wk.
Children. 50,000 units/kg weekly for
3 wk.

SIDE EFFECTS/ADVERSE REACTIONS
Occasional
Lethargy, fever, dizziness, rash, pain
at injection site
Rare
Seizures, interstitial nephritis

PRECAUTIONS AND CONTRAINDICATIONS
Hypersensitivity to any penicillin
Caution
Hypersensitivity to cephalosporins

P

DRUG INTERACTIONS OF CONCERN TO DENTISTRY

- Decreased antimicrobial effect of penicillin: tetracyclines, erythromycins, lincomycins
- Increased penicillin concentrations: aspirin, probenecid
- Suspected increased risk of methotrexate toxicity
- Oral contraceptives: advise patient of a low potential risk for decreased contraceptive action, to maintain compliance with oral contraceptive use while using antibiotics, and to consider the use of additional nonhormonal contraception

SERIOUS REACTIONS

! Hypersensitivity reactions, ranging from chills, fever, and rash to anaphylaxis, may occur.

DENTAL CONSIDERATIONS

General:
- Take precautions regarding allergy to medication.
- Determine why the patient is taking the drug.
- Place on frequent recall to evaluate healing response.

Consultations:
- Medical consultation may be required to assess disease control.

Teach Patient/Family:
- When used for dental infection, advise patient to:
  - Report sore throat, oral burning sensation, fever, fatigue, any of which could indicate superinfection
  - Take at prescribed intervals and complete dosage regimen
  - Immediately notify the dentist if signs or symptoms of infection increase

penicillin G potassium

pen-ih-sil´-lin G poe-tass´-ee-um (Megacillin[CAN], Novepen-G[CAN], Pfizerpen)
Do not confuse penicillin G potassium with penicillin G benzathine or penicillin G procaine.

CATEGORY AND SCHEDULE
Pregnancy Risk Category: B

Drug Class: Antibiotics, penicillins

MECHANISM OF ACTION

A penicillin that inhibits bacterial cell wall synthesis by binding to one or more of the penicillin-binding proteins of bacteria. ***Therapeutic Effect:*** Bactericidal.

USES

Treatment of sepsis, meningitis, pericarditis, endocarditis, pneumonia due to susceptible gram-positive organisms (not *Staphylococcus aureus*), and some gram-negative organisms.

PHARMACOKINETICS

Completely absorbed from intramuscular injection sites. Peak blood levels reached rapidly after intravenous infusion. Bound primarily to albumin. Widely distributed, but has limited penetration into cerebrospinal fluid. 60% excreted within 5 hr by kidney.

INDICATIONS AND DOSAGES

▶ **Sepsis, Meningitis, Pericarditis, Endocarditis, Pneumonia Due to Susceptible Gram-Positive Organisms (not *Staphylococcus Aureus*) and Some Gram-Negative Organisms**
IV, IM
Adults, Elderly. 2–24 million units/kg/day in divided doses q4–6h.

Children. 100,000–400,000 units/kg/day in divided doses q4–6h.
▸ **Dosage in Renal Impairment**
Dosage interval is modified on the basis of creatinine clearance.

Creatinine Clearance	Dosage Interval
10–30 ml/min	Usual dose q8–12h
Less than 10 ml/min	Usual dose q12–18h

SIDE EFFECTS/ADVERSE REACTIONS

Occasional
Lethargy, fever, dizziness, rash, electrolyte imbalance, diarrhea, thrombophlebitis
Rare
Seizures, interstitial nephritis

PRECAUTIONS AND CONTRAINDICATIONS

Hypersensitivity to any penicillin

DRUG INTERACTIONS OF CONCERN TO DENTISTRY

• Increased or prolonged plasma levels: probenecid
• Possible decrease in antimicrobial effectiveness: tetracyclines, erythromycins, lincomycins
• When used for dental infection:
  • Oral contraceptives: advise patient of a potential low risk for decreased contraceptive action, to maintain compliance with oral contraceptive while using antibiotics, and to consider the use of additional nonhormonal contraception

SERIOUS REACTIONS

! Hypersensitivity reactions ranging from rash, fever, and chills to anaphylaxis occur.

DENTAL CONSIDERATIONS

General:
• Determine why patient is taking the drug.
• Caution regarding allergy to medication.
• Use with caution in patients with a history of antibiotic-associated colitis.
Consultations:
• Consult patient's physician if an acute dental infection occurs and another antiinfective is required.
• Medical consultation may be required to assess disease control.
Teach Patient/Family to:
• Use effective oral hygiene to prevent soft tissue inflammation
• Prevent trauma when using oral hygiene aids
• Report sore throat, oral burning sensation, fever, or fatigue, any of which could indicate presence of a superinfection

penicillin V potassium

pen-ih-sil´-in V poe-tass´-ee-um (Abbocillin VK[AUS], Apo-Pen-VK[CAN], Cilicaine VK[AUS], L.P.V.[AUS], Novo-Pen-VK[CAN], Veetids)

CATEGORY AND SCHEDULE

Pregnancy Risk Category: B

Drug Class: Semisynthetic penicillin

MECHANISM OF ACTION

A penicillin that inhibits cell wall synthesis by binding to bacterial cell membranes. *Therapeutic Effect:* Bactericidal.

USES

Effective for treatment of gram-positive cocci (*S. aureus, S. viridans, S. faecalis, S. bovis, S. pneumoniae*), gram-negative cocci (*N. gonorrhoeae, N. meningitidis*), gram-positive bacilli (*B. anthracis, C. perfringens, C. tetani, C. diphtheriae*), gram-negative bacilli (*S. moniliformis*), spirochetes (*T. pallidum*), *Actinomyces, Peptococcus,* and *Peptostreptococcus* species

PHARMACOKINETICS

Moderately absorbed from the GI tract. Protein binding: 80%. Widely distributed. Metabolized in the liver. Primarily excreted in urine. *Half-life:* 1 hr (increased in impaired renal function).

INDICATIONS AND DOSAGES

▸ **Mild-to-Moderate Respiratory Tract or Skin or Skin-Structure Infections, Otitis Media, Necrotizing Ulcerative Gingivitis**

PO

Adults, Elderly, Children 12 yr and older. 125–500 mg q6–8h.
Children younger than 12 yr. 25–50 mg/kg/day in divided doses q6–8h. Maximum: 3 g/day.

▸ **Primary Prevention of Rheumatic Fever**

PO

Adults, Elderly. 500 mg 2–3 times a day for 10 days.
Children. 250 mg 2–3 times a day for 10 days.

SIDE EFFECTS/ADVERSE REACTIONS

Frequent
Mild hypersensitivity reaction (chills, fever, rash), nausea, vomiting, diarrhea

Rare
Bleeding

PRECAUTIONS AND CONTRAINDICATIONS

Hypersensitivity to any penicillin
Caution
Hypersensitivity to cephalosporins, lactation

DRUG INTERACTIONS OF CONCERN TO DENTISTRY

• Decreased antimicrobial effectiveness of penicillin: tetracyclines, erythromycins, lincomycins
• Increased penicillin concentrations: probenecid
• Oral contraceptives: advise patient of a potential low risk for decreased contraceptive action, to maintain compliance with oral contraceptive use while using antibiotics, and to consider the use of additional nonhormonal contraception

SERIOUS REACTIONS

! Severe hypersensitivity reactions, including anaphylaxis, may occur.
! Nephrotoxicity, antibiotic-associated colitis, and other superinfections may result from high dosages or prolonged therapy.

DENTAL CONSIDERATIONS

General:
• Take precautions regarding allergy to medication.
• Determine why the patient is taking the drug.
• If used for dental infection, place on frequent recall to evaluate healing response.

Consultations:
• Medical consultation may be required to assess disease control.
Teach Patient/Family:
• When used for dental infection, advise patient to:
    • Report sore throat, oral burning sensation, fever, fatigue, any of which could indicate superinfection
    • Take at prescribed intervals and complete dosage regimen
    • Immediately notify the dentist if signs or symptoms of infection or allergy occur

pentamidine isethionate

pen-tam´-ih-deen
ice-eth-eyé-oh-nate
(NebuPent, Pentacarinat[CAN], Pentam-300)

CATEGORY AND SCHEDULE
Pregnancy Risk Category: C

Drug Class: Antiprotozoal

MECHANISM OF ACTION
An antiinfective that interferes with nuclear metabolism and incorporation of nucleotides, inhibiting DNA, RNA, phospholipid, and protein synthesis. ***Therapeutic Effect:*** Produces antibacterial and antiprotozoal effects.

USES
Treatment of *Pneumocystis carinii* infections in immunocompromised patients (injection); prevention in high-risk HIV-infected patients (INH)

PHARMACOKINETICS
Well absorbed after IM administration; minimally absorbed after inhalation. Widely distributed. Primarily excreted in urine. Minimally removed by hemodialysis. ***Half-life:*** 6.5 hr (increased in impaired renal function). Powder for Nebulization (Nebupent): 300 mg.

INDICATIONS AND DOSAGES
▶ **Pneumocystis Carinii Pneumonia (PCP)**
IV, IM
Adults, Elderly. 4 mg/kg/day once a day for 14–21 days.
Children. 4 mg/kg/day once a day for 10–14 days.
▶ **Prevention of PCP**
Inhalation
Adults, Elderly. 300 mg once q4wk.
Children 5 yr and older. 300 mg q3–4wks.
Children younger than 5 yr. 8 mg/kg/dose once q3–4wk.

SIDE EFFECTS/ADVERSE REACTIONS
Frequent
Injection: Abscess, pain at injection site
Inhalation: Fatigue, metallic taste, shortness of breath, decreased appetite, dizziness, rash, cough, nausea, vomiting, chills
Occasional
Injection: Nausea, decreased appetite, hypotension, fever, rash, altered taste, confusion
Inhalation: Diarrhea, headache, anemia, muscle pain
Rare
Injection: Neuralgia, thrombocytopenia, phlebitis, dizziness

P

PRECAUTIONS AND CONTRAINDICATIONS

Concurrent use with didanosine

Caution

Blood dyscrasias, hepatic disease, renal disease, diabetes mellitus, cardiac disease, hypocalcemia

DRUG INTERACTIONS OF CONCERN TO DENTISTRY

None reported

SERIOUS REACTIONS

! Rare reactions include life-threatening or fatal hypotension, arrhythmias, hypoglycemia, leukopenia, nephrotoxicity or renal failure, anaphylactic shock, Stevens-Johnson syndrome, and toxic epidural necrolysis.

! Hyperglycemia and insulin-dependent diabetes mellitus (often permanent) may occur even months after therapy has stopped.

DENTAL CONSIDERATIONS

General:

• Monitor vital signs at every appointment because of cardiovascular side effects.

• Patients on chronic drug therapy may rarely have symptoms of blood dyscrasias, which can include infection, bleeding, and poor healing.

• Place on frequent recall to evaluate healing response.

• Assess salivary flow as a factor in caries, periodontal disease, and candidiasis.

• Consider semisupine chair position for patients with respiratory disease.

• For inhalation dosage forms, rinse mouth with water after each dose to prevent dryness.

• Place on frequent recall because of oral side effects.

Consultations:

• In a patient with symptoms of blood dyscrasias, request a medical consultation for blood studies and postpone dental treatment until normal values are reestablished.

• Medical consultation may be required to assess disease control.

Teach Patient/Family to:

• See dentist immediately if secondary oral infection occurs

• Use effective oral hygiene to prevent soft tissue inflammation

• Use caution to prevent injury when using oral hygiene aids

• Use dietary suggestions to maintain oral and systemic health

• When chronic dry mouth occurs, advise patient to:

  • Avoid mouth rinses with high alcohol content because of drying effects

  • Use daily home fluoride products to prevent caries

  • Use sugarless gum, frequent sips of water, or saliva substitutes

pentazocine hydrochloride; naloxone hydrochloride

pen-taz´oh-seen high-droh-klor´-ide; nuh-lok´-sohn high-droh-klor´-ide
(Talwin Nx)

CATEGORY AND SCHEDULE

Pregnancy Risk Category C: Controlled Substance: Schedule IV

Drug Class: Synthetic opioid/ mixed agonist/antagonist

MECHANISM OF ACTION

Pentazocine is both a narcotic agonist and antagonist that induces analgesia by stimulating the kappa and sigma opioid receptors. Naloxone is a narcotic antagonist that displaces opiates at opiate-occupied receptor sites in the CNS. *Therapeutic Effect:* Pentazocine: induces analgesia. Naloxone: blocks narcotic effects; reverses opiate-induced sleep or sedation; increases respiratory rate, returns B/P to normal.

USES

Treatment of moderate-to-severe pain alone or in combination with aspirin or acetaminophen

PHARMACOKINETICS

Well absorbed. Metabolized in liver. Primarily excreted in urine. Minimal excretion in bile and feces. *Half-life:* 2–3 hr.

INDICATIONS AND DOSAGES
▶ **Pain, Moderate-to-Severe**
PO
Adults, Elderly, Children 12 yr and older. 1 tablet every 3–4 hr. May be increased to 2 tablets when needed. Maximum: 12 tablets/day.

SIDE EFFECTS/ADVERSE REACTIONS
Occasional
Confusion, dizziness, fatigue, lightheadedness, drowsiness, mood changes, headache, GI upset, vomiting, constipation, stomach pain, rash, difficulty urinating

PRECAUTIONS AND CONTRAINDICATIONS

Hypersensitivity to pentazocine or naloxone or any component on the formulation
Caution
Addictive personality, lactation, increased intracranial pressure, head injury, MI (acute), severe heart disease, respiratory depression, hepatic disease, renal disease, children 12 yr, acute abdominal conditions, Addison's disease, prostatic hypertrophy, patients taking other narcotics

DRUG INTERACTIONS OF CONCERN TO DENTISTRY
* Increased effects: all CNS depressants, alcohol
* Contraindication: MAOIs
* Do not mix in solutions or syringe with barbiturates
* Additive side effects of opioid agonists
* Increased effects of anticholinergics
* Decreased effects of opioid agonists

SERIOUS REACTIONS
! Respiratory depression and serious skin reactions, such as Stevens-Johnson syndrome, have been reported but occur rarely.

DENTAL CONSIDERATIONS
General:
* Monitor vital signs at every appointment because of cardiovascular and respiratory side effects.
* Assess salivary flow as a factor in caries, periodontal disease, and candidiasis.

- Consider semisupine chair position for patient comfort if GI side effects occur.
- Psychologic and physical dependence may occur with chronic administration.

Teach Patient/Family:
- When chronic dry mouth occurs, advise patient to:
  - Avoid mouth rinses with high alcohol content because of drying effects
  - Use daily home fluoride products to prevent caries
  - Use sugarless gum, frequent sips of water, or saliva substitutes

pentazocine
pen-tah´-zoe-seen
(Talwin)

COMBINATION PRODUCTS
With naloxone, a narcotic antagonist (oral) (Talwin NX); with aspirin (oral) (Talwin Compound); w/acetaminophen (oral) (Talacen)

CATEGORY AND SCHEDULE
Pregnancy Risk Category C: Controlled substance: Schedule IV

Drug Class: Opiod analgesics

MECHANISM OF ACTION
An opioid antagonist that binds with opioid receptors within CNS. **Therapeutic Effect:** Alters processes affecting pain perception, emotional response to pain.

USES
Relief of moderate-to-severe pain associated with surgical procedures

PHARMACOKINETICS
Well absorbed after administration. Widely distributed including in CSF. Metabolized in liver via oxidative and glucuronide conjugation pathways, extensive first-pass effect. Excreted in small amounts as unchanged drug. **Half-life:** 2–3 hr, prolonged with hepatic impairment.

INDICATIONS AND DOSAGES
▶ **Analgesia**
PO
Adults. 50 mg q3–4h. May increase to 100 mg q3–4h, if needed. Maximum: 600 mg/day.
Elderly. 50 mg q4h.
Subcutaneous/IM/IV
Adults. 30 mg q3–4h. Do not exceed 30 mg IV or 60 mg subcutaneous/IM per dose. Maximum: 360 mg/day.
IM
Elderly. 25 mg q4h.
▶ **Obstetric Labor**
IM
Adults. 30 mg as a single dose.
IV
Adults. 20 mg when contractions are regular. May repeat 2–3 times q2–3h.

SIDE EFFECTS/ADVERSE REACTIONS
Frequent
Drowsiness, euphoria, nausea, vomiting
Occasional
Allergic reaction, histamine reaction (decreased B/P, increased sweating, flushing, wheezing), decreased urination, altered vision, constipation, dizziness, dry mouth, headache, hypotension, pain/burning at injection site

PRECAUTIONS AND CONTRAINDICATIONS

Hypersensitivity to pentazocine or any component of the formulation

DRUG INTERACTIONS OF CONCERN TO DENTISTRY

• Increased effects: all CNS depressants, alcohol
• Contraindication: MAOIs
• Do not mix with barbiturates in solutions or syringe
• Additive side effects of opioid agonists
• Increased effects of anticholinergics
• Decreased effects of opioid agonists

SERIOUS REACTIONS

! Overdosage results in severe respiratory depression, skeletal muscle flaccidity, cyanosis, extreme somnolence progressing to convulsions, stupor, and coma.
! Abrupt withdrawal after prolonged use may produce symptoms of narcotic withdrawal (abdominal cramps, rhinorrhea, lacrimation, nausea, vomiting, restlessness, anxiety, increased temperature, piloerection).

DENTAL CONSIDERATIONS

General:
• Monitor vital signs at every appointment because of cardiovascular and respiratory side effects.
• Assess salivary flow as a factor in caries, periodontal disease, and candidiasis.
• Consider semisupine chair position for patient comfort if GI side effects occur.
• Psychologic and physical dependence may occur with chronic administration.

Teach Patient/Family:
• When chronic dry mouth occurs, advise patient to:
  • Avoid mouth rinses with high alcohol content because of drying effects
  • Use daily home fluoride products to prevent caries
  • Use sugarless gum, frequent sips of water, or saliva substitutes

pentobarbital
pen-toe-bar´-bi-tal
(Nembutal, Phenobarbitone[AUS])
Do not confuse with phenobarbital.

CATEGORY AND SCHEDULE
Pregnancy Risk Category: D
Controlled substance: Schedule II (capsules, injection), Schedule III (suppositories)

Drug Class: Sedative-hypnotic barbiturate

MECHANISM OF ACTION
A barbiturate that binds at the gamma-aminobutyric acid (GABA) receptor complex, enhancing GABA activity. **Therapeutic Effect:** Depresses CNS activity and reticular activating system.

USES
Treatment of insomnia, sedation, preoperative medication, increased intracranial pressure (ICP), dental anesthetic

PHARMACOKINETICS
Well absorbed after PO, parenteral administration. Protein binding: 35%–55%. Rapidly, widely distributed. Metabolized in liver. Primarily excreted in urine. Removed by hemodialysis. **Half-life:** 15–48 hr.

INDICATIONS AND DOSAGES
▶ **Preanesthetic**
PO
Adults, Elderly. 100 mg.
Children. 2–6 mg/kg. Maximum:
100 mg/dose.
IM
Adults, Elderly. 150–200 mg.
Children. 2–6 mg/kg. Maximum:
100 mg/dose.
Rectal
Children 12–14 yr. 60 or 120 mg.
Children 5–12 yr. 60 mg.
Children 1–4 yr. 30–60 mg.
Children 1 yr–2 mo. 30 mg.
▶ **Hypnotic**
PO
Adults, Elderly. 100 mg at bedtime.
IM
Adults, Elderly. 150–200 mg at
bedtime.
Children. 2–6 mg/kg. Maximum:
100 mg/dose at bedtime.
IV
Adults, Elderly. 100 mg initially then,
after 1 min, may give additional
small doses at 1-min intervals, up to
500 mg total.
Children. 50 mg initially then, after
1 min, may give additional small
doses at 1-min intervals, up to
desired effect.
Rectal
Adults, Elderly. 120–200 mg at
bedtime.
Children 12–14 yr. 60 or 120 mg at
bedtime.
Children 5–12 yr. 60 mg at bedtime.
Children 1–4 yr. 30–60 mg at
bedtime.
Children 2 mo–1 yr. 30 mg at
bedtime.
▶ **Anticonvulsant**
IV
Adults, Elderly. 2–15 mg/kg loading
dose given slowly over 1–2 hr.
Maintenance infusion:
0.5–5 mg/kg/hr.

Children. 5–15 mg/kg loading dose
given slowly over 1–2 hr.
Maintenance infusion:
0.5–3 mg/kg/hr.

SIDE EFFECTS/ADVERSE REACTIONS
Occasional
Agitation, confusion, dizziness,
somnolence
Rare
Confusion, paradoxic CNS
hyperactivity or nervousness in
children, excitement or restlessness
in elderly

PRECAUTIONS AND CONTRAINDICATIONS
Porphyria, hypersensitivity
to barbiturates
Caution
Anemia, lactation, hepatic disease,
renal disease, hypertension, elderly,
acute/chronic pain

DRUG INTERACTIONS OF CONCERN TO DENTISTRY
• Hepatotoxicity: halogenated-
hydrocarbon anesthetics
• Increased CNS depression: alcohol,
all other CNS depressants
• Increased metabolism of
carbamazepine, tricyclic
antidepressants, corticosteroids
• Decreased half-life of doxycycline

SERIOUS REACTIONS
! Agranulocytosis, megaloblastic
anemia, apnea, hypoventilation,
bradycardia, hypotension,
syncope, hepatic damage, and
Stevens-Johnson syndrome
occur rarely.
! Abrupt withdrawal after prolonged
therapy may produce effects ranging
from markedly increased dreaming,
nightmares or insomnia, tremor,
sweating and vomiting, to

hallucinations, delirium, seizures, and status epilepticus.

! Skin eruptions appear as hypersensitivity reactions.

! Overdosage produces cold or clammy skin, hypothermia, severe CNS depression, cyanosis, and rapid pulse.

DENTAL CONSIDERATIONS

General:

• Determine why the patient is taking the drug.

• Monitor vital signs at every appointment because of cardiovascular side effects. Evaluate respiration characteristics and rate.

• Patients on chronic drug therapy may rarely have symptoms of blood dyscrasias, which can include infection, bleeding, and poor healing.

• When used for sedation in dentistry:

  • Assess vital signs before use and q30min after use as sedative.

  • Observe respiratory dysfunction: respiratory depression, character, rate, rhythm; hold drug if respirations are fewer than 10/min or if pupils are dilated.

  • After supine positioning, have patient sit upright for at least 2 min before standing to avoid orthostatic hypotension.

• Have someone drive patient to and from dental office when drug is used for conscious sedation.

• Barbiturates induce liver microsomal enzymes, which alter the metabolism of other drugs.

• Geriatric patients are more susceptible to drug effects; use lower dose.

Consultations:

• In a patient with symptoms of blood dyscrasias, request a medical consultation for blood studies and postpone dental treatment until normal values are reestablished.

Teach Patient/Family to:

• Avoid driving or other activities requiring alertness

• Avoid alcohol ingestion or CNS depressants; serious CNS depression may result

• Avoid OTC preparations (antihistamines, cold remedies) that contain CNS depressants

pentosan polysulfate

pen´-toe-san poll-ee-sull´-fate
(Elmiron)
Do not confuse with pentostatin.

CATEGORY AND SCHEDULE
Pregnancy Risk Category: B

Drug Class: Anticoagulant

P

MECHANISM OF ACTION
A negatively-charged synthetic sulfated polysaccharide with heparin-like properties that appear to adhere to bladder wall mucosal membrane, may act as a buffering agent to control cell permeability, preventing irritating solutes in the urine. Has anticoagulant/fibrinolytic effects. **Therapeutic Effect:** Relieves bladder pain.

USES
Relief of interstitial cystitis symptoms

PHARMACOKINETICS

Poorly and erratically absorbed from the gastrointestinal tract. Distributed in uroepithelium of GU tract with lesser amount found in the liver, spleen, lung, skin, periosteum, and bone marrow. Metabolized in liver and kidney (secondary). Eliminated in the urine. *Half-life:* 4.8 hr.

INDICATIONS AND DOSAGES
▸ **Interstitial Cystitis**
PO
Adults, Elderly. 100 mg 3 times a day.

SIDE EFFECTS/ADVERSE REACTIONS
Frequent
Alopecia areata (a single area on the scalp), diarrhea, nausea, headache, rash, abdominal pain, dyspepsia
Occasional
Dizziness, depression, increased liver function tests

PRECAUTIONS AND CONTRAINDICATIONS
Hypersensitivity to pentosan polysulfate sodium or structurally related compounds

DRUG INTERACTIONS OF CONCERN TO DENTISTRY
• Potential risk of bleeding: high-dose aspirin

SERIOUS REACTIONS
! Ecchymosis, epistaxis, gum hemorrhage have been reported (drug produces weak anticoagulant effect).
! Overdose may produce liver function abnormalities.

DENTAL CONSIDERATIONS
General:
• Possesses weak anticoagulant activity; question patient about bleeding or bruising.
• Consider semisupine chair position for patient comfort if GI side effects occur.
• Question patient about tolerance of NSAIDs or aspirin related to GI disease.
• Avoid products that affect platelet function, such as aspirin and NSAIDs.
• Consider local hemostasis measures to prevent excessive bleeding.
Consultations:
• Confer with physician if bleeding is a problem; epistaxis, spontaneous gingival bleeding.
• Medical consultation should include routine blood counts, including platelet counts and bleeding time.
Teach Patient/Family to:
• Use effective oral hygiene to prevent soft tissue inflammation
• Prevent trauma when using oral hygiene aids
• Report oral lesions, soreness, or bleeding to dentist
• Importance of updating health and medication history if physician makes any changes in evaluation or drug regimens; include OTC, herbal, and nonherbal drugs in the update

pentostatin
pen-toe-stat´-in
(Nipent)
Do not confuse with pravastatin.

CATEGORY AND SCHEDULE
Pregnancy Risk Category: D

Drug Class: Antineoplastic, enzyme inhibitor

MECHANISM OF ACTION

An antimetabolite that inhibits the enzyme adenosine deaminase (ADA) (increases intracellular levels of adenine deoxynucleotide). Greatest activity in T cells of lymphoid system. Inhibits ADA and RNA synthesis. Produces DNA damage. *Therapeutic Effect:* Leads to death of tumor cells.

USES

Treatment of α-interferon-refractory hairy cell leukemia

PHARMACOKINETICS

After IV administration, rapidly distributed to body tissues (poorly distributed to cerebrospinal fluid). Protein binding: 4%. Excreted primarily in urine unchanged or as active metabolite. *Half-life:* 5.7 hr (2.6–10 hr).

INDICATIONS AND DOSAGES
▸ **Hairy Cell Leukemia**
IV

Adults, Elderly. 4 mg/m² q2wk until complete response attained (without any major toxicity). Discontinue if no response in 6 mo; partial response in 12 mo.
▸ **Dosage in Renal Impairment**
Only when benefits justify risks, give 2–3 mg/m² in patients with creatinine clearance 50–60 ml/min.

SIDE EFFECTS/ADVERSE REACTIONS

Frequent

Nausea, vomiting, fever, fatigue, rash, pain, cough, upper respiratory tract infection, anorexia, diarrhea
Occasional

Headache, pharyngitis, sinusitis, myalgia, chills, arthralgia, peripheral edema, anorexia, blurred vision, conjunctivitis, skin discoloration, sweating, anxiety, depression, dizziness, confusion

PRECAUTIONS AND CONTRAINDICATIONS

Hypersensitivity to pentostatin

SERIOUS REACTIONS

❗ Bone marrow depression is manifested as hematologic toxicity (principally leukopenia, anemia, thrombocytopenia).
❗ Doses higher than recommended (20–50 mg/m² in divided doses for more than 5 days) may produce severe renal, hepatic, pulmonary, or CNS toxicity.

DENTAL CONSIDERATIONS

• Increased susceptibility to infections.
• Increased bleeding.
• Anemia.
• Oral ulcerations, mucositis (use palliative measures for relief).
• Increased nausea, vomiting.
• Consult physician to determine disease control and ability of patient to tolerate dental procedures.

pentoxifylline

P

pen-tox-if´-ih-lin
(Albert[CAN], Apo-Pentoxifylline SR[CAN], Pentoxifylline[CAN], Pentoxyl, Trental)
Do not confuse Trental with Tegretol or Trandate.

CATEGORY AND SCHEDULE

Pregnancy Risk Category: C

Drug Class: Hemorrheologic agent

MECHANISM OF ACTION

A blood viscosity-reducing agent that alters the flexibility of RBCs; inhibits production of tumor necrosis factor, neutrophil activation, and platelet aggregation. *Therapeutic Effect:* Reduces blood viscosity and improves blood flow.

USES
Treatment of intermittent claudication related to chronic occlusive arterial disease of the limbs

PHARMACOKINETICS
Well absorbed after oral administration. Undergoes first-pass metabolism in the liver. Primarily excreted in urine. Unknown if removed by hemodialysis.
Half-life: 24–48 min; metabolite, 60–90 min.

INDICATIONS AND DOSAGES
▶ **Intermittent Claudication**
PO
Adults, Elderly. 400 mg 3 times a day. Decrease to 400 mg twice a day if GI or CNS adverse effects occur. Continue for at least 8 wk.

SIDE EFFECTS/ADVERSE REACTIONS
Occasional
Dizziness, nausea, altered taste, dyspepsia, marked by heartburn, epigastric pain, and indigestion
Rare
Rash, pruritus, anorexia, constipation, dry mouth, blurred vision, edema, nasal congestion, anxiety

PRECAUTIONS AND CONTRAINDICATIONS
History of intolerance to xanthine derivatives, such as caffeine, theophylline, or theobromine; recent cerebral or retinal hemorrhage
Caution
Angina pectoris, cardiac disease, lactation, children, impaired renal function

DRUG INTERACTIONS OF CONCERN TO DENTISTRY
• Increased bleeding: ASA, NSAIDs

SERIOUS REACTIONS
! Angina and chest pain occur rarely and may be accompanied by palpitations, tachycardia, and arrhythmias.
! Signs and symptoms of overdose, such as flushing, hypotension, nervousness, agitation, hand tremor, fever, and somnolence, appear 4–5 hr after ingestion and last for 12 hr.

DENTAL CONSIDERATIONS
General:
• Monitor vital signs at every appointment because of cardiovascular side effects.
• Assess salivary flow as a factor in caries, periodontal disease, and candidiasis.
• Stress from dental procedures may compromise cardiovascular function; determine patient risk.
• Short appointments and a stress-reduction protocol may be required for anxious patients.
• Talk with patient about potential systemic diseases (e.g., diabetes, cardiovascular disease) that may be associated with claudication.
Consultations:
• Medical consultation may be required to assess disease control and patient's ability to tolerate stress.
Teach Patient/Family to:
• Use effective oral hygiene to prevent soft tissue inflammation
• Prevent injury when using oral hygiene aids
• When chronic dry mouth occurs, advise patient to:

• Avoid mouth rinses with high alcohol content because of drying effects
• Use home fluoride products to prevent caries
• Use sugarless gum, frequent sips of water, or saliva substitutes

pergolide mesylate
per´-go-lide mez´-il-ate
(Permax)
Do not confuse Permax with Pentrax or Pernox.

CATEGORY AND SCHEDULE
Pregnancy Risk Category: B

Drug Class: Antiparkinson agent

MECHANISM OF ACTION
A centrally active dopamine agonist that directly stimulates dopamine receptors. *Therapeutic Effect:* Decreases signs and symptoms of Parkinson's disease.

USES
Adjunctive treatment of Parkinson's disease

PHARMACOKINETICS
Well absorbed from the GI tract. Protein binding: 90%. Undergoes extensive first-pass metabolism in the liver. Primarily excreted in urine. Unknown if removed by hemodialysis.

INDICATIONS AND DOSAGES
▸ **Parkinsonism**
PO
Adults, Elderly. Initially, 0.05 mg/day for 2 days. May increase by 0.1–0.15 mg/day every 3 days over the next 12 days; afterward may increase by 0.25 mg/day every 3 days. Range: 2–3 mg/day in 3 divided doses. Maximum: 5 mg/day.

SIDE EFFECTS/ADVERSE REACTIONS
Frequent
Nausea, dizziness, hallucinations, constipation, rhinitis, dystonia, confusion, somnolence
Occasional
Orthostatic hypotension, insomnia, dry mouth, peripheral edema, anxiety, diarrhea, dyspepsia, abdominal pain, headache, abnormal vision, anorexia, tremor, depression, rash
Rare
Urinary frequency, vivid dreams, neck pain, hypotension, vomiting

PRECAUTIONS AND CONTRAINDICATIONS
Hypersensitivity to pergolide or other ergot derivatives
Caution
Symptomatic hypotension, cardiac dysrhythmias, dose adjustment for patients on levodopa, discontinue drug slowly, lactation, children

DRUG INTERACTIONS OF CONCERN TO DENTISTRY
• Decreased action: phenothiazines, haloperidol, droperidol, thiothixenes, and metoclopramide

SERIOUS REACTIONS
! Symptoms of overdose may vary from CNS depression, characterized by sedation, apnea, cardiovascular collapse, and death, to severe paradoxic reactions, such as hallucinations, tremor, and seizures.

DENTAL CONSIDERATIONS

General:
• Monitor vital signs at every appointment because of cardiovascular side effects.
• Short appointments may be required because of disease effects on musculature.
• Use precaution if sedation or general anesthesia is required; risk of hypotensive episode.
• After supine positioning, have patient sit upright for at least 2 min before standing to avoid orthostatic hypotension.
• Assess salivary flow as a factor in caries, periodontal disease, and candidiasis.
• Assess for presence of extrapyramidal motor symptoms, such as tardive dyskinesia and akathisia. Extrapyramidal motor activity may complicate dental treatment.
• Consider semisupine chair position for patient comfort because of GI effects of drug.

Consultations:
• Medical consultation may be required to assess disease control.

Teach Patient/Family to:
• Use electric tooth brush if patient has difficulty holding conventional devices
• Update health history/drug record if physician makes any changes in evaluation or drug regimens; include OTC, herbal, and nonherbal drugs in the update
• When chronic dry mouth occurs, advise patient to:
  • Avoid mouth rinses with high alcohol content because of drying effects
  • Use daily home fluoride products to prevent caries
  • Use sugarless gum, frequent sips of water, or saliva substitutes

perindopril
per-in´-doh-pril
(Aceon)

CATEGORY AND SCHEDULE
Pregnancy Risk Category: C (D if used in second or third trimester)

Drug Class: Angiotensin-converting enzyme (ACE) inhibitor

MECHANISM OF ACTION
An ACE inhibitor that suppresses the renin-angiotensin-aldosterone system and prevents conversion of angiotensin I to angiotensin II, a potent vasoconstrictor; may also inhibit angiotensin II at local vascular and renal sites. *Therapeutic Effect:* Reduces peripheral arterial resistance and B/P.

USES
Treatment of essential hypertension as monotherapy or in combination with other antihypertensive medication

PHARMACOKINETICS
PO: Absolute bioavailability 20%–30%, metabolized to active metabolite, perindoprilat, peak plasma levels 1 hr, active metabolite 3–4 hr; protein binding 10%–20%, hepatic metabolism, excreted mostly in urine (75%)

INDICATIONS AND DOSAGES
▶ Hypertension
PO
Adults, Elderly. 2–8 mg/day as single dose or in 2 divided doses. Maximum: 16 mg/day.

SIDE EFFECTS/ADVERSE REACTIONS

Occasional

Cough, back pain, sinusitis, upper extremity pain, dyspepsia, fever, palpitations, hypotension, dizziness, fatigue, syncope

PRECAUTIONS AND CONTRAINDICATIONS

History of angioedema from previous treatment with ACE inhibitors

Caution

Renal insufficiency, hypertension with CHF, severe CHF, renal artery stenosis, autoimmune disease, collagen vascular disease, pregnancy category C (first trimester); pregnancy category D (second and third trimesters), lactation

DRUG INTERACTIONS OF CONCERN TO DENTISTRY

• Decreased hypotensive effects: NSAIDs, aspirin

• Increased hypotension: caution in use of other drugs that have hypotensive effects

• Suspected reduction in the antihypertensive and vasodilator effects by salicylates; monitor B/P if used concurrently

SERIOUS REACTIONS

! Excessive hypotension ("first-dose syncope") may occur in patients with CHF and in those who are severely salt or volume depleted.

! Angioedema (swelling of face and lips) and hyperkalemia occur rarely.

! Agranulocytosis and neutropenia may be noted in those with collagen vascular disease, including scleroderma and systemic lupus erythematosus, and impaired renal function.

! Nephrotic syndrome may be noted in those with history of renal disease.

DENTAL CONSIDERATIONS

General:

• Monitor vital signs at every appointment because of cardiovascular side effects.

• Limit use of sodium-containing products, such as saline IV fluids, for patients with a dietary salt restriction.

• Short appointments and a stress-reduction protocol may be required for anxious patients.

• Stress from dental procedures may compromise cardiovascular function; determine patient risk.

• After supine positioning, have patient sit upright for at least 2 min before standing to avoid orthostatic hypotension.

• Use precaution if sedation or general anesthesia is required; risk of hypotensive episode.

• Assess salivary flow as a factor in caries, periodontal disease, and candidiasis.

• Consider semisupine chair position for patient comfort if GI or respiratory side effects occur.

• Patients on chronic drug therapy may rarely have symptoms of blood dyscrasias, which can include infection, bleeding, and poor healing.

Consultations:

• In a patient with symptoms of blood dyscrasias, request a medical consultation for blood studies and postpone treatment until normal values are reestablished.

• Medical consultation may be required to assess disease control a nd patient's ability to tolerate stress.

P

Teach Patient/Family to:
• Update health and drug history if physician makes any changes in evaluation or drug regimens; include OTC, herbal, and nonherbal drugs in the update
• Use effective oral hygiene to prevent soft tissue inflammation
• Prevent trauma when using oral hygiene aids
• When chronic dry mouth occurs, advise patient to:
  • Avoid mouth rinses with high alcohol content because of drying effects
  • Use daily home fluoride products for anticaries effect
  • Use sugarless gum, frequent sips of water, or saliva substitutes

perphenazine
per-fen´-ah-zeen
(Trilafon)
Do not confuse perphenazine with promazine.

CATEGORY AND SCHEDULE
Pregnancy Risk Category: C

Drug Class: Phenothiazine antipsychotic

MECHANISM OF ACTION
An antipsychotic agent and antiemetic that blocks postsynaptic dopamine receptor sites in the brain.
Therapeutic Effect: Suppresses behavioral response in psychosis, and relieves nausea and vomiting.

USES
Treatment of psychotic disorders, schizophrenia, alcoholism, nausea, vomiting

PHARMACOKINETICS
PO: Onset erratic, peak 2–4 hr
IM: Onset 10 min, peak 1–2 hr, duration 6 hr, occasionally 12–24 hr
Metabolized by liver, excreted in urine, crosses placenta, excreted in breast milk

INDICATIONS AND DOSAGES
▶ **Severe Schizophrenia**
PO
Adults. 4–16 mg 2–4 times a day.
Maximum: 64 mg/day.
Elderly. Initially, 2–4 mg/day.
May increase at 4–7 day intervals by 2–4 mg/day up to 32 mg/day.
▶ **Severe Nausea and Vomiting**
PO
Adults. 8–16 mg/day in divided doses up to 24 mg/day.

SIDE EFFECTS/ADVERSE REACTIONS
Occasional
Marked photosensitivity, somnolence, dry mouth, blurred vision, lethargy, constipation or diarrhea, nasal congestion, peripheral edema, urine retention
Rare
Ocular changes, altered skin pigmentation, hypotension, dizziness, syncope

PRECAUTIONS AND CONTRAINDICATIONS
Coma, myelosuppression, severe cardiovascular disease, severe CNS depression, subcortical brain damage
Caution
Lactation, seizure disorders, hypertension, hepatic disease, cardiac disease

DRUG INTERACTIONS OF CONCERN TO DENTISTRY

• Increased sedation: other CNS depressants, alcohol, barbiturate anesthetics, opioid analgesics
• Hypotension, tachycardia: epinephrine
• Increased extrapyramidal effects: phenothiazines and related drugs (haloperidol, droperidol), metoclopramide
• Additive photosensitization: tetracyclines, fluoroquinolones
• Increased anticholinergic effects: anticholinergics

SERIOUS REACTIONS

! Extrapyramidal symptoms appear to be dose-related and are divided into 3 categories: akathisia (characterized by inability to sit still, tapping of feet), parkinsonian symptoms (including mask-like face, tremors, shuffling gait, hypersalivation), and acute dystonias (such as torticollis, opisthotonos, and oculogyric crisis).
! Tardive dyskinesia occurs rarely.
! Abrupt withdrawal after long-term therapy may precipitate nausea, vomiting, gastritis, dizziness, and tremors.

DENTAL CONSIDERATIONS

General:
• Monitor vital signs at every appointment because of cardiovascular side effects.
• Patients on chronic drug therapy may rarely have symptoms of blood dyscrasias, which can include infection, bleeding, and poor healing.
• After supine positioning, have patient sit upright for at least 2 min before standing to avoid orthostatic hypotension.
• Assess salivary flow as a factor in caries, periodontal disease, and candidiasis.
• Avoid dental light in patient's eyes; offer dark glasses for patient comfort.
• Assess for presence of extrapyramidal motor symptoms, such as tardive dyskinesia and akathisia. Extrapyramidal motor activity may complicate dental treatment.
• Geriatric patients are more susceptible to drug effects; use lower dose.
• Use vasoconstrictors with caution, in low doses, and with careful aspiration. Avoid use of gingival retraction cord with epinephrine.

Consultations:
• In a patient with symptoms of blood dyscrasias, request a medical consultation for blood studies and postpone dental treatment until normal values are reestablished.
• Take precautions if dental surgery is anticipated and anesthesia is required.
• If signs of tardive dyskinesia or akathisia are present, refer to physician.
• Physician should be informed if significant xerostomic side effects occur (e.g., increased caries, sore tongue, problems eating or swallowing, difficulty wearing prosthesis) so that a medication change can be considered.

Teach Patient/Family to:
• Use effective oral hygiene to prevent soft tissue inflammation
• Use caution to prevent injury when using oral hygiene aids

P

• Use electric tooth brush if patient has difficulty holding conventional devices
• When chronic dry mouth occurs, advise patient to:
  • Avoid mouth rinses with high alcohol content because of drying effects
  • Use daily home fluoride products to prevent caries
  • Use sugarless gum, frequent sips of water, or saliva substitutes

phenazopyridine hydrochloride

fen-az-oh-peer´-ih-deen
high-droh-klor´-ide
(Azo-Gesic, Azo-Standard, Phenazo[CAN], Prodium, Pyridium, Uristat)
Do not confuse phenazopyridine with pyridoxine, or Prodium with Perdiem.

CATEGORY AND SCHEDULE
Pregnancy Risk Category: B

Drug Class: Urinary tract analgesic

MECHANISM OF ACTION
An interstitial cystitis agent that exerts topical analgesic effect on urinary tract mucosa.
Therapeutic Effect: Relieves urinary pain, burning, urgency, and frequency.

USES
Treatment of urinary tract irritation/infection

PHARMACOKINETICS
Well absorbed from the GI tract. Partially metabolized in the liver. Primarily excreted in urine.

INDICATIONS AND DOSAGES
▸ **Urinary Analgesic**
PO
Adults. 100–200 mg 3–4 times a day.
Children 6 yr and older. 12 mg/kg/day in 3 divided doses for 2 days.
▸ **Dosage in Renal Impairment**
Dosage interval is modified on the basis of creatinine clearance.

Creatinine Clearance	Interval
50–80 ml/min	Usual dose q8–16h
Less than 50 ml/min	Avoid use

SIDE EFFECTS/ADVERSE REACTIONS
Occasional
Headache, GI disturbance, rash, pruritus

PRECAUTIONS AND CONTRAINDICATIONS
Hepatic or renal insufficiency
Caution
Renal disease

DRUG INTERACTIONS OF CONCERN TO DENTISTRY
• None reported

SERIOUS REACTIONS
! Overdose may lead to hemolytic anemia, nephrotoxicity, or hepatotoxicity. Patients with renal impairment or severe hypersensitivity to the drug may also develop these reactions.
! A massive and acute overdose may result in methemoglobinemia.

DENTAL CONSIDERATIONS
General:
• Consider semisupine chair position for patient comfort if GI side effects occur.

• Patients on chronic drug therapy may rarely have symptoms of blood dyscrasias, which can include infection, bleeding, and poor healing.
• Be aware that patient might have UTI; question if antiinfectives are also being used.

phendimetrazine
fen-dye-me´-tra-zeen
(Adipost, Bontril PDM, Bontril Slow-Release, Melfiat, Obezine, Phendiet, Phendiet-105, Plegine, Prelu-2)

CATEGORY AND SCHEDULE
Pregnancy Risk Category: C
Controlled Substance: Schedule III, Schedule IV

Drug Class: Anorexiant, amphetamine-like

MECHANISM OF ACTION
A phenylalkylamine sympathomimetic with activity similar to amphetamines that stimulates the CNS and elevates B/P most likely mediated via norepinephrine and dopamine metabolism. Causes stimulation of the hypothalamus. *Therapeutic Effect:* Decreases appetite.

USES
Treatment of exogenous obesity

PHARMACOKINETICS
The pharmacokinetics of phendimetrazine tartrate has not been well established. Metabolized to active metabolite, phendimetrazine. Excreted in urine. *Half-life:* 2–4 hr.

INDICATIONS AND DOSAGES
▶ **Obesity**
PO
Adults, Elderly. 105 mg/day in the morning or before the morning meal (sustained release); 35 mg 2–3 times a day (immediate release).
Maximum: 70 mg 3 times a day.

SIDE EFFECTS/ADVERSE REACTIONS
Occasional
Constipation, nausea, diarrhea, dry mouth, dysuria, libido changes, flushing, hypertension, insomnia, nervousness, headache, dizziness, irritability, agitation, restlessness, palpitations, increased heart rate, sweating, tremor, urticaria

PRECAUTIONS AND CONTRAINDICATIONS
Advanced arteriosclerosis, agitated states, glaucoma, history of drug abuse, history of hypersensitivity to sympathomimetic amines, hyperthyroidism, moderate-to-severe hypertension, symptomatic cardiovascular disease, use within 14 days of discontinuation MAOI, hypersensitivity to phendimetrazine or sympathomimetics
Caution
Drug abuse, anxiety, lactation

DRUG INTERACTIONS OF CONCERN TO DENTISTRY
• Hypertensive crisis: MAOIs or within 14 days of MAOIs
• Increased risk of dysrhythmia: hydrocarbon inhalation, general anesthetics
• Decreased effect: tricyclic antidepressants, ascorbic acid, phenothiazines
• Caffeine or caffeine-containing products: may increase risk of insomnia and dry mouth

P

SERIOUS REACTIONS

! Multivalvular heart disease, primary pulmonary hypertension, and arrhythmias occur rarely.
! Overdose may produce flushing, arrhythmias, and psychosis.
! Abrupt withdrawal following prolonged administration of high doses may produce extreme fatigue and depression.

DENTAL CONSIDERATIONS

General:
• Monitor vital signs at every appointment because of cardiovascular side effects.
• Assess salivary flow as a factor in caries, periodontal disease, and candidiasis.
• Determine why the patient is taking the drug.
• Psychologic and physical dependence may occur with chronic administration.
• Patients on chronic drug therapy may rarely have symptoms of blood dyscrasias, which can include infection, bleeding, and poor healing.
Consultations:
• In a patient with symptoms of blood dyscrasias, request a medical consultation for blood studies and postpone dental treatment until normal values are reestablished.
Teach Patient/Family to:
• Use effective oral hygiene to prevent soft tissue inflammation
• Report oral lesions, soreness, or bleeding to dentist
• Use caution to prevent injury when using oral hygiene aids
• When chronic dry mouth occurs, advise patient to:
  • Avoid mouth rinses with high alcohol content because of drying effects
  • Use daily home fluoride products to prevent caries

• Use sugarless gum, frequent sips of water, or saliva substitutes

---

phenelzine sulfate
fen´-el-zeen sull´-fate
(Nardil)

CATEGORY AND SCHEDULE
Pregnancy Risk Category: C

Drug Class: Antidepressant, MAOI

MECHANISM OF ACTION
An MAOI that inhibits the activity of the enzyme monoamine oxidase at CNS storage sites, leading to increased levels of the neurotransmitters epinephrine, norepinephrine, serotonin, and dopamine at neuronal receptor sites.
Therapeutic Effect: Relieves depression.

USES
Treatment of depression when uncontrolled by other means

PHARMACOKINETICS
Well absorbed from GI tract. Metabolized in the liver. Primarily excreted in urine. **Half-life:** 1.2 hr.

INDICATIONS AND DOSAGES
▶ **Depression Refractory to Other Antidepressants or Electroconvulsive Therapy**
PO
Adults. 15 mg 3 times a day. May increase to 60–90 mg/day.
Elderly. Initially, 7.5 mg/day. May increase by 7.5–15 mg/day q3–4wk up to 60 mg/day in divided doses.

SIDE EFFECTS/ADVERSE REACTIONS

Frequent

Orthostatic hypotension, restlessness, GI upset, insomnia, dizziness, headache, lethargy, asthenia, dry mouth, peripheral edema

Occasional

Flushing, diaphoresis, rash, urinary frequency, increased appetite, transient impotence

Rare

Visual disturbances

PRECAUTIONS AND CONTRAINDICATIONS

Cardiovascular or cerebrovascular disease, hepatic or renal impairment, pheochromocytoma

Caution

Suicidal patients, convulsive disorders, severe depression, schizophrenia, hyperactivity, diabetes mellitus

DRUG INTERACTIONS OF CONCERN TO DENTISTRY

- Increased anticholinergic effect: anticholinergics, haloperidol, phenothiazines, antihistamines
- Hyperpyretic crisis, convulsions, hypertensive episode: meperidine, carbamazepine, cyclobenzaprine
- Cardiac dysrhythmia: caffeine-containing medications
- Increased risk of serotonin syndrome: tricyclic antidepressants, other serotonin reuptake inhibitors
- Increased sedative effects of alcohol, barbiturates, benzodiazepines, CNS depressants
- Increased pressor effects: indirect-acting sympathomimetics, such as ephedrine, amphetamine

SERIOUS REACTIONS

❗ Hypertensive crisis occurs rarely and is marked by severe hypertension, occipital headache radiating frontally, neck stiffness or soreness, nausea, vomiting, diaphoresis, fever or chilliness, clammy skin, dilated pupils, palpitations, tachycardia or bradycardia, and constricting chest pain.

❗ Intracranial bleeding has been reported in association with severe hypertension.

DENTAL CONSIDERATIONS

General:

- Monitor vital signs at every appointment because of cardiovascular side effects.
- Assess salivary flow as a factor in caries, periodontal disease, and candidiasis.
- After supine positioning, have patient sit upright for at least 2 min before standing to avoid orthostatic hypotension.
- Hypertensive episodes are possible even though there are no specific contraindications to vasoconstrictor use in local anesthetics.
- Avoid prescribing caffeine-containing products.
- Take precautions if dental surgery is anticipated and general anesthesia is required.

Consultations:

- Medical consultation may be required to assess disease control and patient's ability to tolerate stress.

Teach Patient/Family to:

- Use electric tooth brush if patient has difficulty holding conventional devices
- When chronic dry mouth occurs, advise patient to:
  - Avoid mouth rinses with high alcohol content because of drying effects
  - Use daily home fluoride products to prevent caries

• Use sugarless gum, frequent sips of water, or saliva substitutes

phenobarbital
fee-noe-bar´-bi-tal
(Luminal, Phenobarbitone[AUS])
Do not confuse phenobarbital with pentobarbital, or Luminal with Tuinal.

CATEGORY AND SCHEDULE
Pregnancy Risk Category: D
Controlled Substance: Schedule IV

Drug Class: Barbiturate anticonvulsant

MECHANISM OF ACTION
A barbiturate that enhances the activity of gamma-aminobutyric acid (GABA) by binding to the GABA receptor complex. ***Therapeutic Effect:*** Depresses CNS activity.

USES
Treatment of all forms of epilepsy, status epilepticus, febrile seizures in children, sedation, insomnia; unapproved: hyperbilirubinemia, chronic cholestasis

PHARMACOKINETICS

Route	Onset	Peak	Duration
PO	20–60 min	N/A	6–10 hr
IV	5 min	30 min	4–10 hr

Well absorbed after PO or parenteral administration. Protein binding: 35%–50%. Rapidly and widely distributed. Metabolized in the liver. Primarily excreted in urine. Removed by hemodialysis.
Half-life: 53–118 hr.

INDICATIONS AND DOSAGES
▶ **Status Epilepticus**
IV
Adults, Elderly, Children, Neonates.
Loading dose of 15–20 mg/kg as a single dose or in divided doses.
▶ **Seizure Control**
PO, IV
Adults, Elderly, Children older than 12 yr. 1–3 mg/kg/day.
Children 6–12 yr. 4–6 mg/kg/day.
Children 1–5 yr. 6–8 mg/kg/day.
Children younger than 1 yr.
5–6 mg/kg/day.
Neonates. 3–4 mg/kg/day.
▶ **Sedation**
PO, IM
Adults, Elderly. 30–120 mg/day
in 2–3 divided doses.
Children. 2 mg/kg 3 times a day.
▶ **Hypnotic**
PO, IV, IM, Subcutaneous
Adults, Elderly. 100–320 mg
at bedtime.
Children. 3–5 mg/kg at bedtime.

SIDE EFFECTS/ADVERSE REACTIONS
Occasional
Somnolence
Rare
Confusion; paradoxic CNS reactions, such as hyperactivity or nervousness in children and excitement or restlessness in the elderly (generally noted during first 2 wk of therapy, particularly in presence of uncontrolled pain)

PRECAUTIONS AND CONTRAINDICATIONS
Porphyria, preexisting CNS depression, severe pain, severe respiratory disease
Caution
Anemia

DRUG INTERACTIONS OF CONCERN TO DENTISTRY

• Increased effects: alcohol, all CNS depressants, saquinavir
• Decreased effects of corticosteroids, doxycycline, carbamazepine

SERIOUS REACTIONS

! Abrupt withdrawal after prolonged therapy may produce increased dreaming, nightmares, insomnia, tremor, diaphoresis, vomiting, hallucinations, delirium, seizures, and status epilepticus.
! Skin eruptions may be a sign of a hypersensitivity reaction.
! Blood dyscrasias, hepatic disease, and hypocalcemia occur rarely.
! Overdose produces cold or clammy skin, hypothermia, severe CNS depression, cyanosis, tachycardia, and Cheyne-Stokes respirations.
! Toxicity may result in severe renal impairment.

DENTAL CONSIDERATIONS

General:
• Determine why the patient is taking the drug.
• Monitor vital signs at every appointment because of cardiovascular side effects. Evaluate respiration characteristics and rate.
• Patients on chronic drug therapy may rarely have symptoms of blood dyscrasias, which can include infection, bleeding, and poor healing.
• When used for sedation in dentistry:
  • Assess vital signs before and during use and after use as sedativey.
  • Observe respiratory dysfunction: respiratory depression, character, rate, rhythm; hold drug if respirations are less frequent than 10/min or if pupils are dilated.

• After supine positioning, have patient sit upright for at least 2 min before standing to avoid orthostatic hypotension.
• Have someone drive patient to and from dental office when drug used for conscious sedation.
• Barbiturates induce liver microsomal enzymes, which alter the metabolism of other drugs.
• Geriatric patients are more susceptible to drug effects; use lower dose.

Consultations:
• In a patient with symptoms of blood dyscrasias, request a medical consultation for blood studies and postpone dental treatment until normal values are reestablished.

Teach Patient/Family to:
• Avoid driving or other activities requiring alertness
• Avoid alcohol ingestion or CNS depressants; serious CNS depression may result
• Use OTC preparations with caution because they may contain other CNS depressants (e.g., antihistamines, cold remedies)

P

phenoxybenzamine
fen-ox-ee-ben´-za-meen
(Dibenzyline)

CATEGORY AND SCHEDULE
Pregnancy Risk Category: C

Drug Class: Antihypertensive, pheochromocytoma

MECHANISM OF ACTION
An antihypertensive that produces long-lasting noncompetitive α-adrenergic blockade of

postganglionic synapses in exocrine glands and smooth muscles. Relaxes urethra and increases opening of the bladder. *Therapeutic Effect:* Controls hypertension.

USES
Treatment of hypertension caused by pheochromocytoma

PHARMACOKINETICS
Well absorbed from the GI tract. Distributed into fatty tissue. Metabolized in liver. Eliminated in urine and feces. Not removed by hemodialysis. *Half-life:* 24 hr.

INDICATIONS AND DOSAGES
▸ **Pheochromocytoma**
PO
Adults. Initially, 10 mg twice daily. May increase dose every other day to 20–40 mg 2–3 times/day
Children. 1–2 mg/kg/day in divided doses.

SIDE EFFECTS/ADVERSE REACTIONS
Frequent
Headache, lethargy, confusion, fatigue
Occasional
Nausea, postural hypotension, syncope, dry mouth
Rare
Palpitations, diarrhea, constipation, inhibition of ejaculation, weakness, altered vision, dizziness

PRECAUTIONS AND CONTRAINDICATIONS
Any condition compromised by hypotension, hypersensitivity to phenoxybenzamine or any component of the formulation

DRUG INTERACTIONS OF CONCERN TO DENTISTRY
● Exaggerated hypotension, tachycardia: epinephrine, other α-adrenergic agonists

SERIOUS REACTIONS
❗ Overdosage produces severe hypotension, irritability, lethargy, tachycardia, dizziness, and shock.

DENTAL CONSIDERATIONS
General:
● Medication may be used in anticipation of surgery to remove the adrenal tumor.
● Hypertension may preclude all dental care except for palliative emergency treatment.
● Question patient about compliance with drug therapy.
● Risk of increased CNS depression when other CNS depressants are used.
● Determine why patient is taking the drug.
● Monitor and record vital signs.
● Use vasoconstrictor with caution, in low doses, and with careful aspiration. Avoid using gingival retraction cord containing epinephrine.
● After supine positioning, have patient sit upright for at least 2 min before standing to avoid orthostatic hypotension.
Consultations:
● Medical consultation may be required to assess disease control and patient's ability to tolerate stress.
Teach Patient/Family to:
● Use effective oral hygiene to prevent soft tissue inflammation
● Not drive or perform other tasks requiring mental alertness

phentermine

fen´-ter-meen

(Adipex-P, Fastin, Ionamin,
Oby-Cap, Phentercot, Pro-Fast HS,
Pro-Fast SA, Pro-Fast SR, T-Diet,
Teramine, Zantryl)

CATEGORY AND SCHEDULE

Pregnancy Risk Category: B
Controlled Substance: Schedule IV

Drug Class: Sympathomimetic,
anorexian

MECHANISM OF ACTION

A sympathomimetic amine
structurally similar to
dextroamphetamine and is most
likely mediated via norephinephrine
and dopamine metabolism. Causes
stimulation of the hypothalamus.
Therapeutic Effect: Decreased
appetite.

USES

Treatment of exogenous obesity

PHARMACOKINETICS

Well absorbed from the GI tract;
resin absorbed slower. Excreted
unchanged in urine. ***Half-life:*** 20 hr.

INDICATIONS AND DOSAGES

▸ **Obesity**
PO
Adults, Children older than 16 yr.
Adipex-P: 37.5 mg as a single daily
dose or in divided doses.
Ionamin: 15–37.5 mg/day before
breakfast or 1–2 hr. after breakfast.
Fastin: 30 mg/day taken in the morning.

SIDE EFFECTS/ADVERSE REACTIONS

Occasional
Restlessness, insomnia, tremor,
palpitations, tachycardia, elevation
in B/P, headache, dizziness, dry
mouth, unpleasant taste, diarrhea or
constipation, changes in libido

PRECAUTIONS AND CONTRAINDICATIONS

Advanced arteriosclerosis, agitated
states, cardiovascular disease, concurrent
use or within 14 days of discontinuation
of MAOI therapy, glaucoma, history of
drug abuse, hypertension (moderate to
severe), hyperthyroidism,
hypersensitivity to phentermine or
sympathomimetic amines
Caution
Lactation, drug abuse, anxiety,
tolerance

DRUG INTERACTIONS OF CONCERN TO DENTISTRY

• Hypertensive crisis: MAOIs or
within 14 days of MAOIs
• Increased risk of dysrhythmia:
hydrocarbon inhalation general
anesthetics
• Decreased effect: tricyclic
antidepressants, ascorbic acid,
phenothiazines
• Caffeine or caffeine-containing
products may increase risk of
insomnia

SERIOUS REACTIONS

❗ Primary pulmonary hypertension
(PPH), psychotic episodes, and
valvular heart disease rarely occur.
❗ Anorectic agents have been
associated with regurgitant
multivalvular heart disease involving
mitral, aortic, and/or tricuspid valves.
❗ Prolonged use may cause physical
or psychological dependence.

DENTAL CONSIDERATIONS

General:
• Monitor vital signs at every
appointment because of
cardiovascular side effects.

- Assess salivary flow as a factor in caries, periodontal disease, and candidiasis.
- Determine why the patient is taking the drug.
- Psychologic and physical dependence may occur with chronic administration.
- Patients on chronic drug therapy may rarely have symptoms of blood dyscrasias, which can include infection, bleeding, and poor healing.

Consultations:
- In a patient with symptoms of blood dyscrasias, request a medical consultation for blood studies and postpone dental treatment until normal values are reestablished.

Teach Patient/Family to:
- Use effective oral hygiene to prevent soft tissue inflammation
- Prevent injury when using oral hygiene aids
- Report oral lesions, soreness, or bleeding to dentist
- When chronic dry mouth occurs, advise patient to:
  - Avoid mouth rinses with high alcohol content because of drying effects
  - Use daily home fluoride products to prevent caries
  - Use sugarless gum, frequent sips of water, or saliva substitutes

phentolamine
fen-tole´-ah-meen
(Regitine)

CATEGORY AND SCHEDULE
Pregnancy Risk Category: C

Drug Class: Antihypertensive

MECHANISM OF ACTION
An α-adrenergic blocking agent that produces peripheral vasodilation and cardiac stimulation. ***Therapeutic Effect:*** Decreases B/P.

USES
Treatment of hypertension, pheochromocytoma, prevention and treatment of dermal necrosis following extravasation of norepinephrine or dopamine; unapproved: with papaverine for intracavernous injection for impotence

PHARMACOKINETICS
Poorly absorbed from the GI tract. Protein binding: 72%. Metabolized in liver. Eliminated in urine and feces. Not removed by hemodialysis. *Half-life:* 19 min.

INDICATIONS AND DOSAGES
▶ **Extravasation—Norepinephrine**
Subcutaneous
Adults, Elderly. Infiltrate area with a small amount (1 ml) of solution (made by diluting 5–10 mg in 10 ml of NS) within 12 hr of extravasation. Do not exceed 0.1–0.2 mg/kg or 5 mg total.
If dose is effective, normal skin color should return to the blanched area within 1 hr.
Children. Infiltrate area with a small amount (1 ml) of solution (made by diluting 5–10 mg in 10 ml of NS) within 12 hr of extravasation. Do not exceed 0.1–0.2 mg/kg or 5 mg total.
▶ **Diagnosis of Pheochromocytoma**
IM/IV
Adults, Elderly. 5 mg as a single dose.
Children. 0.05–0.1 mg/kg/dose. Maximum single dose: 5 mg.

▶ **Surgery for Pheochromocytoma: Hypertension**
IM/IV
Adults, Elderly. 5 mg given 1–2 hr before procedure and repeated as needed every 2–4 hr.
Children. 0.05–0.1 mg/kg/dose given 1–2 hr before procedure. Repeat as needed every 2–4 hr until hypertension is controlled. Maximum single dose: 5 mg.
▶ **Hypertensive Crisis**
IV
Adults, Elderly. 5–20 mg as a single dose.

SIDE EFFECTS/ADVERSE REACTIONS
Occasional
Hypotension, tachycardia, arrhythmia, flushing, orthostatic hypotension, weakness, dizziness, nausea, vomiting, diarrhea, nasal congestion, pulmonary hypertension

PRECAUTIONS AND CONTRAINDICATIONS
Renal impairment, coronary or cerebral arteriosclerosis, concurrent use with phosphodiesterase-5 (PDE-5) inhibitors including sildenafil (more than 25 mg), tadalafil, or vardenafil; hypersensitivity to phentolamine or related compounds
Caution
Lactation

DRUG INTERACTIONS OF CONCERN TO DENTISTRY
• Hypotension, tachycardia: epinephrine
• Decreased pressor effects of epinephrine, ephedrine

SERIOUS REACTIONS
! Symptoms of overdosage include tachycardia, shock, vomiting, and dizziness.
! Mixed agents, such as epinephrine, may cause more hypotension.

DENTAL CONSIDERATIONS
General:
• This is an acute-use drug; hypertension and pheochromocytoma are the immediate concerns.
• Patients with untreated pheochromocytoma or with extreme, uncontrolled hypertension are not candidates for elective dental treatment. Physician consultation is required.
• Short appointments and a stress-reduction protocol may be required for anxious patients.
• Stress from dental procedures may compromise cardiovascular function; determine patient risk.
• Use vasoconstrictors with caution, in low doses, and with careful aspiration. Avoid use of gingival retraction cord with epinephrine.
• Assess vital signs at each appointment because of nature of disease.
Consultations:
• Medical consultation may be required to assess disease control and patient's ability to tolerate stress.

phenylephrine hydrochloride
fen-ill-eh´-frin high-droh-klor´-ide
(AD-Nephrin, AK-Dilate, Isopto Frin[AUS], Mydfrin, Neo-Synephrine, Neo-Synephrine Ophthalmic Viscous 10%[AUS], Prefrin)

CATEGORY AND SCHEDULE
Pregnancy Risk Category: C
OTC (nasal solution, nasal spray, ophthalmic solution)

Drug Class: Nasal decongestant, sympathomimetic

MECHANISM OF ACTION
A sympathomimetic, alpha receptor stimulant that acts on the α-adrenergic receptors of vascular smooth muscle. Causes vasoconstriction of arterioles of nasal mucosa or conjunctiva, activates dilator muscle of the pupil to cause contraction, produces systemic arterial vasoconstriction. *Therapeutic Effect:* Decreases mucosal blood flow and relieves congestion and increases systolic B/P.

USES
Treatment of nasal congestion (temporary relief)

PHARMACOKINETICS

Route	Onset	Peak	Duration
IV	Immediate	N/A	15–20 min
IM	10–15 min	N/A	0.5–2 hr
Subcuta-neous	10–15 min	N/A	1 hr

Minimal absorption after intranasal and ophthalmic administration. Metabolized in the liver and GI tract. Primarily excreted in urine.
Half-life: 2.5 hr.

INDICATIONS AND DOSAGES
▶ **Nasal Decongestant**
Nasal Spray, Nasal Solution
Adults, Elderly, Children 12 yr and older. 2–3 drops or 1–2 sprays of 0.25%–0.5% solution into each nostril.
Children 6–11 yr. 2–3 drops or 1–2 sprays of 0.25% solution into each nostril.
Children younger than 6 yr. 2–3 drops of 0.125% solution (dilute 0.5% solution with 0.9% NaCl to achieve 0.125%) in each nostril. Repeat q4h as needed. Do not use for more than 3 days.

▶ **Conjunctival Congestion, Itching, and Minor Irritation; Whitening of Sclera**
Ophthalmic
Adults, Elderly, Children 12 yr and older. 1–2 drops of 0.12% solution q3–4h.
▶ **Hypotension, Shock**
IM, Subcutaneous
Adults, Elderly. 2–5 mg/dose q1–2h.
Children. 0.1 mg/kg/dose q1–2h.
IV Bolus
Adults, Elderly. 0.1–0.5 mg/dose q10–15min as needed.
Children. 5–20 mcg/kg/dose q10–15min.
IV Infusion
Adults, Elderly. 100–180 mcg/min.
Children. 0.1–0.5 mcg/kg/min.
Titrate to desired effect.

SIDE EFFECTS/ADVERSE REACTIONS
Frequent
Nasal: Rebound nasal congestion due to overuse, especially when used longer than 3 days
Occasional
Mild CNS stimulation (restlessness, nervousness, tremors, headache, insomnia, particularly in those hypersensitive to sympathomimetics, such as elderly patients)
Nasal: Stinging, burning, drying of nasal mucosa
Ophthalmic: Transient burning or stinging, brow ache, blurred vision

PRECAUTIONS AND CONTRAINDICATIONS
Acute pancreatitis, heart disease, hepatitis, narrow-angle glaucoma, pheochromocytoma, severe hypertension, thrombosis, ventricular tachycardia
Caution
Children younger than 6 yr, elderly, diabetes, cardiovascular disease,

hypertension, hyperthyroidism,
increased intraocular pressure,
prostatic hypertrophy, glaucoma,
ischemic heart disease,
excessive use

DRUG INTERACTIONS OF CONCERN TO DENTISTRY

• None reported with normal topical
use
• With systemic absorption, risk of:
bradycardia: β-adrenergic blockers
• Increased dysrhythmias and
hypertension: tricyclic
antidepressants

SERIOUS REACTIONS

! Large doses may produce
tachycardia and palpitations
(particularly in those with cardiac
disease), light-headedness, nausea,
and vomiting.
! Overdose in those older than 60 yr
may result in hallucinations, CNS
depression, and seizures.
! Prolonged nasal use may produce
chronic swelling of nasal mucosa and
rhinitis.

DENTAL CONSIDERATIONS

General:
• Consider semisupine chair position
for patient comfort because of
respiratory effects of disease.
• Assess salivary flow as a factor in
caries, periodontal disease, and
candidiasis.
• Patients with significant nasal
congestion may complicate nasal
administration of nitrous oxide/
oxygen sedation.
Teach Patient/Family:
• That this product is not indicated
for prolonged use because of
congestion rebound

phenylephrine hydrochloride; sulfacetamide sodium

fen-ill-eh´-frin high-droh-klor´-ide;
sul-fa-see´-ta-mide soe´-dee-um
(Vasosulf)

CATEGORY AND SCHEDULE

Pregnancy Risk Category: C

Drug Class: Hydantoin
anticonvulsant

MECHANISM OF ACTION

Phenylephrine is a sympathomimetic
that acts on α-adrenergic receptors of
vascular smooth muscle.
Sulfacetamide is a sulfonamide that
interferes with synthesis of folic acid
that bacteria require for growth.
Therapeutic Effect: Increases
systolic/diastolic B/P, produces
constriction of blood vessels,
conjunctival arterioles, nasal
arterioles. Prevents bacterial growth.

USES

Treatment of generalized tonic-
clonic (grand mal) seizures, status
epilepticus, nonepileptic seizures,
trigeminal neuralgia, cardiac
dysrhythmias (class Ib) caused by
digitalis-type drugs

PHARMACOKINETICS

Minimal absorption following
ophthalmic administration.

INDICATIONS AND DOSAGES

▶ **Topical Application to Conjunctiva
That Relieves Congestion, Itching,
Minor Irritation; Whitens Sclera
of Eye**
Ophthalmic
*Adults, Elderly, Children 12 yr and
older.* Instill 1–2 drops q3–4h.

P

SIDE EFFECTS/ADVERSE REACTIONS
Occasional
Transient burning/stinging, brow ache, blurred vision

PRECAUTIONS AND CONTRAINDICATIONS
Angle-closure glaucoma, those with soft contact lenses, hypersensitivity to phenylephrine, sulfacetamide, or any component of the formulation

DRUG INTERACTIONS OF CONCERN TO DENTISTRY
* None reported with normal topical use
* With systemic absorption, risk of:
  * Bradycardia: β-adrenergic blockers
  * Increased dysrhythmias and hypertension: tricyclic antidepressants

SERIOUS REACTIONS
None reported

DENTAL CONSIDERATIONS
General:
* Consider semisupine chair position for patient comfort because of respiratory effects of disease.
* Assess salivary flow as a factor in caries, periodontal disease, and candidiasis.
* Patients with significant nasal congestion may complicate nasal administration of nitrous oxide/oxygen sedation.
Teach Patient/Family:
* That this product is not indicated for prolonged use because of congestion rebound

physostigmine
fih-zoe-stig´-meen
(Antilirium)
Do not confuse physostigmine with Prostigmin or pyridostigmine.

CATEGORY AND SCHEDULE
Pregnancy Risk Category: C

Drug Class:
Parasympathomimetic (cholinergic)

MECHANISM OF ACTION
A cholinergic that inhibits destruction of acetylcholine by enzyme acetylcholinesterase, thus enhancing impulse transmission across the myoneural junction. *Therapeutic Effect:* Improves skeletal muscle tone, stimulates salivary and sweat gland secretions.

USES
Andtidote for reversal of toxic CNS effects due to anticholinergic drugs, tricyclic antidepressants

INDICATIONS AND DOSAGES
▶ **To Reverse CNS Effects of Anticholinergic Drugs and Tricyclic Antidepressants**
IV, IM
Adults, Elderly. Initially, 0.5–2 mg. If no response, repeat q20min until response or adverse cholinergic effects occur. If initial response occurs, may give additional doses of 1–4 mg q30–60min as life-threatening signs, such as arrhythmias, seizures, and deep coma, recur.
Children. 0.01–0.03 mg/kg. May give additional doses q5–10min until response or adverse cholinergic effects occur or total dose of 2 mg given.

SIDE EFFECTS/ADVERSE REACTIONS
Expected
Miosis, increased GI and skeletal muscle tone, bradycardia
Occasional
Marked drop in B/P (hypertensive patients)
Rare
Allergic reaction

PRECAUTIONS AND CONTRAINDICATIONS
Active uveal inflammation, angle-closure glaucoma before iridectomy, asthma, cardiovascular disease, concurrent use of ganglionic-blocking agents, diabetes, gangrene, glaucoma associated with iridocyclitis, hypersensitivity to cholinesterase inhibitors or their components, mechanical obstruction of intestinal or urogenital tract, vagotonic state

DRUG INTERACTIONS OF CONCERN TO DENTISTRY
• Contraindicated: succinylcholine

SERIOUS REACTIONS
! Parenteral overdose produces a cholinergic crisis manifested as abdominal discomfort or cramps, nausea, vomiting, diarrhea, flushing, facial warmth, excessive salivation, diaphoresis, urinary urgency, and blurred vision. If overdose occurs, stop all anticholinergic drugs and immediately administer 0.6–1.2 mg atropine sulfate IM or IV for adults, or 0.01 mg/kg for infants and children younger than 12 yr.

DENTAL CONSIDERATIONS
General:
• For acute use in hospitals and emergency rooms

Teach Patient/Family to:
• Avoid driving at night or participating in activities requiring visual acuity in the presence of dim lighting

phytonadione
(vitamin K$_1$)
fye-toe-na-dye´-own
(Aqua Mephyton, Mephyton)

CATEGORY AND SCHEDULE
Pregnancy Risk Category: C

Drug Class: Vitamin K1, fat-soluble vitamin

MECHANISM OF ACTION
Needed for adequate blood clotting (factors II, VII, IX, X)

USES
Treatment of vitamin K malabsorption, hypoprothrombinemia, prevention of hypoprothrombinemia caused by oral anticoagulants

PHARMACOKINETICS
PO/Injection: Readily absorbed from duodenum and requires bile salts, rapid hepatic metabolism, onset of action 6–12 hr, normal PT in 12–24 hr, crosses placenta, renal and biliary excretion; because of severe side effects, restrict IV route when other administration routes are not available

INDICATIONS AND DOSAGES
▶ **Hypoprothrombinemia Caused by Vitamin K Malabsorption:**
PO/IM
Adult. 2–25 mg; may repeat or increase to 50 mg.
Child. 5–10 mg.
Infants. 2 mg.

▶ **Prevention of Hemorrhagic Disease of the Newborn:**
Subcutaneous/IM
Neonate. 0.5–1 mg after birth; repeat in 6–8 hr if required.
▶ **Hypoprothrombinemia Caused by Oral Anticoagulants:**
PO/Subcutaneous/IM
Adult. 2.5–10 mg; may repeat 12–48 hr after PO dose or 6–8 hr after subcutaneous/IM dose, based on PT.

SIDE EFFECTS/ADVERSE REACTIONS

Occasional
Taste alterations, headache, cardiac irregularities (tachycardia), nausea, vomiting, hemoglobinuria, rash, urticaria, flushing, erythema, sweating, bronchospasms, dyspnea, cramplike pain
Rare
Hyperbilirubinemia

PRECAUTIONS AND CONTRAINDICATIONS

Hypersensitivity, severe hepatic disease, last few wk of pregnancy

DRUG INTERACTIONS OF CONCERN TO DENTISTRY

• Decreased action: broad-spectrum antibiotics, salicylates (high doses)
• Antagonist to oral anticoagulants

SERIOUS REACTIONS

• Severe hypersensitivity reactions

DENTAL CONSIDERATIONS

General:
• Determine why the patient is taking this drug. Medical consultation should be made before dental treatment.
• Patients on chronic drug therapy may rarely have symptoms of blood dyscrasias, which can include infection, bleeding, and poor healing.
Consultations:
• Medical consultation to determine coagulation stability.

pilocarpine hydrochloride

pye-loe-kar´-peen
high-droh-klor´-ide
(Isopto Carpin[AUS], Ocusert Pilo-20[AUS], Ocusert Pilo-40[AUS], Pilopt Eye Drops[AUS], P.V. Carpine Liquifilm Ophthalmic Solution[AUS], Salagen)

CATEGORY AND SCHEDULE
Pregnancy Risk Category: C

Drug Class: Miotic, cholinergic agonist

MECHANISM OF ACTION

A cholinergic that increases exocrine gland secretions by stimulating cholinergic receptors. *Therapeutic Effect:* Improves symptoms of dry mouth in patients with salivary gland hypofunction.

USES

Treatment of primary glaucoma, early stages of wide-angle glaucoma (less useful in advanced stages), chronic open-angle glaucoma, acute narrow-angle glaucoma before emergency surgery; also used to neutralize mydriatics used during eye exam; may be used alternately with mydriatics to break adhesions between iris and lens

PHARMACOKINETICS

Route	Onset	Peak	Duration
PO	20 min	1 hr	3–5 hr

Absorption decreased if taken with a high-fat meal. Inactivation of pilocarpine thought to occur at neuronal synapses and probably in plasma. Excreted in urine.
Half-life: 4–12 hr.

INDICATIONS AND DOSAGES
▶ **Dry mouth Associated with Radiation Treatment for Head and Neck Cancer**
PO
Adults, Elderly. 5 mg 3 times a day. Range: 15–30 mg/day. Maximum: 2 tablets/dose.
▶ **Dry Mouth Associated with Sjögren's Syndrome**
PO
Adults, Elderly. 5 mg 4 times a day. Range: 20–40 mg/day.
▶ **Dosage in Hepatic Impairment**
Dosage decreased to 5 mg twice a day for adults and elderly with hepatic impairment.

SIDE EFFECTS/ADVERSE REACTIONS
Frequent
Diaphoresis
Occasional
Headache, dizziness, urinary frequency, flushing, dyspepsia, nausea, asthenia, lacrimation, visual disturbances
Rare
Diarrhea, abdominal pain, peripheral edema, chills

PRECAUTIONS AND CONTRAINDICATIONS
Conditions in which miosis is undesirable, such as acute iritis and angle-closure glaucoma; uncontrolled asthma
Caution:
Bronchial asthma, hypertension

DRUG INTERACTIONS OF CONCERN TO DENTISTRY
• Anticholinergic drugs used to reduce salivation antagonize therapeutic action

SERIOUS REACTIONS
! Patients with diaphoresis who don't drink enough fluids may develop dehydration.

DENTAL CONSIDERATIONS
General:
• Avoid drugs with anticholinergic activity, such as antihistamines, opioids, benzodiazepines, propantheline, atropine, and scopolamine.
• Avoid dental light in patient's eyes; offer dark glasses for patient comfort.
• Monitor vital signs at every appointment because of cardiovascular and respiratory side effects.
Consultations:
• Medical consultation may be required to assess disease control.

DENTAL CONSIDERATIONS
Pilocarpine HCl (oral)
General:
• Patients receiving chemotherapy may require palliative treatment for stomatitis.
• Assess salivary flow as a factor in caries, periodontal disease, and candidiasis.
• Monitor vital signs at every appointment because of cardiovascular side effects.
• Place on frequent recall because of oral effects of head and neck radiation.

Consultations:
• Medical consultation may be required to assess disease control.
• Medical consultation may be necessary before prescribing for patients with cardiovascular, retinal, or respiratory disease.

Teach Patient/Family to:
• Use caution when driving at night or performing hazardous activities in reduced lighting (visual blurring)
• Take plenty of fluids, observe for dehydration, or discontinue drug
• When chronic dry mouth occurs, advise patient to:
  • Avoid mouth rinses with high alcohol content because of drying effects
  • Use daily home fluoride products to prevent caries
  • Use sugarless gum, frequent sips of water, or saliva substitutes

pimecrolimus
pim-eh-crow-lee´-mus
(Elidel)

CATEGORY AND SCHEDULE
Pregnancy Risk Category: C

Drug Class: Topical antiinflammatory

MECHANISM OF ACTION
An immunomodulator that inhibits release of cytokine, an enzyme that produces an inflammatory reaction. *Therapeutic Effect:* Produces antiinflammatory activity.

USES
Short-term and intermittent long-term treatment of mild to moderate atopic dermatitis in non-immunocompromised patients age 2 yr and older in whom conventional therapies cannot be used because of potential risks; in patients with an inadequate response; or in patients who are not responsive to conventional therapies

PHARMACOKINETICS
Minimal systemic absorption with topical application. Metabolized in liver. Excreted in feces.

INDICATIONS AND DOSAGES
▶ **Atopic Dermatitis (eczema)**
Topical
Adults, Elderly, Children 2–17 yr.
Apply to affected area twice daily for up to 3 wk (up to 6 wk in adolescents, children 2–17 yr). Rub in gently and completely.

SIDE EFFECTS/ADVERSE REACTIONS
Rare
Transient application-site sensation of burning or feeling of heat

PRECAUTIONS AND CONTRAINDICATIONS
Hypersensitivity to pimecrolimus or any component of the formulation, Netherton's syndrome (potential for increased systemic absorption), application to active cutaneous viral infections
Caution
Do not use for active cutaneous viral infections, infected dermatitis, natural or artificial sunlight exposure, no data on excretion in human milk, children younger than 2 yr

DRUG INTERACTIONS OF CONCERN TO DENTISTRY
• Drug interactions have not been evaluated. Low blood levels were

measured in some patients. Use drugs that inhibit CYP3A4 isoenzymes with caution in patients with widespread and erythrodermic disease.

SERIOUS REACTIONS
! Lymphadenopathy and phototoxicity occur rarely.

DENTAL CONSIDERATIONS
General:
• Determine why the patient is taking this drug.

pimozide
pim´-oh-zide
(Orap)

CATEGORY AND SCHEDULE
Pregnancy Risk Category: C

Drug Class: Antipsychotic, antidyskinetic

MECHANISM OF ACTION
A diphenylbutylpiperidine that blocks dopamine at postsynaptic receptor sites in the brain.
Therapeutic Effect: Suppresses behavioral response in psychosis.

USES
Treatment of motor and phonic tics in Gilles de la Tourette's syndrome; unapproved: psychotic disorders

PHARMACOKINETICS
PO: Onset erratic, peak 6–8 hr. *Half-life:* 50–55 hr; metabolized by liver; excreted in urine, feces.

INDICATIONS AND DOSAGES
▸ **Tourette's Disorder**
PO
Adults, Elderly. 1–2 mg/day in divided doses 3 times a day. Maximum: 10 mg/day.

Children older than 12 yr. Initially, 0.5 mg/kg/day. Maximum: 10 mg/day.

SIDE EFFECTS/ADVERSE REACTIONS
Occasional
Akathisia, dystonic extrapyramidal effects, parkinsonian extrapyramidal effects, tardive dyskinesia, blurred vision, ocular changes, constipation, decreased sweating, dry mouth, nasal congestion, dizziness, drowsiness, orthostatic hypotension, urinary retention, somnolence
Rare
Rash, cholestatic jaundice, priapism

PRECAUTIONS AND CONTRAINDICATIONS
Aggressive schizophrenics when sedation is required; concurrent administration of pemoline; methylphenidate or amphetamines; concurrent administration with dofetilide, sotalol, quinidine, other Class IA and III anti-arrhythmics, mesoridazine, thioridazine, chlorpromazine, droperidol, sparfloxacin, gatifloxacin, moxifloxacin, halofantrine, mefloquine, pentamidine, arsenic trioxide, levomethadyl acetate, dolasetron mesylate, probucol, tacrolimus, ziprasidone, sertraline, macrolide antibiotics, drugs that cause QT prolongation, and less potent inhibitors of CYP3A; congenital or drug-induced long QT syndrome; doses greater than 10 mg daily; history of cardiac arrhythmias, Parkinson's disease; patients with known hypokalemia or hypomagnesemia; severe central nervous system depression; simple tics or tics not associated with Tourette's syndrome; hypersensitivity to pimozide or any of its components.

P

Caution
Children younger than 12 yr,
lactation, hypertension, hepatic
disease, cardiac disease, renal
disease, breast cancer, hypokalemia

DRUG INTERACTIONS OF CONCERN TO DENTISTRY
• Increased CNS depression: alcohol, CNS depressants
• Increased effects of both drugs: phenothiazines
• Increased effects of anticholinergic drugs
• Prolonged QT interval, fatal cardiac arrhythmia; contraindicated: clarithromycin, erythromycin, azithromycin, dirithromycin, itraconazole

SERIOUS REACTIONS
! Serious reactions such as blood dyscrasias, agranulocytosis, leukocytopenia, thrombocytopenia, cholestatic jaundice, neuroleptic malignant syndrome (NMS), constipation or paralytic ileus, priapism, QT prolongation and torsades de pointes, seizure, systemic lupus erythematosus-like syndrome, and temperature regulation dysfunction (heatstroke or hypothermia) occur rarely.
! Abrupt withdrawal following long-term therapy may precipitate nausea, vomiting, gastritis, dizziness, and tremors.

DENTAL CONSIDERATIONS
General:
• Assess salivary flow as a factor in caries, periodontal disease, and candidiasis.
• Monitor vital signs at every appointment because of cardiovascular side effects.
• Assess for presence of extrapyramidal motor symptoms, such as tardive dyskinesia and akathisia. Extrapyramidal motor activity may complicate dental treatment.
• After supine positioning, have patient sit upright for at least 2 min before standing to avoid orthostatic hypotension.
• Consider action of drug in assessment of altered taste.
Consultations:
• Medical consultation may be required to assess disease control.
• If signs of tardive dyskinesia or akathisia are present, refer to physician.
Teach Patient/Family to:
• Use effective oral hygiene to prevent soft tissue inflammation
• Use caution to prevent injury when using oral hygiene aids
• When chronic dry mouth occurs, advise patient to:
  • Avoid mouth rinses with high alcohol content because of drying effects
  • Use daily home fluoride products to prevent caries
  • Use sugarless gum, frequent sips of water, or saliva substitutes

pindolol
pin´-doe-loll
(Apo-Pindol[CAN], Visken)

CATEGORY AND SCHEDULE
Pregnancy Risk Category: B (D if used in second or third trimester)

Drug Class: Nonselective β-adrenergic blocker

MECHANISM OF ACTION
A nonselective beta blocker that blocks β_1- and β_2-adrenergic receptors. **Therapeutic Effect:** Slows

heart rate, decreases cardiac output, decreases B/P, and exhibits antiarrhythmic activity. Decreases myocardial ischemia severity by decreasing oxygen requirements.

USES
Treatment of mild-to-moderate hypertension

PHARMACOKINETICS
Completely absorbed from GI tract. Metabolized in liver. Primarily excreted in urine. *Half-life:* 3–4 hr (half-life increased with impaired renal function, elderly).

INDICATIONS AND DOSAGES
▶ **Mild-to-Moderate Hypertension**
PO
Adults. Initially, 5 mg 2 times a day. Gradually increase dose by 10 mg/day at 2- to 4-wk intervals. Maintenance: 10–30 mg/day in 2–3 divided doses. Maximum: 60 mg/day.
▶ **Usual Elderly Dosage:**
PO
Initially, 5 mg/day. May increase by 5 mg q3–4wk.

SIDE EFFECTS/ADVERSE REACTIONS
Frequent
Decreased sexual ability, drowsiness, trouble sleeping, unusual tiredness or weakness
Occasional
Bradycardia, depression, cold hands/feet, diarrhea, constipation, anxiety, nasal congestion, nausea, vomiting
Rare
Altered taste, dry eyes, itching, numbness of fingers, toes and scalp

PRECAUTIONS AND CONTRAINDICATIONS
Bronchial asthma, COPD, uncontrolled cardiac failure,

sinus bradycardia, heart block greater than first degree, cardiogenic shock, CHF, unless secondary to tachyarrhythmias
Caution
Major surgery, diabetes mellitus, renal disease, thyroid disease, COPD, well-compensated heart failure, CAD, nonallergic bronchospasm, impaired hepatic function, children

DRUG INTERACTIONS OF CONCERN TO DENTISTRY
• Increased hypotension, bradycardia: anticholinergics, hydrocarbon inhalation anesthetics, fentanyl derivatives
• Decreased antihypertensive effects: indomethacin, sympathomimetics
• Increased effect of both drugs: phenothiazines, xanthines
• Decreased bronchodilation: theophyllines
• Hypertension, bradycardia: epinephrine, ephedrine
• Slow metabolism of drug: lidocaine

SERIOUS REACTIONS
! Overdosage may produce profound bradycardia and hypotension.
! Abrupt withdrawal may result in sweating, palpitations, headache, and tremulousness.
! May precipitate CHF or MI in patients with heart disease; thyroid storm in those with thyrotoxicosis; or peripheral ischemia in those with existing peripheral vascular disease.
! Hypoglycemia may occur in previously controlled diabetics.
! Signs of thrombocytopenia, such as unusual bleeding or bruising, occur rarely.

DENTAL CONSIDERATIONS
General:
• Monitor vital signs at every appointment because of cardiovascular side effects.

• Patients on chronic drug therapy may rarely have symptoms of blood dyscrasias, which can include infection, bleeding, and poor healing.
• Stress from dental procedures may compromise cardiovascular function; determine patient risk.
• Use vasoconstrictors with caution, in low doses, and with careful aspiration. Avoid use of gingival retraction cord with epinephrine.
• Consider semisupine chair position for patient comfort if GI side effects occur.
• Assess salivary flow as a factor in caries, periodontal disease, and candidiasis.
• Consider drug effects if taste alteration occurs.
Consultations:
• In a patient with symptoms of blood dyscrasias, request a medical consultation for blood studies and postpone dental treatment until normal values are reestablished.
• Medical consultation may be required to assess disease control and patient's ability to tolerate stress.
Teach Patient/Family to:
• Use effective oral hygiene to prevent soft tissue inflammation
• Use caution to prevent injury when using oral hygiene aids
• When chronic dry mouth occurs, advise patient to:
  • Avoid mouth rinses with high alcohol content because of drying effects
  • Use daily home fluoride products to prevent caries
  • Use sugarless gum, frequent sips of water, or saliva substitutes

pioglitazone
pye-oh-gli´-ta-zone
(Actos)

CATEGORY AND SCHEDULE
Pregnancy Risk Category: C

Drug Class: Antidiabetic, oral

MECHANISM OF ACTION
An antidiabetic that improves target-cell response to insulin without increasing pancreatic insulin secretion. Decreases hepatic glucose output and increases insulin-dependent glucose utilization in skeletal muscle. *Therapeutic Effect:* Lowers blood glucose concentration.

USES
Monotherapy, as an adjunct to diet and exercise in patients with Type 2 diabetes mellitus; may also be used with metformin when metformin, diet, and exercise are not adequate for control

PHARMACOKINETICS
Rapidly absorbed. Highly protein bound (99%), primarily to albumin. Metabolized in the liver. Excreted in urine. Unknown if removed by hemodialysis. *Half-life:* 16–24 hr.

INDICATIONS AND DOSAGES
▸ **Diabetes Mellitus, Combination Therapy**
PO
Adult, Elderly. With insulin: Initially, 15–30 mg once a day. Initially continue current insulin dosage; then decrease insulin dosage by 10%–25% if hypoglycemia occurs or plasma glucose level decreases to less than 100 mg/dl. Maximum: 45 mg/day. With sulfonylureas: Initially, 15–30 mg/day. Decrease

sulfonylurea dosage if hypoglycemia occurs. With metformin: Initially, 15–30 mg/day. As monotherapy: Monotherapy is not to be used if patient is well controlled with diet and exercise alone. Initially, 15–30 mg/day. May increase dosage in increments until 45 mg/day is reached.

SIDE EFFECTS/ADVERSE REACTIONS
Frequent
Headache, upper respiratory tract infection
Occasional
Sinusitis, myalgia, pharyngitis, aggravated diabetes mellitus

PRECAUTIONS AND CONTRAINDICATIONS
Active hepatic disease; diabetic ketoacidosis; increased serum transaminase levels, including ALT (SGPT) greater than 2.5 times normal serum level; Type 1 diabetes mellitus
Caution
Hepatic dysfunction (reduce dose), renal impairment, lactation, children younger than 18 yr

DRUG INTERACTIONS OF CONCERN TO DENTISTRY
None reported

SERIOUS REACTIONS
None known

DENTAL CONSIDERATIONS
General:
• Ensure that patient is following prescribed diet and regularly takes medication.
• Place on frequent recall to evaluate healing response.

• Short appointments and a stress-reduction protocol may be required for anxious patients.
• Diabetics may be more susceptible to infection and have delayed wound healing.
• Question patient about self-monitoring of drug's antidiabetic effect, including blood glucose values or finger-stick records.
• Consider semisupine chair position for patient comfort if GI side effects occur.
Consultations:
• Medical consultation may be required to assess disease control and patient's ability to tolerate stress.
• Medical consultation may include data from patient's blood glucose monitoring, including glycosylated hemoglobin or HbA1c testing.
Teach Patient/Family to:
• Prevent trauma when using oral hygiene aids
• Update health and drug history if physician makes any changes in evaluation or drug regimens; include OTC, herbal, and nonherbal drugs in the update
• Use effective oral hygiene to prevent soft-tissue inflammation

P

pirbuterol
peer-beut´-er-all
(Maxair, Maxair Autohaler)

CATEGORY AND SCHEDULE
Pregnancy Risk Category: C

Drug Class: Bronchodilator

MECHANISM OF ACTION
A sympathomimetic, adrenergic agonist, that stimulates β_2-adrenergic receptors in the lungs, resulting in relaxation of bronchial smooth

muscle. *Therapeutic Effect:* Relieves bronchospasm, reduces airway resistance.

USES

Treatment of reversible bronchospasm (prevention, treatment), including asthma; may be given with theophylline or steroids

PHARMACOKINETICS

Absorbed from bronchi following inhalation. Metabolized in liver. Primarily excreted in urine. Unknown if removed by hemodialysis. *Half-life:* 2–3 hr.

INDICATIONS AND DOSAGES

▶ **Prevention of Bronchospasm**
Inhalation
Adults, Elderly, Children 12 yr and older. 2 inhalations q4–6h. Maximum: 12 inhalations daily.
▶ **Treatment of Bronchospasm**
Inhalation
Adults, Elderly, Children 12 yr and older. 2 inhalations separated by at least 1–3 min, followed by a third inhalation. Maximum: 12 inhalations daily.

SIDE EFFECTS/ADVERSE REACTIONS

Occasional
Nervousness, tremor, headache, palpitations, nausea, dizziness, tachycardia, cough

PRECAUTIONS AND CONTRAINDICATIONS

History of hypersensitivity to pirbuterol, albuterol, or any of its components
Caution
Lactation, cardiac disorders, hyperthyroidism, diabetes mellitus, prostatic hypertrophy

DRUG INTERACTIONS OF CONCERN TO DENTISTRY

• None reported

SERIOUS REACTIONS

! Excessive sympathomimetic stimulation may produce palpitations, extrasystoles, tachycardia, chest pain, slight increases in B/P followed by a substantial decrease, chills, sweating and blanching of skin.
! Too-frequent or excessive use may lead to loss of bronchodilating effectiveness and severe, paradoxical bronchoconstriction.

DENTAL CONSIDERATIONS

General:
• Acute asthmatic episodes may be precipitated in the dental office. Sympathomimetic inhalants should be available for emergency use.
• Be aware that aspirin or sulfite preservatives in vasoconstrictor-containing products can exacerbate asthma.
• Monitor vital signs at every appointment because of cardiovascular and respiratory side effects.
• Assess salivary flow as a factor in caries, periodontal disease, and candidiasis.
• Consider semisupine chair position for patients with respiratory disease.
• Short appointments and a stress reduction protocol may be required for anxious patients.
Consultations:
• Medical consultation may be required to assess disease control and patient's ability to tolerate stress.
Teach Patient/Family to:
• Rinse mouth with water after each dose to prevent dryness (for inhalation dosage forms)

• When chronic dry mouth occurs, advise patient to:
  • Avoid mouth rinses with high alcohol content because of drying effects
  • Use daily home fluoride products to prevent caries
  • Use sugarless gum, frequent sips of water, or saliva substitutes

piroxicam
peer-ox´-ih-kam
(Apo-Piroxicam[CAN], Candyl-D[AUS], Feldene, Fexicam[CAN], Mobilis[AUS], Novopirocam[CAN], Pirohexal-D [AUS], Rosig[AUS], Rosig-D[AUS])
Do not confuse Feldene with Seldane.

CATEGORY AND SCHEDULE
Pregnancy Risk Category: C
(D if used in third trimester or near delivery)

Drug Class: Nonsteroidal antiinflammatory

MECHANISM OF ACTION
An NSAID that produces analgesic and antiinflammatory effects by inhibiting prostaglandin synthesis. *Therapeutic Effect:* Reduces inflammatory response and intensity of pain.

USES
Treatment of osteoarthritis, rheumatoid arthritis; unapproved: gouty arthritis

PHARMACOKINETICS
PO: Peak 2 hr. *Half-life:* 3–3.5 hr; 99% protein binding; metabolized in liver; excreted in urine (metabolites), breast milk.

INDICATIONS AND DOSAGES
▶ **Acute or Chronic Rheumatoid Arthritis and Osteoarthritis**
PO
Adults, Elderly. Initially, 10–20 mg/day as a single dose or in divided doses. Some patients may require up to 30–40 mg/day.
Children. 0.2–0.3 mg/kg/day. Maximum: 15 mg/day.

SIDE EFFECTS/ADVERSE REACTIONS
Frequent
Dyspepsia, nausea, dizziness
Occasional
Diarrhea, constipation, abdominal cramps or pain, flatulence, stomatitis
Rare
Hypertension, urticaria, dysuria, ecchymosis, blurred vision, insomnia, phototoxicity

PRECAUTIONS AND CONTRAINDICATIONS
Active peptic ulcer disease, chronic inflammation of the GI tract, GI bleeding or ulceration, history of hypersensitivity to aspirin or NSAIDs
Caution
Lactation, children, bleeding disorders, GI disorders, cardiac disorders, hypersensitivity to other antiinflammatory agents, hypertension

DRUG INTERACTIONS OF CONCERN TO DENTISTRY
• GI ulceration, bleeding: aspirin, alcohol, corticosteroids
• Nephrotoxicity: acetaminophen (prolonged use and high doses)
• Possible risk of decreased renal function: cyclosporine
• Decreased action: salicylates

P

• First-time users of SSRIs also taking NSAIDs may have a higher risk of GI side effects; until more data are available, it may be advisable to avoid use of NSAIDs in these patients (Br J Clin Pharmacol 55:591–595, 2003)
• When prescribed for dental pain:
  • Risk of increased effects of oral anticoagulants, oral antidiabetics, lithium, methotrexate
  • Decreased antihypertensive effects of diuretics, α-adrenergic blockers, ACE inhibitors

SERIOUS REACTIONS

! Rare reactions with long-term use include peptic ulcer disease, GI bleeding, gastritis, severe hepatic reaction (cholestasis, jaundice), nephrotoxicity (dysuria, hematuria, proteinuria, nephrotic syndrome), hematologic sensitivity (anemia, leukopenia, eosinophilia, thrombocytopenia), and a severe hypersensitivity reaction (fever, chills, bronchospasm).

DENTAL CONSIDERATIONS

General:
• Patients on chronic drug therapy may rarely have symptoms of blood dyscrasias, which can include infection, bleeding, and poor healing.
• Assess salivary flow as a factor in caries, periodontal disease, and candidiasis.
• Avoid prescribing for dental use during pregnancy.
• Minimize use of aspirin-containing products.
• Consider semisupine chair position for patients with arthritic disease or if GI side effects occur.
Consultations:
• In a patient with symptoms of blood dyscrasias, request a medical consultation for blood studies and

postpone dental treatment until normal values are reestablished.
• Medical consultation may be required to assess disease control.
Teach Patient/Family to:
• Use effective oral hygiene to prevent soft tissue inflammation
• Use caution to prevent injury when using oral hygiene aids
• Report oral lesions, soreness, or bleeding to dentist
• When chronic dry mouth occurs, advise patient to:
  • Avoid mouth rinses with high alcohol content because of drying effects
  • Use daily home fluoride products to prevent caries
  • Use sugarless gum, frequent sips of water, or saliva substitutes

podofilox
poe-doe-fil´-ox
(Condyline[CAN], Condyline Paint[AUS], Condylox)

CATEGORY AND SCHEDULE
Pregnancy Risk Category: C

Drug Class: Antimitotic agent

MECHANISM OF ACTION
An active component of podophyllin resin that binds to tubulin to prevent formation of microtubules resulting in mitotic arrest. Exercises many biological effects, such as damages endothelium of small blood vessels, attenuates nucleoside transport, suppresses immune responses, inhibits macrophage metabolism, induces interleukin-1 and interleukin-2, decreases lymphocytes' response to mitogens, and enhances macrophage growth. *Therapeutic Effect:* Removes genital warts.

USES
Removal of certain types of warts on the outside skin of the genital areas (penis or vulva)

PHARMACOKINETICS
Time to peak occurs in 1–2 hr.
Some degree of absorption.
Half-life: 1–4.5 hr.

INDICATIONS AND DOSAGES
▶ **Anogenital Warts**
Topical
Adults. Apply 0.5% gel for 3 days, then withhold for 4 days. Repeat cycle up to 4 times.
▶ **Genital Warts (condylomata acuminate)**
Topical
Adults. Apply 0.5% solution or gel q12h in the morning and evening for 3 days, then withhold for 4 days. Repeat cycle up to 4 times.

SIDE EFFECTS/ADVERSE REACTIONS
Occasional
Erosion, inflammation, itching, pain, burning
Rare
Nausea, vomiting

PRECAUTIONS AND CONTRAINDICATIONS
Bleeding warts, moles, birthmarks or unusual warts with hair, diabetes, poor blood circulation, pregnancy, steroid use, hypersensitivity to podofilox or any component of its formulation

DRUG INTERACTIONS OF CONCERN TO DENTISTRY
None reported

SERIOUS REACTIONS
! Nausea and vomiting occur rarely and usually after cumulative doses.

DENTAL CONSIDERATIONS
General:
• Determine why patient is taking the drug.
• Exam oral mucous membranes for lesions; overuse may be associated with oral ulcers.
• Tactful questions related to STD may be appropriate.
• Explore medical and drug history.
• Not for use on mucous membranes.
Consultations:
• Medical consultation may be required to assess disease control.
Teach Patient/Family to:
• Use effective oral hygiene to prevent soft tissue inflammation
• Prevent trauma when using oral hygiene aids
• Update health and medication history if physician makes any changes in evaluation or drug regimens; include OTC, herbal, and nonherbal drugs in the update

podophyllum resin
po-dof´-fil-um rez-in
(Podocon-25, Pododerm)

CATEGORY AND SCHEDULE
Pregnancy Risk Category: X

Drug Class: Cytotoxic, topical

MECHANISM OF ACTION
A cytotoxic agent that directly affects epithelial cell metabolism by arresting mitosis through binding to a protein subunit of spindle microtubules. *Therapeutic Effect:* Removes soft genital warts.

USES
Removal of benign growths

PHARMACOKINETICS
Topical podophyllum is systemically absorbed. Absorption may be increased if applied to bleeding, friable, or recently biopsied warts.

INDICATIONS AND DOSAGES
▸ **Genital Warts (condylomata acuminate)**
Topical
Adults, Elderly, Children. Apply 10%–25% solution in compound benzoin tincture to dry surface. Use 1 drop at a time allowing drying between drops until area is covered. Total volume should be limited to less than 0.5 ml per treatment session.

SIDE EFFECTS/ADVERSE REACTIONS
Occasional
Pruritus, nausea, vomiting, abdominal pain, diarrhea

PRECAUTIONS AND CONTRAINDICATIONS
Diabetes mellitus, concomitant steroid therapy, circulation disorders, bleeding warts, moles, birthmarks or unusual warts with hair growing from them, pregnancy, hypersensitivity to podophyllum resin preparations

DRUG INTERACTIONS OF CONCERN TO DENTISTRY
None reported

SERIOUS REACTIONS
❗ Paresthesia, polyneuritis, paralytic ileus, pyrexia, leukopenia, thrombocytopenia, coma, and death have been reported with podophyllum resin use.

DENTAL CONSIDERATIONS
General:
• Determine why patient is taking the drug.
• This medication is applied in physician's office.
• Questions related to sexually-transmitted diseases may be appropriate.
Consultations:
• Medical consultation may be required to assess disease control.
Teach Patient/Family to:
• Use effective oral hygiene to prevent soft tissue inflammation
• Prevent trauma when using oral hygiene aids
• Update health and medication history if physician makes any changes in evaluation or drug regimens; include OTC, herbal, and nonherbal drugs in the update

polymyxin B
polly-mix´-in
(Aerosporin)

CATEGORY AND SCHEDULE
Pregnancy Risk Category: B

Drug Class: Antibiotics, polymyxins

MECHANISM OF ACTION
An antibiotic that alters cell membrane permeability in susceptible microorganisms. *Therapeutic Effect:* Bactericidal activity.

USES
Treatment of superficial external infections

PHARMACOKINETICS
Negligible absorption. Protein binding: low. Excreted in urine. Poor removal in hemodialysis. *Half-life:* 6 hr.

INDICATIONS AND DOSAGES
▸ **Mild-to-Moderate Infections**
IV
Adults, Elderly, Children 2 yr and older. 15,000–25,000 units/kg/day in divided doses q12h.
Infants. Up to 40,000 units/kg/day.
IM
Adults, Elderly, Children 2 yr and older. 25,000–30,000 units/kg/day in divided doses q4–6h.
Infants. Up to 40,000 units/kg/day.
▸ **Usual Irrigation Dosage**
Continuous Bladder Irrigation
Adults, Elderly. 1 ml urogenital concentrate (contains 200,000 units polymyxin B, 57 mg neomycin) added to 1000 ml 0.9% NaCl. Give each 1000 ml >24 hr for up to 10 days (may increase to 2000 ml/day when urine output is greater than 2 L/day).
▸ **Usual Ophthalmic Dosage**
Ophthalmic
Adults, Elderly, Children. 1 drop q3–4h.

SIDE EFFECTS/ADVERSE REACTIONS
Frequent
Severe pain, irritation at IM injection sites, phlebitis, thrombophlebitis with IV administration
Occasional
Fever, urticaria

PRECAUTIONS AND CONTRAINDICATIONS
Hypersensitivity to polymyxin B or any component of the formulation
Caution
Hypokalemia, renal disease, hepatic disease, gout, COPD, lupus erythematosus, diabetes mellitus

SERIOUS REACTIONS
❗ Nephrotoxicity, especially with concurrent/sequential use of other nephrotoxic drugs, renal impairment, concurrent/sequential use of muscle relaxants.
❗ Superinfection, especially with fungi, may occur.

DENTAL CONSIDERATIONS
General:
• Avoid dental light in patient's eyes; offer dark glasses for patient comfort and safety during dental treatment.

polymyxin B sulfate; trimethoprim sulfate
pol-ee-mix´-in bee sul´-fate; trye-meth´-oh-prim sul´-fate
(Polytrim)

CATEGORY AND SCHEDULE
Pregnancy Risk Category: C

Drug Class: Antiinfective (ophthalmic)

P

MECHANISM OF ACTION
Polymyxin B damages bacterial cytoplasmic membrane which causes leakage of intracellular components. Trimethoprim is a folate antagonist that blocks bacterial biosynthesis of nucleic acids and proteins by interfering with metabolism of folinic acid. *Therapeutic Effect:* Prevents inflammatory process. Interferes with bacterial protein synthesis. Produces antibacterial activity.

USES
Treatment of superficial external ocular infections

PHARMACOKINETICS
Absorption through intact skin and mucous membranes is insignificant.

INDICATIONS AND DOSAGES
▶ **Treatment of Surface Ocular Bacterial Conjunctivitis and Blepharoconjunctivitis**
Ophthalmic
Adults, Elderly, Children. Instill 1–2 drops in eye(s) every 3 hr for 7–10 days. Maximum: 6 doses/day.

SIDE EFFECTS/ADVERSE REACTIONS
Occasional
Local irritation, redness, burning, stinging, itching

PRECAUTIONS AND CONTRAINDICATIONS
Hypersensitivity to polymyxin B, trimethoprim sulfate, or any component of the formulation

DRUG INTERACTIONS OF CONCERN TO DENTISTRY
• None reported

SERIOUS REACTIONS
! Prolonged use may result in overgrowth of nonsusceptible organisms, including superinfection.
! Hypersensitivity reactions consisting of lid edema, itching, increased redness, tearing, and/or circumocular rash have been reported.
! Photosensitivity has been reported in patients taking oral trimethoprim.

DENTAL CONSIDERATIONS
General:
• Avoid dental light in patient's eyes; offer dark glasses for patient comfort and safety during dental treatment.

posaconazole
poe-sah-kone´-ah-zole
(Noxafil)

CATEGORY AND SCHEDULE
Pregnancy Risk Category: C

Drug Class: Antifungal

MECHANISM OF ACTION
A tirazole antifungal that blocks the synthesis of ergosterol, a key component of fungal cell membrane, through the inhibition of the enzyme lanosterol 14a-α-demethylase and accumulation of methylated sterol precursors. *Therapeutic Effect:* Inhibits fungal cell membrane formation.

USES
Prophylaxis of invasive *Aspergillus* and *Candida* infections in patients who are severely immunocompromised

PHARMACOKINETICS
Food increases absorption. Protein binding: greater than 98%. Not significantly metabolized; undergoes glucuronidation into metabolites. Primarily eliminated in feces (71%, 66% unchanged); partial excretion in urine (13%, less than 0.2% unchanged). *Half-life:* 35 hr.

INDICATIONS AND DOSAGES
▶ **Prophylaxis of Invasive Fungal Infections**
PO
Adults, Children 13 yr and older. 200 mg (5 ml) three times a day.
▶ **Oropharyngeal Candidiasis**
PO
Adults, Children 13 yr and older. Initially, 100 mg (2.5 ml) twice a day

on the first day. Maintenance: 100 mg (2.5 ml) once a day for 13 days.

▸ **Oropharyngeal Candidiasis, Refractory to Itraconazole and/or Fluconazole**
PO
Adults, Children 13 yr and older. 400 mg (10 ml) twice a day.

SIDE EFFECTS/ADVERSE REACTIONS:
Adult
Frequent
Diarrhea
Occasional
Nausea, neutropenia, headache, vomiting, abdominal pain, flatulence, QTc prolongation, rash, hypokalemia, anemia, fever, bilirubin increased, ALT increased, AST increased, GGT increased, dizziness, weakness, anorexia, fatigue, insomnia, mucositis, thrombocytopenia, alkaline phosphatase increased, serum creatinine increased, myalgia, pruritus, dyspepsia, xerostoma
Rare
Hypertension, blurred vision, tremor, hepatocellular damage, taste perversion, constipation, somnolence

PRECAUTIONS AND CONTRAINDICATIONS
Hypersensitivity to azole antifungals, posaconazole or its components; avoid co-administration with ergot alkaloids
Caution
Do not breast-feed, hepatic impairment, patients with an increased risk of arrhythmia, electrolyte abnormalities

DRUG INTERACTIONS OF CONCERN TO DENTISTRY
• Calcium channel blockers: may increase the levels and effects of calcium channel blockers

• Cimetidine: may decrease the levels and effects of posaconazole; avoid concurrent use
• Cyclosporine: may increase the levels and effects of cyclosporine
• CYP3A4 substrates: may increase the levels and effects of CYP3A4 substrates
• Ergot alkaloids: May increase the levels and effects of ergot alkaloids
• HMG-CoA reductase inhibitors: may increase the levels and effects of HMG-CoA reductase inhibitors
• Midazolam: may increase the levels and effects of midazolam
• Phenytoin: may increase the levels and effects of phenytoin; avoid concurrent use
• QT-prolonging agents: increased risk of arrhythmia (torsade de pointes)
• Rifabutin: may increase the levels and effects of rifabutin; avoid concurrent use
• Sirolimus: may increase the levels and effects of sirolimus
• Tacrolimus: may increase the levels and effects of tacrolimus
• Vinca alkaloids: may increase the levels and effects of vinca alkaloids

SERIOUS REACTIONS
! Hepatic dysfunction may occur.
! Arrhythmia (torsade de pointes) has been reported.

DENTAL CONSIDERATIONS
General:
• Monitor vital signs at every appointment due to possible adverse cardiovascular effects.
• Determine why patient is taking the drug.

P

• Consider semisupine chair position for patient comfort due to adverse GI effects of drug.
• To prevent reinoculation of Candidal infection, dispose of toothbrush and other contaminated oral hygiene devices used during period of infection.
• Assess salivary flow as a factor in caries, periodontal disease and candidiasis.
• Disinfect or remake removable prostheses that may harbor residual candidal organisms.
• Consider drug effect in evaluating taste changes versus restorative materials.
Consultations:
• Medical consult may be necessary to determine patient's ability to tolerate dental procedures.
Teach Patient/Family to:
• Avoid mouthrinses with high acohol content due to drying effects.

potassium chloride
poe-tass´-ee-um klor´-ide
(Apo-K[CAN], Cena K; Ed K+10, K+Care; K-10, K-8, Kaochlor, Kaochlor S-F, Kaon-Cl, Kaon-CL 10, Kaon-CL 20%, Kato, Kay Ciel, KCl-20, KCl-40, K-Dur 10, K-Dur 20, K-Lor; Klor-Con, Klor-Con/25, Klor-Con 10, Klor-Con 8, Klor-Con M10, Klor-Con M15, Klor-Con M20, Klotrix, K-Lyte CI, K-Norm, K-Sol, K-Tab, Micro-K, Micro-K 10, Rum-K)
Do not confuse with Cardura or Slow-FE.

CATEGORY AND SCHEDULE
Pregnancy Risk Category: C

Drug Class: Potassium electrolyte

MECHANISM OF ACTION
An electrolyte that is necessary for multiple cellular metabolic processes. Primary action is intracellular. *Therapeutic Effect:* Necessary for nerve impulse conduction, contraction of cardiac, skeletal, and smooth muscle; maintains normal renal function and acid-base balance.

USES
Prevention and treatment of hypokalemia

PHARMACOKINETICS
Well absorbed from the GI tract. Enters cells via active transport from extracellular fluid. Primarily excreted in urine.

INDICATIONS AND DOSAGES
▶ **Prevention of Hypokalemia (on diuretic therapy)**
PO
Adults, Elderly. 20–40 mEq/day in 1–2 divided doses.
Children. 1–2 mEq/kg in 1–2 divided doses.
▶ **Treatment of Hypokalemia**
IV
Adults, Elderly. 5–10 mEq/hr. Maximum: 400 mEq/day.
Children. 1 mEq/kg over 1–2 hr.
PO
Adults, Elderly. 40–80 mEq/day, further doses based on laboratory values.
Children. 1–2 mEq/day, further doses based on laboratory values.

SIDE EFFECTS/ADVERSE REACTIONS
Occasional
Nausea, vomiting, diarrhea, flatulence, abdominal discomfort with distention, phlebitis with IV administration (particularly when

potassium concentration of greater than 40 mEq/L is infused)
Rare
Rash

PRECAUTIONS AND CONTRAINDICATIONS
Digitalis toxicity, heat cramps, hyperkalemia, patients receiving potassium-sparing diuretics, postoperative oliguria, severe burns, severe renal impairment, shock with dehydration or hemolytic reaction, untreated Addison's disease, hypersensitivity to any component of the formulation
Caution
Cardiac disease, potassium-sparing diuretic therapy, systemic acidosis, pregnancy category A, renal impairment

DRUG INTERACTIONS OF CONCERN TO DENTISTRY
• Decreased potassium requirement: corticosteroids
• Increased GI side effects: anticholinergic drugs, NSAIDs
• Increased serum potassium: NSAIDs, cyclosporine

SERIOUS REACTIONS
! Hyperkalemia (observed particularly in elderly or in patients with impaired renal function) manifested as paresthesia of extremities, heaviness of legs, cold skin, grayish pallor, hypotension, mental confusion, irritability, flaccid paralysis, and cardiac arrhythmias.

DENTAL CONSIDERATIONS
General:
• Patients taking potassium supplements will normally be taking a diuretic. Compliance with potassium supplements can be a problem. Verify serum potassium levels as required.

• Consider semisupine chair position for patient comfort if GI side effects occur.

potassium acetate/potassium bicarbonate-citrate/potassium chloride/potassium gluconate
poe-tah´-see-um ass´-eh-tayte
(potassium bicarbonate-citrate: K-Lyte, Klor-Con EF, Effer K, K-Lyte DS; potassium chloride: Apo-K[CAN], Kaochlor, K-Dur, K-Lor, K-Lor-Con M 15, Kaon-Cl, KSR[AUS], KSR-600[AUS], Micro-K, Slow-K[AUS], Span-K[AUS]; potassium gluconate: Kaon)
Do not confuse K-dur with Cardura.

CATEGORY AND SCHEDULE
Pregnancy Risk Category: C (A for potassium chloride)

Drug Class: Potassium electrolyte

MECHANISM OF ACTION
An electrolyte that is necessary for multiple cellular metabolic processes. Primary action is intracellular. ***Therapeutic Effect:*** Is necessary for nerve impulse conduction and contraction of cardiac, skeletal, and smooth muscle; maintains normal renal function and acid-base balance.

USES
Prevention and treatment of hypokalemia

PHARMACOKINETICS

Well absorbed from the GI tract. Enters cells by active transport from extra-cellular fluid. Primarily excreted in urine.

INDICATIONS AND DOSAGES

▸ **Prevention of Hypokalemia (in patients on diuretic therapy)**

PO

Adults, Elderly. 20–40 mEq/day in 1–2 divided doses.
Children. 1–2 mEq/kg/day in 1–2 divided doses.

▸ **Treatment of Hypokalemia**

PO

Adults, Elderly. 40–80 mEq/day; further doses based on laboratory values.
Children. 2–5 mEq/day; further doses based on laboratory values.

IV

Adults, Elderly. 5–10 mEq/hr.
Maximum: 400 mEq/day.
Children. 1 mEq/kg over 1–2 hr.

SIDE EFFECTS/ADVERSE REACTIONS

Occasional

Nausea, vomiting, diarrhea, flatulence, abdominal discomfort with distention, phlebitis with IV administration (particularly when higher concentrations are infused IV)

Rare

Rash

PRECAUTIONS AND CONTRAINDICATIONS

Concurrent use of potassium-sparing diuretics, digitalis toxicity, heat cramps, hyperkalemia, postoperative oliguria, severe burns, severe renal impairment, shock with dehydration or hemolytic reaction, untreated Addison's disease

Caution

Cardiac disease, potassium-sparing diuretic therapy, systemic acidosis, renal impairment

DRUG INTERACTIONS OF CONCERN TO DENTISTRY

• Decreased potassium requirement: corticosteroids
• Increased GI side effects: anticholinergic drugs, NSAIDs
• Increased serum potassium: NSAIDs, cyclosporine

SERIOUS REACTIONS

! Hyperkalemia (more common in elderly patients and those with impaired renal function) may be manifested as paresthesia, feeling of heaviness in the lower extremities, cold skin, grayish pallor, hypotension, confusion, irritability, flaccid paralysis, and cardiac arrhythmias.

DENTAL CONSIDERATIONS

General:

• Patients taking potassium supplements will normally be taking a diuretic. Compliance with potassium supplements can be a problem. Verify serum potassium levels as required.
• Consider semisupine chair position for patient comfort if GI side effects occur.

povidone iodine

poe´vi-done
(ACU-dyne, Aerodine, Betadine, Betagen, Biodine, Efodine, Io-dex-P, Mallisol, Minidyne, Operand, Polydine Proviodine)

CATEGORY AND SCHEDULE

Pregnancy Risk Category: D (vaginal antiseptic)

Drug Class: Iodophor disinfectant

MECHANISM OF ACTION
Destroys a wide variety of microorganisms by local irritation, germicidal action.

USES
Cleansing wounds, disinfection, preoperative skin preparation removal

INDICATIONS AND DOSAGES
Topical
Adults, Children. Use as needed.

SIDE EFFECTS/ADVERSE REACTIONS
Frequent
Skin irritation

PRECAUTIONS AND CONTRAINDICATIONS
Hypersensitivity to iodine
Caution
Extensive burns

DRUG INTERACTIONS OF CONCERN TO DENTISTRY
• Do not use with alcohol or hydrogen peroxide

SERIOUS REACTIONS
• Severe allergic reactions

DENTAL CONSIDERATIONS
General:
• Assess for allergies to seafood; if present, drug should not be used.
• Store in tight, light-resistant container.
• Evaluate area of the body involved for irritation, rash, breaks, dryness, and scales.
Teach Patient/Family to:
• Discontinue use if rash, irritation, or redness occurs

pramipexole
pram-eh-pex´-ol
(Mirapex)
Do not confuse Mirapex with Mifeprex or MiraLax.

CATEGORY AND SCHEDULE
Pregnancy Risk Category: C

Drug Class: Antiparkinson agent

MECHANISM OF ACTION
An antiparkinson agent that stimulates dopamine receptors in the striatum. *Therapeutic Effect:* Relieves signs and symptoms of Parkinson's disease.

USES
Treatment of idiopathic Parkinson's disease

PHARMACOKINETICS
Rapidly and extensively absorbed after PO administration. Protein binding: 15%. Widely distributed. Steady-state concentrations achieved within 2 days. Primarily eliminated in urine. Not removed by hemodialysis. *Half-life:* 8 hr (12 hr in patients older than 65 yr).

INDICATIONS AND DOSAGES
▶ **Parkinson's Disease**
PO
Adults, Elderly. Initially, 0.375 mg/day in 3 divided doses. Do not increase dosage more frequently than every 5–7 days. Maintenance: 1.5–4.5 mg/day in 3 equally divided doses.
▶ **Dosage in Renal Impairment**
Dosage and frequency are modified on the basis of creatinine clearance.

Pramipexole 999

Creatinine Clearance	Initial Dose	Maximum Dose
Greater than 60 ml/min	0.125 mg 3 times a day	1.5 mg 3 times a day
35–59 ml/min	0.125 mg twice a day	1.5 mg twice a day
15–34 ml/min	0.125 mg once a day	1.5 mg once a day

SIDE EFFECTS/ADVERSE REACTIONS

Frequent
Early Parkinson's disease: Nausea, asthenia, dizziness, somnolence, insomnia, constipation
Advanced Parkinson's disease: Orthostatic hypotension, extrapyramidal reactions, insomnia, dizziness, hallucinations
Occasional
Early Parkinson's disease: Edema, malaise, confusion, amnesia, akathisia, anorexia, dysphagia, peripheral edema, vision changes, impotence
Advanced Parkinson's disease: Asthenia, somnolence, confusion, constipation, abnormal gait, dry mouth
Rare
Advanced Parkinson's disease: General edema, malaise, chest pain, amnesia, tremor, urinary frequency or incontinence, dyspnea, rhinitis, vision changes

PRECAUTIONS AND CONTRAINDICATIONS

History of hypersensitivity to pramipexole
Caution
Orthostatic hypotension, hallucination risk higher than 65 yr, renal insufficiency, caution in driving a car (somnolence), risk of falling asleep while performing daily activities, lactation, use not established in children

DRUG INTERACTIONS OF CONCERN TO DENTISTRY

• Increased CNS depression: all CNS depressants
• Possible decreased effects: dopamine antagonists (phenothiazines, butyrophenones, or thioxanthenes) and metoclopramide

SERIOUS REACTIONS

None known

DENTAL CONSIDERATIONS

General:
• Monitor vital signs at every appointment because of cardiovascular side effects.
• Assess salivary flow as factor in caries, periodontal disease, and candidiasis.
• Consider semisupine chair position for patient comfort if GI side effects occur.
• After supine positioning, have patient sit upright for at least 2 min before standing to avoid orthostatic hypotension.
Consultations:
• Medical consultation may be required to assess disease control and patient's ability to tolerate stress.
Teach Patient/Family to:
• Use effective oral hygiene to prevent soft tissue inflammation
• Use caution to prevent trauma when using oral hygiene aids
• Use electric tooth brush if patient has difficulty holding conventional devices
• Update health and drug history if physician makes any changes in evaluation or drug regimens;

include OTC, herbal, and nonherbal drugs in the update
• When chronic dry mouth occurs, advise patient to:
  • Avoid mouth rinses with high alcohol content because of drying effects
  • Use daily home fluoride products for anticaries effect
  • Use sugarless gum, frequent sips of water, or saliva substitutes

pravastatin
prav-ih-sta´-tin
(Pravachol)
Do not confuse pravastatin with Prevacid, or Pravachol with propranolol.

CATEGORY AND SCHEDULE
Pregnancy Risk Category: X

Drug Class: Antihyperlipidemic

MECHANISM OF ACTION
An HMG-CoA reductase inhibitor that interferes with cholesterol biosynthesis by preventing the conversion of HMG-CoA reductase to mevalonate, a precursor to cholesterol. **Therapeutic Effect:** Lowers serum low-density lipoproteins (LDL) and very low-density lipoproteins (VLDL), cholesterol, and plasma triglyceride levels; increases serum high-density lipoprotein (HDL) concentration.

USES
As an adjunct in homozygous or heterozygous familial hypercholesterolemia, mixed hyperlipidemia, elevated serum triglyceride levels, and type IV hyperproteinemia; also reduces total cholesterol LDL-C, apo B, and triglyceride levels; patient should first be placed on cholesterol-lowering diet; primary prevention of coronary events, secondary prevention of cardiovascular events

PHARMACOKINETICS
Poorly absorbed from the GI tract. Protein binding: 50%. Metabolized in the liver (minimal active metabolites). Primarily excreted in feces via the biliary system. Not removed by hemodialysis.
Half-life: 2.7 hr.

INDICATIONS AND DOSAGES
▶ **Hyperlipidemia, Primary and Secondary Prevention of Cardiovascular Events in Patient with Elevated Cholesterol Levels**
PO
Adults, Elderly. Initially, 40 mg/day. Titrate to desired response. Range: 10–80 mg/day.
Children 14–18 yr. 40 mg/day.
Children 8–13 yr. 20 mg/day.
▶ **Dosage in Hepatic and Renal Impairment**
For adults, give 10 mg/day initially. Titrate to desired response.

SIDE EFFECTS/ADVERSE REACTIONS
Pravastatin is generally well tolerated. Side effects are usually mild and transient.
Occasional
Nausea, vomiting, diarrhea, constipation, abdominal pain, headache, rhinitis, rash, pruritus
Rare
Heartburn, myalgia, dizziness, cough, fatigue, flu-like symptoms

PRECAUTIONS AND CONTRAINDICATIONS
Active hepatic disease or unexplained, persistent elevations of liver function test results

Caution
Past liver disease, alcoholics, severe acute infections, trauma, hypotension, uncontrolled seizure disorders, severe metabolic disorders, electrolyte imbalances

DRUG INTERACTIONS OF CONCERN TO DENTISTRY

• Increased risk of myopathy or rhabdomyolysis: erythromycin, itraconazole

SERIOUS REACTIONS

! Malignancy and cataracts may occur.
! Hypersensitivity occurs rarely.

DENTAL CONSIDERATIONS

General:
• Monitor vital signs at every appointment because of possible cardiovascular disease.
• Consider semisupine chair position for patient comfort if GI side effects occur.

prazosin hydrochloride

pra´-zoe-sin high-droh-klor´-ide
(Minipress, Prasig[AUS], Pratisol[AUS], Pressin[AUS])

CATEGORY AND SCHEDULE

Pregnancy Risk Category: C

Drug Class: Antihypertensive, α-adrenergic antagonist

MECHANISM OF ACTION

An antidote, antihypertensive, and vasodilator that selectively blocks α_1-adrenergic receptors, decreasing peripheral vascular resistance.
Therapeutic Effect: Produces vasodilation of veins and arterioles, decreases total peripheral resistance, and relaxes smooth muscle in bladder neck and prostate.

USES

Treatment of hypertension; unapproved: CHF, urinary retention in prostatic hypertrophy, pheochromocytoma

PHARMACOKINETICS

PO: Onset 2 hr, peak 1–3 hr, duration 6–12 hr. **Half-life:** 2–4 hr; metabolized in liver; excreted via bile, feces (greater than 90%), in urine (less than 10%).

INDICATIONS AND DOSAGES

▶ **Mild-to-Moderate Hypertension**
PO
Adults, Elderly. Initially, 1 mg 2–3 times a day. Maintenance: 3–15 mg/day in divided doses. Maximum: 20 mg/day.
Children. 5 mcg/kg/dose q6h. Gradually increase up to 25 mcg/kg/dose.

SIDE EFFECTS/ADVERSE REACTIONS

Frequent
Dizziness, somnolence, headache, asthenia (loss of strength, energy)
Occasional
Palpitations, nausea, dry mouth, nervousness
Rare
Angina, urinary urgency

PRECAUTIONS AND CONTRAINDICATIONS

Hypersensitivity, severe CHF
Caution
Children

DRUG INTERACTIONS OF CONCERN TO DENTISTRY

• Increased effects: epinephrine
• Decreased effect: indomethacin, NSAIDs

SERIOUS REACTIONS

! First-dose syncope (hypotension with sudden loss of consciousness) may occur 30–90 min following initial dose of more than 2 mg, a too-rapid increase in dosage, or addition of another antihypertensive agent to therapy. First-dose syncope may be preceded by tachycardia (pulse rate of 120–160 beats/min).

DENTAL CONSIDERATIONS

General:
• Monitor vital signs at every appointment because of cardiovascular side effects.
• After supine positioning, have patient sit upright for at least 2 min before standing to avoid orthostatic hypotension.
• Assess salivary flow as a factor in caries, periodontal disease, and candidiasis.
• Limit use of sodium-containing products, such as saline IV fluids, for patients with a dietary salt restriction.
• Stress from dental procedures may compromise cardiovascular function; determine patient risk.
• Short appointments and a stress-reduction protocol may be required for anxious patients to.

Consultations:
• Medical consultation may be required to assess disease control.

Teach Patient/Family:
• When chronic dry mouth occurs, advise patient to:
    • Avoid mouth rinses with high alcohol content because of drying effects
    • Use daily home fluoride products to prevent caries
    • Use sugarless gum, frequent sips of water, or saliva substitutes

prednisolone
pred-niss´-oh-lone
(AK-Pred, AK-Tate[CAN], Inflamase Forte, Inflamase Mild, Minims-Prednisolone[CAN], Novo-Prednisolone[CAN], Orapred, Pediapred, Pred Forte, Pred Mild, Prelone, Solone[AUS])
Do not confuse prednisolone with prednisone or primidone.

CATEGORY AND SCHEDULE
Pregnancy Risk Category: C
(D if used in first trimester)

Drug Class: Glucocorticoid, immediate acting

MECHANISM OF ACTION
An adrenocortical steroid that inhibits accumulation of inflammatory cells at inflammation sites, phagocytosis, lysosomal enzyme release and synthesis, and release of mediators of inflammation. *Therapeutic Effect:* Prevents or suppresses cell-mediated immune reactions. Decreases or prevents tissue response to inflammatory process.

USES
Treatment of severe inflammation, immunosuppression, neoplasms, adrenal insufficiency, acute exacerbation of multiple sclerosis

PHARMACOKINETICS
PO: Peak 1–2 hr, duration 2 days.
IM: Peak 3–45 hr.

INDICATIONS AND DOSAGES
▸ **Substitution Therapy for Deficiency States: Acute or Chronic Adrenal Insufficiency, Congenital Adrenal Hyperplasia, and Adrenal Insufficiency Secondary to Pituitary**

Insufficiency; Nonendocrine Disorders: Arthritis; Rheumatic Carditis; Allergic, Collagen, Intestinal Tract, Liver, Ocular, Renal, Skin Diseases; Bronchial Asthma; Cerebral Edema; Malignancies
PO
Adults, Elderly. 5–60 mg/day in divided doses.
Children. 0.1–2 mg/kg/day in 1–4 divided doses.
▶ **Treatment of Conjuctivitis and Corneal Injury**
Ophthalmic
Adults, Elderly. 1–2 drops every hr during day and q2h during night. After response, decrease dosage to 1 drop q4h, then 1 drop 3–4 times a day.

SIDE EFFECTS/ADVERSE REACTIONS
Frequent
Insomnia, heartburn, nervousness, abdominal distention, increased sweating, acne, mood swings, increased appetite, facial flushing, delayed wound healing, increased susceptibility to infection, diarrhea or constipation
Occasional
Headache, edema, change in skin color, frequent urination
Rare
Tachycardia, allergic reaction (such as rash and hives), psychological changes, hallucinations, depression
Ophthalmic: stinging or burning, posterior subcapsular cataracts

PRECAUTIONS AND CONTRAINDICATIONS
Acute superficial herpes simplex keratitis, systemic fungal infections, varicella
Caution
Diabetes mellitus, glaucoma, osteoporosis, seizure disorders, ulcerative colitis, CHF, myasthenia gravis, ulcerative GI disease, rifampin

DRUG INTERACTIONS OF CONCERN TO DENTISTRY
• Decreased action: barbiturates, rifampin, rifabutin
• Increased side effects: alcohol, salicylates, NSAIDs
• Increased action: ketoconazole, macrolide antibiotics (erythromycin, clarithromycin, azithromycin)
• Hepatotoxicity: acetaminophen (chronic use, high doses)

SERIOUS REACTIONS
! Long-term therapy may cause hypocalcemia, hypokalemia, muscle wasting (especially in the arms and legs), osteoporosis, spontaneous fractures, amenorrhea, cataracts, glaucoma, peptic ulcer disease, and CHF.
! Abruptly withdrawing the drug after long-term therapy may cause anorexia, nausea, fever, headache, severe or sudden joint pain, rebound inflammation, fatigue, weakness, lethargy, dizziness, and orthostatic hypotension.
! Suddenly discontinuing prednisolone may be fatal.

DENTAL CONSIDERATIONS
General:
• Monitor vital signs at every appointment because of cardiovascular side effects.
• Patients on chronic drug therapy may rarely have symptoms of blood dyscrasias, which can include infection, bleeding, and poor healing.
• Assess salivary flow as a factor in caries, periodontal disease, and candidiasis.
• Avoid prescribing aspirin-containing products.

- Place on frequent recall to evaluate healing response.
- Prophylactic antibiotics may be indicated to prevent infection if surgery or deep scaling is planned.
- Symptoms of oral infections may be masked.
- Determine dose and duration of steroid therapy for each patient to assess risk for stress tolerance and immunosuppression.
- Patients who have been or are currently on chronic steroid therapy longer than 2 wk may require supplemental steroids for stressful dental treatment.
- Determine why the patient is taking the drug.

Consultations:
- In a patient with symptoms of blood dyscrasias, request a medical consultation for blood studies and postpone dental treatment until normal values are reestablished.
- Medical consultation may be required to assess disease control.
- Consultation may be required to confirm steroid dose and duration of use.

Teach Patient/Family to:
- Use effective oral hygiene to prevent soft tissue inflammation
- Use caution to prevent injury when using oral hygiene aids
- When chronic dry mouth occurs, advise patient to:
  - Avoid mouth rinses with high alcohol content because of drying effects
  - Use daily home fluoride products to prevent caries
  - Use sugarless gum, frequent sips of water, or saliva substitutes

prednisolone acetate

pred-niss´-oh-lone as´-ih-tate
(AK-Pred, Econopred Plus, Inflamase Forte, Inflamase Mild, Ocu-Pred, Ocu-Pred-A, Ocu-Pred Forte, Pred Forte, Pred Mild, Prednisol)

CATEGORY AND SCHEDULE
Pregnancy Risk Category: C

Drug Class: Glucocorticoid, immediate acting

MECHANISM OF ACTION
An adrenal corticosteroid that inhibits accumulation of inflammatory cells at inflammation sites, phagocytosis, lysosomal enzyme release and synthesis, and release of mediators of inflammation. *Therapeutic Effect:* Prevents or suppresses cell-mediated immune reactions. Decreases or prevents tissue response to inflammatory process.

USES
Treatment of severe inflammation, immunosuppression, neoplasms, adrenal insufficiency, acute exacerbation of multiple sclerosis

PHARMACOKINETICS
Absorbed into aqueous humor, cornea, iris, choroids, ciliary body, and retina. Systemic absorption may occur, but significant only at high dosages.

INDICATIONS AND DOSAGES
▶ **Conjunctivitis**
Ophthalmic
Adults, Elderly, Children. 1–2 drops 2–4 times a day.

SIDE EFFECTS/ADVERSE REACTIONS

Occasional

Stinging or burning

PRECAUTIONS AND CONTRAINDICATIONS

Fungal, mycobacterial, or viral infections of the eye, hypersensitivity to prednisolone acetate or any component of the formulation

Caution

Diabetes mellitus, glaucoma, osteoporosis, seizure disorders, ulcerative colitis, CHF, myasthenia gravis, ulcerative GI disease, rifampin

DRUG INTERACTIONS OF CONCERN TO DENTISTRY

• Decreased action: barbiturates, rifampin, rifabutin
• Increased side effects: alcohol, salicylates, NSAIDs
• Increased action: ketoconazole, macrolide antibiotics (erythromycin, clarithromycin, azithromycin)
• Hepatotoxicity: acetaminophen (chronic use, high doses)

SERIOUS REACTIONS

❗ Prolonged use of corticosteroids may result in glaucoma with damage to the optic nerve, defects in visual acuity and fields of vision, posterior subcapsular cataract formation, and delayed wound healing.
❗ Long-term use may cause corneal and scleral thinning.
❗ Systemic effects are uncommon, but systemic hypercorticoidism have been reported.
❗ Acute anterior uveitis and perforation of the globe, keratitis, conjunctivitis, corneal ulcers, mydriasis, conjunctival hyperemia, loss of accommodation, and ptosis have occasionally been reported.

❗ The development of secondary ocular infection has occurred. Fungal and viral infections of the cornea may develop with long-term applications of steroid.

DENTAL CONSIDERATIONS

General:

• Monitor vital signs at every appointment because of cardiovascular side effects.
• Patients on chronic drug therapy may rarely have symptoms of blood dyscrasias, which can include infection, bleeding, and poor healing.
• Assess salivary flow as a factor in caries, periodontal disease, and candidiasis.
• Avoid prescribing aspirin-containing products.
• Place on frequent recall to evaluate healing response.
• Prophylactic antibiotics may be indicated to prevent infection if surgery or deep scaling is planned.
• Symptoms of oral infections may be masked.
• Determine dose and duration of steroid therapy for each patient to assess risk for stress tolerance and immunosuppression.
• Patients who have been or are currently on chronic steroid therapy longer than 2 wk may require supplemental steroids for stressful dental treatment.
• Determine why the patient is taking the drug.

Consultations:

• In a patient with symptoms of blood dyscrasias, request a medical consultation for blood studies and postpone dental treatment until normal values are reestablished.
• Medical consultation may be required to assess disease control.

- Consultation may be required to confirm steroid dose and duration of use.

Teach Patient/Family to:
- Use effective oral hygiene to prevent soft tissue inflammation
- Use caution to prevent injury when using oral hygiene aids
- When chronic dry mouth occurs, advise patient to:
  - Avoid mouth rinses with high alcohol content because of drying effects
  - Use daily home fluoride products to prevent caries
  - Use sugarless gum, frequent sips of water, or saliva substitutes

prednisolone acetate; sulfacetamide sodium

pred-niss´-oh-lone ass´-eh-tate;
sul-fa-see´-ta-mide soe´-dee-um
(AK-Cide; Blephamide;
Blephamide S.O.P.; Medasulf;
Metimyd; Ocu-Lone C; Vasocidin)

CATEGORY AND SCHEDULE
Pregnancy Risk Category: C

Drug Class: Glucocorticoid, immediate acting

MECHANISM OF ACTION
Prednisolone is an adrenal corticosteroid that inhibits accumulation of inflammatory cells at inflammation sites, phagocytosis, lysosomal enzyme release and synthesis, and release of mediators of inflammation. Sulfacetamide is a sulfonamide that interferes with synthesis of folic acid that bacteria require for growth. ***Therapeutic Effect:*** Prevents or suppresses cell-mediated immune reactions. Decreases or prevents tissue response to inflammatory process. Prevents further bacterial growth; bacteriostatic.

USES
Treatment of severe inflammation, immunosuppression, neoplasms, adrenal insufficiency, acute exacerbation of multiple sclerosis

PHARMACOKINETICS
None reported

INDICATIONS AND DOSAGES
▶ **Steroid-Responsive Inflammatory Ocular Conditions for which a Corticosteroid is Indicated and where Superficial Bacterial Ocular Infection or a Risk of Bacterial Ocular Infection Exists**
Ophthalmic ointment
Adults, Elderly, Children. Apply 3 or 4 times a day and once at bedtime.
Ophthalmic suspension
Adults, Elderly, Children. Instill 2–3 drops every 1–2 hr while awake.

SIDE EFFECTS/ADVERSE REACTIONS
Occasional
Local irritation
Rare
Elevation of intraocular pressure

PRECAUTIONS AND CONTRAINDICATIONS
Epithelial herpes simplex keratitis (dendritic keratitis), vaccinia, varicella, and other viral diseases of the cornea or conjunctiva, mycobacterial infection of the eye, and fungal diseases of ocular structure, known or suspected hypersensitivity to other sulfonamides or other corticosteroids or any component of the formulation

P

DRUG INTERACTIONS OF CONCERN TO DENTISTRY
● Decreased action: barbiturates, rifampin, rifabutin
● Increased side effects: alcohol, salicylates, NSAIDs
● Increased action: ketoconazole, macrolide antibiotics (erythromycin, clarithromycin, azithromycin)
● Hepatotoxicity: acetaminophen (chronic use, high doses)

SERIOUS REACTIONS
! Prolonged use of corticosteroids may result in glaucoma with damage to the optic nerve, defects in visual acuity and fields of vision, posterior subcapsular cataract formation, and delayed wound healing.
! Long-term use may cause corneal and scleral thinning.
! Systemic effects are uncommon, but systemic hypercorticoidism has been reported.
! Acute anterior uveitis and perforation of the globe, keratitis, conjunctivitis, corneal ulcers, mydriasis, conjunctival hyperemia, loss of accommodation, and ptosis have occasionally been reported.
! The development of secondary ocular infection has occurred. Fungal and viral infections of the cornea may develop with long-term applications of steroid.
! Fatalities due to reactions to sulfonamides including Stevens-Johnson syndrome, toxic epidermal necrolysis, fulminant hepatic necrosis, agranulocytosis, aplastic anemia, and other blood dyscrasias have occurred.

DENTAL CONSIDERATIONS
General:
● Monitor vital signs at every appointment because of cardiovascular side effects.
● Patients on chronic drug therapy may rarely have symptoms of blood dyscrasias, which can include infection, bleeding, and poor healing.
● Assess salivary flow as a factor in caries, periodontal disease, and candidiasis.
● Avoid prescribing aspirin-containing products.
● Place on frequent recall to evaluate healing response.
● Prophylactic antibiotics may be indicated to prevent infection if surgery or deep scaling is planned.
● Symptoms of oral infections may be masked.
● Determine dose and duration of steroid therapy for each patient to assess risk for stress tolerance and immunosuppression.
● Patients who have been or are currently on chronic steroid therapy longer than 2 wk may require supplemental steroids for stressful dental treatment.
● Determine why the patient is taking the drug.
Consultations:
● In a patient with symptoms of blood dyscrasias, request a medical consultation for blood studies and postpone dental treatment until normal values are reestablished.
● Medical consultation may be required to assess disease control.
● Consultation may be required to confirm steroid dose and duration of use.
Teach Patient/Family to:
● Use effective oral hygiene to prevent soft tissue inflammation
● Use caution to prevent injury when using oral hygiene aids
● When chronic dry mouth occurs, advise patient to:
   ● Avoid mouth rinses with high alcohol content because of drying effects

- Use daily home fluoride products to prevent caries
- Use sugarless gum, frequent sips of water, or saliva substitutes

prednisolone sodium phosphate

pred-nis´-oh-lone soe´-dee-um foss´-fate
(AK-Pred, Inflamase Forte, Inflamase Mild, Orapred, Pediapred)

CATEGORY AND SCHEDULE

Pregnancy Risk Category: C

Drug Class: Glucocorticoid, antiinflammatory

MECHANISM OF ACTION

An adrenal corticosteroid that inhibits accumulation of inflammatory cells at inflammation sites, phagocytosis, lysosomal enzyme release and synthesis, and release of mediators of inflammation. ***Therapeutic Effect:*** Prevents or suppresses cell-mediated immune reactions. Decreases or prevents tissue response to inflammatory process.

USES

Primary or secondary adrenocortical insufficiency; adjunctive therapy of rheumatoid arthritis; collagen diseases; skin inflammatory disorders; allergy; respiratory diseases; hematologic disorders; neoplastic diseases; multiple sclerosis

PHARMACOKINETICS

Rapidly and well absorbed from the GI tract following oral administration. Protein binding: 90%–95%. Widely distributed. Metabolized in the liver. Excreted in the urine as sulfate and glucuronide conjugates.
Half-life: 2–4 hr.
Absorbed into aqueous humor, cornea, iris, choroid, ciliary body, and retina following ocular administration. Systemic absorption occurs, but may be significant only at higher dosages or in extended pediatric therapy.

INDICATIONS AND DOSAGES
▸ **Asthma**
PO
Children. 1–2 mg/kg/day in single or divided doses for 3–10 days.
▸ **Endocrine Disorders, Hematologic and Neoplastic Disorders, Inflammatory Conditions**
PO
Adults, Elderly. 5–60 mg/day.
Children. 0.14–2 mg/kg/day divided into 3 or 4 doses.
▸ **Multiple Sclerosis Exacerbations**
PO
Adults, Elderly. 200 mg/day for 1 wk, followed by 80 mg every other day for 1 mo.
▸ **Nephrotic Syndrome**
PO
Children. 60 mg/m² daily.
Maximum: 80 mg/day divided 3 times a day for 4 wk, then 40 mg/m² every other day for 4 wk.
▸ **Ophthalmic Disorders**
Ophthalmic suspension
Adults, Elderly, Children. Instill 1 or 2 drops up to 6 times a day.

SIDE EFFECTS
Frequent
Insomnia, heartburn, nervousness, abdominal distention, increased sweating, acne, mood swings, increased appetite, facial flushing, delayed wound healing, increased

P

susceptibility to infection, diarrhea or constipation

Occasional

Headache, edema, change in skin color, frequent urination

Rare

Tachycardia, allergic reaction, such as rash and hives, psychic changes, hallucinations, depression

Ophthalmic: stinging or burning, posterior subcapsular cataracts

PRECAUTIONS AND CONTRAINDICATIONS

Systemic fungal infections, live or live attenuated vaccines, hypersensitivity to prednisolone sodium phosphate or any component of the formulation

DRUG INTERACTIONS OF CONCERN TO DENTISTRY

- Decreased action: barbiturates, rifampin, rifabutin
- Increased side effects: alcohol, salicylates, NSAIDs
- Increased action: ketoconazole, macrolide antibiotics (erythromycin, clarithromycin, azithromycin)
- Hepatotoxicity: acetaminophen (chronic use, high doses)

SERIOUS REACTIONS

! Prolonged use of corticosteroids may result in glaucoma with damage to the optic nerve, defects in visual acuity and fields of vision, posterior subcapsular cataract formation, and delayed wound healing.

! Long-term use may cause corneal and scleral thinning.

! Systemic effects are uncommon, but systemic hypercorticoidism has been reported.

! Acute anterior uveitis and perforation of the globe, keratitis, conjunctivitis, corneal ulcers, mydriasis, conjunctival hyperemia, loss of accommodation and ptosis have occasionally been reported.

! The development of secondary ocular infection has occurred. Fungal and viral infections of the cornea may develop with long-term applications of steroid.

DENTAL CONSIDERATIONS

General:

- Monitor vital signs at every appointment because of cardiovascular side effects.
- Patients on chronic drug therapy may rarely have symptoms of blood dyscrasias, which can include infection, bleeding, and poor healing.
- Assess salivary flow as a factor in caries, periodontal disease, and candidiasis.
- Avoid prescribing aspirin-containing products.
- Place on frequent recall to evaluate healing response.
- Prophylactic antibiotics may be indicated to prevent infection if surgery or deep scaling is planned.
- Symptoms of oral infections may be masked.
- Determine dose and duration of steroid therapy for each patient to assess risk for stress tolerance and immunosuppression.
- Patients who have been or are currently on chronic steroid therapy longer than 2 wk may require supplemental steroids for stressful dental treatment.
- Determine why the patient is taking the drug.

Consultations:

- In a patient with symptoms of blood dyscrasias, request a medical consultation for blood studies and postpone dental treatment until normal values are reestablished.
- Medical consultation may be required to assess disease control.

- Consultation may be required to confirm steroid dose and duration of use.

Teach Patient/Family to:
- Use effective oral hygiene to prevent soft tissue inflammation
- Use caution to prevent injury when using oral hygiene aids
- When chronic dry mouth occurs, advise patient to:
  - Avoid mouth rinses with high alcohol content because of drying effects
  - Use daily home fluoride products to prevent caries
  - Use sugarless gum, frequent sips of water, or saliva substitutes

prednisone
pred´-ni-sone
(Apo-Prednisone[CAN], Deltasone, Panafcort[AUS], Prednisone Intensol, Sone[AUS], Sterapred, Sterapred DS, Winpred[CAN])
Do not confuse prednisone with prednisolone or primidone.

CATEGORY AND SCHEDULE
Pregnancy Risk Category: C (D if used in first trimester)

Drug Class: Glucocorticoid, intermediate-acting

MECHANISM OF ACTION
An adrenocortical steroid that inhibits accumulation of inflammatory cells at inflammation sites, phagocytosis, lysosomal enzyme release and synthesis, and release of mediators of inflammation.
Therapeutic Effect: Prevents or suppresses cell-mediated immune reactions. Decreases or prevents tissue response to inflammatory process.

USES
Treatment of severe inflammation, immunosuppression, neoplasms, multiple sclerosis, collagen disorders, dermatologic disorders, acute exacerbation of multiple sclerosis

PHARMACOKINETICS
Well absorbed from the GI tract. Protein binding: 70%–90%. Widely distributed. Metabolized in the liver and converted to prednisolone. Primarily excreted in urine. Not removed by hemodialysis.
Half-life: 3.4–3.8 hr.

INDICATIONS AND DOSAGES
▶ **Substitution Therapy in Deficiency States: Acute or Chronic Adrenal Insufficiency, Congenital Adrenal Hyperplasia, and Adrenal Insufficiency Secondary to Pituitary Insufficiency; Nonendocrine Disorders: Arthritis; Rheumatic Carditis; Allergic, Collagen, Intestinal Tract, Liver, Ocular, Renal, Skin Diseases; Bronchial Asthma; Cerebral Edema; Malignancies**
PO
Adults, Elderly. 5–60 mg/day in divided doses.
Children. 0.05–2 mg/kg/day in 1–4 divided doses.

SIDE EFFECTS/ADVERSE REACTIONS
Frequent
Insomnia, heartburn, nervousness, abdominal distention, increased sweating, acne, mood swings, increased appetite, facial flushing, delayed wound healing, increased susceptibility to infection, diarrhea or constipation
Occasional
Headache, edema, change in skin color, frequent urination

P

Rare

Tachycardia, allergic reaction (including rash and hives), psychological changes, hallucinations, depression

PRECAUTIONS AND CONTRAINDICATIONS

Acute superficial herpes simplex keratitis, systemic fungal infections, varicella

Caution

Diabetes mellitus, glaucoma, osteoporosis, seizure disorders, ulcerative colitis, CHF, myasthenia gravis, renal disease, esophagitis, peptic ulcer, rifampin

DRUG INTERACTIONS OF CONCERN TO DENTISTRY

• Decreased action: barbiturates, rifampin, rifabutin
• Increased side effects: alcohol, salicylates, NSAIDs
• Increased action: ketoconazole, macrolide antibiotics
• Hepatotoxicity: acetaminophen (chronic, high doses)

SERIOUS REACTIONS

❗ Long-term therapy may cause muscle wasting in the arms and legs, osteoporosis, spontaneous fractures, amenorrhea, cataracts, glaucoma, peptic ulcer disease, and CHF.
❗ Abruptly withdrawing the drug following long-term therapy may cause anorexia, nausea, fever, headache, sudden or severe joint pain, rebound inflammation, fatigue, weakness, lethargy, dizziness, and orthostatic hypotension.
❗ Suddenly discontinuing prednisone may be fatal.

DENTAL CONSIDERATIONS

General:

• Monitor vital signs at every appointment because of cardiovascular side effects.
• Patients on chronic drug therapy may rarely have symptoms of blood dyscrasias, which can include infection, bleeding, and poor healing.
• Avoid aspirin-containing products.
• Assess salivary flow as a factor in caries, periodontal disease, and candidiasis.
• Symptoms of oral infections may be masked.
• Place on frequent recall to evaluate healing response.
• Prophylactic antibiotics may be indicated to prevent infection if surgery or deep scaling is planned.
• Determine dose and duration of steroid therapy for each patient to assess risk for stress tolerance and immunosuppression.
• Patients who have been or are currently on chronic steroid therapy longer than 2 wk may require supplemental steroids for stressful dental treatment.
• Determine why the patient is taking the drug.

Consultations:

• In a patient with symptoms of blood dyscrasias, request a medical consultation for blood studies and postpone dental treatment until normal values are reestablished.
• Medical consultation may be required to assess disease control.
• Consultation may be required to confirm steroid dose and duration of use.

Teach Patient/Family to:

• Use effective oral hygiene to prevent soft tissue inflammation
• Use caution to prevent injury when using oral hygiene aids

- When chronic dry mouth occurs, advise patient to:
  - Avoid mouth rinses with high alcohol content because of drying effects
  - Use daily home fluoride products to prevent caries
  - Use sugarless gum, frequent sips of water, or saliva substitutes

prilocaine hydrochloride (local)
pry´lo-kane high-droh-klor´-ide
(Citanest)
With vasoconstrictor:
(Citanest Forte with epinephrine)

CATEGORY AND SCHEDULE
Pregnancy Risk Category: B

Drug Class: Amide local anesthetic

MECHANISM OF ACTION
Inhibits ion fluxes across membranes; decreases rise of depolarization phase of action potential; blocks nerve action potential.

USES
Local dental anesthesia

PHARMACOKINETICS
Injection: Onset 2–10 min, duration 2–4 hr; metabolized in liver; excreted in urine

INDICATIONS AND DOSAGES
▶ **Dental Injection: Infiltration or Conduction Block**
Prilocaine 4% without vasoconstrictor: Maximum dose of 400 mg over a 2-hr period per dental appointment for healthy adult patient*; doses must be adjusted for

medically compromised, debilitated, or elderly and for each individual patient. Doses in excess of 400 mg have caused methemoglobinemia. Always use the lowest effective dose, a slow injection rate, and a careful aspiration technique. In considering the dose of local anesthesia with vasoconstrictor, the dose of epinephrine must also be considered. The recommended dose of epinephrine in a local anesthetic solution is 3 μg/kg, not to exceed a total dose of 0.2 mg per appointment for a healthy adult. For adult patients with clinically significant cardiovascular disease, the dose limit of epinephrine is 0.04 mg per appointment. The dose limits of epinephrine will affect the amount of local anesthetic allowable in a given appointment.

▶ **Example Calculations Illustrating Amount of Drug Administered per Dental Cartridge(s):**

# of Dental Cartridges (1.8 ml)	mg of Prilocaine (4%)
1	72
2	144
3	216
4	288

Prilocaine 4% with epinephrine 1:200,000: Recommended doses are the same; adjust doses for each individual as previously indicated.

P

*Maximum dose cited from Malamed SF: Handbook of local anesthesia, ed 5, 2004, Mosby, as well as manufacturer's package insert. Doses may differ in other published reference resources.

▶ **Example Calculations Illustrating Amount of Drug Administered per Dental Cartridge(s):**

# of Dental Cartridges (1.8 ml)	mg of Prilocaine (4%)	mg (μcg) Vasoconstrictor (1:200,000)
1	72	0.009 (9)
2	144	0.018 (18)
4	288	0.036 (36)

Available forms include: 4% solution, 4% solution with epinephrine 1:200,000.

SIDE EFFECTS/ADVERSE REACTIONS
Occasional
Numbness, tingling, trismus, convulsions, loss of consciousness, drowsiness, disorientation, tremors, shivering, anxiety, restlessness, myocardial depression, cardiac arrest, dysrhythmias, bradycardia, hypotension, hypertension, nausea, vomiting, methemoglobinemia, rash, urticaria, allergic reactions
Rare
Status asthmaticus, respitory arrest, anaphylaxis

PRECAUTIONS AND CONTRAINDICATIONS
Hypersensitivity, cross-sensitivity among amides (rare), severe liver disease
Caution
Elderly, large doses of local anesthetic in myasthenia gravis, risk of methemoglobinemia

DRUG INTERACTIONS OF CONCERN TO DENTISTRY:
• CNS depressants: increased risk of CNS depression with all CNS depressants, especially in children and when larger doses are used

• Avoid placing dental cartridges in disinfection solutions with heavy metals or surface-active agents; may see release of ions into local anesthetic solutions with tissue irritation following injection
• Avoid excessive exposure of dental cartridges to light or heat; hastens deterioration of vasoconstrictor; observe for color change in local anesthetic solution
• Risk of cardiovascular side effects; rapid intravascular administration of local anesthetic containing vasoconstrictor, either alone or in patients taking tricyclic antidepressants, MAOIs, digitalis drugs, cocaine, phenothiazines, β-blockers, and in the presence of halogenated-hydrocarbon general anesthetics; use smallest effective vasoconstrictor dose and careful aspiration technique
• Avoid use of vasoconstrictors in patients with uncontrolled hyperthyroidism, diabetes, angina, or hypertension; refer these patients for medical treatment before elective dental treatment

SERIOUS REACTIONS
• Methemoglobinemia (at higher doses).

DENTAL CONSIDERATIONS
General:
• Monitor vital signs at every appointment because of cardiovascular side effects.
• Often used with vasoconstrictor for increased duration of action.
• Lubricate dry lips before injection or dental treatment as required.
Teach Patient/Family to:
• Use care to prevent injury while numbness exists and to refrain from

chewing gum and eating following dental anesthesia
• Report any signs of infection, muscle pain, or fever to dentist when feeling returns
• Report any unusual soft tissue reactions

primaquine
prim´-ah-kween
(Primacin[AUS])
Do not confuse with primidone.

CATEGORY AND SCHEDULE
Pregnancy Risk Category: C

Drug Class: Antiprotozoal

MECHANISM OF ACTION
An antimalarial and antirheumatic that eliminates tissue exoerythrocytic forms of *Plasmodium falciparum.* Disrupts mitochondria and binds to DNA. *Therapeutic Effect:* Inhibits parasite growth.

USES
Treatment of malaria caused by *P. vivax;* unapproved: with clindamycin in the treatment of *P. carinii* in AIDS

PHARMACOKINETICS
Well absorbed. Metabolized in the liver to the active metabolite, carboxyprimaquine. Excreted in the urine in small amounts as unchanged drug. *Half-life:* 4–6 hr

INDICATIONS AND DOSAGES
▶ **Treatment of Malaria**
PO
Adults, Elderly. 15-mg base daily for 14 days.
Children. 0.3-mg base/kg/wk once daily for 14 days.

▶ **Malaria Prophylaxis**
PO
Adults, Elderly. 30 mg base daily. Begin 1 day before departure and continue for 7 days after leaving malarious area.

SIDE EFFECTS/ADVERSE REACTIONS
Frequent
Abdominal pain, nausea, vomiting
Rare
Leukopenia, hemolytic anemia, methemoglobinemia

PRECAUTIONS AND CONTRAINDICATIONS
Concomitant medications that cause bone marrow suppression, rheumatoid arthritis, lupus erythematosus, glucose-6-phosphate dehydrogenase deficiency, pregnancy, hypersensitivity to primaquine or any of its components

DRUG INTERACTIONS OF CONCERN TO DENTISTRY
None reported

SERIOUS REACTIONS
! Leukopenia, hemolytic anemia, methemoglobinemia occur rarely.
! Overdosage include symptoms of abdominal cramps, vomiting, burning epigastric distress, central nervous system and cardiovascular disturbances, cyanosis, methemoglobinemia, moderate leukocytosis or leukopenia, and anemia.
! Acute hemolysis occurs, but patients recover completely if the dosage is discontinued.

DENTAL CONSIDERATIONS
General:
• Patients on chronic drug therapy may rarely have symptoms of blood

P

dyscrasias, which can include infection, bleeding, and poor healing.
• Avoid dental light in patient's eyes; offer dark glasses for patient comfort.

Consultations:
• In a patient with symptoms of blood dyscrasias, request a medical consultation for blood studies and postpone dental treatment until normal values are reestablished.

Teach Patient/Family to:
• Use effective oral hygiene to prevent soft tissue inflammation
• Use caution to prevent injury when using oral hygiene aids

primidone
prih´-mih-done
(Apo-Primidone[CAN], Mysoline)
Do not confuse primidone with prednisone.

CATEGORY AND SCHEDULE
Pregnancy Risk Category: D
Controlled Substance: Schedule IV

Drug Class: Anticonvulsant, barbiturate derivative

MECHANISM OF ACTION
A barbiturate that decreases motor activity from electrical and chemical stimulation and stabilizes the seizure threshold against hyperexcitability.
Therapeutic Effect: Reduces seizure activity.

USES
Treatment of generalized tonic-clonic (grand mal), complex-partial psychomotor seizures.

PHARMACOKINETICS
PO: Peak 4 hr. ***Half-life:*** 3–24 hr; excreted by kidneys, in breast milk.

INDICATIONS AND DOSAGES
▶ **Seizure Control**
PO
Adults, Elderly, Children 8 yr and older. 125–150 mg/day at bedtime. May increase by 125–250 mg/day every 3–7 days. Maximum: 2 g/day.
Children younger than 8 yr. Initially, 50–125 mg/day at bedtime. May increase by 50–125 mg/day every 3–7 days. Usual dose: 10–25 mg/kg/day in divided doses.
Neonates. 12–20 mg/kg/day in divided doses.

SIDE EFFECTS/ADVERSE REACTIONS
Frequent
Ataxia, dizziness
Occasional
Anorexia, drowsiness, mental changes, nausea, vomiting, paradoxical excitement
Rare
Rash

PRECAUTIONS AND CONTRAINDICATIONS
History of bronchopneumonia, porphyria
Caution
COPD, hepatic disease, renal disease, abrupt withdrawal, lactation, hyperactive children

DRUG INTERACTIONS OF CONCERN TO DENTISTRY
• Increased CNS depression: alcohol, other CNS depressants
• Increased metabolism/hepatotoxicity: halothane, halogenated-hydrocarbon inhalation anesthetics
• Increased seizure threshold: haloperidol, phenothiazines

• Decreased effects of acetaminophen, corticosteroids, doxycycline, fenoprofen
• Lower blood concentrations: carbamazepine

SERIOUS REACTIONS

! Abrupt withdrawal after prolonged therapy may produce effects ranging from increased dreaming, nightmares, insomnia, tremor, diaphoresis, and vomiting to hallucinations, delirium, seizures, and status epilepticus.
! Skin eruptions may may be a sign of a hypersensitivity reaction.
! Blood dyscrasias, hepatic disease, and hypocalcemia occur rarely.
! Overdose produces cold or clammy skin, hypothermia, and severe CNS depression, followed by high fever and coma.

DENTAL CONSIDERATIONS

General:
• Ask about type of epilepsy, seizure frequency, and quality of seizure control.
• After supine positioning, have patient sit upright for at least 2 min before standing to avoid orthostatic hypotension.
• Patients on chronic drug therapy may rarely have symptoms of blood dyscrasias, which can include infection, bleeding, and poor healing.
• Short appointments and a stress reduction protocol may be required for anxious patients.
Consultations:
• Medical consultation may be required to assess disease control and patient's ability to tolerate stress.
• In a patient with symptoms of blood dyscrasias, request a medical consultation for blood studies and postpone dental treatment until normal values are reestablished.

Teach Patient/Family to:
• Use effective oral hygiene to prevent soft tissue inflammation
• Use caution to prevent injury when using oral hygiene aids
• Avoid mouth rinses with high alcohol content because of drying effects

probenecid

proe-ben´-eh-sid
(Benuryl[CAN], Pro-Cid[AUS])
Do not confuse probenecid with procainamide.

CATEGORY AND SCHEDULE
Pregnancy Risk Category: C

Drug Class: Uricosuric

MECHANISM OF ACTION

A uricosuric that competitively inhibits reabsorption of uric acid at the proximal convoluted tubule. Also, inhibits renal tubular secretion of weak organic acids, such as penicillins. **Therapeutic Effect:** Promotes uric acid excretion, reduces serum uric acid level, and increases plasma levels of penicillins and cephalosporins.

USES

Treatment of hyperuricemia in gout, gouty arthritis, adjunct to cephalosporin or penicillin treatment by reducing excretion and maintaining high blood levels

PHARMACOKINETICS

Hyperuricemia in gout, gouty arthritis, adjunct to cephalosporin or penicillin treatment by reducing excretion and maintaining high blood levels.

P

INDICATIONS AND DOSAGES
▸ **Gout**
PO
Adults, Elderly. Initially, 250 mg twice a day for 1 wk; then 500 mg twice a day. May increase by 500 mg q4wk. Maximum: 2–3 g/day. Maintenance: Dosage that maintains normal uric acid level.
▸ **As Adjunct to Penicillin or Cephalosporin Therapy to Prolong Antibiotic Plasma Levels**
PO
Adults, Elderly. 2 g/day in divided doses.
Children weighing more than 50 kg. Receive adult dosage.
Children 2–14 yr. Initially, 25 mg/kg. Maintenance: 40 mg/kg/day in 4 divided doses.
▸ **Gonorrhea**
PO
Adults, Elderly. 1 g 30 min before penicillin, ampicillin, or amoxicillin.

SIDE EFFECTS/ADVERSE REACTIONS
Frequent
Headache, anorexia, nausea, vomiting
Occasional
Lower back or side pain, rash, hives, itching, dizziness, flushed face, frequent urge to urinate, gingivitis

PRECAUTIONS AND CONTRAINDICATIONS
Blood dyscrasias, children younger than 2 yr, concurrent high-dose aspirin therapy, severe renal impairment, uric acid calculi.

Caution
Severe respiratory disease, lactation, cardiac edema

DRUG INTERACTIONS OF CONCERN TO DENTISTRY
● Increased toxicity: dapsone, indomethacin, other NSAIDs, acyclovir
● Increased sedation: benzodiazepines
● Decreased action: alcohol, salicylates
● Increased duration of action: penicillins, cephalosporins
● Contraindicated: ketorolac

SERIOUS REACTIONS
❗ Severe hypersensitivity reactions, including anaphylaxis, occur rarely and usually within a few hr after administration following previous use. If severe hypersensitivity reactions develop, discontinue the drug immediately and contact the physician.
❗ Pruritic maculopapular rash, possibly accompanied by malaise, fever, chills, arthralgia, nausea, vomiting, leukopenia, and aplastic anemias should be considered a toxic reaction.

DENTAL CONSIDERATIONS
General:
● Avoid prescribing aspirin-containing products.
Teach Patient/Family to:
● Use effective oral hygiene to prevent soft tissue inflammation
● Use caution to prevent injury when using oral hygiene aids
● Avoid mouth rinses with high alcohol content because of drying effects

procaine
proe´-kane
(Novocain, Mericaine)

CATEGORY AND SCHEDULE
Pregnancy Risk Category: C

Drug Class: Anesthetics, local

MECHANISM OF ACTION

Procaine causes a reversible blockade of nerve conduction by decreasing nerve membrane permeability to sodium. *Therapeutic Effect:* Local anesthesia.

USES

Treatment of pain by local infiltration, nerve block, spinal

PHARMACOKINETICS

Highly plasma protein-bound and distributed to all body tissues. Excreted in the urine (80%). *Half-life:* 40±9 sec in adults, 84±30 sec in neonates.

INDICATIONS AND DOSAGES

▸ **Spinal Anesthesia**

Intrathecal

Adults. 0.5–1 ml of a 10% solution (50–100 mg) mixed with an equal volume of diluent injected into the third or fourth lumbar interspace (perineum and lower extremeties). 2 ml of a 10% solution (200 mg) mixed with 1 ml of diluent injected into the second, third, or fourth interspace.

▸ **Infiltration Anesthesia, Dental Anesthesia, Control of Severe Pain (post-herpatic neuralgia, cancer pain, or burns)**

Topical

Adults. A single dose of 350–600 mg using a 0.25 or 0.5% solution. Use 0.9% sodium chloride for dilution.

Children. 15 mg/kg of a 0.5% solution is the maximum recommended dose.

▸ **Peripheral or Sympathetic Nerve Block (regional anesthesia)**

Topical

Adults. Up to 200 ml of a 0.5% solution (1 g), 100 ml of a 1% solution (1 g), or 50 ml of a 2% solution (1 g). The 2% solution should only be used when a small volume of anesthetic is required.

SIDE EFFECTS/ADVERSE REACTIONS

Frequent

Numbness or tingling of the face or mouth, pain at the injection site, dizziness, drowsiness, lightheadedness, nausea, vomiting, back pain, headache

Rare

Anxiety, restlessness, difficulty breathing, shortness of breath, seizures (convulsions), skin rash, itching (hives), slow, irregular heartbeat (palpitations), swelling of the face or mouth, tremors, QT prolongation, PR prolongation, atrial fibrillation, sinus bradycardia, hypotension, angina, cardiovascular collapse, fecal or urinary incontinence, loss of perineal sensation and sexual function, persistent motor, sensory, and/or autonomic (sphincter control) deficit

PRECAUTIONS AND CONTRAINDICATIONS

Hypersensitivity to ester local anesthetics, sulfites, PABA, patients on anticoagulant therapy, and in patients with coagulopathy, infection, thrombocytopenia. Should not be given intraarterial, intrathecal, or intravenous

DRUG INTERACTIONS OF CONCERN TO DENTISTRY

- Possible prolonged effects of succinylcholine
- Increased CNS depression with all CNS depressants, especially in children and when larger doses are used
- Risk of cardiovascular side effects: rapid intravascular injection

P

• Suspected interference with antimicrobial activity of sulfonamides

SERIOUS REACTIONS

! Procaine-induced CNS toxicity usually presents with symptoms of stimulation, such as anxiety, apprehension, restlessness, nervousness, disorientation, confusion, dizziness, blurred vision, tremor, nausea/vomiting, shivering, or seizures. Subsequently, depressive symptoms can occur including drowsiness, unconsciousness, and respiratory arrest.

! If higher concentrations are introduced into the bloodstream, depression of cardiac excitability and contractility may cause AV block, ventricular arrhythmias, or cardiac arrest. CNS toxicity including dizziness, tongue numbness, visual impairment and disturbances, and muscular twitching appear to occur before cardiotoxic effects.

Alert

! Procaine should be used with caution in patients that have asthma because there is the increased risk of anaphylactoid reactions including bronchospasm and status asthmaticus.

Alert

! Local anesthetics can cause varying degrees of maternal, fetal, and neonatal toxicities during labor and obstetric delivery. Fetal heart rate should be monitored, as well as the presence of symptoms indicating fetal bradycardia, fetal acidosis, and maternal hypotension. Epidural procaine may cause decreased uterine contractility or maternal expulsion efforts and alter the forces of parturition.

Alert

! Unintentional fetal intracranial injection of procaine occurring during pudenal or paracervical block has been shown to lead to neonatal depression at birth and can lead to seizures within 6 hr as a result of high serum concentrations.

DENTAL CONSIDERATIONS

General:
• Not available for use in dental local anesthetic cartridges.

---

procarbazine hydrochloride

pro-car´-bah-zeen
high-droh-klor´-ide
(Matulane, Natulan[CAN])
Do not confuse procarbazine with dacarbazine.

CATEGORY AND SCHEDULE

Pregnancy Risk Category: D

Drug Class: Antineoplastic, miscellaneous

MECHANISM OF ACTION

A methylhydrazine derivative that inhibits DNA, RNA, and protein synthesis. May also directly damage DNA. Cell cycle–phase specific for S phase of cell division. *Therapeutic Effect:* Causes cell death.

USES

Treatment of lymphoma, Hodgkin's disease, cancers resistant to other therapy

PHARMACOKINETICS

PO: Peak levels 1 hr; concentrates in liver, kidney, skin; metabolized in liver, excreted in urine

INDICATIONS AND DOSAGES
▶ **Advanced Hodgkin's Disease**
PO
Adults, Elderly. Initially, 2–4 mg/kg/day as a single dose or in divided doses for 1 wk, then 4–6 mg/kg/day. Maintenance: 1–2 mg/kg/day.
Children. 50–100 mg/m²/day for 10–14 days of a 28-day cycle. Continue until maximum response occurs, leukocyte count falls below 4000/mm³, or platelet count falls below 100,000/mm³. Maintenance: 50 mg/m²/day.

SIDE EFFECTS/ADVERSE REACTIONS
Frequent
Severe nausea, vomiting, respiratory disorders (cough, effusion), myalgia, arthralgia, drowsiness, nervousness, insomnia, nightmares, diaphoresis, hallucinations, seizures
Occasional
Hoarseness, tachycardia, nystagmus, retinal hemorrhage, photophobia, photosensitivity, urinary frequency, nocturia, hypotension, diarrhea, stomatitis, paraesthesia, unsteadiness, confusion, decreased reflexes, footdrop
Rare
Hypersensitivity reaction (dermatitis, pruritus, rash, urticaria), hyperpigmentation, alopecia

PRECAUTIONS AND CONTRAINDICATIONS
Myelosuppression, hypersensitivity, thrombocytopenia, bone marrow depression
Caution
Renal disease, hepatic disease, radiation therapy

DRUG INTERACTIONS OF CONCERN TO DENTISTRY
• Increased CNS depression: barbiturates, antihistamines, narcotics
• Disulfiram-like reaction: ethyl alcohol
• Hypertension: indirect-acting sympathomimetics
• Increased anticholinergic effect: anticholinergic drugs, antihistamines
• Increased risk of severe toxic reactions: tricyclic antidepressants, meperidine and other opioids, tyramine-containing foods and other MAOIs; may include cyclobenzaprine and carbamazepine

SERIOUS REACTIONS
❗ Procarbazine's major toxic effects are myelosuppression manifested as hematologic toxicity (mainly leukopenia, thrombocytopenia, and anemia) and hepatotoxicity manifested as jaundice and ascites.
❗ UTIs may occur secondary to leukopenia.

DENTAL CONSIDERATIONS
General:
• Patients on chronic drug therapy may rarely have symptoms of blood dyscrasias, which can include infection, bleeding, and poor healing.
• Monitor vital signs at every appointment because of cardiovascular side effects.
• Consider semisupine chair position for patient comfort if GI side effects occur.
• Assess salivary flow as a factor in caries, periodontal disease, and candidiasis.
• After supine positioning, have patient sit upright for at least 2 min before standing to avoid orthostatic hypotension.

P

- Avoid dental light in patient's eyes; offer dark glasses for patient comfort.
- Avoid aspirin-containing products because of bleeding risk.
- Avoid use of gingival retraction cord with epinephrine.
- Patients receiving chemotherapy may require palliative treatment for stomatitis.

Consultations:
- In a patient with symptoms of blood dyscrasias, request a medical consultation for blood studies and postpone dental treatment until normal values are reestablished.
- Take precautions if dental surgery is anticipated and sedation or general anesthesia is required; there is risk of hypotensive episode.

Teach Patient/Family to:
- Use effective oral hygiene to prevent soft tissue inflammation
- Use caution to prevent injury when using oral hygiene aids
- Report oral lesions, soreness, or bleeding to dentist
- When chronic dry mouth occurs, advise patient to:
  - Avoid mouth rinses with high alcohol content because of drying effects
  - Use daily home fluoride products to prevent caries
  - Use sugarless gum, frequent sips of water, or saliva substitutes

prochlorperazine
proe-klor-per´-ah-zeen
(Compazine, Stemetil[CAN], Stemzine[AUS])
Do not confuse prochlorperazine with chlorpromazine, or Compazine with Copaxone.

CATEGORY AND SCHEDULE
Pregnancy Risk Category: C

Drug Class: Antipsychotic

MECHANISM OF ACTION
A phenothiazine that acts centrally to inhibit or block dopamine receptors in the chemoreceptor trigger zone and peripherally to block the vagus nerve in the GI tract. ***Therapeutic Effect:*** Relieves nausea and vomiting and improves psychotic conditions.

PHARMACOKINETICS

Route	Onset*	Peak	Duration
Tablets, oral solution	30–40 min	N/A	3–4 hr
Capsules (extended release)	30–40 min	N/A	10–12 hr
Rectal	60 min	N/A	3–4 hr

*As an antiemetic

Variably absorbed after PO administration. Widely distributed. Metabolized in the liver and GI mucosa. Primarily excreted in urine. Unknown if removed by hemodialysis. ***Half-life:*** 23 hr.

INDICATIONS AND DOSAGES
▶ **Nausea and Vomiting**
PO
Adults, Elderly. 5–10 mg 3–4 times a day.
Children. 0.4 mg/kg/day in 3–4 divided doses.
PO (Extended-Release)
Adults, Elderly. 10 mg twice a day or 15 mg once a day.
IV
Adults, Elderly. 2.5–10 mg. May repeat q3–4h.
Children. 0.1–0.15 mg/kg/dose q8–12h. Maximum: 40 mg/day.
IM
Adults, Elderly. 5–10 mg q3–4h.
Children. 0.1–0.15 mg/kg/dose q8–12h. Maximum: 40 mg/day.

Rectal
Adults, Elderly. 25 mg twice a day.
Children. 0.4 mg/kg/day in
3–4 divided doses.
▶ **Psychosis**
PO
Adults, Elderly. 5–10 mg 3–4 times a
day. Maximum: 150 mg/day.
Children. 2.5 mg 2–3 times a day.
Maximum: 25 mg for children
6–12 yr; 20 mg for children 2–5 yr.
IM
Adults, Elderly. 10–20 mg q4h.
Children. 0.13 mg/kg/dose.

SIDE EFFECTS/ADVERSE REACTIONS

Frequent
Somnolence, hypotension, dizziness,
fainting (commonly occurring after
first dose, occasionally after
subsequent doses, and rarely with
oral form)
Occasional
Dry mouth, blurred vision, lethargy,
constipation, diarrhea, myalgia, nasal
congestion, peripheral edema, urine
retention

PRECAUTIONS AND CONTRAINDICATIONS

Angle-closure glaucoma, CNS
depression, coma, myelosuppression,
severe cardiac or hepatic impairment,
severe hypotension or hypertension
Caution
Children younger than 2 yr, elderly

DRUG INTERACTIONS OF CONCERN TO DENTISTRY

● Increased sedation: other CNS
depressants, alcohol, barbiturate
anesthetics, opioid analgesics
● Hypotension, tachycardia:
epinephrine
● Increased extrapyramidal effects:
phenothiazines and related drugs
(haloperidol, droperidol),
metoclopramide
● Additive photosensitization:
tetracyclines
● Increased anticholinergic effects:
anticholinergics

SERIOUS REACTIONS

! Extrapyramidal symptoms appear
to be dose-related and are divided
into three categories: akathisia
(marked by inability to sit still,
tapping of feet), parkinsonian
symptoms (including mask-like face,
tremors, shuffling gait,
hypersalivation), and acute dystonias
(such as torticollis, opisthotonos, and
oculogyric crisis). A dystonic
reaction may also produce
diaphoresis or pallor.
! Tardive dyskinesia, manifested as
tongue protrusion, puffing of the
cheeks, and puckering of the mouth,
is a rare reaction that may be
irreversible.
! Abrupt withdrawal after long-term
therapy may precipitate nausea,
vomiting, gastritis, dizziness, and
tremors.
! Blood dyscrasias, particularly
agranulocytosis and mild leukopenia,
may occur.
! Prochlorperazine use may lower
the seizure threshold.

DENTAL CONSIDERATIONS

General:
● Monitor vital signs at every
appointment because of
cardiovascular side effects.
● Patients on chronic drug therapy
may rarely have symptoms of blood
dyscrasias, which can include
infection, bleeding, and poor healing.
● After supine positioning, have
patient sit upright for at least 2 min
before standing to avoid orthostatic
hypotension.

• Assess salivary flow as a factor in caries, periodontal disease, and candidiasis.
• Avoid dental light in patient's eyes; offer dark glasses for patient comfort.
• Assess for presence of extrapyramidal motor symptoms, such as tardive dyskinesia and akathisia. Extrapyramidal motor activity may complicate dental treatment.
• Geriatric patients are more susceptible to drug effects; use lower dose.
• Use vasoconstrictors with caution, in low doses, and with careful aspiration.

Consultations:
• In a patient with symptoms of blood dyscrasias, request a medical consultation for blood studies and postpone dental treatment until normal values are reestablished.
• Take precautions if dental surgery is anticipated and anesthesia is required.
• If signs of tardive dyskinesia or akathisia are present, refer to physician.

Teach Patient/Family to:
• Use effective oral hygiene to prevent soft tissue inflammation
• Use caution to prevent injury when using oral hygiene aids
• Use electric tooth brush if patient has difficulty holding conventional devices
• When chronic dry mouth occurs, advise patient to:
    • Avoid mouth rinses with high alcohol content because of drying effects
    • Use daily home fluoride products to prevent caries
    • Use sugarless gum, frequent sips of water, or saliva substitutes

procyclidine
proe-sye′-kli-deen
(Kemadrin)

CATEGORY AND SCHEDULE
Pregnancy Risk Category: C

Drug Class: Anticholinergic, antidyskinetic

MECHANISM OF ACTION
An anticholinergic agent that exerts an atropine-like action and produces an antispasmodic effect on smooth muscle, is a potent mydriatic, and inhibits salivation. ***Therapeutic Effect:*** Relieves symptoms of Parkinson's disease and drug-induced extrapyramidal symptoms.

USES
Treatment of Parkinson symptoms, extrapyramidal symptoms associated with neuroleptic drugs

PHARMACOKINETICS
Well absorbed from the GI tract. Protein binding: extensive. Metabolized in liver, undergoes extensive first-pass effect. Primarily excreted in urine. Unknown if removed by hemodialysis. ***Half-life:*** 7.7–16.1 hr.

INDICATIONS AND DOSAGES
▶ **Drug-Induced Extrapyramidal Reactions**
PO
Adults, Elderly. Initially, 2.5 mg 3 times a day. May increase by 2.5 mg/day as needed. Maintenance: 10–20 mg/day in divided doses 3 times a day.
▶ **Parkinson's Disease**
PO
Adults, Elderly. Initially, 2.5 mg 3 times a day after meals.

Maintenance: 2.5–5 mg mg/day in divided doses 3 times a day after meals.

▶ **Hepatic Function Impairment**
PO
Adults, Elderly. 2.5–5 mg mg/day in divided doses twice a day after meals

SIDE EFFECTS/ADVERSE REACTIONS
Frequent
Blurred vision, mydriasis, disorientation, lightheadedness, nausea, vomiting dry mouth, nose, throat, and lips

PRECAUTIONS AND CONTRAINDICATIONS
Angle-closure glaucoma
Elderly, lactation, tachycardia, prostatic hypertrophy, children, kidney or liver disease, drug abuse, hypotension, hypertension, psychiatric patients

DRUG INTERACTIONS OF CONCERN TO DENTISTRY
• Increased anticholinergic effect: antihistamines, anticholinergics, meperidine
• Increased CNS depression: alcohol, CNS depressants

SERIOUS REACTIONS
! Overdosage may vary from severe anticholinergic effects, such as unsteadiness, severe drowsiness, severe dryness of mouth, nose, or throat, tachycardia, shortness of breath, and skin flushing.
! Also produces severe paradoxical reaction, marked by hallucinations, tremor, seizures, and toxic psychosis.

DENTAL CONSIDERATIONS
General:
• Monitor vital signs at every appointment because of cardiovascular side effects.
• Assess salivary flow as a factor in caries, periodontal disease, and candidiasis.
• After supine positioning, have patient sit upright for at least 2 min before standing to avoid orthostatic hypotension.
• Avoid dental light in patient's eyes; offer dark glasses for patient comfort.
• Do not ingest sodium bicarbonate products, such as the Prophy-Jet air polishing system, until 1 hr after drug use.
• Place on frequent recall because of oral side effects.
Consultations:
• Medical consultation may be required to assess disease control.
• Medical consultation may be required to assess patient's ability to tolerate stress.
Teach Patient/Family to:
• Use electric tooth brush if patient has difficulty holding conventional devices
• Use effective oral hygiene to prevent soft tissue inflammation
• Use caution to prevent injury when using oral hygiene aids
• When chronic dry mouth occurs, advise patient to:
  • Avoid mouth rinses with high alcohol content because of drying effects
  • Use daily home fluoride products for anticaries effect
  • Use sugarless gum, frequent sips of water, or saliva substitutes

P

progesterone

proe-jess´-ter-one
(Crinone, Prochieve, Prometrium)

CATEGORY AND SCHEDULE
Pregnancy Risk Category: D

Drug Class: Contraceptives, hormones/hormone modifiers, progestins

MECHANISM OF ACTION

A natural steroid hormone that promotes mammary gland development and relaxes uterine smooth muscle. *Therapeutic Effect:* Decreases abnormal uterine bleeding; transforms endometrium from proliferative to secretory in an estrogen-primed endometrium.

USES

Prevention of endometrial hyperplasia, secondary amenorrhea, abnormal uterine bleeding, treatment of infertility

PHARMACOKINETICS

IM, Rectal, Vaginal: Duration 24 hr, excreted in urine, feces; metabolized in liver.

INDICATIONS AND DOSAGES
▸ **Amenorrhea**
PO
Adults. 400 mg daily in evening for 10 days.
IM
Adults. 5–10 mg for 6–8 days. Withdrawal bleeding expected in 48–72 hr if ovarian activity produced proliferative endometrium.
Vaginal
Adults. Apply 45 mg (4% gel) every other day for 6 or fewer doses.

▸ **Abnormal Uterine Bleeding**
IM
Adults. 5–10 mg for 6 days. When estrogen given concomitantly, begin progesterone after 2 wk of estrogen therapy; discontinue when menstrual flow begins.
▸ **Prevention of Endometrial Hyperplasia**
PO
Adults. 200 mg in evening for 12 days per 28-day cycle in combination with daily conjugated estrogen.
▸ **Infertility**
Vaginal
Adults. 90 mg (8% gel) once a day (twice a day in women with partial or complete ovarian failure).

SIDE EFFECTS/ADVERSE REACTIONS
Frequent

Breakthrough bleeding or spotting at beginning of therapy, amenorrhea, change in menstrual flow, breast tenderness
Gel: drowsiness
Occasional

Edema, weight gain or loss, rash, pruritus, photosensitivity, skin pigmentation
Rare

Pain or swelling at injection site, acne, depression, alopecia, hirsutism

PRECAUTIONS AND CONTRAINDICATIONS

Breast cancer; history of active cerebral apoplexy; thromboembolic disorders or thrombophlebitis; missed abortion; severe hepatic dysfunction; undiagnosed vaginal bleeding; use as a pregnancy test

DRUG INTERACTIONS OF CONCERN TO DENTISTRY
None reported

Promethazine Hydrochloride   1027

SERIOUS REACTIONS
! Thrombophlebitis, cerebrovascular disorders, retinal thrombosis, and pulmonary embolism occur rarely.

DENTAL CONSIDERATIONS
General:
• Determine why patient is taking the drug.
• Advise patient if dental drugs prescribed have a potential for photosensitivity.
• Monitor vital signs.
• Some patients may experience drowsiness; inquire before using CNS depressants.
Teach Patient/Family to:
• Not drive or perform other tasks requiring mental alertness
• Use effective oral hygiene to prevent soft tissue inflammation
• Prevent trauma when using oral hygiene aids
• Update health and medication history if physician makes any changes in evaluation or drug regimens; include OTC, herbal, and nonherbal drugs in the update

promethazine hydrochloride
proe-meth´-ah-zeen high-droh-klor´-ide
(Insomn-Eze[AUS], Phenadoz, Phenergan)
Do not confuse promethazine with promazine.

CATEGORY AND SCHEDULE
Pregnancy Risk Category: C
Controlled Substance: Schedule V

Drug Class: Antihistamine, H_1-receptor antagonist

MECHANISM OF ACTION
A phenothiazine that acts as an antihistamine, antiemetic, and sedative-hypnotic. As an antihistamine, inhibits histamine at histamine receptor sites. As an antiemetic, diminishes vestibular stimulation, depresses labyrinthine function, and acts on the chemoreceptor trigger zone. As a sedative-hypnotic, produces CNS depression by decreasing stimulation to the brainstem reticular formation.
Therapeutic Effect: Prevents allergic responses mediated by histamine, such as rhinitis, urticaria, and pruritus. Prevents and relieves nausea and vomiting.

USES
Motion sickness, rhinitis, allergy symptoms, sedation, nausea, preoperative or postoperative sedation

PHARMACOKINETICS

Route	Onset	Peak	Duration
PO	20 min	N/A	2–8 hr
IV	3–5 min	N/A	2–8 hr
IM	20 min	N/A	2–8 hr
Rectal	20 min	N/A	2–8 hr

Well absorbed from the GI tract after IM administration. Widely distributed. Metabolized in the liver. Primarily excreted in urine. Not removed by hemodialysis.
Half-life: 16–19 hr.

INDICATIONS AND DOSAGES
▶ **Allergic Symptoms**
PO
Adults, Elderly. 6.25–12.5 mg 3 times a day plus 25 mg at bedtime.
Children. 0.1 mg/kg/dose (maximum: 12.5 mg) 3 times a day plus 0.5 mg/kg/dose (maximum: 25 mg) at bedtime.

IV, IM
Adults, Elderly. 25 mg. May repeat in
2 hr.
▶ **Motion Sickness**
PO
Adults, Elderly. 25 mg 30–60 min
before departure; may repeat in
8–12 hr, then every morning on
rising and before evening meal.
Children. 0.5 mg/kg 30–60 min
before departure; may repeat in
8–12 hr, then every morning on
rising and before evening meal.
▶ **Prevention of Nausea and Vomiting**
PO, IV, IM, Rectal
Adults, Elderly. 12.5–25 mg q4–6h
as needed.
Children. 0.25–1 mg/kg q4–6h as
needed.
▶ **Preoperative and Postoperative
Sedation; Adjunct to Analgesics**
IV, IM
Adults, Elderly. 25–50 mg.
Children. 12.5–25 mg.
▶ **Sedative**
PO, IV, IM, Rectal
Adults, Elderly. 25–50 mg/dose.
May repeat q4–6h as needed.
Children. 0.5–1 mg/kg/dose q6h as
needed. Maximum: 50 mg/dose.

SIDE EFFECTS/ADVERSE REACTIONS
Expected
Somnolence, disorientation; in
elderly, hypotension, confusion,
syncope
Frequent
Dry mouth, nose, or throat; urine
retention; thickening of bronchial
secretions
Occasional
Epigastric distress, flushing, visual
disturbances, hearing disturbances,
wheezing, paresthesia, diaphoresis, chills
Rare
Dizziness, urticaria, photosensitivity,
nightmares

PRECAUTIONS AND CONTRAINDICATIONS
Angle-closure glaucoma, GI or GU
obstruction, severe CNS depression
or coma
Caution
Increased intraocular pressure, renal
disease, cardiac disease,
hypertension, bronchial asthma,
seizure disorder, stenosed peptic
ulcers, hyperthyroidism, prostatic
hypertrophy, bladder neck
obstruction

DRUG INTERACTIONS OF CONCERN TO DENTISTRY
• Increased CNS depression: alcohol,
all CNS depressants
• Hypotension: general anesthetics
• Increased effect of anticholinergic
drugs

SERIOUS REACTIONS
! Children may experience
paradoxical reactions, such as
excitation, nervousness, tremor,
hyperactive reflexes, and seizures.
! Infants and young children have
experienced CNS depression
manifested as respiratory depression,
sleep apnea, and sudden infant death
syndrome.
! Long-term therapy may produce
extrapyramidal symptoms, such as
dystonia (abnormal movements),
pronounced motor restlessness (most
frequently in children), and
parkinsonian symptoms (most
frequently in elderly patients).
! Blood dyscrasias, particularly
agranulocytosis, occur rarely.

DENTAL CONSIDERATIONS
General:
• Determine why the patient is taking
the drug.
• Patients on chronic drug therapy
may rarely have symptoms of blood

dyscrasias, which can include infection, bleeding, and poor healing.
• Monitor vital signs at every appointment because of cardiovascular side effects.
• Assess salivary flow as a factor in caries, periodontal disease, and candidiasis.
• Assess vital signs q30min after use as sedative.
Teach Patient/Family:
• When chronic dry mouth occurs, advise patient to:
  • Avoid mouth rinses with high alcohol content because of drying effects
  • Use daily home fluoride products to prevent caries
  • Use sugarless gum, frequent sips of water, or saliva substitutes

propafenone hydrochloride
proe-pa-fen´-own
high-droh-klor´-ide
(Rythmol, Rythmol SR)

CATEGORY AND SCHEDULE
Pregnancy Risk Category: C

Drug Class: Antidysrhythmic (class Ic)

MECHANISM OF ACTION
An antiarrhythmic that decreases the fast sodium current in Purkinje or myocardial cells. Decreases excitability and automaticity; prolongs conduction velocity and the refractory period.*Therapeutic Effect:* Suppresses dyshythmias.

USES
Treatment of documented life-threatening dysrhythmias;
unapproved: sustained ventricular tachycardia

PHARMACOKINETICS
Peak 3–5 hr. *Half-life:* 2–10 hr; metabolized in liver; excreted in urine (metabolite).

INDICATIONS AND DOSAGES
▸ **Documented, Life-Threatening Ventricular Arrhythmias, such as Sustained Ventricular Tachycardia**
PO (Prompt-Release)
Adults, Elderly. Initially, 150 mg q8h; may increase at 3- to 4-day intervals to 225 mg q8h, then to 300 mg q8h. Maximum: 900 mg/day.
PO (Extended-Release)
Adults, Elderly. Initially, 225 mg q12h. May increase at 5-day intervals. Maximum: 425 mg q12h.

SIDE EFFECTS/ADVERSE REACTIONS
Frequent
Dizziness, nausea, vomiting, altered taste, constipation
Occasional
Headache, dyspnea, blurred vision, dyspepsia (heartburn, indigestion, epigastric pain)
Rare
Rash, weakness, dry mouth, diarrhea, edema, hot flashes

PRECAUTIONS AND CONTRAINDICATIONS
Bradycardia; bronchospastic disorders; cardiogenic shock; electrolyte imbalance; sinoatrial, AV, and intraventricular impulse generation or conduction disorders, such as sick sinus syndrome or AV block, without the presence of a pacemaker; uncontrolled CHF.
Caution
CHF, hypokalemia, hyperkalemia, recent MI, nonallergic

bronchospasm, lactation, children, hepatic or renal disease

DRUG INTERACTIONS OF CONCERN TO DENTISTRY
• No specific interactions are reported; however, any drug that could affect the cardiac action of propafenone (other local anesthetics, vasoconstrictors, anticholinergics) should be used in the lowest effective dose

SERIOUS REACTIONS
! Propafenone may produce or worsen existing arrhythmias.
! Overdose may produce hypotension, somnolence, bradycardia, and atrioventricular conduction disturbances.

DENTAL CONSIDERATIONS
General:
• Monitor vital signs at every appointment because of cardiovascular side effects.
• Patients on chronic drug therapy may rarely have symptoms of blood dyscrasias, which can include infection, bleeding, and poor healing.
• Assess salivary flow as a factor in caries, periodontal disease, and candidiasis.
• Stress from dental procedures may compromise cardiovascular function; determine patient risk.
• Consider semisupine chair position for patients with respiratory distress.
Consultations:
• In a patient with symptoms of blood dyscrasias, request a medical consultation for blood studies and postpone dental treatment until normal values are reestablished.
• Medical consultation may be required to assess disease control and patient's ability to tolerate stress.

Teach Patient/Family to:
• Use effective oral hygiene to prevent soft tissue inflammation
• Use caution to prevent injury when using oral hygiene aids
• When chronic dry mouth occurs, advise patient to:
    • Avoid mouth rinses with high alcohol content because of drying effects
    • Use daily home fluoride products to prevent caries
    • Use sugarless gum, frequent sips of water, or saliva substitutes

propantheline
proe-pan´-the-leen
(Pro-Banthine, Propanthl[CAN])

CATEGORY AND SCHEDULE
Pregnancy Risk Category: C

Drug Class: Anticholinergic

MECHANISM OF ACTION
A quaternary ammonium compound which has anticholinergic properties and that inhibits action of acetylcholine at postganglionic parasympathetic sites. *Therapeutic Effect:* Reduces gastric secretions and urinary frequency, urgency and urge incontinence.

USES
Treatment of peptic ulcer disease, irritable bowel syndrome, duodenography, urinary incontinence; unapproved: reduction in salivary flow

PHARMACOKINETICS
Onset occurs within 90 min. but less than 50% is absorbed from GI tract. Extensive hepatic metabolism.

Excreted in the urine and feces.
Half-life: 2.9 hr.

INDICATIONS AND DOSAGES
▶ **Peptic Ulcer**
PO
Adults, Elderly. 15 mg 3 times a day
30 min. before meals and 30 mg at
bedtime.
Children. 1–2 mg/kg/day, divided
q4–6h and at bedtime.

SIDE EFFECTS/ADVERSE REACTIONS
Frequent

Dry mouth, decreased sweating,
constipation
Occasional

Blurred vision, intolerance to light,
urinary hesitancy, drowsiness,
agitation, excitement
Rare

Confusion, increased intraocular
pressure, orthostatic hypotension,
tachycardia

PRECAUTIONS AND CONTRAINDICATIONS
GI or GU obstruction, myasthenia
gravis, narrow-angle glaucoma, toxic
megacolon, severe ulcerative colitis,
unstable cardiovascular adjustment in
acute hemorrhage, hypersensitivity
to propantheline or other
anticholinergics
Caution

Hyperthyroidism, CAD,
dysrhythmias, CHF, ulcerative colitis,
hypertension, hiatal hernia, hepatic
disease, renal disease, pregnancy
category C, urinary retention,
prostatic hypertrophy

DRUG INTERACTIONS OF CONCERN TO DENTISTRY
• Increased anticholinergic effect:
other anticholinergic drugs

• Constipation, urinary retention:
opioid analgesics
• Decreased absorption of
ketoconazole; take doses 2 hr apart

SERIOUS REACTIONS
! Overdosage may produce
temporary paralysis of ciliary
muscle, pupillary dilation,
tachycardia, palpitations, hot, dry, or
flushed skin, absence of bowel
sounds, hyperthermia, increased
respiratory rate, ECG abnormalities,
nausea, vomiting, rash over face or
upper trunk, CNS stimulation, and
psychosis, marked by agitation,
restlessness, rambling speech, visual
hallucinations, paranoid behavior,
and delusions, followed by
depression.

DENTAL CONSIDERATIONS
General:
• Assess salivary flow as a factor in
caries, periodontal disease, and
candidiasis.
• Avoid dental light in patient's eyes;
offer dark glasses for patient
comfort.
• Place on frequent recall because of
oral side effects.
• Avoid prescribing
aspirin-containing products.
• Consider semisupine chair position
for patient comfort because of GI
effects of disease.
Consultations:
• Physician should be informed if
significant xerostomic side effects
occur (e.g., increased caries, sore
tongue, problems eating or
swallowing, difficulty wearing
prosthesis) so that a medication
change can be considered.
Teach Patient/Family:
• When chronic dry mouth occurs,
advise patient to:

- Avoid mouth rinses with high alcohol content because of drying effects
- Use daily home fluoride products to prevent caries
- Use sugarless gum, frequent sips of water, or saliva substitutes

propofol
pro-poe-fall′
(Diprivan, Recofol[AUS])

CATEGORY AND SCHEDULE
Pregnancy Risk Category: B

Drug Class: General anesthetic

MECHANISM OF ACTION
A rapidly acting general anesthetic that inhibits sympathetic vasoconstrictor nerve activity and decreases vascular resistance. *Therapeutic Effect:* Produces hypnosis rapidly.

USES
Induction or maintenance of anesthesia as part of balanced anesthetic technique, ICU sedation

PHARMACOKINETICS

Route	Onset	Peak	Duration
IV	40 sec	N/A	3–10 min

Rapidly and extensively distributed. Protein binding: 97%–99%. Metabolized in the liver. Primarily excreted in urine. Unknown if removed by hemodialysis. *Half-life:* 3–12 hr.

INDICATIONS AND DOSAGES
▶ Intensive Care Unit Sedation
IV
Adults, Elderly. Initially, 0.3 mg/kg/hr. May increase by 0.3–0.6 mg/kg/hr

q5–10min until desired effect is obtained. Maintenance: 0.3–3 mg/kg/h.
▶ Anesthesia
IV
Adults, American Society of Anesthesiologists (ASA) I and II patients. 2–2.5 mg/kg (about 40 mg q10sec until onset of anesthesia). Maintenance: 0.1–0.2 mg/kg/min. *Elderly, Debilitated, Hypovolemic, ASA III or IV patients.* 1–1.5 mg/kg (about 20 mg q10sec until onset of anesthesia). Maintenance: 0.05–0.1 mg/kg/min. *Children 3 yr and older, ASA I or II patients.* 2.5–3.5 mg/kg (lower dosage for ASA III or IV patients). *Children 2 mo–16 yr.* Maintenance dose: 0.125–0.15 mg/kg/min.

SIDE EFFECTS/ADVERSE REACTIONS
Frequent
Involuntary muscle movements, apnea (common during induction; lasts longer than 60 sec), hypotension, nausea, vomiting, IV site burning or stinging
Occasional
Twitching, bucking, jerking, thrashing, headache, dizziness, bradycardia, hypertension, fever, abdominal cramps, paresthesia, coldness, cough, hiccups, facial flushing, greenish-colored urine
Rare
Rash, dry mouth, agitation, confusion, myalgia, thrombophlebitis

PRECAUTIONS AND CONTRAINDICATIONS
Impaired cerebral circulation, increased intracranial pressure
Caution
Elderly, debilitated, respiratory depression, severe respiratory disorders, cardiac dysrhythmias, pregnancy category B, labor and

delivery, lactation, children younger than 3 yr, epilepsy

DRUG INTERACTIONS OF CONCERN TO DENTISTRY
• Increased CNS depression: alcohol, narcotics, sedative-hypnotics, antipsychotics, skeletal muscle relaxants, inhalational anesthetics

SERIOUS REACTIONS
❗ A continuous infusion or repeated intermittent infusions of propofol may result in extreme somnolence, respiratory depression, and circulatory depression.
❗ Too-rapid IV administration may produce severe hypotension, respiratory depression, and involuntary muscle movements.
❗ The patient may experience an acute allergic reaction, characterized by abdominal pain, anxiety, restlessness, dyspnea, erythema, hypotension, pruritus, rhinitis, and urticaria.

DENTAL CONSIDERATIONS
General:
• Monitor vital signs at regular intervals during recovery after use as anesthetic.
• Have someone drive patient to and from dental office if used for general anesthesia.
• Geriatric patients are more susceptible to drug effects; use lower dose.
• Use only with resuscitative equipment available and only by qualified persons trained in anesthesia.
• Monitor:
  • Injection site: phlebitis, burning/stinging.
  • ECG for changes: PVC, PAC, ST-segment changes.
  • Allergic reactions: hives.
• Administer:
  • After diluting with D5W, use only glass containers when mixing; not stable in plastic.

• By IV injection only.
• Alone; do not mix with other agents before using.
• Perform/provide:
  • Storage in light-resistant area at room temperature.
  • Coughing, turning, deep breathing for postoperative patients.
  • Safety measures: side rails, night light, call bell within reach.
• Evaluate:
  • CNS changes: movement, jerking, tremors, dizziness, LOC, pupil reaction.
  • Respiratory dysfunction: respiratory depression, character, rate, rhythm; notify physician if respirations are <10/min.
• Treatment of overdose:
  • Discontinue drug, artificial ventilation, administer vasopressor agents or anticholinergics.

propoxyphene hydrochloride/propo-xyphene napsylate
pro-pox´-ih-feen high-droh-klor´-ide-naps´-il-ate
propoxyphene hydrochloride: (Darvon);
propoxyphene napsylate: (Darvon-N[CAN] Doloxene[AUS])
Do not confuse Darvon with Diovan.

P

CATEGORY AND SCHEDULE
Pregnancy Risk Category: C (D if used for prolonged periods)
Controlled Substance: Schedule IV

Drug Class: Synthetic opioid narcotic analgesic

MECHANISM OF ACTION
An opioid agonist that binds with opioid receptors in the CNS.
Therapeutic Effect: Alters the

perception of and emotional response to pain.

USES

Treatment of mild-to-moderate pain

PHARMACOKINETICS

Route	Onset	Peak	Duration
PO	15–60 min	N/A	4–6 hr

Well absorbed from the GI tract. Protein binding: High. Widely distributed. Metabolized in the liver. Primarily excreted in urine. Not removed by hemodialysis. *Half-life:* 6–12 hr; metabolite: 30–36 hr.

INDICATIONS AND DOSAGES
▶ **Mild-to-Moderate Pain**
PO (Propoxyphene Hydrochloride)
Adults, Elderly. 65 mg q4h as needed. Maximum: 390 mg/day.
PO (Propoxyphene Napsylate)
Adults, Elderly. 100 mg q4h as needed. Maximum: 600 mg/day.

SIDE EFFECTS/ADVERSE REACTIONS
Frequent

Dizziness, somnolence, dry mouth, euphoria, hypotension (including orthostatic hypotension), nausea, vomiting, fatigue
Occasional

Allergic reaction (including decreased B/P, diaphoresis, flushing, and wheezing), trembling, urine retention, vision changes, constipation, headache
Rare

Confusion, increased B/P, depression, abdominal cramps, anorexia

PRECAUTIONS AND CONTRAINDICATIONS
None known

Caution
Addictive personality, lactation, increased intracranial pressure, MI (acute), severe heart disease, respiratory depression, hepatic disease, renal disease, children under 18 yr, alcoholism

DRUG INTERACTIONS OF CONCERN TO DENTISTRY
* Increased effects with other CNS depressants: alcohol, narcotics, sedative-hypnotics, skeletal muscle relaxants
* Contraindication: MAOIs
* Increased effects of anticholinergics, antihypertensives, carbamazepine

SERIOUS REACTIONS
! Overdose results in respiratory depression, skeletal muscle flaccidity, cold or clammy skin, cyanosis, and extreme somnolence progressing to seizures, stupor, and coma.
! Hepatotoxicity may occur with overdose of the acetaminophen component of fixed-combination products.
! The patient who uses propoxyphene repeatedly may develop a tolerance to the drug's analgesic effect and physical dependence.

DENTAL CONSIDERATIONS
General:
* Monitor vital signs because of cardiovascular and respiratory side effects.
* Consider semisupine chair position for patient comfort if GI side effects occur.
* Assess salivary flow as a factor in caries, periodontal disease, and candidiasis.

• Psychologic and physical dependence may occur with chronic administration.
• When combined with nonopioid analgesics (aspirin, NSAIDs, acetaminophen), permits better-quality pain relief.
Teach Patient/Family:
• When chronic dry mouth occurs, advise patient to:
  • Avoid mouth rinses with high alcohol content because of drying effects
  • Use daily home fluoride products to prevent caries
  • Use sugarless gum, frequent sips of water, or artificial saliva substitutes

propranolol hydrochloride

proe-pran´-oh-lole
high-droh-klor´-ide
(Apo-Propranolol[CAN], Deralin[AUS], Inderal, Inderal LA, InnoPran XL, Nu-Propranolol[CAN], Propranolol Intensol)
Do not confuse Inderal with Adderall or Isordil, or propranolol with Pravachol.

CATEGORY AND SCHEDULE
Pregnancy Risk Category: C (D if used in second or third trimester)

Drug Class: Nonselective β-adrenergic blocker

MECHANISM OF ACTION
An antihypertensive, antianginal, antiarrhythmic, and antimigraine agent that blocks β_1- and β_2-adrenergic receptors. Decreases oxygen requirements. Slows AV conduction and increases refractory period in AV node. Large doses increase airway resistance. **Therapeutic Effect:** Slows sinus heart rate; decreases cardiac output, B/P, and myocardial ischemia severity. Exhibits antiarrhythmic activity.

USES
Treatment of chronic stable angina pectoris, hypertension, supraventricular dysrhythmias (class II), migraine, MI prophylaxis, pheochromocytoma, essential tremor, hypertrophic cardiomyopathy, anxiety

PHARMACOKINETICS

Route	Onset	Peak	Duration
PO	1–2 hr	N/A	6 hr

Well absorbed from the GI tract. Protein binding: 93%. Widely distributed. Metabolized in the liver. Primarily excreted in urine. Not removed by hemodialysis.
Half-life: 3–5 hr.

INDICATIONS AND DOSAGES
▶ **Hypertension**
PO
Adults, Elderly. Initially, 40 mg twice a day. May increase dose q3–7 days. Range: Up to 320 mg/day in divided doses. Maximum: 640 mg/day.
Children. Initially, 0.5–1 mg/kg/day in divided doses q6–12h. May increase at 3- to 5-day intervals. Usual dose: 1–5 mg/kg/day. Maximum: 16 mg/kg/day.
▶ **Angina**
PO
Adults, Elderly. 80–320 mg/day in divided doses. Long acting: Initially, 80 mg/day. Maximum: 320 mg/day.
▶ **Arrhythmias**
IV
Adults, Elderly. 1 mg/dose. May repeat q5min. Maximum: 5 mg total dose.

Children. 0.01–0.1 mg/kg.
Maximum: infants, 1 mg; children,
3 mg.
PO
Adults, Elderly. Initially, 10–20 mg
q6–8h. May gradually increase dose.
Range: 40–320 mg/day.
Children. Initially, 0.5–1 mg/kg/day
in divided doses q6–8h. May
increase q3–5 days. Usual dosage:
2–4 mg/kg/day. Maximum:
16 mg/kg/day or 60 mg/day.

▶ **Life-Threatening Arrhythmias**
IV
Adults, Elderly. 0.5–3 mg. Repeat
once in 2 min. Give additional doses
at intervals of at least 4 hr.
Children. 0.01–0.1 mg/kg.

▶ **Hypertrophic Subaortic Stenosis**
PO
Adults, Elderly. 20–40 mg in
3–4 divided doses. Or 80–160 mg/
day as extended-release capsule.

▶ **Adjunct to α-Blocking Agents to
Treat Pheochromocytoma**
PO
Adults, Elderly. 60 mg/day in divided
doses with α-blocker for 3 days
before surgery. Maintenance
(inoperable tumor): 30 mg/day with
α-blocker.

▶ **Migraine Headache**
PO
Adults, Elderly. 80 mg/day in divided
doses. Or 80 mg once daily as
extended-release capsule. Increase
up to 160–240 mg/day in divided
doses.
Children. 0.6–1.5 mg/kg/day in
divided doses q8h.
Maximum: 4 mg/kg/day.

▶ **Reduction of Cardiovascular
Mortality and Reinfarction in
Patients with Previous MI**
PO
Adults, Elderly. 180–240 mg/day
in divided doses.

▶ **Essential Tremor**
PO
Adults, Elderly. Initially, 40 mg twice
a day increased up to 120–320 mg/
day in 3 divided doses.

SIDE EFFECTS/ADVERSE REACTIONS
Frequent
Diminished sexual ability,
drowsiness, difficulty sleeping,
unusual fatigue or weakness
Occasional
Bradycardia, depression, sensation
of coldness in extremities,
diarrhea, constipation, anxiety,
nasal congestion, nausea,
vomiting
Rare
Altered taste, dry eyes, pruritus,
paraesthesia

PRECAUTIONS AND CONTRAINDICATIONS
Asthma, bradycardia, cardiogenic
shock, COPD, heart block, Raynaud's
syndrome, uncompensated CHF
Caution
Diabetes mellitus, renal disease,
lactation, hyperthyroidism, COPD,
hepatic disease, children, myasthenia
gravis, peripheral vascular disease,
hypotension

DRUG INTERACTIONS OF CONCERN TO DENTISTRY
• Decreased hypotensive effect:
indomethacin, NSAIDs
• Increased hypotension, myocardial
depression: hydrocarbon inhalation
anesthetics
• Hypertension, bradycardia:
sympathomimetics (epinephrine,
ephedrine)
• Suspected increase in plasma
levels: diphenhydramine
• Slow metabolism of lidocaine

- Decreased effects: didanosine (take 2 hr before didanosine tabs)

SERIOUS REACTIONS

! Overdose may produce profound bradycardia and hypotension.

! Abrupt withdrawal may result in sweating, palpitations, headache, and tremors.

! Propranolol administration may precipitate CHF and MI in patients with cardiac disease, thyroid storm in those with thyrotoxicosis, and peripheral ischemia in those with existing peripheral vascular disease.

! Hypoglycemia may occur in patients with previously controlled diabetes.

DENTAL CONSIDERATIONS

General:

- Monitor vital signs at every appointment because of cardiovascular side effects.
- Patients on chronic drug therapy may rarely have symptoms of blood dyscrasias, which can include infection, bleeding, and poor healing.
- Limit use of sodium-containing products, such as saline IV fluids, for patients with a dietary salt restriction.
- Assess salivary flow as a factor in caries, periodontal disease, and candidiasis.
- After supine positioning, have patient sit upright for at least 2 min before standing to avoid orthostatic hypotension.
- Stress from dental procedures may compromise cardiovascular function; determine patient risk.
- Short appointments and a stress-reduction protocol may be required for anxious patients.
- Consider semisupine chair position for patients with respiratory distress.
- Use vasoconstrictors with caution, in low doses, and with careful

aspiration. Avoid use of gingival retraction cord with epinephrine.

Consultations:

- In a patient with symptoms of blood dyscrasias, request a medical consultation for blood studies and postpone dental treatment until normal values are reestablished.
- Medical consultation may be required to assess disease control and patient's ability to tolerate stress.

Teach Patient/Family to:

- Use caution to prevent injury when using oral hygiene aids
- Use effective oral hygiene to prevent soft tissue inflammation
- When chronic dry mouth occurs, advise patient to:
  - Avoid mouth rinses with high alcohol content because of drying effects
  - Use daily home fluoride products to prevent caries
  - Use sugarless gum, frequent sips of water, or saliva substitutes

propylthiouracil

proe-pill-thye-oh-yoor´-ah-sill
(Propylthiouracil,
Propyl-Thyracil[CAN])

CATEGORY AND SCHEDULE
Pregnancy Risk Category: D

Drug Class: Thyroid hormone antagonist

MECHANISM OF ACTION
A thiourea derivative that blocks oxidation of iodine in the thyroid gland and blocks synthesis of thyroxine and triiodothyronine. **Therapeutic Effect:** Inhibits synthesis of thyroid hormone.

USES

Preparation for thyroidectomy, thyrotoxic crisis, hyperthyroidism, thyroid storm

PHARMACOKINETICS

PO: Onset 30–40 min, duration 2–4 hr. *Half-life:* 1–2 hr; excreted in urine, bile, breast milk; crosses placenta.

INDICATIONS AND DOSAGES
▶ **Hyperthyroidism**
PO
Adults, Elderly. Initially: 300–450 mg/day in divided doses q8h. Maintenance: 100–150 mg/day in divided doses q8–12h.
Children. Initially: 5–7 mg/kg/day in divided doses q8h. Maintenance: 33%–66% of initial dose in divided doses q8–12h.
Neonates. 5–10 mg/kg/day in divided doses q8h.

SIDE EFFECTS/ADVERSE REACTIONS
Frequent
Urticaria, rash, pruritus, nausea, skin pigmentation, hair loss, headache, paraesthesia
Occasional
Somnolence, lymphadenopathy, vertigo
Rare
Drug fever, lupus-like syndrome

PRECAUTIONS AND CONTRAINDICATIONS

Infection, bone marrow depression, hepatic disease
Caution
Infection, bone marrow depression, hepatic disease

DRUG INTERACTIONS OF CONCERN TO DENTISTRY

• Increased cardiovascular side effects in uncontrolled patients: anticholinergics and sympathomimetics
• Patients with uncontrolled hyperthyroidism are at risk when vasoconstrictors are used
• Patients with uncontrolled hypothyroidism may be more responsive to CNS depressants

SERIOUS REACTIONS

❗ Agranulocytosis as long as 4 mo after therapy, pancytopenia, and fatal hepatitis have occurred.

DENTAL CONSIDERATIONS

General:
• Patients on chronic drug therapy may rarely have symptoms of blood dyscrasias, which can include infection, bleeding, and poor healing.
• Patients with uncontrolled hyperthyroidism should not be treated in the dental office until thyroid values are normalized.
• Uncontrolled patients should be referred for medical evaluation and treatment.
• Monitor vital signs at every appointment because of cardiovascular side effects.
• Consider semisupine chair position for patient comfort if GI side effects occur.
Consultations:
• Medical consultation may be required to assess disease control and patient's ability to tolerate stress.

protamine sulfate

proe´-ta-meen sull´-fate
(Protamine[CAN], Protamine sulfate)
Do not confuse protamine with
ProAmatine, Protopam, or
Protropin.

CATEGORY AND SCHEDULE
Pregnancy Risk Category: C

Drug Class: Heparin antagonist

MECHANISM OF ACTION
A protein that complexes with
heparin to form a stable salt.
Therapeutic Effect: Reduces
anticoagulant activity of heparin.

USES
Treatment for heparin overdose,
hemorrage

PHARMACOKINETICS
IV: Onset 5 min, duration 2 hr

INDICATIONS AND DOSAGES
▶ **Heparin Overdose (antidote and
treatment)**
IV
Adults, Elderly. 1 mg protamine
sulfate neutralizes 90–115 units of
heparin. Heparin disappears rapidly
from circulation, reducing the dosage
demand for protamine as time elapses.

SIDE EFFECTS/ADVERSE
REACTIONS
Frequent
Decreased B/P, dyspnea
Occasional
Hypersensitivity reaction (urticaria,
angioedema); nausea and vomiting,
which generally occur in those
sensitive to fish and seafood,
vasectomized men, infertile men,
those on isophane (NPH) insulin, or
those previously on protamine therapy

Rare
Back pain

PRECAUTIONS AND
CONTRAINDICATIONS
None known

DRUG INTERACTIONS OF
CONCERN TO DENTISTRY
None reported

SERIOUS REACTIONS
❗ Too rapid IV administration may
produce acute hypotension,
bradycardia, pulmonary
hypertension, dyspnea, transient
flushing, and feeling of warmth.
❗ Heparin rebound may occur several
hr after heparin has been neutralized
(usually 8–9 hr after protamine
administration). Heparin rebound
occurs most often after arterial or
cardiac surgery.

DENTAL CONSIDERATIONS
General
* Acute-use drug for use in hospitals
and emergency rooms; delay any
dental treatment until normal clotting
mechanism is restored.
* Question patient about use of oral
anticoagulants.
* Avoid products that affect platelet
function, such as aspirin and
NSAIDs.
* Determine why patient is taking
the drug.
* Consider local hemostasis
measures to prevent excessive
bleeding.
Consultations:
* Medical consultation may be
required to assess disease control and
patient's ability to tolerate stress.
* Medical consultation should
include routine blood counts
including platelet counts and
bleeding time.

• Medical consultation should include PPT, PT, or INR.

Teach Patient/Family to:

• Inform dentist of unusual bleeding episodes following dental treatment

• Use soft tooth brush to help prevent irritation of oral tissues that could evoke bleeding

protriptyline
proe-trip´-ti-leen
(Vivactil, Triptil[CAN])

CATEGORY AND SCHEDULE
Pregnancy Risk Category: C

Drug Class: Tricyclic antidepressant

MECHANISM OF ACTION
A tricyclic antidepressant that increases synaptic concentration of norepinephrine and/or serotonin by inhibiting their reuptake by presynaptic membranes. *Therapeutic Effect:* Produces antidepressant effect.

USES
Depression; unapproved use: adjunctive use in narcolepsy and attention-deficit disorders

PHARMACOKINETICS
Well absorbed from the GI tract. Protein binding: 92%. Widely distributed. Extensively metabolized in liver. Excreted in urine. Not removed by hemodialysis. *Half-life:* 54–92 hr.

INDICATIONS AND DOSAGES
▶ **Depression**
PO
Adults. 15–40 mg/day divided into 3–4 doses/day. Maximum: 600 mg/day.

Elderly. 5 mg 3 times a day. May increase gradually.

SIDE EFFECTS/ADVERSE REACTIONS
Frequent
Drowsiness, weight gain, fatigue, dry mouth, blurred vision, constipation, delayed micturition, postural hypotension, diaphoresis, disturbed concentration, increased appetite, urinary retention
Occasional
GI disturbances, such as nausea, diarrhea, GI distress, metallic taste sensation
Rare
Paradoxical reaction, marked by agitation, restlessness, nightmares, insomnia, extrapyramidal symptoms, particularly fine hand tremor

PRECAUTIONS AND CONTRAINDICATIONS
Acute recovery period after myocardial infarction, coadministration with cisapride, use of MAOIs within 14 days, hypersensitivity to protriptyline or any component of the formulation.
Caution
Suicidal patients, severe depression, increased intraocular pressure, narrow-angle glaucoma, urinary retention, cardiac disease, hepatic disease, hyperthyroidism, electroshock therapy, elective surgery, MAOIs

DRUG INTERACTIONS OF CONCERN TO DENTISTRY
• Increased anticholinergic effects: muscarinic blockers, antihistamines, phenothiazines
• Increased effects of direct-acting sympathomimetics (epinephrine, levonordefrin)

• Possible risk of increased CNS depression: alcohol, barbiturates, benzodiazepines, and other CNS depressants
• Decreased antihypertensive effects of: clonidine, guanadrel, guanethidine
• Avoid concurrent use with St. John's wort (herb)

SERIOUS REACTIONS

❗ High dosage may produce confusion, seizures, severe drowsiness, arrhythmias, fever, hallucinations, agitation, shortness of breath, vomiting, and unusual tiredness or weakness.
❗ Abrupt withdrawal from prolonged therapy may produce severe headache, malaise, nausea, vomiting, and vivid dreams.

DENTAL CONSIDERATIONS
General:
• Monitor vital signs at every appointment because of cardiovascular side effects.
• Assess salivary flow as a factor in caries, periodontal disease, and candidiasis.
• Patients on chronic drug therapy may rarely have symptoms of blood dyscrasias, which can include infection, bleeding, and poor healing.
• After supine positioning, have patient sit upright for at least 2 min before standing to avoid orthostatic hypotension.
• Use vasoconstrictors with caution, in low doses, and with careful aspiration. Avoid use of gingival retraction cord with epinephrine.
• Place on frequent recall because of oral side effects.
Consultations:
• In a patient with symptoms of blood dyscrasias, request a medical consultation for blood studies and

postpone dental treatment until normal values are reestablished.
• Medical consultation may be required to assess disease control.
• Physician should be informed if significant xerostomic side effects occur (e.g., increased caries, sore tongue, problems eating or swallowing, difficulty wearing prosthesis) so that a medication change can be considered.
Teach Patient/Family to:
• Use effective oral hygiene to prevent soft tissue inflammation
• Use caution to prevent injury when using oral hygiene aids
• When chronic dry mouth occurs, advise patient to:
  • Avoid mouth rinses with high alcohol content because of drying effects
  • Use daily home fluoride products to prevent caries
  • Use sugarless gum, frequent sips of water, or saliva substitutes

pseudoephedrine
soo-doe-eh-fed´-rin
(Balminil Decongestant[CAN], BioContac Cold 12 Hour Relief Non Drowsy[CAN], Decofed, Dimetapp 12 Hour Non Drowsy Extentabs, Dimetapp Decongestant, Dimetapp Sinus Liquid Caps[AUS], Genaphed, PMS-Pseudoephedrine[CAN], Robidrine[CAN], Sudafed, Sudafed 12h[AUS], Sudafed 12 Hour, Sudafed 24 Hour)

P

CATEGORY AND SCHEDULE
Pregnancy Risk Category: C
OTC

Drug Class:
α-adrenergic agonist

MECHANISM OF ACTION

A sympathomimetic that directly stimulates α-adrenergic and β-adrenergic receptors. ***Therapeutic Effect:*** Produces vasoconstriction of respiratory tract mucosa; shrinks nasal mucous membranes; reduces edema and nasal congestion.

USES

Decongestant, treatment of nasal congestion

PHARMACOKINETICS

Route	Onset	Peak	Duration
PO	15–30 min	N/A	4–6 hr
PO	N/A	N/A	8–12 hr

Well absorbed from the GI tract. Partially metabolized in the liver. Primarily excreted in urine. Not removed by hemodialysis. ***Half-life:*** 9–16 hr (children, 3.1 hr).

INDICATIONS AND DOSAGES

▸ **Decongestant**
PO
Adults, Children 12 yr and older.
60 mg q4–6h. Maximum: 240 mg/day.
Children 6–11 yr. 30 mg q6h. Maximum: 120 mg/day.
Children 2–5 yr. 15 mg q6h. Maximum: 60 mg/day.
Children younger than 2 yr.
4 mg/kg/day in divided doses q6h.
Elderly. 30–60 mg q6h as needed.
PO (Extended Release)
Adults, Children 12 yr and older.
120 mg q12h.

SIDE EFFECTS/ADVERSE REACTIONS

Occasional
Nervousness, restlessness, insomnia, tremor, headache

Rare
Diaphoresis, weakness

PRECAUTIONS AND CONTRAINDICATIONS

Breast-feeding women, coronary artery disease, severe hypertension, use within 14 days of MAOIs.
Caution
Cardiac disorders, hyperthyroidism, diabetes mellitus, prostatic hypertrophy

DRUG INTERACTIONS OF CONCERN TO DENTISTRY

• Dysrhythmia: hydrocarbon inhalation anesthetics
• Increased CNS, cardiovascular effects: sympathomimetics

SERIOUS REACTIONS

❗ Large doses may produce tachycardia, palpitations (particularly in patients with cardiac disease), light-headedness, nausea, and vomiting.
❗ Overdose in patients older than 60 yr may result in hallucinations, CNS depression, and seizures.

DENTAL CONSIDERATIONS

General:
• Assess salivary flow as a factor in caries, periodontal disease, and candidiasis.
• Monitor vital signs at every appointment because of cardiovascular side effects.
• Consider semisupine chair position for patient comfort if GI side effects occur.
Teach Patient/Family to:
• Use electric tooth brush if patient has difficulty holding conventional devices
• When chronic dry mouth occurs, advise patient to:
    • Avoid mouth rinses with high alcohol content because of drying effects

- Use daily home fluoride products to prevent caries
- Use sugarless gum, frequent sips of water, or saliva substitutes

pyrazinamide
pye-ra-zin´-ah-mide
(Pyrazinamide, Tebrazid[CAN], Zinamide[AUS])

CATEGORY AND SCHEDULE
Pregnancy Risk Category: C

Drug Class: Antitubercular

MECHANISM OF ACTION
An antitubercular whose exact mechanism of action is unknown. *Therapeutic Effect:* Either bacteriostatic or bactericidal, depending on the drug's concentration at the infection site and the susceptibility of infecting bacteria.

USES
Treatment of tuberculosis (TB), as an adjunct with other drugs

PHARMACOKINETICS
PO: Peak 2 hr. *Half-life:* 9–10 hr; metabolized in liver, excreted in urine (metabolites/unchanged drug).

INDICATIONS AND DOSAGES
▶ **TB (in combination with other antituberculars)**
PO
Adults. 15–30 mg/kg/day in 1–4 doses. Maximum: 3 g/day.
Children. 20–40 mg/kg/day in 1 or 2 doses. Maximum: 2 g/day.

SIDE EFFECTS/ADVERSE REACTIONS
Frequent
Arthralgia, myalgia (usually mild and self-limiting)
Rare
Hypersensitivity reaction (rash, pruritus, urticaria), photosensitivity, gouty arthritis

PRECAUTIONS AND CONTRAINDICATIONS
Severe hepatic dysfunction
Caution
Children younger than 13 yr

DRUG INTERACTIONS OF CONCERN TO DENTISTRY
- None reported.

SERIOUS REACTIONS
! Hepatotoxicity, gouty arthritis, thrombocytopenia, and anemia occur rarely.

DENTAL CONSIDERATIONS
General:
- Determine why the patient is taking the drug (for prophylaxis or active therapy).
- Determine that noninfectious status exists by ensuring that (1) anti-TB drugs have been taken for longer than 3 wk, (2) culture has confirmed TB susceptibility to antiinfectives, (3) patient has had 3 consecutive negative sputum smears, and (4) patient is not in the coughing stage.
Consultations:
- Medical consultation may be required to assess disease control.
Teach Patient/Family to:
- Take medications for full length of regimen to ensure effectiveness of treatment and to prevent the emergence of resistant strains

pyridostigmine bromide
peer-id-oh-stig´-meen broe´-mide
(Mestinon, Mestinon SR[CAN], Mestinon Timespan)
Do not confuse pyridostigmine with physostigmine or Mesitonin with Mesantoin or Metatensin.

CATEGORY AND SCHEDULE
Pregnancy Risk Category: C

Drug Class: Cholinergic

MECHANISM OF ACTION
A cholinergic that prevents destruction of acetylcholine by inhibiting the enzyme acetylcholinesterase, thus enhancing impulse transmission across the myoneural junction. *Therapeutic Effect:* Produces miosis; increases tone of intestinal, skeletal muscle; stimulates salivary and sweat gland secretions.

USES
Nondepolarizing muscle relaxant antagonist, myasthenia gravis

PHARMACOKINETICS
PO: Onset 20–30 min, duration 3–6 hr
IM/IV/Subcutaneous: Onset 2–15 min, duration 2.5–4 hr; metabolized in liver, excreted in urine

INDICATIONS AND DOSAGES
▶ **Myasthenia Gravis**
PO
Adults, Elderly. Initially, 60 mg 3 times a day. Dosage increased at 48 hr intervals. Maintenance: 60 mg–1.5 g a day.
PO (Extended-Release)

Adults, Elderly. 180–540 mg once or twice a day with at least a 6 hr interval between doses.
IV, IM
Adults, Elderly. 2 mg q2–3h.
Children, Neonates. 0.05–0.15 mg/kg/dose. Maximum single dose: 10 mg.
▶ **Reversal of Nondepolarizing Neuromuscular Blockade**
IV
Adults, Elderly. 10–20 mg with, or shortly after, 0.6–1.2 mg atropine sulfate or 0.3–0.6 mg glycopyrrolate.
Children. 0.1–0.25 mg/kg/dose preceded by atropine or glycopyrrolate.

SIDE EFFECTS/ADVERSE REACTIONS
Frequent
Miosis, increased GI and skeletal muscle tone, bradycardia, constriction of bronchi and ureters, diaphoresis, increased salivation
Occasional
Headache, rash, temporary decrease in diastolic B/P with mild reflex tachycardia, short periods of atrial fibrillation (in hyperthyroid patients), marked drop in B/P (in hypertensive patients)

PRECAUTIONS AND CONTRAINDICATIONS
Mechanical GI or urinary tract obstruction
Caution
Seizure disorders, bronchial asthma, coronary occlusion, hyperthyroidism, dysrhythmias, peptic ulcer, megacolon, poor GI motility, elderly, lactation

DRUG INTERACTIONS OF CONCERN TO DENTISTRY
• Decreased effects: atropine, scopolamine, and other

anticholinergic drugs;
methocarbamol
• Reduced rate of metabolism of
ester local anesthetics
• Avoid anticholinergic drugs to
control excessive salivation

SERIOUS REACTIONS

❗ Overdose may produce a
cholinergic crisis, manifested as
increasingly severe muscle weakness
that appears first in muscles
involving chewing and swallowing
and is followed by muscle weakness
of the shoulder girdle and upper
extremities, respiratory muscle
paralysis, and pelvis girdle and leg
muscle paralysis. If overdose occurs,
stop all cholinergic drugs and
immediately administer 1–4 mg
atropine sulfate IV for adults or
0.01 mg/kg for infants and children
younger than 12 yr.

DENTAL CONSIDERATIONS

General:
• Monitor vital signs at every
appointment because of
cardiovascular and respiratory side
effects.
• After supine positioning, have
patient sit upright for at least 2 min
before standing to avoid orthostatic
hypotension.
• Schedule short appointments
because of effects of disease on oral
musculature.
• Avoid dental light in patient's eyes;
offer dark glasses for patient
comfort.
• Place on frequent recall because of
oral side effects.
• Consider semisupine chair position
for patient comfort if GI side effects
occur.
Consultations:
• Medical consultation may be
required to assess disease control.

• Consult with physician about
adjusting dose if excessive salivation
becomes a problem.
Teach Patient/Family to:
• Use electric tooth brush or other
oral hygiene aids if patient has
difficulty in maintaining oral hygiene
• Use effective oral hygiene to
prevent soft tissue inflammation
• Prevent injury when using oral
hygiene aids

pyridoxine hydrochloride (vitamin B6)

peer-ih-dox´-een
high-droh-klor´-ide
(Aminoxin, Beesix, Doxine,
Nestrex, Pryi, Pyroxin[AUS],
Rodex, Vitabee 6)
Do not confuse pyridoxine with
paroxetine, pralidoxime, or
Pyridium.

CATEGORY AND SCHEDULE
Pregnancy Risk Category: A
OTC

Drug Class: Vitamin B$_6$, water
soluble

P

MECHANISM OF ACTION
Acts as a coenzyme for various
metabolic functions, including
metabolism of proteins,
carbohydrates, and fats. Aids in the
breakdown of glycogen and in the
synthesis of gamma-aminobutyric
acid in the CNS. *Therapeutic Effect:*
Prevents pyridoxine deficiency.
Increases the excretion of certain
drugs, such as isoniazid, that are
pyridoxine antagonists.

USES

Treatment of vitamin B6 deficiency associated with inborn errors of metabolism, inadequate diet; unapproved: drug-induced deficiencies

PHARMACOKINETICS

Readily absorbed primarily in jejunum. Stored in the liver, muscle, and brain. Metabolized in the liver. Primarily excreted in urine. Removed by hemodialysis.
Half-life: 15–20 days.

INDICATIONS AND DOSAGES

▸ **Pyridoxine Deficiency**
PO
Adults, Elderly. Initially, 2.5–10 mg/day; then 2.5 mg/day when clinical signs are corrected.
Children. Initially, 5–25 mg/day for 3 wk, then 1.5–2.5 mg/day.
▸ **Pyridoxine Dependent Seizures**
PO, IV, IM
Infants. Initially, 10–100 mg/day. Maintenance: PO: 50–100 mg/day.
▸ **Drug-Induced Neuritis**
PO (treatment)
Adults, Elderly. 100–300 mg/day in divided doses.
Children. 10–50 mg/day.
PO (prophylaxis)
Adults, Elderly. 25–100 mg/day.
Children. 1–2 mg/kg/day.

SIDE EFFECTS/ADVERSE REACTIONS

Occasional
Stinging at IM injection site
Rare
Headache, nausea, somnolence; sensory neuropathy (paresthesia, unstable gait, clumsiness of hands) with high doses

PRECAUTIONS AND CONTRAINDICATIONS

Hypersensitivity, Parkinson's disease

DRUG INTERACTIONS OF CONCERN TO DENTISTRY

• Decreased effectiveness: levodopa
• Decreased serum levels of phenytoin, phenobarbital

SERIOUS REACTIONS

❗ Long-term megadoses (2–6 g over more than 2 mo) may produce sensory neuropathy (reduced deep tendon reflexes, profound impairment of sense of position in distal limbs, gradual sensory ataxia). Toxic symptoms subside when drug is discontinued.
❗ Seizures have occurred after IV megadoses.

DENTAL CONSIDERATIONS

General:
• Vitamin B deficiency and peripheral neuropathy may manifest with oral symptoms of glossitis and cheilosis.

pyrimethamine

pye-ri-meth´-ah-meen
(Daraprim, Malocide[FRANCE])
Do not confuse with Dantrium, Daranide.

CATEGORY AND SCHEDULE

Pregnancy Risk Category: C

Drug Class: Antimalarial

MECHANISM OF ACTION

An antiprotozoal with blood and some tissue schizonticidal activity against malaria parasites of humans. Highly selective activity against plasmodia and *Toxoplasma gondii*.

Therapeutic Effect: Inhibition of tetrahydrofolic acid synthesis.

USES
Malaria prophlaxis

PHARMACOKINETICS
Well absorbed, peak levels occurring between 2 and 6 hr following administration. Protein binding: 87%. Eliminated slowly.
Half-life: approximately 96 hr.

INDICATIONS AND DOSAGES
▸ **Toxoplasmosis**
PO
Adults. Initially, 50–75 mg daily, with 1–4 g daily of a sulfonamide of the sulfapyrimidine type (e.g., sulfadoxine). Continue for 1–3 wk, depending on response of patient and tolerance to therapy, then reduce dose to one-half that previously given for each drug and continue for additional 4–5 wk.
Children. 1 mg/kg/day divided into 2 equal daily doses; after 2–4 days reduce to one-half and continue for approximately 1 month. The usual pediatric sulfonamide dosage is used in conjunction with pyrimethamine.
▸ **Acute Malaria**
PO
Adults (in combination with sulfonamide). 25 mg daily for 2 days with a sulfonamide.
Adults (without concomitant sulfonamide). 50 mg for 2 days
Children 4–10 yr. 25 mg daily for 2 days.
▸ **Chemoprophylaxis of Malaria**
PO
Adults and pediatric patients over 10 yr. 25 mg once a wky.
Children 4–10 yr. 12.5 mg once a wk.
Infants and children under 4 yr. 6.25 mg once a wk.

SIDE EFFECTS/ADVERSE REACTIONS
Frequent
Anorexia, vomiting
Occasional
Hypersensitivity reactions, Stevens-Johnson syndrome, toxic epidermal necrolysis, erythema multiforme, anaphylaxis, hyperphenylalaninemia, megaloblastic anemia, leukopenia, thrombocytopenia, pancytopenia, atrophic glossitis, hematuria, and disorders of cardiac rhythm
Rare
Pulmonary eosinophilia

PRECAUTIONS AND CONTRAINDICATIONS
Hypersensitivity to pyrimethamine, megaloblastic anemia due to folate deficiency, monotherapy for treatment of acute malaria.

DRUG INTERACTIONS OF CONCERN TO DENTISTRY
● Possible mild hepatoxicity: lorazepam

SERIOUS REACTIONS
None known

DENTAL CONSIDERATIONS
General:
● Determine why patient is taking the drug.
● Consider semisupine chair position for patient comfort if GI side effects occur.
● Question patient about tolerance of NSAIDs or aspirin related to GI disease.
● Patient on chronic drug therapy may rarely present with symptoms of blood dyscrasias, which can include infection, bleeding, and poor healing. If dyscrasia is present, advise patient to prevent oral tissue trauma when using oral hygiene aids.

P

• Determine why patient is taking drug (prophylaxis or active therapy).
Consultations:
• Medical consultation may be required to assess disease control and patient's ability to tolerate stress.
Teach Patient/Family to:
• Report sore throat, pallor, purpura, or glossitis, which may be symptoms of serious effects

• Use effective oral hygiene to prevent soft tissue inflammation
• Prevent trauma when using oral hygiene aids
• Update health and medication history if physician makes any changes in evaluation or drug regimens; include OTC, herbal, and nonherbal drug in the update

quazepam
kwaz´-eh-pam
(Doral)

CATEGORY AND SCHEDULE
Pregnancy Risk Category: X
Controlled Substance: Schedule IV

Drug Class: Benzodiazepine,
sedative-hypnotic

MECHANISM OF ACTION
A BZ-1 receptor selective
benzodiazepine with sedative
properties. *Therapeutic Effect:*
Produces sedative effect from its
CNS depressant action.

USES
Treatment of insomnia

PHARMACOKINETICS
Rapidly absorbed from GI tract.
Food increases absorption. Protein
binding: 95%. Extensively
metabolized in liver. Excreted in
urine and feces. Unknown if removed
by hemodialysis. *Half-life:* 25–41 hr.

INDICATIONS AND DOSAGES
▸ **Insomnia**
PO
Adults (older than 18 yr). Initially,
15 mg at bedtime. Adjust dose up or
down from 7.5 mg to 30 mg at bedtime,
depending on initial response.
Elderly, debilitated, liver disease.
Initially, 7.5–15 mg at bedtime. Adjust
dose depending on initial response.

SIDE EFFECTS/ADVERSE REACTIONS
Frequent
Muscular incoordination (ataxia),
lightheadedness, transient mild
drowsiness, slurred speech (particularly
in elderly or debilitated patients)

Occasional
Confusion, depression, blurred
vision, constipation, diarrhea,
dry mouth, headache, nausea
Rare
Behavioral problems such as anger,
impaired memory; paradoxic
reactions, such as insomnia,
nervousness, or irritability

PRECAUTIONS AND CONTRAINDICATIONS
Pregnancy, sleep apnea,
hypersensitivity to quazepam or
any component of the formulation
Caution
Hepatic disease, renal disease,
suicidal individuals, drug abuse,
elderly, psychosis, children younger
than 18 yr, lactation, depression,
pulmonary insufficiency

DRUG INTERACTIONS OF CONCERN TO DENTISTRY
• Increased effects: CNS
depressants, alcohol
• Delayed elimination: erythromycin
• Contraindicated with saquinavir,
ritonavir
• Possible increase in CNS side
effects: kava kava (herb)
• Increased serum levels and
prolonged effect of benzodiazepines:
erythromycin, ketoconazole,
itraconazole, fluconazole,
miconazole (systemic)

SERIOUS REACTIONS
! Abrupt or too-rapid withdrawal
may result in pronounced
restlessness, irritability, insomnia,
hand tremors, abdominal and muscle
cramps, sweating, vomiting, and
seizures.
! Overdosage results in somnolence,
confusion, diminished reflexes, and
coma.
! Blood dyscrasias have been
reported rarely.

DENTAL CONSIDERATIONS
General:
- Assess salivary flow as a factor in caries, periodontal disease, and candidiasis.
- Psychologic and physical dependence may occur with chronic administration.
- Geriatric patients are more susceptible to drug effects; use a lower dose.
- Avoid using this drug in a patient with a history of drug abuse or alcoholism.

Consultations:
- Medical consultation may be required to assess disease control.

Teach Patient/Family:
- When chronic dry mouth occurs, advise patient to:
  - Avoid mouth rinses with high alcohol content because of drying effects
  - Use daily home fluoride products to prevent caries
  - Use sugarless gum, frequent sips of water, or saliva substitutes

quetiapine
kwe-tye´-ah-peen
(Seroquel)

CATEGORY AND SCHEDULE
Pregnancy Risk Category: C

Drug Class: Antipsychotic, atypical

MECHANISM OF ACTION
A dibenzepin derivative that antagonizes dopamine, serotonin, histamine, and α_1-adrenergic receptors. ***Therapeutic Effect:*** Diminishes manifestations of psychotic disorders. Produces moderate sedation, few extrapyramidal effects, and no anticholinergic effects.

USES
Treatment of schizophrenia

PHARMACOKINETICS
Well absorbed after PO administration. Protein binding: 83%. Widely distributed in tissues; CNS concentration exceeds plasma concentration. Undergoes extensive first-pass metabolism in the liver. Primarily excreted in urine. ***Half-life:*** 6 hr.

INDICATIONS AND DOSAGES
▶ **To Manage Manifestations of Psychotic Disorders, Bipolar Disorder**
PO
Adults, Elderly. Initially, 25 mg twice a day, then 25–50 mg 2–3 times a day on the second and third days, up to 300–400 mg/day in divided doses 2–3 times a day by the fourth day. Further adjustments of 25–50 mg twice a day may be made at intervals of 2 days or longer. Maintenance: 300–800 mg/day (adults); 50–200 mg/day (elderly).
▶ **Dosage in Hepatic Impairment, Elderly or Debilitated Patients, and Those Predisposed to Hypotensive Reactions**
These patients should receive a lower initial dose and lower dosage increases.

SIDE EFFECTS/ADVERSE REACTIONS
Frequent
Headache, somnolence, dizziness
Occasional
Constipation, orthostatic hypotension, tachycardia, dry mouth, dyspepsia, rash, asthenia, abdominal pain, rhinitis

Rare
Back pain, fever, weight gain

PRECAUTIONS AND CONTRAINDICATIONS
Renal impairment, hepatic impairment, cardiovascular disease, thyroid disease, hyperprolactinemia, neuromalignant syndrome, tardive dyskinesia, seizure disorders, cataracts, dementia, suicide tendency, lactation; patients should be monitored for signs and symptoms of diabetes mellitus, severe CNS depression.

DRUG INTERACTIONS OF CONCERN TO DENTISTRY
• Risk of increased CNS depression: CNS depressants

SERIOUS REACTIONS
! Overdose may produce heart block, hypotension, hypokalemia, and tachycardia.

DENTAL CONSIDERATIONS
General:
• Monitor vital signs at every appointment because of cardiovascular and respiratory side effects.
• Assess salivary flow as factor in caries, periodontal disease, and candidiasis.
• Assess for presence of extrapyramidal motor symptoms, such as tardive dyskinesia and akathisia. Extrapyramidal motor activity may complicate dental treatment.
• After supine positioning, have patient sit upright for at least 2 min before standing to avoid orthostatic hypotension.
• Consider semisupine chair position for patient comfort if GI side effects occur.

• Patients on chronic drug therapy may rarely have symptoms of blood dyscrasias, which can include infection, bleeding, and poor healing.
• Place on frequent recall because of oral side effects.
Consultations:
• In a patient with symptoms of blood dyscrasias, request a medical consultation for blood studies and postpone treatment until normal values are reestablished.
• Medical consultation may be required to assess disease control and patient's ability to tolerate stress.
• If signs of tardive dyskinesia or akathisia are present, refer to physician.
• Consultation with physician may be necessary if sedation or general anesthesia is required.
• Physician should be informed if significant xerostomic side effects occur (e.g., increased caries, sore tongue, problems eating or swallowing, difficulty wearing prosthesis) so that a medication change can be considered.
Teach Patient/Family to:
• Use caution to prevent trauma when using oral hygiene aids
• Use electric tooth brush if patient has difficulty holding conventional devices
• Use effective oral hygiene to prevent soft tissue inflammation
• Update health and drug history if physician makes any changes in evaluation or drug regimens; include OTC, herbal, and nonherbal drugs in the update
• Be aware of oral side effects and potential sequelae
• When chronic dry mouth occurs, advise patient to:
  • Avoid mouth rinses with high alcohol content because of drying effects

Q

- Use daily home fluoride products for anticaries effect
- Use sugarless gum, frequent sips of water, or saliva substitutes

quinapril
kwin´-ah-pril
(Accupril, Asig[AUS])
Do not confuse Accupril with Accolate or Accutane.

CATEGORY AND SCHEDULE
Pregnancy Risk Category: C (D if used in second or third trimester)

Drug Class: Angiotensin-converting enzyme (ACE) inhibitor

MECHANISM OF ACTION
An ACE inhibitor that suppresses the renin-angiotensin-aldosterone system and prevents the conversion of angiotensin I to angiotensin II, a potent vasoconstrictor; may also inhibit angiotensin II at local vascular and renal sites. *Therapeutic Effect:* Reduces peripheral arterial resistance, B/P, and pulmonary capillary wedge pressure; improves cardiac output.

USES
Treatment of hypertension, alone or in combination with thiazide diuretics, heart failure

PHARMACOKINETICS

Route	Onset	Peak	Duration
PO	1 hr	N/A	24 hr

Readily absorbed from the GI tract. Protein binding: 97%. Metabolized in the liver, GI tract, and extravascular tissue to active metabolite. Primarily excreted in urine. Minimal removal by hemodialysis. *Half-life:* 1–2 hr; metabolite, 3 hr (increased in those with impaired renal function).

INDICATIONS AND DOSAGES
▶ **Hypertension (monotherapy)**
PO
Adults. Initially, 10–20 mg/day. May adjust dosage at intervals of at least 2 wk or longer. Maintenance: 20–80 mg/day as single dose or 2 divided doses. Maximum: 80 mg/day.
Elderly. Initially, 2.5–5 mg/day. May increase by 2.5–5 mg q1–2wk.
▶ **Hypertension (combination therapy)**
PO
Adults. Initially, 5 mg/day titrated to patient's needs.
Elderly. Initially, 2.5–5 mg/day. May increase by 2.5–5 mg q1–2wk.
▶ **Adjunct to Manage Heart Failure**
PO
Adults, Elderly. Initially, 5 mg twice a day. Range: 20–40 mg/day.
▶ **Dosage in Renal Impairment**
Dosage is titrated to the patient's needs after the following initial doses:

Creatinine Clearance	Initial Dose
More than 60 ml/min	10 mg
30–60 ml/min	5 mg
10–29 ml/min	2.5 mg

SIDE EFFECTS/ADVERSE REACTIONS
Frequent
Headache, dizziness
Occasional
Fatigue, vomiting, nausea, hypotension, chest pain, cough, syncope

Rare
Diarrhea, cough, dyspnea, rash, palpitations, impotence, insomnia, drowsiness, malaise

PRECAUTIONS AND CONTRAINDICATIONS

Bilateral renal artery stenosis
Caution
Pregnancy category D, impaired renal/liver function, dialysis patients, hypovolemia, blood dyscrasias, CHF, COPD, asthma, elderly, lactation

DRUG INTERACTIONS OF CONCERN TO DENTISTRY

- Increased hypotension: alcohol, phenothiazines
- Decreased hypotensive effects: indomethacin and possibly other NSAIDs, sympathomimetics
- Suspected reduction in the antihypertensive and vasodilator effects by salicylates; monitor B/P if used concurrently

SERIOUS REACTIONS

! Excessive hypotension ("first-dose syncope") may occur in patients with CHF and in those who are severely salt or volume depleted.
! Angioedema and hyperkalemia occur rarely.
! Agranulocytosis and neutropenia may be noted in those with collagen vascular disease, including scleroderma and systemic lupus erythematosus, and impaired renal function.
! Nephrotic syndrome may be noted in those with history of renal disease.

DENTAL CONSIDERATIONS

General:
- Monitor vital signs at every appointment because of cardiovascular side effects.

- After supine positioning, have patient sit upright for at least 2 min before standing to avoid orthostatic hypotension.
- Patients on chronic drug therapy may rarely have symptoms of blood dyscrasias, which can include infection, bleeding, and poor healing.
- Assess salivary flow as a factor in caries, periodontal disease, and candidiasis.
- Limit use of sodium-containing products, such as saline IV fluids, for patients with a dietary salt restriction.
- Use vasoconstrictors with caution, in low doses, and with careful aspiration.
- Stress from dental procedures may compromise cardiovascular function; determine patient risk.
- Short appointments and a stress reduction protocol may be required for anxious patients.

Consultations:
- Medical consultation may be required to assess disease control and patient's ability to tolerate stress.
- In a patient with symptoms of blood dyscrasias, request a medical consultation for blood studies and postpone dental treatment until normal values are reestablished.
- Take precautions if dental surgery is anticipated and sedation or general anesthesia is required; risk of hypotensive episode.

Teach Patient/Family to:
- Use effective oral hygiene to prevent soft tissue inflammation
- Use caution to prevent injury when using oral hygiene aids
- When chronic dry mouth occurs, advise patient to:
  - Avoid mouth rinses with high alcohol content because of drying effects

• Use daily home fluoride products to prevent caries
• Use sugarless gum, frequent sips of water, or saliva substitutes

quinidine

kwin´-ih-deen
(Apo-Quin-G[CAN], Apo-Quinidine[CAN], BioQuin Durules[CAN], Kinidin Durules[AUS], Quinaglute Dura-Tabs, Quinate[CAN], Quinidex Extentabs)
Do not confuse quinidine with clonidine or quinine.

CATEGORY AND SCHEDULE
Pregnancy Risk Category: C

Drug Class: Antidysrhythmic (class Ia)

MECHANISM OF ACTION
An antidysrhythmic that decreases sodium influx during depolarization, potassium efflux during repolarization, and reduces calcium transport across the myocardial cell membrane. Decreases myocardial excitability, conduction velocity, and contractility. **Therapeutic Effect:** Suppresses cardiac dysrhythmias.

USES
Treatment of premature ventricular contractions (PVCs), atrial flutter and fibrillation, PAT, ventricular tachycardia

PHARMACOKINETICS
PO: Peak 0.5–6 hr (depending on form given), duration 6–8 hr, **Half-life:** 6–7 hr; metabolized in liver; excreted unchanged by kidneys.

INDICATIONS AND DOSAGES
▶ **Maintenance of Normal Sinus Rhythm after Conversion of Atrial Fibrillation or Flutter; Prevention of Premature Atrial, AV, and Ventricular Contractions; Paroxysmal Atrial Tachycardia; Paroxysmal AV Junctional Rhythm; Atrial Fibrillation; Atrial Flutter; Paroxysmal Ventricular Tachycardia not Associated with Complete Heart Block**
PO
Adults, Elderly. 100–600 mg q4–6h. Long-acting: 324–972 mg q8–12h.
Children: 30 mg/kg/day in divided doses q4–6h.
IV
Adults, Elderly. 200–400 mg.
Children. 2–10 mg/kg.

SIDE EFFECTS/ADVERSE REACTIONS
Frequent
Abdominal pain and cramps, nausea, diarrhea, vomiting (can be immediate, intense)
Occasional
Mild cinchonism (ringing in ears, blurred vision, hearing loss) or severe cinchonism (headache, vertigo, diaphoresis, light-headedness, photophobia, confusion, delirium)
Rare
Hypotension (particularly with IV administration), hypersensitivity reaction (fever, anaphylaxis, photosensitivity reaction)

PRECAUTIONS AND CONTRAINDICATIONS
Complete AV block, intraventricular conduction defects (widening of QRS complex)
Caution
Lactation, children, renal disease, potassium imbalance, liver disease, CHF, respiratory depression

DRUG INTERACTIONS OF CONCERN TO DENTISTRY
* May decrease effects of quinidine: barbiturates
* Increased anticholinergic effect: anticholinergic drugs
* Increased effects of neuromuscular blockers, tricyclic antidepressants
* Contraindicated with itraconazole
* Prevention of action: cholinergics

SERIOUS REACTIONS
! Cardiotoxic effects occur most commonly with IV administration, particularly at high concentrations, and are observed as conduction changes (50% widening of QRS complex, prolonged QT interval, flattened T waves, and disappearance of P wave), ventricular tachycardia or flutter, frequent PVCs, or complete AV block.
! Quinidine-induced syncope may occur with the usual dosage.
! Severe hypotension may result from high dosages.
! Patients with atrial flutter and fibrillation may experience a paradoxical, exremely rapid ventricular rate that may be prevented by prior digitalization.
! Hepatotoxicity with jaundice due to drug hypersensitivity may occur.

DENTAL CONSIDERATIONS
General:
* Monitor vital signs at every appointment because of cardiovascular and respiratory side effects.
* Patients on chronic drug therapy may rarely have symptoms of blood dyscrasias, which can include infection, bleeding, and poor healing.
* After supine positioning, have patient sit upright for at least 2 min before standing to avoid orthostatic hypotension.

* Use vasoconstrictors with caution, in low doses, and with careful aspiration. Avoid use of gingival retraction cord with epinephrine.
* Consider semisupine chair position for patient comfort if GI side effects occur.
Consultations:
* In a patient with symptoms of blood dyscrasias, request a medical consultation for blood studies and postpone dental treatment until normal values are reestablished.
* Medical consultation may be required to assess patient's ability to tolerate stress.
Teach Patient/Family to:
* Use effective oral hygiene to prevent soft tissue inflammation

quinine
kwye´-nine
(Quinine)
Do not confuse with quinidine.

CATEGORY AND SCHEDULE
Pregnancy Risk Category: X

Drug Class: Antimalarial

MECHANISM OF ACTION
A cinchone alkaloid that relaxes skeletal muscle by increasing the refractory period, decreasing excitability of motor end plates (curare-like), and affecting distribution of calcium with muscle fiber. Antimalarial: Depresses oxygen uptake, carbohydrate metabolism, elevates pH in intracellular organelles of parasites. *Therapeutic Effect:* Relaxes skeletal muscle; produces parasite death.

USES
Treatment of *P. falciparum* malaria, nocturnal leg cramps

PHARMACOKINETICS
Rapidly absorbed mainly from upper small intestine. Protein binding: 70%–95%. Metabolized in liver. Excreted in feces, saliva, and urine. *Half-life:* 8–14 hr (adults), 6–12 hr (children).

INDICATIONS AND DOSAGES
▸ **Nocturnal Leg Cramps**
PO
Adults, Elderly. 260–300 mg at bedtime as needed.
▸ **Treatment of Malaria**
PO
Adults, Elderly. 260–650 mg 3 times a day for 6–12 days.
Children. 10 mg/kg q8h for 5–7 days.
▸ **Dosage in Renal Impairment**

Creatinine Clearance	Dosage Interval
10–50 ml/min	75% of normal dose or q12h
Less than 10 ml/min	30%–50% of normal dose or q24h

SIDE EFFECTS/ADVERSE REACTIONS
Frequent
Nausea, headache, tinnitus, slight visual disturbances (mild cinchonism)
Occasional
Extreme flushing of skin with intense generalized pruritus is most typical hypersensitivity reaction; also rash, wheezing, dyspnea, angioedema. Prolonged therapy: cardiac conduction disturbances, decreased hearing

PRECAUTIONS AND CONTRAINDICATIONS
Hypersensitivity to quinine (possible cross-sensitivity to quinidine), G-6-PD deficiency, tinnitus, optic neuritis, history of thrombocytopenia during previous quinine therapy, blackwater fever
Caution
Blood dyscrasias, severe GI disease, neurologic disease, severe hepatic disease, psoriasis, cardiac dysrhythmias, tinnitus

DRUG INTERACTIONS OF CONCERN TO DENTISTRY
• Decreased absorption: magnesium or aluminum salts
• Prolonged duration of neuromuscular blocking drugs

SERIOUS REACTIONS
! Overdosage (severe cinchonism) may result in cardiovascular effects, severe headache, intestinal cramps with vomiting and diarrhea, apprehension, confusion, seizures, blindness, and respiratory depression.
! Hypoprothrombinemia, thrombocytopenic purpura, hemoglobinuria, asthma, agranulocytosis, hypoglycemia, deafness, and optic atrophy occur rarely.

DENTAL CONSIDERATIONS
General:
• Patients on chronic drug therapy rarely may have symptoms of blood dyscrasias, which can include infection, bleeding, and poor healing.
• Avoid dental light in patient's eyes; offer dark glasses for patient comfort.
• Monitor vital signs at every appointment because of cardiovascular side effects.

Q

• Consider semisupine chair position for patient comfort if GI side effects occur.

Consultations:
• Medical consultation may be required to assess disease control.
• In a patient with symptoms of blood dyscrasias, request a medical consultation for blood studies and postpone dental treatment until normal values are reestablished.

Teach Patient/Family to:
• Use effective oral hygiene to prevent soft tissue inflammation

Q

rabeprazole sodium

rah-bep′-rah-zole soe′-dee-um
(Aciphex, Pariet[CAN])
Do not confuse Aciphex with
Accupril or Aricept.

CATEGORY AND SCHEDULE
Pregnancy Risk Category: B

Drug Class: Antisecretory,
proton pump inhibitor

MECHANISM OF ACTION
A proton pump inhibitor that
converts to active metabolites that
irreversibly bind to and inhibit
hydrogen-potassium adenosine
triphosphate, an enzyme on the
surface of gastric parietal cells.
Actively secretes hydrogen ions for
potassium ions, resulting in an
accumulation of hydrogen ions in
gastric lumen. *Therapeutic Effect:*
Increases gastric pH, reducing gastric
acid production.

USES
Treatment of gastroesophageal reflux
disease (GERD), duodenal ulcers,
and hypersecretory conditions
(Zollinger-Ellison disease);
eradication of *Helicobacter pylori*
infection (with amoxicillin and
clarithromycin), *H. pylori* eradication
to reduce risk of duodenal ulcer

PHARMACOKINETICS
Rapidly absorbed from the GI tract
after passing through the stomach
relatively intact. Protein binding:
96%. Metabolized extensively in the
liver. Primarily excreted in urine.
Unknown if removed by
hemodialysis. *Half-life:*
1–2 hr (increased with hepatic
impairment).

INDICATIONS AND DOSAGES
▸ **GERD**
PO
Adults, Elderly. 20 mg/day for
4–8 wk. Maintenance: 20 mg/day.
▸ **Duodenal Ulcer**
PO
Adults, Elderly. 20 mg/day after
morning meal for 4 wk.
▸ **NSAID-Induced Ulcer**
PO
Adults, Elderly. 20 mg/day.
▸ **Pathologic Hypersecretory
Conditions**
PO
Adults, Elderly. Initially, 60 mg/day.
May increase to 60 mg twice
a day.
▸ **Helibacter pylori Infection**
PO
Adults, Elderly. 20 mg twice a day
for 7 days (given with amoxicillin
1,000 mg and clarithromycin
500 mg).

SIDE EFFECTS/ADVERSE
REACTIONS
Rare
Headache, nausea, dizziness, rash,
diarrhea, malaise

PRECAUTIONS AND
CONTRAINDICATIONS
Hypersensitivity
Caution
Do not break, crush, or chew tablets,
avoid nursing, pediatric use not
studied

DRUG INTERACTIONS OF
CONCERN TO DENTISTRY
None reported

SERIOUS REACTIONS
! Hyperglycemia, hypokalemia,
hyponatremia, and hyperlipemia
occur rarely.

DENTAL CONSIDERATIONS
General:
• Assess salivary flow as a factor in caries, periodontal disease, and candidiasis.
• Consider semisupine chair position for patient comfort because of GI side effects of disease.
• Patients with gastroesophageal reflux may have oral symptoms, including burning mouth, secondary candidiasis, and signs of tooth erosion.
• Question the patient about tolerance of NSAIDs or aspirin related to GI problems.
Teach Patient/Family to:
• Prevent trauma when using oral hygiene aids
• When chronic dry mouth occurs, advise patient to:
  • Avoid mouth rinses with high alcohol content because of drying effects
  • Use daily home fluoride products for anticaries effect
  • Use sugarless gum, frequent sips of water, or saliva substitutes

raloxifene
ra-lox′-ih-feen
(Evista)
Do not confuse raloxifene with propoxyphene.

CATEGORY AND SCHEDULE
Pregnancy Risk Category: X

Drug Class: Synthetic estrogen

MECHANISM OF ACTION
A selective estrogen receptor modulator that affects some receptors like estrogen. *Therapeutic Effect:* Like estrogen, prevents bone loss and improves lipid profiles.

USES
Prevention and treatment of osteoporosis in postmenopausal women, supplemented with calcium as based on need

PHARMACOKINETICS
Rapidly absorbed after PO administration. Highly bound to plasma proteins (more than 95%) and albumin. Undergoes extensive first-pass metabolism in liver. Excreted mainly in feces and, to a lesser extent, in urine. Unknown if removed by hemodialysis.
Half-life: 27.7 hr.

INDICATIONS AND DOSAGES
▶ **Prevention or Treatment of Osteoporosis**
PO
Adults, Elderly. 60 mg/day.

SIDE EFFECTS/ADVERSE REACTIONS
Frequent
Hot flashes, flu-like symptoms, arthralgia, sinusitis
Occasional
Weight gain, nausea, myalgia, pharyngitis, cough, dyspepsia, leg cramps, rash, depression
Rare
Vaginitis, UTI, peripheral edema, flatulence, vomiting, fever, migraine, diaphoresis

PRECAUTIONS AND CONTRAINDICATIONS
Active or history of venous thromboembolic events, such as deep vein thrombosis, pulmonary embolism, and retinal vein thrombosis; women who are or may become pregnant.

R

Caution
Hepatic impairment, risk of
thromboembolitic events, pregnancy
category X, lactation

DRUG INTERACTIONS OF CONCERN TO DENTISTRY

• Reduced absorption: ampicillin
• Risk of potential drug interactions
with other highly plasma protein-
bound drugs, such as NSAIDs,
aspirin, and diazepam, is unknown

SERIOUS REACTIONS

! Pneumonia, gastroenteritis, chest
pain, vaginal bleeding, and breast
pain occur rarely.

DENTAL CONSIDERATIONS

General:
• Drug should be discontinued
72 hr before prolonged
immobilization, such as
hospitalization, postsurgical
recovery, and bed rest.
• Consider short appointments and
dental chair position if needed for
patient comfort.
Consultations:
• Medical consultation may be
required to assess disease
control and patient's ability to
tolerate stress.

R

ramipril
ram′-ih-pril
(Altace, Ramace[AUS], Tritace[AUS])
Do not confuse Altace with
Alteplase or Artane.

CATEGORY AND SCHEDULE
Pregnancy Risk Category: C (D if
used in second or third trimester)

Drug Class: Angiotensin-
converting enzyme (ACE) inhibitor

MECHANISM OF ACTION
An ACE inhibitor that suppresses the
renin-angiotensin-aldosterone
system. Decreases plasma
angiotensin II, increases plasma
renin activity, and decreases
aldosterone secretion. *Therapeutic
Effect:* Reduces peripheral arterial
resistance and B/P.

USES
Treatment of hypertension; alone or
in combination with thiazide
diuretics; CHF immediately after MI;
reduce risk of MI, stroke, and death
from cardiovascular causes

PHARMACOKINETICS

Route	Onset	Peak	Duration
PO	1–2 hr	3–6 hr	24 hr

Well absorbed from the GI tract.
Protein binding: 73%. Metabolized
in the liver to active metabolite.
Primarily excreted in urine.
Not removed by hemodialysis.
Half-life: 5.1 hr.

INDICATIONS AND DOSAGES
▸ **Hypertension (monotherapy)**
PO
Adults, Elderly. Initially, 2.5 mg/day.
Maintenance: 2.5–20 mg/day as
single dose or in 2 divided doses.
▸ **Hypertension (in combination with
other antihypertensives)**
PO
Adults, Elderly. Initially, 1.25 mg/day
titrated to patient's needs.
▸ **CHF**
PO
Adults, Elderly. Initially, 1.25–2.5 mg
twice a day. Maximum: 5 mg twice a
day.
▸ **Risk Reduction for MI Stroke**
PO
Adults, Elderly. Initially, 2.5 mg/day
for 7 days, then 5 mg/day for

21 days, then 10 mg/day as a single dose or in divided doses.

▸ **Dosage in Renal Impairment**

Creatinine clearance 40 ml/min or less. 25% of normal dose.

Hypertension. Initially, 1.25 mg/day titrated upward.

CHF. Initially, 1.25 mg/day, titrated up to 2.5 mg twice a day.

SIDE EFFECTS/ADVERSE REACTIONS

Frequent

Cough, headache

Occasional

Dizziness, fatigue, nausea, asthenia (loss of strength)

Rare

Palpitations, insomnia, nervousness, malaise, abdominal pain, myalgia

PRECAUTIONS AND CONTRAINDICATIONS

Bilateral renal artery stenosis

Caution

Impaired renal/liver function, dialysis patients, hypovolemia, blood dyscrasias, CHF, COPD, asthma, elderly

DRUG INTERACTIONS OF CONCERN TO DENTISTRY

• Increased hypotension: alcohol, phenothiazines

• Decreased hypotensive effects: indomethacin and possibly other NSAIDs, sympathomimetics

• Suspected reduction in the antihypertensive and vasodilator effects by salicylates; monitor B/P if used concurrently

SERIOUS REACTIONS

❗ Excessive hypotension ("first-dose syncope") may occur in patients with CHF and in those who are severely salt or volume depleted.

❗ Angioedema and hyperkalemia occur rarely.

❗ Agranulocytosis and neutropenia may be noted in those with collagen vascular disease, including scleroderma and systemic lupus erythematosus, and impaired renal function.

❗ Nephrotic syndrome may be noted in those with history of renal disease.

DENTAL CONSIDERATIONS

General:

• Monitor vital signs at every appointment because of cardiovascular and respiratory side effects.

• After supine positioning, have patient sit upright for at least 2 min before standing to avoid orthostatic hypotension.

• Patients on chronic drug therapy may rarely have symptoms of blood dyscrasias, which can include infection, bleeding, and poor healing.

• Assess salivary flow as a factor in caries, periodontal disease, and candidiasis.

• Limit use of sodium-containing products, such as saline IV fluids, for patients with a dietary salt restriction.

• Use vasoconstrictors with caution, in low doses, and with careful aspiration.

• Stress from dental procedures may compromise cardiovascular function; determine patient risk.

• Short appointments and a stress-reduction protocol may be required for anxious patients.

Consultations:

• Medical consultation may be required to assess patient's ability to tolerate stress.

• In a patient with symptoms of blood dyscrasias, request a medical consultation for blood studies and

postpone dental treatment until normal values are reestablished.
• Take precautions if dental surgery is anticipated and sedation or general anesthesia is required; risk of hypotensive episode.
Teach Patient/Family to:
• Use effective oral hygiene to prevent soft tissue inflammation
• Use caution to prevent injury when using oral hygiene aids
• When chronic dry mouth occurs, advise patient to:
  • Avoid mouth rinses with high alcohol content because of drying effects
  • Use daily home fluoride products to prevent caries
  • Use sugarless gum, frequent sips of water, or saliva substitutes

ranitidine hydrochloride/ ranitidine bismuth citrate

ra-ni′-ti-deen high-droh-klor′-ide/ ra-ni′-ti-deen biss′-mooth sih′-trate (ranitidine hydrochloride: Apo-Ranitidine[CAN], Ausran[AUS], Novo-Ranitidine[CAN], Rani-2[AUS], Ranihexal[AUS], Zantac, Zantac-75, Zantac-150, Zantac-300, Zantac EFFERdose, Zantac-25 EFFERdose, Zantac-150 EFFERdose, Zantac-150 Maximum Strength; ranitidine bismuth citrate: Pylorid[AUS], Tritec)
Do not confuse Zantac with Xanax, Ziac, or Zyrtec.

CATEGORY AND SCHEDULE
Pregnancy Risk Category: B
OTC (75 mg tablets)

Drug Class: H_2 histamine receptor antagonist

MECHANISM OF ACTION
An antiulcer agent that inhibits histamine action at histamine 2 receptors of gastric parietal cells. ***Therapeutic Effect:*** Inhibits gastric acid secretion when fasting, at night, or when stimulated by food, caffeine, or insulin. Reduces volume and hydrogen ion concentration of gastric juice.

USES
Treatment of duodenal ulcer, Zollinger-Ellison syndrome, benign gastric ulcers, hypersecretory conditions, gastroesophageal reflux disease, erosive esophagitis, stress ulcers; unapproved: treatment of GI symptoms associated with NSAID use in rheumatoid arthritis

PHARMACOKINETICS
Rapidly absorbed from the GI tract. Protein binding: 15%. Widely distributed. Metabolized in the liver. Primarily excreted in urine. Not removed by hemodialysis. ***Half-life:*** PO, 2.5 hr; IV, 2–2.5 hr (increased with impaired renal function).

INDICATIONS AND DOSAGES
▶ **Duodenal Ulcers, Gastric Ulcers, Gastroesophageal Reflux Disease**
PO
Adults, Elderly. 150 mg twice a day or 300 mg at bedtime. Maintenance: 150 mg at bedtime.
Children. 2–4 mg/kg/day in divided doses twice a day. Maximum: 300 mg/day.
▶ **Duodenal Ulcers Associated with H. Pylori Infection**
PO
Adults, Elderly. 400 mg twice a day for 4 wk in combination with clarithromycin 500 mg 2–3 times a day for the first 2 wk.

▶ **Erosive Esophagitis**
PO
Adults, Elderly. 150 mg 4 times a
day. Maintenance: 150 mg twice a
day or 300 mg at bedtime.
Children. 4–10 mg/kg/day in
2 divided doses. Maximum:
600 mg/day.

▶ **Hypersecretory Conditions**
PO
Adults, Elderly. 150 mg twice a day.
May increase up to 6 g/day.

▶ **OTC Use**
PO
Adults, Elderly. 75 mg 30–60 min
before eating food or drinking
beverages that cause heartburn.
Maximum: 150 mg per 24-hr period
and/or longer than 14 days.

▶ **Usual Parenteral Dosage**
IV, IM
Adults, Elderly. 50 mg/dose q6–8h.
Maximum: 400 mg/day.
Children. 2–4 mg/kg/day in divided
doses q6–8h. Maximum:
200 mg/day.

▶ **Usual Neonatal Dosage**
PO
Neonates. 2 mg/kg/day in divided
doses q12h.
IV
Neonates. Initially, 1.5 mg/kg/dose;
then 1.5–2 mg/kg/day in divided
doses q12h.

▶ **Dosage in Renal Impairment**
For patients with creatinine clearance
less than 50 ml/min, give 150 mg PO
q24h or 50 mg IV or IM q18–24h.

SIDE EFFECTS/ADVERSE REACTIONS
Occasional
Diarrhea
Rare
Constipation, headache (may be
severe)

PRECAUTIONS AND CONTRAINDICATIONS
History of acute porphyria
Caution
Pregnancy category B, lactation,
children younger than 12 yr, hepatic
disease, renal disease

DRUG INTERACTIONS OF CONCERN TO DENTISTRY
• Decreased absorption of diazepam,
anticholinergics, ketoconazole (take
doses 2 hr apart)

SERIOUS REACTIONS
! Reversible hepatitis and blood
dyscrasias occur rarely.

DENTAL CONSIDERATIONS
General:
• Avoid prescribing aspirin-
containing products in patients with
active GI disease.
• Consider semisupine chair position
for patient comfort because of GI
effects of disease.

repaglinide
re-pag′-lih-nide
(GlucoNorm[CAN], NovoNorm[AUS],
Prandin)

CATEGORY AND SCHEDULE
Pregnancy Risk Category: C

Drug Class: Oral antidiabetic,
meglitinide class

MECHANISM OF ACTION
An antihyperglycemic that stimulates
release of insulin from beta cells of
the pancreas by depolarizing beta
cells, leading to an opening of
calcium channels. Resulting calcium
influx induces insulin secretion.

Therapeutic Effect: Lowers blood glucose concentration.

USES

Treatment of type 2 diabetes mellitus when hyperglycemia cannot be controlled by diet and exercise; may also be used in combination with metformin, rosiglitazone maleate, or pioglitazone HCl

PHARMACOKINETICS

Rapidly, completely absorbed from the GI tract. Protein binding: 98%. Metabolized in the liver to inactive metabolites. Excreted primarily in feces with a lesser amount in urine. Unknown if removed by hemodialysis. *Half-life:* 1 hr.

INDICATIONS AND DOSAGES
▸ **Diabetes Mellitus**
PO
Adults, Elderly. 0.5–4 mg 2–4 times a day. Maximum: 16 mg/day.

SIDE EFFECTS/ADVERSE REACTIONS

Frequent
Upper respiratory tract infection, headache, rhinitis, bronchitis, back pain
Occasional
Diarrhea, dyspepsia, sinusitis, nausea, arthralgia, UTI
Rare
Constipation, vomiting, paresthesia, allergy

PRECAUTIONS AND CONTRAINDICATIONS

Diabetic ketoacidosis, type 1 diabetes mellitus
Caution
Increased cardiac mortality risk, hypoglycemia, hypoglycemia in patients taking adrenergic blockers, monitor laboratory values, lactation, pediatric patients

DRUG INTERACTIONS OF CONCERN TO DENTISTRY

● Clinical studies have not been completed; metabolism may be inhibited by ketoconazole, miconazole, erythromycin
● Risk of increased hypoglycemia: NSAIDs, salicylates
● Suspected increase in plasma levels: clarithromycin, erythromycin

SERIOUS REACTIONS

❗ Hypoglycemia occurs in 16% of patients.
❗ Chest pain occurs rarely.

DENTAL CONSIDERATIONS

General:
● If dentist prescribes any of the drugs listed in the drug interactions section, monitor patient blood sugar levels.
● Consider semisupine chair position for patient comfort because of GI side effects of drug.
● Ensure that patient is following prescribed diet and regularly takes medication.
● Place on frequent recall to evaluate healing response.
● Short appointments and a stress-reduction protocol may be required.
● Diabetics may be more susceptible to infection and have delayed wound healing.
Consultations:
● Medical consultation may include data from patient's blood glucose monitoring, including glycosylated hemoglobin or HbA_{1c} testing.
● Medical consultation may be required to assess disease control and patient's ability to tolerate stress.

Teach Patient/Family to:
• Prevent trauma when using oral hygiene aids
• Update health and drug history if physician makes any changes in evaluation or drug regimens; include OTC, herbal, and nonherbal drugs in the update

reserpine
reh-zer′-peen
(Serpalan, Maviserpin[MEX], Novoreserpine[CAN], Rauserpine[TAIWAN], Rauverid[PHILIPPINES], Reserfia[CAN], Serpasil[CAN, INDONESIA], Serpasol[SPAIN])
Do not confuse with Risperdal, risperidone

CATEGORY AND SCHEDULE
Pregnancy Risk Category: C

Drug Class: Antiadrenergic agent, antihypertensive

MECHANISM OF ACTION
An antihypertensive that depletes stores of catecholamines and 5-hydroxytryptamine in many organs, including the brain and adrenal medulla. Depression of sympathetic nerve function results in a decreased heart rate and a lowering of arterial B/P. Depletion of catecholamines and 5-hydroxytryptamine from the brain is thought to be the mechanism of the sedative and tranquilizing properties. ***Therapeutic Effects:*** Decrease B/P and heart rate; sedation.

USES
Treatment of hypertension

PHARMACOKINETICS
Characterized by slow onset of action and sustained effects. Both cardiovascular and CNS effects may persist for a period of time following withdrawal of the drug. Mean maximum plasma levels were attained after a median of 3.5 hr. Bioavailability was approximately 50% of that of a corresponding intravenous dose. Protein binding: 96%. ***Half life:*** 33 hr.

INDICATIONS AND DOSAGES
▶ **Hypertension**
PO
Adults: Usual initial dosage 0.5 mg/day for 1 or 2 wk. For maintenance, reduce to 0.1–0.25 mg/day.
Children: Reserpine is not recommended for use in children. If it is to be used in treating a child, the usual recommended starting dose is 20 μg/kg daily. The maximum recommended dose is 0.25 mg (total) daily.
▶ **Psychiatric Disorders**
PO
Adults: Initial dosage 0.5 mg/day, may range from 0.1 to 1.0 mg. Adjust dosage upward or downward according to response.

SIDE EFFECTS/ADVERSE REACTIONS
Occasional
Burning in the stomach, nausea, vomiting, diarrhea, dry mouth, nosebleed, stuffy nose, dizziness, headache, nervousness, nightmares, drowsiness, muscle aches, weight gain, redness of the eyes
Rare
Irregular heart beat, difficulty breathing, heart problems, feeling faint, swelling, gynecomastia, decreased libido

R

PRECAUTIONS AND CONTRAINDICATIONS

Hypersensitivity, mental depression or history of mental depression (especially with suicidal tendencies), active peptic ulcer, ulcerative colitis, patients receiving electroconvulsive therapy

Caution

Lactation, seizure disorders, renal disease

DRUG INTERACTIONS OF CONCERN TO DENTISTRY

• Increased CNS depression: barbiturates, alcohol, opioids
• Increased pressor effects: epinephrine
• Decreased pressor effects: ephedrine, tricyclic antidepressants
• Decreased hypotensive effect: indomethacin and possibly other NSAIDs

SERIOUS REACTIONS

None known

DENTAL CONSIDERATIONS

General:

• Monitor vital signs at every appointment because of cardiovascular side effects.
• Patients on chronic drug therapy may rarely have symptoms of blood dyscrasias, which can include infection, bleeding, and poor healing.
• Assess salivary flow as a factor in caries, periodontal disease, and candidiasis.
• After supine positioning, have patient sit upright for at least 2 min before standing to avoid orthostatic hypotension.
• Limit use of sodium-containing products, such as saline IV fluids, for patients with a dietary salt restriction.

Consultations:

• Medical consultation may be required to assess disease control.

Teach Patient/Family to:

• Use effective oral hygiene to prevent soft tissue inflammation
• When chronic dry mouth occurs, advise patient to:
   • Avoid mouth rinses with high alcohol content because of drying effects
   • Use daily home fluoride products to prevent caries
   • Use sugarless gum, frequent sips of water, or saliva substitutes

reteplase, recombinant

reh´-te-place
(Rapilysin[AUS], Retavase)
Do not confuse reteplase or Retavase with Restasis.

CATEGORY AND SCHEDULE

Pregnancy Risk Category: C

Drug Class: Thrombolytics

MECHANISM OF ACTION

A tissue plasminogen activator that activates the fibrinolytic system by directly cleaving plasminogen to generate plasmin, an enzyme that degrades the fibrin of the thrombus. **Therapeutic Effect:** Exerts thrombolytic action.

USES

Dissolving of blood clots that have formed in certain blood vessels

PHARMACOKINETICS

Rapidly cleared from plasma. Eliminated primarily by the liver and kidney. **Half-life:** 13–16 min.

INDICATIONS AND DOSAGES
▶ **Acute MI, CHF**
IV Bolus
Adults, Elderly. 10 units over 2 min; repeat in 30 min.

SIDE EFFECTS/ADVERSE REACTIONS
Frequent
Bleeding at superficial sites, such as venous injection sites, catheter insertion sites, venous cutdowns, arterial punctures, and sites of recent surgical procedures, gingival bleeding

PRECAUTIONS AND CONTRAINDICATIONS
Active internal bleeding, AV malformation or aneurysm, bleeding diathesis, history of cerebrovascular accident, intracranial neoplasm, recent intracranial or intraspinal surgery or trauma, severe uncontrolled hypertension

DRUG INTERACTIONS OF CONCERN TO DENTISTRY
• Increased risk of bleeding: drugs that interfere with coagulation or platelet function, such as NSAIDs or aspirin

SERIOUS REACTIONS
! Bleeding at internal sites may occur, including intracranial, retroperitoneal, GI, GU, and respiratory sites.
! Lysis or coronary thrombi may produce atrial or ventricular arrhythmias and stroke.

DENTAL CONSIDERATIONS
General:
• Acute-use drug for use in hospitals or emergency rooms.
• Patients are at risk for bleeding, check for oral signs.

• Monitor and record vital signs.
• Avoid products that affect platelet function, such as aspirin and NSAIDs.
• Patients who have been treated with this drug may present with cardiovascular disease or stroke, review medical and drug history.
Consultations:
• Medical consultation should include routine blood counts including platelet counts and bleeding time.
• In a patient with symptoms of blood dyscrasias, request a medical consultation for blood studies and postpone treatment until normal values are reestablished.
• Medical consultation may be required to assess disease control and patient's ability to tolerate stress.
Teach Patient/Family to:
• Use soft tooth brush to reduce risk of bleeding
• Use effective oral hygiene to prevent soft tissue inflammation
• Report oral lesions, soreness, or bleeding to dentist
• Prevent trauma when using oral hygiene aids
• Update health and medication history if physician makes any changes in evaluation or drug regimens; include OTC, herbal, and nonherbal remedies in the update

ribavirin
rye-ba-vye′-rin
(Copegus, Rebetol, Rebetron, Virazole)
Do not confuse ribavirin with riboflavin.

CATEGORY AND SCHEDULE
Pregnancy Risk Category: X

Drug Class: Antiviral

MECHANISM OF ACTION

A synthetic nucleoside that inhibits influenza virus RNA polymerase activity and interferes with expression of messenger RNA. *Therapeutic Effect:* Inhibits viral protein synthesis and replication of viral RNA and DNA.

USES

Treatment of adults and children with chronic hepatitis C but only in combination with interferon alfa-2b or peginterferon alfa-2a; patients must have compensated liver disease and not previously been treated with interferons; respiratory syncytial virus (RSV) in hospitalized infants and young children, unapproved use in influenza A or B or in lower respiratory tract pneumonia associated with an adenovirus

PHARMACOKINETICS

Rapidly absorbed from the GI tract following oral administration. A small amount is systemically absorbed following inhalation. Primarily excreted in urine. *Half-life:* 298 hr (oral); 9.5 hr (inhalation).

INDICATIONS AND DOSAGES

▶ **Chronic Hepatitis C**

PO (Capsule or Oral Solution in Combination with Interferon Alfa-2b)

Adults, Elderly. 1000–1200 mg/day in 2 divided doses.

Children weighing 60 kg or more. Use adult dosage. (51–60 kg): 400 mg twice a day. (37–50 kg): 200 mg in morning, 400 mg in evening. (24–36 kg): 200 mg twice a day.

PO (Capsules in Combination with Peginterferon Alfa-2b)

Adults, Elderly. 800 mg/day in 2 divided doses.

PO (Tablets in Combination with Peginterferon Alfa-2b)

Adults, Elderly. 800–1200 mg/day in 2 divided doses.

▶ **Severe Lower Respiratory Tract Infection Caused by RSV**

Inhalation

Children, Infants. Use with Viratek small-particle aerosol generator at a concentration of 20 mg/ml (6 g reconstituted with 300 ml sterile water) over 12–18 hr/day for 3–7 days.

SIDE EFFECTS/ADVERSE REACTIONS

Frequent

Dizziness, headache, fatigue, fever, insomnia, irritability, depression, emotional lability, impaired concentration, alopecia, rash, pruritus, nausea, anorexia, dyspepsia, vomiting, decreased hemoglobin, hemolysis, arthralgia, musculoskeletal pain, dyspnea, sinusitis, flu-like symptoms

Occasional

Nervousness, altered taste, weakness

PRECAUTIONS AND CONTRAINDICATIONS

Autoimmune hepatitis, creatinine clearance less than 50 ml/min, hemoglobinopathies, hepatic decompensation, hypersensitivity to ribavirin products, pregnancy, significant or unstable cardiac disease, women of childbearing age who will not use contraception reliably

Caution

Must not be used alone for hepatitis C, severe side effects occur, pregnancy category X, aggravation of sarcoidosis, stop therapy if pancreatitis occurs, use aerosol only for RSV, extra contraception required to prevent pregnancy during use and for up to 6 mo after discontinuing use

DRUG INTERACTIONS OF CONCERN TO DENTISTRY
None reported

SERIOUS REACTIONS
! Cardiac arrest, apnea, and ventilator dependence, bacterial pneumonia, pneumonia, and pneumothorax occur rarely.
! Anemia may occur if ribavirin therapy exceeds 7 days.

DENTAL CONSIDERATIONS
General:
• Patients taking this drug will also be taking an interferon drug; be sure to conduct a thorough drug history.
• Assess salivary flow as a factor in caries, periodontal disease, and candidiasis.
• Patients on chronic drug therapy may rarely have symptoms of blood dyscrasias, which can include infection, bleeding, and poor healing.
• Consider semisupine chair position for patient comfort if GI side effects occur.
• Examine for oral manifestation of opportunistic infection.
• Take precautions if dental surgery is anticipated and general anesthesia is required.
• Monitor vital signs at every appointment because of cardiovascular side effects.
Consultations:
• In a patient with symptoms of blood dyscrasias, request a medical consultation for blood studies and postpone treatment until normal values are reestablished.
• Medical consultation may be required to assess disease control and patient's ability to tolerate stress.

• Consultation with physician may be necessary if sedation or general anesthesia is required.
Teach Patient/Family to:
• Update health and drug history if physician makes any changes in evaluation or drug regimens; include OTC, herbal, and nonherbal drugs in the update
• Use effective oral hygiene to prevent soft tissue inflammation
• Prevent trauma when using oral hygiene aids
• When chronic dry mouth occurs, advise patient to:
    • Avoid mouth rinses with high alcohol content because of drying effects
    • Use daily home fluoride products for anticaries effect
    • Use sugarless gum, frequent sips of water, or saliva substitutes

---

rifabutin
rif′-ah-byoo-ten
(Mycobutin)
Do not confuse rifabutin with rifampin.

CATEGORY AND SCHEDULE
Pregnancy Risk Category: B

Drug Class: Antimycobacterial agent

R

MECHANISM OF ACTION
An antitubercular that inhibits DNA-dependent RNA polymerase, an enzyme in susceptible strains of *Escherichia coli* and Bacillus subtilis. Rifabutin has a broad spectrum of antimicrobial activity, including against mycobacteria such as *Mycobacterium avium* complex (MAC). ***Therapeutic Effect:*** Prevents MAC disease.

USES
Prevention of disseminated MAC disease with advanced HIV infection

PHARMACOKINETICS
Readily absorbed from the GI tract (high-fat meals delay absorption). Protein binding: 85%. Widely distributed. Crosses the blood-brain barrier. Extensive intracellular tissue uptake. Metabolized in the liver to active metabolite. Excreted in urine; eliminated in feces. Unknown if removed by hemodialysis.
Half-life: 16–69 hr.

INDICATIONS AND DOSAGES
▶ **Prevention of MAC Disease (first episode)**
PO
Adults, Elderly. 300 mg as a single dose or in 2 divided doses if GI upset occurs.
▶ **Prevention of Recurrent MAC Disease**
PO
Adults, Elderly. 300 mg/day (in combination)
▶ **Dosage in Renal Impairment**
Dosage is modified on the basis of creatinine clearance. If creatinine clearance is less than 30 ml/min, reduce dosage by 50%.

SIDE EFFECTS/ADVERSE REACTIONS
Frequent
Red-orange or red-brown discoloration of urine, feces, saliva, skin, sputum, sweat, or tears
Occasional
Rash, nausea, abdominal pain, diarrhea, dyspepsia, belching, headache, altered taste, uveitis, corneal deposits
Rare
Anorexia, flatulence, fever, myalgia, vomiting, insomnia

PRECAUTIONS AND CONTRAINDICATIONS
Active tuberculosis; hypersensitivity to other rifamycins, including rifampin
Caution
Pregnancy category B, lactation, concurrent corticosteroid therapy

DRUG INTERACTIONS OF CONCERN TO DENTISTRY
• Decreases plasma concentrations of corticosteroids; may be significant
• May induce CYP3A4 isoenzymes, possible reduction in action of ketoconazole, itraconazole, benzodiazepines, doxycycline, erythromycin, clarithromycin

SERIOUS REACTIONS
! Hepatitis and thrombocytopenia occur rarely. Anemia and neutropenia may also occur.

DENTAL CONSIDERATIONS
General:
• Examine for evidence of oral signs of opportunistic disease.
• Determine why the patient is taking the drug.
• Patients on chronic drug therapy may rarely have symptoms of blood dyscrasias, which can include infection, bleeding, and poor healing.
Consultations:
• Medical consultation may be required to assess patient's ability to tolerate stress.
• In a patient with symptoms of blood dyscrasias, request a medical consultation for blood studies and postpone dental treatment until normal values are reestablished.
Teach Patient/Family to:
• Avoid mouth rinses with high alcohol content because of drying effects

R

• Use effective oral hygiene to prevent soft tissue inflammation

rifampin
rye´-fam-pin
(Rifadin, Rimactane, Rimycin[AUS], Rofact[CAN])
Do not confuse rifampin with rifabutin, Rifamate, rifapentine, or Ritalin.

CATEGORY AND SCHEDULE
Pregnancy Risk Category: C

Drug Class: Antitubercular antiinfective

MECHANISM OF ACTION
An antitubercular that interferes with bacterial RNA synthesis by binding to DNA-dependent RNA polymerase, thus preventing its attachment to DNA and blocking RNA transcription. *Therapeutic Effect:* Bactericidal in susceptible microorganisms.

USES
Pulmonary tuberculosis (TB), meningococcal carriers (prevention); unapproved: leprosy and atypical mycobacterial infections

PHARMACOKINETICS
Well absorbed from the GI tract (food delays absorption). Protein binding: 80%. Widely distributed. Metabolized in the liver to active metabolite. Primarily eliminated by the biliary system. Not removed by hemodialysis. *Half-life:* 3–5 hr (increased in hepatic impairment).

INDICATIONS AND DOSAGES
▸ **Tuberculosis**
PO, IV
Adults, Elderly. 10 mg/kg/day. Maximum: 600 mg/day.
Children. 10–20 mg/kg/day in divided doses q12–24h.
▸ **Prevention of Meningococcal Infections**
PO, IV
Adults, Elderly. 600 mg q12h for 2 days.
Children 1 mo and older. 20 mg/kg/day in divided doses q12–24h. Maximum: 600 mg/dose.
Infants younger than 1 mo. 10 mg/kg/day in divided doses q12h for 2 days.
▸ **Staphylococcal Infections**
PO, IV
Adults, Elderly. 600 mg/day.
Children. 15 mg/kg/day in divided doses q12h.
▸ *Staphylococcus aureus* **Infections (in combination with other antiinfectives)**
PO
Adults, Elderly. 300–600 mg twice a day.
Neonates. 5–20 mg/kg/day in divided doses q12h.
▸ **Prevention of** *Haemophilus influenzae* **Infection**
PO
Adults, Elderly. 600 mg/day for 4 days.
Children 1 mo and older. 20 mg/kg/day in divided doses q12h for 5–10 days.
Children younger than 1 mo. 10 mg/kg/day in divided doses q12h for 2 days.

SIDE EFFECTS/ADVERSE REACTIONS
Expected
Red-orange or red-brown discoloration of urine, feces, saliva, skin, sputum, sweat, or tears

R

Occasional
Hypersensitivity reaction (such as flushing, pruritus, or rash)
Rare
Diarrhea, dyspepsia, nausea, candida as evidenced by sore mouth or tongue

PRECAUTIONS AND CONTRAINDICATIONS
Concomitant therapy with amprenavir, hypersensitivity to rifampin or any other rifamycins
Caution
Lactation, hepatic disease, blood dyscrasias, concurrent therapy with corticosteroids

DRUG INTERACTIONS OF CONCERN TO DENTISTRY
• Increased risk of hepatotoxicity: acetaminophen (chronic use and high doses), alcohol, hydrocarbon inhalation anesthetics (except isoflurane)
• Decreased effects of corticosteroids, dapsone, ketoconazole, fluconazole, itraconazole, oral contraceptives, benzodiazepines, doxycycline, erythromycin, clarithromycin, opioid analgesics
• Suspected decrease in fexofenadine effects
• Induces CYP450 isoenzymes

SERIOUS REACTIONS
! Rare reactions include hepatotoxicity (risk is increased when rifampin is taken with isoniazid), hepatitis, blood dyscrasias, Stevens-Johnson syndrome, and antibiotic-associated colitis.

DENTAL CONSIDERATIONS
General:
• Examine for oral manifestation of opportunistic infections.

• Patients on chronic drug therapy may rarely have symptoms of blood dyscrasias, which can include infection, bleeding, and poor healing.
• Determine why the patient is taking the drug (prophylaxis or active therapy).
• Determine that noninfectious status exists by ensuring that (1) anti-TB drugs have been taken for longer than 3 wk, (2) culture has confirmed TB susceptibility to antiinfectives, (3) patient has had 3 consecutive negative sputum smears, and (4) patient is not in the coughing stage.
Consultations:
• Medical consultation may be required to assess patient's ability to tolerate stress.
• In a patient with symptoms of blood dyscrasias, request a medical consultation for blood studies and postpone dental treatment until normal values are reestablished.
Teach Patient/Family to:
• Avoid mouth rinses with high alcohol content because of drying effects
• Use effective oral hygiene to prevent soft tissue inflammation
• Take medications for full length of regimen to ensure effectiveness of treatment and to prevent the emergence of resistant strains

rifapentine
rif-ah-pen′-teen
(Priftin)
Do not confuse rifapentine with rifampin.

CATEGORY AND SCHEDULE
Pregnancy Risk Category: C

Drug Class: Antimycobacterial agent

• Consider semisupine chair position for patient comfort because of GI side effects of drug.
Consultations:
• Medical consultation may be required to assess disease control and patient's ability to tolerate stress.
• In a patient with symptoms of blood dyscrasias, request a medical consultation for blood studies and postpone treatment until normal values are reestablished.
Teach Patient/Family to:
• Avoid mouth rinses with high alcohol content because of drying effects
• Prevent trauma when using oral hygiene aids
• Use effective oral hygiene to prevent soft tissue inflammation
• Take medication for full length of regimen to ensure effectiveness of treatment and prevent emergence of resistant strains
• Be aware of potential for extrinsic oral staining side effect

riluzole
rye′-loo-zole
(Rilutek)

CATEGORY AND SCHEDULE
Pregnancy Risk Category: C

Drug Class: Glutamate antagonist

MECHANISM OF ACTION
An amyotrophic lateral sclerosis (ALS) agent that inhibits presynaptic glutamate release in the CNS and interferes postsynaptically with the effects of excitatory amino acids.
Therapeutic Effect: Extends survival of ALS patients.

USES
Treatment of ALS (Lou Gehrig's disease)

PHARMACOKINETICS
PO: Well absorbed, extensively metabolized by liver (CYP1A2 isoenzymes), excreted in urine/feces

INDICATIONS AND DOSAGES
▶ **ALS**
PO
Adults, Elderly. 50 mg q12h.

SIDE EFFECTS/ADVERSE REACTIONS
Frequent
Nausea, asthenia, reduced respiratory function
Occasional
Edema, tachycardia, headache, dizziness, somnolence, depression, vertigo, tremor, pruritus, alopecia, abdominal pain, diarrhea, anorexia, dyspepsia, vomiting, stomatitis, increased cough

PRECAUTIONS AND CONTRAINDICATIONS
Hypersensitivity, hepatic impairment, renal impairment, hypertension, other CNS disorders, pregnancy category C, lactation, children

DRUG INTERACTIONS OF CONCERN TO DENTISTRY
• No data reported with dental drugs, but use with caution when given with inducers or inhibitors of CYP1A2 isoenzymes

SERIOUS REACTIONS
None known

DENTAL CONSIDERATIONS
General:
• Short appointments may be required because of nature of disease process.

- Monitor vital signs at every appointment because of cardiovascular and respiratory side effects.
- Consider semisupine chair position for patient comfort.
- Assess salivary flow as factor in caries, periodontal disease, and candidiasis.
- Examine for oral manifestation of opportunistic infection.
- Patients on chronic drug therapy may rarely have symptoms of blood dyscrasias, which can include infection, bleeding, and poor healing.
- After supine positioning, have patient sit upright for at least 2 min before standing to avoid orthostatic hypotension.

Consultations:
- Medical consultation may be required to assess disease control.
- In a patient with symptoms of blood dyscrasias, request a medical consultation for blood studies and postpone treatment until normal values are reestablished.

Teach Patient/Family to:
- Use effective oral hygiene, including use of electric tooth brush if patient has difficulty holding conventional devices or directions for caregiver
- Use caution to prevent trauma when using oral hygiene aids
- When chronic dry mouth occurs, advise patient to:
  - Avoid mouth rinses with high alcohol content because of drying effects
  - Use daily home fluoride products for anticaries effect
  - Use sugarless gum, frequent sips of water, or saliva substitutes

rimantadine hydrochloride
ri-man'-ta-deen high-droh-klor'-ide
(Flumadine)
Do not confuse rimantadine with ranitidine, or Flumadine with flunisolide or flutamide.

CATEGORY AND SCHEDULE
Pregnancy Risk Category: C

Drug Class: Antiviral

MECHANISM OF ACTION
An antiviral that appears to exert an inhibitory effect early in the viral replication cycle. May inhibit uncoating of the virus. ***Therapeutic Effect:*** Prevents replication of influenza A virus.

USES
Adult: prophylaxis and treatment of illnesses caused by strains of influenza A virus; children: prophylaxis against influenza A virus

PHARMACOKINETICS
PO: Peak plasma levels 6 hr; 40% plasma protein binding; hepatic metabolism; renal excretion.

INDICATIONS AND DOSAGES
▶ **Influenza A Virus**
PO
Adults, Elderly. 100 mg twice a day for 7 days.
Elderly nursing home patients, Patients with severe hepatic or renal impairment. 100 mg/day for 7 days.
▶ **Prevention of Influenza A Virus**
PO
Adults, Elderly, Children 10 yr and older. 100 mg twice a day for at least 10 days after known exposure (usually for 6–8 wk).

R

Children younger than 10 yr. 5 mg/kg/day. Maximum: 150 mg.
Elderly nursing home patients, Patients with severe hepatic or renal impairment. 100 mg/day.

SIDE EFFECTS/ADVERSE REACTIONS
Occasional
Insomnia, nausea, nervousness, impaired concentration, dizziness
Rare
Vomiting, anorexia, dry mouth, abdominal pain, asthenia, fatigue

PRECAUTIONS AND CONTRAINDICATIONS
Hypersensitivity to amantadine or rimantadine
Caution
Pregnancy category C, elderly, epilepsy, hepatic or renal impairment, emergence of resistant viral strains

DRUG INTERACTIONS OF CONCERN TO DENTISTRY
• Reduced peak plasma levels: aspirin, acetaminophen

SERIOUS REACTIONS
None known

R DENTAL CONSIDERATIONS
General:
• Monitor vital signs at every appointment because of cardiovascular side effects.
• Determine why the patient is taking the drug (probably will be used only during peak seasons for influenza).
• Assess salivary flow as a factor in caries, periodontal disease, and candidiasis.
Teach Patient/Family to:
• Use effective oral hygiene to prevent soft tissue inflammation

• When chronic dry mouth occurs, advise patient to:
  • Avoid mouth rinses with high alcohol content because of drying effects
  • Use daily home fluoride products to prevent caries
  • Use sugarless gum, frequent sips of water, or saliva substitutes

rimexolone
rye-mex´-oh-lone
(Vexol)
Do not confuse with riluzole.

CATEGORY AND SCHEDULE
Pregnancy Risk Category: C

Drug Class: Corticosteroid

MECHANISM OF ACTION
An ophthalmic agent that suppresses migration of polymorphonuclear leukocytes and reverses increased capillary permeability. ***Therapeutic Effect:*** Decreases inflammation.

USES
Treatment of inflammation of the eye associated with ocular surgery and uveitis

PHARMACOKINETICS
Absorbed through aqueous humor. Metabolized in liver. Excreted in urine and feces.

INDICATIONS AND DOSAGES
▸ **Inflammation after Ocular Surgery, Treatment of Anterior Uveitis**
Ophthalmic
Adults, Elderly. Instill 1 drop 2–4 times a day up to q4h. May use q1–2h during the first 1–2 days.

SIDE EFFECTS/ADVERSE REACTIONS
Occasional
Temporary mild blurred vision

PRECAUTIONS AND CONTRAINDICATIONS
Fungal, viral, or untreated pus-forming bacterial ocular infections, hypersensitivity to rimexolone or any component of the formulation
Caution
Increased intraocular pressure, lactation, children, secondary ocular infections

DRUG INTERACTIONS OF CONCERN TO DENTISTRY
None reported

SERIOUS REACTIONS
! Prolonged use has been associated with the development of corneal or scleral perforation and posterior subcapsular cataracts.
! Cataracts, corneal thinning, glaucoma, increased intraocular pressure, optic nerve damage, secondary ocular infection, and visual acuity defects occur rarely.

DENTAL CONSIDERATIONS
General:
• Determine why the patient is taking the drug.
• Avoid dental light in patient's eyes; offer dark glasses for patient comfort.

risedronate sodium
rye-seh-droe'-nate soe'-dee-um
(Actonel)

CATEGORY AND SCHEDULE
Pregnancy Risk Category: C

Drug Class: Bisphosphonate

MECHANISM OF ACTION
A bisphosphonate that binds to bone hydroxyapatite and inhibits osteoclasts. **Therapeutic Effect:** Reduces bone turnover (the number of sites at which bone is remodeled) and bone resorption.

USES
Treatment of Paget's disease of bone; treatment and prevention of osteoporosis in postmenopausal women and glucocorticoid-induced osteoporosis

INDICATIONS AND DOSAGES
▶ **Paget's Disease**
PO
Adults, Elderly. 30 mg/day for 2 mo. Retreatment may occur after 2-mo post-treatment observation period.
▶ **Prevention and Treatment of Postmenopausal Osteoporosis**
PO
Adults, Elderly. 5 mg/day or 35 mg once a wk.
▶ **Glucocorticoid-Induced Osteoporosis**
PO
Adults, Elderly. 5 mg/day.

SIDE EFFECTS/ADVERSE REACTIONS
Frequent
Arthralgia
Occasional
Rash, flu-like symptoms, peripheral edema

Rare
Bone pain, sinusitis, asthenia, dry eye, tinnitus

PRECAUTIONS AND CONTRAINDICATIONS
Hypersensitivity to other bisphosphonates, including etidronate, tiludronate, risedronate, and alendronate; hypocalcemia; inability to stand or sit upright for at least 20 min; renal impairment when serum creatinine clearance is greater than 5 mg/dl
Caution
Upper GI disease, avoid use in significant renal impairment, pregnancy category C, lactation, pediatric patients

DRUG INTERACTIONS OF CONCERN TO DENTISTRY
• Retarded absorption: calcium, antacids, medications with divalent cations
• Increased GI side effects: NSAIDs, aspirin

SERIOUS REACTIONS
❗ Overdose causes hypocalcemia, hypophosphatemia, and significant GI disturbances.

DENTAL CONSIDERATIONS
General:
• Be aware of the oral manifestations of Paget's disease (macrognathia, alveolar pain).
• Consider semisupine chair position for patient comfort because of GI side effects of drug.
• Short appointments may be required for patient comfort.
Consultations:
• Medical consultation may be required to assess disease control.

Teach Patient/Family to:
• Use electric tooth brush if patient has difficulty holding conventional devices

risperidone
ris-per′-ih-done
(Risperdal, Risperdal Consta, Risperdol M-Tabs)
Do not confuse risperidone with reserpine.

CATEGORY AND SCHEDULE
Pregnancy Risk Category: C

Drug Class: Antipsychotic (benzisoxazole derivative)

MECHANISM OF ACTION
A benzisoxazole derivative that may antagonize dopamine and serotonin receptors. *Therapeutic Effect:* Suppresses psychotic behavior.

USES
Treatment of schizophrenia

PHARMACOKINETICS
Well absorbed from the GI tract; unaffected by food. Protein binding: 90%. Extensively metabolized in the liver to active metabolite. Primarily excreted in urine. *Half-life:* 3–20 hr; metabolite: 21–30 hr (increased in elderly).

INDICATIONS AND DOSAGES
▶ **Psychotic Disorder**
PO
Adults. 0.5–1 mg twice a day. May increase dosage slowly. Range: 2–6 mg/day.
Elderly. Initially, 0.25–2 mg/day in 2 divided doses. May increase dosage slowly. Range: 2–6 mg/day.

IM
Adults, Elderly. 25 mg q2wk.
Maximum: 50 mg q2wk.
▶ **Mania**
PO
Adults, Elderly. Initially, 2–3 mg as a
single daily dose. May increase at
24-hr intervals of 1 mg/day. Range:
2–6 mg/day.
▶ **Dosage in Renal Impairment**
Initial dosage for adults and elderly
patients is 0.25–0.5 mg twice a day.
Dosage is titrated slowly to desired
effect.

SIDE EFFECTS/ADVERSE REACTIONS
Frequent
Agitation, anxiety, insomnia,
headache, constipation
Occasional
Dyspepsia, rhinitis, somnolence,
dizziness, nausea, vomiting, rash,
abdominal pain, dry skin, tachycardia
Rare
Visual disturbances, fever, back pain,
pharyngitis, cough, arthralgia, angina,
aggressive behavior, orthostatic
hypotension, breast swelling

PRECAUTIONS AND CONTRAINDICATIONS
Hypersensitivity, pregnancy category
C, lactation, seizures, suicidal
patients, cardiac diseases, renal or
hepatic impairment, elderly; patients
should be monitored for signs and
symptoms of diabetes mellitus

DRUG INTERACTIONS OF CONCERN TO DENTISTRY
• Increased excretion: chronic use of
carbamazepine
• Increased sedation: other CNS
depressants, alcohol, barbiturate
anesthesia, opioid analgesics
• Increased extrapyramidal effects:
phenothiazines and related drugs

(haloperidol, droperidol),
metoclopramide
• Additive photosensitization:
tetracyclines
• Increased anticholinergic effects:
anticholinergics, such as atropine and
scopolamine

SERIOUS REACTIONS
❗ Rare reactions include tardive
dyskinesia (characterized by tongue
protrusion, puffing of the cheeks, and
chewing or puckering of the mouth)
and neuroleptic malignant syndrome
(marked by hyperpyrexia, muscle
rigidity, change in mental status,
irregular pulse or B/P, tachycardia,
diaphoresis, cardiac arrhythmias,
rhabdomyolysis, and acute renal
failure).

DENTAL CONSIDERATIONS
General:
• Monitor vital signs at every
appointment because of
cardiovascular side effects.
• Patients on chronic drug therapy
may rarely have symptoms of blood
dyscrasias, which can include
infection, bleeding, and poor healing.
• After supine positioning, have
patient sit upright for at least 2 min
before standing to avoid orthostatic
hypotension.
• Assess salivary flow as a factor in
caries, periodontal disease, and
candidiasis.
• Consider semisupine chair position
for patient comfort because of GI
effects of drug.
• Assess for presence of
extrapyramidal motor symptoms, such
as tardive dyskinesia and akathisia.
Extrapyramidal motor activity may
complicate dental treatment.
• Use vasoconstrictors with caution,
in low doses, and with careful
aspiration; avoid use of gingival
retraction cord with epinephrine.

R

Consultations:
- In a patient with symptoms of blood dyscrasias, request a medical consultation for blood studies and postpone dental treatment until normal values are reestablished.
- Take precautions if dental surgery is anticipated and anesthesia is required.
- If signs of tardive dyskinesia or other extrapyramidal symptoms are present, refer to physician.
- Physician should be informed if significant xerostomic side effects occur (e.g., increased caries, sore tongue, problems eating or swallowing, difficulty wearing prosthesis) so that a medication change can be considered.

Teach Patient/Family to:
- Use effective oral hygiene to prevent soft tissue inflammation
- Use caution to prevent injury when using oral hygiene aids
- Use electric tooth brush if patient has difficulty holding conventional devices
- When chronic dry mouth occurs, advise patient to:
  - Avoid mouth rinses with high alcohol content because of drying effects
  - Use daily home fluoride products for anticaries effect
  - Use sugarless gum, frequent sips of water, or saliva substitutes

ritonavir

ri-tone′-ah-veer
(Norvir, Norvisec[CAN])
Do not confuse ritonavir with Retrovir.

CATEGORY AND SCHEDULE
Pregnancy Risk Category: B

Drug Class: Antiviral, protease inhibitor

MECHANISM OF ACTION
Inhibits HIV-1 and HIV-2 proteases, rendering these enzymes incapable of processing the polypeptide precursors; this results in the production of noninfectious, immature HIV particles.
Therapeutic Effect: Impedes HIV replication, slowing the progression of HIV infection.

USES
Treatment of HIV infection in adults and children as single-drug therapy or in combination with nucleoside analogs

PHARMACOKINETICS
Well absorbed after PO administration (absorption increased with food). Protein binding: 98%–99%. Extensively metabolized in the liver to active metabolite. Primarily eliminated in feces. Unknown if removed by hemodialysis. *Half-life:* 2.7–5 hr.

INDICATIONS AND DOSAGES
▶ HIV Infection
PO
Adults, Children 12 yr and older.
600 mg twice a day. If nausea occurs at this dosage, give 300 mg twice a day for 1 day, 400 mg twice a day for 2 days, 500 mg twice a day for 1 day, then 600 mg twice a day thereafter.
Children younger than 12 yr.
Initially, 250 mg/m^2/dose twice a day. Increase by 50 mg/m^2/dose up to 400 mg/m^2/dose. Maximum: 600 mg/dose twice a day.

SIDE EFFECTS/ADVERSE REACTIONS
Frequent
GI disturbances (abdominal pain, anorexia, diarrhea, nausea, vomiting), circumoral and peripheral

paresthesias, altered taste, headache, dizziness, fatigue, asthenia
Occasional
Allergic reaction, flu-like symptoms, hypotension
Rare
Diabetes mellitus, hyperglycemia

PRECAUTIONS AND CONTRAINDICATIONS

Concurrent use of amiodarone, astemizole, bepridil, bupropion, cisapride, clozapine, encainide, flecainide, meperidine, piroxicam, propafenone, propoxyphene, quinidine, rifabutin, or terfenadine (increased risk of serious or life-threatening drug interactions, such as arrhythmias, hematologic abnormalities, and seizures); concurrent use of alprazolam, clorazepate, diazepam, estazolam, flurazepam, midazolam, triazolam, or zolpidem (may produce extreme sedation and respiratory depression)
Caution
Hepatic impairment, lactation, children younger than 12 yr, alters lab chemistry values (triglycerides, ALT, AST, GGT, CPK, uric acid)

DRUG INTERACTIONS OF CONCERN TO DENTISTRY

• Contraindicated with alprazolam, clorazepate, diazepam, bupropion, estazolam, flurazepam, midazolam, triazolam, zolpidem, meperidine, piroxicam, propoxyphene, chlordiazepoxide, halazepam, quazepam
• Increased plasma levels: clarithromycin, fluconazole, fluoxetine, desipramine, theophylline
• Possible alcohol-disulfiram reaction: metronidazole, disulfiram

• Decreased plasma levels with carbamazepine, dexamethasone, phenobarbital, St. John's wort (herb)
• Increased plasma levels of fentanyl
• Note: Multiple drug interactions are reported; check before prescribing dental drugs. This drug is a potent inhibitor of CYP3A4, CYP2D6 isoenzymes.

SERIOUS REACTIONS

None known

DENTAL CONSIDERATIONS

General:
• Monitor vital signs at every appointment because of cardiovascular side effects.
• Examine for oral manifestation of opportunistic infection.
• Place on frequent recall to evaluate healing response.
• Assess salivary flow as a factor in caries, periodontal disease, and candidiasis.
• Consider semisupine chair position for patient comfort because of GI effects of drug.
Consultations:
• Medical consultation may be required to assess disease control.
Teach Patient/Family to:
• Use effective oral hygiene to prevent soft tissue inflammation
• See dentist immediately if secondary oral infection occurs
• When chronic dry mouth occurs, advise patient to:
    • Avoid mouth rinses with high alcohol content because of drying effects
    • Use daily home fluoride products for anticaries effect
    • Use sugarless gum, frequent sips of water, or saliva substitutes

R

rituximab
rye-tucks´-ih-mab
(Mabthera[AUS], Rituxan)

CATEGORY AND SCHEDULE
Pregnancy Risk Category: C

Drug Class: Antineoplastics, monoclonal antibodies

MECHANISM OF ACTION
Binds to CD20, the antigen found on the surface of B lymphocytes and B-cell non-Hodgkin's lymphomas. *Therapeutic Effect:* Produces cytotoxicity, reducing tumor size.

USES
Treatment of a type of cancer called non-Hodgkin's lymphoma. It can be used alone or with other cancer medicines or chemotherapy.

PHARMACOKINETICS
Rapidly depletes B cells. *Half-life:* 59.8 hr after first infusion and 174 hr after fourth infusion.

INDICATIONS AND DOSAGES
▸ **Non-Hodgkin's Lymphoma**
IV
Adults. 375 mg/m² once a wk for 4–8 wk. May administer a second 4-wk course.

SIDE EFFECTS/ADVERSE REACTIONS
Frequent
Fever, chills, nausea, asthenia, headache, angioedema, hypotension, rash or pruritus
Occasional
Myalgia, dizziness, abdominal pain, throat irritation, vomiting, neutropenia, rhinitis, bronchospasm, urticaria

PRECAUTIONS AND CONTRAINDICATIONS
Hypersensitivity to murine proteins

DRUG INTERACTIONS OF CONCERN TO DENTISTRY
None reported

SERIOUS REACTIONS
❗ A hypersensitivity reaction marked by hypotension, bronchospasm, and angioedema may occur.
❗ Arrhythmias may occur, particularly in those with a history of preexisting cardiac conditions.

DENTAL CONSIDERATIONS
General:
• Monitor and record vital signs.
• If additional analgesia is required for dental pain, consider alternative analgesics (NSAIDs) in patients taking narcotics for acute or chronic pain.
• After supine positioning, have patient sit upright for at least 2 min before standing to avoid orthostatic hypotension.
• Patient on chronic drug therapy may rarely present with symptoms of blood dyscrasias, which can include infection, bleeding, and poor healing. If dyscrasia is present, caution patient to prevent oral tissue trauma when using oral hygiene aids.
• Provide emergency dental care only during drug use.
• Hypersensitivity reactions may occur.
• Oral infections should be eliminated and treated aggressively.
Consultations:
• Medical consultation should include routine blood counts including platelet counts and bleeding time.
• Consult physician; prophylactic or therapeutic antiinfectives may be

indicated if surgery or periodontal treatment is required.

• Medical consultation may be required to assess immunologic status during cancer chemotherapy and determine safety risk, if any, posed by the required dental treatment.

• Medical consultation may be required to assess disease control and patient's ability to tolerate stress.

Teach Patient/Family to:

• Use effective oral hygiene to prevent soft tissue inflammation

• Report oral lesions, soreness, or bleeding to dentist

• Prevent trauma when using oral hygiene aids

• Update health and medication history if physician makes any changes in evaluation or drug regimens; include OTC, herbal, and nonherbal remedies in the update

---

rivastigmine tartrate
riv-ah-stig′-meen tar′-trate
(Exelon)

CATEGORY AND SCHEDULE
Pregnancy Risk Category: B

Drug Class: Reversible cholinesterase inhibitor

MECHANISM OF ACTION
A cholinesterase inhibitor that inhibits the enzyme acetylcholinesterase, thus increasing the concentration of acetylcholine at cholinergic synapses and enhancing cholinergic function in the CNS. *Therapeutic Effect:* Slows the progression of symptoms of Alzheimer's disease.

PHARMACOKINETICS
Rapidly and completely absorbed. Protein binding: 60%. Widely distributed throughout the body. Rapidly and extensively metabolized. Primarily excreted in urine.
Half-life: 1.5 hr.

INDICATIONS AND DOSAGES
▸ **Alzheimer's Disease**
PO
Adults, Elderly. Initially, 1.5 mg twice a day. May increase at intervals of at least 2 wk to 3 mg twice a day, then 4.5 mg twice a day, and finally 6 mg twice a day. Maximum: 6 mg twice a day.

SIDE EFFECTS/ADVERSE REACTIONS
Frequent
Nausea, vomiting, dizziness, diarrhea, headache, anorexia
Occasional
Abdominal pain, insomnia, dyspepsia (heartburn, indigestion, epigastric pain), confusion, UTI, depression
Rare
Anxiety, somnolence, constipation, malaise, hallucinations, tremor, flatulence, rhinitis, hypertension, flu-like symptoms, weight loss, syncope

PRECAUTIONS AND CONTRAINDICATIONS
Hypersensitivity to this drug or other carbamate derivatives
Caution
Significant GI reactions, nausea, vomiting, and weight-loss occur; history of GI ulcers or GI bleeding, patients taking NSAIDs, seizures, asthma, COPD, lactation, pediatric patients (no studies); smoking increases renal clearance

R

DRUG INTERACTIONS OF CONCERN TO DENTISTRY

- Caution in use of NSAIDs if GI side effects are significant
- Decreased response to neuromuscular blocking agents used in general anesthesia
- Increased cholinergic response: other cholinergic drugs
- Decreased cholinergic response: anticholinergics or other drugs with anticholinergic actions

SERIOUS REACTIONS

! Overdose may result in cholinergic crisis, characterized by severe nausea and vomiting, increased salivation, diaphoresis, bradycardia, hypotension, respiratory depression, and seizures.

DENTAL CONSIDERATIONS

General:

- Determine why patient is taking the drug.
- Monitor vital signs at every appointment because of cardiovascular side effects.
- Drug is used early in the disease; ensure that patient or caregiver understands informed consent.
- Place on frequent recall because early attention to dental health is important for Alzheimer's patients.
- Assess salivary flow as a factor in caries, periodontal disease, and candidiasis.
- Use precaution if sedation or general anesthesia is required; risk of hypotensive episode.
- Consider semisupine chair position for patient comfort if GI side effects occur.
- Patients on chronic drug therapy may rarely have symptoms of blood dyscrasias, which can include

infection, bleeding, and poor healing.

Consultations:

- Consultation with physician may be necessary if sedation or general anesthesia is required.
- In a patient with symptoms of blood dyscrasias, request a medical consultation for blood studies and postpone treatment until normal values are reestablished.
- Medical consultation may be required to assess disease control and patient's ability to tolerate stress.

Teach Patient/Family to:

- Use electric tooth brush if patient has difficulty holding conventional devices
- Prevent trauma when using oral hygiene aids
- Use effective oral hygiene to prevent soft tissue inflammation

rizatriptan benzoate

rize-ah-trip′-tan ben′-zoe-ate
(Maxalt, Maxalt-MLT)

CATEGORY AND SCHEDULE

Pregnancy Risk Category: C

Drug Class: Serotonin agonist

MECHANISM OF ACTION

A serotonin receptor agonist that binds selectively to vascular receptors, producing a vasoconstrictive effect on cranial blood vessels. *Therapeutic Effect:* Relieves migraine headache.

USES

Acute treatment of migraine attacks with or without aura

PHARMACOKINETICS

Well absorbed after PO administration. Protein binding: 14%. Crosses the blood-brain barrier. Metabolized by the liver to inactive metabolite. Eliminated primarily in urine and, to a lesser extent, in feces. *Half-life:* 2–3 hr.

INDICATIONS AND DOSAGES

▶ **Acute Migraine Attack**

PO

Adults older than 18 yr, Elderly. 5–10 mg. If headache improves, but then returns, dose may be repeated after 2 hr. Maximum: 30 mg/24 hr.

SIDE EFFECTS/ADVERSE REACTIONS

Frequent
Dizziness, somnolence, paraesthesia, fatigue
Occasional
Nausea, chest pressure, dry mouth
Rare
Headache; neck, throat, or jaw pressure; photosensitivity

PRECAUTIONS AND CONTRAINDICATIONS

Basilar or hemiplegic migraine, coronary artery disease, ischemic heart disease (including angina pectoris, history of MI, silent ischemia, and Prinzmetal's angina), uncontrolled hypertension, use within 24 hr of ergotamine-containing preparations or another serotonin receptor agonist, use within 14 days of MAOIs
Caution
Risk of serious cardiovascular events, renal/hepatic impairment, SSRI antidepressants, lactation, use in children not established, orally disintegrating tabs contain aspartame

DRUG INTERACTIONS OF CONCERN TO DENTISTRY

• No specific interactions with dental drugs reported
• Increased plasma levels: propranolol
• Should not be used within 24 hr of another 5-HT agonist

SERIOUS REACTIONS

❗ Cardiac reactions (such as ischemia, coronary artery vasospasm, and MI) and noncardiac vasospasm-related reactions (including hemorrhage and CVA) occur rarely, particularly in patients with hypertension, diabetes, or a strong family history of coronary artery disease; obese patients; smokers; males older than 40 yr; and postmenopausal women.

DENTAL CONSIDERATIONS

General:
• This is an acute-use drug; it is doubtful that patients will be treated in the office if acute migraine is present.
• Be aware of patient's disease, its severity, and its frequency, when known.
• Avoid dental light in patient's eyes; offer dark glasses for patient comfort.
• Short appointments and a stress-reduction protocol may be required for anxious patients.
• After supine positioning, have patient sit upright for at least 2 min before standing to avoid orthostatic hypotension.
Consultations:
• If treating chronic orofacial pain, consult with physician of record.
• Medical consultation may be required to assess disease control and patient's ability to tolerate stress.

R

Teach Patient/Family to:
• Update health and drug history if physician makes any changes in evaluation or drug regimens; include OTC, herbal, and nonherbal drugs in the update

ropinirole hydrochloride
roe-pin'-ih-role high-droh-klor'-ide (Requip)

CATEGORY AND SCHEDULE
Pregnancy Risk Category: C

Drug Class: Antiparkinson agent

MECHANISM OF ACTION
An antiparkinson agent that stimulates dopamine receptors in the striatum. *Therapeutic Effect:* Relieves signs and symptoms of Parkinson's disease.

USES
Treatment of Parkinson's disease

PHARMACOKINETICS
Rapidly absorbed after PO administration. Protein binding: 40%. Extensively distributed throughout the body. Extensively metabolized. Steady-state concentrations achieved within 2 days. Eliminated in urine. Unknown if removed by hemodialysis. *Half-life:* 6 hr.

INDICATIONS AND DOSAGES
▶ **Parkinson's Disease**
PO
Adults, Elderly. Initially, 0.25 mg 3 times a day. May increase dosage every 7 days.

SIDE EFFECTS/ADVERSE REACTIONS
Frequent
Nausea, dizziness, somnolence
Occasional
Syncope, vomiting, fatigue, viral infection, dyspepsia, diaphoresis, asthenia, orthostatic hypotension, abdominal discomfort, pharyngitis, abnormal vision, dry mouth, hypertension, hallucinations, confusion
Rare
Anorexia, peripheral edema, memory loss, rhinitis, sinusitis, palpitations, impotence

PRECAUTIONS AND CONTRAINDICATIONS: HYPERSENSITIVITY
Cardiovascular disease, severely impaired renal or hepatic function, lactation, pregnancy category C, syncope, hypotension

DRUG INTERACTIONS OF CONCERN TO DENTISTRY
• Possible increase in sedation with all CNS depressants
• Possible diminished effects: dopamine antagonists, phenothiazines, haloperidol, droperidol, and metoclopramide

SERIOUS REACTIONS
None known

DENTAL CONSIDERATIONS
General:
• Monitor vital signs at every appointment because of cardiovascular side effects.
• Assess salivary flow as factor in caries, periodontal disease, and candidiasis.
• After supine positioning, have patient sit upright for at least 2 min

R

before standing to avoid orthostatic hypotension.
• Patients on chronic drug therapy may rarely have symptoms of blood dyscrasias, which can include infection, bleeding, and poor healing.
• Consider semisupine chair position for patient comfort if GI side effects occur.

Consultations:
• In a patient with symptoms of blood dyscrasias, request a medical consultation for blood studies and postpone treatment until normal values are reestablished.
• Medical consultation may be required to assess disease control and patient's ability to tolerate stress.

Teach Patient/Family to:
• Use caution to prevent trauma when using oral hygiene aids
• Use electric tooth brush if patient has difficulty holding conventional devices
• Use effective oral hygiene to prevent soft tissue inflammation
• Update health and drug history if physician makes any changes in evaluation or drug regimens; include OTC, herbal, and nonherbal drugs in the update
• When chronic dry mouth occurs, advise patient to:
    • Avoid mouth rinses with high alcohol content because of drying effects
    • Use daily home fluoride products for anticaries effect
    • Use sugarless gum, frequent sips of water, or saliva substitutes

rosiglitazone maleate
roz-ih-gli′-tah-zone mal′-ee-ate
(Avandia)
Do not confuse Avandia with Avalide, Avinza, or Prandin.

CATEGORY AND SCHEDULE
Pregnancy Risk Category: C

Drug Class: Oral antidiabetic

MECHANISM OF ACTION
An antidiabetic that improves target-cell response to insulin without increasing pancreatic insulin secretion. Decreases hepatic glucose output and increases insulin-dependent glucose utilization in skeletal muscle.
Therapeutic Effect: Lowers blood glucose concentration.

USES
Monotherapy, as an adjunct to diet and exercise in patients with Type 2 diabetes mellitus; may also be used with metformin when metformin, diet, and exercise are not adequate for control

PHARMACOKINETICS
Rapidly absorbed. Protein binding: 99%. Metabolized in the liver. Excreted primarily in urine, with a lesser amount in feces. Not removed by hemodialysis. *Half-life:* 3–4 hr.

INDICATIONS AND DOSAGES
▸ **Diabetes Mellitus, Combination Therapy**
PO
Adults, Elderly. Initially, 4 mg as a single daily dose or in divided doses twice a day. May increase to 8 mg/day after 12 wk of therapy if fasting

glucose level is not adequately controlled.

▶ **Diabetes Mellitus, Monotherapy**
Adults, Elderly. Initially, 4 mg as single daily dose or in divided doses twice a day. May increase to 8 mg/day after 12 wk of therapy.

SIDE EFFECTS/ADVERSE REACTIONS

Frequent
Upper respiratory tract infection
Occasional
Headache, edema, back pain, fatigue, sinusitis, diarrhea

PRECAUTIONS AND CONTRAINDICATIONS

Active hepatic disease, diabetic ketoacidosis, increased serum transaminase levels, including ALT (SGPT) greater than 2.5 times the normal serum level, Type 1 diabetes mellitus
Caution
May cause resumption of ovulation in premenopausal anovulatory women (risk of pregnancy), patients with edema, advanced heart failure, hepatic impairment, monitor liver enzymes, lactation

DRUG INTERACTIONS OF CONCERN TO DENTISTRY

None reported

SERIOUS REACTIONS

None known

DENTAL CONSIDERATIONS

General:
• Ensure that patient is following prescribed diet and regularly takes medication.
• Place on frequent recall to evaluate healing response.

• Short appointments and a stress-reduction protocol may be required for anxious patients.
• Diabetics may be more susceptible to infection and have delayed wound healing.
• Question patient about self-monitoring of drug's antidiabetic effect, including blood glucose values or finger-stick records.
Consultations:
• Medical consultation may include data from patient's blood glucose monitoring, including glycosylated hemoglobin or HbA1c testing.
• Medical consultation may be required to assess disease control and patient's ability to tolerate stress.
Teach Patient/Family to:
• Prevent trauma when using oral hygiene aids
• Update health and drug history if physician makes any changes in evaluation or drug regimens; include OTC, herbal, and nonherbal drugs in the update

rosuvastatin calcium
ross-uh-vah-stah′-tin kal′-see-um
(Crestor)

CATEGORY AND SCHEDULE
Pregnancy Risk Category: X

Drug Class: Antihyperlipidemic

MECHANISM OF ACTION

An antihyperlipidemic that interferes with cholesterol biosynthesis by inhibiting the conversion of the enzyme HMG-CoA to mevalonate, a precursor to cholesterol. *Therapeutic Effect:* Decreases low-density lipoprotein (LDL) cholesterol, very low-density lipoprotein (VLDL), and plasma triglyceride levels; increases high-density lipoprotein (HDL) concentration.

USES
An adjunct to diet in primary hypercholesterolemia, mixed lipidemia (Fredricksen types IIa and IIb), and homogygous familial hypercholesterolemia and to lower triglycerides in Fredrickson type IV hyperlipidemia

PHARMACOKINETICS
Protein binding: 88%. Minimal hepatic metabolism. Primarily eliminated in the feces. *Half-life:* 19 hr (increased in patients with severe renal dysfunction).

INDICATIONS AND DOSAGES
▶ **Hyperlipidemia, Dyslipidemia**
PO
Adults, Elderly. 5 to 40 mg/day. Usual starting dosage is 10 mg/day, with adjustments based on lipid levels; monitor q2–4wk until desired level is achieved.
▶ **Renal Impairment (creatinine clearance less than 30 ml/min)**
PO
Adults, Elderly. 5 mg/day; do not exceed 10 mg/day.
▶ **Concurrent Cyclosporine Use**
PO
Adults, Elderly. 5 mg/day.
▶ **Concurrent Lipid-Lowering Therapy**
PO
Adults, Elderly. 10 mg/day.

SIDE EFFECTS/ADVERSE REACTIONS
Rosuvastatin is generally well tolerated. Side effects are usually mild and transient.

Occasional
Pharyngitis, headache, diarrhea, dyspepsia, including heartburn and epigastric distress, nausea
Rare
Myalgia, asthenia or unusual fatigue and weakness, back pain

PRECAUTIONS AND CONTRAINDICATIONS
Active hepatic disease, breast-feeding, pregnancy, unexplained, persistent elevations of serum transaminase levels
Caution
Severe renal impairment, hepatic impairment, pregnancy category X, liver function test recommended, alcoholics, efficacy and safety in pediatric patients unknown

DRUG INTERACTIONS OF CONCERN TO DENTISTRY
• No dental drug interactions reported; however, interactions with cyclosporine, warfarin, and gemfibrozil are noted
• Does not inhibit CYP3A4

SERIOUS REACTIONS
! Lens opacities may occur.
! Hypersensitivity reaction and hepatitis occur rarely.

R

DENTAL CONSIDERATIONS
General:
• Monitor vital signs because patients with high cholesterol levels are predisposed to cardiovascular disease.
• Consider semisupine chair position for patient comfort if GI side effects occur.

salmeterol
sal-me′-teh-rol
(Serevent Diskus, Serevent Inhaler and Disks[AUS])
Do not confuse Serevent with Serentil.

CATEGORY AND SCHEDULE
Pregnancy Risk Category: C

Drug Class: Long-acting selective β_2-adrenergic receptor agonist

MECHANISM OF ACTION
An adrenergic agonist that stimulates β_2-adrenergic receptors in the lungs, resulting in relaxation of bronchial smooth muscle. *Therapeutic Effect:* Relieves bronchospasm and reduces airway resistance.

USES
Treatment of bronchospasm associated with COPD, maintenance treatment of bronchospasm associated with COPD, asthma, and exercise-induced bronchospasm

PHARMACOKINETICS

Route	Onset	Peak	Duration
Inhalation	10–20 min	3 hr	12 hr

Low systemic absorption; acts primarily in the lungs. Protein binding: 95%. Metabolized by hydroxylation. Primarily eliminated in feces. *Half-life:* 3–4 hr.

INDICATIONS AND DOSAGES
▶ **Prevention and Maintenance Treatment of Asthma**
Inhalation (Diskus)
Adults, Elderly, Children 4 yr and older. 1 inhalation (50 mcg) q12h.

▶ **Prevention of Exercise-Induced Bronchospasm**
Inhalation
Adults, Elderly, Children 4 yr and older. 1 inhalation at least 30 min before exercise.
▶ **COPD**
Inhalation
Adults, Elderly. 1 inhalation q12h.

SIDE EFFECTS/ADVERSE REACTIONS
Frequent
Headache
Occasional
Cough, tremor, dizziness, vertigo, throat dryness or irritation, pharyngitis
Rare
Palpitations, tachycardia, nausea, heartburn, GI distress, diarrhea

PRECAUTIONS AND CONTRAINDICATIONS
History of hypersensitivity to sympathomimetics
Caution
Lactation, children younger than 12 yr, hepatic impairment, coronary insufficiency, dysrhythmias, hypertension, convulsive disorders; not for acute symptoms, not to exceed recommended dose, paradoxic bronchospasm may occur with use; not recommended for use with a spacer or other aerosol device

DRUG INTERACTIONS OF CONCERN TO DENTISTRY
• Increased cardiovascular effects: tricyclic antidepressants

SERIOUS REACTIONS
❗ Salmeterol may prolong the QT interval, which may precipitate ventricular arrhythmias.
❗ Hypokalemia and hyperglycemia may occur.

S

DENTAL CONSIDERATIONS

General:

• Monitor vital signs at every appointment because of cardiovascular and respiratory side effects.

• Be aware that aspirin or sulfite preservatives in vasoconstrictor-containing products can exacerbate asthma.

• Acute asthmatic episodes may be precipitated in the dental office. Rapid-acting sympathomimetic inhalants should be available for emergency use. Salmeterol is not a rapid-acting drug and is not intended for use in acute asthmatic attacks.

• Consider semisupine chair position for patients with respiratory disease.

• Midmorning appointments and a stress reduction protocol may be required for anxious patients.

Consultations:

• Medical consultation may be required to assess disease control and patient's ability to tolerate stress.

Teach Patient/Family to:

• Use effective oral hygiene to prevent soft tissue inflammation

salsalate

sal′-sa-late
(Amigesic, Disalcid, Mono-Gesic, Salflex)

CATEGORY AND SCHEDULE

Pregnancy Risk Category: C

Drug Class: Salicylate, nonnarcotic analgesic

MECHANISM OF ACTION

An NSAID that inhibits prostaglandin synthesis, reducing the inflammatory response and the intensity of pain stimuli reaching the sensory nerve endings.
Therapeutic Effect: Produces analgesic and antiinflammatory effects.

USES

Treatment of mild-to-moderate pain or fever, including arthritis, juvenile rheumatoid arthritis

PHARMACOKINETICS

Half-life: 7–8 hr.

INDICATIONS AND DOSAGES

▶ **Rheumatoid Arthritis, Osteoarthritis Pain**
PO
Adults, Elderly. Initially, 3 g/day in 2–3 divided doses. Maintenance: 2–4 g/day.

SIDE EFFECTS/ADVERSE REACTIONS

Occasional
Nausea, dyspepsia (including heartburn, indigestion, and epigastric pain)

PRECAUTIONS AND CONTRAINDICATIONS

Bleeding disorders, hypersensitivity to salicylates or NSAIDs
Caution
Anemia, hepatic disease, renal disease, Hodgkin's disease, lactation

DRUG INTERACTIONS OF CONCERN TO DENTISTRY

• Increased risk of GI complaints and occult blood loss: alcohol, NSAIDs, corticosteroids

• Increased risk of bleeding: oral anticoagulants, valproic acid, dipyridamole

• Avoid prolonged or concurrent use with NSAIDs, corticosteroids, acetaminophen

S

• Increased risk of hypoglycemia: oral antidiabetics
• Increased risk of toxicity: methotrexate, lithium, zidovudine
• Decreased effects of probenecid, sulfinpyrazone
• Suspected reduction in the antihypertensive and vasodilator effects of ACE inhibitors; monitor B/P if used concurrently

SERIOUS REACTIONS

! Tinnitus may be the first indication that the serum salicylic acid concentration is reaching or exceeding the upper therapeutic range.
! Salsalate use may also produce vertigo, headache, confusion, drowsiness, diaphoresis, hyperventilation, vomiting, and diarrhea.
! Reye's syndrome may occur in children with chickenpox or the flu.
! Severe overdose may result in electrolyte imbalance, hyperthermia, dehydration, and blood pH imbalance.
! GI bleeding, peptic ulcer, and Reye's syndrome rarely occur.

DENTAL CONSIDERATIONS
General:
• Patients on chronic drug therapy rarely have symptoms of blood dyscrasias, which can include infection, bleeding, and poor healing.
• Potential cross-allergies with other salicylates such as aspirin.
• Consider semisupine chair position for patients with inflammatory joint diseases.
• Avoid prescribing aspirin-containing products because this drug is a salicylate.
• If used for dental patients, take with food or milk to decrease GI complaints; give 30 min before

meals or 2 hr after meals; take with a full glass of water.
Consultations:
• In a patient with symptoms of blood dyscrasias, request a medical consultation for blood studies and postpone dental treatment until normal values are reestablished.
• Medical consultation may be required to assess disease control.
Teach Patient/Family to:
• Not place directly on a tooth or oral mucosa because of risk of chemical burns
• Not exceed recommended dosage; acute toxicity may result
• Read label on other OTC drugs; many contain aspirin
• Avoid alcohol ingestion; GI bleeding may occur
• Use effective oral hygiene to prevent soft tissue inflammation
• Use caution to prevent injury when using oral hygiene aids

saquinavir
sa-kwin′-ah-veer
(Fortovase, Invirase)
Do not confuse saquinavir with Sinequan.

CATEGORY AND SCHEDULE
Pregnancy Risk Category: B

Drug Class: Antiviral

MECHANISM OF ACTION
Inhibits HIV protease, rendering the enzyme incapable of processing the polyprotein precursors needed to generate functional proteins in HIV-infected cells.
Therapeutic Effect: Interferes with HIV replication, slowing the progression of HIV infection.

USES
Treatment of AIDS in combination with nucleoside analogs, zidovudine, or zalcitabine

PHARMACOKINETICS
Poorly absorbed after PO administration (absorption increased with high-calorie and high-fat meals). Protein binding: 99%. Metabolized in the liver to inactive metabolite. Primarily eliminated in feces. Unknown if removed by hemodialysis. *Half-life:* 13 hr.

INDICATIONS AND DOSAGES
▶ **HIV Infection in Combination with Other Antiretrovirals**
PO
Adults, Elderly. 1,200 mg Fortovase 3 times a day or 600 mg Invirase 3 times a day within 2 hr after a full meal.
▶ **Dosage Adjustments When Given in Combination Therapy:**
Delavirdine: Fortovase 800 mg 3 times a day.
Lopinavir/ritonavir: Fortovase 800 mg 2 times a day.
Nelfinavir: Fortovase 800 mg 3 times/day or 1200 mg 2 times a day.
Ritonavir: Fortovase or Invirase 1000 mg 2 times a day.

SIDE EFFECTS/ADVERSE REACTIONS
Occasional
Diarrhea, abdominal discomfort and pain, nausea, photosensitivity, stomatitis
Rare
Confusion, ataxia, asthenia, headache, rash

PRECAUTIONS AND CONTRAINDICATIONS
Clinically significant hypersensitivity to saquinavir; concurrent use with ergot medications, lovastatin, midazolam, simvastatin, or triazolam
Caution
Hepatic impairment, children younger than 16 yr, pregnancy category B, lactation (unknown), bone marrow suppression, renal impairment

DRUG INTERACTIONS OF CONCERN TO DENTISTRY
• Increased plasma levels of clindamycin, troleandomycin, ketoconazole, itraconazole, fentanyl, clarithromycin, midazolam, triazolam
• Increased metabolism of carbamazepine, dexamethasone, phenobarbital
• Inhibits CYP3A4 isoenzymes: use with caution or avoid use with drugs metabolized by these enzymes

SERIOUS REACTIONS
! Ketoacidosis occurs rarely.

DENTAL CONSIDERATIONS
General:
• Examine for oral manifestations of opportunistic infections.
• Patients on chronic drug therapy may rarely have symptoms of blood dyscrasias, which can include infection, bleeding, and poor healing.
• Palliative medication may be required for management of oral side effects.
Consultations:
• Medical consultation may be required to assess disease control.
• In a patient with symptoms of blood dyscrasias, request a medical consultation for blood studies and postpone dental treatment until normal values are reestablished.
Teach Patient/Family to:
• Use effective oral hygiene to prevent soft tissue inflammation
• Use caution to prevent trauma when using oral hygiene aids

• See dentist immediately if secondary oral infection occurs
• Update medical/drug history if physician makes any changes in evaluation or drug regimen; include OTC, herbal, and nonherbal drugs in the update

sargramostim (granulocyte macrophage colony-stimulating factor, GM-CSF)

sar-gra-moh'-stim
(Leukine)
Do not confuse Leukine with Leukeran.

CATEGORY AND SCHEDULE

Pregnancy Risk Category: C

Drug Class: Chemotherapeutic

MECHANISM OF ACTION

A colony-stimulating factor that stimulates proliferation and differentiation of hematopoietic cells to activate mature granulocytes and macrophages. **Therapeutic Effect:** Assists bone marrow in making new WBCs and increases their chemotactic, antifungal, and antiparasitic activity. Increases cytoneoplastic cells and activates neutrophils to inhibit tumor cell growth.

USES

Acute myelogenous leukemia; myeloid reconstitution after bone-marrow transplantation

PHARMACOKINETICS

Effect	Onset	Peak	Duration
Increase WBCs	7–14 days	N/A	1 wk

Detected in serum within 5 min after subcutaneous administration.
Half-life: IV, 1 hr; subcutaneous, 3 hr.

INDICATIONS AND DOSAGES
▶ **Myeloid Recovery Following Bone Marrow Transplant (BMT)**
IV Infusion
Adults, Elderly. Usual parenteral dosage: 250 mcg/m^2/day for 21 days (as 2-hr infusion). Begin 2–4 hr after autologous bone marrow infusion and not less than 24 hr after last dose of chemotherapy or not less than 12 hr after last radiation treatment. Discontinue if blast cells appear or underlying disease progresses.
▶ **BMT Failure, Engraftment Delay**
IV Infusion
Adults, Elderly. 250 mcg/m^2/day for 14 days. Infuse over 2 hr. May repeat after 7 days off therapy if engraftment has not occurred with 500 mcg/m^2/day for 14 days.
▶ **Stem Cell Transplant**
IV, Subcutaneous
Adults. 250 mcg/m^2/day.

SIDE EFFECTS/ADVERSE REACTIONS
Frequent
GI disturbances, including nausea, diarrhea, vomiting, stomatitis, anorexia, and abdominal pain; arthralgia or myalgia; headache; malaise; rash; pruritus
Occasional
Peripheral edema, weight gain, dyspnea, asthenia, fever, leukocytosis, capillary leak syndrome (such as fluid retention, irritation at local injection site, and peripheral edema)
Rare
Rapid or irregular heartbeat, thrombophlebitis

PRECAUTIONS AND CONTRAINDICATIONS

Use 12 hr before or after radiation therapy; 24 hr before or after chemotherapy; excessive leukemic myeloid blasts in bone marrow or peripheral blood (10%); known hypersensitivity to GM-CSF, yeast-derived products, or components of drug

DRUG INTERACTIONS OF CONCERN TO DENTISTRY

• Potentiation of myeloproliferative effects: corticosteroids

SERIOUS REACTIONS

! Pleural or pericardial effusion occurs rarely after infusion.

DENTAL CONSIDERATIONS
General:
• Caution: graft patients or myelosuppressed patients may be at high risk for infection.
• Provide palliative care for dental emergencies only.
• Oral infections should be eliminated and/or treated aggressively.
• If additional analgesia is required for dental pain, consider alternative analgesics (NSAIDs) in patients taking narcotics for acute or chronic pain.
• Monitor and record vital signs.
• Avoid products that affect platelet function, such as aspirin and NSAIDs.
• Patient on chronic drug therapy may rarely present with symptoms of blood dyscrasias, which can include infection, bleeding, and poor healing. If dyscrasia is present, caution patient to prevent oral tissue trauma when using oral hygiene aids.
• Examine for oral manifestation of opportunistic infection.

• Palliative medication may be required for management of oral side effects.
Consultations:
• Medical consultation should include routine blood counts, including platelet counts and bleeding time.
• Consult physician; prophylactic or therapeutic antiinfectives may be indicated if surgery or periodontal treatment is required.
• In a patient with symptoms of blood dyscrasias, request a medical consultation for blood studies and postpone treatment until normal values are reestablished.
• Medical consultation may be required to assess disease control and patient's ability to tolerate stress.
Teach Patient/Family to:
• Use soft tooth brush to reduce risk of bleeding
• Use effective oral hygiene to prevent soft tissue inflammation
• Prevent trauma when using oral hygiene aids
• Report oral lesions, soreness, or bleeding to dentist

scopolamine
skoe-pol′-ah-meen
(Trans-Derm Scop, Transderm-V)

CATEGORY AND SCHEDULE
Pregnancy Risk Category: C

Drug Class: Antiemetic, anticholinergic

MECHANISM OF ACTION
An anticholinergic that reduces excitability of labyrinthine receptors, depressing conduction in the vestibular cerebellar pathway.
Therapeutic Effect: Prevents

motion-induced nausea and vomiting.

USES
Prevention of motion sickness; prevention of nausea, vomiting associated with anesthesia or opiate analgesia

PHARMACOKINETICS
Patch: Onset 4–5 hr, duration 72 hr.

INDICATIONS AND DOSAGES
▶ **Prevention of Motion Sickness**
Transdermal
Adults. 1 system q72h.
▶ **Postoperative Nausea or Vomiting**
Transdermal
Adults, Elderly. 1 system no sooner than 1 h before surgery and removed 24 h after surgery.

SIDE EFFECTS/ADVERSE REACTIONS
Frequent
Dry mouth, somnolence, blurred vision
Rare
Dizziness, restlessness, hallucinations, confusion, difficulty urinating, rash

PRECAUTIONS AND CONTRAINDICATIONS
Angle-closure glaucoma, GI or GU obstruction, myasthenia gravis, paralytic ileus, tachycardia, thyrotoxicosis
Caution
Children, elderly, pyloric, urinary, bladder neck, intestinal obstruction; liver, kidney disease

DRUG INTERACTIONS OF CONCERN TO DENTISTRY
• Increased anticholinergic effects: propantheline and other anticholinergic drugs

• Increased risk of CNS depression: alcohol, all CNS depressants

SERIOUS REACTIONS
None known

DENTAL CONSIDERATIONS
General:
• Avoid dental light in patient's eyes; offer dark glasses for patient comfort.
• Caution patients about driving or performing other tasks requiring mental alertness.
Teach Patient/Family to:
• Avoid mouth rinses with high alcohol content because of drying effects

secobarbital
see-koe-bar'-bih-tal
Schedule II
(Seconal)

CATEGORY AND SCHEDULE
Pregnancy Risk Category: D
Controlled Substance: Schedule II

Drug Class: Sedative-hypnotic barbiturate

MECHANISM OF ACTION
A barbiturate that depresses the CNS activity by binding to barbiturate site at the gamma-aminobutyric acid (GABA)-receptor complex, enhancing GABA activity and depressing the reticular activity system. ***Therapeutic Effect:*** Produces hypnotic effect due to CNS depression.

USES
Treatment of insomnia, sedation, preoperative medication, status epilepticus, acute tetanus convulsions

PHARMACOKINETICS
Well absorbed from the GI tract.
Protein binding: 52%–57%. Crosses
blood–brain barrier. Widely
distributed. Metabolized in liver by
microsomal enzyme system to
inactive and active metabolites.
Primarily excreted in urine.
Not removed by hemodialysis.
Half-life: 15–40 hr.

INDICATIONS AND DOSAGES
▶ **Insomnia**
PO
Adults. 100 mg at bedtime.
▶ **Preoperative Sedation**
PO
Adults. 100–300 mg 1–2 hr.
before procedure.
Children. 2–6 mg/kg 1–2 hr. before
procedure. Maximum: 100 mg/dose.
▶ **Sedation, Daytime**
PO
Adults. 30–50 mg 3–4 times a day.
Children. 2 mg/kg 3 times a day.

SIDE EFFECTS/ADVERSE REACTIONS
Frequent
Somnolence
Occasional
Agitation, confusion, hyperkinesia,
ataxia, CNS depression, nightmares,
nervousness, psychiatric disturbance,
hallucinations, insomnia, anxiety,
dizziness, abnormality in thinking,
hypoventilation, apnea, bradycardia,
hypotension, syncope, nausea,
vomiting, constipation, headache
Rare
Hypersensitivity reactions, fever,
liver damage, megaloblastic anemia

PRECAUTIONS AND CONTRAINDICATIONS
History of manifest or latent
porphyria, marked liver dysfunction,
marked respiratory disease in which

dyspnea or obstruction is evident,
and hypersensitivity to secobarbital
or barbiturates
Caution
Anemia, lactation, hepatic disease,
renal disease, hypertension, elderly,
acute/chronic pain

DRUG INTERACTIONS OF CONCERN TO DENTISTRY
• Hepatotoxicity: halogenated
hydrocarbon anesthetics
• Increased CNS depression: alcohol,
all CNS depressants
• Increased metabolism of
carbamazepine, tricyclic
antidepressants, corticosteroids
• Decreased half-life of doxycycline

SERIOUS REACTIONS
❗ Agranulocytosis, megaloblastic
anemia, apnea, hypoventilation,
bradycardia, hypotension, syncope,
hepatic damage, and Stevens-
Johnson syndrome rarely occur.
❗ Tolerance and physical dependence
may occur with repeated use.

DENTAL CONSIDERATIONS
General:
• Determine why the patient is taking
the drug.
• Monitor vital signs at every
appointment because of
cardiovascular side effects. Evaluate
respiration characteristics and rate.
• Patients on chronic drug therapy
may rarely have symptoms of
blood dyscrasias, which can
include infection, bleeding, and poor
healing.
• When used for sedation in
dentistry:
  • Assess vital signs before and
  q30min after use as sedative.
  • Observe respiratory dysfunction:
  respiratory depression, character,
  rate, rhythm; hold drug if

S

respirations are less than 10/min or if pupils are dilated.
• After supine positioning, have patient sit upright for at least 2 min before standing to avoid orthostatic hypotension.
• Have someone drive patient to and from dental office when drug used for conscious sedation.
• Barbiturates induce liver microsomal enzymes, which alter the metabolism of other drugs.
• Geriatric patients are more susceptible to drug effects; use a lower dose.
Consultations:
• In a patient with symptoms of blood dyscrasias, request a medical consultation for blood studies and postpone dental treatment until normal values are reestablished.
Teach Patient/Family to:
• Avoid driving or other activities requiring mental alertness
• Avoid alcohol ingestion and CNS depressants; serious CNS depression may result
• Use caution when using OTC preparations (antihistamines, cold remedies) that contain CNS depressants

selegiline hydrochloride

seh-leg′-ill-ene high-droh-klor′-ide
(Apo-Selegiline[CAN], Eldepryl, Novo-Selegiline[CAN], Selgene[AUS])
Do not confuse selegiline with Stelazine, or Eldepryl with enalapril.

CATEGORY AND SCHEDULE
Pregnancy Risk Category: C

Drug Class: Antiparkinson agent

MECHANISM OF ACTION
An antiparkinson agent that irreversibly inhibits the activity of monoamine oxidase type B, the enzyme that breaks down dopamine, thereby increasing dopaminergic action. *Therapeutic Effect:* Relieves signs and symptoms of Parkinson's disease.

USES
Adjunct management of Parkinson's disease in patients being treated with levodopa or carbidopa

PHARMACOKINETICS
Rapidly absorbed from the GI tract. Crosses the blood–brain barrier. Metabolized in the liver to the active metabolites. Primarily excreted in urine. *Half-life:* 17 hr (amphetamine), 20 hr (methamphetamine).

INDICATIONS AND DOSAGES
▶ **Adjunctive Treatment for Parkinsonism**
PO
Adults. 10 mg/day in divided doses, such as 5 mg at breakfast and lunch, given concomitantly with each dose of carbidopa and levodopa.
Elderly. Initially, 5 mg in the morning. May increase up to 10 mg/day.

SIDE EFFECTS/ADVERSE REACTIONS
Frequent
Nausea, dizziness, light-headedness, syncope, abdominal discomfort
Occasional
Confusion, hallucinations, dry mouth, vivid dreams, dyskinesia
Rare
Headache, myalgia, anxiety, diarrhea, insomnia

PRECAUTIONS AND CONTRAINDICATIONS

Hypersensitivity: fluoxetine, meperidine

Caution

Lactation, children

DRUG INTERACTIONS OF CONCERN TO DENTISTRY

• Fatal interaction: opioids (especially meperidine); do not administer together
• Risk of serotonin syndrome: serotonin uptake inhibitors (fluoxetine, sertraline, paroxetine)

SERIOUS REACTIONS

! Symptoms of overdose may vary from CNS depression, characterized by sedation, apnea, cardiovascular collapse, and death, to severe paradoxic reactions, such as hallucinations, tremor, and seizures.
! Other serious effects may include involuntary movements, impaired motor coordination, loss of balance, blepharospasm, facial grimaces, feeling of heaviness in the lower extremities, depression, nightmares, delusions, overstimulation, sleep disturbance, and anger.

DENTAL CONSIDERATIONS

General:

• Monitor vital signs at every appointment because of cardiovascular side effects.
• After supine positioning, have patient sit upright for at least 2 min before standing to avoid orthostatic hypotension.
• Assess for presence of extrapyramidal motor symptoms, such as tardive dyskinesia and akathisia. Extrapyramidal motor activity may complicate dental treatment.
• Assess salivary flow as a factor in caries, periodontal disease, and candidiasis.

Consultations:

• Medical consultation may be required to assess disease control and patient's ability to tolerate stress.
• If signs of tardive dyskinesia or akathisia are present, refer to physician.

Teach Patient/Family to:

• Use electric tooth brush if patient has difficulty holding conventional devices
• When chronic dry mouth occurs, advise patient to:
  • Avoid mouth rinses with high alcohol content because of drying effects
  • Use daily home fluoride products to prevent caries
  • Use sugarless gum, frequent sips of water, or saliva substitutes

sertaconazole

sir-tah-con′-ah-zole
(Ertaczo)

CATEGORY AND SCHEDULE

Pregnancy Risk Category: C

Drug Class: Antifungal

MECHANISM OF ACTION

An imidazole derivative that inhibits synthesis of ergosterol, a vital component of fungal cell formation. **Therapeutic Effect:** Damages the fungal cell membrane, altering its function.

USES

Fungal infections

PHARMACOKINETICS

Half-life: 60 hr.

INDICATIONS AND DOSAGES

▶ **Tinea Pedis**

Topical

Adults, Elderly, Children 12 yr and older. Apply to affected area twice a day for 4 wk.

SIDE EFFECTS/ADVERSE REACTIONS
Rare
Burning, tenderness, erythema, dryness, pruritus, hyperpigmentation, and contact dermatitis at application site

PRECAUTIONS AND CONTRAINDICATIONS
None known.

DRUG INTERACTIONS OF CONCERN TO DENTISTRY
None reported

SERIOUS REACTIONS
None known.

DENTAL CONSIDERATIONS
General:
• Determine why patient is taking this drug.

sertraline
sir'-trall-een
(Apo-Sertraline[CAN], Novo-Sertraline[CAN], PMS-Sertraline[CAN], Zoloft)
Do not confuse sertraline with Serentil.

CATEGORY AND SCHEDULE
Pregnancy Risk Category: B

Drug Class: Antidepressant

MECHANISM OF ACTION
An antidepressant, anxiolytic, and obsessive-compulsive disorder adjunct that blocks the reuptake of the neurotransmitter serotonin at CNS neuronal presynaptic membranes,
increasing its availability at postsynaptic receptor sites. *Therapeutic Effect:* Relieves depression, reduces obsessive-compulsive behavior, decreases anxiety.

USES
Treatment of major depression, obsessive-compulsive disorder (OCD), panic disorder, posttraumatic stress disorder, premenstrual dysphoric mood disorder, social anxiety disorder

PHARMACOKINETICS
Incompletely and slowly absorbed from the GI tract; food increases absorption. Protein binding: 98%. Widely distributed. Undergoes extensive first-pass metabolism in the liver to active compound. Excreted in urine and feces. Not removed by hemodialysis. *Half-life:* 26 hr.

INDICATIONS AND DOSAGES
▶ **Depression**
PO
Adults. Initially, 50 mg/day.
May increase by 50 mg/day at 7-day intervals up to 200 mg/day.
Elderly. Initially, 25 mg/day.
May increase by 25–50 mg/day at 7-day intervals up to 200 mg/day.
▶ **OCD**
PO
Adults, Children 13–17 yr. Initially, 50 mg/day with morning or evening meal. May increase by 50 mg/day at 7-day intervals.
Elderly, Children 6–12 yr. Initially, 25 mg/day. May increase by 25–50 mg/day at 7-day intervals.
Maximum: 200 mg/day.
▶ **Panic Disorder, Posttraumatic Stress Disorder, Social Anxiety Disorder**
PO
Adults, Elderly. Initially, 25 mg/day.
May increase by 50 mg/day at 7-day intervals. Range: 50–200 mg/day.
Maximum: 200 mg/day.

▶ **Premenstrual Dysphoric Disorder**
PO
Adults. Initially, 50 mg/day. May increase up to 150 mg/day in 50-mg increments.

SIDE EFFECTS/ADVERSE REACTIONS
Frequent
Headache, nausea, diarrhea, insomnia, somnolence, dizziness, fatigue, rash, dry mouth
Occasional
Anxiety, nervousness, agitation, tremor, dyspepsia, diaphoresis, vomiting, constipation, abnormal ejaculation, visual disturbances, altered taste
Rare
Flatulence, urinary frequency, paraesthesia, hot flashes, chills

PRECAUTIONS AND CONTRAINDICATIONS
User within 14 days of MAOIs
Caution
Lactation, elderly, hepatic/renal disease, epilepsy

DRUG INTERACTIONS OF CONCERN TO DENTISTRY
• Increased CNS depression: alcohol, CNS depressants, St. John's wort (herb)
• Increased side effects: highly protein-bound drugs (aspirin), tricyclic antidepressants
• Increased half-life of diazepam
• Possible inhibition of sertraline metabolism: erythromycin, clarithromycin
• Potent inhibitor of CYP2D6 isoenzymes; use drugs metabolized by the enzyme only with caution
• Possible risk of serotonin syndrome with tramadol, oxycodone
• Decreased effects: carbamazepine
• First-time users of SSRIs also taking NSAIDs may have a higher

risk of GI side effects; until more data are available, it may be advisable to avoid use of NSAIDs in these patients (Br J Clin Pharmacol 55:591–595, 2003)

SERIOUS REACTIONS
None known

DENTAL CONSIDERATIONS
General:
• Monitor vital signs at every appointment because of cardiovascular side effects.
• After supine positioning, have patient sit upright for at least 2 min before standing to avoid orthostatic hypotension.
• Assess salivary flow as a factor in caries, periodontal disease, and candidiasis.
• Avoid dental light in patient's eyes; offer dark glasses for patient comfort.
• Consider semisupine chair position for patient comfort if GI side effects occur.
Consultations:
• Medical consultation may be required to assess patient's ability to tolerate stress.
• Physician should be informed if significant xerostomic side effects occur (e.g., increased caries, sore tongue, problems eating or swallowing, difficulty wearing prosthesis) so that a medication change can be considered.
Teach Patient/Family to:
• Use electric tooth brush if patient has difficulty holding conventional devices
• When chronic dry mouth occurs, advise patient to:
  • Avoid mouth rinses with high alcohol content because of drying effects
  • Use daily home fluoride products to prevent caries

- Use sugarless gum, frequent sips of water, or saliva substitutes

sevelamer hydrochloride

seh-vel′-ah-mer high-droh-klor′-ide
(Renagel)
Do not confuse Renagel with Reglan or Regonol.

CATEGORY AND SCHEDULE

Pregnancy Risk Category: C

Drug Class: Chelating agent

MECHANISM OF ACTION

An antihyperphosphatemia agent that binds with dietary phosphorus in the GI tract, thus allowing phosphorus to be eliminated through the normal digestive process and decreasing the serum phosphorus level. *Therapeutic Effect:* Decreases incidence of hypercalcemic episodes in patients receiving calcium acetate treatment.

USES

Adjunct to peritoneal dialysis

PHARMACOKINETICS

Not absorbed systemically. Unknown if removed by hemodialysis.

INDICATIONS AND DOSAGES

▶ **Hyperphosphatemia**
PO
Adults, Elderly. 800–1600 mg with each meal, depending on severity of hyperphosphatemia.

SIDE EFFECTS/ADVERSE REACTIONS

Frequent
Infection, pain, hypotension, diarrhea, dyspepsia, nausea, vomiting

Occasional
Headache, constipation, hypertension, thrombosis, increased cough

PRECAUTIONS AND CONTRAINDICATIONS

Bowel obstruction, hypophosphatemia

DRUG INTERACTIONS OF CONCERN TO DENTISTRY

- Possible decrease in bioavailability: orally administered, rapidly absorbed drugs; give at least 1 hr before or 3 hr after sevelamer doses

SERIOUS REACTIONS

None known

DENTAL CONSIDERATIONS

General:
- Patients taking this drug may be undergoing renal dialysis; confirm the medical and drug history to plan appropriate management.
- If you prescribe medications for dental needs, have patient take medication 1 hr before or 3 hr after sevelamer doses.
- Monitor and record vital signs.
- Consider semisupine chair position for patient comfort if GI side effects occur.
- Patient may need assistance getting into and out of dental chair. Adjust chair position for patient comfort.
- Consultation with physician may be necessary if sedation or general anesthesia is required.
Consultations:
- Medical consultation may be required to assess disease control and patient's ability to tolerate stress.
Teach Patient/Family to:
- Report oral lesions, soreness, or bleeding to dentist

S

• Use effecive oral hygiene to prevent soft tissue inflammation
• Prevent trauma when using oral hygiene aids
• Update health and medication history if physician makes any changes in evaluation or drug regimens; include OTC, herbal, and nonherbal remedies in the update

sibutramine
sih-byoo'-tra-meen
(Meridia)

CATEGORY AND SCHEDULE
Pregnancy Risk Category: C
Controlled Substance: Schedule IV

Drug Class: Amphetamine analog anorexiant

MECHANISM OF ACTION
A CNS stimulant that inhibits reuptake of serotonin (enhancing satiety) and norepinephrine (raises metabolic rate) centrally.
Therapeutic Effect: Induces and maintains weight loss.

USES
Treatment of obesity

PHARMACOKINETICS
Rapidly absorbed from the GI tract. Protein binding: 95%–97%. Metabolized in liver, undergoes first-pass metabolism. Primarily excreted in urine, minimal elimination in feces. *Half-life:* 1.1 hr.

INDICATIONS AND DOSAGES
▶ **Weight Loss**
PO
Adults 16 yr and older. Initially, 10 mg/day. May increase up to *15 mg/day.* Maximum: 20 mg/day.

SIDE EFFECTS/ADVERSE REACTIONS
Frequent
Headache, dry mouth, anorexia, constipation, insomnia, rhinitis, pharyngitis
Occasional
Back pain, flu syndrome, dizziness, nausea, asthenia (loss of strength, energy), arthralgia, nervousness, dyspepsia, sinusitis, abdominal pain, anxiety, dysmenorrhea
Rare
Depression, rash, cough, sweating, tachycardia, migraine, increased B/P, paresthesia, altered taste

PRECAUTIONS AND CONTRAINDICATIONS
Anorexia nervosa, concomitant MAOI use, concomitant use of centrally acting appetite suppressants, hypersensitivity to sibutramine or any component of the formulation
Caution
Requires monitoring of B/P, risk of serotonin syndrome with other serotonin reuptake inhibitors, glaucoma, lactation, children younger than 16 yr, elderly, seizures

DRUG INTERACTIONS OF CONCERN TO DENTISTRY
• Avoid use of meperidine: risk of serotonin syndrome

SERIOUS REACTIONS
! Seizures, thrombocytopenia, and deaths have been reported.
! Serotonin syndrome can occur with concomitant use of drugs that increase serotonin.
! Large doses may produce extreme nervousness and tachycardia.

S

DENTAL CONSIDERATIONS

General:

• Monitor vital signs at every appointment because of cardiovascular side effects.

• Assess salivary flow as factor in caries, periodontal disease, and candidiasis.

• Information on any abuse liability is unknown.

• Determine why patient is taking the drug.

Teach Patient/Family:

• When chronic dry mouth occurs, advise patient to:
  • Avoid mouth rinses with high alcohol content because of drying effects
  • Use daily home fluoride products to prevent caries
  • Use sugarless gum, frequent sips of water, or saliva substitutes

sildenafil citrate

sill-den´-ah-fill sih´-trate

(Viagra)

Do not confuse Viagra with Vaniqa.

CATEGORY AND SCHEDULE

Pregnancy Risk Category: B

Drug Class: Impotence therapy

MECHANISM OF ACTION

An erectile dysfunction agent that inhibits phosphodiesterase type 5, the enzyme responsible for degrading cyclic guanosine monophosphate in the corpus cavernosum of the penis, resulting in smooth muscle relaxation and increased blood flow. *Therapeutic Effect:* Facilitates an erection.

USES

Treatment of male erectile dysfunction

PHARMACOKINETICS:

PO: Rapid oral absorption, bioavailability 40%, peak plasma levels 30 min–2 hr, hepatic metabolism by CYP3A4 (major) and CYP2C9 (minor) isoenzymes, active metabolite, highly plasma protein bound (96%), major excretion route in feces, lesser route in urine.

INDICATIONS AND DOSAGES
▶ **Erectile Dysfunction**

PO

Adults. 50 mg (30 min–4 hr before sexual activity). Range: 25–100 mg. Maximum dosing frequency is once daily.

Elderly older than 65 yr. Consider starting dose of 25 mg.

SIDE EFFECTS/ADVERSE REACTIONS

Frequent

Headache, flushing

Occasional

Dyspepsia, nasal congestion, UTI, abnormal vision, diarrhea

Rare

Dizziness, rash

PRECAUTIONS AND CONTRAINDICATIONS

Concurrent use of sodium nitroprusside or nitrates in any form

Caution

Complete medical and physical exam to determine cause of erectile dysfunction; because of cardiac risk associated with sexual activity, cardiovascular status should be evaluated; anatomic deformation of penis, conditions predisposing to priapism (sickle cell anemia, anemia, multiple myeloma, leukemia), retinitis pigmentosa, not indicated for women, children, or newborns, pregnancy category B; hepatic or renal impairment, men 65 yr or older

DRUG INTERACTIONS OF CONCERN TO DENTISTRY
• Avoid use of nitroglycerin within 24 hr
• Increased plasma levels caused by interference with metabolism: cimetidine, erythromycin, ketoconazole, itraconazole
• Inhibitors of CYP3A4 or CYP2C9 isoenzymes: should be used with caution

SERIOUS REACTIONS
! Prolonged erections (lasting over 4 hr) and priapism (painful erections lasting over 6 hr) occur rarely.

DENTAL CONSIDERATIONS
General:
• This is an acute-use drug intended to be taken just before sexual activity, and the reported incidence of oral side effects does not differ from a placebo. However, the potential interacting drugs should be avoided.

silver sulfadiazine
sul-fah-dye′-ah-zeen
(Flamazine[CAN], SSD, SSD AF, Silvadene)

CATEGORY AND SCHEDULE
Pregnancy Risk Category: B

Drug Class: Antimicrobial

MECHANISM OF ACTION
An antiinfective that acts upon the cell wall and cell membrane. Releases silver slowly in concentrations selectively toxic to bacteria. *Therapeutic Effect:* Produces bactericidal effect.

USES
Treatment of urinary tract infections

PHARMACOKINETICS
Variably absorbed. Significant systemic absorption may occur if applied to extensive burns. Absorbed medication excreted unchanged in urine. *Half-life:* 10 hr (half-life increased with impaired renal function).

INDICATIONS AND DOSAGES
▶ **Burns**
Topical
Adults, Elderly Children. Apply 1–2 times daily.

SIDE EFFECTS/ADVERSE REACTIONS
Side effects characteristic of all sulfonamides may occur when systemically absorbed, such as extensive burn areas, anorexia, nausea, vomiting, headache, diarrhea, dizziness, photosensitivity, joint pain
Frequent
Burning feeling at treatment site
Occasional
Brown-gray skin discoloration, rash, itching
Rare
Increased sensitivity of skin to sunlight

PRECAUTIONS AND CONTRAINDICATIONS
Hypersensitivity to silver sulfadiazine or any component of the formulation

DRUG INTERACTIONS OF CONCERN TO DENTISTRY
None reported

SERIOUS REACTIONS
! If significant systemic absorption occurs, less often but serious are

S

hemolytic anemia, hypoglycemia, diuresis, peripheral neuropathy, Stevens-Johnson syndrome, agranulocytosis, disseminated lupus erythematosus, anaphylaxis, hepatitis, and toxic nephrosis.
! Fungal superinfections may occur.
! Interstitial nephritis occurs rarely.

DENTAL CONSIDERATIONS
General:
• Dental management depends on extent and severity of burns and patient's ability to cooperate; above all use aseptic techniques.
• Provide palliative dental care for dental emergencies only.
Consultations:
• Medical consultation may be required to assess disease control and patient's ability to tolerate stress.
• Consult patient's physician if an acute dental infection occurs and another antiinfective is required.
Teach Patient/Family to:
• Use effective oral hygiene to prevent soft tissue inflammation
• Prevent trauma when using oral hygiene aids

simethicone
sih-meth′-ih-kone
(Alka-Seltzer Gas Relief, Gas-X, Genasym, Infant Mylicon, Mylanta Gas, Ovol[CAN], Phazyme)

CATEGORY AND SCHEDULE
Pregnancy Risk Category: C
OTC

Drug Class: Antiflatulent

MECHANISM OF ACTION
An antiflatulent that changes surface tension of gas bubbles, allowing easier elimination of gas.

Therapeutic Effect: Drug dispersal, prevents formation of gas pockets in the GI tract.

USES
Relief of bloating, discomfort, and pain caused by excessive gas in the stomach

PHARMACOKINETICS
Does not appear to be absorbed from GI tract. Excreted unchanged in feces.

INDICATIONS AND DOSAGES
▶ **Antiflatulent**
PO
Adults, Elderly, Children 12 yr and older. 40–250 mg after meals and at bedtime. Maximum: 500 mg/day.
Children 2–11 yr. 40 mg 4 times a day.
Children younger than 2 yr. 20 mg 4 times a day.

SIDE EFFECTS/ADVERSE REACTIONS
None known

PRECAUTIONS AND CONTRAINDICATIONS
None known

DRUG INTERACTIONS OF CONCERN TO DENTISTRY
None reported

SERIOUS REACTIONS
None known

DENTAL CONSIDERATIONS
General:
• Determine why patient is taking the drug.
• Consider semisupine chair position for patient comfort because of GI effects of disease.
• Question patient about tolerance of NSAIDs or aspirin related to GI disease.

• Patients with gastroesophageal reflux may present with oral symptoms, including burning mouth, secondary candidiasis, and signs of tooth erosion.
• Patients using this drug may have GI disease; review medical and drug history.

Teach Patient/Family to:
• Update health and medication history if physician makes any changes in evaluation or drug regimens; include OTC, herbal, and nonherbal remedies in the update
• Use effective oral hygiene to prevent soft tissue inflammation

---

simvastatin

sim′-vah-sta-tin
(Apo-Simvastatin[CAN], Lipex[AUS], Zocor)
Do not confuse Zocor with Cozaar.

CATEGORY AND SCHEDULE
Pregnancy Risk Category: X

Drug Class: Antihyperlipidemic

MECHANISM OF ACTION
A HMG-CoA reductase inhibitor that interferes with cholesterol biosynthesis by inhibiting the conversion of the enzyme HMG-CoA to mevalonate. ***Therapeutic Effect:*** Decreases serum low-density lipoproteins (LDL), cholesterol, very low-density lipoproteins (VLDL), and plasma triglyceride levels; slightly increases serum high-density lipoprotein (HDL) concentration.

USES
An adjunct in homozygous familial hypercholesterolemia, mixed hyperlipidemia, elevated serum triglyceride levels, and type IV hyperproteinemia; also reduces total cholesterol LDL-C, apo B, and triglyceride levels; patient should first be placed on cholesterol-lowering diet; effective in reducing risk of heart attacks and strokes

PHARMACOKINETICS

Route	Onset	Peak	Duration
PO to reduce cholesterol	3 days	14 days	N/A

Well absorbed from the GI tract. Protein binding: 95%. Undergoes extensive first-pass metabolism. Hydrolyzed to active metabolite. Primarily eliminated in feces. Unknown if removed by hemodialysis.

INDICATIONS AND DOSAGES
▶ **Adjunct to Diet to Decrease Heterozygous Familial Hypercholesterolemia in Adolescents 10–17 yr of Age (girls at least 1-yr post-menarche)**
▶ **Heterozygous Familial Hypercholesterolemia**
PO
Pediatric. 10 mg once daily in evening. Range: 10–40 mg/day. Maximum: 40 mg/day.
▶ **To Decrease Elevated Total and LDL Cholesterol in Hypercholesterolemia (types IIa and IIb), Lower Triglyceride Levels, and Increase HDL Levels; to Reduce Risk of Death and Prevent MI in Patients with Heart Disease and Elevated Cholesterol Level; to Reduce Risk of Revascularization Procedures; to Decrease Risk of Stroke or Transient Ischemic Attack; to Prevent Cardiovascular Events**
PO
Adults. Initially, 10–40 mg/day in evening. Dosage adjusted at 4-wk intervals.

S

Elderly. Initially, 10 mg/day. May increase by 5–10 mg/day q4wk. Range: 5–80 mg/day. Maximum: 80 mg/day.

SIDE EFFECTS/ADVERSE REACTIONS
Simvastatin is generally well tolerated; side effects are usually mild and transient
Occasional
Headache, abdominal pain or cramps, constipation, upper respiratory tract infection
Rare
Diarrhea, flatulence, asthenia (loss of strength and energy), nausea or vomiting

PRECAUTIONS AND CONTRAINDICATIONS
Active hepatic disease or unexplained, persistent elevations of liver function test results, age younger than 18 yr, pregnancy
Caution
Past liver disease, alcoholics (first-pass metabolism with CYP3A4 isoenzymes); severe acute infections, trauma, hypotension, uncontrolled seizure disorders, severe metabolic disorders, electrolyte imbalances

DRUG INTERACTIONS OF CONCERN TO DENTISTRY
• Increased myalgia, myositis: erythromycin, cyclosporine, itraconazole, ketoconazole
• Caution with use of drugs that are strong inhibitors of CYP3A4 isoenzymes

SERIOUS REACTIONS
❗ Lens opacities may occur.
❗ Hypersensitivity reaction and hepatitis occur rarely.

General:
• Consider semisupine chair position for patient comfort because of GI side effects.
• Assess patient for possible cardiovascular disease.

sirolimus
sir-oh-leem′-us
(Rapamune)

CATEGORY AND SCHEDULE
Pregnancy Risk Category: C

Drug Class: Immunosuppressant

MECHANISM OF ACTION
An immunosuppressant that inhibits T-lymphocyte proliferation induced by stimulation of cell surface receptors, mitogens, alloantigens, and lymphokines. Prevents activation of the enzyme target of rapamycin, a key regulatory kinase in cell cycle progression. *Therapeutic Effect:* Inhibits proliferation of T and B cells, essential components of the immune response; prevents organ transplant rejection.

USES
Adjunct to organ transplantation

PHARMACOKINETICS
Rapidly absorbed from the GI tract. Peak levels 1 hr (inhibited by food). Protein binding: 92%. Extensively metabolized by the CYP 3A4 isoenzyme in the intestinal wall and liver. Primarily excreted in feces.

INDICATIONS AND DOSAGES
▶ **Prevention of Organ Transplant Rejection**
PO
Adults. Loading dose: 6 mg.
Maintenance: 2 mg/day.
Children 13 yr and older weighing less than 40 kg. Loading dose: 3 mg/m^2.
Maintenance: 1 mg/m^2/day.

SIDE EFFECTS/ADVERSE REACTIONS
Occasional
Hypercholesterolemia, hyperlipidemia, hypertension, rash; with high doses (5 mg/day): anemia, arthralgia, diarrhea, hypokalemia, and thrombocytopenia

PRECAUTIONS AND CONTRAINDICATIONS
Hypersensitivity to sirolimus, malignancy

DRUG INTERACTIONS OF CONCERN TO DENTISTRY
• Increased blood levels: potent inhibitors of CYP3A4 isoenzymes (clarithromycin, clotrimazole, erythromycin, fluconazole, itraconazole, ritonavir, indinavir, grapefruit juice)
• Decreased blood levels: potent inducers of CYP3A4 isoenzymes (phenobarbital, carbamazepine, St. John's wort [herb])

SERIOUS REACTIONS
None known

DENTAL CONSIDERATIONS
General:
• Caution: patients on immunosuppressive therapy may be at high risk for infection.
• Provide palliative dental care for dental emergencies only.
• Oral infections should be eliminated and/or treated aggressively.

• Patients may be at risk for bleeding; check oral signs.
• Examine for evidence of oral candidiasis. Topically acting antifungals may be preferred: note potential drug interactions.
• Monitor and record vital signs.
• Avoid products that affect platelet function, such as aspirin and NSAIDs.
• Patient on chronic drug therapy may rarely present with symptoms of blood dyscrasias, which can include infection, bleeding, and poor healing. If dyscrasia is present, caution patient to prevent oral tissue trauma when using oral hygiene aids.
• Consider local hemostasis measures to prevent excessive bleeding.
Consultations:
• Medical consultation should include routine blood counts, including platelet counts and bleeding time.
• Consult physician; prophylactic or therapeutic antiinfectives may be indicated if surgery or periodontal treatment is required.
• In a patient with symptoms of blood dyscrasias, request a medical consultation for blood studies and postpone treatment until normal values are reestablished.
• Medical consultation may be required to assess disease control and patient's ability to tolerate stress.
Teach Patient/Family to:
• Use soft tooth brush to reduce risk of bleeding
• Use effective oral hygiene to prevent soft tissue inflammation
• Prevent trauma when using oral hygiene aids
• Report oral lesions, soreness, or bleeding to dentist
• Use electric tooth brush if patient has difficulty holding conventional devices

S

sodium fluoride

soe′-dee-um flor′-ide
(Fluoritabs, Flura-Drops, Fluor-
A-Day, Fluotic, Flurodex Karidium,
Luride Lozi-Tabs, Pediaflor,
PediDent, Solu-Flur; also found in
pediatric vitamin formulas)

CATEGORY AND SCHEDULE

Pregnancy Risk Category: Not
established

Drug Class: Fluoride ion

MECHANISM OF ACTION

Interacts with tooth structure to
increase resistance to acid
dissolution; promotes enamel
remineralization and inhibits
dental plaque microorganisms

USES

Prevention of dental caries

PHARMACOKINETICS

PO: Efficient oral absorption
(75–90%); distributed to
calcified tissues (bones and
teeth); excreted in urine, feces;
crosses placenta, excreted in
breast milk.

INDICATIONS AND DOSAGES

▶ **Prevention of Dental Caries**
Topical
Adult, Children older than 12 yr. 10 ml
0.2% solution daily after brushing
teeth; rinse mouth for at least 1 min
with solution.
PO
Children 6–12 yr. 5 ml 0.2%
solution.
Must ascertain fluoride concentration
in patient's drinking water before

prescribing, as shown in the
following tables:
▶ **USA–Fluoride Supplementation Schedule**
Drinking Water [F⁻]

Child's Age	Less than 0.3 ppm	0.3–0.6 ppm	More than 0.6 ppm
Birth–6 mo	0	0	0
6 mo–3 yr	0.25 mg/day		0
3–6 yr	0.50 mg/day	0.25 mg/day	0
6–16 yr	1.0 mg/day	0.50 mg/day	0

▶ **Canada–Fluoride Supplementation Schedule**

Age	Canadian Paediatric Society (Applies to all Children)	Canadian Dental Association (Applies to Children with High Risk of Caries)
6 mo–2 yr	0.25 mg/day	0
3–5 yr	0.50 mg/day	0.25 mg/day (0.5 mg/day if fluoridated toothpaste is not used regularly)
6–12 yr	Not applicable	1.00 mg/day
6–16 yr	1.0 mg/day	Not applicable

SIDE EFFECTS/ADVERSE REACTIONS

Occasional
Mottled, stained enamel (chronic
use), stomatitis
Acute overdose: Black tarry stools,
bloody vomit, diarrhea, decreased
respiration, increased salivation,
watery eyes

Chronic overdose: Hypocalcemia, tetany, respiratory arrest, constipation, loss of appetite, nausea, vomiting, weight loss

PRECAUTIONS AND CONTRAINDICATIONS
Hypersensitivity, renal insufficiency, GI ulcerations
Caution
Children younger than 6 yr (must evaluate total fluoride ingestion)

DRUG INTERACTIONS OF CONCERN TO DENTISTRY:
● Avoid use with dairy products and gastric alkalinizers

SERIOUS REACTIONS
● Cardiac arrhythmias, renal failure

DENTAL CONSIDERATIONS
General:
● Determine fluoride concentration in water supply, then calculate dosage.
● In the United States, the use of fluoride supplements is not recommended when community drinking water contains at least 0.6 ppm fluoride or after age 16.
● Recommended dose should not be exceeded or dental fluorosis and osseous changes may occur.
● To reduce risk of accidental ingestion and overdosage, ADA recommends that a limit of 264 mg sodium fluoride be dispensed in prepackaged containers.
● Give drops after meals with fluids or undiluted tablets; may be chewed; do not swallow whole; may be given with water or juice; avoid milk.
● Systemic fluoride use during pregnancy has not been shown to prevent tooth decay in children.
● Treatment of acute overdose:
  ● Gastric lavage with calcium chloride or calcium hydroxide solution to precipitate fluoride.

● Maintenance of high urine output.
● Refer to hospital emergency facility.
Teach Patient/Family to:
● Monitor children using gel or rinse; not to be swallowed
● Not drink, eat, or rinse mouth for at least 0.5 hr after topical use
● Apply after brushing and flossing at bedtime
● Store out of children's reach

sodium fluoride (topical)
soe'-dee-um flor'-ide
(nonabrasive: Karigel, Neutracare, Prevident; with abrasive: PreviDent 5000 Plus)

CATEGORY AND SCHEDULE
Pregnancy Risk Category: Not established

Drug Class: Fluoride ion

MECHANISM OF ACTION
Interacts with enamel surface to increase resistance to acid dissolution; promotes enamel remineralization and inhibits dental plaque microorganisms

USES
Prevention of dental caries, hypersensitive root surfaces

PHARMACOKINETICS
PO: Efficient oral absorption (75–90%); distributed to calcified tissues (bones and teeth); excreted in urine, feces; crosses placenta, excreted in breast milk.

INDICATIONS AND DOSAGES
▸ **Prevention of Dental Caries**
Topical
Adults, Children older than 6 yr.
Nonabrasive gels—use daily; apply thin ribbon to tooth brush for at least 1 min after regular brushing,

preferably at bedtime; expectorate and refrain from eating, drinking, and rinsing; children should use under parental supervision.
Available forms include: Gel or cream 2 oz (56 g) squeeze tube 0.5% (as 1.1% sodium fluoride) with and without mild abrasive.
Other fluoride topical products include the following daily-use gels.
1.1% APF (Thera-Flur); 0.4% Sn F2 (Control, Easy-Gel, Flocare, Flo-Gel, Florentine, Gel-Kam, Gel-Pro, Gel-Tin, Perfect Choice, Quick-Gel, Stan-Gard, Stop Gel).
Rinses: 0.05% APF daily use (NaFrinse, Phos-Flur) and 0.2% NaF weekly use (NaFrinse, Point-Two, Preventive, Prevident).

Product Strength	F- Ion (%)	ppm F Equivalence
1.1% NaF	0.5	4950
0.4% SnF2	0.10	970
0.2% NaF	0.10	910
0.05% NaF	0.02	230

SIDE EFFECTS
Occasional
Mottled, stained enamel (chronic use), stomatitis
Acute overdose: Black tarry stools, bloody vomit, diarrhea, decreased respiration, increased salivation, watery eyes
Chronic overdose: Hypocalcemia, tetany, respiratory arrest, constipation, loss of appetite, nausea, vomiting, weight loss

PRECAUTIONS AND CONTRAINDICATIONS
Hypersensitivity; may be used in areas of fluoridated drinking water.
Caution
Children younger than 6 yr (repeated swallowing of agent could cause dental fluorosis); do not use in pediatric patients younger than 6 yr, infants. Supervise children younger than 6 yr.

A 2-oz tube of 1.1% NaF contains 250 mg fluoride, more than twice the amount that the ADA recommends to be dispensed in 1 container. Ingestion of as little as 0.29 oz could cause acute toxicity in a 1-yr-old child. Repeated swallowing could cause fluorosis.

DRUG INTERACTIONS OF CONCERN TO DENTISTRY
• None reported

SERIOUS REACTIONS
• Cardiac arrhythmias, renal failure

DENTAL CONSIDERATIONS
General:
• Neutral sodium fluoride preparations are recommended for patients with exposed root surfaces, which may be hypersensitive.
Teach Patient/Family to:
• Apply daily a thin ribbon of dental cream or gel to toothbrush and brush thoroughly for 2 min, preferably at bedtime
• Expectorate after use and not to eat, drink, or rinse for 30 min
• Have children use under parental supervision

sotalol hydrochloride
soe′-tah-lole high-droh-klor′-ide
(Apo-Sotalol[CAN], Betapace, Betapace AF, Cardol[AUS], Novo-Sotalol[CAN], PMS-Sotalol[CAN], Solavert[AUS], Sorine, Sotab[AUS], Sotacor[AUS], Sotahexal[AUS])
Do not confuse sotalol with Stadol.

CATEGORY AND SCHEDULE
Pregnancy Risk Category: B (D if used in second or third trimester)

Drug Class: Nonselective β-adrenergic blocker

MECHANISM OF ACTION

A β-adrenergic blocking agent that prolongs action potential, effective refractory period, and QT interval. Decreases heart rate and AV node conduction; increases AV node refractoriness. *Therapeutic Effect:* Produces antiarrhythmic activity.

USES

Treatment of life-threatening ventricular dysrhythmias (class II), atrial fibrillation (Betapace AF only)

PHARMACOKINETICS

Well absorbed from the GI tract. Protein binding: None. Widely distributed. Primarily excreted unchanged in urine. Removed by hemodialysis. *Half-life:* 12 hr (increased in the elderly and patients with impaired renal function).

INDICATIONS AND DOSAGES
▶ **Documented, Life-Threatening Arrhythmias**
PO
Adults, Elderly. Initially, 80 mg twice a day. May increase gradually at 2- to 3-day intervals. Range: 240–320 mg/day.
▶ **Dosage in Renal Impairment**
Dosage interval is modified on the basis of creatinine clearance.

Creatinine Clearance	Dosage Interval
31–60 ml/min	24 hr
10–30 ml/min	36–48 hr
Less than 10 ml/min	Individualized

SIDE EFFECTS/ADVERSE REACTIONS
Frequent
Diminished sexual function, drowsiness, insomnia, unusual fatigue or weakness

Occasional
Depression, cold hands or feet, diarrhea, constipation, anxiety, nasal congestion, nausea, vomiting
Rare
Altered taste, dry eyes, itching, numbness of fingers, toes, or scalp

PRECAUTIONS AND CONTRAINDICATIONS

Bronchial asthma, cardiogenic shock, prolonged QT syndrome (unless functioning pacemaker is present), second- and third-degree heart block, sinus bradycardia, uncontrolled cardiac failure
Caution
Lactation, diabetes mellitus, renal disease before initiating doses place patient in cardiac care facility to monitor for drug-induced arrhythmia

DRUG INTERACTIONS OF CONCERN TO DENTISTRY

• Decreased hypotensive effect: NSAIDs, indomethacin
• Increased hypotension, myocardial depression: hydrocarbon inhalation anesthetics
• Hypertension, bradycardia: sympathomimetics
• Slow metabolism of lidocaine

SERIOUS REACTIONS

! Bradycardia, CHF, hypotension, bronchospasm, hypoglycemia, prolonged QT interval, torsades de pointes, ventricular tachycardia, and premature ventricular complexes may occur.

S

DENTAL CONSIDERATIONS
General:
• Monitor vital signs at every appointment because of cardiovascular side effects.
• After supine positioning, have patient sit upright for at least 2 min

before standing to avoid orthostatic hypotension.

• Stress from dental procedures may compromise cardiovascular function; determine patient risk.

• Use vasoconstrictors with caution, in low doses, and with careful aspiration. Avoid use of gingival retraction cord with epinephrine.

• Short appointments and a stress-reduction protocol may be required for anxious patients.

Consultations:

• Medical consultation should be made to assess disease control and patient's ability to tolerate stress.

sparfloxacin

spar-floks′-ah-sin
(Zagam)
Not available in U.S.

CATEGORY AND SCHEDULE

Pregnancy Risk Category: C

Drug Class: Fluoroquinolone antiinfective

MECHANISM OF ACTION

A fluoroquinolone that interferes with DNA-gyrase in susceptible microorganisms. *Therapeutic Effect:* Inhibits DNA replication and repair. Bactericidal.

USES

Community-acquired pneumonia and acute bacterial exacerbations of chronic bronchitis caused by susceptible microorganisms (*C. pneumoniae, H. influenzae, M. pneumoniae, S. pneumoniae, K. pneumoniae, M. catarrhalis, S. aureus, E. cloacae*)

PHARMACOKINETICS

Well absorbed from the GI tract after PO administration. Widely distributed. Metabolized in liver. Primarily excreted in urine with a lesser amount eliminated in the feces. *Half-life:* 16–30 hr.

INDICATIONS AND DOSAGES
▶ **Bronchitis, Pneumonia**
PO
Adults 18 yr and older, Elderly.
Initially, 2 200 mg tablets as a loading dose on first day. Then 1 200 mg tablet q24h for a total of 10 days.

▶ **Dosage in Renal Impairment (creatinine clearance less than 50 ml/min)**
PO
Adults 18 yr and older, Elderly.
Initially, 2 200 mg tablets as a loading dose on first day. Then 1 200 mg tablet q48h for a total of 9 days.

SIDE EFFECTS/ADVERSE REACTIONS

Occasional
Photosensitivity, diarrhea, nausea, headache
Rare
Dyspepsia, dizziness, insomnia, abdominal pain, change in taste

PRECAUTIONS AND CONTRAINDICATIONS

Hypersensitivity to fluoroquinolones, cinoxacin, nalidixic acid
Caution
Antacids retard absorption, renal impairment, avoid exposure to sun, artificial ultraviolet light, patients younger than 18 yr, seizures, cardiovascular arrhythmics, MI, CHF, lactation

DRUG INTERACTIONS OF CONCERN TO DENTISTRY
• Avoid concurrent use with erythromycin, pentamidine, tricyclic antidepressants, phenothiazines
• Concurrent administration with antacids greatly reduces oral absorption, can increase warfarin levels
• Increased risk of life-threatening arrhythmias: procainamide

SERIOUS REACTIONS
! Superinfection (particularly enterococcal or fungal overgrowth of nonsusceptible organisms) caused by altered bacterial balance may occur (genital-anal pruritus, ulceration or changes in oral mucosa, moderate to severe diarrhea, new or increased fever).
! Hypersensitivity reactions have occurred in those receiving fluoroquinolone therapy.

DENTAL CONSIDERATIONS
General:
• Contraindicated for patients whose lifestyle or employment will not permit compliance with photosensitivity precautions.
• Determine why patient is taking the drug.
• Assess salivary flow as factor in caries, periodontal disease, and candidiasis.
• Consider semisupine chair position for patient comfort if GI side effects occur.
• Avoid dental light in patient's eyes; offer dark glasses for patient comfort.
Consultations:
• Consult with patient's physician if an acute dental infection occurs and another antiinfective is required.

Teach Patient/Family to:
• Avoid exposure to sunlight and wear sunscreen if sun exposure is planned during treatment and for 5 days after treatment is stopped

spironolactone
speer-on-oh-lak′-tone
(Aldactone, Novo-Spiroton[CAN], Spiractin[AUS])
Do not confuse Aldactone with Aldactazide.

CATEGORY AND SCHEDULE
Pregnancy Risk Category: C
(D if used in pregnancy-induced hypertension)

Drug Class: Potassium-sparing diuretic

MECHANISM OF ACTION
A potassium-sparing diuretic that interferes with sodium reabsorption by competitively inhibiting the action of aldosterone in the distal tubule, thus promoting sodium and water excretion and increasing potassium retention. ***Therapeutic Effect:*** Produces diuresis; lowers B/P; diagnostic aid for primary aldosteronism.

USES
Edema, hypertension, diuretic-induced hypokalemia, primary hyperaldosteronism (diagnosis, short-term treatment, long-term treatment), nephrotic syndrome, cirrhosis of the liver with ascites

PHARMACOKINETICS

Route	Onset	Peak	Duration
PO	24–48 hr	48–72 hr	48–72 hr

Well absorbed from the GI tract (absorption increased with food). Protein binding: 91%–98%. Metabolized in the liver to active metabolite. Primarily excreted in urine. Unknown if removed by hemodialysis. *Half-life:* 0–24 hr (metabolite, 13–24 hr).

INDICATIONS AND DOSAGES
▸ **Edema**
PO
Adults, Elderly. 25–200 mg/day as a single dose or in 2 divided doses.
Children. 1.5–3.3 mg/kg/day in divided doses.
Neonates. 1–3 mg/kg/day in 1–2 divided doses.
▸ **Hypertension**
PO
Adults, Elderly. 25–50 mg/day in 1–2 doses/day.
Children. 1.5–3.3 mg/kg/day in divided doses.
▸ **Hypokalemia**
PO
Adults, Elderly. 25–200 mg/day as a single dose or in 2 divided doses.
▸ **Male Hirsutism**
PO
Adults, Elderly. 50–200 mg/day as a single dose or in 2 divided doses.
▸ **Primary Aldosteronism**
PO
Adults, Elderly. 100–400 mg/day as a single dose or in 2 divided doses.
Children. 100–400 mg/m^2/day as a single dose or in 2 divided doses.
▸ **Dosage in Renal Impairment**
Dosage interval is modified on the basis of creatinine clearance.

Creatinine Clearance	Interval
10–50 ml/min	Usual dose q12–24h
Less than 10 ml/min	Avoid use

SIDE EFFECTS/ADVERSE REACTIONS
Frequent
Hyperkalemia (in patients with renal insufficiency and those taking potassium supplements), dehydration, hyponatremia, lethargy
Occasional
Nausea, vomiting, anorexia, abdominal cramps, diarrhea, headache, ataxia, somnolence, confusion, fever
Male: Gynecomastia, impotence, decreased libido
Female: Menstrual irregularities (including amenorrhea and postmenopausal bleeding), breast tenderness
Rare
Rash, urticaria, hirsutism

PRECAUTIONS AND CONTRAINDICATIONS
Acute renal insufficiency, anuria, BUN and serum creatinine levels more than twice normal values, hyperkalemia
Caution
Dehydration, hepatic disease, lactation, hyponatremia

DRUG INTERACTIONS OF CONCERN TO DENTISTRY
• Nephrotoxicity: indomethacin and possibly other NSAIDs
• Decreased antihypertensive effect: indomethacin and possibly other NSAIDs

SERIOUS REACTIONS
! Severe hyperkalemia may produce arrhythmias, bradycardia, and ECG changes (tented T waves, widening QRS complex and ST segment depression). These may proceed to cardiac standstill or ventricular fibrillation.
! Cirrhosis patients are at risk for hepatic decompensation if dehydration or hyponatremia occurs.

! Patients with primary aldosteronism may experience rapid weight loss and severe fatigue during high-dose therapy.

DENTAL CONSIDERATIONS

General:
• Monitor vital signs at every appointment because of cardiovascular side effects.
• Assess salivary flow as a factor in caries, periodontal disease, and candidiasis.
• If dry mouth occurs, follow usual preventive and palliative measures, but consider hyponatremia as a contributing factor.
• Consider semisupine chair position for patient comfort if GI side effects occur.
Consultations:
• Medical consultation may be required to assess disease control and patient's ability to tolerate stress.
Teach Patient/Family:
• When chronic dry mouth occurs, advise patient to:
  • Avoid mouth rinses with high alcohol content because of drying effects
  • Use daily home fluoride products to prevent caries
  • Use sugarless gum, frequent sips of water, or saliva substitutes

sucralfate

soo-kral'-fate
(Apo-Sucralate[CAN], Carafate, Novo-Sucralate[CAN], Ulcyte[AUS])
Do not confuse Carafate with Cafergot.

CATEGORY AND SCHEDULE

Pregnancy Risk Category: B

Drug Class: Protectant, aluminum salt of a sulfated sucrose

MECHANISM OF ACTION

An antiulcer agent that forms an ulcer-adherent complex with proteinaceous exudate, such as albumin, at ulcer site. Also forms a viscous adhesive barrier on the surface of intact mucosa of the stomach or duodenum. ***Therapeutic Effect:*** Protects damaged mucosa from further destruction by absorbing gastric acid, pepsin, and bile salts.

USES

Treatment of duodenal ulcer

PHARMACOKINETICS

Minimally absorbed from the GI tract. Eliminated in feces, with small amount excreted in urine. Not removed by hemodialysis.

INDICATIONS AND DOSAGES

▶ **Active Duodenal Ulcers**
PO
Adults, Elderly. 1 g 4 times a day (before meals and at bedtime) for up to 8 wk.
▶ **Maintenance Therapy after Healing of Acute Duodenal Ulcers**
PO
Adults, Elderly. 1 g twice a day.

SIDE EFFECTS/ADVERSE REACTIONS

Frequent
Constipation
Occasional
Dry mouth, backache, diarrhea, dizziness, somnolence, nausea, indigestion, rash, hives, itching, abdominal discomfort

PRECAUTIONS AND CONTRAINDICATIONS

Caution
Lactation, children

S

DRUG INTERACTIONS OF CONCERN TO DENTISTRY

- Gastric irritation: chloral hydrate
- Decreased absorption of tetracyclines, fluoroquinolones
- Decreased effects of diclofenac, ketoconazole

SERIOUS REACTIONS

None known

DENTAL CONSIDERATIONS

General:
- Prescribe acetaminophen for analgesia if needed. ASA and NSAIDs are contraindicated in active upper GI disease.
- Consider semisupine chair position for patient comfort because of GI effects of disease.
- Tetracycline doses should be given 2 hr before or after the sucralfate dose.

Teach Patient/Family to:
- Avoid mouth rinses with high alcohol content because of drying effects

sulconazole nitrate

sul-kon´-ah-zole nye-trate
(Exelderm)

CATEGORY AND SCHEDULE

Pregnancy Risk Category: C

Drug Class: Topical antifungal

MECHANISM OF ACTION

An imidazole derivative that inhibits synthesis of ergosterol (a vital component of fungal cell formation), the damaging cell membrane.
Therapeutic Effect: Fungistatic.

USES

Treatment of tinea pedis, tinea corporis, tinea cruris, tinea versicolor; unapproved: cutaneous candidiasis

PHARMACOKINETICS

Minimal systemic absorption following topical administration. Excreted in urine. **Half-life:** Unknown.

INDICATIONS AND DOSAGES

▸ **Tinea pedis**
Topical
Adults, Elderly, Children 12 yr and older. Apply 2 times a day until signs and symptoms significantly improve.

▸ **Tinea corporis, Tinea cruris, Tinea versicolor**
Topical
Adults, Elderly, Children 12 yr and older. Apply 1–2 times a day until signs and symptoms significantly improve.

SIDE EFFECTS/ADVERSE REACTIONS

Occasional
Headache, nausea
Rare
Burning or stinging, pruritus, redness

PRECAUTIONS AND CONTRAINDICATIONS

Hypersensitivity to sulconazole nitrate or any component of the formulation
Caution
Pregnancy category C

DRUG INTERACTIONS OF CONCERN TO DENTISTRY

None reported

SERIOUS REACTIONS

None known

DENTAL CONSIDERATIONS

General:
• There are no significant dental considerations. One possible concern is the few patients with topical candidiasis, in whom broad-spectrum antiinfectives could potentially contribute to a superinfection.

sulfacetamide

sul-fa-see'-ta-mide
(AK-Sulf, Bleph-10, Isopto Cetamide, Diosulf[CAN], Ophthacet, Sodium Sulamyd, Sulfair)

CATEGORY AND SCHEDULE

Pregnancy Risk Category: C

Drug Class: Antibacterial sulfonamide

MECHANISM OF ACTION

Interferes with synthesis of folic acid that bacteria require for growth. **Therapeutic Effect:** Prevents further bacterial growth. Bacteriostatic.

USES

Treatment of conjunctivitis, superficial eye infections, corneal ulcers, trachoma

PHARMACOKINETICS

Small amounts may be absorbed into the cornea. Excreted rapidly in urine. **Half-life:** 7–13 hr.

INDICATIONS AND DOSAGES

▶ **Treatment of Corneal Ulcers, Conjunctivitis, and Other Superficial Infections of the Eye, Prophylaxis after Injuries to the Eye/Removal of Foreign Bodies, Adjunctive Therapy for Trachoma and Inclusion Conjunctivitis**
Ophthalmic

Adults, Elderly. Ointment: Apply small amount in lower conjunctival sac 1–4 times a day and at bedtime. Solution: 1–3 drops to lower conjunctival sac q2–3h. Seborrheic dermatitis, seborrheic sicca (dandruff), secondary bacterial skin infections
Topical
Adults, Elderly. Apply 1–4 times a day.

SIDE EFFECTS/ADVERSE REACTIONS

Frequent
Transient ophthalmic burning, stinging
Occasional
Headache
Rare
Hypersensitivity (erythema, rash, itching, swelling, photosensitivity)

PRECAUTIONS AND CONTRAINDICATIONS

Hypersensitivity to sulfonamides or any component of preparation (some products contain sulfite), use in combination with silver-containing products
Caution
Cross-sensitivity with other sulfas; pregnancy category C

DRUG INTERACTIONS OF CONCERN TO DENTISTRY

None reported

SERIOUS REACTIONS

! Superinfection, drug-induced lupus erythematosus, Stevens-Johnson syndrome occur rarely; nephrotoxicity with high dermatologic concentrations.

DENTAL CONSIDERATIONS

General:
• Avoid dental light in patient's eyes; offer dark glasses for patient comfort.

sulfasalazine

sul-fa-sal'-ah-zeen
(Alti-Sulfasalazine[CAN],
Azulfidine, Azulfidine EN-tabs,
Pyralin EN[AUS], Salazopyrin[CAN],
Salazopyrin EN[AUS], Salazopyrin
EN-Tabs[CAN])
Do not confuse Azulfidine with
azathioprine, or sulfasalazine with
sulfadiazine or sulfisoxazole.

CATEGORY AND SCHEDULE

Pregnancy Risk Category: B
(D if given near term)

Drug Class: Sulfonamide
derivative with antiinflammatory
action

MECHANISM OF ACTION

A sulfonamide that inhibits
prostaglandin synthesis, acting
locally in the colon. ***Therapeutic
Effect:*** Decreases inflammatory
response, interferes with GI
secretion.

USES

Treatment of ulcerative colitis,
Crohn's disease, rheumatoid
arthritis, juvenile rheumatoid
arthritis; unapproved: ankylosing
spondylitis

PHARMACOKINETICS

Poorly absorbed from the GI
tract. Cleaved in colon by
intestinal bacteria, forming
sulfapyridine and mesalamine
(5-ASA). Absorbed in colon.
Widely distributed. Metabolized in
the liver. Primarily excreted
in urine.
Half-life: sulfapyridine, 6–14 hr;
5-ASA, 0.6–1.4 hr.

INDICATIONS AND DOSAGES

▶ **Ulcerative Colitis**
PO
Adults, Elderly. 1 g 3–4 times
a day in divided doses q4–6h.
Maintenance: 2 g/day in divided
doses q6–12h. Maximum:
6 g/day.
Children. 40–75 mg/kg/day in
divided doses q4–6h. Maintenance:
30–50 mg/kg/day in divided doses
q4–8h. Maximum: 2 g/day.
Maximum: 6 g/day.
▶ **Rheumatoid Arthritis**
PO
Adults, Elderly. Initially, 0.5–1 g/day
for 1 wk. Increase by 0.5 g/wk, up to
3 g/day.
▶ **Juvenile Rheumatoid Arthritis**
PO
Children. Initially, 10 mg/kg/day.
May increase by 10 mg/kg/day at
weekly intervals. Range: 30–50 mg/
kg/day. Maximum: 2 g/day.

SIDE EFFECTS/ADVERSE REACTIONS

Frequent
Anorexia, nausea, vomiting,
headache, oligospermia
(generally reversed by withdrawal
of drug)
Occasional
Hypersensitivity reaction
(rash, urticaria, pruritus, fever,
anemia)
Rare
Tinnitus, hypoglycemia, diuresis,
photosensitivity

PRECAUTIONS AND CONTRAINDICATIONS

Children younger than 2 yr;
hypersensitivity to carbonic
anhydrase inhibitors, local
anesthetics, salicylates,
sulfonamides, sulfonylureas,
sunscreens containing PABA, or

thiazide or loop diuretics; intestinal or urinary tract obstruction; porphyria; pregnancy at term; severe hepatic or renal dysfunction
Caution
Lactation, impaired hepatic function, severe allergy, bronchial asthma, impaired renal function, intolerance to aspirin

DRUG INTERACTIONS OF CONCERN TO DENTISTRY
• Increased photosensitizing effects: tetracycline
• Decreased absorption: folic acid

SERIOUS REACTIONS
! Anaphylaxis, Stevens-Johnson syndrome, hematologic toxicity (leukopenia, agranulocytosis), hepatotoxicity, and nephrotoxicity occur rarely.

DENTAL CONSIDERATIONS
General:
• Patients on chronic drug therapy may rarely have symptoms of blood dyscrasias, which can include infection, bleeding, and poor healing.
• Question patient about response to antibiotics to avoid responses that might provoke pseudomembranous colitis.
• Palliative medication may be required for management of oral side effects.
• Consider semisupine chair position for patient comfort because of GI effects of disease.
Consultations:
• Medical consultation may be required to assess disease control and patient's ability to tolerate stress.
• In a patient with symptoms of blood dyscrasias, request a medical consultation for blood studies and postpone dental treatment until normal values are reestablished.

Teach Patient/Family to:
• Use caution to prevent injury when using oral hygiene aids

sulfinpyrazone
sul-fin-pyr´-ah-zone
(Anturane, Apo-Sulfinpyrazone[CAN], Nu-Sufinpyrazone[CAN])
Do not confuse with Accutane.

CATEGORY AND SCHEDULE
Pregnancy Risk Category: C/D (near term)

Drug Class: Uricosuric

MECHANISM OF ACTION
A uricosuric that increases urinary excretion of uric acid, thereby decreasing blood urate levels. ***Therapeutic Effect:*** Promotes uric acid excretion and reduces serum uric acid levels.

USES
Treatment of chronic gouty arthritis

PHARMACOKINETICS
Rapidly and completely absorbed from GI tract. Widely distributed. Metabolized in liver to 2 active metabolite, p-hydroxy-sulfinpyrazone and a sulfide analog. Excreted primarily in urine. Not removed by hemodialysis. ***Half-life:*** 2.7–6 hr.

INDICATIONS AND DOSAGES
▸ **Gout**
PO
Adults, Elderly. 100–200 mg 2 times a day. Maximum: 800 mg/day.

SIDE EFFECTS/ADVERSE REACTIONS

Frequent
Nausea, vomiting, stomach pain
Occasional
Flushed face, headache, dizziness, frequent urge to urinate, rash
Rare
Increased bleeding time, hepatic necrosis, nephrotic syndrome, uric acid stones

PRECAUTIONS AND CONTRAINDICATIONS

Active peptic ulcer, blood dyscrasias, GI inflammation, pregnancy (near term), hypersensitivity to sulfinpyrazone or any of its components, phenylbutazone, or other pyrazoles

DRUG INTERACTIONS OF CONCERN TO DENTISTRY

- Increased bleeding: NSAIDs, aspirin
- Decreased effects of salicylates

SERIOUS REACTIONS

! Hematological toxicity including anemia, leucopenia, agranulocytosis, thrombocytopenia, and aplastic anemia occur rarely.
! Overdose causes a drowsiness, dizziness, anorexia, abdominal pain, hemolytic anemia, acidosis, jaundice, fever, and agranulocytosis.

DENTAL CONSIDERATIONS

General:
- Consider local hemostasis measures to prevent excessive bleeding.
- Avoid prescribing aspirin-containing products.
- Patients on chronic drug therapy may rarely have symptoms of blood dyscrasias, which can include infection, bleeding, and poor healing.
- Consider semisupine chair position for patient comfort if GI side effects occur.
- Evaluate respiration characteristics and rate.

Consultations:
- In a patient with symptoms of blood dyscrasias, request a medical consultation for blood studies and postpone dental treatment until normal values are reestablished.

Teach Patient/Family to:
- Use caution to prevent injury when using oral hygiene aids

---

sulfisoxazole

sul-fi-sox′-ah-zole
(Gantrisin, Novo-Soxazole[CAN], Sulfizole[CAN], Truxazole)
Do not confuse with sulfadiazine, sulfamethoxazole, sulfasalazine, Gastrosed

CATEGORY AND SCHEDULE

Pregnancy risk category: B/D (near term)

Drug Class: Sulfonamide, antiinfective

MECHANISM OF ACTION

An antibacterial sulphonamide that inhibits bacterial synthesis of dihydrofolic acid by preventing condensation of pteridine with aminobenzoic acid through competitive inhibition of the enzyme dihydropteroate synthetase.
Therapeutic Effect: Bacteriostatic.

USES

Treatment of urinary tract, systemic infections; chancroid; trachoma; toxoplasmosis; acute otitis media; lymphogranuloma venereum; eye infections

PHARMACOKINETICS

Rapidly and completely absorbed. Small intestine is major site of absorption, but some absorption occurs in the stomach. Exists in the blood as unbound, protein-bound, and conjugated forms. Sulfisoxazole is metabolized primarily by acetylation and oxidation in the liver. The free form is considered to be the therapeutically active form. Protein binding: 85%. *Half-life:* 5–8 hr.

INDICATIONS AND DOSAGES
▶ **Acute, Recurrent or Chronic UTI, Meningococcal Meningitis, Acute Otitis Media due to Haemophilus Influenzae**
PO
Infants older than 2 mo, Children.
One-half of the 24-hr dose initially then 150 mg/kg daily or 4 g/M^2 daily for maintenance divided q4–6h. Maximum dose: 6 g daily.
Adults. 2–4 g initially then 4–8 g daily divided q4–6h.

SIDE EFFECTS/ADVERSE REACTIONS

Anaphylaxis, erythema multiforme (Stevens-Johnson syndrome), toxic epidermal necrolysis, exfoliative dermatitis, angioedema, arteritis and vasculitis, allergic myocarditis, serum sickness, rash, urticaria, pruritus, photosensitivity, conjunctival and scleral injection, generalized allergic reactions, generalized skin eruptions, tachycardia, palpitations, syncope, cyanosis, goiter, diuresis, hypoglycemia, arthralgia, myalgia, headache, dizziness, peripheral neuritis, paresthesia, convulsions, tinnitus, vertigo, ataxia, intracranial hypertension, cough, shortness of breath, pulmonary infiltrates

PRECAUTIONS AND CONTRAINDICATIONS

Patients with a known hypersensitivity to sulfonamides, children younger than 2 mo (except in the treatment of congenital toxoplasmosis as adjunctive therapy with pyrimethamine), pregnant women at term, and mothers nursing infants younger than 2 mo of age
Caution
Lactation, impaired hepatic function, severe allergy, bronchial asthma

DRUG INTERACTIONS OF CONCERN TO DENTISTRY

• Decreased effect: ester-type local anesthetics (procaine, tetracaine)
• Increased photosensitizing effect: tetracycline
• Decreased effect of penicillins, cephalosporins

SERIOUS REACTIONS

! Fatalities associated with the administration of sulfonamides, including Stevens-Johnson syndrome toxic epidermal necrolysis; fulminant hepatic necrosis, agranulocytosis, aplastic anemia, and other blood dyscrasias occur rarely.
! Clinical signs, such as rash, sore throat, fever, arthralgia, pallor, purpura, or jaundice, may be early indications of serious reactions.

DENTAL CONSIDERATIONS
General:
• Patients on chronic drug therapy may rarely have symptoms of blood dyscrasias, which can include infection, bleeding, and poor healing.
• Determine why the patient is taking the drug.
• Palliative medication may be required for management of oral side effects.

S

• Consider semisupine chair position for patient comfort if GI side effects occur.

Consultations:

• Medical consultation may be required to assess disease control.

• In a patient with symptoms of blood dyscrasias, request a medical consultation for blood studies and postpone dental treatment until normal values are reestablished.

Teach Patient/Family to:

• Use effective oral hygiene to prevent soft tissue inflammation

sulindac

sul-in'-dak

(Aclin[AUS], Apo-Sulin[CAN], Clinoril, Novo Sundac[CAN])

Do not confuse Clinoril with Clozaril.

CATEGORY AND SCHEDULE

Pregnancy Risk Category: B (D if used in third trimester or near delivery)

Drug Class: Nonsteroidal antiinflammatory

MECHANISM OF ACTION

An NSAID that produces analgesic and antiinflammatory effects by inhibiting prostaglandin synthesis. *Therapeutic Effect:* Reduces inflammatory response and intensity of pain.

USES

Treatment of osteoarthritis, rheumatoid arthritis, acute gouty arthritis, tendinitis, bursitis, ankylosing spondylitis

PHARMACOKINETICS

Route	Onset	Peak	Duration
PO (Antirheumatic)	7 days	2–3 wk	N/A

Well absorbed from the GI tract. Metabolized in liver to active metabolite. Primarily excreted in urine. Not removed by hemodialysis. *Half-life:* 7.8 hr; metabolite: 16.4 hr.

INDICATIONS AND DOSAGES

▸ **Rheumatoid Arthritis, Osteoarthritis, Ankylosing Spondylitis**

PO

Adults, Elderly. Initially, 150 mg twice a day; may increase up to 400 mg/day.

▸ **Acute Shoulder Pain, Gouty Arthritis, Bursitis, Tendinitis**

PO

Adults, Elderly. 200 mg twice a day.

SIDE EFFECTS/ADVERSE REACTIONS

Frequent

Diarrhea or constipation, indigestion, nausea, maculopapular rash, dermatitis, dizziness, headache

Occasional

Anorexia, abdominal cramps, flatulence

PRECAUTIONS AND CONTRAINDICATIONS

Active peptic ulcer disease, chronic inflammation of GI tract, GI bleeding or ulceration, history of hypersensitivity to aspirin or NSAIDs

Caution

Lactation, children, bleeding disorders, GI disorders, cardiac disorders, hypersensitivity to other NSAIDs, geriatric patients

DRUG INTERACTIONS OF CONCERN TO DENTISTRY
• Increased bleeding, GI effects: alcohol, aspirin, steroids, other NSAIDs
• Renal toxicity: acetaminophen (prolonged use)
• Possible risk of decreased renal function: cyclosporine
• Increased photosensitizing effect: tetracycline
• Increased toxicity of methotrexate, cyclosporine
• Decreased plasma levels: diflunisal
• First-time users of SSRIs also taking NSAIDs may have a higher risk of GI side effects; until more data are available, it may be advisable to avoid use of NSAIDs in these patients (Br J Clin Pharmacol 55:591–595, 2003)

SERIOUS REACTIONS
! Rare reactions with long-term use include peptic ulcer disease, GI bleeding, gastritis, nephrotoxicity (glomerular nephritis, interstitial nephritis, nephrotic syndrome), severe hepatic reactions (cholestasis, jaundice), and severe hypersensitivity reactions (fever, chills, and joint pain).

DENTAL CONSIDERATIONS
General:
• Patients on chronic drug therapy may rarely have symptoms of blood dyscrasias, which can include infection, bleeding, and poor healing.
• Assess salivary flow as a factor in caries, periodontal disease, and candidiasis.
• Avoid prescribing in last trimester of pregnancy.
• Should oral inflammation or lesions occur, refer to physician and consider palliative treatment for the lesions.

• Consider semisupine chair position for patient comfort because of GI side effects.
Consultations:
• Medical consultation may be required to assess disease control.
• In a patient with symptoms of blood dyscrasias, request a medical consultation for blood studies and postpone dental treatment until normal values are reestablished.
Teach Patient/Family to:
• Report oral lesions, soreness, or bleeding to dentist
• Use caution to prevent injury in use of oral hygiene aids
• Use effective oral hygiene to prevent soft tissue inflammation
• When chronic dry mouth occurs, advise patient to:
  • Avoid mouth rinses with high alcohol content because of drying effects
  • Use daily home fluoride products to prevent caries
  • Use sugarless gum, frequent sips of water, or saliva substitutes

sumatriptan
soo-ma-trip'-tan
(Imigran[AUS], Imitrex, Suvalan[AUS])
Do not confuse sumatriptan with somatropin.

CATEGORY AND SCHEDULE
Pregnancy Risk Category: C

Drug Class: Serotonin agonist

MECHANISM OF ACTION
A serotonin receptor agonist that binds selectively to vascular receptors, producing a vasoconstrictive effect on cranial

blood vessels. *Therapeutic Effect:* Relieves migraine headache.

USES

Treatment of migraine headaches; cluster headaches

PHARMACOKINETICS

Route	Onset	Peak	Duration
Nasal	15 min	N/A	24–48 h
PO	30 min	2 h	24–48 h
Subcutaneous	10 min	1 h	24–48 h

Rapidly absorbed after subcutaneous administration. Absorption after PO administration is incomplete, with significant amounts undergoing hepatic metabolism, resulting in low bioavailability (about 14%). Protein binding: 10%–21%. Widely distributed. Undergoes first-pass metabolism in the liver. Excreted in urine. *Half-life:* 2 hr.

INDICATIONS AND DOSAGES
▶ **Acute Migraine Attack**
PO
Adults, Elderly. 25–50 mg. Dose may be repeated after at least 2 hr. Maximum: 100 mg/single dose; 200 mg/24 hr.
Subcutaneous
Adults, Elderly. 6 mg. Maximum: Two 6-mg injections/24 hr (separated by at least 1 hr).
Intranasal
Adults, Elderly. 5–20 mg; may repeat in 2 hr. Maximum: 40 mg/24 hr.

SIDE EFFECTS/ADVERSE REACTIONS
Frequent
Oral: Tingling, nasal discomfort
Subcutaneous: Injection site reactions, tingling, warm or hot sensation, dizziness, vertigo
Nasal: Bad or unusual taste, nausea, vomiting
Occasional
Oral: Flushing, asthenia, visual disturbances
Subcutaneous: Burning sensation, numbness, chest discomfort, drowsiness, asthenia
Nasal: Nasopharyngeal discomfort, dizziness
Rare
Oral: Agitation, eye irritation, dysuria
Subcutaneous: Anxiety, fatigue, diaphoresis, muscle cramps, myalgia
Nasal: Burning sensation

PRECAUTIONS AND CONTRAINDICATIONS
CVA, ischemic heart disease (including angina pectoris, history of MI, silent ischemia, and Prinzmetal's angina), severe hepatic impairment, transient ischemic attack, uncontrolled hypertension, use within 14 days of MAOIs, use within 24 hr of ergotamine preparations
Caution
Hepatic and renal impairment, elderly, lactation, children

DRUG INTERACTIONS OF CONCERN TO DENTISTRY
• None reported; avoid ergot-containing medications

SERIOUS REACTIONS
! Excessive dosage may produce tremor, red extremities, reduced respirations, cyanosis, seizures, and paralysis.
! Serious arrhythmias occur rarely, especially in patients with hypertension, diabetes, or a strong

family history of coronary artery disease; obese patients; and smokers.

DENTAL CONSIDERATIONS

General

• Be aware of the patient's disease, its severity, and its frequency, when known.

• Monitor vital signs at every appointment because of cardiovascular side effects.

• Avoid dental light in patient's eyes; offer dark glasses for patient comfort.

Consultations:

• If treating chronic orofacial pain, consult with physician of record.

Teach Patient/Family:

• That oral symptoms rarely occur and will disappear when drug is discontinued

---

sunitinib
soo-nih´-tih-nib
(Sutent)

CATEGORY AND SCHEDULE
Pregnancy Risk Category: D

Drug Class: Antineoplastic (tyrosine kinase inhibitor)

MECHANISM OF ACTION
An antineoplastic agent that inhibits multiple receptor tyrosine kinases (RTK) inducing platelet-derived growth factor (PDGF), vascular endothelial growth factor receptors (VEGFR1, VEGFR2, and VEGFR3), stem cell factor receptor (KIT), Fms-like tyrosine kinase-3 (FLT3), colony stimulation factor receptor Type 1 (CSF-1R), and glial cell-line derived neurotrophic factor receptor (RET). **Therapeutic Effect:** Decreases tumor cell growth.

USES
Treatment of GI stromal tumor after disease progression on or intolerance to imatinib; also used for treatment of advanced renal cell carcinoma

PHARMACOKINETICS
Protein binding: 95% and 90% (primary metabolite). Primarily metabolized in liver by CYP450 3A4. Primarily eliminated in feces (61%); partial excretion in urine (16%). **Half-life:** 40–60 hr; 80–110 hr (primary metabolite).

INDICATIONS AND DOSAGES
▶ **GI Stromal Tumor after Disease Progression on or Intolerance to Imatinib**
PO
Adults. 50 mg once a day, on a schedule of 4 wk on treatment followed by 2 wk off.
▶ **Renal Cell Carcinoma, Advanced**
PO
Adults. 50 mg once a day, on a schedule of 4 wk on treatment followed by 2 wk off.
▶ **Dosage Adjustment**
Concurrent CYP3A4 inhibitor (such as ketoconazole). Reduce sunitinib to a minimum of 37.5 mg daily.
Concurrent CYP3A4 inducer (such as rifampin). Increase sunitinib to a maximum of 87.5 mg daily

SIDE EFFECTS/ADVERSE REACTIONS:
Frequent
Fatigue, diarrhea, nausea, mucositis/stomatitis, neutropenia, dyspepsia, taste perversion, AST/ALT increased, lymphopenia, rash, thrombocytopenia, vomiting, constipation, anorexia, hyperpigmentation, abdominal pain, hypertension, arthralgia, dyspnea, bleeding, anemia, hyperlipasemia, headache, alkaline phosphatase

S

increased, weakness, limb pain, fever, edema, dry skin, myalgia, back pain, cough, hair color changes, amylase increased, dizziness, hyperbilirubinemia, glossodynia, hyperuricemia, flatulence, hand-foot syndrome, hypokalemia, creatinine increased, alopecia, dehydration, hypernatremia, neuropathy, hypophosphatemia, LVEF decreased
Occasional
Appetite disturbance, skin blistering, periorbital edema, hypothyroidism, lacrimation increased, oral pain, hyperkalemia, hyponatremia, DVT
Rare
Myocardial ischemia, pulmonary embolism

PRECAUTIONS AND CONTRAINDICATIONS
Hypersensitivity to sunitinib or its components
Caution
Do not breast-feed, left ventricular dysfunction, hypertension

DRUG INTERACTIONS OF CONCERN TO DENTISTRY
• CYP3A4 inducers: may decrease the levels and effects of sunitinib
• CYP3A4 inhibitors (e.g., macrolide antibiotics, azole antifungal agents): may increase the levels and effects of sunitinib

SERIOUS REACTIONS
! Severe GI complications have been reported.
! Hemorrhagic events have been reported.
! Hypertension may occur.
! Left ventricular dysfunction has been reported.
! Adrenal toxicity have been noted.

DENTAL CONSIDERATIONS
General:
• Avoid aspirin and NSAIDs to prevent GI irritation and excessive bleeding.
• Examine patient carefully for signs of opportunistic infections, mucositis, blood dyscrasias, stomatitis and bleeding.
• Confirm patient's disease status and treatment regimen.
• Chlorhexidine mouthrinse prior to and during chemotherapy may reduce severity of oral inflammation.
• Palliative medication may be required for management of oral adverse effects of drug.
• Patient may be taking prophylactic antiinfective drug.
• Place patient on frequent recall because of adverse oral effects of drug.
Consultations:
• Consult physician to determine control of disease and ability of patient to tolerate dental procedures.
• Consult physician to determine need for prophylactic or therapeutic antiinfective medications if oral surgery or periodontal treatment is planned.
• Consult physician to determine patient's immunologic and coagulation status and determine safety risk, if any, posed by the required dental treatment.
Teach Patient/Family to:
• Be aware of oral adverse effects of drugs
• Use effective, atraumatic oral hygiene measures to prevent soft tissue inflammation
• Report oral lesions, soreness or bleeding to dentist
• Update health and medication history if physician makes any changes in evaluation or drug

regimen; include OTC, herbal, and nonherbal drugs in update

suprofen
soo-proe´-fen
(Profenal)

CATEGORY AND SCHEDULE
Pregnancy Risk Category: C

Drug Class: Ophthalmic, antiinflammatory

MECHANISM OF ACTION
A nonsteroidal antiinflammatory that inhibits prostaglandin synthesis and the intensity of pain stimulus reaching sensory nerve endings. Constricts iris sphincter. **Therapeutic Effect:** Produces analgesic and antiinflammatory effect. Prevents miosis during cataract surgery.

USES
Adjunct to ophthalmic surgery

PHARMACOKINETICS
No data available on systemic absorption.

INDICATIONS AND DOSAGES
▶ **Miosis Inhibitor in Ophthalmic Surgery**
Ophthalmic
Adults, Elderly. Apply 2 drops 3, 2, and 1 hr prior to surgery. If desired, 2 drops may be applied q4h while the patient is awake on the day prior to surgery.

SIDE EFFECTS/ADVERSE REACTIONS
Frequent
Burning, stinging on instillation, ocular discomfort

Occasional
Itching, tearing
Rare
Headache, trouble sleeping, weakness

PRECAUTIONS AND CONTRAINDICATIONS
Rhinitis, urticaria, asthma, allergic reactions to aspirin or other antiinflammatory agents, epithelial herpes keratitis, hypersensitivity to suprofen or any component of the formulation.

DRUG INTERACTIONS OF CONCERN TO DENTISTRY
None reported

SERIOUS REACTIONS
❗ Nausea or vomiting, pain, sensitivity to light, trouble breathing, and shortness of breath occur rarely.

DENTAL CONSIDERATIONS
General:
• Avoid dental light in patient's eyes; offer dark glasses for patient comfort.

S

tacrine hydrochloride

tack´-rin high-droh-klor´-ide
(Cognex)

CATEGORY AND SCHEDULE
Pregnancy Risk Category: C

Drug Class: Cholinesterase inhibitor

MECHANISM OF ACTION
A cholinesterase inhibitor that inhibits the enzyme acetylcholinesterase, thus increasing the concentration of acetylcholine at cholinergic synapses and enhancing cholinergic function in the CNS. *Therapeutic Effect:* Slows the progression of Alzheimer's disease.

USES
Treatment of mild-to-moderate cognitive defects associated with Alzheimer's disease

PHARMACOKINETICS
PO: Peak plasma levels 1–2 hr; plasma levels are higher in females; hepatic metabolism (CYP1A2 isoenzymes); renal excretion.

INDICATIONS AND DOSAGES
▶ **Alzheimer's Disease**
PO
Adults, Elderly. Initially, 10 mg 4 times a day for 6 wk, followed by 20 mg 4 times a day for 6 wk, 30 mg 4 times a day for 12 wk, then 40 mg 4 times a day if needed.
▶ **Dosage in Hepatic Impairment**
For patients with ALT (SGPT) greater than 3–5 times normal, decrease the dose by 40 mg/day and resume the normal dose when ALT (SGPT) returns to normal. For patients with ALT (SGPT) greater than 5 times normal, stop treatment and resume it when ALT (SGPT) returns to normal.

SIDE EFFECTS/ADVERSE REACTIONS
Frequent
Headache, nausea, vomiting, diarrhea, dizziness
Occasional
Fatigue, chest pain, dyspepsia, anorexia, abdominal pain, flatulence, constipation, confusion, agitation, rash, depression, ataxia, insomnia, rhinitis, myalgia
Rare
Weight loss, anxiety, cough, facial flushing, urinary frequency, back pain, tremor

PRECAUTIONS AND CONTRAINDICATIONS
Known hypersensitivity to tacrine, patients previously treated with tacrine who developed jaundice
Caution
Cardiovascular disease, GI ulcers, general anesthesia, smokers, liver disease, seizures, asthma, lactation, children, decrease in absolute neutrophil count; liver enzyme monitoring required

DRUG INTERACTIONS OF CONCERN TO DENTISTRY
• Potential increase in GI complaints: NSAIDs
• Action inhibited by anticholinergic drugs
• Increased effects with succinylcholine and other cholinergic agonists

SERIOUS REACTIONS
❗ Overdose can cause cholinergic crisis, marked by increased salivation, lacrimation, bradycardia, respiratory depression, hypotension, and increased muscle weakness.

Treatment usually consists of supportive measures and an anticholinergic, such as atropine.

DENTAL CONSIDERATIONS
General:
• Patients on chronic drug therapy may rarely have symptoms of blood dyscrasias, which can include infection, bleeding, and poor healing.
• Monitor vital signs at every appointment because of cardiovascular and respiratory side effects.
• After supine positioning, have patient sit upright for at least 2 min before standing to avoid orthostatic hypotension.
• Assess salivary flow as a factor in caries, periodontal disease, and candidiasis.
• Take precautions if dental surgery is anticipated and anesthesia is required.
• Consider semisupine chair position for patient comfort because of GI effects of drug.
• Place on frequent recall because early attention to dental health is important for Alzheimer's patients.
Consultations:
• Medical consultation may be required to assess disease control.
• In a patient with symptoms of blood dyscrasias, request a medical consultation for blood studies and postpone dental treatment until normal values are reestablished.
Teach Patient/Family to:
• Use effective oral hygiene to prevent soft tissue inflammation
• Prevent injury when using oral hygiene aids
• Use electric tooth brush if patient has difficulty holding conventional devices
• When chronic dry mouth occurs, advise patient to:

• Avoid mouth rinses with high alcohol content because of drying effects
• Use daily home fluoride to prevent caries
• Use sugarless gum, frequent sips of water, or saliva substitutes

tacrolimus
tak-roe-leem´-us
(Prograf, Protopic)
Do not confuse Protopic with Protonix, Protopam, Protropin.

CATEGORY AND SCHEDULE
Pregnancy Risk Category: C

Drug Class: Immunosuppressant

MECHANISM OF ACTION
An immunologic agent that inhibits T-lymphocyte activation by binding to intracellular proteins, forming a complex and inhibiting phosphatase activity. **Therapeutic Effect:** Suppresses the immunologically mediated inflammatory response; prevents organ transplant rejection.

USES
Treatment of short-term and intermittent long-term treatment of moderate-to-severe atopic dermatitis in patients not able to use or who do not respond to alternative, conventional therapies

PHARMACOKINETICS
Variably absorbed after PO administration (food reduces absorption). Protein binding: 75%–97%. Extensively metabolized in the liver. Excreted in urine. Not removed by hemodialysis. **Half-life:** 11.7 hr.

INDICATIONS AND DOSAGES
▶ **Prevention of Liver Transplant Rejection**
PO
Adults, Elderly. 0.1–0.15 mg/kg/day in 2 divided doses 12 hr apart.
Children. 0.15–0.2 mg/kg/day in 2 divided doses 12 hr apart.
IV
Adults, Elderly, Children. 0.03–0.15 mg/kg/day as a continuous infusion.
▶ **Prevention of Kidney Transplant Rejection**
PO
Adults, Elderly. 0.2 mg/kg/day in 2 divided doses 12 hr apart
IV
Adults, Elderly. 0.03–0.15 mg/kg/day as continuous infusion.
▶ **Atopic Dermatitis**
Topical
Adults, Elderly, Children 2 yr and older. Apply 0.03% ointment to affected area twice a day. 0.1% ointment may be used in adults and the elderly. Continue until 1 wk after symptoms have cleared.

SIDE EFFECTS/ADVERSE REACTIONS
Frequent
Headache, tremor, insomnia, paresthesia, diarrhea, nausea, constipation, vomiting, abdominal pain, hypertension
Occasional
Rash, pruritus, anorexia, asthenia, peripheral edema, photosensitivity

PRECAUTIONS AND CONTRAINDICATIONS
Concurrent use with cyclosporine (increases the risk of nephrotoxicity), hypersensitivity to HCO-60 polyoxyl 60 hydrogenated castor oil (used in solution for injection), hypersensitivity to tacrolimus

Caution
Infections at treatment site; lymphadenopathy, acute infections, mononucleosis, reduce exposure to sunlight or artificial sunlight, lactation, use has not been established in children younger than 2 yr

DRUG INTERACTIONS OF CONCERN TO DENTISTRY
Topical
• No drug interactions are documented, but use with caution in patients taking CYP3A4 isoenzyme inhibitors: erythromycin, itraconazole, ketoconazole, fluconazole tacrolimus (FK506)
• No confirmed studies to date: avoid drugs with potential for renal impairment
• Risk of increased blood levels with clotrimazole, fluconazole, ketoconazole, clarithromycin, erythromycin, and methylprednisolone
• Risk of decreased blood levels with carbamazepine, phenobarbital, St. John's wort (herb)

SERIOUS REACTIONS
! Nephrotoxicity (characterized by increased serum creatinine level and decreased urine output), neurotoxicity (including tremor, headache, and mental status changes), and pleural effusion are common adverse reactions.
! Thrombocytopenia, leukocytosis, anemia, atelectasis, sepsis, and infection occur occasionally.

DENTAL CONSIDERATIONS

Topical
General:
• Advise patient if dental drugs prescribed have a potential for photosensitivity.

FK506

General:
- Patients on immunosuppressant therapy have increased susceptibility to infection.
- Patients on chronic drug therapy may rarely have symptoms of blood dyscrasias, which can include infection, bleeding, and poor healing.
- Monitor vital signs at every appointment because of cardiovascular side effects.
- Prophylactic antibiotics may be indicated to prevent infection if surgery or deep scaling is planned.
- Examine for evidence of oral candidiasis. Topically acting antifungals may be preferred.

Consultations:
- Medical consultation may be required to assess disease control.
- In a patient with symptoms of blood dyscrasias, request a medical consultation for blood studies and postpone dental treatment until normal values are reestablished.
- Consult with patient's physician for recommendations on possible antibiotic prophylaxis before dental treatment or when considering use of systemic antifungals.

Teach Patient/Family to:
- Use effective oral hygiene to prevent soft tissue inflammation
- Use caution to prevent injury when using oral hygiene aids
- Use electric tooth brush if patient has difficulty holding conventional devices
- See dentist immediately if secondary oral infection occurs
- Report oral lesions, soreness, or bleeding to dentist

tadalafil

tah-dal´-ah-fill
(Cialis)

CATEGORY AND SCHEDULE
Pregnancy Risk Category: B

Drug Class: Impotence therapy

MECHANISM OF ACTION
An erectile dysfunction agent that inhibits phosphodiesterase type 5, the enzyme responsible for degrading cyclic guanosine monophosphate in the corpus cavernosum of the penis, resulting in smooth muscle relaxation and increased blood flow. ***Therapeutic Effect:*** Facilitates an erection.

USES
Treatment of male erectile dysfunction

PHARMACOKINETICS

Route	Onset	Peak	Duration
PO	16 min	2 hr	36 hr

Rapidly absorbed after PO administration. Drug has no effect on penile blood flow without sexual stimulation. ***Half-life:*** 17.5 hr.

INDICATIONS AND DOSAGES
▸ **Erectile Dysfunction**
PO
Adults, Elderly. 10 mg 30 min before sexual activity. Dose may be increased to 20 mg or decreased to 5 mg based on patient tolerance. Maximum dosing frequency is once daily.
▸ **Dosage in Renal Impairment**
For patients with a creatinine clearance of 31–50 ml/min, the

starting dose is 5 mg before sexual activity once a day and the maximum dose is 10 mg no more frequently than once q48h.

For patients with a creatinine clearance of less than 31 ml/min, the starting dose is 5 mg before sexual activity once a day.

▶ **Dosage in Mild or Moderate Hepatic Impairment**

Patients with Child-Pugh class A or B hepatic impairment should take no more than 10 mg once a day.

SIDE EFFECTS/ADVERSE REACTIONS

Occasional

Headache, dyspepsia, back pain, myalgia, nasal congestion, flushing

PRECAUTIONS AND CONTRAINDICATIONS

Concurrent use of α-adrenergic blockers (other than the minimum dose tamsulosin), concurrent use of sodium nitroprusside or nitrates in any form, severe hepatic impairment

Caution

Renal impairment, hepatic dysfunction, risk of hypotension in cardiovascular disease, ischemic heart disease, patients at risk of priapism, penile deformities, safety and efficacy for use in women not established

DRUG INTERACTIONS OF CONCERN TO DENTISTRY

• Maximum dose in patients taking CYP3A4 isoenzyme inhibitors is 10 mg: includes ketoconazole, erythromycin, itraconazole, and other potent inhibitors of CYP3A4
• Avoid use of nitroglycerin within 24–36 hr

SERIOUS REACTIONS

! Prolonged erections (lasting longer than 4 hr) and priapism (painful erections lasting longer than 6 hr) occur rarely.

DENTAL CONSIDERATIONS

General:

• This is an acute-use drug intended to be taken just before sexual activity. Be mindful of the drug interactions when prescribing potent inhibitors of CYP3A4 isoenzymes and warn patient.

tamoxifen citrate
ta-mox´-ih-fen sih´-trate
(Apo-Tamox[CAN], Genox[AUS], Istubol, Nolvadex, Nolvadex-D[CAN], Novo-Tamoxifen[CAN], Tamofen[CAN], Tamosin[AUS])

CATEGORY AND SCHEDULE
Pregnancy Risk Category: D

Drug Class: Antineoplastic, antiestrogen hormone

MECHANISM OF ACTION
A nonsteroidal antiestrogen that competes with estradiol for estrogen-receptor binding sites in the breasts, uterus, and vagina. ***Therapeutic Effect:*** Inhibits DNA synthesis and estrogen response.

USES
Advanced breast carcinoma that has not responded to other therapy in estrogen receptor–positive patients (usually postmenopausal), to reduce the incidence of breast cancer in healthy women with high risk of developing the disease; ductal carcinoma in situ

PHARMACOKINETICS
Well absorbed from the GI tract. Metabolized in the liver. Primarily

eliminated in feces by biliary system. *Half-life:* 7 days.

INDICATIONS AND DOSAGES
▸ **Adjunctive Treatment of Breast Cancer**
PO
Adults, Elderly. 20–40 mg/day. Give doses greater than 20 mg/day in divided doses.
▸ **Prevention of Breast Cancer in High-Risk Women**
PO
Adults, Elderly. 20 mg/day.

SIDE EFFECTS/ADVERSE REACTIONS
Frequent
Women: Hot flashes, nausea, vomiting
Occasional
Women: Changes in menstruation, genital itching, vaginal discharge, endometrial hyperplasia or polyps
Men: Impotence, decreased libido
Men and women: Headache, nausea, vomiting, rash, bone pain, confusion, weakness, somnolence

PRECAUTIONS AND CONTRAINDICATIONS
Concomitant coumarin-type therapy when used in the treatment of breast cancer in high-risk women, history of deep vein thrombosis or pulmonary embolism in high-risk women, pregnancy
Caution
Leukopenia, thrombocytopenia, lactation, cataracts, risk of stroke, pulmonary emboli, and uterine malignancy

DRUG INTERACTIONS OF CONCERN TO DENTISTRY
None reported

SERIOUS REACTIONS
❗ Retinopathy, corneal opacity, and decreased visual acuity have been noted in patients receiving extremely high dosages (240–320 mg/day) for longer than 17 mo.
❗ There have been an increased number of incidences of endometrial changes, thromboembolic events, and uterine malignancies while using tamoxifen.

DENTAL CONSIDERATIONS
General:
• Patients on chronic drug therapy may rarely have symptoms of blood dyscrasias, which can include infection, bleeding, and poor healing.
• Consider semisupine chair position for patient comfort if GI side effects occur.
Consultations:
• Medical consultation may be required to assess disease control.
• In a patient with symptoms of blood dyscrasias, request a medical consultation for blood studies and postpone dental treatment until normal values are reestablished.
Teach Patient/Family:
• Importance of good oral hygiene to prevent soft tissue inflammation

tamsulosin hydrochloride
tam-sool′-oh-sin
high-droh-klor′-ide
(Flomax)
Do not confuse Flomax with Fosamax or Volmax.

T

CATEGORY AND SCHEDULE
Pregnancy Risk Category: B (not indicated for use in women)

Drug Class: Adrenoreceptor antagonist

MECHANISM OF ACTION

An α_1 antagonist that targets receptors around bladder neck and prostate capsule. *Therapeutic Effect:* Relaxes smooth muscle and improves urinary flow and symptoms of prostatic hyperplasia.

USES

Treatment of benign prostatic hyperplasia (BPH)

PHARMACOKINETICS

Well absorbed and widely distributed. Protein binding: 94%–99%. Metabolized in the liver. Primarily excreted in urine. Unknown if removed by hemodialysis. *Half-life:* 9–13 hr.

INDICATIONS AND DOSAGES
▸ **BPH**
PO
Adults. 0.4 mg once a day, approximately 30 min after same meal each day. May increase dosage to 0.8 mg if inadequate response in 2–4 wk.

SIDE EFFECTS/ADVERSE REACTIONS

Frequent
Dizziness, somnolence
Occasional
Headache, anxiety, insomnia, orthostatic hypotension
Rare
Nasal congestion, pharyngitis, rhinitis, nausea, vertigo, impotence

PRECAUTIONS AND CONTRAINDICATIONS

History of sensitivity to tamsulosin
Caution
Potential syncope risk caused by hypotension, vertigo, dizziness, carcinoma of prostate; avoid use with other-adrenoreceptor antagonists; not for use in women, children; lactation

DRUG INTERACTIONS OF CONCERN TO DENTISTRY

• No interactions reported with usual dental drugs; it is possible but not known whether risk of orthostatic hypotension could be increased with conscious sedation techniques
• Opioids and anticholinergic drugs may enhance urinary retention; use alternative analgesics (NSAIDs)
• Caution in use or avoid concurrent use with other adrenergic antagonists

SERIOUS REACTIONS

! First-dose syncope (hypotension with sudden loss of consciousness) may occur within 30–90 min after administration of initial dose and may be preceded by tachycardia (pulse rate of 120–160 beats/min).

DENTAL CONSIDERATIONS

General:
• Monitor vital signs at every appointment because of cardiovascular and respiratory side effects.
• Consider semisupine chair position for patient comfort when GI side effects occur.
• After supine positioning, have patient sit upright for at least 2 min before standing to avoid orthostatic hypotension.

tazarotene
ta-zare´-oh-teen
(Tazorac, Avage)

CATEGORY AND SCHEDULE
Pregnancy Risk Category: X

Drug Class: Topical retinoid

MECHANISM OF ACTION

Modulates differentiation and proliferation of epithelial tissue, binds selectively to retinoic acid receptors. *Therapeutic Effect:* Restores normal differentiation of the epidermis and reduction in epidermal inflammation.

USES

Topical treatment in stable plaque psoriasis, mild to moderate facial acne vulgaris

PHARMACOKINETICS

Minimal systemic absorption occurs through the skin. Binding to plasma proteins is greater than 99%. Metabolism is in the skin and liver. Elimination occurs through the fecal and renal pathways. *Half-life:* 18 hr.

INDICATIONS AND DOSAGES

▶ **Psoriasis**
Topical
Adults, Adolescents, Children older than 12 yr. Thin film applied once daily in the evening; only cover the lesions, and area should be dry before application

▶ **Acne Vulgaris**
Topical
Adults, Adolescents, Children older than 12 yr. Thin film applied to affected areas once daily in the evening after face is gently cleansed and dried.

▶ **Fine Facial Wrinkles, Facial Mottled Hyperpigmentation (liver spots), Hypopigmentation Associated with Photoaging**
Topical
Adults. Thin film applied to affected areas once daily in the evening after face is gently cleansed and dried.

SIDE EFFECTS/ADVERSE REACTIONS

Frequent
Desquamation, burning or stinging, dry skin, itching, erythema, worsening of psoriasis, irritation, skin pain, pruritus, xerosis, photosensitivity
Occasional
Irritation, skin pain, fissuring, localized edema, skin discoloration, rash, desquamation, contact dermatitis, skin inflammation, bleeding, dry skin, hypertriglyceridemia, peripheral edema, acne vulgaris, cheilitis

PRECAUTIONS AND CONTRAINDICATIONS

Should not be used in pregnant women, patients with hypersensitivity to tazarotene, benzyl alcohol, or any one of its components
Caution
Pregnancy category X, use birth control measures in women of childbearing age, avoid contact with eyes, eyelids, mouth; exposure to tanning (sun, sun lamps) or drugs that cause photosensitivity, lactation, children younger than 12 yr

DRUG INTERACTIONS OF CONCERN TO DENTISTRY

• Increased risk of photosensitivity: tetracyclines, fluoroquinolones, phenothiazines
• Caution in use with systemic vitamin A

T

DENTAL CONSIDERATIONS

General:
• Apply lubricant to dry lips for patient comfort before dental procedures.
• Advise patient if dental drugs prescribed have a potential for photosensitivity.

Teach Patient/Family:
• That this drug should not be used if the patient is pregnant
• To avoid application to oral mucous membranes or lips

As of March 2007, this drug was removed from the U.S. market by the FDA.

tegaserod
teh-gas´-er-od
(Zelnorm)

CATEGORY AND SCHEDULE
Pregnancy Risk Category: B

Drug Class: Serotonin agonist, a prokinetic drug

MECHANISM OF ACTION
An anti-irritable bowel syndrome agent that binds to 5-HT4 receptors in the GI tract. *Therapeutic Effect:* Triggers a peristaltic reflex in the gut, increasing bowel motility.

USES
Short-term treatment of irritable bowel syndrome in women whose primary bowel symptom is constipation

PHARMACOKINETICS
Rapidly absorbed. Widely distributed. Protein binding: 98%. Metabolized by hydrolysis in the stomach and by oxidation and conjugation of the primary metabolite. Primarily excreted in feces. *Half-life:* 11 hr.

INDICATIONS AND DOSAGES
▶ **Irritable Bowel Syndrome**
PO
Adults, Elderly women. 6 mg twice a day for 4–6 wk.

▶ **Chronic Constipation**
PO
Adults. 6 mg twice a day.

SIDE EFFECTS/ADVERSE REACTIONS
Frequent
Headache, abdominal pain, diarrhea, nausea, flatulence
Occasional
Dizziness, migraine, back pain, extremity pain

PRECAUTIONS AND CONTRAINDICATIONS
Abdominal adhesions, diarrhea, history of bowel obstruction, moderate to severe hepatic impairment, severe renal impairment, suspected sphincter of Oddi dysfunction, symptomatic gallbladder disease
Caution
Avoid use in patients with diarrhea, pregnancy category B, lactation (discontinue drug or discontinue nursing), safety and usefulness in children younger than 18 yr not established

DRUG INTERACTIONS OF CONCERN TO DENTISTRY
• No dental drug interactions reported; does not induce CYP450 isoenzymes
• Avoid use of drugs (opioids, anticholinergics) that could lead to risk of constipation
• Use NSAIDs or acetaminophen for mild or moderate pain

SERIOUS REACTIONS
None known

DENTAL CONSIDERATIONS
General:
• Monitor vital signs at every appointment because of cardiovascular side effects.

- Consider semisupine chair position for patient comfort if GI side effects occur.
- Short appointments and a stress-reduction protocol may be required for anxious patients.
- Avoid drugs with anticholinergic activity, such as antihistamines, opioids, benzodiazepines, propantheline, atropine, and scopolamine.
- Question patient about tolerance of NSAIDs or aspirin related to GI disease.

Consultations:
- Consult with physician before prescribing drugs that can cause constipation (opioids).
- Consultation with physician may be necessary if sedation or general anesthesia is required.
- Medical consultation may be required to assess disease control and patient's ability to tolerate stress.

Teach Patient/Family to:
- Update health and drug history if physician makes any changes in evaluation or drug regimens; include OTC, herbal, and nonherbal drugs in the update

telmisartan
tel-meh-sar´-tan
(Micardis, Pritor[AUS])

CATEGORY AND SCHEDULE
Pregnancy Risk Category: C (D if used in second or third trimester)

Drug Class: Angiotensin II (AT1) receptor antagonist

MECHANISM OF ACTION
An angiotensin II receptor, type AT1, antagonist that blocks vasoconstrictor and aldosterone-secreting effects of angiotensin II, inhibiting the binding of angiotensin II to the AT1 receptors. *Therapeutic Effect:* Causes vasodilation, decreases peripheral resistance, and decreases B/P.

USES
Treatment of hypertension as a single drug or in combination with other antihypertensives

PHARMACOKINETICS
Rapidly and completely absorbed after PO administration. Protein binding: greater than 99%. Undergoes metabolism in the liver to inactive metabolite. Excreted in feces. Unknown if removed by hemodialysis. *Half-life:* 24 hr.

INDICATIONS AND DOSAGES
▶ **Hypertension**
PO
Adults, Elderly. 40 mg once a day. Range: 20–80 mg/day.

SIDE EFFECTS/ADVERSE REACTIONS
Occasional
Upper respiratory tract infection, sinusitis, back or leg pain, diarrhea
Rare
Dizziness, headache, fatigue, nausea, heartburn, myalgia, cough, peripheral edema

PRECAUTIONS AND CONTRAINDICATIONS
Hypersensitivity, discontinue if pregnancy occurs, risk of fetal and neonatal injury, correct volume depletion if present, hepatic impairment, impaired renal function
Caution
Discontinue if pregnancy occurs, risk of fetal and neonatal injury, correct volume depletion if present, hepatic impairment, impaired renal function; lactation

DRUG INTERACTIONS OF CONCERN TO DENTISTRY
• None reported; CYP450 isoenzymes are not involved with metabolism of this drug

SERIOUS REACTIONS
! Overdosage may manifest as hypotension and tachycardia. Bradycardia occurs less often.

DENTAL CONSIDERATIONS
General:
• Monitor vital signs at every appointment because of cardiovascular side effects.
• Stress from dental procedures may compromise cardiovascular function; determine patient risk.
• Use precaution if sedation or general anesthesia is required; risk of hypotensive episode.
• Short appointments and a stress-reduction protocol may be required for anxious patients.
• Limit use of sodium-containing products, such as saline IV fluids, for patients with a dietary salt restriction.
Consultations:
• Medical consultation may be required to assess disease control and patient's ability to tolerate stress.

temazepam
te-maz´-eh-pam
(Apo-Temazepam[CAN], Novo-Temazepam[CAN], PMS-Temazepam[CAN], Restoril)
Do not confuse Restoril with Vistaril or Zestril.

CATEGORY AND SCHEDULE
Pregnancy Risk Category: X
Controlled Substance: Schedule IV

Drug Class: Benzodiazepine, sedative-hypnotic

MECHANISM OF ACTION
A benzodiazepine that enhances the action of the inhibitory neurotransmitter gamma-aminobutyric acid (GABA), resulting in CNS depression. *Therapeutic Effect:* Induces sleep.

USES
A sedative and hypnotic for treatment of insomnia

PHARMACOKINETICS
Well absorbed from the GI tract. Protein binding: 96%. Widely distributed. Crosses the blood–brain barrier. Metabolized in the liver. Primarily excreted in urine. Not removed by hemodialysis. *Half-life:* 4–18 hr.

INDICATIONS AND DOSAGES
▶ Insomnia
PO
Adults, Children 18 yr and older. 15–30 mg at bedtime.
Elderly, Debilitated. 7.5–15 mg at bedtime.

SIDE EFFECTS/ADVERSE REACTIONS
Frequent
Somnolence, sedation, rebound insomnia (may occur for 1–2 nights after drug is discontinued), dizziness, confusion, euphoria
Occasional
Asthenia, anorexia, diarrhea
Rare
Paradoxic CNS excitement or restlessness (particularly in elderly or debilitated patients)

PRECAUTIONS AND CONTRAINDICATIONS
Angle-closure glaucoma; CNS depression; pregnancy or breast-feeding; severe, uncontrolled pain; sleep apnea

Caution
Anemia, hepatic disease, renal disease, suicidal individuals, drug abuse, elderly, psychosis, children younger than 18 yr, acute narrow-angle glaucoma

DRUG INTERACTIONS OF CONCERN TO DENTISTRY
• Increased action: alcohol, all CNS depressants
• Increased bioavailability: macrolide antibiotics

SERIOUS REACTIONS
! Abrupt or too-rapid withdrawal may result in pronounced restlessness, irritability, insomnia, hand tremor, abdominal or muscle cramps, vomiting, diaphoresis, and seizures.
! Overdose results in somnolence, confusion, diminished reflexes, respiratory depression, and coma.

DENTAL CONSIDERATIONS
General:
• Psychologic and physical dependence may occur with chronic administration.
• Geriatric patients are more susceptible to drug effects; use lower dose.
Teach Patient/Family to:
• Use effective oral hygiene to prevent soft tissue inflammation

temozolomide
teh-moe-zoll´-oh-mide
(Temodal[AUS], Temodar)

CATEGORY AND SCHEDULE
Pregnancy Risk Category: D

Drug Class: Antineoplastic

MECHANISM OF ACTION
An imidazotetrazine derivative that acts as a prodrug and is converted to a highly active cytotoxic metabolite. Its cytotoxic effect is associated with methylation of DNA. ***Therapeutic Effect:*** Inhibits DNA replication, causing cell death.

USES
Treatment of specific types of cancer of the brain

PHARMACOKINETICS
Rapidly and completely absorbed after PO administration. Protein binding: 15%. Peak plasma concentration occurs in 1 hr. Penetrates the blood-brain barrier. Eliminated primarily in urine and, to a much lesser extent, in feces. ***Half-life:*** 1.6–1.8 hr.

INDICATIONS AND DOSAGES
▸ **Anaplastic Astrocytoma**
PO
Adults, Elderly. Initially, 150 mg/m^2/day for 5 consecutive days of a 28-day treatment cycle. Subsequent doses based on platelet count and ANC during previous cycle. ANC greater than 1500 per microliter and platelet: more than 100,000 per microliter. Maintenance: 200 mg/m^2/day for 5 days q4wk. Minimum:100 mg/m^2/day for 5 days q4wk.

SIDE EFFECTS/ADVERSE REACTIONS
Frequent
Nausea, vomiting, headache, fatigue, constipation
Occasional
Diarrhea, asthenia, fever, dizziness, peripheral edema, incoordination, insomnia

T

Rare
Paraesthesia, drowsiness, anorexia, urinary incontinence, anxiety, pharyngitis, cough

PRECAUTIONS AND CONTRAINDICATIONS
Hypersensitivity to dacarbazine, pregnancy

DRUG INTERACTIONS OF CONCERN TO DENTISTRY
None reported

SERIOUS REACTIONS
! Elderly patients and women are at increased risk for developing severe myelosuppression, characterized by neutropenia and thrombocytopenia and usually occurring within the first few cycles. Neutrophil and platelet counts reach their nadirs approximately 26–28 days after administration and recover within 14 days of the nadir.

DENTAL CONSIDERATIONS
General:
• Caution: patients may be at high risk for infection.
• Provide palliative dental care for dental emergencies only.
• Oral infections should be eliminated and/or treated aggressively.
• Patients may be at risk for bleeding; check oral signs.
• Caution: potential drug interactions with drugs used in dentistry.
• Monitor and record vital signs.
• If additional analgesia is required for dental pain, consider alternative analgesics (NSAIDs) in patients taking narcotics for acute or chronic pain.
• Avoid products that affect platelet function, such as aspirin and NSAIDs.
• Patient on chronic drug therapy may rarely present with symptoms of blood dyscrasias, which can include infection, bleeding, and poor healing. If dyscrasia is present, caution patient to prevent oral tissue trauma when using oral hygiene aids.
• Consider local hemostasis measures to prevent excessive bleeding.
• Consider semisupine chair position for patient comfort if GI side effects occur.
Consultations:
• Medical consultation should include routine blood counts including platelet counts and bleeding time.
• Consult physician; prophylactic or therapeutic antiinfectives may be indicated if surgery or periodontal treatment is required.
• In a patient with symptoms of blood dyscrasias, request a medical consultation for blood studies and postpone treatment until normal values are reestablished.
• Medical consultation may be required to assess disease control and patient's ability to tolerate stress.
Teach Patient/Family to:
• Use soft tooth brush to reduce risk of bleeding
• Use effective oral hygiene to prevent soft tissue inflammation
• Prevent trauma when using oral hygiene aids
• Report oral lesions, soreness, or bleeding to dentist
• Use electric tooth brush if patient has difficulty holding conventional devices

tenecteplase
ten-eck´-teh-place
(Metalyse[AUS], TNKase)

CATEGORY AND SCHEDULE
Pregnancy Risk Category: C

Drug Class: Thrombolytic

MECHANISM OF ACTION

A tissue plasminogen activator produced by recombinant DNA that binds to fibrin and converts plasminogen to plasmin. Initiates fibrinolysis by degrading fibrin clots, fibrinogen, other plasma proteins. *Therapeutic Effect:* Exerts thrombolytic action.

USES

Dissolving blood clots

PHARMACOKINETICS

Extensively distributed to tissues. Completely eliminated by hepatic metabolism. *Half-life:* 11–20 min.

INDICATIONS AND DOSAGES
▸ **Acute MI**
IV

Adults. Dosage is based on patient's weight. Treatment should be initiated as soon as possible after onset of symptoms.

Weight (kg)	(mg)	(ml)
90 or more	50	10
80 to less than 90	45	9
70 to less than 80	40	8
60 to less than 70	35	7
Less than 60	30	6

SIDE EFFECTS/ADVERSE REACTIONS

Frequent
Bleeding (major, 4.7%; minor, 21.8%)

PRECAUTIONS AND CONTRAINDICATIONS

Active internal bleeding, aneurysm, AV malformation, bleeding diathesis, history of cerebrovascular accident, intracranial or intraspinal surgery or trauma within past 2 mo, intracranial neoplasm, severe uncontrolled hypertension

DRUG INTERACTIONS OF CONCERN TO DENTISTRY

• Increased risk of bleeding: drugs that interfere with coagulation or platelet function, such as NSAIDs and aspirin, ginkgo biloba (herb)

SERIOUS REACTIONS

❗ Bleeding at internal sites may occur, including intracranial, retroperitoneal, GI, GU, and respiratory sites.
❗ Lysis or coronary thrombi may produce atrial or ventricular arrhythmias and stroke.

DENTAL CONSIDERATIONS

General:
• An acute use drug for use in hospitals or emergency departments.
• Patients are at risk for bleeding; check for oral signs.
• Avoid products that affect platelet function, such as aspirin and NSAIDs.
• Monitor and record vital signs.
• Review medical and drug history.
Consultations:
• Medical consultation should include routine blood counts, including platelet counts and bleeding time.
• In a patient with symptoms of blood dyscrasias, request a medical consultation for blood studies and postpone treatment until normal values are reestablished.
• Medical consultation may be required to assess disease control and patient's ability to tolerate stress.
Teach Patient/Family to:
• Use soft tooth brush to reduce risk of bleeding
• Use effective oral hygiene to prevent soft tissue inflammation
• Report oral lesions, soreness, or bleeding to dentist

T

• Prevent trauma when using oral hygiene aids
• Update health and medication history if physician makes any changes in evaluation or drug regimens; include OTC, herbal, and nonherbal remedies in the update

teniposide
ten-ih´-poe-side
(Vumon)

CATEGORY AND SCHEDULE
Pregnancy Risk Category: D

Drug Class: Antineoplastics, epipodophyllotoxins

MECHANISM OF ACTION
An epipodophyllotoxin that induces single- and double-strand breaks in DNA, inhibiting or altering DNA synthesis. Acts in the late S and early G2 phases of cell cycle. *Therapeutic Effect:* Prevents cells from entering mitosis.

USES
Treatment of childhood acute lymphocytic leukemia

PHARMACOKINETICS
Plasma levels decline biexponentially over 1-2.5 hr, with a mean terminal half-life of 5 hr. Protein binding: >99%, excreted in the urine, primarily as metabolites.

INDICATIONS AND DOSAGES
▶ **Induction Therapy in Patients with Refractory Childhood Acute Lymphoblastic Leukemia (in combination with other antineoplastic agents)**
Children. Dosage is individualized on the basis of the patient's clinical

response and tolerance of the drug's adverse effects. When used in combination therapy, consult specific protocols for optimum dosage or sequence of drug administration.

SIDE EFFECTS/ADVERSE REACTIONS
Frequent
Mucositis, nausea, vomiting, diarrhea, anemia
Occasional
Alopecia, rash
Rare
Hepatic dysfunction, fever, renal dysfunction, peripheral neurotoxicity

PRECAUTIONS AND CONTRAINDICATIONS
Absolute neutrophil count less than 500/mm³; hypersensitivity to Cremophor EL (polyoxyethylated castor oil), etoposide, or teniposide; platelet count less than 50,000/mm³

DRUG INTERACTIONS OF CONCERN TO DENTISTRY
None reported

SERIOUS REACTIONS
❗ Myelosuppression manifested as hematologic toxicity (principally leukopenia, neutropenia, and thrombocytopenia) may be severe and may increase the risk of infection or bleeding.
❗ Hypersensitivity reaction may include anaphylaxis (marked by chills, fever, tachycardia, bronchospasm, dyspnea, and facial flushing).

DENTAL CONSIDERATIONS
General:
• If additional analgesia is required for dental pain, consider alternative analgesics (NSAIDs) in patients taking narcotics for acute or chronic pain.

• Examine for oral manifestation of opportunistic infection.
• Avoid products that affect platelet function, such as aspirin and NSAIDs.
• This drug may be used in the hospital or on an outpatient basis. Confirm the patient's disease and treatment status.
• Chlorhexidine mouth rinse prior to and during chemotherapy may reduce severity of mucositis.
• Patient on chronic drug therapy may rarely present with symptoms of blood dyscrasias, which can include infection, bleeding, and poor healing. If dyscrasia is present, caution patient to prevent oral tissue trauma when using oral hygiene aids.
• Palliative medication may be required for management of oral side effects.
• Short appointments and a stress reduction protocol may be required for anxious patients.
• Consider semisupine chair position for patient comfort if GI side effects occur.
• Caution: patients may be at high risk for infection.
• Patients may be at risk for bleeding; check oral signs.
• Oral infections should be eliminated and/or treated aggressively.

Consultations:
• Medical consultation should include routine blood counts, including platelet counts and bleeding time.
• Consult physician; prophylactic or therapeutic antiinfectives may be indicated if surgery or periodontal treatment is required.
• Medical consultation may be required to assess immunologic status during cancer chemotherapy and determine safety risk, if any, posed by the required dental treatment.

• Medical consultation may be required to assess disease control and patient's ability to tolerate stress.
• In a patient with symptoms of blood dyscrasias, request a medical consultation for blood studies and postpone treatment until normal values are reestablished.

Teach Patient/Family to:
• See dentist immediately if secondary oral infection occurs.
• Be aware of oral side effects
• Use effective oral hygiene to prevent soft tissue inflammation
• Report oral lesions, soreness, or bleeding to dentist
• Prevent trauma when using oral hygiene aids
• Update health and medication history if physician makes any changes in evaluation or drug regimens; include OTC, herbal, and nonherbal remedies in the update

tenofovir
ten-oh´-foh-veer
(Viread)

CATEGORY AND SCHEDULE
Pregnancy Risk Category: B

Drug Class: Antiviral

MECHANISM OF ACTION
A nucleotide analog that inhibits HIV reverse transcriptase by being incorporated into viral DNA, resulting in DNA chain termination. *Therapeutic Effect:* Slows HIV replication and reduces HIV RNA levels (viral load).

USES
Treatment of HIV-1 infection in combination with other antiretroviral drugs

PHARMACOKINETICS

PO: Bioavailability 5% (improves with meal); maximum serum levels 0.6–1.4 hr; low plasma protein binding less than 7%; minimal systemic metabolism; excreted by glomerular filtration and active tubular secretion; use in children not evaluated.

INDICATIONS AND DOSAGES

▶ **HIV Infection (in combination with other antiretrovirals)**
PO
Adults, Elderly, Children 18 yr and older. 300 mg once a day.

SIDE EFFECTS/ADVERSE REACTIONS

Occasional
GI disturbances (diarrhea, flatulence, nausea, vomiting)

PRECAUTIONS AND CONTRAINDICATIONS

Hypersensitivity; avoid breast-feeding; obesity and prolonged nucleoside use; risk of lactic acidosis/severe hepatomegaly with steatosis; no data on hepatic impairment; redistribution of body fat
Caution
Obesity and prolonged nucleoside use; risk of lactic acidosis/severe hepatomegaly with steatosis; no data on hepatic impairment; redistribution of body fat

DRUG INTERACTIONS OF CONCERN TO DENTISTRY

• Potential for competition for renal clearance: acyclovir, valacyclovir

SERIOUS REACTIONS

❗ Lactic acidosis and hepatomegaly with steatosis occur rarely, but may be severe.

General:
• Examine for oral manifestation of opportunistic infection.
Consultations:
• Medical consultation may be required to assess disease control and patient's ability to tolerate stress.
Teach Patient/Family to:
• Use effective oral hygiene to prevent soft tissue inflammation/infection

terazosin hydrochloride

ter-ah´-zoe-sin high-droh-klor´-ide
(Apo-Terazosin[CAN], Hytrin, Novo-Terazosin[CAN])

CATEGORY AND SCHEDULE
Pregnancy Risk Category: C

Drug Class: Antihypertensive, antiadrenergic

MECHANISM OF ACTION

An antihypertensive and benign prostatic hyperplasia agent that blocks α-adrenergic receptors. Produces vasodilation, decreases peripheral resistance, and targets receptors around bladder neck and prostate. *Therapeutic Effect:* In hypertension, decreases B/P. In benign prostatic hyperplasia, relaxes smooth muscle and improves urine flow.

USES

Treatment of hypertension as a single agent or in combination with diuretics or β-blockers; benign prostatic hypertrophy

PHARMACOKINETICS

Rapidly, completely absorbed from the GI tract. Protein binding: 90%–94%.

Metabolized in the liver to active metabolite. Primarily eliminated in feces via biliary system; excreted in urine. Not removed by hemodialysis. *Half-life:* 12 hr.

Route	Onset	Peak	Duration
PO	15 min	1–2 hr	12–24 hr

INDICATIONS AND DOSAGES
▶ **Mild-to-Moderate Hypertension**
PO
Adults, Elderly. Initially, 1 mg at bedtime. Slowly increase dosage to desired levels. Range: 1–5 mg/day as single or 2 divided doses. Maximum: 20 mg.
▶ **Benign Prostatic Hyperplasia**
PO
Adults, Elderly. Initially, 1 mg at bedtime. May increase up to 10 mg/day. Maximum: 20 mg/day.

SIDE EFFECTS/ADVERSE REACTIONS
Frequent
Dizziness, headache, unusual tiredness
Rare
Peripheral edema, orthostatic hypotension, myalgia, arthralgia, blurred vision, nausea, vomiting, nasal congestion, somnolence

PRECAUTIONS AND CONTRAINDICATIONS
Hypersensitivity, children, lactation

DRUG INTERACTIONS OF CONCERN TO DENTISTRY
• Decreased antihypertensive effects: NSAIDs, indomethacin

SERIOUS REACTIONS
❗ First-dose syncope (hypotension with sudden loss of consciousness) may occur 30 to 90 min after initial dose of 2 mg or more, a too-rapid increase in dosage, or addition of another antihypertensive agent to

therapy. First-dose syncope may be preceded by tachycardia (pulse rate of 120–160 beats/min).

DENTAL CONSIDERATIONS
General:
• Monitor vital signs at every appointment because of cardiovascular side effects.
• After supine positioning, have patient sit upright for at least 2 min before standing to avoid orthostatic hypotension.
• Assess salivary flow as a factor in caries, periodontal disease, and candidiasis.
• Limit use of sodium-containing products, such as saline IV fluids, for patients with a dietary salt restriction.
• Consider semisupine chair position for patient comfort if GI side effects occur.
Teach Patient/Family:
• When chronic dry mouth occurs, advise patient to:
  • Avoid mouth rinses with high alcohol content because of drying effects
  • Use daily home fluoride to prevent caries
  • Use sugarless gum, frequent sips of water, or saliva substitutes

terbinafine hydrochloride
ter-been´-ah-feen
high-droh-klor´-ide
(Apo-Terbinafine[CAN], Lamisil, Lamisil AT, Novo-Terbinafine[CAN])
Do not confuse terbinafine with terbutaline or Lamisil with Lamictal.

CATEGORY AND SCHEDULE
Pregnancy Risk Category: B

Drug Class: Antifungal

MECHANISM OF ACTION
A fungicidal antifungal that inhibits the enzyme squalene epoxidase, thereby interfering with fungal biosynthesis. *Therapeutic Effect:* Results in death of fungal cells.

USES
Treatment of tinea pedis, tinea cruris, tinea corporis; unapproved uses: treatment of cutaneous candidiasis, tinea versicolor; treatment of onychomycosis of the toenail or fingernail caused by dermatophytes (tinea unguium)

PHARMACOKINETICS
PO: Bioavailability 40%, peak plasma levels approximately 2 hr; highly plasma protein bound (99%), extensive metabolism, excreted in urine (70%).

INDICATIONS AND DOSAGES
▶ **Tinea Pedis**
Topical
Adults, Elderly, Children 12 yr and older. Apply twice a day until signs and symptoms significantly improve.
▶ **Tinea Cruris, Tinea Corporis**
Topical
Adults, Elderly, Children 12 yr and older. Apply 1–2 times a day until signs and symptoms significantly improve.
▶ **Onychomycosis**
PO
Adults, Elderly, Children 12 yr and older. 250 mg/day for 6 wk (fingernails) or 12 wk (toenails).
▶ **Tinea Versicolor**
Topical Solution
Adults, Elderly. Apply to the affected area twice a day for 7 days.
▶ **Systemic Mycosis**
PO
Adults, Elderly. 250–500 mg/day for up to 16 mo.

SIDE EFFECTS/ADVERSE REACTIONS
Frequent
Oral: Headache
Occasional
Oral: Diarrhea, rash, dyspepsia, pruritus, taste disturbance, nausea, abdominal pain, flatulence, urticaria, visual disturbance
Topical: Irritation, burning, pruritus, dryness

PRECAUTIONS AND CONTRAINDICATIONS
Oral: Children younger than 12 yr, preexisting hepatic or renal impairment (creatinine clearance of less than 50 ml/min).
Caution
Preexisting liver or renal disease, use not recommended during nursing, pediatric patients

DRUG INTERACTIONS OF CONCERN TO DENTISTRY
None reported

SERIOUS REACTIONS
! Hepatobiliary dysfunction (including cholestatic hepatitis), serious skin reactions, and severe neutropenia occur rarely.
! Ocular lens and retinal changes have been noted.

DENTAL CONSIDERATIONS
General:
• Determine why patient is taking the drug.
• Consider semisupine chair position for patient comfort if GI side effects occur.
• Patients on chronic drug therapy may rarely have symptoms of blood dyscrasias, which can include infection, bleeding, and poor healing.

Consultations:
• In a patient with symptoms of blood dyscrasias, request a medical consultation for blood studies and postpone treatment until normal values are reestablished.
Teach Patient/Family to:
• Use effective oral hygiene to prevent soft tissue inflammation
• Prevent trauma when using oral hygiene aids

terconazole
ter-kon´-ah-zole
(Terazol[CAN], Terazol 3, Terazol 7)

CATEGORY AND SCHEDULE
Pregnancy Risk Category: C

Drug Class: Local antifungal

MECHANISM OF ACTION
An antifungal that disrupts fungal cell membrane permeability.
Therapeutic Effect: Produces antifungal activity.

USES
Treatment of vaginal, vulval, vulvovaginal candidiasis (moniliasis)

PHARMACOKINETICS
Extent of systemic absorption after vaginal administration may be dependent on presence of a uterus, 5%–8% in women who had a hysterectomy versus 12%–16% in nonhysterectomy women.

INDICATIONS AND DOSAGES
▸ **Vulvovaginal Candidiasis**
Intravaginal
Adults, Elderly. 1 suppository vaginally at bedtime for 3 days.
Adults, Elderly. 1 applicatorful at bedtime for 7 days (0.4% cream) or for 3 days (0.8% cream).

SIDE EFFECTS/ADVERSE REACTIONS
Frequent
Headache, vulvovaginal burning
Occasional
Dysmenorrhea, pain in female genitalia, abdominal pain, fever, itching
Rare
Chills

PRECAUTIONS AND CONTRAINDICATIONS
Hypersensitivity to terconazole or any component of the formulation
Caution
Children younger than 2 yr, pregnancy, lactation

DRUG INTERACTIONS OF CONCERN TO DENTISTRY
• None reported.

SERIOUS REACTIONS
❗ Flu-like syndrome has been reported.

DENTAL CONSIDERATIONS
General:
• Broad-spectrum antibiotics can exacerbate vaginal candidiasis.

teriparatide
ter-ih-par´-ah-tide
(Forteo)

CATEGORY AND SCHEDULE
Pregnancy Risk Category: C

Drug Class: Bone resorption inhibitor (a synthetic polypeptide of rDNA origin, contains recombinant human parathyroid hormone [rhPTH(1-34)])

MECHANISM OF ACTION
A synthetic polypeptide hormone that acts on bone to mobilize

calcium; also acts on kidney to reduce calcium clearance, increase phosphate excretion. ***Therapeutic Effect:*** Promotes an increased rate of release of calcium from bone into blood, stimulates new bone formation.

USES
Treatment of postmenopausal women with osteoporosis at high risk for fracture; to increase bone mass in men with primary or hypogonadal osteoporosis at high risk for fracture

PHARMACOKINETICS
Subcutaneous: Absolute bioavailability 95%, peak serum levels 30 min. ***Half-life:*** 1 hr, no excretion or metabolism studies have been done, may be the same as PTH with hepatic metabolism and renal excretion.

INDICATIONS AND DOSAGES
▶ **Osteoporosis**
Subcutaneous
Adults, Elderly. 20 mcg once daily into the thigh or abdominal wall.

SIDE EFFECTS/ADVERSE REACTIONS
Occasional
Leg cramps, nausea, dizziness, headache, orthostatic hypotension, increased heart rate

PRECAUTIONS AND CONTRAINDICATIONS
Serum calcium above normal level, those at increased risk for osteosarcoma (Paget's disease, unexplained elevations of alkaline phosphatase, open epiphyses, prior radiation therapy that includes the skeleton), hypercalcemic disorder (e.g., hyperparathyroidism), hypersensitivity to teriparatide or any of the components of the formulation
Caution
Active or recent urolithiasis, use longer than 2 yr, postinjection

orthostatic hypotension, symptoms of hypercalcemia, pregnancy category C, avoid in nursing mothers, not for use in children

DRUG INTERACTIONS OF CONCERN TO DENTISTRY
None reported

SERIOUS REACTIONS
None known

DENTAL CONSIDERATIONS
General:
• Patients with osteoporosis and risk of fracture should be asked if they use this drug; otherwise some patients may not report its use.
• Patients may need special assistance in the dental office to avoid risk of falling.
Teach Patient/Family to:
• Update health and drug history, reporting changes in health status, drug regimen, or disease/treatment status
• Contact physician if symptoms of hypercalcemia appear (nausea, vomiting, constipation, lethargy, muscle weakness)

testosterone
tess-toss´-ter-one
(Andriol[CAN], Androderm, AndroGel, Andropository[CAN], Delatestryl, Depotest[CAN], Depo-Testosterone, Everone[CAN], Striant, Testim, Testoderm, Testoprel, Virilon IM[CAN])
Do not confuse testosterone with testolactone.

CATEGORY AND SCHEDULE
Pregnancy Risk Category: X
Controlled Substance: Schedule III

Drug Class: Androgen, anabolic steroid

MECHANISM OF ACTION

A primary endogenous androgen that promotes growth and development of male sex organs and maintains secondary sex characteristics in androgen-deficient males. ***Therapeutic Effect:*** Helps relieve androgen deficiency.

USES

Treatment of androgen deficiency, delayed puberty, female breast cancer, certain anemias, gender changes, hypogonadism, cryptorchidism

PHARMACOKINETICS

Well absorbed after IM administration. Protein binding: 98%. Undergoes first-pass metabolism in the liver. Primarily excreted in urine. Unknown if removed by hemodialysis. ***Half-life:*** 10–20 min.

INDICATIONS AND DOSAGES
▸ **Male Hypogonadism**
IM
Adults. 50–400 mg q2–4wk.
Adolescents. Initially 40–50 mg/m^2/dose monthly until growth rate falls to prepubertal levels. 100 mg/m^2/dose until growth ceases.
Maintenance virilizing dose: 100 mg/m^2/dose twice a mo.
Subcutaneous (Pellets)
Adults, Adolescents. 150–450 mg q3–6mo.
Transdermal (Patch [Testoderm])
Adults, Elderly. Start therapy with 6 mg/day patch. Apply patch to scrotal skin.
Transdermal (Patch [Testoderm TTS])
Adults, Elderly. Apply TTS patch to arm, back, or upper buttocks.
Transdermal (Patch [Androderm])
Adults, Elderly. Start therapy with 5 mg/day patch applied at night. Apply patch to abdomen, back, thighs, or upper arms.

Transdermal (Gel [AndroGel])
Adults, Elderly. Initial dose of 5 mg delivers 50 mg testosterone and is applied once daily to the abdomen, shoulders, or upper arms. May increase to 7.5 g, then to 10 g, if necessary.
Transdermal (Gel [Testim])
Adults, Elderly. Initial dose of 5 g delivers 50 mg testosterone and is applied once a day to the shoulders or upper arms. May increase to 10 g.
Buccal System (Striant)
Adults, Elderly: 30 mg q12h.
▸ **Delayed Puberty**
IM
Adults. 50–200 mg q2–4wk.
Adolescents. 40–50 mg/m^2/dose every mo for 6 mo.
Subcutaneous (Pellets)
Adults, Adolescents. 150–450 mg q3–6mo.
▸ **Breast Carcinoma**
IM (testosterone aqueous)
Adults. 50–100 mg 3 times a wk.
IM (testosterone cypionate or testosterone ethanate)
Adults. 200–400 mg q2–4wk.
IM (testosterone propionate)
Adults. 50–100 mg 3 times a wk.

SIDE EFFECTS/ADVERSE REACTIONS

Frequent
Gynecomastia, acne
Females: Hirsutism, amenorrhea or other menstrual irregularities, deepening of voice, clitoral enlargement that may not be reversible when drug is discontinued
Occasional
Edema, nausea, insomnia, oligospermia, priapism, male-pattern baldness, bladder irritability, hypercalcemia (in immobilized patients or those with breast cancer), hypercholesterolemia, inflammation and pain at IM injection site

T

Transdermal: Pruritus, erythema, skin irritation
Rare
Polycythemia (with high dosage), hypersensitivity

PRECAUTIONS AND CONTRAINDICATIONS
Cardiac impairment, hypercalcemia, pregnancy, prostate or breast cancer in males, severe hepatic or renal disease
Caution
Diabetes mellitus, cardiovascular disease, MI, increased risk of prostatic hypertrophy, prostatic carcinoma, virilization (women), increased PT

DRUG INTERACTIONS OF CONCERN TO DENTISTRY
• Edema: ACTH, adrenal steroids

SERIOUS REACTIONS
! Peliosis hepatitis (presence of blood-filled cysts in parenchyma of liver), hepatic neoplasms, and hepatocellular carcinoma have been associated with prolonged high-dose therapy.
! Anaphylactic reactions occur rarely.

DENTAL CONSIDERATIONS
General:
• Determine why the patient is taking the drug.
• Consider local hemostasis measures to prevent excessive bleeding.
• Short appointments and a stress-reduction protocol may be required for anxious patients.
• Prophylactic antibiotics may be indicated to prevent infection if surgery or deep scaling is planned.
Consultations:
• Physician consultation may be required if signs of anemia are observed in oral tissues.

• Medical consultation may be required to assess disease control and patient's ability to tolerate stress.
• Medical consultation should include PPT or PT.
Teach Patient/Family to:
• Use effective oral hygiene to prevent soft tissue inflammation
• Be aware of the possibility of secondary oral infection and the need to see dentist immediately if infection occurs

tetracaine
tet´-ra-cane
(AK-T Caine, Cepacol, Opticaine, Pontocaine, Viractin)
Do not confuse with procaine, lidocaine.

CATEGORY AND SCHEDULE
Pregnancy Risk Category: C

Drug Class: Topical anesthetic (ester group)

MECHANISM OF ACTION
Tetracaine causes a reversible blockade of nerve conduction by decreasing nerve membrane permeability to sodium. *Therapeutic Effect:* Local anesthetic.

USES
Local anesthesia of mucous membranes, pruritus, sunburn, sore throat, cold sores, oral pain, rectal pain and irritation, control of gagging

PHARMACOKINETICS
Systemic absorption of tetracaine is variable. Metabolized by plasma pseudocholinesterases. Excreted in the urine.

INDICATIONS AND DOSAGES
▸ **Anesthetize Lower Abdomen**
Spinal
Adults. 3–4 ml (9–12 mg) of a
0.3% solution.
▸ **Anesthetize Perineum**
Spinal
Adults. 1–2 ml (3–6 mg) of a
0.3% solution.
▸ **Anesthetize Upper Abdomen**
Spinal
Adults. 5 ml (15 mg) of a
0.3% solution.
▸ **Obstetric Anesthesia, Low Spinal (saddle block) Anesthesia**
Spinal
Adults. 1–2 ml (2–14 mg) of a
0.2% solution.
▸ **Anesthesia of the Perineum**
Intrathecal
Adults. 0.5 ml (5 mg) as a 1%
solution, diluted with equal amount
of CSF or 10% dextrose injection.
▸ **Anesthesia of the Perineum and Lower Extremeties**
Intrathecal
Adults. 1 ml (10 mg) as a 1%
solution, diluted with equal amount
of CSF or 10% dextrose injection.
▸ **Anesthesia up to the Costal Margin**
Intrathecal
Adults. 1.5–2 ml (15–20 mg) as a 1%
solution, diluted with equal amount
of CSF.
▸ **Topical Anesthesia**
Topical
Adults. Apply to the affected areas
as needed. Maximum dosage is
28 g/24 hr.
Children. Apply to the affected areas
as needed. Maximum dosage is 7 g
in a 24-hr period.
▸ **Topical Anesthesia of Nose and Throat, Abolish Laryngeal and Esophageal Reflexes Prior to Diagnostic Procedure**
Topical
Adults. Direct application of a 0.25%
or 0.5% topical solution or by oral

inhalation of a nebulized 0.5%
solution. Total dose should not
exceed 20 mg.
▸ **Mild Pain, Burning and/or Pruritis Associated with Herpes Labialis (cold sores or fever blisters)**
Topical
Adults, Children 2 yr and older.
Apply to the affected area no more
than 3–4 times a day.
▸ **Ophthalmic Anesthesia**
Topical
Adults. 1–2 drops of a 0.5% solution.

SIDE EFFECTS/ADVERSE REACTIONS
Frequent
Burning stinging, or tenderness, skin
rash, itching, redness, or inflammation,
numbness or tingling of the face or
mouth, pain at the injection site,
sensitivity to light, swelling of the
eye or eyelid, watering of the eyes,
acute ocular pain and ocular
irritation (burning, stinging,
or redness)
Occasional
Paresthesias, weakness and paralysis
of lower extremity, hypotension,
high or total spinal block, urinary
retention or incontinence, fecal
incontinence, headache, back pain,
septic meningitis, meningismus,
arachnoiditis, shivering, cranial
nerve palsies due to traction on
nerves from loss of CSF, and loss of
perineal sensation and sexual
function
Rare
Anxiety; restlessness; difficulty
breathing; shortness of
breath; dizziness; drowsiness;
lightheadedness; nausea; vomiting;
seizures (convulsions); slow,
irregular heartbeat (palpitations);
swelling of the face or mouth;
skin rash; itching (hives); tremors;
visual impairment

T

PRECAUTIONS AND CONTRAINDICATIONS

Hypersensitivity to ester local anesthetics, sulfites, PABA; infection or inflammation at the injection site, bacteremia, platelet abnormalities, thrombocytopenia, increased bleeding time, uncontrolled coagulopathy, anticoagulant therapy, sulfonamide therapy

Caution

Children younger than 12 yr, sepsis, lactation, local infection, geriatric, debilitated patient

DRUG INTERACTIONS OF CONCERN TO DENTISTRY

• Specific drug interactions are not listed; it would be wise to use with caution in patients taking tocainide, mexiletine; significant systemic absorption could lead to synergistic and potentially toxic effects

SERIOUS REACTIONS

! Tetracaine-induced CNS toxicity usually presents with symptoms of CNS stimulation, such as anxiety, apprehension, restlessness, nervousness, disorientation, confusion, dizziness, tinnitus, blurred vision, tremor, and/or seizures. Subsequently, depressive symptoms may occur, including drowsiness, respiratory arrest, or coma.

! Depression or cardiac excitability and contractility may cause AV block, ventricular arrhythmias, or cardiac arrest. Symptoms of local anesthetic CNS toxicity, such as dizziness, tongue numbness, visual impairment or disturbances, and muscular twitching appear to occur before cardiotoxic effects. Cardiotoxic effects include angina, QT prolongation, PR prolongation, atrial fibrillation, sinus bradycardia, hypotension, palpitations, and

cardiovascular collapse. Maternal seizures and cardiovascular collapse may occur following paracervical block in early pregnancy due to rapid systemic absorption.

Alert

! Tetracaine is more likely than any other topical anesthetic to cause contact reactions, including skin rash (unspecified), mucous membrane irritation, erythema, pruritus, urticaria, burning, stinging, edema, or tenderness.

Alert

! During labor and obstetric delivery, local anesthetics can cause varying degrees of maternal, fetal, and neonatal toxicities. Fetal heart rate should be monitored continuously because fetal bradycardia may occur in patients receiving tetracaine anesthesia and may be associated with fetal acidosis. Maternal hypotension can result from regional anesthesia; patient position can alleviate this problem. Spinal tetracaine may cause decreased uterine contractility or maternal expulsion efforts and alter the forces of parturition.

DENTAL CONSIDERATIONS

General:

• Apply smallest effective dose; apply to small area because significant absorption can occur, especially from denuded areas.
• Absorption of excessive amounts of drug may lead to signs of local anesthetic toxicity; with correct use, toxicity is a rare event.
• Use for topical anesthesia or temporary relief of symptoms; reevaluate if symptoms persist.
• Toxic amounts can be absorbed from denuded mucosa or skin.

• Apply with cotton-tipped applicator by pressing, not rubbing, paste on lesion.

Teach Patient/Family to:

• Apply correctly

• Not chew gum or eat while numbness is present after dental treatment

• Recognize the symptoms of systemic toxicity, which can include nervousness, nausea, excitement followed by drowsiness, convulsions, and cardiac and respiratory depression

• Be aware that symptoms may vary because they depend on the amount of drug actually absorbed

tetracycline hydrochloride

tet-ra-sye´-kleen
high-droh-klor´-ide
(Apo-Tetra[CAN], Latycin[AUS],
Mysteclin[AUS], Novotetra[CAN],
Nu-Tetra[CAN], Sumycin,
Tetrex[AUS])

CATEGORY AND SCHEDULE

Pregnancy Risk Category:
D (B with topical form)

Drug Class: Tetracycline, broad-spectrum antibiotic

MECHANISM OF ACTION

A tetracycline antibiotic that inhibits bacterial protein synthesis by binding to ribosomes. ***Therapeutic Effect:*** Bacteriostatic.

USES

Treatment of syphilis, *C. trachomatis*, gonorrhea, lymphogranuloma venereum, *M. pneumoniae*, rickettsial infections, acne, actinomycosis, anthrax, bronchitis, GU infections, sinusitis, and many other infections produced by susceptible organisms; *H. pylori*–associated duodenal ulcer

PHARMACOKINETICS

Readily absorbed from the GI tract. Protein binding: 30%–60%. Widely distributed. Excreted in urine; eliminated in feces through biliary system. Not removed by hemodialysis. ***Half-life:*** 6–11 hr (increased in impaired renal function).

INDICATIONS AND DOSAGES

▶ **Inflammatory Acne Vulgaris, Lyme Disease, Mycoplasmal Disease, Legionella Infections, Rocky Mountain Spotted Fever, Chlamydial Infections in Patients with Gonorrhea**
PO
Adults, Elderly. 250–500 mg q6–12h.
Children 8 yr and older. 25–50 mg/kg/day in 4 divided doses.
Maximum: 3 g/day.
▶ ***H. pylori* Infections**
PO
Adults, Elderly. 500 mg 2–4 times a day (in combination).
Topical
Adults, Elderly. Apply twice a day (once in the morning, once in the evening).
▶ **Dosage in Renal Impairment**
Dosage interval is modified on the basis of creatinine clearance.

Creatinine Clearance	Dosage Interval
50–80 ml/min	Usual dose q8–12h
10–50 ml/min	Usual dose q12–24h
Less than 10 ml/min	Usual dose q24h

T

SIDE EFFECTS/ADVERSE REACTIONS

Frequent
Dizziness, light-headedness, diarrhea, nausea, vomiting, abdominal cramps, possibly severe photosensitivity
Topical: Dry, scaly skin; stinging or burning sensation
Occasional
Pigmentation of skin or mucous membranes, rectal or genital pruritus, stomatitis
Topical: Pain, redness, swelling, or other skin irritation.

PRECAUTIONS AND CONTRAINDICATIONS

Children 8 yr and younger, hypersensitivity to tetracyclines or sulfites.
Caution
Renal disease, hepatic disease

DRUG INTERACTIONS OF CONCERN TO DENTISTRY

- Decreased absorption: $NaHCO_3$, other antacids
- Decreased effect of penicillins, cephalosporins
- Possible increase in serum levels of methotrexate
- Suspected increase in effects of warfarin, theophylline

SERIOUS REACTIONS

! Superinfection (especially fungal), anaphylaxis, and benign intracranial hypertension may occur.
! Bulging fontanelles occur rarely in infants.

DENTAL CONSIDERATIONS

General:
- Determine why the patient is taking tetracycline.

- Broad-spectrum antibiotics may be a factor in oral or vaginal *Candida* infections.
- Advise patient if dental drugs prescribed have a potential for photosensitivity.

Consultations:
- Medical consultation may be required to assess disease control.

Teach Patient/Family to:
- Use effective oral hygiene to prevent soft tissue inflammation
- Prevent injury when using oral hygiene aids
- Avoid milk products; to take with a full glass of water
- Take tetracycline doses 1 hr before or 2 hr after air polishing device (Prophy-Jet), if used
- When used for dental infection, advise patient to:
  - Use additional method of contraception for duration of cycle if taking birth control pill
  - Report sore throat, oral burning sensation, fever, fatigue, any of which could indicate superinfection
  - Take at prescribed intervals and complete dosage regimen
  - Immediately notify the dentist if signs or symptoms of infection increase

tetracycline periodontal fiber
tet-ra-sye′-kleen pare-ee-oh
-don′-tal fye′-ber
(Actisite)

CATEGORY AND SCHEDULE
Pregnancy Risk Category: C

Drug Class: Tetracycline, broad-spectrum antiinfective

MECHANISM OF ACTION

Antimicrobial effect related to inhibition of protein synthesis; decreases incidence of postsurgical inflammation and edema; suppresses bacteria and acts as a barrier to bacterial entry; acts on cementum or fibroblasts to enhance periodontal ligament regeneration.

USES

Adjunctive treatment in adult periodontitis.

PHARMACOKINETICS

Topical: In vitro release rate 2 μg/cm/hr; gingival concentration maintained over 10 days; plasma levels below detectable limits

INDICATIONS AND DOSAGES

Fiber: Adjust length to fit pocket depth and contour of teeth treated; fiber should contact base of pocket; apply cyanoacrylate adhesive to secure fiber for 10 days; replace if lost before 7 days; up to 11 teeth can be treated.

SIDE EFFECTS/ADVERSE REACTIONS

Oral: Gingival inflammation and pain, glossitis, local erythema, candidiasis, staining of tongue
EENT: Minor throat irritation
INTEG: Photosensitivity

PRECAUTIONS AND CONTRAINDICATIONS

Hypersensitivity, children younger than 8 yr, acutely abscessed periodontal pocket
Caution
Lactation, children, superinfection, patients with predisposition to candidiasis; must remove fibers after 10 days

DRUG INTERACTIONS OF CONCERN TO DENTISTRY:

It is not known if the tetracycline fiber will decrease the effectiveness of oral contraceptives; however, manufacturer recommends suggesting the use of an alternative form of contraception during the remaining cycle to female patients taking oral contraceptives

SERIOUS REACTIONS

• Serious systemic toxicity unlikely by this route of administration

DENTAL CONSIDERATIONS

General:
• Take precautions regarding allergy to tetracyclines.
• Examine oral mucosa for candidiasis before placing fiber.
Teach Patient/Family to:
• Not chew hard, crusty, or sticky foods
• Not brush or floss near treated area but clean other teeth
• Avoid other oral hygienic practices that could dislodge fibers, such as the use of toothpicks
• Not probe or pick at the treated area
• Notify dentist if fiber dislodges or falls out
• Notify dentist if pain, swelling, or other symptoms occur

thalidomide
thah-lid´-owe-mide
(Thalomid)

CATEGORY AND SCHEDULE
Pregnancy Risk Category: X

Drug Class: Immunomodulators, tumor necrosis factor modulators

MECHANISM OF ACTION

An immunomodulator whose exact mechanism is unknown. Has sedative, antiinflammatory, and immunosuppressive activity, which may be due to selective inhibition of the production of tumor necrosis factor-α. *Therapeutic Effect:* Improves muscle wasting in HIV patients; reduces local and systemic effects of leprosy.

USES

Treatment of and prevention of erythema nodosum leprosum (ENL)

PHARMACOKINETICS

Slowly absorbed from GI tract; peak blood level in 2.9–5.7 hr. Protein binding 55–66%; metabolized in plasma. *Half-life:* 5–7 hr; elimination in urine and by other routes.

INDICATIONS AND DOSAGES

▶ **AIDS-Related Muscle Wasting**
PO
Adults. 100–300 mg a day.

▶ **Leprosy**
PO
Adults, Elderly. Initially, 100–300 mg/day as single bedtime dose, at least 1 hr after the evening meal. Continue until active reaction subsides, then reduce dose q2–4 wk in 50 mg increments.

SIDE EFFECTS/ADVERSE REACTIONS

Frequent
Somnolence, dizziness, mood changes, constipation, dry mouth, peripheral neuropathy
Occasional
Increased appetite, weight gain, headache, loss of libido, edema of face and limbs, nausea, alopecia, dry skin, rash, hypothyroidism

PRECAUTIONS AND CONTRAINDICATIONS

Neutropenia, peripheral neuropathy; pregnancy, sensitivity to thalidomide

DRUG INTERACTIONS OF CONCERN TO DENTISTRY

• Increased sedative effects of: alcohol, barbiturates, phenothiazines
• Increased risk of peripheral neuropathy: metronidazole
• May interfere with hormonal contraceptives: patient must use two alternative methods of contraception

SERIOUS REACTIONS

! Neutropenia, peripheral neuropathy, and thromboembolism occur rarely.

DENTAL CONSIDERATIONS

General:
• Determine why patient is taking the drug.
• Consider semisupine chair position for patient comfort if GI side effects occur.
• Assess salivary flow as a factor in caries, periodontal disease, and candidiasis.
• Examine for oral manifestation of opportunistic infection.
• Patient on chronic drug therapy may rarely present with symptoms of blood dyscrasias, which can include infection, bleeding, and poor healing. If dyscrasia is present, caution patient to prevent oral tissue trauma when using oral hygiene aids.
• After supine positioning, have patient sit upright for at least 2 min before standing to avoid orthostatic hypotension.
• Can be prescribed only by S.T.E.P.S. (System for Thalidomide Education and Prescribing Safety) registered prescribers.
• Absolutely contraindicated in pregnancy.

Consultations:
• Refer patients to attending physician if symptoms of peripheral neuropathy are present (numbness, tingling or pain in hands or feet).
• Consultation with physician may be necessary if sedation or general anesthesia is required.
• Medical consultation may be required to assess disease control and patient's ability to tolerate stress.
• In a patient with symptoms of blood dyscrasias, request a medical consultation for blood studies and postpone treatment until normal values are reestablished.
• Precaution if dental surgery is anticipated or general anesthesia required.

Teach Patient/Family to:
• Not drive or perform other tasks requiring mental alertness.
• When chronic dry mouth occurs, advise patient to:
  • Avoid mouth rinses with high alcohol content due to drying effects
  • Use daily home fluoride products for anticaries effect
  • Use sugarless gum, frequent sips of water or saliva substitutes
• Use effective oral hygiene to prevent soft tissue inflammation
• Prevent trauma when using oral hygiene aids
• Report oral lesions, soreness, or bleeding to dentist
• Update health and medication history if physician makes any changes in evaluation or drug regimens; include OTC, herbal, and nonherbal remedies in the update

theophylline

thee-off´-ih-lin

(Accubron, Aquaphyllin, Asmalix, Broncodyl, Elixomin, Elixophyllin, Lanophyllin, Quibron-T, Respbid, Slo-Bid, Slo-Phyllin, Sustaire, T-Phyl, Theobid, Theoclear LA, Theolair, Theo-Dur, Theo-24, Theolair-24, Theochron, TheoSav, Theovent, Theo-X, Uni-Dur, Uniphyl)

CATEGORY AND SCHEDULE
Pregnancy risk category: C

Drug Class: Xanthine

MECHANISM OF ACTION
An antiasthmatic medication with two distinct actions in the airways of patients with reversible obstruction; smooth muscle relaxation and suppression of the response of airways to stimuli. Mechanisms of action are not known with certainty. It is known that theophylline increases force of contraction of diaphragmatic muscles by enhancing calcium uptake through adenosine-mediated channels. *Therapeutic Effect:* Causes bronchodilation and decreased airway reactivity.

USES
Treatment of bronchial asthma, bronchospasm of COPD, chronic bronchitis; unapproved use: apnea in the neonate

PHARMACOKINETICS
The pharmacokinetics of theophylline vary widely among similar patients and cannot be predicted by age, sex, body weight or other demographic characteristics. Rapidly and completely absorbed after oral administration in solution

or immediate-release solid oral dosage form. Distributed freely into fat-free tissues. Extensively metabolized in liver. *Half-life:* 4–8 hr.

INDICATIONS AND DOSAGES
▸ **Chronic Asthma/Lung Diseases**
PO
Adults. Acute symptoms: 5 mg/kg as a loading dose, maintenance 3 mg/kg every 8 hr (nonsmokers), 3 mg/kg every 6 hr (smokers), 2 mg/kg every 8 hr (older patients), 1–2 mg/kg every 12 hr (CHF); IV 5 mg/kg load over 20 min, maintenance 0.2 mg/kg/hr (CHF, elderly), 0.43 mg/kg/hr (nonsmokers), 0.7 mg/kg/hr (young adult smokers).
Slow titration. Initial dose 16 mg/kg/day or 400 mg daily, whichever is less, doses divided every 6–8 hr.

SIDE EFFECTS/ADVERSE REACTIONS
Anxiety, dizziness, headache, insomnia, lightheadedness, muscle twitching, restlessness, seizures, dysrhythmias, fluid retention with tachycardia, hypotension, palpitations, pounding heartbeat, sinus tachycardia, anorexia, bitter taste, diarrhea, dyspepsia, gastroesophageal reflux, nausea, vomiting, urinary frequency, increased respiratory rate, flushing, urticaria

PRECAUTIONS AND CONTRAINDICATIONS
Hypersensitivity to theophylline or any component of the formulation, active peptic ulcer disease, underlying seizure disorders unless receiving appropriate anticonvulsant medication

Caution
Elderly, CHF, cor pulmonale, hepatic disease, active peptic ulcer disease, diabetes mellitus, hyperthyroidism, hypertension, children

DRUG INTERACTIONS OF CONCERN TO DENTISTRY
• Increased action: erythromycin, ciprofloxacin, glucocorticoids
• Increased risk of cardiac dysrhythmia: halothane inhalation anesthesia, CNS stimulants
• Decreased effect: barbiturates, carbamazepine, ketoconazole
• May decrease sedative effects of benzodiazepines

SERIOUS REACTIONS
! Severe toxicity from theophylline overdose is a relatively rare event.

DENTAL CONSIDERATIONS
General:
• Consider semisupine chair position for patients with respiratory disease.
• Monitor vital signs at every appointment because of cardiovascular side effects.
• Assess salivary flow as a factor in caries, periodontal disease, and candidiasis.
• Be aware that aspirin or sulfite preservatives in vasoconstrictor-containing products can exacerbate asthma.
• Acute asthmatic episodes may be precipitated in the dental office. Sympathomimetic inhalants should be available for emergency use.
• Midday appointments and a stress-reduction protocol may be required for anxious patients.

Consultations:
• Medical consultation may be required to assess disease control.
Teach Patient/Family:
• When chronic dry mouth occurs, advise patient to:
 • Avoid mouth rinses with high alcohol content because of drying effects
 • Use daily home fluoride products to prevent caries
 • Use sugarless gum, frequent sips of water, or saliva substitutes

thiabendazole
thye-ah-ben´-da-zole
(Mintezol)

CATEGORY AND SCHEDULE
Pregnancy Risk Category: C

Drug Class: Anthelmintic, systemic

MECHANISM OF ACTION
An anthelmintic agent that inhibits helminth-specific mitochondrial fumarate reductase. *Therapeutic Effect:* Suppresses parasite production.

USES
Treatment of worm infections

PHARMACOKINETICS
Rapidly and well absorbed from the GI tract. Rapidly metabolized in liver. Primarily excreted in urine; partially eliminated in feces. *Half-life:* 1.2 hr.

INDICATIONS AND DOSAGES
Dose is based on patient's body weight

▶ **Cutaneous Lava Migrans (creeping eruption)**
PO
Adults, Elderly, Children. 50 mg/kg/day q12h for 2 days. Maximum: 3 g/day.
▶ **Intestinal Roundworms**
PO
Adults, Elderly, Children. 50 mg/kg/day q12h for 2 days. Maximum: 3 g/day.
▶ **Strongloidiasis (thread worms)**
PO
Adults, Elderly, Children. 50 mg/kg/day q12h for 2 days. Maximum: 3 g/day.
▶ **Trichinosis**
PO
Adults, Elderly, Children. 50 mg/kg/day q12h for 2–4 days. Maximum: 3 g/day.
▶ **Visceral Larva Migrans**
PO
Adults, Elderly, Children. 50 mg/kg/day q12h for 7 days. Maximum: 3 g/day.

SIDE EFFECTS/ADVERSE REACTIONS
Occasional
Dizziness, drowsiness, nausea, vomiting, diarrhea
Rare
Erythema multiforme, liver damage

PRECAUTIONS AND CONTRAINDICATIONS
Prophylactic treatment of pinworm infestation, hypersensitivity to thiabendazole or its components

DRUG INTERACTIONS OF CONCERN TO DENTISTRY
• Suspected interference with xanthine metabolism

SERIOUS REACTIONS

! Overdose includes symptoms of altered mental status and visual problems.
! Erythema multiform, liver damage, and Stevens-Johnson's syndrome occur rarely.

DENTAL CONSIDERATIONS

General:
- Determine why patient is taking the drug.
- Patient on chronic drug therapy may rarely present with symptoms of blood dyscrasias, which can include infection, bleeding, and poor healing. If dyscrasia is present, caution patient to prevent oral tissue trauma when using oral hygiene aids.
- Assess salivary flow as a factor in caries, periodontal disease, and candidiasis.
- Pinworm infections are easily spread to persons in close contact.
- Question patients about other drugs they may be using.

Consultations:
- In a patient with symptoms of blood dyscrasias, request a medical consultation for blood studies and postpone treatment until normal values are reestablished.
- Medical consultation may be required to assess disease control in the patient.

Teach Patient/Family:
- When chronic dry mouth occurs, advise patient to:
  - Avoid mouth rinses with high alcohol content due to drying effects
  - Use daily home fluoride products for anticaries effect
  - Use sugarless gum, frequent sips of water, or saliva substitutes

thiamine hydrochloride (vitamin B₁)

thy´-ah-min high-droh-klor´-ide
(Beta-Sol[AUS], Betaxin[CAN], Thiamilate)

CATEGORY AND SCHEDULE

Pregnancy Risk Category: A (C if used in doses above recommended daily allowance)
OTC (tablets)

Drug Class: Vitamin B₁, water soluble

MECHANISM OF ACTION

A water-soluble vitamin that combines with adenosine triphosphate in the liver, kidneys, and leukocytes to form thiamine diphosphate, a coenzyme that is necessary for carbohydrate metabolism. **Therapeutic Effect:** Prevents and reverses thiamine deficiency.

USES

Treatment of vitamin B₁ deficiency or prophylaxis, beriberi, Wernicke-Korsakoff syndrome

PHARMACOKINETICS

Readily absorbed from the GI tract, primarily in duodenum, after IM administration. Widely distributed. Metabolized in the liver. Primarily excreted in urine.

INDICATIONS AND DOSAGES

▸ Dietary Supplement
PO
Adults, Elderly. 1–2 mg/day.
Children. 0.5–1 mg/day.
Infants. 0.3–0.5 mg/day.
▸ Thiamine Deficiency
PO

Adults, Elderly. 5–30 mg/day, as a single dose or in 3 divided doses, for 1 mo.
Children. 10–50 mg/day in 3 divided doses.
▶ **Thiamine Deficiency in Patients Who Are Critically Ill or Have Malabsorption Syndrome**
IV, IM
Adults, Elderly. 5–100 mg, 3 times a day.
Children. 10–25 mg/day.
▶ **Metabolic Disorders**
PO
Adults, Elderly, Children. 10–20 mg/day; increased up to 4 g/day in divided doses.

SIDE EFFECTS/ADVERSE REACTIONS
Frequent
Pain, induration, and tenderness at IM injection site

PRECAUTIONS AND CONTRAINDICATIONS
Sensitivity to thiamin, Wernicke's encephalopathy

DRUG INTERACTIONS OF CONCERN TO DENTISTRY
• None reported.

SERIOUS REACTIONS
! IV administration may result in a rare, severe hypersensitivity reaction marked by a feeling of warmth, pruritus, urticaria, weakness, diaphoresis, nausea, restlessness, tightness in throat, angioedema, cyanosis, pulmonary edema, GI tract bleeding, and cardiovascular collapse.

DENTAL CONSIDERATIONS
General:
• Determine why the patient is taking this vitamin.

Teach Patient/Family:
• Food sources to be included in diet: yeast, whole grain, beef, liver, legumes

thiethylperazine
thye-eth-il-per´-ah-zeen
(Torecan)
Do not confuse with thioridazine.

CATEGORY AND SCHEDULE
Pregnancy Risk Category: X

Drug Class: Phenothiazine-type, antiemetic

MECHANISM OF ACTION
A piperazine phenothiazine that acts centrally to block dopamine receptors in chemoreceptor trigger zone (CTZ) in CNS. *Therapeutic Effect:* Relieves nausea and vomiting.

USES
Treatment of nausea, vomiting

PHARMACOKINETICS
PO: Onset 45–60 min. Rectal: Onset 45–60 min. Metabolized by liver; excreted by kidneys; crosses placenta; excreted in breast milk.

INDICATIONS AND DOSAGES
▶ **Nausea or Vomiting**
PO/Rectal/IM
Adults, Elderly. 10 mg 1–3 times a day.

SIDE EFFECTS/ADVERSE REACTIONS
Frequent
Drowsiness, dizziness
Occasional
Blurred vision, decreased color/night vision, fever, headache, orthostatic hypotension, rash, ringing in ears,

constipation, dry mouth, decreased sweating

PRECAUTIONS AND CONTRAINDICATIONS
Comatose states, severe CNS depression, pregnancy, hypersensitivity to phenothiazines
Caution
Children younger than 12 yr, elderly

DRUG INTERACTIONS OF CONCERN TO DENTISTRY
• Increased anticholinergic action: anticholinergics
• Increased CNS depression, hypotension: alcohol, CNS depressants

SERIOUS REACTIONS
! Extrapyramidal symptoms manifested as torticollis (neck muscle spasm), oculogyric crisis (rolling back of eyes), and akathisia (motor restlessness, anxiety) occur rarely.

DENTAL CONSIDERATIONS
General:
• Postpone elective dental treatment when symptoms are present.
Consultations:
• Medical consultation may be required to assess disease control.

thioridazine
thye-oh-rid´-ah-zeen
(Aldazine[AUS], Apo-Thioridazine [CAN], Mellaril, Mellaril [AUS], Thioridazine Intensol)
Do not confuse thioridazine with thiothixene or Thorazine, or Mellaril with Mebaral.

CATEGORY AND SCHEDULE
Pregnancy Risk Category: C

Drug Class: Phenothiazine antipsychotic

MECHANISM OF ACTION
A phenothiazine that blocks dopamine at postsynaptic receptor sites. Possesses strong anticholinergic and sedative effects. *Therapeutic Effect:* Suppresses behavioral response in psychosis; reduces locomotor activity and aggressiveness.

USES
Treatment of psychotic disorders, schizophrenia, behavioral problems in children, alcohol withdrawal as adjunct, anxiety, major depressive disorders, organic brain syndrome

PHARMACOKINETICS
PO: Onset erratic, peak 2–4 hr. *Half-life:* 26–36 hr; metabolized by liver; excreted in urine; crosses placenta; excreted in breast milk.

INDICATIONS AND DOSAGES
▶ **Psychosis**
PO
Adults, Elderly, Children 12 yr and older. Initially, 25–100 mg 3 times a day; dosage increased gradually. Maximum: 800 mg/day.
Children 2–11 yr. Initially, 0.5 mg/kg/day in 2–3 divided doses. Maximum: 3 mg/kg/day.

SIDE EFFECTS/ADVERSE REACTIONS
Occasional
Drowsiness during early therapy, dry mouth, blurred vision, lethargy, constipation or diarrhea, nasal congestion, peripheral edema, urine retention
Rare
Ocular changes, altered skin pigmentation (in those taking high doses for prolonged periods), photosensitivity, darkening of urine

PRECAUTIONS AND CONTRAINDICATIONS

Angle-closure glaucoma, blood dyscrasias, cardiac arrhythmias, cardiac or hepatic impairment, concurrent use of drugs that prolong QT interval, severe CNS depression
Caution
Lactation, seizure disorders, hypertension, hepatic disease, cardiac disease

DRUG INTERACTIONS OF CONCERN TO DENTISTRY

• Increased sedation: other CNS depressants, alcohol, barbiturate anesthetics, opioid analgesics
• Hypotension, tachycardia: epinephrine (systemic)
• Increased extrapyramidal effects: phenothiazines and related drugs (haloperidol, droperidol), metoclopramide
• Additive photosensitization: tetracyclines
• Increased anticholinergic effects: anticholinergics

SERIOUS REACTIONS

! Prolonged QT interval may produce torsades de pointes, a form of ventricular tachycardia, and sudden death.

DENTAL CONSIDERATIONS

General:
• Monitor vital signs at every appointment because of cardiovascular side effects.
• Patients on chronic drug therapy may rarely have symptoms of blood dyscrasias, which can include infection, bleeding, and poor healing.
• After supine positioning, have patient sit upright for at least 2 min before standing to avoid orthostatic hypotension.

• Assess salivary flow as a factor in caries, periodontal disease, and candidiasis.
• Avoid dental light in patient's eyes; offer dark glasses for patient comfort.
• Assess for presence of extrapyramidal motor symptoms, such as tardive dyskinesia and akathisia. Extrapyramidal motor activity may complicate dental treatment.
• Geriatric patients are more susceptible to drug effects; use lower dose.
• Use vasoconstrictors with caution, in low doses, and with careful aspiration.
Consultations:
• In a patient with symptoms of blood dyscrasias, request a medical consultation for blood studies and postpone dental treatment until normal values are reestablished.
• Take precautions if dental surgery is anticipated and anesthesia is required.
• Refer to physician if signs of tardive dyskinesia or akathisia are present.
• Physician should be informed if significant xerostomic side effects occur (e.g., increased caries, sore tongue, problems eating or swallowing, difficulty wearing prosthesis) so that a medication change can be considered.
Teach Patient/Family to:
• Use effective oral hygiene to prevent soft tissue inflammation
• Use caution to prevent injury when using oral hygiene aids
• Use electric tooth brush if patient has difficulty holding conventional devices
• When chronic dry mouth occurs, advise patient to:
  • Avoid mouth rinses with high alcohol content because of drying effects

T

• Use daily home fluoride products to prevent caries
• Use sugarless gum, frequent sips of water, or saliva substitutes

thiotepa
thigh-oh-teh´-pah
(Thioplex)

CATEGORY AND SCHEDULE
Pregnancy Risk Category: D

Drug Class: Antineoplastic

MECHANISM OF ACTION
An alkylating agent that inhibits DNA and RNA protein synthesis by cross-linking with DNA and RNA strands, preventing cell growth. Cell cycle-phase nonspecific. *Therapeutic Effect:* Interferes with DNA and RNA function.

USES
Treatment of some kinds of cancer

PHARMACOKINETICS
Peak serum levels reached rapidly; elimination half-life of 2.4 hr. Excreted in urine primarily as TEPA metabolite and parent drug.

INDICATIONS AND DOSAGES
▸ **Adenocarcinoma of Breast and Ovary, Hodgkin's Disease, Lymphosarcoma, Superficial Papillary Carcinoma of Urinary Bladder**
IV
Adults, Elderly. Initially, 0.3–0.4 mg/kg every 1–4 wk. Maintenance dose adjusted weekly on the basis of blood counts.
Children. 25–65 mg/m² as a single dose every 3–4 wk.

▸ **Control of Pericardial, Peritoneal, or Pleural Effusions Due to Metastatic Tumors**
Intracavitary Injection
Adults, Elderly. 0.6–0.8 mg/kg every 1–4 wk.

SIDE EFFECTS/ADVERSE REACTIONS
Occasional
Pain at injection site, headache, dizziness, urticaria, rash, nausea, vomiting, anorexia, stomatitis
Rare
Alopecia, cystitis, hematuria (after intravesical dose)

PRECAUTIONS AND CONTRAINDICATIONS
Pregnancy, severe myelosuppression (leukocyte count less than 3000/mm³ or platelet count less than 150,000/mm³)

DRUG INTERACTIONS OF CONCERN TO DENTISTRY
• Suspected decrease in effects: probenecid
• Prolonged neuromuscular blockade: pancuronium

SERIOUS REACTIONS
! Hematologic toxicity, manifested as leukopenia, anemia, thrombocytopenia, and pancytopenia, may occur from bone marrow depression.
! Although the WBC count falls to its lowest point 10–14 days after initial therapy, the initial effects on bone marrow may not evident for 30 days.
! Stomatitis and ulceration of intestinal mucosa may occur.

DENTAL CONSIDERATIONS
General:
• If additional analgesia is required for dental pain, consider alternative

analgesics (NSAIDs) in patients taking narcotics for acute or chronic pain.
• Examine for oral manifestation of opportunistic infection.
• Avoid products that affect platelet function, such as aspirin and NSAIDs.
• This drug may be used in the hospital or on an outpatient basis. Confirm the patient's disease and treatment status.
• Patient on chronic drug therapy may rarely present with symptoms of blood dyscrasias, which can include infection, bleeding, and poor healing. If dyscrasia is present, caution patient to prevent oral tissue trauma when using oral hygiene aids.
• Palliative medication may be required for management of oral side effects.
• Patient may need assistance in getting into and out of dental chair. Adjust chair position for patient comfort.
• Consider semisupine chair position for patient comfort if GI side effects occur.
• Caution: patients may be at high risk for infection.
• Patients may be at risk for bleeding; check oral signs.
• Oral infections should be eliminated and/or treated aggressively.
Consultations:
• Medical consultation should include routine blood counts including platelet counts and bleeding time.
• In a patient with symptoms of blood dyscrasias, request a medical consultation for blood studies and postpone treatment until normal values are reestablished.
• Consult physician; prophylactic or therapeutic antiinfectives may be indicated if surgery or periodontal treatment is required.

• Medical consultation may be required to assess immunologic status during cancer chemotherapy and determine safety risk, if any, posed by the required dental treatment.
• Medical consultation may be required to assess disease control and patient's ability to tolerate stress.
Teach Patient/Family to:
• Use effective oral hygiene to prevent soft tissue inflammation
• Report oral lesions, soreness, or bleeding to dentist
• Prevent trauma when using oral hygiene aids
• Update health and medication history if physician makes any changes in evaluation or drug regimens; include OTC, herbal, and nonherbal remedies in the update

thiothixene
thye-oh-thix´-een
(Navane)
Do not confuse thiothixene with thioridazine.

CATEGORY AND SCHEDULE
Pregnancy Risk Category: C

Drug Class:
Thioxanthene/antipsychotic

MECHANISM OF ACTION
An antipsychotic that blocks postsynaptic dopamine receptor sites in brain. Has α-adrenergic blocking effects, and depresses the release of hypothalamic and hypophyseal hormones. *Therapeutic Effect:* Suppresses psychotic behavior.

USES
Treatment of psychotic disorders, schizophrenia, acute agitation

PHARMACOKINETICS

Well absorbed from the GI tract after IM administration. Widely distributed. Metabolized in the liver. Primarily excreted in urine. Unknown if removed by hemodialysis. *Half-life:* 34 hr.

INDICATIONS AND DOSAGES
▶ **Psychosis**

PO

Adults, Elderly, Children older than 12 yr. Initially, 2 mg 3 times a day. Maximum: 60 mg/day.

IM

Adults, Elderly, Children older than 12 yr. Initially, 4 mg 2–4 times a day. Maximum: 30 mg/day.

SIDE EFFECTS/ADVERSE REACTIONS

Expected

Hypotension, dizziness, syncope (occur frequently after first injection, occasionally after subsequent injections, and rarely with oral form)

Frequent

Transient drowsiness, dry mouth, constipation, blurred vision, nasal congestion

Occasional

Diarrhea, peripheral edema, urine retention, nausea

Rare

Ocular changes, altered skin pigmentation (in those taking high doses for prolonged periods), photosensitivity

PRECAUTIONS AND CONTRAINDICATIONS

Blood dyscrasias, circulatory collapse, CNS depression, coma, history of seizures

Caution

Lactation, seizure disorders, hypertension, hepatic disease

DRUG INTERACTIONS OF CONCERN TO DENTISTRY

• Increased sedation: other CNS depressants, alcohol, barbiturate anesthetics, opioid analgesics
• Hypotension, tachycardia: epinephrine (systemic)
• Increased extrapyramidal effects: phenothiazines and related drugs (haloperidol, droperidol), metoclopramide
• Additive photosensitization: tetracyclines
• Increased anticholinergic effects: anticholinergics

SERIOUS REACTIONS

! The most common extrapyramidal reaction is akathisia, characterized by motor restlessness and anxiety. Akinesia, marked by rigidity, tremor, increased salivation, mask-like facial expression, and reduced voluntary movements, occurs less frequently. Dystonias, including torticollis, opisthotonos, and oculogyric crisis, occur rarely.

! Tardive dyskinesia, characterized by tongue protrusion, puffing of the cheeks, and chewing or puckering of the mouth, occurs rarely but may be irreversible. Elderly female patients have a greater risk of developing this reaction.

! Grand mal seizures may occur in epileptic patients, especially those receiving the drug by IM administration.

! Neuroleptic malignant syndrome occurs rarely.

DENTAL CONSIDERATIONS

General:

• Monitor vital signs at every appointment because of cardiovascular side effects.
• Patients on chronic drug therapy may rarely have symptoms of blood

dyscrasias, which can include infection, bleeding, and poor healing.
• After supine positioning, have patient sit upright for at least 2 min before standing to avoid orthostatic hypotension.
• Assess salivary flow as a factor in caries, periodontal disease, and candidiasis.
• Assess for presence of extrapyramidal motor symptoms, such as tardive dyskinesia and akathisia. Extrapyramidal motor activity may complicate dental treatment.
• Use vasoconstrictors with caution, in low doses, and with careful aspiration.
• Avoid dental light in patient's eyes; offer dark glasses for patient comfort.
• Geriatric patients are more susceptible to drug effects; use lower dose.
Consultations:
• In a patient with symptoms of blood dyscrasias, request a medical consultation for blood studies and postpone dental treatment until normal values are reestablished.
• Take precautions if dental surgery is anticipated and anesthesia is required.
• If signs of tardive dyskinesia or akathisia are present, refer to physician.
Teach Patient/Family to:
• Use effective oral hygiene to prevent soft tissue inflammation
• Use caution to prevent injury when using oral hygiene aids
• Use electric tooth brush if patient has difficulty holding conventional devices
• When chronic dry mouth occurs, advise patient to:

• Avoid mouth rinses with high alcohol content because of drying effects
• Use daily home fluoride products to prevent caries
• Use sugarless gum, frequent sips of water, or saliva substitutes

---

thrombin, topical (thrombinar, thrombin-JMI, thrombostat, etc.)
throm´-bin

CATEGORY AND SCHEDULE
Pregnancy Risk Category: C

Drug Class: Thrombolytic

MECHANISM OF ACTION
A protein substance produced through a conversion reaction in which prothrombin of bovine origin is activated by tissue thromboplastin in the presence of calcium chloride. It directly clots fibrinogen in the blood. *Therapeutic Effect:* Controls bleeding.

USES
Dissolving blood clots that have formed in certain blood vessels

PHARMACOKINETICS
The speed with which thrombin clots blood is dependent upon the concentration of both thrombin and fibrinogen.

INDICATIONS AND DOSAGES
▶ **Hemorrhage, Mild**
Topical
Adults. Apply 100 units/ml as needed.
▶ **Hemorrhage, Severe**
Topical

Adults. Apply 1000 units/ml as needed.

SIDE EFFECTS/ADVERSE REACTIONS
Occasional
Allergic reaction

PRECAUTIONS AND CONTRAINDICATIONS
Sensitivity to thrombin, any of its components and/or to material of bovine origin

DRUG INTERACTIONS OF CONCERN TO DENTISTRY
None reported

SERIOUS REACTIONS
! Because of its action in the clotting mechanism, thrombin must not be injected or otherwise allowed to enter large blood vessels. Extensive intravascular clotting and even death may result.

DENTAL CONSIDERATIONS
General:
• Solutions (approximately 100 U/ml) are prepared with sterile normal saline or sterile distilled water.
• Can be used with absorbable gelatin sponge but not microfibrillar collagen.
Teach Patient/Family to:
• Report oral lesions, soreness, or bleeding to dentist

thyroid
thye´-roid
(Armour Thyroid, Nature-Throid NT, Westhroid)

CATEGORY AND SCHEDULE
Pregnancy Risk Category: A

Drug Class: Thyroid hormone

MECHANISM OF ACTION
A natural hormone derived from animal sources, usually beef or pork, that is involved in normal metabolism, growth, and development, especially the CNS of infants. Possesses catabolic and anabolic effects. Provides both levothyroxine and liothyronine hormones. *Therapeutic Effect:* Increases basal metabolic rate, enhances gluconeogenesis, stimulates protein synthesis.

USES
Treatment of hypothyroidism, cretinism, myxedema

PHARMACOKINETICS
Partially absorbed from the GI tract. Protein binding: 99%. Widely distributed. Metabolized in liver to active liothyronine (T3), and inactive reverse triiodothyronine (rT3), metabolites. Eliminated by biliary excretion. *Half-life:* 2–7 days.

INDICATIONS AND DOSAGES
▶ **Hypothyroidism**
PO
Adults, Elderly. Initially, 15–30 mg. May increase by 15 mg increments q2–4wk. Maintenance: 60–120 mcg/day. Use 15 mg in patients with cardiovascular disease or myxedema.
Children 12 yr and older. 90 mg/day.
Children 6–12 yr. 60–90 mg/day.
Children older than 1yr–5 yr. 45–60 mg/day.
Children older than 6–12 mo. 30–45 mg/day.
Children 3 mo and younger. 15–30 mg/day.

SIDE EFFECTS/ADVERSE REACTIONS
Rare
Dry skin, GI intolerance, skin rash, hives, severe headache

PRECAUTIONS AND CONTRAINDICATIONS
Uncontrolled adrenal cortical insufficiency, untreated thyrotoxicosis, treatment of obesity, uncontrolled angina, uncontrolled hypertension, uncontrolled MI, and hypersensitivity to any component of the formulations
Caution
Lactation, seizure disorders, hypertension, hepatic disease

DRUG INTERACTIONS OF CONCERN TO DENTISTRY
• Increased effects of sympathomimetics when thyroid doses are not carefully monitored or with coronary artery disease

SERIOUS REACTIONS
! Excessive dosage produces signs and symptoms of hyperthyroidism including weight loss, palpitations, increased appetite, tremors, nervousness, tachycardia, hypertension, headache, insomnia, and menstrual irregularities.
! Cardiac arrhythmias occur rarely.

DENTAL CONSIDERATIONS
General:
• Increased nervousness, excitability, sweating, or tachycardia may indicate uncontrolled hyperthyroidism or a dose of medication that is too high. Uncontrolled patients should be referred for medical treatment.
Consultations:
• Medical consultation may be required to assess disease control.

---

tiagabine
tih-ah-ga´-bean
(Gabitril)

CATEGORY AND SCHEDULE
Pregnancy Risk Category: C

Drug Class: Anticonvulsant

MECHANISM OF ACTION
An anticonvulsant that enhances the activity of gamma-aminobutyric acid, the major inhibitory neurotransmitter in the CNS. **Therapeutic Effect:** Inhibits seizures.

USES
Adjunctive therapy for partial seizures

PHARMACOKINETICS
PO: Rapid absorption, peak plasma levels 0.5–1 hr; highly plasma protein bound (95%), hepatic metabolism (CYP 3A isoenzymes), some enterohepatic circulation

INDICATIONS AND DOSAGES
▶ **Adjunctive Treatment of Partial Seizures**
PO
Adults, Elderly. Initially, 4 mg once a day. May increase by 4–8 mg/day at weekly intervals. Maximum: 56 mg/day.
Children 12–18 yr. Initially, 4 mg once a day. May increase by 4 mg at wk 2 and by 4–8 mg at weekly intervals thereafter. Maximum: 32 mg/day.

SIDE EFFECTS/ADVERSE REACTIONS
Frequent
Dizziness, asthenia, somnolence, nervousness, confusion, headache, infection, tremor

T

Occasional
Nausea, diarrhea, abdominal pain,
impaired concentration

PRECAUTIONS AND CONTRAINDICATIONS
Hepatic disease, Alzheimer's disease,
dementia, organic brain disease,
stroke

DRUG INTERACTIONS OF CONCERN TO DENTISTRY
• Increased tiagabine clearance:
carbamazepine, phenobarbital
• Use CNS depressants with caution
because of possible additional
effects

SERIOUS REACTIONS
❗ Overdose is characterized by
agitation, confusion, hostility, and
weakness. Full recovery occurs
within 24 hr.

DENTAL CONSIDERATIONS
General:
• Monitor vital signs at every
appointment because of
cardiovascular and respiratory
side effects.
• Consider semisupine chair position
for patient comfort when GI side
effects occur.
• Short appointments and a stress
reduction protocol may be required
for anxious patients.
• Determine type of epilepsy, seizure
frequency, and quality of seizure
control.
• Assess salivary flow as factor in
caries, periodontal disease, and
candidiasis.
• Place on frequent recall if oral side
effects occur.
Consultations:
• Consultation with physician may
be necessary if sedation or general
anesthesia is required.

Teach Patient/Family to:
• Use caution to prevent trauma
when using oral hygiene aids
• Use electric tooth brush if patient
has difficulty holding conventional
devices
• Use effective oral hygiene to
prevent soft tissue inflammation
• Update health and drug history if
physician makes any changes in
evaluation or drug regimens; include
OTC, herbal, and nonherbal drugs in
the update
• Be aware of oral side effects and
potential sequelae
• When chronic dry mouth occurs,
advise patient to:
  • Avoid mouth rinses with high
  alcohol content because of drying
  effects
  • Use daily home fluoride products
  for anticaries effect
  • Use sugarless gum, frequent sips
  of water, or saliva substitutes

ticarcillin
tye-kar-sill′-in
(Ticar)

CATEGORY AND SCHEDULE
Pregnancy Risk Category: B

Drug Class: Antibiotic,
penicillin

MECHANISM OF ACTION
Binds to bacterial cell wall,
inhibiting bacterial cell wall
synthesis. ***Therapeutic Effect:***
Causes cell lysis, death. Bactericidal.

USES
Treatment of infections caused by
bacteria

PHARMACOKINETICS
Well absorbed. Widely distributed.
Protein binding: 45%–60%.
Minimal metabolism in liver.
Primarily excreted unchanged
in urine. Moderately dialyzable.
Half-life: 1.2 hr (half-life is
increased in those with impaired
renal function).

INDICATIONS AND DOSAGES
▶ **Septicemia; Skin and Skin-
Structure, Bone, Joint, and Lower
Respiratory Tract Infections;
and Endometriosis**
IV
Adults, Elderly, Children over 40 kg.
200–300 mg/kg/day q4–6h or 3 g
q4h or 4 g q6h. Maximum: 18 g/day.
Children and infants under 40 kg.
200–300 mg/kg/day q4–6h.
Maximum: 18 g/day.
Neonates over 2000 g. 75 mg/kg IV
q8h under 7 days old; 100 mg/kg IV
q8h over 7 old.
Neonates under 2000 g. 75 mg/kg IV
q12h under 7 days old; 75 mg/kg q8h
over 7 days old.
▶ **UTI, Complicated**
IV
Adults, Elderly, Children over 40 kg.
150–200 mg/kg/day divided q4–6h
or 3 g q6h.
Children under 40 kg. 150–200 mg/
kg/day in divided doses q6–8h.
▶ **UTI, Uncomplicated**
IV/IM
Adults, Elderly, Children over 40 kg.
1 g q6h.
Children under 40 kg. 50–100 mg/
kg/day in divided doses q6–8h.
▶ **Dosage in Renal Impairment**

Creatinine Clearance	Dosage Interval
30–60 ml/min	2 g q4h
10–30 ml/min	2 g q8h
Less than 10 ml/min	2 g q12h

SIDE EFFECTS/ADVERSE REACTIONS
Frequent
Phlebitis, thrombophlebitis with IV
dose, rash, urticaria, pruritus, smell
or taste disturbances
Occasional
Nausea, diarrhea, vomiting
Rare
Headache, fatigue, hallucinations,
bleeding or bruising

PRECAUTIONS AND CONTRAINDICATIONS
Hypersensitivity to any penicillin

DRUG INTERACTIONS OF CONCERN TO DENTISTRY
• Possible increase in bleeding:
anticoagulants, thrombolytic drugs,
diflunisal (high doses), platelet
aggregation inhibitors
• Decreased antimicrobial
effectiveness: erythromycins,
sulfonamides, tetracyclines
• Oral contraceptives: advise patient
of a potential low risk for decreased
contraceptive action, to maintain
compliance with oral contraceptive
while using antibiotics, and to
consider the use of additional
nonhormonal contraception
• Possible increase in methotrexate
toxicity
• Increased or prolonged plasma
levels: probenecid

SERIOUS REACTIONS
! Overdosage may produce seizures
and neurologic reactions.
! Superinfections including
potentially fatal antibiotic-associated
colitis, may result from bacterial
imbalance.
! Severe hypersensitivity reactions,
including anaphylaxis, occur
rarely.

General:
• For selected infections in the hospital setting; provide emergency dental treatment only.
• Caution regarding allergy to medication.
• Examine for oral manifestation of opportunistic infection.
• Determine why patient is taking the drug.

Consultations:
• Medical consultation may be required to assess disease control.
• CONIF

Teach Patient/Family to:
• Use effective oral hygiene to prevent soft tissue inflammation
• Report oral lesions, soreness, or bleeding to dentist
• Prevent trauma when using oral hygiene aids

ticarcillin disodium/ clavulanate potassium

tie-car-sill´-in dye-soe´-dee-um/ klah-view-lan´-ate poh-tass´-ee-um
(Timentin)

CATEGORY AND SCHEDULE
Pregnancy Risk Category: B

Drug Class: Antibiotics, penicillin

MECHANISM OF ACTION
Ticarcillin binds to bacterial cell walls, inhibiting cell wall synthesis. Clavulanate inhibits the action of bacterial β-lactamase. *Therapeutic Effect:* Ticarcillin is bactericidal in susceptible organisms. Clavulanate protects ticarcillin from enzymatic degradation.

USES
Treatment of infections caused by bacteria

PHARMACOKINETICS
Widely distributed. Protein binding: ticarcillin 45%–60%, clavulanate 9%–30%. Minimally metabolized in the liver. Primarily excreted unchanged in urine. Removed by hemodialysis. *Half-life:* 1–1.2 hr (increased in impaired renal function).

INDICATIONS AND DOSAGES
▸ **Skin and Skin-Structure, Bone, Joint, and Lower Respiratory Tract Infections; Septicemia; Endometriosis**
IV
Adults, Elderly. 3.1 g (3 g ticarcillin) q4–6h. Maximum: 18–24 g/day.
Children 3 mo and older. 200–300 mg (as ticarcillin) q4–6h.
▸ **UTIs**
IV
Adults, Elderly. 3.1 g q6–8h.
▸ **Dosage in Renal Impairment**
Dosage interval is modified on the basis of creatinine clearance.

Creatinine Clearance	Dosage Interval
10–30 ml/min	Usual dose q8h
Less than 10 ml/min	Usual dose q12h

SIDE EFFECTS/ADVERSE REACTIONS
Frequent
Phlebitis or thrombophlebitis (with IV dose), rash, urticaria, pruritus, altered smell or taste
Occasional
Nausea, diarrhea, vomiting
Rare
Headache, fatigue, hallucinations, bleeding, or ecchymosis

PRECAUTIONS AND CONTRAINDICATIONS
Hypersensitivity to any penicillin

DRUG INTERACTIONS OF CONCERN TO DENTISTRY
• Possible increase in bleeding: anticoagulants, thrombolytic drugs, diflunisal (high doses), platelet aggregation inhibitors
• Decreased antimicrobial effectiveness: erythromycins, sulfonamides, tetracyclines
• Oral contraceptives: advise patient of a potential risk for decreased contraceptive action, to maintain compliance with oral contraceptive while using antibiotics, and to consider the use of additional nonhormonal contraception
• Possible increase in methotrexate toxicity
• Increased or prolonged plasma levels: probenecid

SERIOUS REACTIONS
! Overdosage may produce seizures and other neurologic reactions.
! Antibiotic-associated colitis and other superinfections may result from bacterial imbalance.
! Severe hypersensitivity reactions including anaphylaxis occur rarely.

DENTAL CONSIDERATIONS
General:
• For selected infections in the hospital setting; provide emergency dental treatment only.
• Caution regarding allergy to medication.
• Examine for oral manifestation of opportunistic infection.
• Determine why patient is taking the drug.
Consultations:
• Medical consultation may be required to assess disease control.

Teach Patient/Family to:
• Use effective oral hygiene to prevent soft tissue inflammation
• Report oral lesions, soreness, or bleeding to dentist
• Prevent trauma when using oral hygiene aids

ticlopidine hydrochloride
tye-klo´-pa-deen
high-droh-klor´-ide
(Apo-Ticlopidine[CAN], Ticlid, Tilodene[AUS])

CATEGORY AND SCHEDULE
Pregnancy Risk Category: B

Drug Class: Platelet aggregation inhibitor

MECHANISM OF ACTION
An aggregation inhibitor that inhibits the release of adenosine diphosphate from activated platelets, which prevents fibrinogen from binding to glycoprotein IIb/IIIa receptors on the surface of activated platelets. **Therapeutic Effect:** Inhibits platelet aggregation and thrombus formation.

USES
Reduction of the risk of stroke in high-risk patients

PHARMACOKINETICS
Peak 1–3 hr, half-life increases with repeated dosing; metabolized by the liver; excreted in urine, feces.

INDICATIONS AND DOSAGES
▶ **Prevention of Stroke**
PO
Adults, Elderly. 250 mg twice a day.

T

SIDE EFFECTS/ADVERSE REACTIONS

Frequent
Diarrhea, nausea, dyspepsia including heartburn, indigestion GI discomfort, and bloating
Rare
Vomiting, flatulence, pruritus, dizziness

PRECAUTIONS AND CONTRAINDICATIONS

Active pathologic bleeding, such as bleeding peptic ulcer and intracranial bleeding, hematopoietic disorders including neutropenia and thrombocytopenia; presence of hemostatic disorder; severe hepatic impairment
Caution
Past liver disease, renal disease, elderly, lactation, children; increased bleeding risk requires hematologic monitoring every 2 wk for the first 3 mo of therapy

DRUG INTERACTIONS OF CONCERN TO DENTISTRY

• Increased bleeding tendencies: aspirin, NSAIDs

SERIOUS REACTIONS

! Neutropenia occurs in approximately 2% of patients.
! Thrombotic thrombocytopenia purpura, agranulocytosis, hepatitis, cholestatic jaundice, and tinnitus occur rarely.

DENTAL CONSIDERATIONS

General:
• Patients on chronic drug therapy may rarely have symptoms of blood dyscrasias, which can include infection, bleeding, and poor healing.

• Consider local hemostatic measures to prevent excessive bleeding.
Consultations:
• Medical consultation may be required to assess disease control and patient's ability to tolerate stress. Consultation should include data on hematologic profile.
Teach Patient/Family to:
• Prevent injury when using oral hygiene aids

tiludronate
ti-loo´-dro-nate
(Skelid)

CATEGORY AND SCHEDULE
Pregnancy Risk Category: C

Drug Class: Bisphosphonate derivative

MECHANISM OF ACTION
A calcium regulator that inhibits functioning osteoclasts through disruption of cytoskeletal ring structure and inhibition of osteoclastic proton pump.
Therapeutic Effect: Inhibits bone resorption.

USES
Treatment of Paget's disease of bone in patients with twice normal upper limit values for serum alkaline phosphatase (SAP) and who are symptomatic and at risk for future complications

PHARMACOKINETICS
PO: Rapid but incomplete absorption, bioavailability 6% (fasted), peak plasma levels 2 hr, little or no metabolism, excreted in urine.

INDICATIONS AND DOSAGES
▶ **Paget's Disease**
PO
Adults, Elderly. 400 mg once a day
for 3 mo. Must take with 6–8 oz
plain water. Do not give within 2 hr
of food intake. Avoid giving aspirin,
calcium supplements, mineral
supplements, or antacids within
2 hr of tiludronate administration.

SIDE EFFECTS/ADVERSE REACTIONS
Frequent
Nausea, diarrhea, generalized body
pain, back pain, headache
Occasional
Rash, dyspepsia, vomiting, rhinitis,
sinusitis, dizziness

PRECAUTIONS AND CONTRAINDICATIONS
GI disease, such as dysphagia and
gastric ulcer, impaired renal function
Caution
Lactation, safety in children younger
than 18 yr not established

DRUG INTERACTIONS OF CONCERN TO DENTISTRY
• Bioavailability decreased by
calcium, food, aluminum or
magnesium antacids
• Do not take indomethacin, aspirin,
or calcium supplements 2 hr before
or after tiludronate

SERIOUS REACTIONS
Acute renal failure associated with
hypocalcemia

DENTAL CONSIDERATIONS
General:
• Potential for osteonecrosis of the
jaw (emphasize preventative care and
avoid invasive procedures).
• Be aware of oral manifestations
of Paget's disease (macrognathia,
alveolar pain).
• Consider semisupine chair position
for patient comfort when GI side
effects occur.

• Consider short appointments for
patient comfort.
• Assess salivary flow as a factor
in caries, periodontal disease, and
candidiasis.
Consultations:
• Medical consultation may be
required to assess disease control.
Teach Patient/Family to:
• Use caution to prevent trauma
when using oral hygiene aids
• Use effective oral hygiene to
prevent soft tissue inflammation
• Update health and drug history if
physician makes any changes in
evaluation or drug regimens; include
OTC, herbal, and nonherbal drugs in
the update
• When chronic dry mouth occurs,
advise patient to:
  • Avoid mouth rinses with high
  alcohol content because of drying
  effects
  • Use daily home fluoride products
  for anticaries effect
  • Use sugarless gum, frequent sips
  of water, or saliva substitutes

---

timolol maleate
tim´-oh-lole mal´-ee-ate
(Apo-Timol[CAN], Apo-
Timop[CAN], Betimol, Blocadren,
Gen-Timolol[CAN], Istalol,
Optimol[AUS], PMS-Timolol[CAN],
Tenopt[AUS], Timoptic, Timoptic
OccuDose, Timoptic XE,
Timoptol[AUS], Timoptol XE[AUS])
Do not confuse timolol with
atenolol, or Timoptic with Viroptic.

CATEGORY AND SCHEDULE
Pregnancy Risk Category: C (D if
used in second or third trimester)

Drug Class: Nonselective
β-adrenergic blocker

MECHANISM OF ACTION

An antihypertensive, antimigraine, and antiglaucoma agent that blocks β_1- and β_2-adrenergic receptors. *Therapeutic Effect:* Reduces intraocular pressure (IOP) by reducing aqueous humor production, lowers B/P, slows the heart rate, and decreases myocardial contractility.

USES

Treatment of mild-to-moderate hypertension, reduction of mortality risk after MI, migraine prophylaxis; unapproved uses: essential tremors, angina, cardiac dysrhythmias, anxiety

PHARMACOKINETICS

Route	Onset	Peak	Duration
PO	15–45 min	0.5–2.5 hr	4 hr
Ophthalmic	30 min	1–2 hr	12–24 hr

Well absorbed from the GI tract. Protein binding: 60%. Minimal absorption after ophthalmic administration. Metabolized in the liver. Primarily excreted in urine. Not removed by hemodialysis. *Half-life:* 4 hr. Systemic absorption may occur with ophthalmic administration.

INDICATIONS AND DOSAGES

▶ **Mild-to-Moderate Hypertension**
PO
Adults, Elderly. Initially, 10 mg twice a day, alone or in combination with other therapy. Gradually increase at intervals of not less than 1 wk. Maintenance: 20–60 mg/day in 2 divided doses.

▶ **Reduction of Cardiovascular Mortality in Definite or Suspected Acute MI**
PO

Adults, Elderly. 10 mg twice a day, beginning 1–4 wk after infarction.

▶ **Migraine Prevention**
PO
Adults, Elderly. Initially, 10 mg twice a day. Range: 10–30 mg/day.

▶ **Reduction of IOP in Open-Angle Glaucoma, Aphakic Glaucoma, Ocular Hypertension, and Secondary Glaucoma**
Ophthalmic
Adults, Elderly, Children. 1 drop of 0.25% solution in affected eye(s) twice a day. May be increased to 1 drop of 0.5% solution in affected eye(s) twice a day. When IOP is controlled, dosage may be reduced to 1 drop once a day. If patient is switched to timolol from another antiglaucoma agent, administer concurrently for 1 day. Discontinue other agent on following day.
Ophthalmic (Timoptic XE)
Adults, Elderly. 1 drop/day.
Ophthalmic (Istalol)
Adults, Elderly. Apply once a day.

SIDE EFFECTS/ADVERSE REACTIONS

Frequent
Diminished sexual function, drowsiness, difficulty sleeping, unusual tiredness or weakness
Ophthalmic: Eye irritation, visual disturbances
Occasional
Depression, cold hands or feet, diarrhea, constipation, anxiety, nasal congestion, nausea, vomiting
Rare
Altered taste, dry eyes, itching, numbness of fingers, toes, or scalp

PRECAUTIONS AND CONTRAINDICATIONS

Bronchial asthma, cardiogenic shock, CHF unless secondary to tachyarrhythmias, COPD, patients

receiving MAOI therapy, second-
or third-degree heart block, sinus
bradycardia, uncontrolled cardiac
failure
Caution
Major surgery, lactation, diabetes
mellitus, renal disease, thyroid
disease, COPD, well-compensated
heart failure, CAD, nonallergic
bronchospasm

DRUG INTERACTIONS OF CONCERN TO DENTISTRY
• Increased hypotension,
bradycardia: anticholinergics,
sympathomimetics (epinephrine)
• Decreased antihypertensive effects:
indomethacin and other NSAIDs
• Suspected increase in plasma
levels: diphenhydramine
• May slow metabolism of lidocaine
Optic
• Avoid use of anticholinergic drugs,
atropine-like drugs, propantheline,
and diazepam (benzodiazepines)

SERIOUS REACTIONS
! Overdose may produce profound
bradycardia, hypotension, and
bronchospasm.
! Abrupt withdrawal may result in
diaphoresis, palpitations, headache,
and tremors.
! Timolol administration may
precipitate CHF and MI in patients
with cardiac disease; thyroid storm
in those with thyrotoxicosis; and
peripheral ischemia in those with
existing peripheral vascular disease.
! Hypoglycemia may occur in
patients with previously controlled
diabetes.
! Ophthalmic overdose may
produce bradycardia, hypotension,
bronchospasm, and acute cardiac
failure.

DENTAL CONSIDERATIONS
General:
• Potentially reduced effectiveness of
epinephrine administer for anaphylaxis
• Monitor vital signs at every
appointment because of
cardiovascular side effects.
• Patients on chronic drug therapy
may rarely have symptoms of blood
dyscrasias, which can include
infection, bleeding, and poor healing.
• Assess salivary flow as a factor in
caries, periodontal disease, and
candidiasis.
• Limit use of sodium-containing
products, such as saline IV fluids, for
patients with a dietary salt restriction.
• After supine positioning, have
patient sit upright for at least 2 min
before standing to avoid orthostatic
hypotension.
• Stress from dental procedures may
compromise cardiovascular function;
determine patient risk.
• Short appointments and a stress-
reduction protocol may be required
for anxious patients.
• Consider semisupine chair
position for patients with nausea
or respiratory distress.
Consultations:
• In a patient with symptoms of
blood dyscrasias, request a medical
consultation for blood studies and
postpone dental treatment until
normal values are reestablished.
• Medical consultation may be
required to assess disease control
and patient's ability to tolerate stress.
Teach Patient/Family to:
• Use effective oral hygiene
to prevent soft tissue inflammation
• Use caution to prevent injury when
using oral hygiene aids
• When chronic dry mouth occurs,
advise patient to:
  • Avoid mouth rinses with high
  alcohol content because of drying
  effects

T

- Use daily home fluoride products to prevent caries
- Use sugarless gum, frequent sips of water, or saliva substitutes

Optic
General:
- Check compliance of patient with prescribed drug regimen for glaucoma.
- Avoid dental light in patient's eyes; offer dark glasses for patient comfort.

Consultations:
- Consultation with physician may be necessary if sedation or anesthesia is required.

tinzaparin sodium
tin-za´-pair-in soe´-dee-um
(Innohep)

CATEGORY AND SCHEDULE
Pregnancy Risk Category: B

Drug Class: Anticoagulants

MECHANISM OF ACTION
A low-molecular-weight heparin that inhibits factor Xa. Causes less inactivation of thrombin, inhibition of platelets, and bleeding than standard heparin. Does not significantly influence bleeding time, PT, aPTT. **Therapeutic Effect:** Produces anticoagulation.

USES
Prevention and/or treatment of deep venous thrombosis (DVT), a condition in which harmful blood clots form in the blood vessels of the legs

PHARMACOKINETICS
Well absorbed after subcutaneous administration. Primarily eliminated in urine. **Half-life:** 3–4 hr.

INDICATIONS AND DOSAGES
▸ **DVT**
Subcutaneous
Adults, Elderly. 175 anti-Xa international units/kg once a day. Continue for at least 6 days and until patient is sufficiently anticoagulated with warfarin (INR of 2 or more for 2 consecutive days).

SIDE EFFECTS/ADVERSE REACTIONS
Frequent
Injection site reaction, such as inflammation, oozing, nodules, and skin necrosis
Rare
Nausea, asthenia, constipation, epistaxis

PRECAUTIONS AND CONTRAINDICATIONS
Active major bleeding, concurrent heparin therapy, hypersensitivity to heparin or pork products, thrombocytopenia associated with positive in vitro test for antiplatelet antibody

DRUG INTERACTIONS OF CONCERN TO DENTISTRY
- Increased risk of bleeding: drugs that interfere with coagulation or platelet function, such as NSAIDs and aspirin

SERIOUS REACTIONS
! Overdose may lead to bleeding complications ranging from local ecchymoses to major hemorrhage. Antidote: Dose of protamine sulfate (1% solution) should be equal to dose of tinzaparin injected. One mg protamine sulfate neutralizes 100 units of tinzaparin. A second dose of 0.5 mg tinzaparin per 1 mg protamine sulfate may be given if aPTT tested 2–4 hr after the initial infusion remains prolonged.

DENTAL CONSIDERATIONS

General:
- Determine why patient is taking the drug.
- Consider local hemostasis measures to prevent excessive bleeding.
- Avoid products that affect platelet function, such as aspirin and NSAIDs.
- Antibiotic prophylaxis prior to dental treatment may be required for joint prosthesis (see 1997 ADA guidelines).
- Patient may need assistance in getting into and out of dental chair. Adjust chair position for patient comfort.
- Product may be used in outpatient therapy. Delay elective dental treatment until patient completes tinzaparin therapy.

Consultations:
- Medical consultation should include routine blood counts including platelet counts and bleeding time.

Teach Patient/Family to:
- Prevent trauma when using oral hygiene aids
- Report oral lesions, soreness, or bleeding to dentist
- Use effective oral hygiene to prevent soft tissue inflammation

tioconazole
tyo-con´-ah-zole
(Gynecure[CAN], Monistat-1, Trosyd[CAN], Vagistat)

CATEGORY AND SCHEDULE
Pregnancy Risk Category: C

Drug Class: Antifungals, topical, dermatologics

MECHANISM OF ACTION
An imidazole derivative that inhibits synthesis of ergosterol (vital component of fungal cell formation). *Therapeutic Effect:* Damaging fungal cell membrane. Fungistatic.

USES
Treatment of infections caused by a fungus or yeast

PHARMACOKINETICS
Negligible absorption from vaginal application.

INDICATIONS AND DOSAGES
▶ **Vulvovaginal Candidiasis**
Intravaginal
Adults, Elderly. 1 applicatorful just before bedtime as a single dose.

SIDE EFFECTS/ADVERSE REACTIONS
Frequent
Headache
Occasional
Burning, itching
Rare
Irritation, vaginal pain, dysuria, dryness of vaginal secretions, vulvar edema/swelling

PRECAUTIONS AND CONTRAINDICATIONS
Hypersensitivity to tioconazole or other imidazole antifungal agents

DRUG INTERACTIONS OF CONCERN TO DENTISTRY
None reported

SERIOUS REACTIONS
None reported

DENTAL CONSIDERATIONS
General:
- Be aware that broad-spectrum antibiotics can exacerbate vaginal candidiasis.

tiotropium bromide
tee-oh-trow´-pea-um broe´-mide
(Spiriva)

CATEGORY AND SCHEDULE
Pregnancy Risk Category: C

Drug Class: Anticholinergics,
bronchodilators

MECHANISM OF ACTION
An anticholinergic that binds to
recombinant human muscarinic
receptors at the smooth muscle,
resulting in long-acting bronchial
smooth-muscle relaxation.
Therapeutic Effect: Relieves
bronchospasm.

USES
Treatment of bronchospasm (wheezing
or difficulty in breathing) that is
associated with chronic obstructive
pulmonary disease (COPD)

PHARMACOKINETICS

Route	Onset	Peak	Duration
Inhalation	N/A	N/A	24–36 hr

Binds extensively to tissue. Protein
binding: 72%. Metabolized by
oxidation. Excreted in urine.
Half-life: 5–6 days.

INDICATIONS AND DOSAGES
▶ COPD
Inhalation
Adults, Elderly. 18 mcg (1 capsule)/
day via HandiHaler inhalation device.

SIDE EFFECTS/ADVERSE
REACTIONS
Frequent
Dry mouth, sinusitis, pharyngitis,
dyspepsia, UTI, rhinitis

Occasional
Abdominal pain, peripheral edema,
constipation, epistaxis, vomiting,
myalgia, rash, oral candidiasis

PRECAUTIONS AND
CONTRAINDICATIONS
History of hypersensitivity to atropine
or its derivatives, including ipratropium

DRUG INTERACTIONS OF
CONCERN TO DENTISTRY
• Dental drug interactions have not
been studied

SERIOUS REACTIONS
! Angina pectoris, depression, and
flu-like symptoms occur rarely.

DENTAL CONSIDERATIONS
General:
• Monitor vital signs, especially
respiration.
• Ask patient about exercise and
activity tolerance.
• Caution: Not for acute episodes
or emergency use.
• Assess salivary flow as a factor
in caries, periodontal disease, and
candidiasis.
• Place on frequent recall due to oral
side effects.
• Acute asthmatic episodes may be
precipitated in the dental office.
A rapid-acting sympathomimetic
inhalant (rescue inhaler) should
be available for emergency use.
Many patients may already have
a prescribed rescue inhaler they
normally use for acute asthmatic
events.
• Consider semisupine chair position
for patients with respiratory disease.
Consultations:
• Medical consultation may be
required to assess disease control
and patient's ability to tolerate
stress.

Teach Patient/Family to:
• Gargle, rinse mouth with water, and expectorate after each aerosol dose
• When chronic dry mouth occurs, advise patient to:
  • Avoid mouth rinses with high alcohol content due to drying effects
  • Use daily home fluoride products for anticaries effect
  • Use sugarless gum, frequent sips of water, or saliva substitutes

tirofiban
tye-roe-fye´-ban
(Aggrastat)
Do not confuse Aggrastat with Aggrenox.

CATEGORY AND SCHEDULE
Pregnancy Risk Category: B

Drug Class: Platelet inhibitors

MECHANISM OF ACTION
An antiplatelet and antithrombotic agent that binds to platelet receptor glycoprotein IIb/IIIa, preventing binding of fibrinogen. *Therapeutic Effect:* Inhibits platelet aggregation and thrombus formation.

USES
An antiplatelet in combination with heparin, treatment of acute coronary syndrome, including those to be managed medically and those undergoing percutaneous transluminal coronary angioplasty (PTCA) or atherectomy

PHARMACOKINETICS
Poorly bound to plasma proteins; unbound fraction in plasma: 35%. Limited metabolism. Primarily eliminated in the urine (65%) and, to a lesser amount, in the feces. Removed by hemodialysis. *Half-life:* 2 hr. Clearance is significantly decreased in severe renal impairment (creatinine clearance less than 30 ml/min).

INDICATIONS AND DOSAGES
▶ **Inhibition of Platelet Aggregation**
IV
Adults, Elderly. Initially, 0.4 mcg/kg/min for 30 min; then continue at 0.1 mcg/kg/min through procedure and for 12–24 hr after procedure.
▶ **Severe Renal Insufficiency (creatinine clearance less than 30 ml/min)**
Adults, Elderly. Half the usual rate of IV infusion.

SIDE EFFECTS/ADVERSE REACTIONS
Occasional
Pelvis pain, bradycardia, dizziness, leg pain
Rare
Edema and swelling, vasovagal reaction, diaphoresis, nausea, fever, headache

PRECAUTIONS AND CONTRAINDICATIONS
Active internal bleeding or a history of bleeding diathesis within previous 30 days, arteriovenous malformation or aneurysm, history of intracranial hemorrhage, history of thrombocytopenia after prior exposure to tirofiban, intracranial neoplasm, major surgical procedure within previous 30 days, severe hypertension, stroke

DRUG INTERACTIONS OF CONCERN TO DENTISTRY
• Increased risk of bleeding: drugs that interfere with coagulation or

platelet function, such as NSAIDs
and aspirin

SERIOUS REACTIONS

❗ Signs and symptoms of
overdose include generally minor
mucocutaneous bleeding and
bleeding at the femoral artery
access site.
❗ Thrombocytopenia occurs rarely.

DENTAL CONSIDERATIONS
General:
• An acute-use drug for use in
hospitals or emergency departments.
If a patient should report this drug
in his/her medical history, question
about cardiovascular disease and
drugs he or she may be taking.
• Patients are at risk for bleeding
while receiving this drug; provide
palliative dental care for dental
emergencies only.
• Avoid products that affect platelet
function, such as aspirin and
NSAIDs.
Consultations:
• Medical consultation should
include routine blood counts,
including platelet counts and
bleeding time.
• Medical consultation may be
required to assess disease control
and patient's ability to tolerate stress.
Teach Patient/Family:
• To inform dentist of unusual
bleeding episodes following dental
treatment

tobramycin
toe-bra-mye´-sin
(Nebcin, Nebcin Pediatric, Tobi)

CATEGORY AND SCHEDULE
Pregnancy Risk Category: C

Drug Class: Antiinfective

MECHANISM OF ACTION
An aminoglycoside antibiotic that
irreversibly binds to protein on
bacterial ribosomes. *Therapeutic
Effect:* Interferes in protein synthesis
of susceptible microorganisms.

USES
Treatment of serious bacterial
infections

PHARMACOKINETICS
Rapid, complete absorption after
IM administration. Protein binding:
less than 30%. Widely distributed
but does not cross the blood-brain
barrier and is in low concentrations
in CSF. Excreted unchanged in urine.
Removed by hemodialysis. *Half-life:*
2 hr. Half-life is increased with
impaired renal function and in
neonates. Half-life is decreased
in cystic fibrosis, febrile, or burn
patients.

INDICATIONS AND DOSAGES
▶ Skin/Skin-Structure, Bone, Joint,
Respiratory Tract, Postoperative,
Burn, Intraabdominal Infections;
Complicated UTI; Septicemia;
Meningitis
IM/IV
Adults, Elderly. 3mg/kg/day in
3 divided doses. May use up to
5 mg/kg/day in 3 to 4 equal doses.
▶ Cystic Fibrosis
Inhalation
*Adult, Elderly, Children 6 yr and
older.* 1 ampule (300 mg) via
nebulizer twice daily (28 days on,
28 days off). Consider starting
elderly patients at 3 mg/kg IV q8h.
▶ Dosage in Renal Impairment
Dosage and frequency are modified
on the basis of degree of renal
impairment and the serum
concentration of the drug. After
a loading dose of 1–2 mg/kg, the

maintenance dose and frequency are based on serum creatinine levels and creatinine clearance. Dosage should be reduced to 3 mg/kg/day as soon as clinically indicated. Dosage should not exceed 5 mg/kg/day.

SIDE EFFECTS/ADVERSE REACTIONS

Occasional
IM: Pain, induration at IM injection site
IV: Phlebitis, thrombophlebitis
Rare
Hypotension, nausea, vomiting

PRECAUTIONS AND CONTRAINDICATIONS

Hypersensitivity to aminoglycosides (cross-sensitivity)

DRUG INTERACTIONS OF CONCERN TO DENTISTRY

• Increased risk of nephrotoxicity: cephalosporins, enflurane, vancomycin
• Increased neuromuscular blocking effects: neuromuscular blockers

SERIOUS REACTIONS

! Nephrotoxicity, as evidenced by increased BUN and serum creatinine and decreased creatinine clearance, may be reversible if the drug is stopped at the first sign of nephrotoxic symptoms.
! Irreversible ototoxicity, manifested as tinnitus, dizziness, ringing or roaring in ears, impaired hearing and neurotoxicity, as evidenced by headache, dizziness, lethargy, tremors, and visual disturbances, occur occasionally. The risk of irreversible neurotoxicity and ototoxicity is greater with higher dosages, prolonged therapy, or if the solution is applied directly to the mucosa.
! Superinfections, particularly with fungi, may result from bacterial

imbalance with any route of administration.
! Anaphylaxis may occur.

DENTAL CONSIDERATIONS

General:
• For selected infections in the hospital setting; provide emergency dental treatment only.
• Caution regarding allergy to medication.
• Examine for oral manifestation of opportunistic infection.
• Determine why patient is taking the drug.
Consultations:
• Medical consultation may be required to assess disease control in the patient.
Teach Patient/Family to:
• Use effective oral hygiene to prevent soft tissue inflammation
• Report oral lesions, soreness, or bleeding to dentist
• Prevent trauma when using oral hygiene aids

tobramycin sulfate
tow-bra-my´-sin sull´-fate
(AK-Tob, Apo-Tobramycin[CAN], Nebcin, PMS-Tobramycin, TOBI, Tobrex)

CATEGORY AND SCHEDULE
Pregnancy Risk Category: C
(B, ophthalmic form)

Drug Class: Antiinfective

T

MECHANISM OF ACTION
An aminoglycoside antibiotic that irreversibly binds to protein on bacterial ribosomes. ***Therapeutic Effect:*** Interferes with protein synthesis of susceptible microorganisms.

USES
Treatment of serious bacterial infections

PHARMACOKINETICS
Rapid, complete absorption after IM administration. Protein binding: less than 30%. Widely distributed (doesn't cross the blood–brain barrier; low concentrations in CSF. Excreted unchanged in urine. Removed by hemodialysis. *Half-life:* 2–4 hr (increased in impaired renal function and neonates; decreased in cystic fibrosis and febrile or burn patients).

INDICATIONS AND DOSAGES
▶ **Skin and Skin-Structure, Bone, Joint, Respiratory Tract, Postoperative, Intraabdominal, and Burn Wound Infections; Complicated UTIs; Septicemia; Meningitis**
IV, IM
Adults, Elderly. 3–6 mg/kg/day in 3 divided doses or 4–6.6 mg/kg once a day.
▶ **Superficial Eye Infections Including Blepharitis, Conjunctivitis, Keratitis, and Corneal Ulcers**
Ophthalmic Ointment
Adults, Elderly. Usual dosage, apply a thin strip to conjunctiva q8–12h (q3–4h for severe infections).
Ophthalmic Solution
Adults, Elderly. Usual dosage, 1–2 drops in affected eye q4h (2 drops/hr for severe infections).
▶ **Bronchopulmonary Infections in Patients with Cystic Fibrosis**
Inhalation Solution
Adults. Usual dosage, 60–80 mg twice a day for 28 days, then off for 28 days.
Children. 40–80 mg 2–3 times a day.
▶ **Dosage in Renal Impairment**
Dosage and frequency are modified on the basis of the degree of renal impairment and the serum drug concentration. After a loading dose of 1–2 mg/kg, the maintenance dose and frequency are based on serum creatinine levels and creatinine clearance.

SIDE EFFECTS/ADVERSE REACTIONS
Occasional
IM: Pain, induration
IV: Phlebitis, thrombophlebitis
Topical: Hypersensitivity reaction (fever, pruritus, rash, urticaria)
Ophthalmic: Tearing, itching, redness, eyelid swelling
Rare
Hypotension, nausea, vomiting

PRECAUTIONS AND CONTRAINDICATIONS
Hypersensitivity to tobramycin, other aminoglycosides (cross-sensitivity), and their components

DRUG INTERACTIONS OF CONCERN TO DENTISTRY
• Antibiotics: potentially reduced effectiveness

SERIOUS REACTIONS
! Nephrotoxicity (as evidenced by increased BUN and serum creatinine levels and decreased creatinine clearance) may be reversible if the drug is stopped at the first sign of nephrotoxic symptoms.
! Irreversible ototoxicity (manifested as tinnitus, dizziness, ringing or roaring in ears, and hearing loss) and neurotoxicity (manifested as headache, dizziness, lethargy, tremor, and visual disturbances) occur occasionally. The risk of these reactions increases with higher dosages or prolonged therapy and when the solution is applied directly to the mucosa.
! Superinfections, particularly fungal infections, may result from bacterial imbalance with any administration route.
! Anaphylaxis may occur.

DENTAL CONSIDERATIONS

General:
• Avoid directing dental light into patient's eyes; provide dark glasses during treatment to avoid irritation.
• Protect patient's eyes from accidental spatter during dental treatment.

tocainide hydrochloride

toe´-kay-nide high-droh-klor´-ide
(Tonocard)

CATEGORY AND SCHEDULE

Pregnancy Risk Category: C

Drug Class: Antidysrhythmic (class IB), lidocaine analog

MECHANISM OF ACTION

An amide-type local anesthetic that shortens the action potential duration and decreases the effective refractory period and automaticity in the His-Purkinje system of the myocardium by blocking sodium transport across myocardial cell membranes.
Therapeutic Effect: Suppresses ventricular arrhythmias.

USES

Treatment of documented life-threatening ventricular dysrhythmias

PHARMACOKINETICS

PO: Peak 0.5–3 hr. **Half-life:** 10–17 hr; metabolized by liver; excreted in urine.

INDICATIONS AND DOSAGES

▶ **Suppression and Prevention of Ventricular Arrhythmias**
PO
Adults, Elderly. Initially, 400 mg q8h. Maintenance: 1.2–1.8 g/day in divided doses q8h. Maximum: 2400 mg/day.

SIDE EFFECTS/ADVERSE REACTIONS

Tocainide is generally well tolerated
Frequent
Minor, transient light-headedness, dizziness, nausea, paraesthesia, rash, tremor
Occasional
Clammy skin, night sweats, myalgia
Rare
Restlessness, nervousness, disorientation, mood changes, ataxia (muscular incoordination), visual disturbances

PRECAUTIONS AND CONTRAINDICATIONS

Hypersensitivity to local anesthetics, second- or third-degree AV block
Caution
Lactation, children, renal disease, liver disease, CHF, respiratory depression, myasthenia gravis, blood dyscrasias

DRUG INTERACTIONS OF CONCERN TO DENTISTRY

• No specific interactions are reported with dental drugs; however, any drug that could affect the cardiac action of tocainide (local anesthetics, vasoconstrictors, and anticholinergics) should be used in the least effective dose

SERIOUS REACTIONS

! High dosage may produce bradycardia or tachycardia, hypotension, palpitations, increased ventricular arrhythmias, premature ventricular contractions (PVCs), chest pain, and exacerbation of CHF.

T

DENTAL CONSIDERATIONS

General:
- Monitor vital signs at every appointment because of cardiovascular and respiratory side effects.
- After supine positioning, have patient sit upright for at least 2 min before standing to avoid orthostatic hypotension.
- Patients on chronic drug therapy may rarely have symptoms of blood dyscrasias, which can include infection, bleeding, and poor healing.
- Assess salivary flow as a factor in caries, periodontal disease, and candidiasis.
- Stress from dental procedures may compromise cardiovascular function; determine patient risk.

Consultations:
- In a patient with symptoms of blood dyscrasias, request a medical consultation for blood studies and postpone dental treatment until normal values are reestablished.
- Medical consultation may be required to assess disease control and patient's ability to tolerate stress.

Teach Patient/Family to:
- Use effective oral hygiene to prevent soft tissue inflammation
- Use caution to prevent injury when using oral hygiene aids
- When chronic dry mouth occurs, advise patient to:
  - Avoid mouth rinses with high alcohol content because of drying effects
  - Use daily home fluoride products to prevent caries
  - Use sugarless gum, frequent sips of water, or saliva substitutes

tolazamide
tole-az´-ah-mide
(Tolinase)
Do not confuse with tolubutamide, tocainide, or tolazine.

CATEGORY AND SCHEDULE
Pregnancy Risk Category: D

Drug Class: Sulfonylurea (first-generation) oral antidiabetic

MECHANISM OF ACTION
A first-generation sulfonylurea that promotes release of insulin from beta cells of pancreas. **Therapeutic Effect:** Lowers blood glucose concentration.

USES
Treatment of type 2 diabetes mellitus

PHARMACOKINETICS
Well absorbed from the GI tract. Extensively metabolized in liver to 5 metabolites, 3 of which are active. Primarily excreted in urine. Unknown if removed by hemodialysis. **Half-life:** 7 hr.

INDICATIONS AND DOSAGES
▸ **Diabetes Mellitus**
PO
Adults, Elderly. Initially, 100–250 mg once a day, with breakfast or first main meal. Maintenance: 100–1000 mg once a day. May increase by increments of 100–250 mg weekly on the basis of blood glucose response. May increase by 100–250 mg/day at weekly intervals. Maximum: 1000 mg/day. Doses more than 500 mg/day should be given in 2 divided doses with meals.

SIDE EFFECTS/ADVERSE REACTIONS

Frequent

Altered taste sensation, dizziness, drowsiness, weight gain, constipation, diarrhea, heartburn, nausea, vomiting, stomach fullness, headache

Occasional

Increased sensitivity of skin to sunlight, peeling of skin, itching, rash

PRECAUTIONS AND CONTRAINDICATIONS

Diabetic complications, such as ketosis, acidosis, and diabetic coma, sole therapy for type 1 diabetes mellitus, hypersensitivity to tolazamide or its components

Caution

Elderly, cardiac disease, thyroid disease, severe hypoglycemic reactions, renal disease, hepatic disease

DRUG INTERACTIONS OF CONCERN TO DENTISTRY

• Increased hypoglycemic reaction: NSAIDs, salicylates, ketoconazole, miconazole

• Decreased action of tolazamide: corticosteroids, sympathomimetics (epinephrine)

SERIOUS REACTIONS

! Severe hypoglycemia may occur due to overdosage and insufficient food intake, especially with increased glucose demands.

! GI hemorrhage, cholestatic hepatic jaundice, leukopenia, thrombocytopenia, pancytopenia, agranulocytosis, and aplastic or hemolytic anemia occur rarely.

DENTAL CONSIDERATIONS

General:

• Patients on chronic drug therapy may rarely have symptoms of blood dyscrasias, which can include infection, bleeding, and poor healing.

• Place on frequent recall to evaluate healing response.

• Short appointments and a stress-reduction protocol may be required for anxious patients.

• Diabetics may be more susceptible to infection and have delayed wound healing.

• Ensure that patient is following prescribed diet and regularly takes medication.

• Question patient about self-monitoring of drug's antidiabetic effect.

• Avoid prescribing aspirin-containing products.

Consultations:

• In a patient with symptoms of blood dyscrasias, request a medical consultation for blood studies and postpone dental treatment until normal values are reestablished.

• Medical consultation may be required to assess disease control.

Teach Patient/Family to:

• Use effective oral hygiene to prevent soft tissue inflammation

• Avoid mouth rinses with high alcohol content because of drying effects

tolbutamide

tole-byoo´-ta-mide

(Apo-Tolbutamide[CAN], Orinase, Orinase Diagnostic, Rastinon[AUS], Tol-Tab)

Do not confuse with tolazamide, tocainide, or tolazine.

T

CATEGORY AND SCHEDULE

Pregnancy Risk Category: C

Drug Class: Sulfonylurea (first-generation) oral antidiabetic

MECHANISM OF ACTION

A first-generation sulfonylurea that promotes the release of insulin from β cells of pancreas. *Therapeutic Effect:* Lowers blood glucose concentration.

USES

Treatment of Type 2 diabetes mellitus

PHARMACOKINETICS

Route	Onset	Peak	Duration
PO	1 hr	5–8 hr	12–24 hr
IV	N/A	30–45 min	90–180 min

Well absorbed from the GI tract. Protein binding: 80%–99%. Extensively metabolized in liver to 2 inactive metabolites, primarily via oxidation. Excreted in urine. Removed by hemodialysis. *Half-life:* 4.5–6.5 hr.

INDICATIONS AND DOSAGES
▸ **Diabetes Mellitus**
PO
Adults. Initially, 1 g daily, with breakfast or first main meal, or in divided doses. Maintenance: 0.25–3 g once a day. After dose of 2 g is reached, dosage should be increased in increments of up to 2 mg q1–2wk, based on blood glucose response. Maximum: 3 g/day.
▸ **Endocrine Tumor Diagnosis**
IV
Adults. 1 g infused over 2–3 min.

SIDE EFFECTS/ADVERSE REACTIONS
Frequent
Increased sensitivity of skin to sunlight, peeling of skin, itching, rash, dizziness, drowsiness, weight gain, constipation, diarrhea, heartburn, nausea, headache, pain at injection site, oral lichenoid reaction
Occasional
Altered taste sensation, constipation, vomiting, stomach fullness

PRECAUTIONS AND CONTRAINDICATIONS

Diabetic ketoacidosis with or without coma, sole therapy for Type 1 diabetes mellitus, use in children, hypersensitivity to tolbutamide or any component of its formulation
Caution
Elderly, cardiac disease, thyroid disease, severe hypoglycemic reactions, renal disease, hepatic disease

DRUG INTERACTIONS OF CONCERN TO DENTISTRY
• Increased hypoglycemic reactions: NSAIDs, salicylates, ketoconazole, miconazole
• Decreased effects: corticosteroids, sympathomimetics

SERIOUS REACTIONS
! Severe hypoglycemia may occur because of overdosage or insufficient food intake, especially with increased glucose demands.
! Cardiovascular mortality has been reported higher in patients treated with tolbutamide.
! GI hemorrhage, cholestatic hepatic jaundice, leukopenia, thrombocytopenia, pancytopenia, agranulocytosis and aplastic or hemolytic anemia occur rarely.

DENTAL CONSIDERATIONS
General:
• Patients on chronic drug therapy may rarely have symptoms of blood dyscrasias, which can include infection, bleeding, and poor healing.

T

- Ensure that patient is following prescribed diet and regularly takes medication.
- Question patient about self-monitoring of drug's antidiabetic effect including blood glucose values or finger-stick records.
- Place on frequent recall to evaluate healing response.
- Short appointments and a stress reduction protocol may be required for anxious patients.
- Diabetics may be more susceptible to infection and have delayed wound healing.
- Avoid prescribing aspirin-containing products.

Consultations:
- In a patient with symptoms of blood dyscrasias, request a medical consultation for blood studies and postpone dental treatment until normal values are reestablished.
- Medical consultation may be required to assess disease control.
- Medical consultation may include data from patient's blood glucose monitoring including glycosylated hemoglobin or HbA$_{1c}$ testing.

Teach Patient/Family to:
- Use effective oral hygiene to prevent soft tissue inflammation
- Avoid mouth rinses with high alcohol content because of drying effects

tolcapone
toll´-ka-pone
(Tasmar)

CATEGORY AND SCHEDULE
Pregnancy Risk Category: C

Drug Class: Antiparkinsonian

MECHANISM OF ACTION
An antiparkinson agent that inhibits the enzyme catechol-O-methyltransferase (COMT), potentiating dopamine activity and increasing the duration of action of levodopa. *Therapeutic Effect:* Relieves signs and symptoms of Parkinson's disease.

USES
An adjunct to levodopa and carbidopa in the treatment of Parkinson's disease

PHARMACOKINETICS
Rapidly absorbed after PO administration. Protein binding: 99%. Metabolized in the liver. Eliminated primarily in urine (60%) and, to a lesser extent, in feces (40%). Unknown if removed by hemodialysis. *Half-life:* 2–3 hr.

INDICATIONS AND DOSAGES
▶ **Adjunctive Treatment of Parkinson's Disease**
PO
Adults, Elderly. Initially, 100–200 mg 3 times a day concomitantly with each dose of carbidopa and levodopa. Maximum: 600 mg/day.
▶ **Dosage in Hepatic Impairment**
Patients with moderate to severe cirrhosis should not receive more than 200 mg tolcapone 3 times a day.

SIDE EFFECTS/ADVERSE REACTIONS
Alert
Frequency of side effects increases with dosage. The following effects are based on a 200-mg dose
Frequent
Nausea, insomnia, somnolence, anorexia, diarrhea, muscle cramps, orthostatic hypotension, excessive dreaming, dry mouth
Occasional
Headache, vomiting, confusion, hallucinations, constipation, diaphoresis, bright yellow urine,

dry eyes, abdominal pain, dizziness, flatulence
Rare
Dyspepsia, neck pain, hypotension, fatigue, chest discomfort

PRECAUTIONS AND CONTRAINDICATIONS
Hypersensitivity, patients with SGPT/ALT and SGOT/AST exceeding upper limit of normal or other signs of hepatic impairment; informed consent required; history of nontraumatic rhabdomyolysis, hyperpyrexia, and confusion related to medication
Caution
Discontinue drug with signs of hepatocellular injury, MAOIs, hypotension, dyskinesia, lactation

DRUG INTERACTIONS OF CONCERN TO DENTISTRY
• Increased sedation: alcohol and all CNS depressants
• No other data for dental drugs reported

SERIOUS REACTIONS
! Upper respiratory tract infection and UTI occur in 7%–5% of patients.
! Too-rapid withdrawal from therapy may produce withdrawal-emergent hyperpyrexia, characterized by fever, muscular rigidity, and altered LOC.
! Dyskinesia and dystonia occur frequently.

DENTAL CONSIDERATIONS
General:
• Notify physician immediately if symptoms of liver failure are observed (bleeding, jaundice, etc.).
• Assess salivary flow as a factor in caries, periodontal disease, and candidiasis.
• After supine positioning, have patient sit upright for at least 2 min

before standing to avoid orthostatic hypotension.
• Consider semisupine chair position for patient comfort because of GI side effects of drug.
Consultations:
• Medical consultation may be required to assess disease control.
• Take precaution if dental surgery is anticipated and general anesthesia is required.
Teach Patient/Family to:
• Use electric tooth brush if patient has difficulty holding conventional devices
• When chronic dry mouth occurs, advise patient to:
   • Avoid mouth rinses with high alcohol content because of drying effects
   • Use daily home fluoride products for anticaries effect
   • Use sugarless gum, frequent sips of water, or saliva substitutes

tolmetin
tole´-met-in
(Novo-Tolmetin[CAN], Tolectin, Tolectin DS)

CATEGORY AND SCHEDULE
Pregnancy Risk Category: C (D if used in third trimester or near delivery)

Drug Class: Nonsteroidal antiinflammatory

MECHANISM OF ACTION
A nonsteroidal antiinflammatory that produces analgesic and antiinflammatory effects by inhibiting prostaglandin synthesis.
Therapeutic Effect: Reduces inflammatory response and intensity of pain stimulus reaching sensory nerve endings.

USES
Treatment of osteoarthritis, rheumatoid arthritis, juvenile rheumatoid arthritis

PHARMACOKINETICS
Rapidly absorbed from the GI tract. Metabolized in liver. Excreted in urine. Minimally removed by hemodialysis. *Half-life:* 5 hr.

INDICATIONS AND DOSAGES
▸ **Rheumatoid Arthritis, Osteoarthritis**
PO
Adults, Elderly. Initially, 400 mg 3 times a day (including 1 dose upon arising, 1 dose at bedtime). Adjust dose at 1- to 2-wk intervals. Maintenance: 600–1800 mg/day in 3–4 divided doses.
▸ **Juvenile Rheumatoid Arthritis**
PO
Children more than 2 yr. Initially, 20 mg/kg/day in 3–4 divided doses. Maintenance: 15–30 mg/kg/day in 3–4 divided doses.

SIDE EFFECTS/ADVERSE REACTIONS
Occasional
Nausea, vomiting, diarrhea, abdominal cramping, dyspepsia (heartburn, indigestion, epigastric pain), flatulence, dizziness, headache, weight decrease or increase
Rare
Constipation, anorexia, rash, pruritus

PRECAUTIONS AND CONTRAINDICATIONS
Severely incapacitated, bedridden, wheelchair bound, hypersensitivity to aspirin or other NSAIDs
Caution
Lactation, children, bleeding disorders, GI disorders, cardiac disorders, hypersensitivity to aspirin, NSAIDs, peptic ulcer disease, geriatric patients

DRUG INTERACTIONS OF CONCERN TO DENTISTRY
• Increased risk of GI side effects: ASA, NSAIDs, ethanol (alcohol)
• Nephrotoxicity: acetaminophen (prolonged use and high doses)
• Possible risk of decreased renal function: cyclosporine
• Decreased antihypertensive effect of diuretics, α-adrenergic blockers, and ACE inhibitors
• First-time users of SSRIs also taking NSAIDs may have a higher risk of GI side effects; until more data are available, it may be advisable to avoid use of NSAIDs in these patients (Br J Clin Pharmacol 55:591–595, 2003)

SERIOUS REACTIONS
! Peptic ulcer, GI bleeding, gastritis, and severe hepatic reaction (cholestasis, jaundice) occur rarely.
! Nephrotoxicity (dysuria, hematuria, proteinuria, nephrotic syndrome) and severe hypersensitivity reaction (fever, chills, bronchospasm) occur rarely.

DENTAL CONSIDERATIONS
General:
• Patients on chronic drug therapy may rarely have symptoms of blood dyscrasias, which can include infection, bleeding, and poor healing.
• Monitor vital signs at every appointment because of cardiovascular side effects.
• Assess salivary flow as a factor in caries, periodontal disease, and candidiasis.
• Avoid prescribing for dental use in last trimester of pregnancy.
• Possibility of cross-allergenicity when patient is allergic to aspirin.
Consultations:
• Medical consultation may be required to assess disease control.

• In a patient with symptoms of blood dyscrasias, request a medical consultation for blood studies and postpone dental treatment until normal values are reestablished.

Teach Patient/Family to:
• Use effective oral hygiene to prevent soft tissue inflammation
• Use caution to prevent injury when using oral hygiene aids
• When chronic dry mouth occurs, advise patient to:
  • Avoid mouth rinses with high alcohol content because of drying effects
  • Use daily home fluoride products to prevent caries
  • Use sugarless gum, frequent sips of water, or saliva substitutes

tolterodine tartrate
tol-tare´-oh-deen tar´-trate
(Detrol, Detrol LA)

CATEGORY AND SCHEDULE
Pregnancy Risk Category: C

Drug Class: Antispasmodic

MECHANISM OF ACTION
An antispasmodic that exhibits potent antimuscarinic activity by interceding via cholinergic muscarinic receptors, thereby inhibiting urinary bladder contraction. *Therapeutic Effect:* Decreases urinary frequency, urgency.

USES
Treatment of overactive bladder with symptoms of urinary frequency or incontinence

PHARMACOKINETICS
Rapidly and well absorbed after PO administration. Protein binding: 96%. Extensively metabolized in the liver to active metabolite. Primarily excreted in urine. Unknown if removed by hemodialysis.
Half-life: 1.9–3.7 hr.

INDICATIONS AND DOSAGES
▶ **Overactive Bladder**
PO
Adults, Elderly. 1–2 mg twice a day.
▶ **Dosage in Severe Renal or Hepatic Impairment**
PO
Adults, Elderly. 1 mg twice a day.
PO (Extended-Release)
Adults, Elderly. 2–4 mg once a day.

SIDE EFFECTS/ADVERSE REACTIONS
Frequent
Dry mouth
Occasional
Headache, dizziness, fatigue, constipation, dyspepsia (heartburn, indigestion, epigastric discomfort), upper respiratory tract infection, UTI, dry eyes, abnormal vision (accommodation problems), nausea, diarrhea
Rare
Somnolence, chest or back pain, arthralgia, rash, weight gain, dry skin

PRECAUTIONS AND CONTRAINDICATIONS
Uncontrolled angle-closure glaucoma, urine retention
Caution
Bladder obstruction, pyloric stenosis, GI obstructive disorders, treated narrow-angle glaucoma, significant hepatic dysfunction, renal impairment, lactation, pediatric use

DRUG INTERACTIONS OF CONCERN TO DENTISTRY
• Studies not available; however, drugs that inhibit cytochrome P-450

3A4 enzymes, such as erythromycin, clarithromycin, ketoconazole, itraconazole, and fluoxetine, require a dose reduction to 1 mg twice daily
• Increased anticholinergic effects: possibly with other anticholinergic drugs

SERIOUS REACTIONS
! Overdose can result in severe anticholinergic effects including abdominal cramps, facial warmth, excessive salivation or lacrimation, diaphoresis, pallor, urinary urgency, blurred vision, and prolonged QT interval.

DENTAL CONSIDERATIONS
General:
• Assess salivary flow as a factor in caries, periodontal disease, and candidiasis.
• Consider semisupine chair position for patient comfort because of GI side effects of drug.
• Avoid dental light in patient's eyes; offer dark glasses for patient comfort.
• Avoid drugs with anticholinergic activity, such as antihistamines, opioids, benzodiazepines, propantheline, atropine, and scopolamine.
Consultations:
• Physician should be informed if significant xerostomic side effects occur (e.g., increased caries, sore tongue, problems eating or swallowing, difficulty wearing prosthesis) so that a medication change can be considered.
Teach Patient/Family to:
• Use effective oral hygiene to prevent soft tissue inflammation
• When chronic dry mouth occurs, advise patient to:
  • Avoid mouth rinses with high alcohol content because of drying effects

• Use daily home fluoride products for anticaries effect
• Use sugarless gum, frequent sips of water, or saliva substitutes

topiramate
toe-peer´-ah-mate
(Topamax)
Do not confuse topiramate or Topamax with Toprol XL.

CATEGORY AND SCHEDULE
Pregnancy Risk Category: C

Drug Class: Anticonvulsant

MECHANISM OF ACTION
An anticonvulsant that blocks repetitive, sustained firing of neurons by enhancing the ability of gamma-aminobutyric acid to induce an influx of chloride ions into the neurons; may also block sodium channels. *Therapeutic Effect:* Decreases seizure activity.

USES
Adjunctive therapy for adult patients with partial-onset seizures or for primary generalized tonic-clonic seizures; Lennox-Gastaut syndrome

PHARMACOKINETICS
Rapidly absorbed after PO administration. Protein binding: 13%–17%. Not extensively metabolized. Primarily excreted unchanged in urine. Removed by hemodialysis. *Half-life:* 21 hr.

INDICATIONS AND DOSAGES
▶ **Adjunctive Treatment of Partial Seizures, Lennox-Gastant Syndrome**
PO
Adults, Elderly, Children older than 17 yr. Initially, 25–50 mg for 1 wk.

May increase by 25–50 mg/day at weekly intervals. Maximum: 1,600 mg/day.

Children 2–16 yr. Initially, 1–3 mg/kg/day to maximum of 25 mg. May increase by 1–3 mg/kg/day at weekly intervals. Maintenance: 5–9 mg/kg/day in 2 divided doses.

▸ **Tonic-Clonic Seizures**
PO
Adults, Elderly, Children. Dosage is individualized and titrated.

▸ **Migraine Prevention**
PO
Adults, Elderly. 100 mg/day in 2 divided doses.

▸ **Dosage in Renal Impairment**
Expect to reduce drug dosage by 50% in patients with tonic-clonic seizures who have a creatinine clearance of less than 70 ml/min.

SIDE EFFECTS/ADVERSE REACTIONS

Frequent
Somnolence, dizziness, ataxia, nervousness, nystagmus, diplopia, paresthesia, nausea, tremor
Occasional
Confusion, breast pain, dysmenorrhea, dyspepsia, depression, asthenia, pharyngitis, weight loss, anorexia, rash, musculoskeletal pain, abdominal pain, difficulty with coordination, sinusitis, agitation, flu-like symptoms
Rare
Mood disturbances, such as irritability and depression; dry mouth; aggressive behavior

PRECAUTIONS AND CONTRAINDICATIONS

Renal impairment, hepatic impairment, rapid drug withdrawal, kidney stones, lactation, children
Caution
Renal impairment, hepatic impairment, rapid drug withdrawal, kidney stones, lactation, children

DRUG INTERACTIONS OF CONCERN TO DENTISTRY

• Increased CNS depression: opioids, sedatives, ethanol, and other CNS depressants
• Decreased serum levels: carbamazepine

SERIOUS REACTIONS

! Psychomotor slowing, impaired concentration, language problems (such as word-finding difficulties), and memory disturbances occur occasionally. These reactions are generally mild to moderate but may be severe enough to require discontinuation of drug therapy.

DENTAL CONSIDERATIONS

General:
• Patients on chronic drug therapy may rarely have symptoms of blood dyscrasias, which can include infection, bleeding, and poor healing.
• Short appointments and a stress reduction protocol may be required for anxious patients.
• Assess salivary flow as factor in caries, periodontal disease, and candidiasis.
• Avoid dental light in patient's eyes; offer dark glasses for patient comfort.
• Determine type of epilepsy, seizure frequency, and quality of seizure control. A stress reduction protocol may be required.
Consultations:
• In a patient with symptoms of blood dyscrasias, request a medical consultation for blood studies and postpone dental treatment until normal values are reestablished.
• Medical consultation may be required to assess disease control.

Teach Patient/Family to:
• Use effective oral hygiene to prevent soft tissue inflammation
• Use caution to prevent trauma when using oral hygiene aids
• Use electric tooth brush if patient has difficulty holding conventional devices
• Update health and drug history if physician makes any changes in evaluation or drug regimens; include OTC, herbal, and nonherbal drugs in the update
• When chronic dry mouth occurs, advise patient to:
  • Avoid mouth rinses with high alcohol content because of drying effects
  • Use daily home fluoride products for anticaries effect
  • Use sugarless gum, frequent sips of water, or saliva substitutes

topotecan
toe-poh´-teh-can
(Hycamtin)

CATEGORY AND SCHEDULE
Pregnancy Risk Category: D

Drug Class: Antineoplastic

MECHANISM OF ACTION
A DNA topoisomerase inhibitor that interacts with topoisomerase I, an enzyme that allows DNA replication by producing reversible single-strand breaks in DNA that relieve torsional strain. Topotecan prevents religation of the DNA strand, resulting in damage to double-strand DNA and cell death. **Therapeutic Effect:** Kills cancer cells.

USES
Treatment of breast cancer that has spread to other parts of the body

PHARMACOKINETICS
Hydrolyzed to active form after IV administration. Protein binding: 35%. Excreted in urine. **Half-life:** 2–3 hr (increased in impaired renal function).

INDICATIONS AND DOSAGES
▶ **Ovarian Carcinoma, Small-Cell Lung Cancer**
IV
Adults, Elderly. 1.5 mg/m^2/day over 30 min for 5 consecutive days, beginning on day 1 of a 21-day course. Minimum of 4 courses recommended. If severe neutropenia (neutrophil count less than 1500/mm^2) occurs during treatment, reduce dose for subsequent courses by 0.25 mg/m^2 or administer filgrastim (G-CSF) no sooner than 24 hr after the last dose of topotecan.
▶ **Dosage in Renal Impairment**
No dosage adjustment is necessary in patients with mild renal impairment (creatinine clearance of 40–60 ml/min). For moderate renal impairment (creatinine clearance of 20–39 ml/min), give 0.75 mg/m^2.

SIDE EFFECTS/ADVERSE REACTIONS
Frequent
Nausea, vomiting, diarrhea, total alopecia, headache, dyspnea
Occasional
Paraesthesia, constipation, abdominal pain
Rare
Anorexia, malaise, arthralgia, asthenia, myalgia

PRECAUTIONS AND CONTRAINDICATIONS
Baseline neutrophil count less than 1500 cells/mm^3, breast-feeding, pregnancy, severe myelosuppression

DRUG INTERACTIONS OF CONCERN TO DENTISTRY
None reported

SERIOUS REACTIONS
! Severe neutropenia (neutrophil count less than 500 cells/mm^3) occurs in 60% of patients, usually during the first course of therapy. The neutrophil nadir usually occurs at a median of 11 days after starting therapy.

! Thrombocytopenia (platelet countless than 25,000/mm^3) occurs in 26% of patients, and severe anemia (RBC count less than 8 g/dl) occurs in 40% of patients. The platelet and RBC nadirs usually occur at a median of 15 days after starting the first course of therapy.

DENTAL CONSIDERATIONS

General:
• If additional analgesia is required for dental pain, consider alternative analgesics (NSAIDs) in patients taking narcotics for acute or chronic pain.
• Examine for oral manifestations of opportunistic infection.
• This drug may be used in the hospital or on an outpatient basis. Confirm the patient's disease and treatment status.
• Chlorhexidine mouth rinse prior to and during chemotherapy may reduce severity of mucositis.
• Patient on chronic drug therapy may rarely present with symptoms of blood dyscrasias, which can include infection, bleeding, and poor healing. If dyscrasia is present, caution patient to prevent oral tissue trauma when using oral hygiene aids.
• Palliative medication may be required for management of oral side effects.
• Short appointments and a stress-reduction protocol may be required for anxious patients.

• Consider semisupine chair position for patient comfort if GI side effects occur.
• Caution: patients may be at high risk for infection.
• Patients may have received other chemotherapy or radiation; confirm medical and drug history.
• Oral infections should be eliminated and/or treated aggressively.

Consultations:
• Medical consultation should include routine blood counts including platelet counts and bleeding time.
• Consult physician; prophylactic or therapeutic antiinfectives may be indicated if surgery or periodontal treatment is required.
• Medical consultation may be required to assess immunologic status during cancer chemotherapy and determine safety risk, if any, posed by the required dental treatment.
• Medical consultation may be required to assess disease control and patient's ability to tolerate stress.
• In a patient with symptoms of blood dyscrasias, request a medical consultation for blood studies and postpone treatment until normal values are reestablished.

Teach Patient/Family to:
• See dentist immediately if secondary oral infection occurs.
• Be aware of oral side effects.
• Use effective oral hygiene to prevent soft tissue inflammation.
• Report oral lesions, soreness, or bleeding to dentist.
• Prevent trauma when using oral hygiene aids.
• Update health and medication history if physician makes any changes in evaluation or drug

regimens; include OTC, herbal, and nonherbal remedies in the update.
• Use soft tooth brush to reduce risk of bleeding.

toremifene citrate
toe-ref´-ah-meen sih´-trate
(Fareston)

CATEGORY AND SCHEDULE
Pregnancy Risk Category: D

Drug Class: Antineoplastic, antiestrogen agent

MECHANISM OF ACTION
A nonsteroidal antiestrogen and antineoplastic agent that binds to estrogen receptors on tumors, producing a complex that decreases DNA synthesis and inhibits estrogen effects. *Therapeutic Effect:* Blocks growth-stimulating effects of estrogen in breast cancer.

USES
Treatment of metastatic breast cancer in postmenopausal women with estrogen receptor–positive or unknown tumors

PHARMACOKINETICS
Well absorbed after PO administration. Metabolized in the liver. Eliminated in feces. *Half-life:* Approximately 5 days.

INDICATIONS AND DOSAGES
▶ **Breast Cancer**
PO
Adults. 60 mg/day until disease progression is observed.

SIDE EFFECTS/ADVERSE REACTIONS
Frequent
Hot flashes, diaphoresis, nausea, vaginal discharge, dizziness, dry eyes
Occasional
Edema, vomiting, vaginal bleeding
Rare
Fatigue, depression, lethargy, anorexia

PRECAUTIONS AND CONTRAINDICATIONS
History of thromboembolic disease
Caution
Thromboembolic diseases, endometrial hyperplasia, hypercalcemia with bone metastases, monitor leukocyte and platelet counts, tumor flare

DRUG INTERACTIONS OF CONCERN TO DENTISTRY
None reported

SERIOUS REACTIONS
! Ocular toxicity (cataracts, glaucoma, decreased visual acuity) and hypercalcemia may occur.

DENTAL CONSIDERATIONS
General:
• Patients on chronic drug therapy may rarely have symptoms of blood dyscrasias, which can include infection, bleeding, and poor healing.
• Consider semisupine chair position for patient comfort because of GI side effects of drug.
Consultations:
• Medical consultation may be required to assess disease control.
Teach Patient/Family to:
• Use effective oral hygiene to prevent soft tissue inflammation

T

torsemide
tor´-se-mide
(Demadex)
Do not confuse torsemide with
furosemide.

CATEGORY AND SCHEDULE
Pregnancy Risk Category: B

Drug Class: Loop diuretic

MECHANISM OF ACTION
A loop diuretic that enhances
excretion of sodium, chloride,
potassium, and water at the
ascending limb of the loop of Henle;
also reduces plasma and extracellular
fluid volume. *Therapeutic Effect:*
Produces diuresis; lowers B/P.

USES
Treatment of hypertension and
edema associated with CHF, liver
disease, chronic renal failure

PHARMACOKINETICS

Route	Onset	Peak	Duration
PO	1 hr	1–2 hr	6–8 hr
IV	10 min	1 hr	6–8 hr

Rapidly and well absorbed from
the GI tract. Protein binding:
97%–99%. Metabolized in the liver.
Primarily excreted in urine.
Not removed by hemodialysis.
Half-life: 3.3 hr.

INDICATIONS AND DOSAGES
▶ **Hypertension**
PO
Adults, Elderly. Initially, 5 mg/day.
May increase to 10 mg/day if no
response in 4–6 wk. If no response,
additional antihypertensive
added.

▶ **CHF**
PO, IV
Adults, Elderly. Initially, 10–20 mg/
day. May increase by approximately
doubling dose until desired
therapeutic effect is attained.
Doses greater than 200 mg have
not been adequately studied.
▶ **Chronic Renal Failure**
PO, IV
Adults, Elderly. Initially, 20 mg/day.
May increase by approximately
doubling dose until desired therapeutic
effect is attained. Doses greater than
200 mg have not been adequately
studied.
▶ **Hepatic Cirrhosis**
PO, IV
Adults, Elderly. Initially, 5 mg/day
given with aldosterone antagonist
or potassium-sparing diuretic. May
increase by approximately doubling
dose until desired therapeutic effect
is attained. Doses greater than 40 mg
have not been adequately studied.

SIDE EFFECTS/ADVERSE
REACTIONS
Frequent
Headache, dizziness, rhinitis
Occasional
Asthenia, insomnia, nervousness,
diarrhea, constipation, nausea,
dyspepsia, edema, ECG changes,
pharyngitis, cough, arthralgia,
myalgia
Rare
Syncope, hypotension, arrhythmias

PRECAUTIONS AND
CONTRAINDICATIONS
Anuria, hepatic coma, severe
electrolyte depletion
Caution
Lactation, children younger than
18 yr, dehydration, systemic lupus
erythematosus, ototoxicity,
electrolyte imbalance

T

DRUG INTERACTIONS OF CONCERN TO DENTISTRY
- Increased electrolyte imbalance: systemic corticosteroids
- Masked ototoxicity: phenothiazines
- Decreased antihypertensive effects: NSAIDs, especially indomethacin
- Increased sweating, hot flashes, weakness, cardiovascular symptoms: chloral hydrate (rare)

SERIOUS REACTIONS
! Ototoxicity may occur with high doses or a too-rapid IV administration.
! Overdose produces acute, profound water loss; volume and electrolyte depletion; dehydration; decreased blood volume; and circulatory collapse.

DENTAL CONSIDERATIONS
General:
- Monitor vital signs at every appointment because of cardiovascular side effects.
- After supine positioning, have patient sit upright for at least 2 min before standing to avoid orthostatic hypotension.
- Patients on high-potency loop diuretics should be questioned about serum potassium levels or potassium supplement use.
- Short appointments and a stress reduction protocol may be required for anxious patients.
- Consider semisupine chair position for patient comfort if GI side effects occur.
Consultations:
- Medical consultation may be required to assess disease control and patient's ability to tolerate stress.
Teach Patient/Family to:
- Update health history/drug record if physician makes any changes in

evaluation or drug regimens; include OTC, herbal, and nonherbal drugs in the update

tramadol hydrochloride
tram´-ah-dole high-droh-klor´-ide
(Tramal[AUS], Tramal SR[AUS], Ultram, Zydol[AUS])
Do not confuse tramadol with Toradol, or Ultram with Ultane.

CATEGORY AND SCHEDULE
Pregnancy Risk Category: C

Drug Class: Synthetic opioid analgesic

MECHANISM OF ACTION
An analgesic that binds to μ-opioid receptors and inhibits reuptake of norepinephrine and serotonin. Reduces the intensity of pain stimuli reaching sensory nerve endings. ***Therapeutic Effect:*** Alters the perception of and emotional response to pain.

USES
Treatment of moderate-to-severe pain

PHARMACOKINETICS

Route	Onset	Peak	Duration
PO	Less than 1 hr	2–3 hr	4–6 hr

Rapidly and almost completely absorbed after PO administration. Protein binding: 20%. Extensively metabolized in the liver to active metabolite (reduced in patients with advanced cirrhosis). Primarily excreted in urine. Minimally removed by hemodialysis.
Half-life: 6–7 hr.

INDICATIONS AND DOSAGES
▶ **Moderate to Moderately Severe Pain**
PO
Adults, Elderly. 50–100 mg q4–6h. Maximum: 400 mg/day for patients 75 yr and younger; 300 mg/day for patients older than 75 yr.
▶ **Dosage in Renal Impairment**
For patients with creatinine clearance of less than 30 ml/min, increase dosing interval to q12h. Maximum: 200 mg/day.
▶ **Dosage in Hepatic Impairment**
Dosage is decreased to 50 mg q12h.

SIDE EFFECTS/ADVERSE REACTIONS
Frequent
Dizziness or vertigo, nausea, constipation, headache, somnolence
Occasional
Vomiting, pruritus, CNS stimulation (such as nervousness, anxiety, agitation, tremor, euphoria, mood swings, and hallucinations), asthenia, diaphoresis, dyspepsia, dry mouth, diarrhea
Rare
Malaise, vasodilation, anorexia, flatulence, rash, blurred vision, urine retention or urinary frequency, menopausal symptoms

PRECAUTIONS AND CONTRAINDICATIONS
Acute alcohol intoxication; concurrent use of centrally acting analgesics, hypnotics, opioids, or psychotropic drugs
Caution
Not a controlled substance, but dependence and abuse are possible

DRUG INTERACTIONS OF CONCERN TO DENTISTRY
• Increased risk of respiratory depression: anesthetics, alcohol

• Significant increase in metabolism: carbamazepine
• Increased serum concentrations: quinidine
• Increased risk of seizures: MAOIs, tricyclic antidepressants, selective serotonin reuptake inhibitors
• Increased risk of sedation: other CNS depressant drugs, alcohol

SERIOUS REACTIONS
! Overdose results in respiratory depression and seizures.
! Tramadol may have a prolonged duration of action and cumulative effect in patients with hepatic or renal impairment.

DENTAL CONSIDERATIONS
General:
• Determine why the patient is taking the drug.
• Patients taking opioids for acute or chronic pain should be given alternative analgesics for dental pain.
• Geriatric patients are more susceptible to drug effects; use lower dose.
• Assess salivary flow as a factor in caries, periodontal disease, and candidiasis.
• Take precautions if dental surgery is anticipated and general anesthesia is required.
• Risk of cross-hypersensitivity to other opioid analgesics.
Teach Patient/Family to:
• Use caution to prevent trauma when using oral hygiene aids
• Use caution when driving or operating complex equipment
• When chronic dry mouth occurs, advise patient to:
    • Avoid mouth rinses with high alcohol content because of drying effects
    • Use daily home fluoride products for anticaries effect

- Use sugarless gum, frequent sips of water, or saliva substitutes

trandolapril
tran-doe´-la-pril
(Gopten[AUS], Mavik, Odrik[AUS])
Do not confuse trandolapril with tramadol.

CATEGORY AND SCHEDULE
Pregnancy Risk Category: C (D if used in second or third trimester)

Drug Class: Angiotensin-converting enzyme (ACE) inhibitor

MECHANISM OF ACTION
An ACE inhibitor that suppresses the renin-angiotensin-aldosterone system and prevents the conversion of angiotensin I to angiotensin II, a potent vasoconstrictor; may also inhibit angiotensin II at local vascular and renal sites. Decreases plasma angiotensin II, increases plasma renin activity, and decreases aldosterone secretion. *Therapeutic Effect:* Reduces peripheral arterial resistance and pulmonary capillary wedge pressure; improves cardiac output and exercise tolerance.

USES
Treatment of hypertension alone or in combination with other antihypertensive medications; maintenance therapy to prevent CHF after MI; ventricular dysfunction after MI

PHARMACOKINETICS
Slowly absorbed from the GI tract. Protein binding: 80%. Metabolized in the liver and GI mucosa to active metabolite. Primarily excreted in urine. Removed by hemodialysis. *Half-life:* 24 hr.

INDICATIONS AND DOSAGES
▶ **Hypertension (without diuretic)**
PO
Adults, Elderly. Initially, 1 mg once a day in nonblack patients, 2 mg once a day in African-American patients. Adjust dosage at least at 7-day intervals. Maintenance: 2–4 mg/day. Maximum: 8 mg/day.
▶ **CHF**
PO
Adults, Elderly. Initially, 0.5–1 mg, titrated to target dose of 4 mg/day.

SIDE EFFECTS/ADVERSE REACTIONS
Frequent
Dizziness, cough
Occasional
Hypotension, dyspepsia (heartburn, epigastric pain, indigestion), syncope, asthenia (loss of strength), tinnitus
Rare
Palpitations, insomnia, drowsiness, nausea, vomiting, constipation, flushed skin

PRECAUTIONS AND CONTRAINDICATIONS
History of angioedema from previous treatment with ACE inhibitors
Caution
Angioedema (higher rate in African-American patients), CHF, ischemic heart disease, aortic stenosis, cerebrovascular disease, monitor WBC count in SLE or scleroderma, impaired renal function, hyperkalemia, pediatric patients, potassium-sparing diuretics

DRUG INTERACTIONS OF CONCERN TO DENTISTRY
- Decreased absorption of tetracycline

T

• Drugs that lower B/P could possibly exaggerate hypotensive effects

SERIOUS REACTIONS

! Excessive hypotension ("first-dose syncope") may occur in patients with CHF and in those who are severely salt or volume depleted.

! Angioedema and hyperkalemia occur rarely.

! Agranulocytosis and neutropenia may be noted in those with collagen vascular disease including scleroderma and systemic lupus erythematosus and impaired renal function.

! Nephrotic syndrome may be noted in those with history of renal disease.

DENTAL CONSIDERATIONS

General:

• Monitor vital signs at every appointment because of cardiovascular disease.

• Limit use of sodium-containing products, such as saline IV fluids, for patients with a dietary salt restriction.

• Stress from dental procedures may compromise cardiovascular function; determine patient risk.

• Short appointments and a stress-reduction protocol may be required for anxious patients.

• Use precaution if sedation or general anesthesia is required; risk of hypotensive episode.

• After supine positioning, have patient sit upright for at least 2 min before standing to avoid orthostatic hypotension.

• Consider semisupine chair position for patient comfort because of respiratory side effects of drug.

• Patients on chronic drug therapy may rarely have symptoms of blood dyscrasias, which can include infection, bleeding, and poor healing.

Consultations:

• Medical consultation may be required to assess disease control and patient's ability to tolerate stress.

Teach Patient/Family to:

• Use effective oral hygiene to prevent soft tissue inflammation

• Use caution to prevent trauma when using oral hygiene aids

• Update health and drug history if physician makes any changes in evaluation or drug regimens; include OTC, herbal, and nonherbal drugs in the update

tranexamic acid
tran-ex-am´-ik ass-id
(Cyklokapron)

CATEGORY AND SCHEDULE
Pregnancy Risk Category: B

Drug Class: Hemostatic, antithrombolytic

MECHANISM OF ACTION

A competitive inhibitor of plasminogen activation and, at much higher concentrations, a noncompetitive inhibitor of plasmin (i.e., actions similar to aminocaproic acid), which exerts its antifibrinolytic effects primarily by forming a reversible complex with a modified plasminogen. **Therapeutic Effect:** Prevents fibrin clots from forming.

USES

Prophylaxis and treatment of hemophilia patients to reduce or prevent hemorrhage during and after extractions; unapproved uses: in hyperfibrinolysis-induced hemorrhage, angioedema; oral rinse (with systemic therapy) to reduce bleeding in oral surgery patients who are also taking anticoagulants

PHARMACOKINETICS

Absorption after PO administration represents 30%–50% of the ingested dose, and bioavailability is not affected by food intake. Protein binding: 3%. Site of metabolism is not established. Excreted in urine. *Half-life:* Unknown.

INDICATIONS AND DOSAGES
▶ **Hemorrhage Prophylaxis, Tooth Extraction**
IV/PO
Adults, Children. 10 mg/kg body weight immediately before dental extraction. Following surgery, a dose of 25 mg/kg body weight can be given orally 3 or 4 times daily for 2–8 days. Alternatively, tranexamic acid can be administered entirely orally, 25 mg/kg body weight 3–4 times per day beginning 1 day before surgery.
▶ **Dosage in Renal Impairment**

Serum Creatinine	IV Dosage	Tablets
120–250 μmol/L (1.36–2.83 mg/dl)	10 mg/kg twice daily	15 mg/kg twice daily
250–500 μmol/L (2.83–5.66 mg/dl)	10 mg/kg daily	15 mg/kg daily
More than 500 μmol/L (2–5.66 mg/dl)	10 mg/kg q48h or 5 mg/kg q24h	15 mg/kg q48h or 7.5 mg/kg q24h

SIDE EFFECTS/ADVERSE REACTIONS
Occasional
Hypotension, diarrhea, nausea, vomiting, dizziness

PRECAUTIONS AND CONTRAINDICATIONS
Acquired defective color vision, subarachnoid hemorrhage, active intravascular clotting process, hypersensitivity to tranexamic acid or any component of the formulation
Caution
Lactation, reduce dose in renal impairment, limited use experience in children

DRUG INTERACTIONS OF CONCERN TO DENTISTRY
• Increased risk of bleeding: drugs that affect coagulation
• Factor IX complex: increased risk of thrombotic complications when used concurrently

SERIOUS REACTIONS
! Thromboembolic events (e.g., deep vein thrombosis, pulmonary embolism, cerebral thrombosis, acute renal cortical necrosis, central retinal artery and vein obstruction) have been reported.

DENTAL CONSIDERATIONS
General:
• Has been used as an antifibrinolytic mouthwash following oral surgery to prevent hemorrhage in patients taking oral anticoagulants.
Consultations:
• Hematologist consultation is strongly recommended.
Teach Patient/Family to:
• Update health and drug history if physician makes any changes in evaluation or drug regimens; include OTC, herbal, and nonherbal drugs in the update
• Report hemorrhage or bleeding not responding to postsurgical hemostasis
• Use caution to prevent trauma when using oral hygiene aids

T

tranylcypromine sulfate
tran-ill-sip´-roe-meen sull´-fate
(Parnate)

CATEGORY AND SCHEDULE
Pregnancy Risk Category: C

Drug Class: Antidepressant, MAOI

MECHANISM OF ACTION
An MAOI that inhibits the activity of the enzyme monoamine oxidase at CNS storage sites, leading to increased levels of the neurotransmitters epinephrine, norepinephrine, serotonin, and dopamine at neuronal receptor sites. **Therapeutic Effect:** Relieves depression.

USES
Treatment of depression (when uncontrolled by other means)

PHARMACOKINETICS
Well absorbed from GI tract. Metabolized in the liver. Primarily excreted in urine. Removed by hemodialysis. **Half-life:** 1.5–3.5 hr.

INDICATIONS AND DOSAGES
▶ **Depression Refractory to or Intolerant of Other Therapy**
PO
Adults, Elderly. Initially, 10 mg twice a day. May increase by 10 mg/day at 1- to 3-wk intervals up to 60 mg/day in divided doses.

SIDE EFFECTS/ADVERSE REACTIONS
Frequent
Orthostatic hypotension, restlessness, GI upset, insomnia, dizziness, lethargy, weakness, dry mouth, peripheral edema

Occasional
Flushing, diaphoresis, rash, urinary frequency, increased appetite, transient impotence
Rare
Visual disturbances

PRECAUTIONS AND CONTRAINDICATIONS
CHF, children younger than 16 yr, pheochromocytoma, severe hepatic or renal impairment, uncontrolled hypertension
Caution
Suicidal patients, convulsive disorders, severe depression, schizophrenia, hyperactivity, diabetes mellitus

DRUG INTERACTIONS OF CONCERN TO DENTISTRY
• Increased pressor effects: indirect-acting sympathomimetics (ephedrine)
• Hyperpyretic crisis, convulsions, hypertensive episode, and death: carbamazepine, meperidine, and possibly other opioids
• Increased anticholinergic effects: anticholinergics and antihistamines
• Increased effects of alcohol, barbiturates, benzodiazepines, CNS depressants, fluoxetine, tricyclic antidepressants

SERIOUS REACTIONS
! Hypertensive crisis occurs rarely and is marked by severe hypertension, occipital headache radiating frontally, neck stiffness or soreness, nausea, vomiting, diaphoresis, fever or chills, clammy skin, dilated pupils, palpitations, tachycardia or bradycardia, and constricting chest pain.
! Intracranial bleeding has been reported in association with severe hypertension.

DENTAL CONSIDERATIONS
General:
• After supine positioning, have patient sit upright for at least 2 min before standing to avoid orthostatic hypotension.
• Monitor vital signs at every appointment because of cardiovascular side effects.
• Assess salivary flow as a factor in caries, periodontal disease, and candidiasis.
• Hypertensive episodes are possible even though there are no specific contraindications to vasoconstrictor use in local anesthetics.
Consultations:
• Medical consultation may be required to assess patient's ability to tolerate stress.
Teach Patient/Family to:
• Use electric tooth brush if patient has difficulty holding conventional devices
• When chronic dry mouth occurs, advise patient to:
  • Avoid mouth rinses with high alcohol content because of drying effects
  • Use daily home fluoride products to prevent caries
  • Use sugarless gum, frequent sips of water, or saliva substitutes

---

trastuzumab
traz-two´-zoo-mab
(Herceptin)

CATEGORY AND SCHEDULE
Pregnancy Risk Category: B

Drug Class: Antineoplastic, monoclonal antibody

MECHANISM OF ACTION
Binds to the HER-2 protein, which is overexpressed in 25%–30% of primary breast cancers, thereby inhibiting proliferation of tumor cells. **Therapeutic Effect:** Inhibits the growth of tumor cells and mediates antibody-dependent cellular cytotoxicity.

USES
Treatment of breast cancer that has spread to other parts of the body

PHARMACOKINETICS
Half-life: 5.8 days (range: 1–32 days).

INDICATIONS AND DOSAGES
▶ **Breast Cancer**
IV
Adults, Elderly. Initially, 4 mg/kg as a 30–90-min infusion, then 2 mg/kg weekly as a 30-min infusion.

SIDE EFFECTS/ADVERSE REACTIONS
Frequent
Pain, asthenia, fever, chills, headache, abdominal pain, back pain, infection, nausea, diarrhea, vomiting, cough, dyspnea
Occasional
Tachycardia, CHF, flu-like symptoms, anorexia, edema, bone pain, arthralgia, insomnia, dizziness, paresthesia, depression, rhinitis, pharyngitis, sinusitis
Rare
Allergic reaction, anemia, leukopenia, neuropathy, herpes simplex

PRECAUTIONS AND CONTRAINDICATIONS
Preexisting cardiac disease

DRUG INTERACTIONS OF CONCERN TO DENTISTRY
• Dental drug interactions have not been studied

SERIOUS REACTIONS
❗ Cardiomyopathy, ventricular dysfunction, and CHF occur rarely.
❗ Pancytopenia may occur.

DENTAL CONSIDERATIONS

General:

- If additional analgesia is required for dental pain, consider alternative analgesics (NSAIDs) in patients taking narcotics for acute or chronic pain.
- Monitor and record vital signs.
- Avoid products that affect platelet function, such as aspirin and NSAIDs.
- This drug may be used in the hospital or on an outpatient basis. Confirm the patient's disease and treatment status.
- Patient on chronic drug therapy may rarely present with symptoms of blood dyscrasias, which can include infection, bleeding, and poor healing. If dyscrasia is present, caution patient to prevent oral tissue trauma when using oral hygiene aids.
- Consider semisupine chair position for patient comfort if GI side effects occur.
- Caution: patients may be at high risk for infection.
- Patients may be at risk for bleeding; check oral signs.
- Oral infections should be eliminated and/or treated aggressively.

Consultations:

- Medical consultation should include routine blood counts including platelet counts and bleeding time.
- In a patient with symptoms of blood dyscrasias, request a medical consultation for blood studies and postpone treatment until normal values are reestablished.
- Consult physician; prophylactic or therapeutic antiinfectives may be indicated if surgery or periodontal treatment is required.
- Medical consultation may be required to assess immunologic status during cancer chemotherapy and determine safety risk, if any, posed by the required dental treatment.
- Medical consultation may be required to assess disease control and patient's ability to tolerate stress.

Teach Patient/Family to:

- Inform dentist of unusual bleeding episodes following dental treatment
- See dentist immediately if secondary oral infection occurs.
- Use effective oral hygiene to prevent soft tissue inflammation
- Report oral lesions, soreness, or bleeding to dentist
- Prevent trauma when using oral hygiene aids
- Update health and medication history if physician makes any changes in evaluation or drug regimens; include OTC, herbal, and nonherbal remedies in the update

travoprost

tra´-voe-prost

(Apo-Timop[CAN], Gen-Timolol[CAN], Optimol[AUS], Tenopt[AUS], Travatan)

CATEGORY AND SCHEDULE

Pregnancy Risk Category: C

Drug Class: Synthetic prostaglandin F_2-α analog

MECHANISM OF ACTION

An ophthalmic agent that is a prostanoid-selective FP receptor agonist. **Therapeutic Effect:** Reduces intraocular pressure (IOP) by reducing aqueous humor production.

USES

Reduction of elevated IOP in patients with open-angle glaucoma or ocular hypertension in patients intolerant to, or who show insufficient response to, other IOP-reducing drugs

PHARMACOKINETICS

Absorbed through the cornea and hydrolyzed to the active free acid form. Metabolized in cornea and liver. Metabolites are inactive. Excreted in urine. *Half-life:* 17–86 min.

INDICATIONS AND DOSAGES
▶ **Open-Angle Glaucoma, Ocular Hypertension**
Ophthalmic
Adults, Elderly. 1 drop in affected eye(s) once daily, in the evening.

SIDE EFFECTS/ADVERSE REACTIONS
Frequent
Ocular hyperemia
Occasional
Ocular pain, pruritus, eye discomfort, decreased visual acuity, foreign body sensation
Rare
Abnormal vision, cataract, conjunctivitis, dry eye, eye disorder, flare, iris discoloration, keratitis, lid margin crusting, photophobia, subconjunctival hemorrhage, and tearing

PRECAUTIONS AND CONTRAINDICATIONS
Hypersensitivity to travoprost or benzalkonium chloride, or any other component of the formulation
Caution
May cause changes in pigmented tissues (iris, eyelid) and growth of eyelashes (length, thickness, color); do not administer with contact lens in place; renal or hepatic impairment, lactation, pediatric use, macular edema

DRUG INTERACTIONS OF CONCERN TO DENTISTRY
None reported

SERIOUS REACTIONS

❗ Ocular adverse events including accidental injury, angina pectoris, anxiety, arthritis, back pain, bradycardia, bronchitis, chest pain, cold syndrome, depression, dyspepsia, gastrointestinal disorder, headache, hypercholesterolemia, hypertension, hypotension, infection, pain, prostate disorder, sinusitis, urinary incontinence, and UTI, occur rarely.

DENTAL CONSIDERATIONS
General:
• Monitor vital signs at every appointment because of cardiovascular and respiratory side effects and question patient about occurrence of cardiovascular side effects.
• Avoid drugs with anticholinergic activity, such as antihistamines, opioids, benzodiazepines, propantheline, atropine, and scopolamine.
• Protect patient's eyes from accidental spatter during dental treatment.
• Avoid dental light in patient's eyes; offer dark glasses for patient comfort.
Consultations:
• Medical consultation may be required to assess disease control.
Teach Patient/Family to:
• Update health and drug history if physician makes any changes in evaluation or drug regimens

trazodone hydrochloride
tray´-zoe-done high-droh-klor´-ide
(Apo-Trazodone[CAN], Desyrel, Novo-Trazodone[CAN], PMS-Trazodone[CAN])
Do not confuse Desyrel with Delsym or Zestril.

CATEGORY AND SCHEDULE
Pregnancy Risk Category: C

Drug Class: Antidepressant

changes in evaluation or drug regimens; include OTC, herbal, and nonherbal drugs in the update

MECHANISM OF ACTION

An antidepressant that blocks the reuptake of serotonin at neuronal presynaptic membranes, increasing its availability at postsynaptic receptor sites. *Therapeutic Effect:* Relieves depression.

USES

Treatment of depression

PHARMACOKINETICS

Well absorbed from the GI tract. Protein binding: 85%–95%. Metabolized in the liver. Primarily excreted in urine. Unknown if removed by hemodialysis. *Half-life:* 5–9 hr.

INDICATIONS AND DOSAGES
▶ **Depression**
PO
Adults. Initially, 150 mg/day in equally divided doses. Increase by 50 mg/day at 3- to 4-day intervals until therapeutic response is achieved. Maximum: 600 mg/day.
Elderly. Initially, 25–50 mg at bedtime. May increase by 25–50 mg every 3–7 days. Range: 75–150 mg/day.
Children 6–18 yr. Initially, 1.5–2 mg/kg/day in divided doses. May increase gradually to 6 mg/kg/day in 3 divided doses.

SIDE EFFECTS/ADVERSE REACTIONS

Frequent
Somnolence, dry mouth, light-headedness, dizziness, headache, blurred vision, nausea, vomiting
Occasional
Nervousness, fatigue, constipation, generalized aches and pains, mild hypotension

Rare
Photosensitivity reaction

PRECAUTIONS AND CONTRAINDICATIONS

Hypersensitivity to tricyclic antidepressants, recovery phase of MI, convulsive disorders, prostatic hypertrophy
Caution
Suicidal patients, severe depression, increased intraocular pressure, narrow-angle glaucoma, urinary retention, cardiac disease, hepatic disease, hyperthyroidism, electroshock therapy, elective surgery

DRUG INTERACTIONS OF CONCERN TO DENTISTRY

• Increased anticholinergic effects: anticholinergic drugs
• Increased CNS depression: alcohol, all other CNS depressants

SERIOUS REACTIONS

! Priapism, diminished or improved libido, retrograde ejaculation, and impotence occur rarely.
! Trazodone appears to be less cardiotoxic than other antidepressants, although arrhythmias may occur in patients with preexisting cardiac disease.

DENTAL CONSIDERATIONS

General:
• Monitor vital signs at every appointment because of cardiovascular side effects.
• Patients on chronic drug therapy may rarely have symptoms of blood dyscrasias, which can include infection, bleeding, and poor healing.
• Assess salivary flow as a factor in caries, periodontal disease, and candidiasis.
• After supine positioning, have patient sit upright for at least 2 min before standing to avoid orthostatic hypotension.

Consultations:
• In a patient with symptoms of blood dyscrasias, request a medical consultation for blood studies and postpone dental treatment until normal values are reestablished.
• Medical consultation may be required to assess disease control.
• Physician should be informed if significant xerostomic side effects occur (e.g., increased caries, sore tongue, problems eating or swallowing, difficulty wearing prosthesis) so that a medication change can be considered.
Teach Patient/Family to:
• Report oral lesions, soreness, or bleeding to dentist
• When chronic dry mouth occurs, advise patient to:
  • Avoid mouth rinses with high alcohol content because of drying effects
  • Use daily home fluoride products to prevent caries
  • Use sugarless gum, frequent sips of water, or saliva substitutes

---

treprostinil sodium
treh-prost´-in-ill soe´-dee-um
(Remodulin)

CATEGORY AND SCHEDULE
Pregnancy Risk Category: B

Drug Class: Antihypertensive (pulmonary), vasodilator

MECHANISM OF ACTION
An antiplatelet that directly dilates pulmonary and systemic arterial vascular beds, inhibiting platelet aggregation. **Therapeutic Effect:** Reduces symptoms of pulmonary arterial hypertension associated with exercise.

USES
Treatment of the symptoms of primary pulmonary hypertension or high B/P

PHARMACOKINETICS
Rapidly, completely absorbed after subcutaneous infusion; 91% bound to plasma protein. Metabolized by the liver. Excreted mainly in the urine with a lesser amount eliminated in the feces. **Half-life:** 2–4 hr.

INDICATIONS AND DOSAGES
▸ **Pulmonary Arterial Hypertension**
Continuous subcutaneous infusion
Adults, Elderly. Initially, 1.25 ng/kg/min. Reduce infusion rate to 0.625 ng/kg/min if initial dose cannot be tolerated. Increase infusion rate in increments of no more than 1.25 ng/kg/min per week for the first 4 wk and then no more than 2.5 ng/kg/min per wk for the duration of infusion.
▸ **Hepatic Impairment (mild to moderate)**
Adults, Elderly. Decrease the initial dose to 0.625 ng/kg/min on the basis of ideal body weight and increase cautiously.

SIDE EFFECTS/ADVERSE REACTIONS
Frequent
Infusion site pain, erythema, induration, rash
Occasional
Headache, diarrhea, jaw pain, vasodilation, nausea
Rare
Dizziness, hypotension, pruritus, edema

PRECAUTIONS AND CONTRAINDICATIONS
None known

DRUG INTERACTIONS OF CONCERN TO DENTISTRY
• Increased risk of bleeding: drugs that interfere with coagulation or platelet function, such as NSAIDs and aspirin

T

SERIOUS REACTIONS

! Abrupt withdrawal or sudden large reductions in dosage may result in worsening of pulmonary arterial hypertension symptoms.

DENTAL CONSIDERATIONS

General:

• An acute use drug for use in hospitals or emergency departments.
• If a patient reports this drug in his or her medical history, question about cardiovascular disease and drugs he or she may be taking.
• Patients are at risk for bleeding while receiving this drug; provide palliative dental care for dental emergencies only.
• Avoid products that affect platelet function, such as aspirin and NSAIDs.

Consultations:

• Medical consultation should include routine blood counts including platelet counts and bleeding time.
• Medical consultation may be required to assess disease control and patient's ability to tolerate stress.

Teach Patient/Family to:

• Inform dentist of unusual bleeding episodes following dental treatment

tretinoin

tret´-ih-noyn
(Altinac, Avita, Renova, Retin-A, Retin-A Micro, Vesanoid)

CATEGORY AND SCHEDULE

Pregnancy Risk Category: D (oral), C (topical)

Drug Class: Vitamin A acid

MECHANISM OF ACTION

A retinoid that decreases cohesiveness of follicular epithelial cells. Increases turnover of follicular epithelial cells. Bacterial skin counts are not altered. Transdermal: Exerts its effects on growth and differentiation of epithelial cells. Antineoplastic: Induces maturation, decreases proliferation of acute promyelocytic leukemia (APL) cells
Therapeutic Effect: Causes expulsion of blackheads; alleviates fine wrinkles, hyperpigmentation; causes repopulation of bone marrow and blood by normal hematopoietic cells.

USES

Treatment of acne vulgaris, reducing fine facial wrinkles associated with sun exposure and aging; unlabeled uses: skin cancer, lichen planus (Renova: not for use in acne)

PHARMACOKINETICS

Topical: Minimally absorbed. Oral: Well absorbed following oral administration. Protein binding: 95%. Metabolized in liver. Primarily excreted in urine, minimal excretion in feces. **Half-life:** 0.5–2 hr.

INDICATIONS AND DOSAGES

▶ **Acne**
Topical
Adults. Apply once daily at bedtime.
Transdermal
Adults. Apply to face once daily at bedtime.

▶ **Acute Promyelocytic Leukemia**
PO
Adults. 45 mg/m^2/day given as two evenly divided doses until complete remission is documented.
Discontinue therapy 30 days after complete remission or after 90 days of treatment, whichever comes first.

SIDE EFFECTS/ADVERSE REACTIONS

Expected
Topical: Temporary change in pigmentation, photosensitivity. Local inflammatory reactions

(peeling, dry skin, stinging, erythema, pruritus) are to be expected and are reversible with discontinuation of tretinoin
Frequent
PO: Headache, fever, dry skin/oral mucosa, bone pain, nausea, vomiting, rash
Occasional
PO: Mucositis, earache or feeling of fullness in ears, flushing, pruritus, increased sweating, visual disturbances, hypo-/hypertension, dizziness, anxiety, insomnia, alopecia, skin changes
Rare
PO: Change in visual acuity, temporary hearing loss

PRECAUTIONS AND CONTRAINDICATIONS
Sensitivity to parabens (used as preservative in gelatin capsule)
Caution
Pregnancy category C, lactation, eczema, sunburn

DRUG INTERACTIONS OF CONCERN TO DENTISTRY
• Increased peeling: medication-containing agents, such as alcohol or astringents
• Avoid concurrent use with photosensitizing drugs: tetracycline, fluoroquinolones, sulfonamides

SERIOUS REACTIONS
PO
! Retinoic acid syndrome (fever, dyspnea, weight gain, abnormal chest auscultatory findings, episodic hypotension) occurs commonly, as does leukocytosis.
! Syndrome generally occurs during first month of therapy (sometimes occurs following first dose).
! Pseudo tumor cerebri may be noted, especially in children (headache, nausea, vomiting, visual disturbances).
! Possible tumorigenic potential when combined with ultraviolet radiation.

Topical
! Possible tumorigenic potential when combined with ultraviolet radiation.

DENTAL CONSIDERATIONS
General:
• May cause dry, peeling skin if used around lips; provide lip lubricant for patient comfort during dental treatment.
• Advise patient if dental drugs prescribed have a potential for photosensitivity.
Teach Patient/Family to:
• Avoid application on normal skin or getting cream in eyes, mouth, or other mucous membranes

triamcinolone/ triamcinolone acetonide/ triamcinolone diacetate/ triamcinolone hexacetonide

trye-am-sin´-oh-lone/ trye-am-sin´-oh-lone ah-set´-oh-nide/ trye-am-sin´-oh-lone dye-ass´-ih-tate/ trye-am-sin´-oh-lone hex-ah-set´-oh-nide
triamcinolone
(Aristocort)
triamcinolone acetonide:
(Aristocort, Azmacort, Kenacort A[AUS], Kenalog, Kenalog in Orabase[AUS], Nasacort AQ, Triaderm[CAN])
triamcinolone diacetate:
(Amcort, Aristocort Intralesional)
triamcinolone hexacetonide:
(Aristospan)
Do not confuse triamcinolone with Triaminicin or Triaminicol.

CATEGORY AND SCHEDULE
Pregnancy Risk Category: C (D if used in first trimester)

Drug Class: Glucocorticoid, intermediate acting

MECHANISM OF ACTION

An adrenocortical steroid that inhibits accumulation of inflammatory cells at inflammation sites, phagocytosis, lysosomal enzyme release and synthesis, and release of mediators of inflammation. *Therapeutic Effect:* Prevents or suppresses cell-mediated immune reactions. Decreases or prevents tissue response to inflammatory process.

USES

Maintenance treatment of chronic asthma

PHARMACOKINETICS

PO/IM: Peak 1–2 hr. *Half-life:* 2–5 hr.

INDICATIONS AND DOSAGES

▶ **Immunosuppression, Relief of Acute Inflammation**
PO
Adults, Elderly. 4–60 mg/day.
IM (Triamcinolone Acetonide)
Adults, Elderly. Initially, 2.5–60 mg/day.
IM (Triamcinolone Diacetate)
Adults, Elderly. 40 mg/wk.
IM (Triamcinolone Hexacetonide)
Adults, Elderly. Initially, 2.5–40 mg up to 100 mg; 2–20 mg.
Intraarticular, Intralesional
Adults, Elderly. 5–40 mg.

▶ **Control of Bronchial Asthma**
Inhalation
Adults, Elderly. 2 inhalations 3–4 times a day.
Children 6–12 yr. 1–2 inhalations 3–4 times a day. Maximum: 12 inhalations/day.

▶ **Rhinitis**
Intranasal
Adults, Children 6 yr and older. 2 sprays each nostril each day.

▶ **Relief of Inflammation or Pruritus Associated with Corticoid-Responsive Dermatoses**
Topical
Adults, Elderly. 2–4 times a day. May give 1–2 times a day or as intermittent therapy.

SIDE EFFECTS/ADVERSE REACTIONS

Frequent
Insomnia, dry mouth, heartburn, nervousness, abdominal distention, diaphoresis, acne, mood swings, increased appetite, facial flushing, delayed wound healing, increased susceptibility to infection, diarrhea or constipation

Occasional
Headache, edema, change in skin color, frequent urination

Rare
Tachycardia, allergic reaction (including rash and hives), mental changes, hallucinations, depression
Topical: Allergic contact dermatitis

PRECAUTIONS AND CONTRAINDICATIONS

Administration of live-virus vaccines, especially smallpox vaccine; hypersensitivity to corticosteroids or tartrazine; IM injection or oral inhalation in children younger than 6 yr; peptic ulcer disease (except life-threatening situations); systemic fungal infection
Topical: Marked circulation impairment

Caution
Tuberculosis; untreated fungal, bacterial or viral infections of respiratory tract; lactation, children younger than 6 yr; different doses may be required for patients on systemic glucocorticoids or patients

with chickenpox, measles; transfer from systemic glucocorticoid therapy to inhalation must be done cautiously to avoid adrenal insufficiency response

DRUG INTERACTIONS OF CONCERN TO DENTISTRY

Triamcinolone/Triamcinolone Acetonide/Triamcinolone Hexacetonide

- Decreased action: barbiturates, rifampin, rifabutin
- Increased GI side effects: alcohol, salicylates, NSAIDs
- Increased action: ketoconazole, macrolide antibiotics

SERIOUS REACTIONS

! Long-term therapy may cause muscle wasting in the arms or legs, osteoporosis, spontaneous fractures, amenorrhea, cataracts, glaucoma, peptic ulcer disease, and CHF.

! Abruptly withdrawing the drug following long-term therapy may cause anorexia, nausea, fever, headache, arthralgia, rebound inflammation, fatigue, weakness, lethargy, dizziness, and orthostatic hypotension.

! Anaphylaxis occurs rarely with parenteral administration.

! Suddenly discontinuing triamcinolone may be fatal.

! Blindness has occurred rarely after intralesional injection around face and head.

DENTAL CONSIDERATIONS

General:
- Place on frequent recall because of oral side effects.
- Evaluate respiration characteristics and rate.

- Midday appointments and a stress reduction protocol may be required for anxious patients.
- Acute asthmatic episodes may be precipitated in the dental office. Rapid-acting sympathomimetic inhalants should be available for emergency use. Triamcinolone is not a rapid-acting drug and is not intended for use in acute asthmatic attacks.
- Be aware that aspirin or sulfite preservatives in vasoconstrictor-containing products can exacerbate asthma.
- Examine for oral manifestation of opportunistic infection.

Consultations:
- Medical consultation may be required to assess disease control.

Teach Patient/Family to:
- Use effective oral hygiene to prevent soft tissue inflammation
- Gargle, rinse mouth with water, and expectorate after each aerosol dose

DENTAL CONSIDERATIONS

Triamcinolone/Triamcinolone Acetonide/Triamcinolone Diacetate/Triamcinolone Hexacetonide

General:
- Symptoms of oral infections may be masked.
- Examine for oral manifestation of opportunistic infections.
- Oral side effects may be more common with inhalation products; significant steroid side effects are more likely to occur with chronic systemic doses.
- Acute asthmatic episodes may be precipitated in the dental office. Rapid-acting sympathomimetic inhalants should be available for emergency use. A stress reduction protocol may be required.

T

• Monitor vital signs at every appointment because of cardiovascular side effects.
• Assess salivary flow as a factor in caries, periodontal disease, and candidiasis.
• Prophylactic antibiotics may be indicated to prevent infection.
• Place on frequent recall to monitor healing response.
• Determine dose and duration of steroid therapy for each patient to assess risk for stress tolerance and immunosuppression.
• Be aware that aspirin or sulfite preservatives in vasoconstrictor-containing products can exacerbate asthma.
• Patients who have been or are currently on chronic steroid therapy longer than 2 wk may require supplemental steroids for dental treatment.
Consultations:
• Medical consultation may be required to assess disease control.
• Consultation may be required to confirm steroid dose and duration of use.
Teach Patient/Family to:
• Use effective oral hygiene to prevent soft tissue inflammation
• Report oral lesions, soreness, or bleeding to dentist
• When chronic dry mouth occurs, advise patient to:
  • Avoid mouth rinses with high alcohol content because of drying effects
  • Use daily home fluoride products for anticaries effect
  • Use sugarless gum, frequent sips of water, or saliva substitutes

Triamcinolone Acetonide (Topical)
General:
• Apply approximately 0.25 inch; measure with cotton-tipped applicator; press on lesion, do not rub.

Use after brushing and eating and at bedtime for optimal effect.
• When used for oral lesions, return for oral evaluation if response of oral tissues has not occurred in 7–14 days.
Teach Patient/Family to:
• Avoid sunlight on affected area; burns may occur
• Not use on herpetic lesions

triamterene
try-am´-ter-een
(Dyrenium)
Do not confuse triamterene with trimipramine.

CATEGORY AND SCHEDULE
Pregnancy Risk Category: C
(D if used in pregnancy-induced hypertension)

Drug Class: Potassium-sparing diuretic

MECHANISM OF ACTION
A potassium-sparing diuretic that inhibits sodium, potassium, ATPase. Interferes with sodium and potassium exchange in distal tubule, cortical collecting tubule, and collecting duct. Increases sodium and decreases potassium excretion. Also increases magnesium, decreases calcium loss. ***Therapeutic Effect:*** Produces diuresis and lowers B/P.

USES
Edema; hypertension; more commonly used in combination with a thiazide diuretic

PHARMACOKINETICS

Route	Onset	Peak	Duration
PO	2–4 hr	N/A	7–9 hr

Incompletely absorbed from the GI tract. Widely distributed. Metabolized in the liver. Primarily eliminated in feces via biliary route. *Half-life:* 1.5–2.5 hr (increased in renal impairment).

INDICATIONS AND DOSAGES
▶ **Edema, Hypertension**
PO
Adults, Elderly. 25–100 mg/day as a single dose or in 2 divided doses. Maximum: 300 mg/day. *Children.* 2–4 mg/kg/day as a single dose or in 2 divided doses. Maximum: 6 mg/kg/day or 300 mg/day.

SIDE EFFECTS/ADVERSE REACTIONS
Occasional
Fatigue, nausea, diarrhea, abdominal pain, leg cramps, headache
Rare
Anorexia, asthenia, rash, dizziness

PRECAUTIONS AND CONTRAINDICATIONS
Drug-induced or preexisting hyperkalemia, progressive or severe renal disease, severe hepatic disease
Caution
Dehydration, hepatic disease, lactation, CHF, renal disease, cirrhosis

DRUG INTERACTIONS OF CONCERN TO DENTISTRY
• Nephrotoxicity: possible risk with NSAIDs, indomethacin
• Decreased antihypertensive effect: possible risk with NSAIDs, indomethacin
• Decreased effect of folic acid

SERIOUS REACTIONS
! Triamterene use may result in hyponatremia (somnolence, dry mouth, increased thirst, lack of energy) or severe hyperkalemia (irritability, anxiety, heaviness of legs, paresthesia, hypotension, bradycardia, ECG changes [tented T waves, widening QRS complex, ST segment depression]).
! Agranulocytosis, nephrolithiasis, and thrombocytopenia occur rarely.

DENTAL CONSIDERATIONS
General:
• Limit use of sodium-containing products, such as saline IV fluids, for patients with a dietary salt restriction.
• Assess salivary flow as a factor in caries, periodontal disease, and candidiasis.
• Monitor vital signs at every appointment because of cardiovascular effects and possible hyperkalemia.
• Patients on chronic drug therapy may rarely have symptoms of blood dyscrasias, which can include infection, bleeding, and poor healing.
Consultations:
• In a patient with symptoms of blood dyscrasias, request a medical consultation for blood studies and postpone dental treatment until normal values are reestablished.
• Medical consultation may be required to assess disease control.
Teach Patient/Family to:
• Use effective oral hygiene to prevent soft tissue inflammation
• Use caution to prevent injury when using oral hygiene aids
• Report oral lesions, soreness, or bleeding to dentist
• When chronic dry mouth occurs, advise patient to:
  • Avoid mouth rinses with high alcohol content because of drying effects

T

- Use daily home fluoride products to prevent caries
- Use sugarless gum, frequent sips of water, or saliva substitutes

triazolam
trye-ay´-zoe-lam
(Apo-Triazo[CAN], Halcion)
Do not confuse Halcion with Haldol or Healon.

CATEGORY AND SCHEDULE
Pregnancy Risk Category: X
Controlled Substance: Schedule IV

Drug Class: Benzodiazepine, sedative-hypnotic

MECHANISM OF ACTION
A benzodiazepine that enhances the action of the inhibitory neurotransmitter gamma-aminobutyric acid, resulting in CNS depression. *Therapeutic Effect:* Induces sleep.

USES
Treatment of insomnia

PHARMACOKINETICS
PO: Onset 30–45 min, duration 6–8 hr. *Half-life:* 2–3 hr; metabolized by liver (CYP3A4 isoenzymes); excreted by kidneys (inactive metabolites); crosses placenta; excreted in breast milk.

INDICATIONS AND DOSAGES
▶ Insomnia
PO
Adults, Children 18 yr and older.
0.125–0.5 mg at bedtime.
Elderly. 0.0625–0.125 mg at bedtime.

SIDE EFFECTS/ADVERSE REACTIONS
Frequent
Somnolence, sedation, dry mouth, headache, dizziness, nervousness, lightheadedness, incoordination, nausea, rebound insomnia (may occur for 1–2 nights after drug is discontinued)
Occasional
Euphoria, tachycardia, abdominal cramps, visual disturbances
Rare
Paradoxic CNS excitement or restlessness (particularly in elderly or debilitated patients)

PRECAUTIONS AND CONTRAINDICATIONS
Angle-closure glaucoma; CNS depression; pregnancy or breast-feeding; severe, uncontrolled pain; sleep apnea
Caution
Anemia, hepatic disease, renal disease, suicidal individuals, drug abuse, elderly, psychosis, children younger than 15 yr, acute narrow-angle glaucoma, seizure disorders

DRUG INTERACTIONS OF CONCERN TO DENTISTRY
- Increased effects: erythromycin, clarithromycin
- Increased sedation: alcohol, CNS depressants, opioid analgesics, diltiazem, anesthetics
- Avoid use with ketoconazole, itraconazole, ritonavir, indinavir, nelfinavir
- Caution if used with fluvoxamine, reduce dose by 50%
- Caution when used with drugs that are strong inhibitors of CYP3A4 isoenzymes (e.g., erythromycin)

SERIOUS REACTIONS

! Abrupt or too-rapid withdrawal may result in pronounced restlessness, irritability, insomnia, hand tremors, abdominal or muscle cramps, vomiting, diaphoresis, and seizures.

! Overdose results in somnolence, confusion, diminished reflexes, respiratory depression, and coma.

DENTAL CONSIDERATIONS

General:
• Assess salivary flow as a factor in caries, periodontal disease, and candidiasis.
• If dizziness occurs, provide assistance when escorting patient to and from dental chair.
• When used for conscious sedation, have someone drive patient to and from dental office.
• Avoid the use of this drug in a patient with a history of drug abuse or alcoholism.
• Geriatric patients are more susceptible to drug effects; use a lower dose.
• Psychologic and physical dependence may occur with chronic administration.
• Determine why the patient is taking the drug.
• Patients on chronic drug therapy may rarely have symptoms of blood dyscrasias, which can include infection, bleeding, and poor healing.

Teach Patient/Family:
• When chronic dry mouth occurs, advise patient to:
  • Avoid mouth rinses with high alcohol content because of drying effects
  • Use daily home fluoride products to prevent caries
  • Use sugarless gum, frequent sips of water, or saliva substitutes

trifluoperazine hydrochloride

trye-floo-oh-per´-ah-zeen
high-droh-klor´-ide
(Apo-Trifluoperazine[CAN], Nono-Trifluzine[CAN], PMS-Trifluoperazine[CAN], Stelazine)
Do not confuse trifluoperazine with triflupromazine, or Stelazine with selegiline.

CATEGORY AND SCHEDULE
Pregnancy Risk Category: C

Drug Class: Phenothiazine antipsychotic

MECHANISM OF ACTION
A phenothiazine derivative that blocks dopamine at postsynaptic receptor sites. Possesses strong extrapyramidal and antiemetic effects and weak anticholinergic and sedative effects. ***Therapeutic Effect:*** Suppresses behavioral response in psychosis; reduces locomotor activity and aggressiveness.

USES
Treatment of psychotic disorders, nonpsychotic anxiety, schizophrenia

PHARMACOKINETICS
PO: Onset rapid, peak 2–3 hr, duration 12 hr. IM: Onset immediate, peak 1 hr, duration 12 hr. Metabolized by liver, excreted in urine, crosses placenta, excreted in breast milk.

INDICATIONS AND DOSAGES
▶ **Psychotic Disorders**
PO
Adults, Elderly, Children 12 yr and older. Initially, 2–5 mg once or twice

a day. Range: 15–20 mg/day.
Maximum: 40 mg/day.
Children 6–11 yr. Initially, 1 mg once
or twice a day. Maintenance: Up to
15 mg/day.
IM
Adults. 1–2 mg q4–6h. Maximum:
10 mg/24h.
Elderly. 1 mg q4–6h. Maximum:
6 mg/24h.
Children. 1 mg 2 times a day.

SIDE EFFECTS/ADVERSE REACTIONS

Frequent
Hypotension, dizziness, and syncope
(occur frequently after first injection,
occasionally after subsequent
injections, and rarely with oral form)
Occasional
Drowsiness during early therapy,
dry mouth, blurred vision, lethargy,
constipation or diarrhea, nasal
congestion, peripheral edema,
urine retention
Rare
Ocular changes, altered skin
pigmentation (in those taking high
doses for prolonged periods),
photosensitivity

PRECAUTIONS AND CONTRAINDICATIONS

Angle-closure glaucoma, circulatory
collapse, myelosuppression, severe
cardiac or hepatic disease, severe
hypertension or hypotension
Caution
Breast cancer, seizure disorders,
lactation, diabetes mellitus,
respiratory conditions, prostatic
hypertrophy

DRUG INTERACTIONS OF CONCERN TO DENTISTRY

• Increased sedation: other CNS
depressants, alcohol, barbiturate
anesthetics, opioid analgesics

• Hypotension, tachycardia:
epinephrine
• Increased extrapyramidal effects:
phenothiazines and related drugs
(haloperidol, droperidol),
metoclopramide
• Additive photosensitization:
tetracyclines
• Increased anticholinergic effects:
anticholinergics

SERIOUS REACTIONS

! Extrapyramidal symptoms appear
to be dose related (particularly
high doses) and are divided into
3 categories: akathisia (inability to
sit still, tapping of feet), parkinsonian
symptoms (such as mask-like
face, tremors, shuffling gait, and
hypersalivation), and acute dystonias
(such as torticollis, opisthotonos, and
oculogyric crisis). Dystonic reactions
may also produce diaphoresis and
pallor.
! Tardive dyskinesia, marked by
tongue protrusion, puffing of the
cheeks, and chewing or puckering
of the mouth, occurs rarely but may
be irreversible.
! Abrupt withdrawal after long-term
therapy may precipitate nausea,
vomiting, gastritis, dizziness,
and tremors.
! Blood dyscrasias, particularly
agranulocytosis, and mild leukopenia
may occur.
! Trifluoperazine may lower the
seizure threshold.

DENTAL CONSIDERATIONS

General:
• Monitor vital signs at every
appointment because of
cardiovascular side effects.
• Patients on chronic drug therapy
may rarely have symptoms of blood
dyscrasias, which can include
infection, bleeding, and poor healing.

- After supine positioning, have patient sit upright for at least 2 min before standing to avoid orthostatic hypotension.
- Assess salivary flow as a factor in caries, periodontal disease, and candidiasis.
- Avoid dental light in patient's eyes; offer dark glasses for patient comfort.
- Assess for presence of extrapyramidal motor symptoms, such as tardive dyskinesia and akathisia. Extrapyramidal motor activity may complicate dental treatment.
- Geriatric patients are more susceptible to drug effects; use lower dose.
- Use vasoconstrictors with caution, in low doses, and with careful aspiration.

Consultations:
- In a patient with symptoms of blood dyscrasias, request a medical consultation for blood studies and postpone dental treatment until normal values are reestablished.
- Take precautions if dental surgery is anticipated and anesthesia is required.
- Physician should be informed if significant xerostomic side effects occur (e.g., increased caries, sore tongue, problems eating or swallowing, difficulty wearing prosthesis) so that a medication change can be considered.
- If signs of tardive dyskinesia or akathisia are present, refer to physician.

Teach Patient/Family to:
- Use effective oral hygiene to prevent soft tissue inflammation
- Use caution to prevent injury when using oral hygiene aids
- Use electric tooth brush if patient has difficulty holding conventional devices

- When chronic dry mouth occurs, advise patient to:
  - Use daily home fluoride products for anticaries effect
  - Avoid mouth rinses with high alcohol content because of drying effects
  - Use sugarless gum, frequent sips of water, or saliva substitutes

trifluridine
trye-flure´-ih-deen
(Viroptic)
Do not confuse with Zostrix.

CATEGORY AND SCHEDULE
Pregnancy Risk Category: C

Drug Class: Antiviral

MECHANISM OF ACTION
An antiviral agent that incorporates into DNS causing increased rate of mutation and errors in protein formation. *Therapeutic Effect:* Prevents viral replication.

USES
Treatment of primary keratoconjunctivitis, recurring epithelial keratitis, keratitis associated with human herpes virus types 1 and 2, and vicciniavirus

PHARMACOKINETICS
Intraocular solution is undetectable in serum. *Half-life:* 12 min.

INDICATIONS AND DOSAGES
▶ **Herpes Simplex Virus Ocular Infections**
Ophthalmic
Adults, Elderly, Children older than 6 yr. 1 drop onto cornea q2h while awake. Maximum: 9 drops/day.

Continue until corneal ulcer has completely reepithelialized, then 1 drop q4h while awake (minimum: 5 drops/day) for an additional 7 days.

SIDE EFFECTS/ADVERSE REACTIONS
Frequent
Transient stinging or burning with instillation
Occasional
Edema of eyelid
Rare
Hypersensitivity reaction

PRECAUTIONS AND CONTRAINDICATIONS
Hypersensitivity to trifluridine or any component of the formulation
Caution
Antibiotic hypersensitivity

DRUG INTERACTIONS OF CONCERN TO DENTISTRY
None reported

SERIOUS REACTIONS
! Ocular toxicity may occur if used longer than 21 days.

DENTAL CONSIDERATIONS
General:
* Avoid dental light in patient's eyes; offer dark glasses for patient comfort.
* Evaluate:
  * Therapeutic response: absence of redness, inflammation, tearing
  * Allergy: itching, lacrimation, redness, swelling

trihexyphenidyl
trye-hex-ee-fen´-ih-dill
(Artane, Apo-Trihex[CAN])

CATEGORY AND SCHEDULE
Pregnancy Risk Category: C

Drug Class: Antiparkinsonian, anticholinergic

MECHANISM OF ACTION
An anticholinergic agent that blocks central cholinergic receptors (aids in balancing cholinergic and dopaminergic activity). ***Therapeutic Effect:*** Decreases salivation, relaxes smooth muscle.

USES
Treatment of Parkinson symptoms

PHARMACOKINETICS
Well absorbed from GI tract. Primarily excreted in urine. ***Half-life:*** 3.3–4.1 hr.

INDICATIONS AND DOSAGES
▸ **Parkinsonism**
PO
Adults, Elderly. Initially, 1 mg on first day. May increase by 2 mg/day at 3–5-day intervals up to 6–10 mg/day (12–15 mg/day in patients with postencephalitic parkinsonism).
▸ **Drug-Induced Extrapyramidal Symptoms**
PO
Adults, Elderly. Initially, 1 mg/day. Range: 5–15 mg/day.

SIDE EFFECTS/ADVERSE REACTIONS
Elderly (older than 60 yr) tend to develop mental confusion, disorientation, agitation, psychotic-like symptoms

Frequent
Drowsiness, dry mouth
Occasional
Blurred vision, urinary retention, constipation, dizziness, headache, muscle cramps
Rare
Seizures, depression, rash

PRECAUTIONS AND CONTRAINDICATIONS
Angle closure glaucoma, GI obstruction, paralytic ileus, intestinal atony, severe ulcerative colitis, prostatic hypertrophy, myasthenia gravis, megacolon, hypersensitivity to trihexyphenidyl or any component of the formulation
Caution
Children, gastric ulcer

DRUG INTERACTIONS OF CONCERN TO DENTISTRY
• Increased anticholinergic effects: scopolamine, atropine, phenothiazines, antihistamines, and other anticholinergics
• Increased CNS depression: alcohol, CNS depressants
• Decreased effects of phenothiazines

SERIOUS REACTIONS
❗ Hypersensitivity reaction (eczema, pruritus, rash, cardiac disturbances, photosensitivity) may occur.
❗ Overdosage may vary from CNS depression (sedation, apnea, cardiovascular collapse, death) to severe paradoxic reaction (hallucinations, tremor, seizures).

DENTAL CONSIDERATIONS
General:
• Assess salivary flow as a factor in caries, periodontal disease, and candidiasis.

• Place on frequent recall because of oral side effects.
• After supine positioning, have patient sit upright for at least 2 min before standing to avoid orthostatic hypotension.
• Avoid dental light in patient's eyes; offer dark glasses for patient comfort.
Teach Patient/Family to:
• Use effective oral hygiene to prevent soft tissue inflammation
• Use electric tooth brush if patient has difficulty holding conventional devices
• When chronic dry mouth occurs, advise patient to:
  • Avoid mouth rinses with high alcohol content because of drying effects
  • Use daily home fluoride products to prevent caries
  • Use sugarless gum, frequent sips of water, or saliva substitutes

trimethobenzamide hydrochloride
trye-meth-oh-ben´-za-mide
high-droh-klor´-ide
(Tigan)

CATEGORY AND SCHEDULE
Pregnancy Risk Category: C

Drug Class: Antiemetic

MECHANISM OF ACTION
An anticholinergic that acts at the chemoreceptor trigger zone in the medulla oblongata. *Therapeutic Effect:* Relieves nausea and vomiting.

USES
Treatment of nausea, vomiting

PHARMACOKINETICS

Route	Onset	Peak	Duration
PO	10–40 min	N/A	3–4 hr
IM	15–30 min	N/A	2–3 hr

Partially absorbed from the GI tract. Distributed primarily to the liver. Metabolic fate unknown. Excreted in urine. *Half-life:* 7–9 hr.

INDICATIONS AND DOSAGES
▸ **Nausea and Vomiting**
PO
Adults, Elderly. 300 mg 3–4 times a day.
Children weighing 30–100 lb. 100–200 mg 3–4 times a day.
IM
Adults, Elderly. 200 mg 3–4 times a day.
Rectal
Adults, Elderly. 200 mg 3–4 times a day.
Children weighing 30–100 lb. 100–200 mg 3–4 times a day.
Children weighing less than 30 lb. 100 mg 3–4 times a day.

SIDE EFFECTS/ADVERSE REACTIONS
Frequent
Somnolence
Occasional
Blurred vision, diarrhea, dizziness, headache, muscle cramps
Rare
Rash, seizures, depression, opisthotonos, parkinsonian syndrome, Reye's syndrome (marked by vomiting, seizures)

PRECAUTIONS AND CONTRAINDICATIONS
Hypersensitivity to benzocaine or similar local anesthetics; use of parenteral form in children or suppositories in premature infants or neonates
Caution
Children, cardiac dysrhythmias, elderly, asthma, prostatic hypertrophy, bladder neck obstruction, narrow-angle glaucoma, stenosing
peptic ulcer, pyloroduodenal obstruction

DRUG INTERACTIONS OF CONCERN TO DENTISTRY
• Increased effect: CNS depressants
• May mask ototoxic symptoms associated with antibiotics or large doses of salicylates

SERIOUS REACTIONS
! A hypersensitivity reaction, manifested as extrapyramidal symptoms such as muscle rigidity and allergic skin reactions, occurs rarely.
! Children may experience paradoxic reactions, marked by restlessness, insomnia, euphoria, nervousness, and tremor.
! Overdose may produce CNS depression (manifested as sedation, apnea, cardiovascular collapse, and death) or severe paradoxic reactions (such as hallucinations, tremor, and seizures).

DENTAL CONSIDERATIONS
General:
• Nausea and vomiting may be accompanied by dehydration and electrolyte imbalance and should be corrected as part of treatment.
• Postpone elective dental treatment when symptoms are present.

trimetrexate

try-meh-trex´-ate
(Neutrexin)
Do not confuse with Amicar.

CATEGORY AND SCHEDULE
Pregnancy Risk Category: D

Drug Class: Folate antagonist

MECHANISM OF ACTION
A folate antagonist that inhibits the enzyme dihydrofolate reductase (DHFR). *Therapeutic Effect:* Disrupts purine, DNA, RNA, protein synthesis, with consequent cell death.

USES
Alternative therapy for *P. carinii* pneumonia (PCP) in immunocompromised patients, including patients with AIDS; unapproved uses: treatment of lung, prostate, colon cancer

PHARMACOKINETICS
Following IV administration, distributed readily into ascitic fluid. Metabolized in liver. Eliminated in urine. *Half-life:* 11–20 hr.

INDICATIONS AND DOSAGES
▶ PCP

IV Infusion

Adults. Trimetrexate: 45 mg/m^2 once daily over 60–90 min. Leucovorin: 20 mg/m^2 over 5–10 min q6h for total daily dose of 80 mg/m^2, or orally as 4 doses of 20 mg/m^2 spaced equally throughout the day. Round up the oral dose to the next higher 25-mg increment. Recommended course of therapy: 21 days trimetrexate, 24 days leucovorin.

SIDE EFFECTS/ADVERSE REACTIONS
Occasional
Fever, rash, pruritus, nausea, vomiting, confusion
Rare
Fatigue

PRECAUTIONS AND CONTRAINDICATIONS
Clinically significant hypersensitivity to trimetrexate, leucovorin, or methotrexate
Caution
Lactation, children younger than 18 yr; impaired hematologic, renal, or hepatic function; serious bone marrow depression can occur if leucovorin is not used concurrently

DRUG INTERACTIONS OF CONCERN TO DENTISTRY
• Alteration of plasma levels: concurrent use with erythromycin, ketoconazole, and fluconazole
• Alteration in trimetrexate metabolites: acetaminophen
• Caution with use of drugs that are strong inhibitors of CYP3A4 isoenzymes

SERIOUS REACTIONS
❗ Trimetrexate given without concurrent leucovorin may result in serious or fatal hematologic, hepatic, and/or renal complications, including bone marrow suppression, oral and GI mucosal ulceration, and renal and hepatic dysfunction.
❗ In event of overdose, stop trimetrexate and give leucovorin 40 mg/m^2 q6h for 3 days.
❗ Anaphylaxis occurs rarely.

DENTAL CONSIDERATIONS
General:
• Examine for evidence of oral manifestations of blood dyscrasia (infection, bleeding, poor healing).

T

- Place on frequent recall because of oral side effects.
- Determine why the patient is taking the drug.
- Examine for oral manifestations of opportunistic infections.
- Consider local hemostasis measures to prevent excessive bleeding.
- Palliative treatment may be required for stomatitis.
- Refer to physician if oral ulcerative lesions occur.
- Consider semisupine chair position for patient comfort because of GI effects of disease.

Consultations:
- Obtain a medical consultation for blood studies (CBC) because leukopenic or thrombocytopenic side effects may result in infection, delayed healing, and excessive bleeding. Postpone elective dental treatment until normal values are maintained.
- Medical consultation may be required to assess disease control.

Teach Patient/Family to:
- Use effective oral hygiene to prevent soft tissue inflammation
- Use caution to prevent injury when using oral hygiene aids
- See dentist immediately if secondary oral infection occurs

---

trimipramine

trye-mih-prah´-meen
(Apo-Trimip[CAN], Novo-Tripramine[CAN], Nu-Trimipramine[CAN], Rhotrimine[CAN], Surmontil)
Do not confuse with desipramine.

CATEGORY AND SCHEDULE

Pregnancy Risk Category: C

Drug Class:

Antidepressant–tricyclic

MECHANISM OF ACTION

A tricyclic antibulimic, anticataplectic, antidepressant, antinarcoleptic, antineuralgic, antineuritic, and antipanic agent that blocks the reuptake of neurotransmitters, such as norepinephrine and serotonin, at presynaptic membranes, increasing their concentration at postsynaptic receptor sites. May demonstrate less autonomic toxicity than other tricyclic antidepressants. *Therapeutic Effect:* Results in antidepressant effect. Anticholinergic effect controls nocturnal enuresis.

USES

Treatment of depression

PHARMACOKINETICS

Rapidly, completely absorbed after PO administration, and not affected by food. Protein binding: 95%. Metabolized in liver (significant first-pass effect). Primarily excreted in urine. Not removed by hemodialysis. *Half-life:* 16–40 hr.

INDICATIONS AND DOSAGES
▶ **Depression**
PO
Adults. 50–150 mg/day at bedtime. Maximum: 200 mg/day for outpatients, 300 mg/day for inpatients.
Elderly. Initially, 25 mg/day at bedtime. May increase by 25 mg q3–7days. Maximum: 100 mg/day.

SIDE EFFECTS/ADVERSE REACTIONS

Frequent
Drowsiness, fatigue, dry mouth, blurred vision, constipation, delayed micturition, postural hypotension, diaphoresis, disturbed concentration,

increased appetite, urinary retention, photosensitivity
Occasional
GI disturbances, such as nausea, and a metallic taste sensation
Rare
Paradoxic reaction marked by agitation and restlessness, nightmares, insomnia, and extrapyramidal symptoms, particularly fine hand tremors

PRECAUTIONS AND CONTRAINDICATIONS
Acute recovery period after MI, within 14 days of MAOI ingestion, hypersensitivity to trimipramine or any component of the formulation
Caution
Suicidal patients, severe depression, increased intraocular pressure, narrow-angle glaucoma, urinary retention, cardiac disease, hepatic disease, hyperthyroidism, electroshock therapy, elective surgery, MAOIs

DRUG INTERACTIONS OF CONCERN TO DENTISTRY
• Increased anticholinergic effects: muscarinic blockers, antihistamines, phenothiazines
• Increased effects of direct-acting sympathomimetics (epinephrine, levonordefrin)
• Possible risk of increased CNS depression: alcohol, barbiturates, benzodiazepines, and other CNS depressants
• Decreased antihypertensive effects: clonidine, guanadrel, guanethidine

SERIOUS REACTIONS
! High dosage may produce cardiovascular effects, such as severe postural hypotension, dizziness, tachycardia, palpitations, arrhythmias and seizures. High dosage may also result in altered temperature regulation, including hyperpyrexia or hypothermia.
! Abrupt withdrawal from prolonged therapy may produce headache, malaise, nausea, vomiting, and vivid dreams.

DENTAL CONSIDERATIONS
General:
• Monitor vital signs at every appointment because of cardiovascular side effects.
• Assess salivary flow as a factor in caries, periodontal disease, and candidiasis.
• Patients on chronic drug therapy may rarely have symptoms of blood dyscrasias, which can include infection, bleeding, and poor healing.
• After supine positioning, have patient sit upright for at least 2 min before standing to avoid orthostatic hypotension.
• Use vasoconstrictors with caution, in low doses, and with careful aspiration. Avoid use of gingival retraction cord with epinephrine.
• Place on frequent recall because of oral side effects.
Consultations:
• In a patient with symptoms of blood dyscrasias, request a medical consultation for blood studies and postpone dental treatment until normal values are reestablished.
• Medical consultation may be required to assess disease control.
• Physician should be informed if significant xerostomic side effects occur (e.g., increased caries, sore tongue, problems eating or swallowing, difficulty wearing prosthesis) so that a medication change can be considered.

Teach Patient/Family:
• Importance of good oral hygiene to prevent soft tissue inflammation
• To use caution to prevent injury when using oral hygiene aids
• When chronic dry mouth occurs, advise patient:
  • To avoid mouth rinses with high alcohol content because of drying effects
  • To use daily home fluoride products to prevent caries
  • To use sugarless gum, frequent sips of water, or saliva substitutes

triptorelin pamoate
trip-toe-ree´-linn pam´-oh-ate
(Trelstar Depot, Trelstar LA)

CATEGORY AND SCHEDULE
Pregnancy Risk Category: X

Drug Class: Antineoplastic

MECHANISM OF ACTION
A gonadotropin-releasing hormone (GnRH) analog and antineoplastic agent that inhibits gonadotropin hormone secretion through a negative feedback mechanism. Circulating levels of luteinizing hormone, follicle-stimulating hormone, testosterone, and estradiol rise initially, then subside with continued therapy. *Therapeutic Effect:* Suppresses growth of abnormal prostate tissue.

USES
Decreasing testosterone levels

PHARMACOKINETICS
Metabolism may be by CYP450, eliminated by liver, kidneys; terminal half-life is 3 hr in healthy males

INDICATIONS AND DOSAGES
▶ **Prostate Cancer**
IM (Trelstar Depot)
Adults, Elderly. 3.75 mg once q28 days.
IM (Trelstar LA)
Adults, Elderly. 11.25 mg q84 days.

SIDE EFFECTS/ADVERSE REACTIONS
Frequent
Hot flashes, skeletal pain, headache, impotence
Occasional
Insomnia, vomiting, leg pain, fatigue
Rare
Dizziness, emotional lability, diarrhea, urine retention, UTIs, anemia, pruritus

PRECAUTIONS AND CONTRAINDICATIONS
Hypersensitivity to luteinizing hormone-releasing hormone (LHRH) or LHRH agonists

DRUG INTERACTIONS OF CONCERN TO DENTISTRY
• Dental drug interactions have not been studied

SERIOUS REACTIONS
! Bladder outlet obstruction, skeletal pain, hematuria, and spinal cord compression (with weakness or paralysis of the lower extremities) may occur.

DENTAL CONSIDERATIONS
General:
• If additional analgesia is required for dental pain, consider alternative analgesics (NSAIDs) in patients taking narcotics for acute or chronic pain.
• This drug may be used in the hospital or on an outpatient basis.

Confirm the patient's disease and treatment status.
• Patients may have received other chemotherapy or radiation; confirm medical and drug history.
• When urinary retention is a problem, use anticholinergic drugs with care.
Consultations:
• Consult patient's physician if an acute dental infection occurs and another antiinfective is required.
• Medical consultation may be required to assess disease control and patient's ability to tolerate stress.
Teach Patient/Family to:
• Use effective oral hygiene to prevent soft tissue inflammation
• Prevent trauma when using oral hygiene aids
• Update health and medication history if physician makes any changes in evaluation or drug regimens; include OTC, herbal, and nonherbal remedies in the update

tropicamide
troe-pik´-ah-mide
(Diotrope[CAN], Mydriacyl, Opticyl, Tropicacyl)

CATEGORY AND SCHEDULE
Pregnancy Risk Category: C

Drug Class: Mydriatic, cycloplegic

MECHANISM OF ACTION
An antimuscarinic agent that produces competitive antagonism of the actions of acetylcholine.
Therapeutic Effect: Produces dilation of pupil (mydriasis); produces paralysis of accommodation (cycloplegia).

USES
Dilation of the pupil

PHARMACOKINETICS
Onset of action occurs within 20–40 min. The duration is about 6 hr.

INDICATIONS AND DOSAGES
▶ **Ocular Diagnostic Procedure, Examination of Fundus**
Ophthalmic
Adults, Elderly, Children. 1–2 drops in the eye(s) 15–20 min prior to exam
▶ **Ocular Diagnostic Procedure, Refractive Procedures**
Ophthalmic
Adults, Elderly, Children. 1–2 drops in the eye(s). May be repeated in 5 min.

SIDE EFFECTS/ADVERSE REACTIONS
Occasional
Blurred vision, ocular irritation, headache
Rare
Photophobia, increased intraocular pressure

PRECAUTIONS AND CONTRAINDICATIONS
Primary glaucoma or tendency toward glaucoma, hypersensitivity to tropicamide or any component of the formulation

DRUG INTERACTIONS OF CONCERN TO DENTISTRY
None reported

SERIOUS REACTIONS
❗ Cardiorespiratory collapse has been reported.
❗ Systemic absorption, including behavioral disturbances, confusion, dry mouth, fast heartbeat, and psychotic reactions, occurs rarely.

DENTAL CONSIDERATIONS

General:
- An acute use drug for diagnostic purposes.
- Protect patient's eyes from accidental spatter during dental treatment.
- Avoid dental light in patient's eyes; offer dark glasses for patient comfort.

trovafloxacin mesylate/ alatrofloxacin mesylate

troe-va-flox´-ah-sin meh´-sil-ate/ ala-troe-flox´-ah-sin meh´-sil-ate
Trovafloxacin mesylate oral: (Trovan)
Alatrofloxacin mesylate injection: (Trovan I.V.)

CATEGORY AND SCHEDULE

Pregnancy Risk Category: C

Drug Class: A fluoronaphthyridone antiinfective (related to the fluoroquinolones)

MECHANISM OF ACTION

A broad-spectrum bactericidal agent that inhibits the enzymes topoisomerase II (DNA gyrase) and topoisomerase IV required for bacterial DNA replication, transcription repair, and recombination.

USES

Treatment of infections caused by susceptible microorganisms in nosocomial pneumonia, community-acquired pneumonia, acute bacterial exacerbated chronic bronchitis, acute sinusitis, abdominal infections, gynecologic infections, UTI, bacterial prostatitis, skin and skin-structure infections, and selected STDs

PHARMACOKINETICS

PO: Good oral absorption, bioavailability 88%, can be administered with food, peak serum levels 1.7 hr, plasma protein binding 76%, wide tissue distribution, excreted in breast milk, hepatic metabolism, excretion in feces and urine, 50% of dose is excreted unchanged in feces. IV: Alatrofloxacin is a prodrug converted to trovafloxacin.

INDICATIONS AND DOSAGES

PO: Skin infections
Adults older than 18 yr. Dose depends on type of infection; 200 mg daily for 1–14 days.
IV: Nosocomial pneumonia
Adults older than 18 yr. IV dose depends on type of infection; range 300 mg daily; single IV doses can be followed by appropriate oral doses for 10–14 days.

SIDE EFFECTS/ADVERSE REACTIONS

Oral: Dry mouth, stomatitis, angular cheilitis
CNS: Dizziness, headache, light-headedness, confusion, anxiety, hallucinations
CV: Hypotension, palpitation, flushing, peripheral edema, chest pain
GI: Vomiting, nausea, diarrhea, abdominal pain, flatulence, antibiotic-associated pseudomembranous colitis, hepatic toxicity
Resp: Dyspnea, bronchospasm, coughing
Hema: Anemia, leukopenia, thrombocytopenia

GU: Vaginitis, frequency of urination, abnormal renal function
EENT: Rhinitis, sinusitis
Integ: Pruritus, rash, photosensitization
Meta: Increased liver enzymes
MS: Arthralgia, myalgia, muscle cramps
Misc: Pain on injection, increased sweating, fatigue, fever, anaphylaxis

PRECAUTIONS AND CONTRAINDICATIONS

Hypersensitivity and allergy to the fluoroquinolones
Serious liver injury

Caution

Children younger than 18 yr, mild to moderate cirrhosis, potential for liver damage, exposure to sunlight, visible or ultraviolet radiation, seizure disorders, cerebral atherosclerosis, lactation, warning associated with possible serious hepatic injury leading to death or transplant

DRUG INTERACTIONS OF CONCERN TO DENTISTRY:

• Reduction in absorption: magnesium or aluminum antacid products, iron salts, sucralfate, and morphine within 30 min of oral trovafloxacin; separate doses by at least 2 hr
• Increases serum levels of caffeine

SERIOUS REACTIONS

Serious liver injury

DENTAL CONSIDERATIONS

General:
• Determine why patient is taking the drug; specific infection.
• Do not use ingestible sodium bicarbonate products, such as the air polishing system Prophy-Jet, within 2 hr of drug use.
• Examine for oral manifestation of opportunistic infection.
• Avoid dental light in patient's eyes; offer dark glasses for patient comfort.
• Use caution in prescribing caffeine-containing analgesics.

Consultations:
• Medical consultation may be required to assess disease control in the patient.
• Consult with patient's physician if an acute dental infection occurs and another antiinfective is required.

Teach Patient/Family to:
• Prevent trauma when using oral hygiene aids
• Use effective oral hygiene to prevent soft tissue inflammation
• Avoid mouth rinses with high alcohol content because of drying effects

T

unoprostone isopropyl

yoo-noh-prost′-ohn
eye-seh-pro′-pel
(Rescula)

CATEGORY AND SCHEDULE

Pregnancy Risk Category: C

Drug Class: Prostaglandin agonist

MECHANISM OF ACTION

An ophthalmic agent that increases the outflow of aqueous humor. *Therapeutic Effect:* Decreases intraocular pressure.

USES

Indicated for lowering intraocular pressure (IOP) in patients with open-angle glaucoma or ocular hypertension who are intolerant to other medications or who failed to achieve a targeted IOP

PHARMACOKINETICS

Peak response occurs in 4–8 wk. The duration of a single dose is about 10 hr. Hydrolyzed to unoprostone free acid form in the cornea. Rapidly eliminated from plasma. Excreted as metabolites in urine. *Half-life:* 14 min.

INDICATIONS AND DOSAGES

▶ **Glaucoma, Ocular Hypertension**
Ophthalmic
Adults, Elderly. Instill 1 drop in affected eye(s) 2 times a day.

SIDE EFFECTS/ADVERSE REACTIONS

Frequent
Burning, stinging, dry eyes, itching, increased eyelash length and redness

Occasional
Abnormal vision, eyelid disorder, foreign body sensation

PRECAUTIONS AND CONTRAINDICATIONS

Hypersensitivity to unoprostone isopropyl, benzalkonium chloride, or any other component of the formulation
Caution
Permanent changes in pigmented tissues of eye, bacterial keratitis, do not use while wearing contact lens, no data on use in renal or hepatic failure or pediatric patients

DRUG INTERACTIONS OF CONCERN TO DENTISTRY

• None reported; avoid use of anticholinergic drugs: atropine-like drugs, propantheline, diazepam, other benzodiazepines

SERIOUS REACTIONS

! Elevated IOP occurs rarely.

DENTAL CONSIDERATIONS

General:
• Check compliance of patient with prescribed drug regimen for glaucoma.
• Avoid dental light in patient's eyes; offer dark glasses for patient comfort.
Consultations:
• Medical consultation may be required to assess disease control.

ursodiol
your-soo´-dee-ol
(Actigall, Urso)

CATEGORY AND SCHEDULE
Pregnancy Risk Category: B

Drug Class: Gallstone
solubilizing agent

MECHANISM OF ACTION
A gallstone solubilizing agent that
suppresses hepatic synthesis and
secretion of cholesterol; inhibits
intestinal absorption of cholesterol.
Therapeutic Effect: Changes the bile
of patients with gallstones from
precipitating (capable of forming
crystals) to cholesterol solubilizing
(capable of being dissolved).

USES
Dissolution of radiolucent,
noncalcified gallbladder stones
(<20 mm in diameter) in which
surgery is not indicated; prevent
gallstones in obese patients
experiencing rapid weight loss

INDICATIONS AND DOSAGES
▶ **Dissolution of Radiolucent,
Noncalcified Gallstones When
Cholecystectomy Is not
Recommended; Treatment of
Biliary Cirrhosis**
PO
Adults, Elderly. 8–10 mg/kg/day in
2–3 divided doses. Treatment may
require months. Obtain ultrasound
image of gallbladder at 6-mo
intervals for first yr. If gallstones
have dissolved, continue therapy and
repeat ultrasound within 1–3 mo.

▶ **Prevention of Gallstones**
PO
Adults, Elderly. 300 mg twice a day.

SIDE EFFECTS/ADVERSE REACTIONS
Occasional
Diarrhea

PRECAUTIONS AND CONTRAINDICATIONS
Allergy to bile acids, calcified
cholesterol stones, chronic hepatic
disease, radiolucent bile pigment
stones, radiopaque stones
Caution
Lactation, children

DRUG INTERACTIONS OF CONCERN TO DENTISTRY
• Reduced action: aluminum-based
antacids

SERIOUS REACTIONS
None significant

DENTAL CONSIDERATIONS
General:
• Consider semisupine chair position
for patient comfort because of GI
effects of disease.
• Some opioids can cause spasm of
bile duct leading to epigastric
distress. Use caution in use for
sedation or pain control. NSAIDs
may be better choice.
• Consider drug as a factor in the
diagnosis of altered taste.

U

valacyclovir
val-ah-sye´-kloe-ver
(Valtrex)

CATEGORY AND SCHEDULE
Pregnancy Risk Category: B

Drug Class: Antiviral

MECHANISM OF ACTION
A virustatic antiviral that is converted to acyclovir triphosphate, becoming part of the viral DNA chain. *Therapeutic Effect:* Interferes with DNA synthesis and replication of herpes simplex virus and varicella-zoster virus.

USES
Treatment of herpes zoster in immunocompetent patients, genital herpes, recurrent genital herpes; treatment of herpes labialis

PHARMACOKINETICS
Rapidly absorbed after PO administration. Protein binding: 13%–18%. Rapidly converted by hydrolysis to the active compound acyclovir. Widely distributed to tissues and body fluids (including CSF). Primarily eliminated in urine. Removed by hemodialysis. *Half-life:* 2.5–3.3 hr (increased in impaired renal function).

INDICATIONS AND DOSAGES
▶ **Herpes Zoster (shingles)**
PO
Adults, Elderly. 1 g 3 times a day for 7 days.
▶ **Herpes Simplex (cold sores)**
PO
Adults, Elderly. 2 g twice a day for 1 day.

▶ **Initial Episode of Genital Herpes**
PO
Adults, Elderly. 1 g twice a day for 10 days.
▶ **Recurrent Episodes of Genital Herpes**
PO
Adults, Elderly. 500 mg twice a day for 3 days.
▶ **Prevention of Genital Herpes**
PO
Adults, Elderly. 500–1000 mg/day.
▶ **Dosage in Renal Impairment**
Dosage and frequency are modified on the basis of creatinine clearance.

Creatinine Clearance	Herpes Zoster	Genital Herpes
50 ml/min or higher	1 g q8h	500 mg q12h
30–49 ml/min	1 g q12h	500 mg q12h
10–29 ml/min	1 g q24h	500 mg q24h
Less than 10 ml/min	500 mg q24h	500 mg q24h

SIDE EFFECTS/ADVERSE REACTIONS
Frequent
Herpes zoster: Nausea, headache
Genital herpes: Headache
Occasional
Herpes zoster: Vomiting, diarrhea, constipation (50 yr and older), asthenia, dizziness (50 yr and older)
Genital herpes: Nausea, diarrhea, dizziness
Rare
Herpes zoster: Abdominal pain, anorexia
Genital herpes: Asthenia, abdominal pain

V

PRECAUTIONS AND CONTRAINDICATIONS

Hypersensitivity to or intolerance of acyclovir, valacyclovir, or their components
Caution
Renal impairment, lactation, children; reduce dose in renal impairment

DRUG INTERACTIONS OF CONCERN TO DENTISTRY

None reported in otherwise uncompromised patients

SERIOUS REACTIONS

None known

DENTAL CONSIDERATIONS

General:
• Determine why the patient is taking the drug.
• Be aware of general discomfort associated with shingles; acute symptoms may preclude patient's routine dental visit or mandate short appointments.
• Patients on chronic drug therapy may rarely have symptoms of blood dyscrasias, which can include infection, bleeding, and poor healing.
Consultations:
• Medical consultation may be required to assess disease control.
• In a patient with symptoms of blood dyscrasias, request a medical consultation for blood studies and postpone dental treatment until normal values are reestablished.
Teach Patient/Family to:
• Use effective oral hygiene to prevent soft tissue inflammation
• Use caution to prevent trauma when using oral hygiene aids

valganciclovir hydrochloride
val-gan-sye´-kloh-veer
high-droh-klor´-ide
(Valcyte)

CATEGORY AND SCHEDULE
Pregnancy Risk Category: C

Drug Class: Antiviral

MECHANISM OF ACTION
A synthetic nucleoside that competes with viral DNA esterases and is incorporated directly into growing viral DNA chains. *Therapeutic Effect:* Interferes with DNA synthesis and viral replication.

USES
Treatment of cytomegalovirus (CMV) retinitis in patients with AIDS

PHARMACOKINETICS
Well absorbed and rapidly converted to ganciclovir by intestinal and hepatic enzymes. Widely distributed. Slowly metabolized intracellularly. Primarily excreted unchanged in urine. Removed by hemodialysis. *Half-life:* 18 hr (increased in impaired renal function).

INDICATIONS AND DOSAGES
▶ **CMV Retinitis in Patients with Normal Renal Function**
PO
Adults. Initially, 900 mg (two 450-mg tablets) twice a day for 21 days. Maintenance: 900 mg once a day.

V

▶ **Prevention of CMV after Transplant**
PO
Adults, Elderly. 900 mg once a day
beginning within 10 days of
transplant and continuing until
100 days post-transplant.
▶ **Dosage in Renal Impairment**
Dosage and frequency are modified
on the basis of creatinine clearance.

Creatinine Clearance	Induction Dosage	Maintenance Dosage
60 ml/min or more	900 mg twice a day	900 mg once a day
40–59 ml/min	450 mg twice a day	450 mg once a day
25–36 ml/min	450 mg once a day	450 mg every 2 days
10–24 ml/min	450 mg every 2 days	450 mg twice a wk

PRECAUTIONS AND CONTRAINDICATIONS

Hypersensitivity to acyclovir or
ganciclovir
Caution
Renal impairment (requires
dose adjustment), preexisting
cytopenias, cannot be substituted
for ganciclovir capsules on a one-
to-one basis, patients older than
65 yr, pediatric use

DRUG INTERACTIONS OF CONCERN TO DENTISTRY

• Increased risk of blood dyscrasias:
dapsone, carbamazepine,
phenothiazines
• Increased risk of seizures:
imipenem/cilastatin (Primaxin)
• Low platelet counts may prevent
the use of aspirin, NSAIDs

SERIOUS REACTIONS

! Hematologic toxicity including
severe neutropenia (most common),
anemia, and thrombocytopenia may
occur.
! Retinal detachment occurs rarely.
! An overdose may result in renal
toxicity.
! Valganciclovir may decrease sperm
production and fertility.

DENTAL CONSIDERATIONS

General:
    Patients on chronic drug therapy
may rarely have symptoms of blood
dyscrasias, which can include
infection, bleeding, and poor healing.
• Examine for oral manifestation of
opportunistic infection.
• Place on frequent recall to evaluate
healing response.
• Consider local hemostasis measures
to control excessive bleeding.
Consultations:
• Medical consultation for blood
studies (CBC); leukopenic or
thrombocytopenic side effects may
result in infection, delayed healing,
and excessive bleeding. Postpone
elective dental treatment until normal
values are maintained.
• Medical consultation may be
required to assess disease control.
Teach Patient/Family to:
• Prevent trauma when using oral
hygiene aids
• See dentist immediately if signs of
secondary oral infection occur
• Use effective oral hygiene to
prevent soft tissue inflammation

V

valproic acid/ valproate sodium/ divalproex sodium

val-pro´-ick

valproic acid
(Depakene)
valproate sodium
(Depakene syrup, Epilim[AUS]
Valpro[AUS])
divalproex sodium
(Depacon, Depakote, Depakote ER,
Depakote Sprinkle)

CATEGORY AND SCHEDULE

Pregnancy Risk Category: D

Drug Class: Anticonvulsant

MECHANISM OF ACTION

An anticonvulsant, antimanic, and antimigraine agent that directly increases concentration of the inhibitory neurotransmitter gamma-aminobutyric acid. *Therapeutic Effect:* Reduces seizure activity.

USES

Treatment of simple, complex (petit mal) absence, mixed seizures; divalproex for manic episodes in bipolar disorder, complex partial seizures, migraine prophylaxis; unapproved: tonic-clonic (grand mal) seizures

PHARMACOKINETICS

Well absorbed from the GI tract. Protein binding: 80%–90%. Metabolized in the liver. Primarily excreted in urine. Not removed by hemodialysis. *Half-life:* 6–16 hr (may be increased in hepatic impairment, the elderly, and children younger than 18 mo).

INDICATIONS AND DOSAGES
▶ **Seizures**
PO
Adults, Elderly, Children 10 yr and older. Initially, 10–15 mg/kg/day in 1–3 divided doses. May increase by 5–10 mg/kg/day at weekly intervals up to 30–60 mg/kg/day. Usual adult dosage: 1000–2500 mg/day.
IV
Adults, Elderly, Children. Same as oral dose but given q6h.
▶ **Manic Episodes**
PO
Adults, Elderly. Initially, 750 mg/day in divided doses. Maximum: 60 mg/kg/day.
▶ **Prevention of Migraine Headaches**
PO (Extended Release)
Adults, Elderly. Initially, 500 mg/day for 7 days. May increase up to 1000 mg/day.
PO (Delayed Release)
Adults, Elderly. Initially, 250 mg twice a day. May increase up to 1000 mg/day.

SIDE EFFECTS/ADVERSE REACTIONS

Frequent
Epilepsy: Abdominal pain, irregular menses, diarrhea, transient alopecia, indigestion, nausea, vomiting, tremors, weight gain or loss
Mania: Nausea, somnolence
Occasional
Epilepsy: Constipation, dizziness, drowsiness, headache, skin rash, unusual excitement, restlessness
Mania: Asthenia, abdominal pain, dyspepsia (heartburn, indigestion, epigastric distress), rash
Rare
Epilepsy: Mood changes, diplopia, nystagmus, spots before eyes, unusual bleeding or ecchymosis

V

PRECAUTIONS AND CONTRAINDICATIONS

Active hepatic disease

Caution

MI (recovery phase), hepatic disease, renal disease, Addison's disease, pancreatitis, lactation, children younger than 2 yr have higher risk for hepatotoxicity, urea cycle disorders, thrombocytopenia, acute head injury

DRUG INTERACTIONS OF CONCERN TO DENTISTRY

• Increased effects: CNS depressants; carbamazepine, phenobarbital levels may be increased; phenothiazines can lower the seizure threshold
• Increased bleeding and toxicity: salicylates, NSAIDs
• Increased blood levels: erythromycin
• Increased serum levels of amitriptyline, nortriptyline (start with low dose and monitor)
• Decreased effects of diazepam

SERIOUS REACTIONS

! Hepatotoxicity may occur, particularly in the first 6 months of valproic acid therapy. It may be preceded by loss of seizure control, malaise, weakness, lethargy, anorexia, and vomiting rather than abnormal serum liver function test results.
! Blood dyscrasias may occur.

DENTAL CONSIDERATIONS

General:
• Patients on chronic drug therapy may rarely have symptoms of blood dyscrasias, which can include infection, bleeding, and poor healing.
• Evaluate for clotting ability during gingival instrumentation because

inhibition of platelet aggregation may occur.
• Consider semisupine chair position for patient comfort if GI side effects occur.
• Place on frequent recall if gingival overgrowth occurs.
• Ask about type of epilepsy, seizure frequency, and quality of seizure control.

Consultations:
• In a patient with symptoms of blood dyscrasias, request a medical consultation for blood studies and postpone dental treatment until normal values are reestablished.
• Medical consultation may be required to assess disease control.

Teach Patient/Family to:
• Use effective oral hygiene to prevent soft tissue inflammation and minimize gingival overgrowth
• Use caution to prevent injury when using oral hygiene aids
• Use electric tooth brush if patient has difficulty holding conventional devices
• Schedule frequent oral prophylaxis if gingival overgrowth occurs
• Report oral lesions, soreness, or bleeding to dentist

valrubicin
val-rue´-bih-sin
(VaHaxan[CAN], Valstar)
Do not confuse valrubicin with valsartan.

CATEGORY AND SCHEDULE
Pregnancy Risk Category: C

Drug Class: Antineoplastic

MECHANISM OF ACTION
An anthracycline antibiotic that inhibits incorporation of nucleosides into nucleic acids after penetrating

cells. *Therapeutic Effect:* Causes chromosomal damage, arresting cells in the G_2 phase of cell division, and interferes with DNA synthesis.

USES
Treatment of bladder cancer

PHARMACOKINETICS
Concentrated in bladder wall; not absorbed into circulation. Excreted in urine

INDICATIONS AND DOSAGES
▶ **Bladder Cancer**
Intravesical
Adults, Elderly. 800 mg once weekly for 6 wk.

SIDE EFFECTS/ADVERSE REACTIONS
Frequent
Local intravesical reaction: Local bladder symptoms, urinary frequency or urgency, dysuria, hematuria, bladder pain, cystitis, bladder spasms
Systemic: Abdominal pain, nausea, UTI
Occasional
Local intravesical reaction: Nocturia, local burning, urethral pain, pelvic pain, gross hematuria
Systemic: Diarrhea, vomiting, urine retention, microscopic hematuria, asthenia, headache, malaise, back pain, chest pain, dizziness, rash, anemia, fever, vasodilation
Rare
Systemic: Flatus, peripheral edema, hyperglycemia, pneumonia, myalgia

PRECAUTIONS AND CONTRAINDICATIONS
Perforated bladder, sensitivity to valrubicin, severe irritated bladder, small bladder capacity, UTI

DRUG INTERACTIONS OF CONCERN TO DENTISTRY
None reported

SERIOUS REACTIONS
Serious systemic toxicity if bladder wall perforated

DENTAL CONSIDERATIONS
General:
• If additional analgesia is required for dental pain, consider alternative analgesics (NSAIDs) in patients taking narcotics for acute or chronic pain.
• This drug may be used in the hospital or on an outpatient basis. Confirm the patient's disease and treatment status.
• Offer patient frequent breaks if urinary frequency is a concern.
• Avoid prescribing drugs that could cause urinary retention, such as drugs with anticholinergic activity.
Consultations:
• Medical consultation may be required to assess disease control and patient's ability to tolerate stress.
Teach Patient/Family to:
• Use effective oral hygiene to prevent soft tissue inflammation
• Update health and medication history if physician makes any changes in evaluation or drug regimens; include OTC, herbal, and nonherbal remedies in the update

valsartan
val-sar´-tan
(Diovan)
Do not confuse valsartan with Valstan.

CATEGORY AND SCHEDULE
Pregnancy Risk Category: C (D if used in second or third trimester)

Drug Class: Angiotensin II receptor (AT1) antagonist

V

MECHANISM OF ACTION

An angiotensin II receptor, type AT_1, antagonist that blocks vasoconstrictor and aldosterone-secreting effects of angiotensin II, inhibiting the binding of angiotensin II to the AT_1 receptors. *Therapeutic Effect:* Causes vasodilation, decreases peripheral resistance, and decreases B/P.

USES

Treatment of hypertension as a single drug or in combination with other antihypertensive medications, heart failure

PHARMACOKINETICS

Poorly absorbed after PO administration. Food decreases peak plasma concentration. Protein binding: 95%. Metabolized in the liver. Recovered primarily in feces and, to a lesser extent, in urine. Unknown if removed by hemodialysis. *Half-life:* 6 hr.

INDICATIONS AND DOSAGES
▶ **Hypertension**
PO
Adults, Elderly. Initially, 80–160 mg/day in patients who are not volume depleted. May increase up to a maximum of 320 mg/day.
▶ **CHF**
PO
Adults, Elderly. Initially, 40 mg twice a day. May increase up to 160 mg twice a day. Maximum: 320 mg/day.

SIDE EFFECTS/ADVERSE REACTIONS
Rare
Insomnia, fatigue, heartburn, abdominal pain, dizziness, headache, diarrhea, nausea, vomiting, arthralgia, edema

PRECAUTIONS AND CONTRAINDICATIONS

Bilateral renal artery stenosis, biliary cirrhosis or obstruction, hypoaldosteronism, severe hepatic impairment
Caution
Volume depletion, less effect in African-Americans, liver impairment, lactation, children younger than 18 yr, elevated labs for liver function, BUN, and potassium

DRUG INTERACTIONS OF CONCERN TO DENTISTRY
• Possible reduction in effect: ketoconazole

SERIOUS REACTIONS
! Overdosage may manifest as hypotension and tachycardia. Bradycardia occurs less often.
! Viral infection and upper respiratory tract infection (cough, pharyngitis, sinusitis, rhinitis) occur rarely.

DENTAL CONSIDERATIONS
General:
• Monitor vital signs at every appointment because of cardiovascular side effects.
• Limit use of sodium-containing products, such as saline IV fluids, for patients with a dietary salt restriction.
• Stress from dental procedures may compromise cardiovascular function; determine patient risk.
• Short appointments and a stress-reduction protocol may be required for anxious patients.
• Use precaution if sedation or general anesthesia is required; risk of hypotensive episode.

Consultations:
• Medical consultation may be required to assess disease control and patient's ability to tolerate stress.

vancomycin hydrochloride
van-koe-mye´-sin
high-droh-klor´-ide
(Vancocin, Vancocin CP[AUS], Vancocin HCl Pulvules[AUS])

CATEGORY AND SCHEDULE
Pregnancy Risk Category: B

Drug Class: Glycopeptide-type antiinfective

MECHANISM OF ACTION
A tricyclic glycopeptide antibiotic that binds to bacterial cell walls, altering cell membrane permeability and inhibiting RNA synthesis. *Therapeutic Effect:* Bactericidal.

USES
Treatment of resistant staphylococcal infections, pseudomembranous colitis, staphylococcal enterocolitis, endocarditis

PHARMACOKINETICS
PO: Poorly absorbed from the GI tract. Primarily eliminated in feces. Parenteral: Widely distributed. Protein binding: 55%. Primarily excreted unchanged in urine. Not removed by hemodialysis. *Half-life:* 4–11 hr (increased in impaired renal function).

INDICATIONS AND DOSAGES
▶ **Treatment of Bone, Respiratory Tract, Skin, and Soft Tissue Infections; Endocarditis, Peritonitis, and Septicemia; Prevention of Bacterial Endocarditis in Those at Risk (if Penicillin Is Contraindicated) When Undergoing Biliary, Dental, GI, GU, or Respiratory Surgery or Invasive Procedures**
IV
Adults, Elderly. 500 mg q6h or 1 g q12h.
Children older than 1 mo. 40 mg/kg/day in divided doses q6–8h. Maximum: 3–4 g/day.
Neonates. Initially, 15 mg/kg, then 10 mg/kg q8–12h.
▶ **Staphylococcal Enterocolitis, Antibiotic-Associated Pseudomembranous Colitis Caused by *Clostridium Difficile***
PO
Adults, Elderly. 0.5–2 g/day in 3–4 divided doses for 7–10 days.
Children. 40 mg/kg/day in 3–4 divided doses for 7–10 days. Maximum: 2 g/day.
▶ **Dosage in Renal Impairment**
After a loading dose, subsequent dosages and frequency are modified on the basis of creatinine clearance, the severity of the infection, and the serum concentration of the drug.

SIDE EFFECTS/ADVERSE REACTIONS
Frequent
PO: Bitter or unpleasant taste, nausea, vomiting, mouth irritation (with oral solution)
Rare
Parenteral: Phlebitis, thrombophlebitis, or pain at peripheral IV site; dizziness; vertigo; tinnitus; chills; fever; rash; necrosis with extravasation
PO: Rash

V

PRECAUTIONS AND CONTRAINDICATIONS

Hypersensitivity, decreased hearing
Caution
Renal disease, lactation, elderly

DRUG INTERACTIONS OF CONCERN TO DENTISTRY

• Ototoxicity or nephrotoxicity: aminoglycosides and high-dose salicylates
• Increased effects of nondepolarizing muscle relaxants

SERIOUS REACTIONS

! Nephrotoxicity and ototoxicity may occur.
! "Red-neck" syndrome (redness on face, neck, arms, and back; chills; fever; tachycardia; nausea or vomiting; pruritus; rash; unpleasant taste) may result from too-rapid injection.

DENTAL CONSIDERATIONS

General:
• Monitor vital signs at every appointment because of cardiovascular side effects.
• Administer IV slowly over 1 hr; administration that is too rapid can lead to a fall in B/P (monitor) and a red rash on the face, neck, and chest caused by local histamine release. No specific treatment is required for this reaction; evaluate recovery progress.
• Determine why the patient is taking the drug.
Consultations:
• Medical consultation may be required to assess disease control.

---

vardenafil
var-den´-ah-fill
(Levitra)
Do not confuse Levitra with Lexiva.

CATEGORY AND SCHEDULE
Pregnancy Risk Category: B

Drug Class: Impotence therapy

MECHANISM OF ACTION
An erectile dysfunction agent that inhibits phosphodiesterase type 5, the enzyme responsible for degrading cyclic guanosine monophosphate in the corpus cavernosum of the penis, resulting in smooth muscle relaxation and increased blood flow. **Therapeutic Effect:** Facilitates an erection.

USES
Treatment of male erectile dysfunction

PHARMACOKINETICS
Rapidly absorbed after PO administration. Extensive tissue distribution. Protein binding: 95%. Metabolized in the liver. Excreted primarily in feces; a lesser amount eliminated in urine. Drug has no effect on penile blood flow without sexual stimulation. **Half-life:** 4–5 hr.

INDICATIONS AND DOSAGES
▶ **Erectile Dysfunction**
PO
Adults. 10 mg approximately 1 hr before sexual activity. Dose may be increased to 20 mg or decreased to 5 mg, based on patient tolerance. Maximum dosing frequency is once daily.
Elderly, older than 65 yr. 5 mg.

▶ **Dosage in Moderate Hepatic Impairment**
PO
For patients with Child-Pugh class B hepatic impairment. 5 mg 60 min before sexual activity.

▶ **Dosage with Concurrent Ritonavir**
PO
Adults. 2.5 mg in a 72-hr period.

▶ **Dosage with Concurrent Ketoconazole or Itraconazole (at 400 mg/day), or Indinavir**
PO
Adults. 2.5 mg in a 24-hr period.

▶ **Dosage with Concurrent Ketoconazole or Itraconazole (at 200 mg/day), or Erythromycin**
PO
Adults. 5 mg in a 24-hr period.

SIDE EFFECTS/ADVERSE REACTIONS
Occasional
Headache, flushing, rhinitis, indigestion
Rare
Dizziness, changes in color vision, blurred vision

PRECAUTIONS AND CONTRAINDICATIONS
Concurrent use of α-adrenergic blockers, sodium nitroprusside, or nitrates in any form
Caution
Men with cardiovascular disease in whom sexual activity is not recommended, left ventricular outflow destruction, vasodilator effects on B/P, strong inhibitors of CYP3A4 isoenzymes, anatomic deformation of penis, not approved for use in women or children

DRUG INTERACTIONS OF CONCERN TO DENTISTRY
• Dose adjustments caused by potential drug interactions—do not exceed the maximum single dose of 2.5 mg in a 72-hr period: ritonavir
• Do not exceed 2.5 mg in a 24-hr period: indinavir, ketoconazole (400 mg), itraconazole (400 mg)
• Do not exceed 5 mg in a 24-hr period: ketoconazole (200 mg), itraconazole (200 mg), erythromycin
• Increased plasma levels: drugs that are potent inhibitors of CYP3A4 isoenzymes (e.g., erythromycin, ketoconazole)
• Avoid nitroglycerin within a 24-hr period

SERIOUS REACTIONS
! Prolonged erections (lasting longer than 4 hr) and priapism (painful erections lasting longer than 6 hr) occur rarely.

DENTAL CONSIDERATIONS
General:
• This is an acute-use drug intended to be taken just before sexual activity. Be sure to include drug use in medical history and avoid use of potentially interacting drugs or warn patient of the interaction when CYP3A4 isoenzyme inhibitors are required.
• If signs of angina pectoris occur during dental treatment, do not use sublingual nitroglycerin.

vasopressin
vay-soe-press´-in
(Pitressin, Pressyn[CAN])
Do not confuse Pitressin with Pitocin.

CATEGORY AND SCHEDULE
Pregnancy Risk Category: B

Drug Class: Antidiuretic

V

MECHANISM OF ACTION

A posterior pituitary hormone that increases reabsorption of water by the renal tubules. Increases water permeability at the distal tubule and collecting duct. Directly stimulates smooth muscle in the GI tract. *Therapeutic Effect:* Causes peristalsis and vasoconstriction.

USES

Control of frequent urination, increased thirst, and loss of water associated with diabetes insipidus

PHARMACOKINETICS

Route	Onset	Peak	Duration
IV	N/A	N/A	0.5–1 hr
IM, Subcutaneous	1–2 hr	N/A	2–8 hr

Distributed throughout extracellular fluid. Metabolized in the liver and kidney. Primarily excreted in urine. *Half-life:* 10–20 min.

INDICATIONS AND DOSAGES
▶ **Cardiac Arrest**
IV
Adults, Elderly. 40 units as a one-time bolus.
▶ **Diabetes Insipidus**
IV Infusion
Adults, Children. 0.5 mUnits/kg/hr. May double dose q30min. Maximum: 10 mUnits/kg/hr.
IM, Subcutaneous
Adults, Elderly. 5–10 units 2–4 times a day. Range: 5–60 unit/day.
Children. 2.5–10 units, 2–4 times a day.
▶ **Abdominal Distention, Intestinal Paresis**
IM
Adults, Elderly. Initially, 5 units. Subsequent doses, 10 units q3–4h.

▶ **GI Hemorrhage**
IV Infusion
Adults, Elderly. Initially, 0.2–0.4 unit/min progressively increased to 0.9 unit/min.
Children. 0.002–0.005 unit/kg/min. Titrate as needed. Maximum: 0.01 unit/kg/min.
▶ **Vasodilatory Shock**
IV
Adults, Elderly. Initially, 0.04–0.1 unit/min. Titrate to desired effect.

SIDE EFFECTS/ADVERSE REACTIONS
Frequent
Pain at injection site (with vasopressin tannate)
Occasional
Abdominal cramps, nausea, vomiting, diarrhea, dizziness, diaphoresis, pale skin, circumoral pallor, tremors, headache, eructation, flatulence
Rare
Chest pain; confusion; allergic reaction, including rash or hives, pruritus, wheezing or difficulty breathing, facial and peripheral edema; sterile abscess (with vasopressin tannate)

PRECAUTIONS AND CONTRAINDICATIONS
Hypersensitivity, patients taking nitrates or β-adrenergic blockers, unstable cardiovascular disease, severe hepatic impairment, ESRD, degenerative retinal disorders
Men with cardiovascular disease in whom sexual activity is not recommended, left ventricular outflow destruction, vasodilator effects on B/P, strong inhibitors of CYP3A4 isoenzymes, anatomic deformation of penis, not approved for use in women or children

DRUG INTERACTIONS OF CONCERN TO DENTISTRY
• Decreased effects: demeclocycline, alcohol
• Increased effects: carbamazepine

SERIOUS REACTIONS
! Anaphylaxis, MI, and water intoxication have occurred.
! The elderly and very young are at higher risk for water intoxication.

DENTAL CONSIDERATIONS
General:
• Normally for acute use in the hospital or emergency department setting.
• Determine why patient is taking the drug.
Consultations:
• Medical consultation may be required to assess disease control and patient's ability to tolerate stress.

venlafaxine
ven-la-fax´-een
(Effexor, Effexor XR)

CATEGORY AND SCHEDULE
Pregnancy Risk Category: C

Drug Class: Bicyclic antidepressant

MECHANISM OF ACTION
A phenethylamine derivative that potentiates CNS neurotransmitter activity by inhibiting the reuptake of serotonin, norepinephrine and, to a lesser degree, dopamine.
Therapeutic Effect: Relieves depression.

USES
Treatment of depression, prevention of major depressive disorder relapse; generalized anxiety disorder (XR product only)

PHARMACOKINETICS
Well absorbed from the GI tract. Protein binding: 25%–30%. Metabolized in the liver to active metabolite. Primarily excreted in urine. Not removed by hemodialysis. *Half-life:* 3–7 hr; metabolite, 9–13 hr (increased in hepatic or renal impairment).

INDICATIONS AND DOSAGES
▸ Depression
PO
Adults, Elderly. Initially, 75 mg/day in 2–3 divided doses with food. May increase by 75 mg/day at intervals of 4 days or longer. Maximum: 375 mg/day in 3 divided doses.
PO (Extended-Release)
Adults, Elderly. 75 mg/day as a single dose with food. May increase by 75 mg/day at intervals of 4 days or longer. Maximum: 225 mg/day.
▸ Anxiety Disorder
PO (Extended-Release)
Adults. 37.5–225 mg/day.
▸ Dosage in Renal and Hepatic Impairment
Expect to decrease venlafaxine dosage by 50% in patients with moderate hepatic impairment, 25% in patients with mild to moderate renal impairment, and 50% in patients on dialysis (withhold dose until completion of dialysis).

SIDE EFFECTS/ADVERSE REACTIONS
Frequent
Nausea, somnolence, headache, dry mouth
Occasional
Dizziness, insomnia, constipation, diaphoresis, nervousness, asthenia, ejaculatory disturbance, anorexia

Rare

Anxiety, blurred vision, diarrhea, vomiting, tremor, abnormal dreams, impotence

PRECAUTIONS AND CONTRAINDICATIONS

Use within 14 days of MAOIs

Caution

Lactation, children younger than 18 yr, sustained hypertension with use, renal or hepatic impairment, elderly, long-term use (longer than 4–6 wk), history of seizures, suicidal patients, mania, hyperthyroidism, impairment of driving, avoid use of alcohol

DRUG INTERACTIONS OF CONCERN TO DENTISTRY

• None reported; however, because this drug is similar in action to other antidepressants, it would be wise to avoid excessive amounts of vasoconstrictors, especially in gingival retraction cords
• Increased CNS depression: all CNS depressants
• Risk of serotonin syndrome: St. John's wort (herb)

SERIOUS REACTIONS

! A sustained increase in diastolic B/P of 10–15 mm Hg occurs occasionally.

DENTAL CONSIDERATIONS

General:
• Monitor vital signs at every appointment because of cardiovascular side effects.
• After supine positioning, have patient sit upright for at least 2 min before standing to avoid orthostatic hypotension.

• Assess salivary flow as a factor in caries, periodontal disease, and candidiasis.
• Examine for evidence of oral manifestations of blood dyscrasias (infection, bleeding, poor healing).
• Place on frequent recall to evaluate healing response.
• Consider semisupine chair position for patient comfort because of GI effects of disease.

Consultations:
• Medical consultation may be required to assess disease control.
• Physician should be informed if significant xerostomic side effects occur (e.g., increased caries, sore tongue, problems eating or swallowing, difficulty wearing prosthesis) so that a medication change can be considered.
• Obtain a medical consultation for blood studies (CBC) because leukopenic or thrombocytopenic side effects may result in infection, delayed healing, and excessive bleeding. Postpone elective dental treatment until normal values are maintained.

Teach Patient/Family to:
• Use effective oral hygiene to prevent soft tissue inflammation
• Use caution to prevent injury when using oral hygiene aids
• When chronic dry mouth occurs, advise patient to:
  • Avoid mouth rinses with high alcohol content because of drying effects
  • Use home fluoride products daily to prevent caries
  • Use sugarless gum, frequent sips of water, or saliva substitutes

V

verapamil hydrochloride

ver-ap´-ah-mill high-droh-klor´-ide
(Anpec[AUS], Apo-Verap[CAN],
Calan, Calan SR, Chronovera[CAN],
Cordilox SR[AUS], Covera-HS,
Isoptin[AUS], Isoptin SR,
Novo-Veramil[CAN], Novo-Veramil
SR[CAN], Veracaps SR[AUS],
Verahexal[AUS], Verelan,
Verelan PM)
Do not confuse Isoptin with
Intropin, or Verelan with Virilon,
Vivarin, or Voltaren.

CATEGORY AND SCHEDULE

Pregnancy Risk Category: C

Drug Class: Calcium channel
blocker

MECHANISM OF ACTION

A calcium channel blocker and
antianginal, antiarrhythmic, and
antihypertensive agent that inhibits
calcium ion entry across cardiac and
vascular smooth-muscle cell
membranes. This action causes the
dilation of coronary arteries,
peripheral arteries, and arterioles.
Therapeutic Effect: Decreases heart
rate and myocardial contractility and
slows SA and AV conduction.
Decreases total peripheral vascular
resistance by vasodilation.

USES

Treatment of chronic stable angina
pectoris, vasospastic angina,
dysrhythmias (class IV),
hypertension; unapproved: migraine
headache, cardiomyopathy

PHARMACOKINETICS

Route	Onset	Peak	Duration
PO	30 min	1–2 hr	6–8 hr
PO (extended release)	30 min	N/A	N/A
IV	1–2 min	3–5 min	10–60 min

Well absorbed from the GI tract.
Protein binding: 90% (60% in
neonates). Undergoes first-pass
metabolism in the liver to active
metabolite. Primarily excreted in
urine. Not removed by hemodialysis.
Half-life: 2–8 hr.

INDICATIONS AND DOSAGES

▸ **Supraventricular
Tachyarrhythmias, Temporary
Control of Rapid Ventricular Rate
with Atrial Fibrillation or Flutter**
IV
Adults, Elderly. Initially, 5–10 mg;
repeat in 30 min with 10-mg dose.
Children 1–15 yr. 0.1 mg/kg. May
repeat in 30 min up to a maximum
second dose of 10 mg. Not
recommended in children younger
than 1 yr.
▸ **Arrhythmias, Including Prevention
of Recurrent Paroxysmal
Supraventricular Tachycardia and
Control of Ventricular Resting Rate
in Chronic Atrial Fibrillation or
Flutter (with digoxin)**
PO
Adults, Elderly. 240–480 mg/day in
3–4 divided doses.
▸ **Vasospastic Angina (prinzmetal's
variant), Unstable (crescendo or
preinfarction) Angina, Chronic
Stable (effort-associated) Angina**
PO
Adults. Initially, 80–120 mg 3 times
a day. For elderly patients and those
with hepatic dysfunction, 40 mg
3 times a day. Titrate to optimal dose.
Maintenance: 240–480 mg/day in
3–4 divided doses.

V

PO (Covera-HS)
Adults, Elderly. 180–480 mg/day at
bedtime.
▶ **Hypertension**
PO
Adults, Elderly. Initially, 40–80 mg
3 times a day. Maintenance: 480 mg
or less a day.
PO (Covera-HS)
Adults, Elderly. 180–480 mg/day at
bedtime.
PO (Extended-Release)
Adults, Elderly. 120–240 mg/day.
May give 480 mg or less a day in
2 divided doses.
PO (Verelan PM)
Adults, Elderly. 100–300 mg/day.

SIDE EFFECTS/ADVERSE REACTIONS
Frequent
Constipation
Occasional
Dizziness, light-headedness,
headache, asthenia (loss of strength,
energy), nausea, peripheral edema,
hypotension
Rare
Bradycardia, dermatitis, or rash

PRECAUTIONS AND CONTRAINDICATIONS
Atrial fibrillation or flutter and an
accessory bypass tract, cardiogenic
shock, heart block, sinus bradycardia,
ventricular tachycardia
Caution
CHF, hypotension, hepatic
injury, lactation, children, renal
disease, concomitant-blocker
therapy

DRUG INTERACTIONS OF CONCERN TO DENTISTRY
• Decreased effect: indomethacin,
possibly other NSAIDs,
phenobarbital

• Increased effect: parenteral and
inhalation general anesthetics or
other drugs with hypotensive actions,
benzodiazepines
• Increased effects of nondepolarizing
muscle relaxants
• Increased effects of carbamazepine
• Caution in use of strong inhibitors
of CYP3A4 isoenzymes,
itraconazole

SERIOUS REACTIONS
! Rapid ventricular rate in atrial
flutter or fibrillation, marked
hypotension, extreme bradycardia,
CHF, asystole, and second- and third-
degree AV block occur rarely.

DENTAL CONSIDERATIONS
General:
• Monitor cardiac status; take vital
signs at every appointment because
of cardiovascular side effects.
Consider a stress-reduction protocol
to prevent stress-induced angina
during the dental appointment.
• After supine positioning, have
patient sit upright for at least 2 min
before standing to avoid orthostatic
hypotension.
• Place on frequent recall to monitor
gingival condition.
• Limit use of sodium-containing
products, such as saline IV fluids, for
patients with a dietary salt
restriction.
• Assess salivary flow as a factor in
caries, periodontal disease, and
candidiasis.
• Use vasoconstrictors with caution,
in low doses, and with careful
aspiration. Avoid use of gingival
retraction cord with epinephrine.
Consultations:
• In a patient with symptoms of
blood dyscrasias, request a medical
consultation for blood studies and

postpone dental treatment until normal values are reestablished.
• Medical consultation may be required to assess disease control and patient's ability to tolerate stress.
Teach Patient/Family to:
• Use effective oral hygiene to prevent soft tissue inflammation and minimize gingival overgrowth
• Schedule frequent oral prophylaxis if gingival overgrowth occurs
• When chronic dry mouth occurs, advise patient to:
  • Avoid mouth rinses with high alcohol content because of drying effects
  • Use daily home fluoride products to prevent caries
  • Use sugarless gum, frequent sips of water, or saliva substitutes

vidarabine
vye-dare´-ah-been
(Ara-A, Vira-A)
Do not confuse with Zostrix.

CATEGORY AND SCHEDULE
Pregnancy Risk Category: C

Drug Class: Antiviral

MECHANISM OF ACTION
An antiviral agent that appears to interfere with viral DNS synthesis.
Therapeutic Effect: Regenerates corneal epithelium.

USES
Treatment of keratoconjunctivitis caused by human herpes virus, recurrent epithelial keratitis

PHARMACOKINETICS
None reported

INDICATIONS AND DOSAGES
▶ **Treatment of Keratitis, Keratoconjunctivitis Caused by Human Herpes Virus, Types 1 and 2**
Ophthalmic
Adults, Elderly. Apply 0.5 inch into lower conjunctival sac 5 times a day at 3-hr intervals. After re-epithelialization, treat for additional 7 days at dosage of 2 times a day.

SIDE EFFECTS/ADVERSE REACTIONS
Frequent
Burning, itching, irritation
Occasional
Foreign body sensation, tearing, sensitivity to light, pain, photophobia

PRECAUTIONS AND CONTRAINDICATIONS
Hypersensitivity to vidarabine or any component of the formulation
Caution
Antibiotic hypersensitivity

DRUG INTERACTIONS OF CONCERN TO DENTISTRY
None reported

SERIOUS REACTIONS
None significant

DENTAL CONSIDERATIONS
General:
• Avoid dental light in patient's eyes; offer dark glasses for patient comfort.
Teach Patient/Family to:
• Seek evaluation if healing has not occurred in 7–10 days.

vinblastine sulfate

vin-blass´-teen sull´-fate
(Oncovin[AUS], Velban, Velbe[AUS])
Do not confuse vinblastine with
vincristine or vinorelbine.

CATEGORY AND SCHEDULE

Pregnancy Risk Category: D

Drug Class: Antineoplastic

MECHANISM OF ACTION

A vinca alkaloid that binds to
microtubular protein of mitotic
spindle, causing metaphase arrest.
Therapeutic Effect: Inhibits cell
division.

USES

Treatment of certain kinds of cancer,
including lymphoma and cancer of
the breast or testicles

PHARMACOKINETICS

Does not cross the blood-brain
barrier. Protein binding: 75%.
Metabolized in the liver to active
metabolite. Primarily eliminated in
feces by biliary system.
Half-life: 24.8 hr.

INDICATIONS AND DOSAGES

▸ Remission Induction in Advanced
Testicular Carcinoma, Advanced
Mycosis Fungoides, Breast
Carcinoma, Choriocarcinoma,
Disseminated Hodgkin's Disease,
Non-Hodgkin's Lymphoma, Kaposi's
Sarcoma (KS), or Letterer-Siwe
Disease
IV
Adults, Elderly. Initially, 3.7 mg/m²
as a single dose. Increase dose by
about 1.8 mg/m² at weekly intervals
until desired therapeutic response is
attained, WBC count falls below
3000/mm³, or maximum weekly dose
of 18.5 mg/m² is reached.
Children. Initially, 2.5 mg/m² as a
single dose. Increase dose by about
1.25 mg/m² at weekly intervals until
desired therapeutic response is
attained, WBC count falls below
3000/mm³, or maximum weekly dose
of 7.5–12.5 mg/m² is reached.
▸ Maintenance Dose for Treatment of
Advanced Testicular Carcinoma,
Advanced Mycosis Fungoides,
Breast Carcinoma, Choriocarcinoma,
Disseminated Hodgkin's Disease,
Non-Hodgkin's Lymphoma, KS, or
Letterer-Siwe Disease
IV
Adults, Elderly, Children. Administer
one increment less than dose
required to produce WBC count of
3000/mm³. Each subsequent dose
given when WBC count returns to
4000/mm³ and at least 7 days have
elapsed since previous dose.

SIDE EFFECTS/ADVERSE REACTIONS

Frequent
Nausea, vomiting, alopecia
Occasional
Constipation or diarrhea, rectal
bleeding, headache, paraesthesia
(occur 4–6 hr after administration
and persist for 2–10 hr); malaise;
asthenia; dizziness; pain at tumor
site; jaw or face pain; depression;
dry mouth
Rare
Dermatitis, stomatitis, phototoxicity,
hyperuricemia

PRECAUTIONS AND CONTRAINDICATIONS

Bacterial infection, severe
leukopenia, significant
granulocytopenia (unless it stems
from disease being treated)

DRUG INTERACTIONS OF CONCERN TO DENTISTRY
• Suspected increase in metabolism: strong inhibitors of CYP3A4 isoenzymes (erythromycin, clarithromycin, fluconazole, itraconazole, ketoconazole, metronidazole)

SERIOUS REACTIONS
! Hematologic toxicity is manifested as leukopenia and, less commonly, anemia. The WBC count reaches its nadir 4–10 days after initial therapy and recovers within 7–14 days (21 days with high vinblastine dosages).
! Thrombocytopenia is usually mild and transient, with recovery occurring in a few days.
! Hepatic insufficiency may increase the risk of toxic drug effects.
! Acute shortness of breath or bronchospasm may occur, particularly when vinblastine is administered concurrently with mitomycin.

DENTAL CONSIDERATIONS
General:
• If additional analgesia is required for dental pain, consider alternative analgesics (NSAIDs) in patients taking narcotics for acute or chronic pain.
• This drug may be used in the hospital or on an outpatient basis. Confirm the patient's disease and treatment status.
• Short appointments and a stress reduction protocol may be required for anxious patients.
• Patient on chronic drug therapy may rarely present with symptoms of blood dyscrasias, which can include infection, bleeding, and poor healing. If dyscrasia is present, caution patient to prevent oral tissue trauma when using oral hygiene aids.

• Examine for oral manifestation of opportunistic infection.
• Palliative medication may be required for management of oral side effects.
• Chlorhexidine mouth rinse prior to and during chemotherapy may reduce severity of mucositis.
• Advise patient if dental drugs prescribed have a potential for photosensitivity.
• Assess salivary flow as a factor in caries, periodontal disease, and candidiasis.
• Patients may have received other chemotherapy and radiation; confirm medical and drug history.
• Patients presenting with KS also may be HIV positive.
• Patients may be at risk for infection.
Consultations:
• Medical consultation may be required to assess immunologic status during cancer chemotherapy and determine safety risk, if any, posed by the required dental treatment.
• Medical consultation may be required to assess disease control and patient's ability to tolerate stress.
• In a patient with symptoms of blood dyscrasias, request a medical consultation for blood studies and postpone treatment until normal values are reestablished.
Teach Patient/Family to:
• Maintain fastidious oral hygiene
• Use effective oral hygiene to prevent soft tissue inflammation
• Report oral lesions, soreness, or bleeding to dentist
• Prevent trauma when using oral hygiene aids
• When chronic dry mouth occurs, advise patient to:
  • Avoid mouth rinses with high alcohol content due to drying effects

V

- Use daily home fluoride products for anticaries effect
- Use sugarless gum, frequent sips of water or saliva substitutes
- Update health and medication history if physician makes any changes in evaluation or drug regimens; include OTC, herbal, and nonherbal remedies in the update

vincristine sulfate

vin-cris´-teen sull´-fate
(Oncovin, Vincasar PFS)
Do not confuse vincristine with vinblastine, or Oncovin with Ancobon.

CATEGORY AND SCHEDULE
Pregnancy Risk Category: D

Drug Class: Antineoplastic

MECHANISM OF ACTION
A vinca alkaloid that binds to microtubular protein of mitotic spindle, causing metaphase arrest. **Therapeutic Effect:** Inhibits cell division.

USES
Treatment of acute Leukemia, advanced non-Hodgkin's Lymphoma, disseminated Hodgkin's disease, neuroblastoma, rhabdomyosarcoma, Wilms' tumor

PHARMACOKINETICS
Does not cross the blood-brain barrier. Protein binding: 75%. Metabolized in the liver. Primarily eliminated in feces by biliary system. **Half-life:** 10–37 hr.

INDICATIONS AND DOSAGES
▶ **Acute Leukemia, Advanced Non-Hodgkin's Lymphoma, Disseminated Hodgkin's Disease, Neuroblastoma, Rhabdomyosarcoma, Wilms' Tumor**
IV
Adults, Elderly. 0.4–1.4 mg/m^2 once a wk.
Children. 1–2 mg/m^2 once a wk.
Children weighing less than 10 kg or with a body surface area less than 1 m^2. 0.05 mg/kg. Maximum: 2 mg.
▶ **Dosage in Hepatic Impairment**
Reduce dosage by 50% in patients with a direct serum bilirubin concentration more than 3 mg/dl.

SIDE EFFECTS/ADVERSE REACTIONS
Expected
Peripheral neuropathy (occurs in nearly every patient; first clinical sign is depression of Achilles tendon reflex)
Frequent
Peripheral paraesthesia, alopecia, constipation or obstipation (upper colon impaction with empty rectum), abdominal cramps, headache, jaw pain, hoarseness, diplopia, ptosis or drooping of eyelid, urinary tract disturbances
Occasional
Nausea, vomiting, diarrhea, abdominal distention, stomatitis, fever
Rare
Mild leukopenia, mild anemia, thrombocytopenia

PRECAUTIONS AND CONTRAINDICATIONS
Patients receiving radiation therapy through ports that include the liver

DRUG INTERACTIONS OF CONCERN TO DENTISTRY
None reported

SERIOUS REACTIONS

! Acute shortness of breath and bronchospasm may occur, especially when vincristine is administered concurrently with mitomycin.

! Prolonged or high-dose therapy may produce foot or wrist drop, difficulty walking, slapping gait, ataxia, and muscle wasting.

! Acute uric acid nephropathy may occur.

DENTAL CONSIDERATIONS

General:

• If additional analgesia is required for dental pain, consider alternative analgesics (NSAIDs) in patients taking narcotics for acute or chronic pain.

• This drug may be used in the hospital or on an outpatient basis. Confirm the patient's disease and treatment status.

• Short appointments and a stress reduction protocol may be required for anxious patients.

• Patient on chronic drug therapy may rarely present with symptoms of blood dyscrasias, which can include infection, bleeding, and poor healing. If dyscrasia is present, caution patient to prevent oral tissue trauma when using oral hygiene aids.

• Examine for oral manifestation of opportunistic infection.

• Assess salivary flow as a factor in caries, periodontal disease, and candidiasis.

• Palliative medication may be required for management of oral side effects.

• Chlorhexidine mouth rinse prior to and during chemotherapy may reduce severity of mucositis.

• Patients may have received other chemotherapy or radiation; confirm medical and drug history.

• Patients may be at risk for infection.

Consultations:

• Medical consultation may be required to assess immunologic status during cancer chemotherapy and determine safety risk, if any, posed by the required dental treatment.

• Medical consultation may be required to assess disease control and patient's ability to tolerate stress.

• In a patient with symptoms of blood dyscrasias, request a medical consultation for blood studies and postpone treatment until normal values are reestablished.

• Refer patients to attending physician if symptoms of peripheral neuropathy are present (numbness, tingling, or pain in hands and feet).

Teach Patient/Family to:

• Use effective oral hygiene to prevent soft tissue inflammation

• Report oral lesions, soreness, or bleeding to dentist

• Prevent trauma when using oral hygiene aids

• Update health and medication history if physician makes any changes in evaluation or drug regimens; include OTC, herbal, and nonherbal remedies in the update

• When chronic dry mouth occurs, advise patient to:

  • Avoid mouth rinses with high alcohol content due to drying effects

  • Use daily home fluoride products for anticaries effect

  • Use sugarless gum, frequent sips of water, or saliva substitutes

V

vinorelbine
vin-oh-rell´-bean
(Navelbine)
Do not confuse vinorelbine with
vinblastine.

CATEGORY AND SCHEDULE
Pregnancy Risk Category: D

Drug Class: Antineoplastic

MECHANISM OF ACTION
A semisynthetic vinca alkaloid that
interferes with mitotic microtubule
assembly. *Therapeutic Effect:*
Prevents cell division.

USES
Treatment of some kinds of lung
cancer

PHARMACOKINETICS
Widely distributed after IV
administration. Protein binding:
80%–90%. Metabolized in the liver.
Primarily eliminated in feces by
biliary system. *Half-life:* 28–43 hr.

INDICATIONS AND DOSAGES
▶ **Unresectable, Advanced
Non–Small-Cell Lung Cancer
(as monotherapy or in combination
with cisplatin)**
IV
Adults, Elderly. 30 mg/m²
administered weekly over 6–10 min.
▶ **Dosage Adjustment Guidelines**
Dosage adjustments should be based
on granulocyte count obtained on the
day of treatment, as follows:

Granulocyte Count (cells/mm³) on Day of Treatment	Dose
More than 1500	30 mg/m²
1000–1499	15 mg/m²
Less than 1000	Do not administer

▶ **Combination Therapy (with cisplatin)**
IV Injection
Adults, Elderly. 25 mg/m² every wk
or 30 mg/m² on days 1 and 29,
then q6wk.

SIDE EFFECTS/ADVERSE REACTIONS
Frequent
Asthenia; mild or moderate
nausea; constipation; erythema,
pain, or vein discoloration at
injection site; fatigue; peripheral
neuropathy manifested as paresthesia
and hyperesthesia; diarrhea;
alopecia
Occasional
Phlebitis, dyspnea, loss of deep
tendon reflexes
Rare
Chest pain, jaw pain, myalgia,
arthralgia, rash

PRECAUTIONS AND CONTRAINDICATIONS
Granulocyte count before treatment
of fewer than 1000 cells/mm³

DRUG INTERACTIONS OF CONCERN TO DENTISTRY
None reported

SERIOUS REACTIONS
❗ Bone marrow depression is
manifested mainly as
granulocytopenia, which may be
severe. Other hematologic toxicities,
including neutropenia,
thrombocytopenia, leukopenia, and
anemia, increase the risk of infection
and bleeding.
❗ Acute shortness of breath and
severe bronchospasm occur
infrequently, particularly in patients
with preexisting pulmonary
dysfunction and in those receiving
mitomycin concurrently.

DENTAL CONSIDERATIONS

General:
• If additional analgesia is required for dental pain, consider alternative analgesics (NSAIDs) in patients taking narcotics for acute or chronic pain.
• Avoid products that affect platelet function, such as aspirin and NSAIDs.
• This drug may be used in the hospital or on an outpatient basis. Confirm the patient's disease and treatment status.
• Patient on chronic drug therapy may rarely present with symptoms of blood dyscrasias, which can include infection, bleeding, and poor healing. If dyscrasia is present, caution patient to prevent oral tissue trauma when using oral hygiene aids.
• Consider semisupine chair position for patients with respiratory disease.
• Caution: patients may be at high risk for infection.
• Patient may have received other chemotherapy or radiation; confirm medical and drug history.
• Oral infections should be eliminated and/or treated aggressively.

Consultations:
• Medical consultation should include routine blood counts including platelet counts and bleeding time.
• Consult physician; prophylactic or therapeutic antiinfectives may be indicated if surgery or periodontal treatment is required.
• Medical consultation may be required to assess immunologic status during cancer chemotherapy and determine safety risk, if any, posed by the required dental treatment.
• Medical consultation may be required to assess disease control and patient's ability to tolerate stress.

Teach Patient/Family to:
• See dentist immediately if secondary oral infection occurs
• Use effective oral hygiene to prevent soft tissue inflammation
• Report oral lesions, soreness, or bleeding to dentist
• Prevent trauma when using oral hygiene aids
• Update health and medication history if physician makes any changes in evaluation or drug regimens; include OTC, herbal, and nonherbal remedies in the update

vitamin A

vight´-ah-min A
(Aquasol A, Palmitate A)
Do not confuse Aquasol A with Anusol.

CATEGORY AND SCHEDULE

Pregnancy Risk Category: A (X if used in doses greater than recommended daily allowance)

Drug Class: Fat-soluble vitamin

MECHANISM OF ACTION

A fat-soluble vitamin that may act as a cofactor in biochemical reactions. *Therapeutic Effect:* Is essential for normal function of retina, visual adaptation to darkness, bone growth, testicular and ovarian function, and embryonic development; preserves integrity of epithelial cells.

USES

Treatment of vitamin A deficiency

PHARMACOKINETICS
Rapidly absorbed from the GI tract if bile salts, pancreatic lipase, protein, and dietary fat are present. Transported in blood to the liver, where it's metabolized; stored in parenchymal hepatic cells, then transported in plasma as retinol, as needed. Excreted primarily in bile and, to a lesser extent, in urine.

INDICATIONS AND DOSAGES
▶ Severe Vitamin A Deficiency
PO
Adults, Elderly, Children 8 yr and older. 500,000 units/day for 3 days; then 50,000 units/day for 14 days, then 10,000–20,000 units/day for 2 mo.
Children 1–7 yr. 5000 units/kg/day for 5 days, then 5000–10,000 units/day for 2 mo.
Children younger than 1 yr. 5000–10,000 units/day for 2 mo.
IM
Adults, Elderly, Children 8 yr and older. 100,000 units/day for 3 days; then 50,000 units/day for 14 days.
Children 1–7 yr. 17,500–35,000 units/day for 10 days.
Children younger than 1 yr. 7500–15,000 units/day.
▶ Malabsorption Syndrome
PO
Adults, Elderly, Children 8 yr and older. 10,000–50,000 units/day.
▶ Dietary Supplement
PO
Adults, Elderly. 4000–5000 units/day.
Children 7–10 yr. 3300–3500 units/day.
Children 4–6 yr. 2500 units/day.
Children 6 mo–3 yr. 1500–2000 units/day.
Neonates younger than 5 mo. 1500 units/day.

SIDE EFFECTS/ADVERSE REACTIONS
None known

PRECAUTIONS AND CONTRAINDICATIONS
Hypervitaminosis A
Caution
Impaired renal function; pregnancy category A (RDA doses), otherwise pregnancy category C

DRUG INTERACTIONS OF CONCERN TO DENTISTRY
None listed

SERIOUS REACTIONS
! Chronic overdose produces malaise, nausea, vomiting, drying or cracking of skin or lips, inflammation of tongue or gums, irritability, alopecia, and night sweats.
! Bulging fontanelles have occurred in infants.

DENTAL CONSIDERATIONS
General:
• Oral manifestation of side effects could indicate hypervitaminosis.
• May cause dry or peeling skin around lips; provide lip lubricant for patient comfort during dental treatment.

vitamin D
vight´-ah-min D
(Calciferol, Drisdol, Ostoforet[CAN])

CATEGORY AND SCHEDULE
Pregnancy Risk Category: A (D if used in doses above recommended daily allowance)

Drug Class: Fat-soluble vitamin

MECHANISM OF ACTION

A fat-soluble vitamin that stimulates calcium and phosphate absorption from the small intestine, promotes secretion of calcium from bone to blood, and promotes resorption of phosphate in renal tubules; also acts on bone cells to stimulate skeletal growth and on parathyroid gland to suppress hormone synthesis and secretion. *Therapeutic Effect:* Essential for absorption and utilization of calcium and phosphate and normal bone calcification. Reduces parathyroid hormone level. Improves phosphorus and calcium homeostasis in chronic renal failure.

USES

Varies with the type of vitamin D selected, but generally includes vitamin D deficiency, rickets, renal osteodystrophy, tetany, hypoparathyroidism, and hypophosphatemia; doxercalciferol is indicated for reduction of elevated intact parathyroid hormone (iPTH) levels for secondary hyperparathyroidism in patients receiving chronic renal dialysis

PHARMACOKINETICS

Readily absorbed from small intestine. Concentrated primarily in liver and fat deposits. Activated in the liver and kidneys. Eliminated by biliary system; excreted in urine. *Half-life:* 19–48 hr for ergocalciferol.

INDICATIONS AND DOSAGES

AlertOral dosing is preferred. Administer the drug IM only in patients with GI, hepatic, or biliary disease associated with malabsorption of vitamin D.

▸ **Dietary Supplement**
PO
Adults, Elderly, Children. 10 mcg (400 units)/day.
Neonates. 10–20 mcg (400–800 units)/day.
▸ **Renal Failure**
PO
Adults, Elderly. 0.5 mg/day.
Children. 0.1–1 mg/day.
▸ **Hypoparathyroidism**
PO
Adults, Elderly. 625 mcg–5 mg/day (with calcium supplements).
Children. 1.25–5 mg/day (with calcium supplements).
▸ **Nutritional Rickets, Osteomalacia**
PO
Adults, Elderly, Children. 25–125 mcg/day for 8–12 wk.
Adults, Elderly (with malabsorption syndrome). 250–7500 mcg/day.
Children (with malabsorption syndrome). 250–625 mcg/day.
▸ **Vitamin D–Dependent Rickets**
PO
Adults, Elderly. 250 mcg–1.5 mg/day.
Children. 75–125 mcg/day.
Maximum: 1500 mcg/day.
▸ **Vitamin D–Resistant Rickets**
PO
Adults, Elderly. 250–1500 mcg/day (with phosphate supplements).
Children. Initially 1000–2000 mcg/day (with phosphate supplements). May increase in 250- to 600-mcg increments q3–4mo.

SIDE EFFECTS/ADVERSE REACTIONS

None known

PRECAUTIONS AND CONTRAINDICATIONS

Hypercalcemia, malabsorption syndrome, vitamin D toxicity

V

Caution
Cardiovascular disease, renal calculi,
hyperphosphatemia

DRUG INTERACTIONS OF CONCERN TO DENTISTRY
• Reduction in calcitriol levels:
ketoconazole

SERIOUS REACTIONS
! Early signs and symptoms of
overdose are weakness, headache,
somnolence, nausea, vomiting, dry
mouth, constipation, muscle and
bone pain, and metallic taste.
! Later signs and symptoms of
overdose include polyuria, polydipsia,
anorexia, weight loss, nocturia,
photophobia, rhinorrhea, pruritus,
disorientation, hallucinations,
hyperthermia, hypertension, and
cardiac arrhythmias.

DENTAL CONSIDERATIONS
General:
• Sensitivity of eyes to dental light
may indicate late toxicity.
Teach Patient/Family to:
• Be aware that oral side effects are
associated with early symptoms of
overdose

vitamin E
vight´-ah-min E
(Aqua Gem E, Aquasol E, E-Gems,
Key-E, Key-E Kaps)
Do not confuse Aquasol E with
Anusol.

CATEGORY AND SCHEDULE
Pregnancy Risk Category: A (C if
used in doses above recommended
daily allowance)
OTC

Drug Class: Vitamin E
(fat-soluble vitamin)

MECHANISM OF ACTION
An antioxidant that prevents
oxidation of vitamins A and C,
protects fatty acids from attack by
free radicals, and protects RBCs
from hemolysis by oxidizing agents.
Therapeutic Effect: Prevents and
treats vitamin E deficiency.

USES
Treatment of vitamin E deficiency,
hemolytic anemia in premature
neonates, prevention of retrolental
fibroplasia

PHARMACOKINETICS
Variably absorbed from the GI tract
(requires bile salts, dietary fat, and
normal pancreatic function).
Primarily concentrated in adipose
tissue. Metabolized in the liver.
Primarily eliminated by biliary
system.

INDICATIONS AND DOSAGES
▶ Vitamin E Deficiency
PO
Adults, Elderly. 60–75 units/day.
Children. 1 unit/kg/day.

SIDE EFFECTS/ADVERSE REACTIONS
CNS: Headache, fatigue
CV: Increased risk of
thrombophlebitis
GI: Nausea, cramps, diarrhea
GU: Gonadal dysfunction
EENT: Blurred vision
Integ: Sterile abscess, contact
dermatitis
MS: Weakness
Meta: Altered metabolism of
hormones (thyroid, pituitary,
adrenal), altered immunity

V

PRECAUTIONS AND CONTRAINDICATIONS

None significant

DRUG INTERACTIONS OF CONCERN TO DENTISTRY

• With doses greater than 400 international units: increased action of oral anticoagulants

SERIOUS REACTIONS

! Chronic overdose may produce fatigue, weakness, nausea, headache, blurred vision, flatulence, and diarrhea.

DENTAL CONSIDERATIONS

General:
• Determine why the patient is taking the drug.

V

warfarin sodium
war´-far-in soe´-dee-um
(Apo-Warfarin[CAN], Coumadin,
Gen-Warfarin[CAN], Jantoven,
Marevan[AUS], Tar-Warfarin[CAN])
Do not confuse Coumadin with
Kemadrin.

CATEGORY AND SCHEDULE
Pregnancy Risk Category: D

Drug Class: Oral anticoagulant

MECHANISM OF ACTION
A coumarin derivative that interferes
with hepatic synthesis of vitamin K-
dependent clotting factors, resulting
in depletion of coagulation factors II,
VII, IX, and X. *Therapeutic Effect:*
Prevents further extension of formed
existing clot; prevents new clot
formation or secondary
thromboembolic complications.

USES
Treatment of pulmonary emboli,
deep vein thrombosis (DVT), MI,
atrial dysrhythmias, to reduce risk of
recurrent MI and thromboembolic
events

PHARMACOKINETICS

Route	Onset	Peak	Duration
PO	1.5–3 days	5–7 days	N/A

Well absorbed from the GI tract.
Metabolized in the liver. Primarily
excreted in urine. Not removed by
hemodialysis. *Half-life:* 1.5–2.5 days.

INDICATIONS AND DOSAGES
▶ Anticoagulant
PO
Adults, Elderly. Initially, 5–15 mg/day
for 2–5 days; then adjust based on
INR. Maintenance: 2–10 mg/day.

Children. Initially, 0.1–0.2 mg/kg
(maximum 10 mg). Maintenance:
0.05–0.34 mg/kg/day.
▶ Usual Elderly Dosage
(Maintenance)
PO, IV
Elderly. 2–5 mg/day.

SIDE EFFECTS/ADVERSE REACTIONS
Occasional
GI distress, such as nausea, anorexia,
abdominal cramps, diarrhea
Rare
Hypersensitivity reaction including
dermatitis and urticaria, especially in
those sensitive to aspirin

PRECAUTIONS AND CONTRAINDICATIONS
Neurosurgical procedures, open
wounds, pregnancy, severe
hypertension, severe hepatic or renal
damage, uncontrolled bleeding,
ulcers
Caution
Alcoholism, elderly

DRUG INTERACTIONS OF CONCERN TO DENTISTRY
• Increased action: diflunisal,
salicylates, propoxyphene,
metronidazole, erythromycin,
clarithromycin, ketoconazole,
itraconazole, fluconazole, NSAIDs,
indomethacin, chloral hydrate,
tetracyclines, fluoroquinolones,
acetaminophen, ciprofloxacin,
levofloxacin
• If NSAIDs must be used, monitor
patient (avoid aspirin)
• Decreased action: barbiturates,
carbamazepine
• Possible increase in anticoagulant
effects with celecoxib, rofecoxib,
acetaminophen (monitor INR levels)
• Herbal products with some
anticoagulant activity: feverfew,
garlic, ginger, ginkgo, ginseng

SERIOUS REACTIONS

! Bleeding complications ranging from local ecchymoses to major hemorrhage may occur. Drug should be discontinued immediately and vitamin K or phytonadione administered. Mild hemorrhage: 2.5–10 mg PO, IM, or IV. Severe hemorrhage: 10–15 mg IV and repeated q4h as necessary.

! Hepatotoxicity, blood dyscrasias, necrosis, vasculitis, and local thrombosis occur rarely.

DENTAL CONSIDERATIONS

General:

• Reports on concomitant use of acetaminophen and warfarin seem to suggest a possible increase in anticoagulant effects, especially in patients with other diseases or contributing factors (diarrhea, age, debilitation, etc.). Patients taking warfarin should be questioned about recent use of acetaminophen and current INR values. Acetaminophen has been shown to increase the INR, depending on the amount of acetaminophen taken and duration of use. A new PT or INR value may be required if surgical procedures are planned. Data from one study indicated that use of 4 regular-strength acetaminophen tablets (325 mg) every day for 1 wk can increase INR values. Use of acetaminophen over a long duration and in higher doses suggests that it is important to closely monitor INR values (JAMA 279:657–662, 1998).

• Patients on chronic drug therapy may rarely have symptoms of blood dyscrasias, which can include infection, bleeding, and poor healing.

• Consider local hemostasis measures to prevent excessive bleeding.

• Increased bleeding may occur with IM injections.

Consultations:

• Medical consultation should include PPT, PT, or INR.

• For dental surgical procedures that may result in excessive bleeding, consider requesting physician to make dose reduction before dental treatment so that PT is no more than twice normal.

• In a patient with symptoms of blood dyscrasias, request a medical consultation for blood studies and postpone dental treatment until normal values are reestablished.

Teach Patient/Family to:

• Use effective oral hygiene to prevent soft tissue inflammation

• Use caution to prevent injury when using oral hygiene aids

• Report oral lesions, soreness, or bleeding to dentist

W

zafirlukast
za-feer´-loo-kast
(Accolate)
Do not confuse Accolate with
Accupril or Aclovate.

CATEGORY AND SCHEDULE
Pregnancy Risk Category: B

Drug Class: Selective
leukotriene receptor antagonist

MECHANISM OF ACTION
An antiasthmic that binds to
leukotriene receptors, inhibiting
bronchoconstriction caused by sulfur
dioxide, cold air, and specific
antigens, such as grass, cat dander,
and ragweed. *Therapeutic Effect:*
Reduces airway edema and smooth
muscle constriction; alters cellular
activity associated with the
inflammatory process.

USES
Prophylaxis and chronic treatment
of asthma

PHARMACOKINETICS
Rapidly absorbed after PO
administration (food reduces
absorption). Protein binding: 99%.
Extensively metabolized in the liver.
Primarily excreted in feces.
Unknown if removed by
hemodialysis. *Half-life:* 10 hr.

INDICATIONS AND DOSAGES
▶ **Bronchial Asthma**
PO
*Adults, Elderly, Children 12 yr and
older.* 20 mg twice a day.
Children 5–11 yr. 10 mg twice a day.

SIDE EFFECTS/ADVERSE
REACTIONS
Frequent
Headache

Occasional
Nausea, diarrhea
Rare
Generalized pain, asthenia, myalgia,
fever, dyspepsia, vomiting,
dizziness

PRECAUTIONS AND
CONTRAINDICATIONS
Hypersensitivity, hepatic
dysfunction with prior use of
zafirlukast
Caution
Not for acute bronchospasm, food
decreases bioavailability, pregnancy
category B, lactation, patients
younger than 7 yr, hepatic
impairment, liver enzyme elevation,
elderly (increased infection); if liver
dysfunction suspected, discontinue
use and measure liver enzymes,
serum ALT (SPGT)

DRUG INTERACTIONS OF
CONCERN TO DENTISTRY
• Increased PT with concurrent use
of warfarin
• Reduced plasma levels:
erythromycin, terfenadine,
theophylline
• Increased plasma levels with
aspirin
• Inhibits CYP2C9 and CYP3A4
isoenzymes: use with caution when
drugs metabolized by these enzymes
are used

SERIOUS REACTIONS
! Concurrent administration of
inhaled corticosteroids increases the
risk of upper respiratory tract
infection.

DENTAL CONSIDERATIONS
General:
• Midday appointments and a stress-
reduction protocol may be required
for anxious patients.

Z

• Avoid prescribing aspirin-containing products.

• Acute asthmatic episodes may be precipitated in the dental office. Sympathomimetic inhalants should be available for emergency use. A stress reduction protocol may be required.

• Be aware that aspirin or sulfite preservatives in vasoconstrictor-containing products can exacerbate asthma.

• Consider semisupine chair position for patients with respiratory disease or if GI side effects occur.

Consultations:

• Medical consultation may be required to assess disease control.

Teach Patient/Family to:

• Use electric tooth brush if patient has difficulty holding conventional devices

• Update health and drug history if physician makes any changes in evaluation or drug regimens; include OTC, herbal, and nonherbal remedies in the update

zalcitabine
zal-site´-ah-been
(Hivid)

CATEGORY AND SCHEDULE
Pregnancy Risk Category: C

Drug Class: Synthetic pyrimidine antiviral

MECHANISM OF ACTION
A nucleoside reverse transcriptase inhibitor that inhibits viral DNA synthesis. ***Therapeutic Effect:*** Prevents replication of HIV-1.

USES
Treatment of advanced HIV infection in combination with zidovudine

PHARMACOKINETICS
Readily absorbed from the GI tract (absorption decreased by food). Protein binding: less than 4%. Undergoes phosphorylation intracellularly to the active metabolite. Primarily excreted in urine. Removed by hemodialysis. ***Half-life:*** 1–3 hr; metabolite, 2.6–10 hr (increased in impaired renal function).

INDICATIONS AND DOSAGES
▸ **HIV Infection (in combination with other antiretrovirals)**
PO
Adults, Children 13 yr and older.
0.75 mg q8h.
Children younger than 13 yr.
0.01 mg/kg q8h.
Range: 0.005–0.01 mg/kg q8h.
▸ **Dosage in Renal Impairment**
Dosage and frequency are modified on the basis of creatinine clearance.

Creatinine Clearance	Dose
10–40 ml/min	0.75 mg q12h
Less than 10 ml/min	0.75 mg q24h

SIDE EFFECTS/ADVERSE REACTIONS
Frequent
Peripheral neuropathy, fever, fatigue, headache, rash
Occasional
Diarrhea, abdominal pain, oral ulcers, cough, pruritus, myalgia, weight loss, nausea, vomiting
Rare
Nasal discharge, dysphagia, depression, night sweats, confusion

PRECAUTIONS AND CONTRAINDICATIONS
Moderate or severe peripheral neuropathy

Caution
Lactation, children younger than 13
yr, renal impairment, hepatic
impairment, risk of serious
peripheral neuropathy, risk of severe
hepatic impairment, CHF

DRUG INTERACTIONS OF CONCERN TO DENTISTRY

• Increased peripheral neuropathy:
metronidazole, dapsone, or other
drugs associated with peripheral
neuropathy

SERIOUS REACTIONS

❗ Peripheral neuropathy
(characterized by numbness, tingling,
burning, and pain in the lower
extremities) occurs in 17% to 31% of
patients. These symptoms may be
followed by sharp, shooting pain and
progress to a severe, continuous,
burning pain that may be irreversible
if the drug is not discontinued in
time.
❗ Pancreatitis, leukopenia,
neutropenia, eosinophilia, and
thrombocytopenia occur rarely.

DENTAL CONSIDERATIONS

General:
• Examine oral cavity for side effects
if on long-term drug therapy.
• Monitor vital signs at every
appointment because of
cardiovascular side effects.
• Palliative medication may be
required for management of oral side
effects.
• Assess salivary flow as a factor in
caries, periodontal disease, and
candidiasis.
• Prophylactic antibiotics may be
indicated to prevent infection if
surgery or deep scaling is planned.
• Patients may be more susceptible
to infection and have delayed wound
healing.

Consultations:
• Medical consultation may be
required to assess disease control and
patient's ability to tolerate stress.
Teach Patient/Family to:
• Use effective oral hygiene to
prevent soft tissue inflammation
• Use caution to prevent injury when
using oral hygiene aids
• See dentist immediately if
secondary oral infection occurs
• When chronic dry mouth occurs,
advise patient to:
  • Avoid mouth rinses with high
  alcohol content because of drying
  effects
  • Use daily home fluoride products
  to prevent caries
  • Use sugarless gum, frequent sips
  of water, or saliva substitutes

zaleplon
zal´-eh-plon
(Sonata, Stamoc[CAN])

CATEGORY AND SCHEDULE
Pregnancy Risk Category: C
Controlled Substance Schedule IV

Drug Class: Hypnotic

MECHANISM OF ACTION
A nonbenzodiazepine that
enhances the action of the
inhibitory neurotransmitter
gamma-aminobutyric acid.
Therapeutic Effect: Induces
sleep.

USES
Short-term treatment of insomnia

PHARMACOKINETICS
PO: Rapid absorption,
bioavailability 30%, peak plasma
levels 1 hr, wide tissue distribution,

rapid hepatic metabolism
(CYP3A4 minor pathway), excretion
in urine; heavy, high-fat meal
significantly delays absorption

INDICATIONS AND DOSAGES
▶ **Insomnia**
PO
Adults. 10 mg at bedtime. Range:
5–20 mg.
Elderly. 5 mg at bedtime.

SIDE EFFECTS/ADVERSE REACTIONS
Expected
Somnolence, sedation, mild rebound
insomnia (on first night after drug is
discontinued)
Frequent
Nausea, headache, myalgia,
dizziness
Occasional
Abdominal pain, asthenia, dyspepsia,
eye pain, paresthesia
Rare
Tremors, amnesia, hyperacusis
(acute sense of hearing), fever,
dysmenorrhea

PRECAUTIONS AND CONTRAINDICATIONS
Severe hepatic impairment
Caution
Abuse potential similar to
benzodiazepines, elderly, debilitated,
smaller patients adjust dose
downward; lactation, children

DRUG INTERACTIONS OF CONCERN TO DENTISTRY
• Caution when using dental drugs
that inhibit or induce cytochrome
P-450 enzymes; this drug is a minor
substrate for CYP3A4; however, use
caution (see Appendix I)
• CNS depression: all CNS
depressant drugs

SERIOUS REACTIONS
! Zaleplon may produce altered
concentration, behavior changes, and
impaired memory.
! Taking the drug while up and about
may result in adverse CNS effects,
such as hallucinations, impaired
coordination, dizziness, and
light-headedness.
! Overdose results in somnolence,
confusion, diminished reflexes, and
coma.

DENTAL CONSIDERATIONS
General:
• Assess salivary flow as a factor in
caries, periodontal disease, and
candidiasis.
• Determine why patient is taking
the drug.
• Consider semisupine chair position
for patient comfort if GI side effects
occur.
Consultations:
• Medical consultation may be
required to assess disease control and
patient's ability to tolerate stress.
Teach Patient/Family:
• When chronic dry mouth occurs,
advise patient to:
  • Avoid mouth rinses with high
  alcohol content because of drying
  effects
  • Use daily home fluoride products
  for anticaries effect
  • Use sugarless gum, frequent sips
  of water, or saliva substitutes

zanamivir
za-na´-mi-veer
(Relenza)

CATEGORY AND SCHEDULE
Pregnancy Risk Category: B

Drug Class: Antiviral

MECHANISM OF ACTION

An antiviral that appears to inhibit the influenza virus enzyme neuraminidase, which is essential for viral replication. ***Therapeutic Effect:*** Prevents viral release from infected cells.

USES

Treatment of uncomplicated influenza in adults and children older than 7 yr with symptoms of no more than 2 days; more effective against influenza type A virus

PHARMACOKINETICS

Inhalation: 4%–17% of inhaled dose is absorbed, peak serum levels 1–2 hr, low plasma protein binding (less than 10%), excreted unchanged in urine.

INDICATIONS AND DOSAGES

▶ **Influenza Virus**
Inhalation
Adults, Elderly, Children 7 yr and older. 2 inhalations (one 5-mg blister per inhalation for a total dose of 10 mg) twice a day (about 12 hr apart) for 5 days.
▶ **Prevention of Influenza Virus**
Inhalation
Adults, Elderly. 2 inhalations once a day for the duration of the exposure period.

SIDE EFFECTS/ADVERSE REACTIONS

Occasional
Diarrhea, sinusitis, nausea, bronchitis, cough, dizziness, headache
Rare
Malaise, fatigue, fever, abdominal pain, myalgia, arthralgia, urticaria

PRECAUTIONS AND CONTRAINDICATIONS

Hypersensitivity
Caution
Teach use of inhaler to patient; chronic obstructive pulmonary disease or asthma does not preclude influenza vaccine, safety in children younger than 12 yr not established

DRUG INTERACTIONS OF CONCERN TO DENTISTRY

None reported

SERIOUS REACTIONS

! Neutropenia may occur.
! Bronchospasm may occur in those with a history of COPD or bronchial asthma.

DENTAL CONSIDERATIONS

General:
• Acute influenza patients are unlikely to be seen in the dental office except for dental emergencies.

ziconotide
zi-koe´-no-tide
(Prialt)

CATEGORY AND SCHEDULE
Pregnancy Risk Category: C

Drug Class: Analgesic

MECHANISM OF ACTION

A synthetic peptide that selectively binds to *N*-type voltage-sensitive calcium channels located on afferent nerves in the spinal cord. This binding is thought to block *N*-type calcium channels. ***Therapeutic Effect:*** Blocks excitatory neurotransmitter release, reducing sensitivity to painful stimuli.

USES
Reduction of chronic pain in the body

PHARMACOKINETICS
Elimination Half-life: 4.6 hr
after intrathecal administration.
50% bound to plasma proteins;
metabolized in multiple organs.
Excreted in urine as proteolytic
degradation products.

INDICATIONS AND DOSAGES
▶ **Pain control**
Intrathecal
Adults, Elderly. Initially, 2.4 mcg/day
(0.1 mcg/hr). May titrate to maximum
of 19.2 mcg/day (0.8 mcg/hr).

SIDE EFFECTS/ADVERSE REACTIONS
Frequent
Dizziness, nausea, somnolence,
weakness, diarrhea, confusion,
ataxia, headache, vomiting, gait
disturbance, memory impairment,
hypertonia
Occasional
Anorexia, visual disturbances,
anxiety, urinary retention, speech
disorder, aphasia, nystagmus,
paresthesia, fever, hallucinations,
nervousness, vertigo
Rare
Insomnia, dry skin, constipation,
arthralgia, myalgia, tremor

PRECAUTIONS AND CONTRAINDICATIONS
History of psychosis, presence of
infection at the injection site,
uncontrolled bleeding, or spinal
canal obstruction that impairs CSF
circulation, IV administration

DRUG INTERACTIONS OF CONCERN TO DENTISTRY
• Enhanced CNS depression: all
CNS depressants

SERIOUS REACTIONS
❗ Atrial fibrillation, cerebral vascular
accident, seizures, kidney failure
(acute), myoclonus, and psychosis
occur rarely.

DENTAL CONSIDERATIONS
General:
• Determine why patient is taking
the drug.
• For use in the hospital setting.
Consultations:
• Medical consultation may be
required to assess disease control and
patient's ability to tolerate stress.
Teach Patient/Family to:
• Use effective oral hygiene to
prevent soft tissue inflammation
• Update health and medication
history if physician makes any
changes in evaluation or drug
regimens; include OTC, herbal, and
nonherbal remedies in the update

zidovudine
zyde-oh´-vue-deen
(Apo-Zidovudine[CAN], AZT,
Novo-AZT[CAN], Retrovir)
Do not confuse Retrovir with
ritonavir.

CATEGORY AND SCHEDULE
Pregnancy Risk Category: C

Drug Class: Antiviral thymidine
analog

MECHANISM OF ACTION
A nucleoside reverse transcriptase
inhibitor that interferes with viral
RNA-dependent DNA polymerase,
an enzyme necessary for viral HIV
replication. *Therapeutic Effect:*
Interferes with HIV replication,
slowing the progression of HIV
infection.

USES

Treatment of symptomatic HIV infections (AIDS, ARC), confirmed *P. carinii* pneumonia (PCP), or absolute CD4 lymphocytes less than 200/mm^3; prevention of maternal-fetal transmission

PHARMACOKINETICS

Rapidly and completely absorbed from the GI tract. Protein binding: 25%–38%. Undergoes first-pass metabolism in the liver. Crosses the blood-brain barrier and is widely distributed, including to CSF. Primarily excreted in urine. Minimal removal by hemodialysis. *Half-life:* 0.8–1.2 hr (increased in impaired renal function).

INDICATIONS AND DOSAGES
▸ **HIV Infection**
PO
Adults, Elderly, Children older than 12 yr. 200 mg q8h or 300 mg q12h.
Children 12 yr and younger. 160 mg/m2/dose q8h.
Range: 90–180 mg/m^2/dose q6–8h.
Neonates. 2 mg/kg/dose q6h.
IV
Adults, Elderly, Children older than 12 yr. 1–2 mg/kg/dose q4h.
Children 12 yr and younger. 120 mg/m^2/dose q6h.
Neonates. 1.5 mg/kg/dose q6h.

SIDE EFFECTS/ADVERSE REACTIONS
Expected
Nausea, headache
Frequent
Abdominal pain, asthenia, rash, fever, acne
Occasional
Diarrhea, anorexia, malaise, myalgia, somnolence
Rare
Dizziness, paresthesia, vomiting, insomnia, dyspnea, altered taste

PRECAUTIONS AND CONTRAINDICATIONS

Life-threatening allergic reactions to zidovudine or its components
Caution
Granulocyte count less than 1000/mm^3 or Hgb less than 9.5 g/dl, lactation, children, severe renal disease, severe hepatic function, risk of severe neutropenia and anemia

DRUG INTERACTIONS OF CONCERN TO DENTISTRY
• Decreased blood levels: acetaminophen, clarithromycin
• Increased serum levels: fluconazole

SERIOUS REACTIONS
! Serious reactions include anemia, which occurs most commonly after 4–6 wk of therapy, and granulocytopenia; both effects are more likely to occur in patients who have a low Hgb level or granulocyte count before beginning therapy.
! Neurotoxicity (as evidenced by ataxia, fatigue, lethargy, nystagmus, and seizures) may occur.

DENTAL CONSIDERATIONS
General:
• Examine for oral manifestations of opportunistic infections.
• Patients on chronic drug therapy may rarely have symptoms of blood dyscrasias, which can include infection, bleeding, and poor healing.
• Avoid dental light in patient's eyes; offer dark glasses for patient comfort.
• Place on frequent recall because of oral side effects.
Consultations:
• In a patient with symptoms of blood dyscrasias, request a medical consultation for blood studies and postpone dental treatment until normal values are reestablished.

• Medical consultation may be required to assess disease control.
Teach Patient/Family to:
• Use effective oral hygiene to prevent soft tissue inflammation
• Use caution to prevent injury when using oral hygiene aids
• See dentist immediately if secondary oral infection occurs

zileuton
zye-lew´-ton
(zyelo)
Do not confuse Zyflo with Zyban.

CATEGORY AND SCHEDULE
Pregnancy Risk Category: C

Drug Class: Leukotriene pathway inhibitor

MECHANISM OF ACTION
A leukotriene inhibitor that inhibits the enzyme responsible for producing inflammatory response. Prevents formation of leukotrienes (leukotrienes induce bronchoconstriction response, enhances vascular permeability, stimulates mucus secretion).
Therapeutic Effect: Prevents airway edema, smooth muscle contraction, and the inflammatory process, relieving signs and symptoms of bronchial asthma.

USES
Prophylaxis and chronic treatment of asthma

PHARMACOKINETICS
Rapidly absorbed from GI tract. Protein binding: 93%. Metabolized in liver. Primarily excreted in urine. Unknown if removed by hemodialysis. **Half-life:** 2.1–2.5 hr.

INDICATIONS AND DOSAGES
▶ **Bronchial Asthma**
PO
Adults, Elderly, Children 12 yr and older. 600 mg 4 times a day.
Total daily dosage: 2400 mg.

SIDE EFFECTS/ADVERSE REACTIONS
Frequent
Headache
Occasional
Dyspepsia, nausea, abdominal pain, asthenia (loss of strength), myalgia
Rare
Conjunctivitis, constipation, dizziness, flatulence, insomnia

PRECAUTIONS AND CONTRAINDICATIONS
Active liver disease, impaired liver function, hypersensitivity to zileuton or any component of the formulation.
Caution
Not for acute bronchospasm, status asthmaticus; theophylline, warfarin, propranolol; hepatic impairment, lactation, children younger than 12 yr, monitor ALT (SGPT) levels

DRUG INTERACTIONS OF CONCERN TO DENTISTRY
• Increased plasma levels of theophylline, propranolol
• Significant increase in PT when taking warfarin
• Use caution when prescribing dental drugs that are strong inhibitors of CYP1A2 isoenzymes

SERIOUS REACTIONS
! Liver dysfunction occurs rarely and may be manifested as right upper quadrant pain, nausea, fatigue,

Z

lethargy, pruritus, jaundice or flu-like symptoms.

DENTAL CONSIDERATIONS
General:
• Consider semisupine chair position for patient comfort because of GI side effects of disease.
• Acute asthmatic episodes may be precipitated in the dental office. Sympathomimetic inhalants should be available for emergency use.
• Midday appointments and a stress reduction protocol may be required for anxious patients.
• Be aware that aspirin or sulfite preservatives in vasoconstrictor-containing products can exacerbate asthma.
Consultations:
• Medical consultation may be required to assess disease control.
Teach Patient/Family to:
• Update health and drug history if physician makes any changes in evaluation or drug regimens; include OTC, herbal, and nonherbal remedies in the update

zinc oxide/zinc sulfate
zink´ox´-eyed/zink´sul´-fate
(zinc oxide: Balmex, Desitin; zinc sulfate: Orazinc, Zincaps[AUS])

CATEGORY AND SCHEDULE
Pregnancy Risk Category: C

Drug Class: Mineral

MECHANISM OF ACTION
A mineral that acts as a cofactor for enzymes that are important for protein and carbohydrate metabolism. ***Therapeutic Effect:*** Zinc oxide acts as a mild astringent

and skin protectant. Zinc sulfate helps maintain normal growth and tissue repair, as well as skin hydration.

USES
Treatment of zinc deficiency

INDICATIONS AND DOSAGES
▶ **Mild Skin Irritations and Abrasions (such as chapped skin, diaper rash)**
Topical (zinc oxide)
Adults, Elderly, Children. Apply as needed.
▶ **Treatment and Prevention of Zinc Deficiency, Wound Healing**
PO (zinc sulfate)
Adults, Elderly. 220 mg 3 times a day.

SIDE EFFECTS/ADVERSE REACTIONS
None known

PRECAUTIONS AND CONTRAINDICATIONS
None known

DRUG INTERACTIONS OF CONCERN TO DENTISTRY
• Decreased absorption: tetracyclines, fluoroquinolones

SERIOUS REACTIONS
None known

DENTAL CONSIDERATIONS
General:
• Determine why patient is taking the drug.

ziprasidone
zye-pray´-za-done
(geodon)

CATEGORY AND SCHEDULE
Pregnancy Risk Category: C

Drug Class: Antipsychotic, atypical

Z

MECHANISM OF ACTION

A piperazine derivative that antagonizes β-adrenergic, dopamine, histamine, and serotonin receptors; also inhibits reuptake of serotonin and norepinephrine. *Therapeutic Effect:* Diminishes symptoms of schizophrenia and depression.

USES

Treatment of schizophrenia

PHARMACOKINETICS

Well absorbed after PO administration. Food increases bioavailability. Protein binding: 99%. Extensively metabolized in the liver. Not removed by hemodialysis. *Half-life:* 7 hr.

INDICATIONS AND DOSAGES

▶ **Schizophrenia**
PO
Adults, Elderly. Initially, 20 mg twice a day with food. Titrate at intervals of no less than 2 days. Maximum: 80 mg twice a day.
IM
Adults, Elderly. 10 mg q2h or 20 mg q4h. Maximum: 40 mg/day.
▶ **Bipolar Mania**
PO
Adults, Elderly. 40 mg 2 times a day.

SIDE EFFECTS/ADVERSE REACTIONS

Frequent
Headache, somnolence, dizziness
Occasional
Rash, orthostatic hypotension, weight gain, restlessness, constipation, dyspepsia

PRECAUTIONS AND CONTRAINDICATIONS

Conditions that prolong the QT interval, such as congenital long QT syndrome

Caution
May antagonize levodopa, dopamine agonists; QT prolongation and risk of sudden death, bradycardia, hypokalemia, hypomagnesemia, electrolyte depletion caused by diarrhea, diuretics, or vomiting, neuromalignant syndrome, tardive dyskinesia, seizures, suicide, lactation, pediatric use

DRUG INTERACTIONS OF CONCERN TO DENTISTRY

• Avoid use of any drug that prolongs the QT interval
• Caution in use of other CNS depressants: increased risk of CNS depressant effects
• Reduced plasma levels: carbamazepine
• Increased plasma levels: ketoconazole and other strong inhibitors of CYP3A4 isoenzymes (see Appendix I)
• Drugs that lower B/P: increased risk of hypotension
• Increased extrapyramidal effects: phenothiazines and related drugs (haloperidol, droperidol), metoclopramide

SERIOUS REACTIONS

! Prolongation of QT interval may produce torsades de pointes, a form of ventricular tachycardia. Patients with bradycardia, hypokalemia, or hypomagnesemia are at increased risk.

DENTAL CONSIDERATIONS

General:
• Monitor vital signs at every appointment because of cardiovascular side effects.
• After supine positioning, have patient sit upright for at least 2 min

before standing to avoid orthostatic hypotension.
• Assess salivary flow as a factor in caries, periodontal disease, and candidiasis.
• Consider semisupine chair position for patient comfort if GI side effects occur.
• Assess for presence of extrapyramidal motor symptoms, such as tardive dyskinesia and akathisia. Extrapyramidal motor activity may complicate dental treatment.
• Use vasoconstrictors with caution, in low doses, and with careful aspiration; avoid use of epinephrine-impregnated gingival retraction cord.
Consultations:
• Consultation with physician may be necessary if sedation or general anesthesia is required.
• Physician should be informed if significant xerostomic side effects occur (e.g., increased caries, sore tongue, problems eating or swallowing, difficulty wearing prosthesis) so that a medication change can be considered.
• Medical consultation may be required to assess disease control and patient's ability to tolerate stress.
Teach Patient/Family to:
• Use effective oral hygiene to prevent soft tissue inflammation
• Prevent trauma when using oral hygiene aids
• Use electric tooth brush if patient has difficulty holding conventional devices
• When chronic dry mouth occurs, advise patient to:
  • Avoid mouth rinses with high alcohol content because of drying effects
  • Use daily home fluoride products for anticaries effect
  • Use sugarless gum, frequent sips of water, or saliva substitutes

zoledronic acid
zole-eh-drone´-ick ass´-id
(zometa)

CATEGORY AND SCHEDULE
Pregnancy Risk Category: C

Drug Class: Osteoporosis therapy adjunct, bisphosphonate

MECHANISM OF ACTION
A bisphosphonate that inhibits the resorption of mineralized bone and cartilage; inhibits increased osteoclastic activity and skeletal calcium release induced by stimulatory factors produced by tumors. *Therapeutic Effect:* Increases urinary calcium and phosphorus excretion; decreases serum calcium and phosphorus levels.

USES
Treatment of hypercalcemia from malignancy, bone metastases associated with prostate and lung cancer; multiple myeloma, bone metastases from solid tumors

PHARMACOKINETICS
IV Infusion: Shows triphasic half-life; plasma protein binding 22%; little to no metabolism; excreted mainly in urine; a high percentage of the dose remains bound to bone

INDICATIONS AND DOSAGES
▶ **Hypercalcemia**
IV Infusion
Adults, Elderly. 4 mg IV infusion given over no less than 15 min. Retreatment may be considered, but at least 7 days should elapse to allow for full response to initial dose.

Z

▶ **Multiple Myeloma**
IV
Adults, Elderly. 4 mg q3–4wk.

SIDE EFFECTS/ADVERSE REACTIONS
Frequent
Fever, nausea, vomiting, constipation
Occasional
Hypotension, anxiety, insomnia, flu-like symptoms (fever, chills, bone pain, myalgia, and arthralgia)
Rare
Conjunctivitis

PRECAUTIONS AND CONTRAINDICATIONS
Hypersensitivity to other bisphosphonates, including alendronate, etidronate, pamidronate, risedronate, and tiludronate. Dental implants are contraindicated for patients taking this drug.
Caution
Data for use in children not available, monitor hypercalcemic parameters, ensure good hydration, renal impairment, bronchospasm in aspirin-sensitive asthmatics, hypocalcemia, hypoparathyroidism, lactation

DRUG INTERACTIONS OF CONCERN TO DENTISTRY
None reported

SERIOUS REACTIONS
! Renal toxicity may occur if IV infusion is administered in less than 15 min.

DENTAL CONSIDERATIONS
General:
• This drug is used only in oncology units or hospitals.
• Examine for oral manifestation of opportunistic infection.

• Consider semisupine chair position for patient comfort if GI side effects occur.
• Short appointments may be required.
• If oral candidiasis occurs, treat with suitable antifungal drug.
Consultations:
• Medical consultation may be required to assess disease control.

zolmitriptan
zohl-mih-trip´-tan
(Zomig, Zomig Rapimelt[CAN], Zomig-ZMT)

CATEGORY AND SCHEDULE
Pregnancy Risk Category: C

Drug Class: Serotonin agonist

MECHANISM OF ACTION
A serotonin receptor agonist that binds selectively to vascular receptors, producing a vasoconstrictive effect on cranial blood vessels. ***Therapeutic Effect:*** Relieves migraine headache.

USES
Acute treatment of migraine with or without aura in adults

PHARMACOKINETICS
Rapidly but incompletely absorbed after PO administration. Protein binding: 15%. Undergoes first-pass metabolism in the liver to active metabolite. Eliminated primarily in urine (60%) and, to a lesser extent, in feces (30%). ***Half-life:*** 3 hr.

INDICATIONS AND DOSAGES
▶ **Acute Migraine Attack**
PO
Adults, Elderly, Children older than 18 yr. Initially, 2.5 mg or less.

If headache returns, may repeat dose in 2 hr. Maximum: 10 mg/24 hr.
Intranasal
Adults, Elderly. 5 mg. May repeat in 2 hr. Maximum: 10 mg/24hr.

SIDE EFFECTS/ADVERSE REACTIONS
Frequent
Oral: Dizziness; tingling; neck, throat, or jaw pressure; somnolence
Nasal: Altered taste, paraesthesia
Occasional
Oral: Warm or hot sensation, asthenia, chest pressure
Nasal: Nausea, somnolence, nasal discomfort, dizziness, asthenia, dry mouth
Rare
Diaphoresis, myalgia, paresthesia

PRECAUTIONS AND CONTRAINDICATIONS
Arrhythmias associated with conduction disorders, basilar or hemiplegic migraine, coronary artery disease, ischemic heart disease (including angina pectoris, history of MI, silent ischemia, and Prinzmetal's angina), uncontrolled hypertension, use within 24 hr of ergotamine-containing preparations or another serotonin receptor agonist, use within 14 days of MAOIs, Wolff-Parkinson-White syndrome
Caution
Renal impairment, hepatic impairment, may cause coronary vasospasm, lactation, children, elderly

DRUG INTERACTIONS OF CONCERN TO DENTISTRY
• Potential serotonin crises: selective serotonin reuptake inhibitors, ergot-containing drugs (avoid use within 24 hr of taking this drug)

• Decreased plasma levels: cimetidine

SERIOUS REACTIONS
! Cardiac reactions (including ischemia, coronary artery vasospasm, and MI) and noncardiac vasospasm-related reactions (such as hemorrhage and CVA) occur rarely, particularly in patients with hypertension, diabetes, or a strong family history of coronary artery disease; obese patients; smokers; males older than 40 yr; and postmenopausal women.

DENTAL CONSIDERATIONS
General:
• This is an acute-use drug; thus it is doubtful that patients will come to the office if acute migraine is present.
• Be aware of patient's disease, its severity, and its frequency, when known.
• Advise patient if dental drugs prescribed have potential for photosensitivity.
Consultations:
• If treating chronic orofacial pain, consult with physician of record.
• Medical consultation may be required to assess disease control and patient's ability to tolerate stress.
Teach Patient/Family to:
• Be aware that dryness of the mouth may occur when taking this drug
• Avoid mouth rinses with high alcohol content because of drying effects
• Update health and drug history if physician makes any changes in evaluation or drug regimens; include OTC, herbal, and nonherbal remedies in the update

zolpidem tartrate
zole-pi´-dem tar´-trate
(Ambien, Stilnox[AUS])
Do not confuse Ambien with Amen.

CATEGORY AND SCHEDULE
Pregnancy Risk Category: B
Controlled Substance: Schedule IV

Drug Class: Nonbarbiturate,
nonbenzodiazepine
sedative-hypnotic

MECHANISM OF ACTION
A nonbenzodiazepine that enhances
the action of the inhibitory
neurotransmitter gamma-
aminobutyric acid. *Therapeutic
Effect:* Induces sleep and improves
sleep quality.

USES
Treatment of insomnia

PHARMACOKINETICS

Route	Onset	Peak	Duration
PO	30 min	N/A	6–8 hr

Rapidly absorbed from the GI tract.
Protein binding: 92%. Metabolized
in the liver; excreted in urine.
Not removed by hemodialysis.
Half-life: 1.4–4.5 hr (increased in
hepatic impairment).

INDICATIONS AND DOSAGES
▶ **Insomnia**
PO
Adults. 10 mg at bedtime.
Elderly, Debilitated. 5 mg at
bedtime.

SIDE EFFECTS/ADVERSE REACTIONS
Occasional
Headache

Rare
Dizziness, nausea, diarrhea, muscle
pain

PRECAUTIONS AND CONTRAINDICATIONS
Hypersensitivity, ritonavir
Caution
Discontinue if skin rash occurs,
pediatric patients at risk for
oligohidrosis, hyperthermia;
seizures with abrupt withdrawal; use
contraception in women of
childbearing age; hepatic or renal
dysfunction; lactation, kidney stones

DRUG INTERACTIONS OF CONCERN TO DENTISTRY
• Increased CNS depression: alcohol,
all CNS depressants, fluconazole,
ketoconazole, itraconazole

SERIOUS REACTIONS
! Overdose may produce severe
ataxia, bradycardia, altered
vision (such as diplopia), severe
drowsiness, nausea and vomiting,
difficulty breathing, and
unconsciousness.
! Abrupt withdrawal of the drug
after long-term use may produce
asthenia, facial flushing, diaphoresis,
vomiting, and tremor.
! Drug tolerance or dependence may
occur with prolonged, high-dose
therapy.

DENTAL CONSIDERATIONS
General:
• Assess salivary flow as a factor in
caries, periodontal disease, and
candidiasis.
• Monitor vital signs at every
appointment because of
cardiovascular side effects.
Consultations:
• Medical consultation may be
required to assess disease control.

Teach Patient/Family:
• When chronic dry mouth occurs, advise patient to:
  • Avoid mouth rinses with high alcohol content because of drying effects
  • Use daily home fluoride products to prevent caries
  • Use sugarless gum, frequent sips of water, or saliva substitutes

zonisamide
zoh-nis´-ah-mide
(Zonegran)

CATEGORY AND SCHEDULE
Pregnancy Risk Category: C

Drug Class: Anticonvulsant (sulfonamide derivative)

MECHANISM OF ACTION
A succinimide that may stabilize neuronal membranes and suppress neuronal hypersynchronization by blocking sodium and calcium channels. *Therapeutic Effect:* Reduces seizure activity.

USES
Adjunctive therapy in partial seizures in adults with epilepsy

PHARMACOKINETICS
Well absorbed after PO administration. Extensively bound to RBCs. Protein binding: 40%. Primarily excreted in urine. *Half-life:* 63 hr (plasma), 105 hr (RBCs).

INDICATIONS AND DOSAGES
▶ **Partial Seizures**
PO
Adults, Elderly, Children older than 16 yr. Initially, 100 mg/day for 2 wk. May increase by 100 mg/day at intervals of 2 wk or longer. Range: 100–600 mg/day.

SIDE EFFECTS/ADVERSE REACTIONS
Frequent
Somnolence, dizziness, anorexia, headache, agitation, irritability, nausea
Occasional
Fatigue, ataxia, confusion, depression, impaired memory or concentration, insomnia, abdominal pain, diplopia, diarrhea, speech difficulty
Rare
Paresthesia, nystagmus, anxiety, rash, dyspepsia, weight loss

PRECAUTIONS AND CONTRAINDICATIONS
Allergy to sulfonamides
Caution
Discontinue if skin rash occurs, pediatric patients at risk for oligohidrosis, hyperthermia; seizures with abrupt withdrawal; use contraception in women of childbearing age; hepatic or renal dysfunction; lactation, kidney stones

DRUG INTERACTIONS OF CONCERN TO DENTISTRY
• No dental drug interactions reported; it has been proposed that drugs which either induce or inhibit CYP3A4 enzymes may not significantly alter serum levels
• Carbamazepine increases renal clearance

SERIOUS REACTIONS
! Overdose is characterized by bradycardia, hypotension, respiratory depression, and coma.
! Leukopenia, anemia, and thrombocytopenia occur rarely.

DENTAL CONSIDERATIONS

General:

• Determine type of epilepsy, seizure frequency, and quality of seizure control.

• Patients on chronic drug therapy may rarely have symptoms of blood dyscrasias, which can include infection, bleeding, and poor healing.

• Short appointments and a stress reduction protocol may be required for anxious patients.

• Place on frequent recall to evaluate gingival condition and self-care.

• Consider semisupine chair position for patient comfort if GI side effects occur.

• Warn patient of increased CNS side effects when sedation is used. Advise not to drive a car to and from dental appointment.

Consultations:

• Consultation with physician may be necessary if sedation or general anesthesia is required.

• In a patient with symptoms of blood dyscrasias, request a medical consultation for blood studies and postpone treatment until normal values are reestablished.

• Medical consultation may be required to assess disease control and patient's ability to tolerate stress.

Teach Patient/Family to:

• Use effective oral hygiene to prevent soft tissue inflammation

• Prevent trauma when using oral hygiene aids

• Update health and drug history if physician makes any changes in evaluation or drug regimens; include OTC, herbal, and nonherbal remedies in the update

• See physician immediately if rash develops because of drug

Z

Appendix A   Abbreviations

ā   before

aa   of each

ab   antibody

abd   abdomen

ABGs   arterial blood gases

ac   before meals (ante cibum)

ACE   angiotensin-converting enzyme

ACEI   angiotensin-converting enzyme inhibitor

ACh   acetylcholine

ACT   activated clotting time

ACTH   adrenocorticotropic hormone

ad lib   as desired

ADH   antidiuretic hormone

ADP   adenosine diphosphate

ADR   adverse drug reaction

AIDS   acquired immunodeficiency syndrome

aka   also known as

ALT   alanine aminotransferase, serum

ama   against medical advice

amb   ambulation

amp   ampule

ANA   antinuclear antibody

ant   anterior

ANUG   acute necrotizing ulcerative gingivitis

AP   anteroposterior

APAP   N-acetyl-para-aminophenol (acetaminophen)

APB   atrial premature beat

aPTT   activated partial thromboplastin time

ARC   AIDS-related complex

AROM   active range of motion

ASA   acetylsalicylic acid (aspirin)

asap   as soon as possible

ASHD   arteriosclerotic heart disease

AST   aspartate aminotransferase, serum

AV   atrioventricular

BAC   blood alcohol concentration

bid   twice per day (bis in die)

BM   bowel movement

BMR   basal metabolic rate

bol   bolus

B/P   blood pressure

BPH   benign prostatic hypertrophy

bpm   beats per minute

BS   blood sugar

BUN   blood urea nitrogen

Bx   biopsy

c̄   with

C   Celsius (centigrade)

C section   cesarean section

CA   cancer

Ca   calcium

CAD   coronary artery disease

cAMP   cyclic adenosine monophosphate

cap   capsule

cath   catheterization or catheterize

CBC   complete blood count

CC   chief complaint

cc   cubic centimeter

CCB   calcium channel blocker

cGMP   cyclic guanosine monophosphate

CHD   coronary heart disease

CHF   congestive heart failure

cm   centimeter

CML   chronic myeloid leukemia

CMV   cytomegalovirus I

CNS   central nervous system

CO   cardiac output

CO_2 carbon dioxide

CoA   coenzyme A

c/o   complains of

COMT   catechol-O-methyltransferase

con rel   controlled release

conc   concentration

COPD   chronic obstructive pulmonary disease

COX-1   cyclooxygenase-1

COX-2   cyclooxygenase-2

CPAP   continuous positive airway pressure

CPK   creatinine phosphokinase

CPR   cardiopulmonary resuscitation

CrCl   creatinine clearance

CRD   chronic respiratory disease

CRF   chronic renal failure

C&S   culture and sensitivity

CSF   cerebrospinal fluid

CTZ   chemoreceptor trigger zone

CV   cardiovascular

CVA   cerebrovascular accident

CVP   central venous pressure

$CysLT_1$ cysteinyl leukotriene receptor

D&C   dilation and curettage

del rel   delayed release

DIC   disseminated intravascular coagulation

DM   diabetes mellitus

DMARD   disease-modifying antirheumatic drug

DNA   deoxyribonucleic acid

DOB   date of birth

dr   dram

dsg   dressing

DVT   deep vein thrombosis

D_5W 5% glucose in distilled water

dx   diagnosis

EBV   Epstein-Barr virus

ECG   electrocardiogram (EKG)

EEG   electroencephalogram

EENT   ear, eye, nose, and throat

elix   elixir, hydroalcoholic solution containing an active drug(s)

ENDO   endocrine systems

EPO   erythropoietin

EPS   extrapyramidal symptoms

ESR   erythrocyte sedimentation rate

ext rel   extended release

F   Fahrenheit

FBS   fasting blood sugar

FHT   fetal heart tones

FIO$_2$ inspired oxygen concentration

FSH   follicle-stimulating hormone

fx   fracture

g   gram

GABA   gamma-aminobutyric acid

gal   gallon

GERD   gastroesophageal reflux disease

GGTP   gamma-glutamyl transpeptidase

GHb   glycosylated hemoglobin

GI   gastrointestinal

G6PD   glucose-6-phosphate dehydrogenase

GR   glucocorticoid receptor

gr   grain

GTT   glucose tolerance test

gtt   drop

GU   genitourinary

Gyn   gynecology

HbA1c   laboratory test for glycosylated hemoglobin

HCG   human chorionic gonadotropin

Hct   hematocrit

HDL   high-density lipoprotein

HEMA   hematologic system

Hgb   hemoglobin

H&H   hematocrit and hemoglobin

5-HIAA   5-hydroxyindole-acetic acid

HIV   human immunodeficiency virus

HMG-CoA   3-hydroxy-3-methyl-glutaryl–coenzyme A reductase

H$_2$O   water

H&P   history and physical examination

HPA   hypothalamic-pituitary-adrenocortical axis

HR   heart rate

hr   hour

HRT   hormone replacement therapy

hs   at bedtime

HSV   herpes simplex virus

HSV-2   herpes genitalis

5-HT   5-hydroxytryptamine (serotonin)

hypo   hypodermically

Hx   history

IBS   irritable bowel syndrome

ICP   intracranial pressure

ICU   intensive care unit

I&D   incision and drainage

IDDM insulin-dependent diabetes mellitus

IgG immunoglobulin G

IL-2 interleukin-2

IM intramuscular

immed rel immediate release

inf infusion

inh inhalation

inj injection

INR international normalized ratio

INTEG relating to integumentary structures

IOP intraocular pressure

IPPB intermittent positive-pressure breathing

ITP idiopathic thrombocytopenic purpura

IU international unit

IUD intrauterine contraceptive device

IV intravenous

IVP intravenous piggyback

K potassium

kg kilogram

L or l left; liter

lat lateral

lb pound

LDH lactic dehydrogenase

LDL low-density lipoprotein

LDL-C low-density lipoprotein–cholesterol

LE lupus erythematosus

LFT liver function test

LH luteinizing hormone

LHRH luteinizing hormone-releasing hormone

liq liquid

LLQ left lower quadrant

LMP last menstrual period

LOC loss of consciousness

lot lotion

loz lozenge

LR lactated Ringer's solution

LRI lower respiratory infection

LVD left ventricular dysfunction

m meter

m^2 square meter

MAC mycobacterium avium complex

MAO monoamine oxidase

MAOI monoamine oxidase inhibitor

max maximum

mEq milliequivalent

META metabolic

mg milligram

μg microgram

MI myocardial infarction

min minute

mixt mixture

ml milliliter

mm millimeter

mo month

MPA mycophenolic acid

MS musculoskeletal

MVA motor vehicle accident

Na sodium

NC nasal cannula

neg negative

ng nanogram

NIDDM non–insulin-dependent diabetes mellitus

NKA no known allergies

NMDA N-methyl-D-aspartate

NMI no middle initial

noc nocturnal (night)

NPH neutral protamine Hagedorn

NPO nothing by mouth (nil per os)

NS normal saline

NSAID nonsteroidal antiinflammatory drug

NV neurovascular

O_2 oxygen

OBS organic brain syndrome

OC oral contraceptive

OD right eye (oculus dexter)

oint ointment

OOB out of bed

ophth ophthalmic

OR operating room

ORIF open reduction, internal fixation

OS left eye (ocular sinister)

OTC over the counter

ou each eye (oculus uterque)

oz ounce

p̄ after (post)

p pulse

PABA para-aminobenzoic acid

PAC premature atrial contraction

PAT paroxysmal atrial tachycardia

PBI protein-bound iodine

PBP penicillin binding protein

pc after meals (post cibum)

PCA patient-controlled analgesia

PCN penicillin

pCO_2 arterial carbon dioxide tension (pressure tore)

PE physical examination

PG prostaglandin

pH hydrogen ion concentration

PMDD premenstrual dysphoric disorder

PMS premenstrual syndrome

PNS peripheral nervous system

PO by mouth (per os)

pO_2 arterial oxygen tension (pressure tore)

postop postoperatively

PP postprandial

ppm parts per million

preop preoperatively

prep preparation

prn   as needed (pro re nata)

PSA   prostate-specific antigen

PT   prothrombin time

PTSD   posttraumatic stress disorder

PTT   partial thromboplastin time

PVC   premature ventricular contraction

PVD   peripheral vascular disease

q   every

qAM   every morning

qd   every day

qh   every hour

qid   four times per day

qod   every other day

qPM   every night

qt   quart

q2h   every 2 hours

q3h   every 3 hours

q4h   every 4 hours

q6h   every 6 hours

q12h   every 12 hours

qwk   every week

r   right

rap disintegr   rapidly disintegrating

RAR   retinoic acid receptor

RBC   red blood count or cell

RDA   recommended dietary allowance

rec   rectal

REM   rapid eye movement

RESP   respiratory system

rhPDGF-BB   recombinant human platelet-derived growth factor

RNA   ribonucleic acid

R/O   rule out

ROAD   reversible obstructive airway disease

ROM   range of motion

RTI   respiratory tract infection

Rx   therapy, treatment, or prescription

s̄   without

SA   sinoatrial

SAN   sinoatrial node

SC   subcutaneous

sec   second

SERM   selective estrogen receptor modulator

SGOT   serum glutamic-oxaloacetic transaminase (now AST)

SGPT   serum glutamic pyruvate transaminase (now ALT)

SIADH   syndrome of inappropriate antidiuretic hormone

sig   patient dosing instructions on prescription label

SL   sublingual

SLE   systemic lupus erythematosus

slow rel   slow release

SMBG   self-monitored blood glucose

SMZ   sulfamethoxazole

SOB   shortness of breath

sol   solution

ss   semis (one half)

SSRI   selective serotonin reuptake inhibitor

stat   at once

STD   sexually transmitted disease

supp   suppository

surg   surgical

sus rel   sustained-release dose form

Sx   symptoms

syr   syrup, a highly concentrated sucrose solution containing a drug(s)

T   temperature

$T_{1/2}$ drug half-life

T_3 triiodothyronine

T_4 thyroxine

tab   tablet

TB   tuberculosis

TBG   thyroxine-binding globulin

tbsp   tablespoon

TCA   tricyclic antidepressant

TD   transdermal

temp   temperature

TG   total triglycerides

TIA   transient ischemic attack

tid   three times per day (ter in die)

time rel   time-release dose form

tinc   tincture, alcoholic solution of a drug

TMD   temporomandibular dysfunction

TMJ   temporomandibular joint

TMP   trimethoprim

TNF   tumor necrosis factor

top   topical

tPA   tissue plasminogen activator

TPN   total parenteral nutrition

TPR   temperature, pulse, respirations

TSH   thyroid-stimulating hormone

tsp   teaspoon

TT   thrombin time

Tx   treatment

U   unit

UA   urinalysis

ULDL   ultra-low-density lipoprotein

URI   upper respiratory infection

USP   United States Pharmacopeia

UTI   urinary tract infection

UV   ultraviolet

vag   vaginal

visc   viscous

VD   venereal disease

VHDL   very-high-density lipoprotein

VLDL   very-low-density lipoprotein

VO   verbal order

vol	volume	wt	weight
VPB	ventricular premature beat	yr	year
VS	vital signs	>	greater than
WBC	white blood cell, white blood cell count	<	less than
		≠	not equal
WHO	World Health Organization	↑	increase
wk	week	↓	decrease
WNL	within normal limits	2°	secondary

Appendix B   Anesthetics

ANESTHETICS: GENERAL

Uses

IV anesthetic agents are used to induce general anesthesia. The general anesthetic state consists of unconsciousness, amnesia, analgesia, immobility, and attenuation of autonomic responses to noxious stimuli.

Volatile inhalation agents produce all of the components of the anesthetic state but are administered through the lungs via an anesthesia machine. Agents for use include desflurane, enflurane, halothane, isoflurane, and sevoflurane. They are used in practice to maintain general anesthesia.

Mechanisms of Action

IV anesthetic agents act on the gamma-aminobutyric acid (GABA) receptor complex to produce CNS depression. GABA is the primary inhibitory neurotransmitter in the CNS. Ketamine produces dissociation between the thalamus and the limbic system.

The specific actions of volatile inhalation agents are not all fully understood but may disrupt neuronal transmission throughout the CNS. These agents may either block excitatory transmission or enhance inhibitory transmission through axons or synapses.

TABLE B-1
Anesthetics: General

Name	Availability	Uses	Dosage Range	Side Effects
Etomidate (Amidate)	I: 2 mg/ml	IV induction	0.2–0.6 mg/kg	Myoclonus, pain on injection, nausea, vomiting, respiratory depression
Ketamine (Ketalar)	I: 10 mg/ml, 50 mg/ml, 100 mg/ml	Analgesia, sedation, IV induction	1–4.5 mg/kg	Delirium, euphoria, nausea, vomiting
Methohexital (Brevital)	Powder for injection: 500 mg	IV induction, sedation	50–120 mg	Cardiovascular depression, myoclonus, nausea, vomiting, respiratory depression
Midazolam (Versed)	I: 1 mg/ml, 5 mg/ml	Anxiolytic, amnesic, sedation	1–5 mg titrated slowly	Respiratory depression
Propofol (Diprivan)	I: 10 mg/ml	Sedation IV induction maintenance	0.5 mg/kg 2–2.5 mg/kg 100–200 mcg/kg/min	Cardiovascular depression, delirium, euphoria, pain on injection, respiratory depression
Thiopental (Pentothal)	Powder for injection: 2.5% (25 mg/ml)	IV induction	Titrate vs. pt response. Average: 50–75 mg	Cardiovascular depression, nausea, vomiting, respiratory depression

I, injection; pt, patient.

ANESTHETICS: LOCAL

Uses

Local anesthetics suppress pain by blocking impulses along axons. When carefully administered, they do not cause generalized depression of the entire nervous system. Local anesthetics may be given topically and by injection (local infiltration, peripheral nerve block [axillary], IV regional [Bier block], epidural, and spinal).

Action

Most local anesthetics fall into one of two groups: esters or amides. Both provide anesthesia and analgesia by reversibly binding to and blocking sodium (Na) channels. This slows the rate of depolarization of the nerve action potential; thus, propagation of the electrical impulses needed for nerve conduction is prevented.

TABLE B-2
Anesthetics: Local

Name	Uses	Onset (min)	Duration (hr)	Side Effects
Esters				
Chloroprocaine (Nesacaine)	Local infiltrate Nerve block Spinal	6–12	0.25–0.5	Excitation (e.g., seizures) followed by decreased level of consciousness (drowsiness to unconsciousness), bradycardia, heart block, decreased myocardial contractile force, hypotension, hypersensitivity reaction
Procaine (Novocaine)	Local infiltrate Nerve block Spinal	2–5	0.25–1	Same as above
Tetracaine	Topical Spinal	15	2–3	Same as above
Amides				
Bupivacaine (Marcaine, Sensorcaine)	Local infiltrate Nerve block Epidural Spinal	5	2–4	Same as above
Etidocaine (Duranest)	Nerve block Epidural	3–5	5–10	Same as above
Levobupivacaine (Chirocaine)	Nerve block Epidural	–	–	Same as above

TABLE B-2—cont'd
Anesthetics: Local

Name	Uses	Onset (min)	Duration (hr)	Side Effects
Lidocaine	Local infiltrate Nerve block Spinal Epidural Topical IV regional	Less than 2	0.5–1	Same as above
Mepivacaine (Carbocaine, Polocaine)	Local infiltrate Nerve block Epidural	3–5	0.75–1.5	Same as above
Ropivacaine (Naropin)	Local infiltrate Nerve block Epidural Spinal	1–15	2–6	Same as above

Note: Most side effects are manifestations of excessive plasma concentrations.
From Mosby's 2006 drug consult for nurses, St. Louis, 2006, Mosby.

TABLE B-3
Contraindications for Local Anesthetics

Medical Problem	Drugs to Avoid	Type of Contraindication	Alternative Drug
Local anesthetic allergy, documented	All local anesthetics in same chemical class (e.g., esters)	Absolute	Local anesthetics in a different chemical class (e.g., amides)
Bisulfite allergy	Vasoconstrictor-containing local anesthetics	Absolute	Any local anesthetic without vasoconstrictor
Atypical plasma cholinesterase	Esters	Relative	Amides
Methemoglobinemia, idiopathic or congenital	Prilocaine	Relative	Other amides or esters
Significant liver dysfunction (ASA III–IV)	Amides	Relative	Amides or esters, but judiciously
Significant renal dysfunction (ASA III–IV)	Amides or esters	Relative	Amides or esters, but judiciously
Significant cardiovascular disease (ASA III–IV)	High concentrations of vasoconstrictors	Relative	Local anesthetics with epinephrine concentrations of 1:200,000 or 1:100,000 or mepivacaine 3% or prilocaine 4% (nerve blocks)
Clinical hyperthyroidism (ASA III–IV)	High concentrations of vasoconstrictors	Relative	Local anesthetics with epinephrine concentrations of 1:200,000 or 1:100,000 or mepivacaine 3% or prilocaine 4% (nerve blocks)

ASA, American Society of Anesthesiologists' classification.
From Malamed SF: Handbook of local anesthesia, ed 5, St. Louis, 2004, Mosby.

TABLE B-4
Hydrochloride

Proprietary Name	Manufacturer	Percent Local Anesthetic	Vaso-constrictor	Duration of Analgesia (min)		MRD-m and MRD-a
				Pulpal	Soft Tissue	
Articaine Hydrochloride						
(United States) Septocaine	Septodont	4	Epinephrine 1:100,000; 1:200,000	60–75	180–360	7 mg/kg 3.2 mg/lb 500 mg absolute maximum
(Canada) Septanest SP	Septodont					
Astracaine	Dentsply					
Ultracaine D-S forte	Hoechst					
(Canada) Septanest N	Septodont	4	Epinephrine 1:200,000	45–60	120–300	7 mg/kg 3.2 mg/lb 500 mg absolute maximum
Astracaine	Dentsply					
Ultracaine D-S	Hoechst					
Bupivacaine Hydrochloride						
Marcaine	Kodak	0.5	Epinephrine 1:200,000	90–180	240–540 (reports up to 720)	1.3 mg/kg 0.6 mg/lb 90 mg absolute maximum

Continued

TABLE B-4—cont'd
Hydrochloride

Proprietary Name	Manufacturer	Percent Local Anesthetic	Vaso-constrictor	Duration of Analgesia (min)		MRD-m and MRD-a	
				Pulpal	Soft Tissue		
Lidocaine Hydrochloride							
Lidocaine HCl	Many generics	2	—	5–10	60–120	4.4 mg/kg 2.0 mg/lb 300 mg absolute maximum	
Alphacaine	Carlisle Labs						
Xylocaine	Dentsply						
Lidocaine HCl	Many generics	2	Epinephrine 1:50,000	60	180–300	6.6 mg/kg 3.0 mg/lb 500 mg absolute maximum	4.4 mg/kg 2.0 mg/lb 300 mg absolute maximum
Alphacaine	Carlisle Labs						
Lignospan	Septodont						
Octocaine	Novocol Chemical						
Xylocaine	Dentsply						
Mepivacaine Hydrochloride							
Mepivacaine HCl	Many generics	3	—	20–40 (20 for infiltration; 40 for nerve block)	120–180	6.6 mg/kg 3.0 mg/lb 400 absolute maximum	4.4 mg/kg 2.0 mg/lb 300 absolute maximum
Arestocaine	Carlisle Labs						
Carbocaine	Kodak						
Isocaine	Novocol						
Polocaine	Dentsply						
Scandonest	Septodont						

Drug	Manufacturer	mL	Vasoconstrictor			MRD	
Mepivacaine HCl Arestocaine Isocaine Polocaine Scandonest Carbocaine	Many generics Carlisle Labs Dentsply Kodak Septodont Novocol	2	Levonordefrin 1:20,000 Neo-Cobefrin 1:20,000	60	180–300	6.6 mg/kg 3.0 mg/lb 400 absolute maximum	4.4 mg/kg 2.0 mg/lb 300 absolute maximum
Carbocaine	Kodak	2	Epinephrine 1:200,000	45–60	120–240	6.6 mg/kg 3.0 mg/lb 400 absolute maximum	4.4 mg/kg 2.0 mg/lb 300 absolute maximum
Scandonest 2% Special	Septodont	2	Epinephrine 1:200,000	60	120–300	6.6 mg/kg 3.0 mg/lb 400 absolute maximum	4.4 mg/kg 2.0 mg/lb 300 absolute maximum
Prilocaine Hydrochloride							
Prilocaine HCl Citanest Plain	Generic Dentsply	4		10–15 (infil- tration) 40–60 (nerve block)	90–120 (inf) 120–240 (nb)	6 mg/kg 2.7 mg/lb 400 mg absolute maximum	
Prilocaine HCl+ epinephrine 1:200,000 Citanest Forte	Generic Dentsply	4	Epinephrine 1:200,000	60–90	180–480	6 mg/kg 2.7 mg/lb 400 mg absolute maximum	

MRD, maximum recommended dose.
From Malamed SF: Handbook of local anesthesia, ed 5, St. Louis, 2004, Mosby.

TABLE B-5
Mandibular Teeth and Available Local Anesthetic Techniques

Teeth	Pulpal Anesthesia	Soft Tissue	
		Buccal	Palatal
Incisors	Inc IANB GG VA PDL injection IS IO Inf (lateral incisor only)	IANB GG VA Inc IS Mental PDL injection Inf IO	IANB GG VA PDL injection IS Inf IO
Canines	IANB GG VA Inc PDL injection IS IO	IANB GG VA Inc PDL injection IS IO Mental Inf	IANB GG VA PDL injection IS IO Inf
Premolars	IANB GG VA Inc PDL injection IS IO	IANB GG VA Inc PDL injection IS IO Mental Inf	IANB GG VA PDL injection IS IO Inf
Molars	IANB GG VA PDL injection IS IO	IANB GG VA PDL injection IS IO Inf	IANB GG VA PDL injection IS IO Inf

GG, Gow-Gates; IANB, inferior alveolar; Inc, incisive; Inf, infiltration; IO, intraosseous; IS, intraseptal; PDL, periodontal ligament; VA, Vazirani-Akinosi.
From Malamed SF: Handbook of local anesthesia, ed 5, St. Louis, 2004, Mosby.

TABLE B-6

Maxillary Teeth and Available Local Anesthetic

Teeth	Pulpal Anesthesia	Soft Tissue	
		Buccal	Palatal
Incisors	IO	IO	Nasopalatine
	Infiltration	Infiltration	Infiltration
	AMSA	AMSA	AMSA
	P–ASA	P–ASA	P–ASA
	V2	V2	V2
Canines	Infraorbital	Infraorbital	Nasopalatine
	Infiltration	Infiltration	Infiltration
	AMSA	AMSA	AMSA
	P–ASA	P–ASA	P–ASA
	V2	V2	V2
Premolars	Infraorbital	Infraorbital	Greater palatine
	Infiltration	Infiltration	Infiltration
	MSA	MSA	AMSA
	ASA	ASA	V2
	V2	V2	
Molars	PSA	PS	Greater palatine
	Infiltration	Infiltration	Infiltration
	V2	V2	V2

IO, infraorbital

From Malamed SF: Handbook of local anesthesia, ed 5, St. Louis, 2004, Mosby.

Appendix C   Combination Drugs by Trade Name

Many drugs are available in fixed combinations of two or more medications. Some of the most common trade names for combination drugs in the United States are listed, along with their generic components and classifications. The list is alphabetical by the brand name of the combination product. Brand names for identical drug combinations are listed together. When the patient's drug history includes one of these combination products, it can be easily accessed through the index.

Combination Product Name	Generic Components
AC Gel	Cocaine (an anesthetic)/epinephrine (a vasopressor)
Accuretic	Quinapril (an ACE inhibitor)/hydrochlorothiazide (a diuretic)
Activella	Estradiol (an estrogen)/norethindrone (a hormone)
Advair	Fluticasone (a corticosteroid)/salmeterol (a bronchodilator)
Advil Cold	Pseudoephedrine (a sympathomimetic)/ibuprofen (an NSAID)
Aggrenox	Aspirin (an antiplatelet and nonnarcotic analgesic)/dipyridamole (an antiplatelet)
Aldactazide	Spironolactone (a potassium-sparing diuretic)/ hydrochlorothiazide (a diuretic)
Aldoril	Methyldopa (an antihypertensive)/hydrochlorothiazide (a diuretic)
Allegra-D	Fexofenadine (an antihistamine)/pseudoephedrine (a sympathomimetic nasal decongestant)
Allegra-D 24 Hour	Fexofenadine (an antihistamine)/pseudoephedrine (a sympathomimetic nasal decongestant)
Anexsia	Hydrocodone (a narcotic analgesic)/acetaminophen (a nonnarcotic analgesic)
Apresazide	Hydralazine (a vasodilator)/hydrochlorothiazide (a diuretic)
Arthrotec	Diclofenac (an NSAID)/misoprostol (an antisecretory gastric protectant)
Atacand HCT	Candesartan (an angiotensin II receptor antagonist)/ hydrochlorothiazide (a diuretic)
Avalide	Irbesartan (an angiotensin II receptor antagonist)/ hydrochlorothiazide (a diuretic)
Avandamet	Rosiglitazone (an antidiabetic)/metformin (an antidiabetic)
Bactrim	Sulfamethoxazole (a sulfonamide)/trimethoprim (an antiinfective)
Bellergal-S	Ergotamine (an antimigraine)/belladonna (an anticholinergic)/ phenobarbital (an anticonvulsant)
Benicar HCT	Olmesartan (an angiotensin II receptor antagonist)/ hydrochlorothiazide (a diuretic)

Combination Product Name	Generic Components
Bicillin CR	Penicillin G benzathine (a penicillin)/penicillin procaine (a penicillin)
Blephamide	Sulfacetamide (an antiinfective)/prednisolone (an adrenocortical steroid)
Caduet	Amlodipine (a calcium channel blocker)/atorvastatin (an antihyperlipidemic)
Caladryl	Calamine (an astringent)/diphenhydramine (an antihistamine)/camphor (a counterirritant)
Capital with Codeine	Acetaminophen (a nonnarcotic analgesic)/codeine (a narcotic analgesic)
Capozide	Captopril (an ACE inhibitor)/hydrochlorothiazide (a diuretic)
Children's Advil Cold	Ibuprofen (an NSAID)/pseudoephedrine (a sympathomimetic nasal decongestant)
Cipro HC Otic	Ciprofloxacin (an antiinfective)/hydrocortisone (an adrenocortical steroid)
Ciprodex Otic	Ciprofloxacin (an antiinfective)/dexamethasone (an adrenocortical steroid)
Claritin-D	Loratadine (an antihistamine)/pseudoephedrine (a nasal decongestant)
CombiPatch	Estradiol (an estrogen)/norethindrone (a hormone)
Combipres	Clonidine (an antihypertensive)/chlorthalidone (a diuretic)
Combivent	Ipratropium (a bronchodilator)/albuterol (a bronchodilator)
Combivir	Lamivudine (an antiretroviral)/zidovudine (an antiretroviral)
Combunox	Ibuprofen (an NSAID)/oxycodone (a narcotic analgesic)
Cortisporin	Neomycin (an antiinfective)/polymyxin B (an antiinfective)/hydrocortisone (an adrenocortical steroid)
Corzide	Nadolol (a β-blocker)/bendroflumethiazide (a diuretic)
Cosopt	Dorzolamide (a carbonic anhydrase inhibitor)/timolol (a β-blocker)
Darvocet A500	Propoxyphene (a narcotic analgesic)/acetaminophen (a nonnarcotic analgesic)
Darvocet-N	Propoxyphene (a narcotic analgesic)/acetaminophen (a nonnarcotic analgesic)
Dexacidin	Neomycin (an antiinfective)/polymyxin (an antiinfective)/dexamethasone (an adrenocortical steroid)
Dilantin with PB	Phenobarbital (an anticonvulsant)/phenytoin (an anticonvulsant)
Diovan HCT	Valsartan (an angiotensin II receptor antagonist)/hydrochlorothiazide (a diuretic)
Donnatal	Atropine (an anticholinergic)/hyoscyamine (an anticholinergic)/phenobarbital (a sedative)/scopolamine (an anticholinergic)
Duocet	Acetaminophen (a nonnarcotic analgesic)/hydrocodone (a narcotic analgesic)

Continued

Combination Product Name	Generic Components
DuoNeb	Ipratropium (a bronchodilator)/albuterol base (a bronchodilator)
Dyazide	Triamterene (a potassium-sparing diuretic)/hydrochlorothiazide (a diuretic)
EMLA	Lidocaine (a local anesthetic)/prilocaine (an anesthetic)
Epzicom	Abacavir (an antiretroviral)/lamivudine (an antiretroviral)
Eryzole	Erythromycin (a macrolide)/sulfisoxazole (a sulfonamide)
Etrafon	Perphenazine (an antipsychotic)/amitriptyline (an antidepressant)
Extra Strength Maalox	Magnesium hydroxide (an antacid)/simethicone Maalox (an antiflatulent)
Femhrt	Norethindrone (a hormone)/estradiol (an estrogen)
Ferro-Sequels	Ferrous fumarate (a hematinic)/docusate (a laxative)
Fioricet	Butabarbital (a sedative-hypnotic)/acetaminophen (a nonnarcotic analgesic)/caffeine (a CNS stimulant)
Fiorinal	Butabarbital (a sedative-hypnotic)/aspirin (a nonnarcotic analgesic)/caffeine (a CNS stimulant)
Gaviscon (oral suspension)	Aluminum hydroxide (an antacid)/magnesium carbonate (an antacid)
Gaviscon (tablets)	Aluminum hydroxide (an antacid)/magnesium trisilicate (an antacid)
Gelusil	Aluminum hydroxide (an antacid)/magnesium hydroxide (a laxative)/simethicone (an antiflatulent)
Gentlax-S	Senna (a laxative)/docusate (a laxative)
Glucovance	Glyburide (an antidiabetic)/metformin (an antidiabetic)
Haley's M-O	Magnesium (a laxative)/mineral oil (a lubricant laxative)
Helidac	Bismuth (an antidiarrheal)/metronidazole (an antiinfective)/tetracycline (an antiinfective)
Humalog Mix 75/25	Insulin: lispro suspension 75% and lispro solution 25%
Humulin 50/50	Insulin: NPH 50% and regular 50%
Humulin 70/30	Insulin: NPH 70% and rapid-acting regular 30%
Hyzaar	Losartan (an angiotensin II receptor antagonist)/hydrochlorothiazide (a diuretic)
Imodium Advanced	Loperamide (an antidiarrheal)/simethicone (an antiflatulent)
Inderide	Propranolol (a β-blocker)/hydrochlorothiazide (a diuretic)
Inderide LA	Propranolol (a β-blocker)/hydrochlorothiazide (a diuretic)
Lexxel	Enalapril (an ACE inhibitor)/felodipine (a calcium channel blocker)
Librax	Chlordiazepoxide (an antianxiety agent)/clidinium (an anticholinergic)

Combination Product Name	Generic Components
Lidocaine with Epinephrine	Lidocaine (a local anesthetic)/epinephrine (a vasoconstrictor)
LidoSite	Epinephrine (a sympathomimetic)/lidocaine (an anesthetic)
Limbitrol	Chlordiazepoxide (an antianxiety agent)/amitriptyline (an antidepressant)
Lomotil	Diphenoxylate (an antidiarrheal)/atropine (an anticholinergic/antispasmodic)
Lopressor HCT	Metoprolol (a β-blocker)/hydrochlorothiazide (a diuretic)
Lorcet	Acetaminophen (a nonnarcotic analgesic)/hydrocodone (a narcotic analgesic)
Lortab	Hydrocodone (a narcotic analgesic)/acetaminophen (a nonnarcotic analgesic)
Lortab Elixir	Hydrocodone (a narcotic analgesic)/acetaminophen (a nonnarcotic analgesic)
Lortab/ASA	Hydrocodone (a narcotic analgesic)/aspirin (a nonnarcotic analgesic)
Lotensin HCT	Benazepril (an ACE inhibitor)/hydrochlorothiazide (a diuretic)
Lotrel	Amlodipine (a calcium channel blocker)/benazepril (an ACE inhibitor)
Lotrisone	Clotrimazole (an antifungal)/betamethasone (an adrenocortical steroid)
Lunelle	Medroxyprogesterone (a progestin)/estradiol (an estrogen)
Maalox	Aluminum hydroxide (an antacid)/magnesium hydroxide (an antacid)
Maalox Plus	Aluminum hydroxide (an antacid)/magnesium hydroxide (an antacid)/simethicone (an antiflatulent)
Maxitrol	Neomycin (an antiinfective)/polymyxin (an antiinfective)/dexamethasone (an adrenocortical steroid)
Maxzide	Triamterene (a potassium-sparing diuretic)/hydrochlorothiazide (a diuretic)
Metaglip	Glipizide (an antidiabetic)/metformin (an antidiabetic)
Micardis HCT	Telmisartan (an angiotensin II receptor antagonist)/hydrochlorothiazide (a diuretic)
Minizide	Prazosin (an antihypertensive)/polythiazide (a diuretic)
Moduretic	Amiloride (a potassium-sparing diuretic)/hydrochlorothiazide (a diuretic)
Motrin Cold	Pseudoephedrine (a sympathomimetic nasal decongestant)/ibuprofen (an NSAID)
Mucinex D	Guaifenesin (an expectorant)/pseudoephedrine (a sympathomimetic nasal decongestant)
Mucinex DM	Guaifenesin (an expectorant)/dextromethorphan (an expectorant)

Continued

Combination Product Name	Generic Components
Mycitracin	Neomycin (an aminoglycoside)/polymyxin B (an antiinfective)/bacitracin (an antiinfective)
Myco II	Nystatin (an antifungal)/triamcinolone (an adrenocortical steroid)
Mycolog II	Nystatin (an antifungal)/triamcinolone (an adrenocortical steroid)
Myco-Triacet	Nystatin (an antifungal)/triamcinolone (an adrenocortical steroid)
Mylanta	Aluminum hydroxide (an antacid)/magnesium hydroxide (oral suspension) (an antacid)/simethicone (an antiflatulent)
Mylanta (tablets)	Calcium carbonate/magnesium hydroxide
Naphcon-A	Naphazoline (a nasal decongestant)/pheniramine (an antihistamine)
Neosporin GU	Neomycin (an aminoglycoside)/polymyxin B (an antiinfective)
Neosporin Ointment, Triple Antibiotic	Neomycin (an aminoglycoside)/polymyxin B (an antiinfective)/bacitracin (an antiinfective)
Norco	Hydrocodone (a narcotic analgesic)/acetaminophen (a nonnarcotic analgesic)
Normozide	Labetalol (a β-blocker)/hydrochlorothiazide (a diuretic)
Novolin 70/30	Insulin: NPH 70% and rapid-acting regular 30%
NovoLog 70/30	Insulin: aspart suspension 70% and aspart solution 30%
Pediazole	Erythromycin (a macrolide)/sulfisoxazole (a sulfonamide)
Pepcid Complete	Famotidine (an H_2 antagonist)/calcium chloride (an antacid)/magnesium hydroxide (an antacid)
Percocet	Oxycodone (a narcotic analgesic)/acetaminophen (a nonnarcotic analgesic)
Percodan	Oxycodone (a narcotic analgesic)/aspirin (a nonnarcotic analgesic)
Phenergan with Codeine	Promethazine (an antihistamine)/codeine (a cough suppressant)
Phenergan VC	Promethazine (an antihistamine)/phenylephrine (a vasopressor)
Phenergan VC with Codeine	Promethazine (an antihistamine)/phenylephrine (a vasopressor)/codeine (a cough suppressant)
Polysporin	Polymyxin B (an antiinfective)/bacitracin (an antiinfective)
Pravigard	Aspirin (an antiplatelet)/pravastatin (an antihyperlipidemic)
Premphase	Conjugated estrogens (an estrogen)/medroxyprogesterone (an androgen)
Prempro	Conjugated estrogens (an estrogen)/medroxyprogesterone (an androgen)

Combination Product Name	Generic Components
Prevacid NapraPAC	Lansoprazole (a proton pump inhibitor)/naproxen (an NSAID)
Prinzide	Lisinopril (an ACE inhibitor)/hydrochlorothiazide (a diuretic)
Rebetron	Ribavirin (an antiviral)/interferon alfa 2b (an immunologic agent)
Reprexain CIII	Ibuprofen (an NSAID)/hydrocodone (a narcotic analgesic)
Rifamate	Rifampin (an antitubercular)/isoniazid (an antitubercular)
Rifater	Rifampin (an antitubercular)/isoniazid (an antitubercular)/ pyrazinamide (an antitubercular)
Robitussin AC	Guaifenesin (an antitussive)/codeine (a narcotic analgesic)
Robitussin DM	Dextromethorphan (a cough suppressant)/guaifenesin (an antitussive)
Roxicet	Oxycodone (a narcotic analgesic)/acetaminophen (a nonnarcotic analgesic)
Senokot-S	Senna (a laxative)/docusate (a laxative)
Septra	Sulfamethoxazole (a sulfonamide)/trimethoprim (an antiinfective)
Silain-Gel	Magnesium hydroxide (an antacid)/aluminum hydroxide (an antacid)/simethicone (an antiflatulent)
Stalevo	Carbidopa-levodopa (an antiparkinson agent)/entacapone (an antiparkinson agent)
Suboxone	Buprenorphine (a nonnarcotic analgesic)/naloxone (a narcotic antagonist)
Symbyax	Fluoxetine (an antidepressant)/olanzapine (an antipsychotic)
TAC	Tetracaine (an anesthetic)/epinephrine (a vasoconstrictor)/ cocaine (an anesthetic)
Tarka	Trandolapril (an ACE inhibitor)/verapamil (a calcium blocker)
Teczem	Enalapril (an ACE inhibitor)/diltiazem (a calcium channel blocker)
Tenoretic	Atenolol (a β-blocker)/chlorthalidone (a diuretic)
Teveten HCT	Eprosartan (an angiotensin II receptor antagonist)/ hydrochlorothiazide (a diuretic)
Thyrolar	Liothyronine (a thyroid agent)/levothyroxine (a thyroid agent)
Timolide	Timolol (a β-blocker)/hydrochlorothiazide (a diuretic)
TobraDex	Tobramycin (an aminoglycoside)/dexamethasone (an adrenocortical steroid)
Triavil	Perphenazine (an antipsychotic)/amitriptyline (an antidepressant)
Trizivir	Abacavir (an antiretroviral)/lamivudine (an antiretroviral)/ zidovudine (an antiretroviral)
Truvada	Emtricitabine (an antiretroviral)/tenofovir (an antiretroviral)
Tylenol with Codeine	Acetaminophen (a nonnarcotic analgesic)/codeine (a narcotic analgesic)

Continued

Combination Product Name	Generic Components
Tylox	Acetaminophen (a nonnarcotic analgesic)/oxycodone (a narcotic analgesic)
Ultracet	Tramadol (a nonnarcotic analgesic)/acetaminophen (a nonnarcotic analgesic)
Uniretic	Moexipril (an ACE inhibitor)/hydrochlorothiazide (a diuretic)
Vaseretic	Enalapril (an ACE inhibitor)/hydrochlorothiazide (a diuretic)
Vasocidin	Sulfacetamide (an antiinfective)/prednisolone (an adrenocortical steroid)
Vicodin	Hydrocodone (a narcotic analgesic)/acetaminophen (a nonnarcotic analgesic)
Vicodin ES	Hydrocodone (a narcotic analgesic)/acetaminophen (a nonnarcotic analgesic)
Vicodin HP	Hydrocodone (a narcotic analgesic)/acetaminophen (a nonnarcotic analgesic)
Vicoprofen	Hydrocodone (a narcotic analgesic)/ibuprofen (an NSAID)
Vytorin	Ezetimibe (an antihyperlipidemic)/simvastatin (an antihyperlipidemic)
Zestoretic	Lisinopril (an ACE inhibitor)/hydrochlorothiazide (a diuretic)
Ziac	Bisoprolol (a β-blocker)/hydrochlorothiazide (a diuretic)
Zotrim	Trimethoprim (an antiinfective)/sulfamethoxazole (a sulfonamide)/phenazopyridine (a spasmolytic)
Zydone	Hydrocodone (a narcotic analgesic)/acetaminophen (a nonnarcotic analgesic)
Zyrtec D 12 Hour Tablets	Cetirizine (an antihistamine)/pseudoephedrine (a nasal decongestant)

ACE, angiotensin-converting enzyme inhibitor.
From Mosby's 2006 drug consult for nurses, St. Louis, 2006, Mosby.

Appendix D Controlled Substances Chart

Drugs	United States	Canada
Heroin, LSD, peyote, marijuana, mescaline, phencyclidine	Schedule I (CI)	Schedule H
Opium, fentanyl, morphine, meperidine, methadone, oxycodone (and its combinations), hydromorphone, codeine (single-drug entity), and cocaine	Schedule II (CII)	Schedule N
Short-acting barbiturates	Schedule II (CII)	Schedule C
Amphetamine and methylphenidate	Schedule II (CII)	Schedule G
Codeine combinations, hydrocodone combinations, glutethimide, paregoric, phendimetrazine, thiopental, testosterone, and other androgens	Schedule III (CIII)	Schedule F
Benzodiazepines (diazepam, midazolam, etc.), chloral hydrate, meprobamate, phenobarbital, propoxyphene (and combinations), pentazocine (and combinations), and methohexital	Schedule IV (CIV)	Schedule F
Antidiarrheals and antitussives with opioid derivatives	Schedule V (CV)	

Appendix E   Disorders and Conditions

TABLE E-1
Asthma Medications

Agent	Indication	Mechanism of Action	Example
Inhaled β_2-agonist (short-acting)	Acute exacerbation, used in all categories.	Bronchodilator: smooth muscle relaxation following adenylate cyclase activation, resulting in an increase in cyclic AMP activating protein kinase A, which lowers needed intracellular calcium for smooth muscle contraction.	Albuterol Metaproterenol
Inhaled β_2-agonist (long-acting)	Longer-term prevention usually added to antiinflammatory therapy.	Bronchodilator (see above).	Salmeterol
Oral β_2-agonist (long-lasting)	Longer term prevention usually added to antiinflammatory therapy.	Bronchodilator (see above).	Albuterol (sustained-release)
Inhaled corticosteroids	Longer-term prevention. Daily medication in all persistent forms. Low-, medium-, high-dose formulations depending on asthma severity/control.	Antiinflammatory: inhibits cytokine production and adhesion protein activation. Reserves β_2 down-regulation. Suppresses recruitment of airway eosinophils.	Beclomethasone Flunisolide Fluticasone Budesonide Triamcinolone

Systemic corticosteroids	Acute exacerbation, used in all categories. Long-term prevention in severe, persistent asthma.	Antiinflammatory (see above).	Methylprednisolone Prednisolone Prednisone
Anticholinergics	Acute exacerbation, used in patients intolerant to short-acting β_2-agonists.	Bronchodilator: competitive inhibition of muscarinic cholinergic receptors.	Ipratropium bromide Cromolyn Nedocromil Theophylline (sustained-release)
Leukotriene modifiers	Long-term control and prevention in Step 2 mild, persistent asthma.	Antiinflammatory: Leukotriene receptor antagonist (competitive inhibition) = Zafirlukast/Montelukast 5-Lipooxygenase inhibitor interfering with leukotriene synthesis = Zileuton.	Zafirlukast Montelukast Zileuton

All medications have side effects with which the dentist should be familiar.
Medication usage/discontinuance based on step-up, step-down fashion relating to symptoms.
Specific dosage/delivery of medication tailored to patient/severity.
Children younger than 5 years old have different regimens.
(Sollecito TP, Tino G: Oral Surg Oral Med Oral Pathol Radiol Endod 92:486–487, 2001).

TABLE E-2

Drugs Used for Treatment of Seizure Disorder

Drug	Pharmacologic Category	Adverse Effects
Carbamazepine (Epitol, Tegretol)	Tricyclic	Sedation, dizziness, fatigue, confusion, ataxia, nausea, blood dyscrasias, hepatotoxicity
Clonazepam (Klonopin)	Benzodiazepine	Tachycardia, drowsiness, fatigue, anxiety, ataxia, headache, dizziness, blurred vision, xerostomia
Ethosuximide (Zarontin)	Succinimide	Ataxia, sedation, dizziness, hallucinations, behavioral changes, headache, Stevens-Johnson syndrome, systemic lupus erythematosus, nausea, anorexia
Gabapentin (Neurontin)	Neurotransmitter	Somnolence, dizziness, ataxia, fatigue, nystagmus
Phenobarbital (Barbita, Luminal, Solfoton)	Barbiturate	Dizziness, light-headedness, sedation, ataxia, impaired judgment, skin rashes
Phenytoin (Mysoline)	Barbiturate derivative	Drowsiness, vertigo, ataxia, behavioral changes, headache, nausea
Primidone (Mysoline)	Barbiturate derivative	Drowsiness, vertigo, ataxia, behavioral changes, headache, nausea
Topiramate (Topamax)	Sulfamate-substituted monosaccharide	Acidosis (may decrease serum bicarbonate concentrations), increased risk of kidney stones, hyperthermia, paresthesias, sedation, confusion, psychomotor slowing, mood disturbances
Valproic acid, sodium valproate (Depakene, Depakote)	Carboxylic acid	Anorexia, diarrhea, nausea, drowsiness, ataxia, irritability, confusion, headache, hepatotoxicity, leucopenia, thrombocytopenia resulting in prolonged bleeding time

From Hupp JR, Williams TP, Firriolo FJ: Dental clinical advisor, ed 1, St. Louis, 2006, Elsevier.

TABLE E-3
Drugs Used for Management of Oral Candidosis

Medication	Dosage and Directions*
Chlorhexidine 0.12% oral rinse (Peridex, PerioGard)† or 0.2% alcohol-free aqueous‡	15 ml mouthrinse and expectorate 3 times a day. NPO $\frac{1}{2}$ hr after use.
Nystatin oral suspension 100,000 units/ml§	5 ml mouthrinse and 1 min expectorate 4 times a day (before breakfast and at bedtime). NPO $\frac{1}{2}$ hr after use.
Clotrimazole 10 mg/ml suspension¶	Swab 1–2 ml on affected area 4 times a day (pc and hs). NPO $\frac{1}{2}$ hr after use.
Ketoconazole 2% cream (Nizoral) or clotrimazole 1% cream (Lotrimin)	Apply thin film to inner surface of denture(s) and/or corners of mouth 4 times a day (before breakfast and at bedtime). NPO $\frac{1}{2}$ hr after use.
Clotrimazole 200-mg vaginal tablets (Gyne-Lotrimin)	Dissolve $\frac{1}{2}$ tablet slowly in mouth 2 times a day. NPO $\frac{1}{2}$ hr after use.
Clotrimazole 10-mg oral troches (Nizoral)	Dissolve 1 troche slowly in mouth 5 times a day. NPO $\frac{1}{2}$ hr after use.
Ketoconazole 200-mg tablets (Nizoral)	1 tablet PO 4 times a day for 7–10 days. Do not take antacids within 2 hr of this medication.**
Fluconazole 100-mg tablets (Diflucan)	1 tablet PO 2 times a day for first day, then 1 tablet PO 4 times a day for 10–14 days.

*In most patients, decreased frequency and dosages can be used if maintenance therapy is required.
†High alcohol content (11.6%) will irritate mucosa and enhance xerostomia. Should not be prescribed for recovering alcoholics.
‡Must be prepared by experienced compounding pharmacist. Many formulas include flavorings that decrease efficacy.
§High sucrose content. Not first-line choice.
¶May be swallowed for pharyngeal involvement.
‖Compounded in confectioners glycerin.
**Acidic environment is required for absorption.
From Klienegger CL: Diseases of the mouth. In Rakel RE, Bope ET, editors: Conn's Current Therapy 2002. Philadelphia, 2002, WB Saunders.

Appendix F   Drugs Causing Dry Mouth

Drug Category	Brand Name	Generic Name
Alcohol Abuse Deterrent	Campral	acamprosate calcium
Anorexiant	Adipex-P, Fastin, Ionamin Anorex Mazanor, Sanorex Tenuate, Tepanil	phentermine phendimetrazine mazindol diethylpropion
Antiacne	Accutane	isotretinoin
Antianemic	Revlimid	lenalidomide
Antianxiety	Atarax, Vistaril Ativan BuSpar Equanil, Miltown Librium Paxipam Serax Sonata Valium Xanax	hydroxyzine lorazepam buspirone meprobamate chlordiazepoxide halazepam oxazepam zaleplon diazepam alprazolam
Antiarthritic	Arava	leflunomide

Anticholinergic/Antispasmodic	Anaspaz
	Sal-Tropine
	Bellergal
	Bentyl
	Ditropan
	Donnatal, Kinesed
	
	Librax
	
	Pro-Banthine
	Transderm-Scop
		hyoscyamine
		atropine
		belladonna alkaloids
		dicyclomine
		oxybutynin
		hyoscyamine atropine,
		  phenobarbital,
		  scopolamine
		chlordiazepoxide,
		  clidinium
		propantheline
		scopolamine

Anticonvulsant	Felbatol Lamictal Lyrica Neurontin Tegretol	felbamate lamotrigine pregabalin gabapentin carbamazepine
Antidepressant	Anafranil Asendin Celexa Cymbalta Effexor Elavil Luvox Marplan Nardil Norpramin Parnate Paxil Prozac	clomipramine amoxapine citalopram duloxetine venlafaxine amitriptyline fluvoxamine isocarboxazid phenelzine desipramine tranylcypromine paroxetine fluoxetine

Drug Category	Brand Name	Generic Name
	Replax	eletriptan
	Sinequan	doxepin
	Tofranil	imipramine
	Wellbutrin, Zyban	bupropion
	Zoloft	sertraline
Antidiarrheal	Imodium AD	loperamide
	Lomotil	diphenoxylate, atropine
	Motofen	difenoxin
Antifungal	Noxafil	posaconazole
Antihistamine	Actifed	triprolidine with pseudoephedrine
	Atarax	hydroxyzine
	Benadryl	diphenhydramine
	Chlor-Trimeton	chlorpheniramine
	Claritin	loratadine
	Dimetapp	pseudoephedrine
	Phenergan	promethazine
Antihypertensive	Capoten	captopril
	Catapres	clonidine
	Coreg	carvedilol
	Ismelin	guanethidine
	Aceon	perindopril
	Minipress	prazosin
	Serpasil	reserpine
	Wytensin	guanabenz
	Vasotec	enalapril
Antiinflammatory Analgesic	Celebrex	celecoxib
	Dolobid	diflunisal
	Feldene	piroxicam
	Motrin	ibuprofen
	Nalfon	fenoprofen
	Naprosyn	naproxen
	Vioxx	rofecoxib
Antiinflammatory GI	Colazal	balsalazide
Antinauseant	Antivert	meclizine
	Dramamine	dimenhydrinate
	Emend	aprepitant
	Marezine	cyclizine
Anti-parkinsonian	Akineton	biperiden
	Artane	trihexyphenidyl
	Cogentin	benztropine mesylate
	Larodopa	levodopa
	Paridol	ethopropazine
	Sinemet	carbidopa, levodopa
	Tasmar	tolcapone

Continued

Drug Category	Brand Name	Generic Name
Antipsychotic	Abilify	aripiprazole
	Clozaril	clozapine
	Compazine	prochlorperazine
	Eskalith	lithium
	Haldol	haloperidol
	Mellaril	thioridazine
	Navane	thiothixene
	Orap	pimozide
	Risperdal	risperidone
	Sparine	promazine
	Thorazine	chlorpromazine
	Triavil	amitriptyline, perphenazine
	Zyprexa	olanzapine
Antisecretory	Aciphex	rabeprazole
	Nexium	esomeprazole
Antispasmodic	Detrol	tolterodine
	Sanctura	trospium chloride
Antiviral	Copegus	ribavirin
	Sustiva	efavirenz
Bronchodilator	(generic)	ephedrine
	Isuprel	isoproterenol
	Proventil, Ventolin	albuterol
	Xopenex	levalbuterol
CNS Stimulant	Desoxyn	methamphetamine
	Dexedrine	dextroamphetamine
Decongestant	Sudafed	pseudoephedrine
Diuretic	Aldactone	spironolactone
	Diuril	chlorothiazide
	Dyazide, Maxzide, Dyrenium	triamterene
	Esidrix, HydroDIURIL	hydrochlorothiazide
	Lasix	furosemide
	Midamor	amiloride
Migraine	Amerge	naratriptan
	Axert	almotriptan
	Frova	frovatriptan
	Maxalt	rizatriptan
	Replax	eletriptan
Multikinase Inhibitor	Nexavar	sorafenib
Muscle Relaxant	Flexeril	cyclobenzaprine
	Lioresal	baclofen
	Norflex	orphenadrine
Antinarcoleptic	Provigil	modafinil
Nicotine Receptor Agonist	Chantix	varenicline

Drug Category	Brand Name	Generic Name
Opioid Analgesic	Buprenex Demerol MS Contin Synalgos DC	buprenorphine meperidine morphine dihydrocodeine combinations
Ophthalmic	Azopt	brinzolamide
Sedative	Dalmane Halcion Lunesta Restoril	flurazepam triazolam eszopiclone temazepam

Appendix G Drugs That Affect Taste

ALCOHOL DETOXIFICATION
disulfiram (Antabuse)

ALZHEIMER'S
donepezil (Aricept)

ANALGESICS (NSAIDs)
diclofenac (Voltaren)
etodolac (Lodine)
ketoprofen (Orudis)
meclofenamate (Meclofen)
sulindac (Clinoril)

ANESTHETICS (GENERAL)
midazolam (Versed)
propofol (Diprivan)

ANESTHETICS (LOCAL)
lidocaine transoral delivery system
(Dentipatch)

ANOREXIANTS
diethylpropion (Tenuate)
mazindol (Mazanor)
phendimetrazine (Adipost)
phentermine (Ionamin)

ANTACIDS
aluminum hydroxide (Amphojel)
calcium carbonate (Tums)
lansoprazole (Prevacid)
magaldrate (Riopan)
omeprazole (Prilosec)
sucralfate (Carafate)

ANTAGONISTS
azelastine (Astelin)
cetirizine (Zyrtec)
famotidine (Pepcid)

ANTIANEMIC
lenalidomide (Revlimid)

ANTIANXIETY
buspirone (BuSpar)

ANTIARTHRITIC
leflunomide (Arava)

ANTICHOLINERGICS
clidinium (Quarzan)
mepenzolate (Cantil)
propantheline (Pro-Banthine)

ANTICONVULSANTS
fosphenytoin (Cerebyx)
phenytoin (Dilantin)
topiramate (Topamax)

ANTIDEPRESSANTS
amitriptyline (Elavil)
clomipramine (Anafranil)
desipramine (Norpramin)
doxepin (Sinequan)
fluoxetine (Prozac)
imipramine (Tofranil)
nefazodone (Serzone)
nortriptyline (Pamelor)
protriptyline (Vivactil)
sertraline (Zoloft)

ANTIDIABETICS
metformin (Glucophage)
tolbutamide (Orinase)

ANTIDIARRHEALS
bismuth subsalicylate
(Pepto-Bismol)

ANTIEMETICS
aprepitant (Emend)
dolasetron mesylate (Anzemet)

ANTIFUNGALS
terbinafine (Lamisil)

ANTIGOUT
allopurinol (Zyloprim)
colchicine

ANTIHISTAMINE (H$_1$)

ANTIHISTAMINE (H$_2$)

ANTIHYPERLIPIDEMICS
clofibrate (Atromid-S)
fluvastatin (Lescol)

ANTIINFECTIVES

ciprofloxacin (Ciloxan)
daptomycin (Cubicin)
ethionamide (Trecator-SC)
gatifloxacin (Zymar)
gemifloxacin (Factive)
levofloxacin (Levaquin)
lincomycin (Lincocin)
metronidazole (Flagyl)
ofloxacin (Floxin)

ANTIINFLAMMATORY/ ANTIARTHRITIC

auranofin (Ridaura)
aurothioglucose (Solganal)
celecoxib (Celebrex)
sulfasalazine (Azulfidine)

ANTIMIGRAINE

almotriptan (Axert)
frovatriptan (Frova)

ANTIPARKINSON

apomorphine (Apokyn)
entacapone (Comtan)
levodopa (Larodopa)
levodopa-carbidopa (Sinemet)
pergolide (Permax)
pramipexole dihydrochloride (Mirapex)

ANTIPROTOZOAL

tinidazole (Tindamax)

ANTIPSYCHOTICS

lithium (Eskalith)
pimozide (Orap)
prochlorperazine (Compazine)
quetiapine fumarate (Seroquel)
risperidone (Risperdal)

ANTITHYROID

methimazole (Tapazole)
propylthiouracil

ANTIVIRALS

acyclovir (Zovirax)
amprenavir (Agenerase)
atazanavir (Reyataz)
delavirdine mesylate (Rescriptor)
didanosine (Videx)
efavirenz (Sustiva)
foscarnet (Foscavir)
indinavir (Crixivan)
penciclovir (Denavir)
ribavirin (Copegus)
rimantadine (Flumadine)
ritonavir (Norvir)
saquinavir (Invirase)
valacyclovir (Valtrex)
zidovudine (Retrovir)

ANXIOLYTIC/SEDATIVES

chloral hydrate
estazolam (ProSom)
quazepam (Doral)
zolpidem (Ambien)

ASTHMA PREVENTIVES

cromolyn (Intal)
nedocromil (Tilade)

BRONCHODILATORS

albuterol (Proventil)
bitolterol (Tornalate)
formoterol fumarate (Foradil)
ipratropium (Atrovent)
isoproterenol (Isuprel)
metaproterenol (Alupent)
pirbuterol (Maxair)
terbutaline (Brethine)

CALCIUM-AFFECTING DRUGS

alendronate (Fosamax)
calcitonin (Calcimar)
etidronate (Didronel)

CANCER

CHEMOTHERAPEUTICS

capecitabine (Xeloda)
fluorouracil (Efudex)
levamisole (Ergamisol)
tamoxifen (Nolvadex)

CARDIOVASCULAR

amiodarone (Cordarone)
amlodipine (Norvasc)
bepridil (Vascor)
captopril (Capoten)
clonidine (Catapres)

diltiazem (Cardizem)
enalapril (Vasotec)
flecainide (Tambocor)
fosinopril (Monopril)
guanfacine (Tenex)
labetalol (Trandate)
losartan (Cozaar)
mecamylamine (Inversine)
mexiletine (Mexitil)
moricizine (Ethmozine)
nadolol (Corgard)
nifedipine (Procardia XL)
penbutolol (Levatol)
perindopril (Aceon)
propafenone (Rythmol)
quinidine (Cardioquin)
valsartan (Diovan)

CNS STIMULANTS
dextroamphetamine (Dexedrine)
methamphetamine (Desoxyn)

DECONGESTANT
phenylephrine (Neo-Synephrine)

DIURETICS
acetazolamide (Diamox)
methazolamide (Neptazane)
polythiazide (Renese)

GLUCOCORTICOIDS
budesonide (Rhinocort)
flunisolide (Aerobid)
rimexolone (Vexol)

GALLSTONE SOLUBILIZATION
ursodiol (Actigall)

HEMORHEOLOGIC
pentoxifylline (Trental)

IMMUNOMODULATORS
interferon alfa (Roferon-A)
levamisole (Ergamisol)
tacrolimus (Protopic)

IMMUNOSUPPRESSANTS
azathioprine (Imuran)

IRRITABLE BOWEL SYNDROME
alosetron (Lotronex)
telithromycin (Ketek)

MELATONIN RECEPTOR AGONIST HYPNOTIC
ramelteon (Rozerem)

METHYLXANTHINES
aminophylline (Somophyllin)
dyphylline (Dilor)
oxtriphylline (Choledyl)
theophylline (Theo-Dur)

NICOTINE CESSATION
nicotine polacrilex (Nicorette)
varenicline (Chantix)

OPHTHALMICS
apraclonidine (Iopidine)
brimonidine (Alphagan)
brinzolamide (Azopt)
dorzolamide (Trusopt)
olopatadine (Patanol)

PROTON PUMP INHIBITORS
esomeprazole (Nexium)
lansoprazole (Prevacid)
omeprazole (Prilosec)

RETINOID, SYSTEMIC
acitretin (Soriatane)

SALIVARY STIMULANT
pilocarpine (Salagen)

SEDATIVE-HYPNOTIC
eszopiclone (Lunesta)

SKELETAL MUSCLE RELAXANTS
baclofen (Lioresal)
cyclobenzaprine (Flexeril)
methocarbamol (Robaxin)

VITAMINS
calcifediol (vitamin D)
calcitriol (vitamin D)
dihydrotachysterol (vitamin D)
phytonadione (vitamin K)

Appendix H   Herbal and Nonherbal Remedies

aloe vera
(Aloe vera, *Aloe barbadensis*)

OTHER NAMES:
Burn plant, curaçao aloes

Class: Herbal remedy

MAJOR INGREDIENTS
The term aloe vera conventionally refers to the gel within the aloe leaf. (the glands in the leaf surface contain a different and unsafe substance called drug aloe, which is not present, except in trace amounts, in aloe gel products.) The major active ingredients of aloe vera gel are thought to be its polysaccharides, especially one called acemannan. Other potentially important constituents include sitosterols and lignins.

CLAIMED ACTIONS
Aloe vera juice is widely credited with the ability to enhance skin regeneration after burns or wounds, but randomized controlled trials (RCTs) of aloe for speeding resolution of sunburn, skin damage caused by radiation therapy, and wounds have generally failed to find benefit. On the basis of the same putative tissue healing effect, aloe has been recommended for treatment of stomach ulcers and other GI tract diseases, but no meaningful evidence supports these uses. Other claimed effects that lack supporting evidence from properly designed RCTs include immune stimulation and suppression of HIV infection (however, acemannan is approved by the U.S. Food and Drug Administration for treatment of fibrosarcoma in cats and dogs). Two RCTs indicate that oral aloe gel might have a hypoglycemic effect in patients with Type 2 diabetes, but it has been suggested that these benefits were due to trace contamination of the aloe gel with parts of the leaf glands, supplying some drug aloe.

USES
Preliminary RCTs of moderate-to-low quality suggest that aloe vera cream offers benefit for treatment of seborrhea, psoriasis, and genital herpes, reducing symptoms and speeding resolution. Other uses based on the claimed actions noted previously lack RCT support.

ADMINISTRATION
In most of the studies that produced positive results for seborrhea, psoriasis, and genital herpes, aloe was applied as a cream containing 0.5% of aloe extract administered 3 times a day. One study used a cream containing 30% aloe gel. Whole aloe gel (rather than cream) applied topically has generally shown less benefit. A typical oral dose of aloe vera juice is 1 tablespoon twice a day. Maximum safe doses in pregnant or nursing women, young children, and individuals with severe hepatic or renal disease are not established.

SIDE EFFECTS
Use of aloe gel, either internally or externally, has not been associated with any significant side effects other than nonspecific GI distress or allergic reactions. Drug aloe (made from the leaf glands and not generally available in the United States) is a strong laxative and should not be used.

DENTAL CONSIDERATIONS
Some people may swish or gargle with aloe preparation in hopes of

treating periodontal disease. There is no evidence for or against this use.

DRUG INTERACTIONS

If aloe vera products can, in fact, reduce blood sugar in type 2 diabetes, potentiation interactions with oral hypoglycemics are a possibility. However, no such interactions have yet been reported.

bilberry fruit
(Vaccinium myrtillus)

OTHER NAMES:
Blueberry, huckleberry, hurtleberry, Myrtilli fructus

Class: Herbal remedy

MAJOR INGREDIENTS

The fruit is the medicinal part under discussion. (Bilberry leaf is an entirely different and much less common product, with different uses, often proposed for glucose control.) The proposed active ingredients of bilberry fruit are its anthocyanosides. Other constituents include flavone glycosides, iridoids, tannins, caffeic acid derivatives, and fruit acids.

CLAIMED ACTIONS

The anthocyanosides in bilberry have antioxidant properties. In vitro and other highly preliminary evidence suggests that they influence collagen metabolism by increasing cross-linkage of collagen fibers, inhibiting collagen degradation, promoting collagen biosynthesis, reducing inflammatory activity, and scavenging free radicals. The net effect may be decreased capillary permeability

and hence reduced capillary leakage in venous insufficiency and ischemia reperfusion. Other in vitro studies hint that anthocyanosides have an affinity for the retina, where they speed recovery of rhodopsin and alter enzymatic reactions in retinal tissues. At very high doses, anthocyanosides inhibit platelet aggregation.

USES

Bilberry fruit is widely used in the belief that it enhances night vision, but the basis for this use rests largely on anecdotes and a few poorly controlled studies performed in the 1960s. More recent and better-designed randomized controlled trials (RCTs) have failed to find any benefit. However, weak evidence from small, poor-quality clinical trials hints at benefits in diabetic or hypertensive retinopathy, as well as venous insufficiency.

ADMINISTRATION

Typical dose of bilberry fruit is 160 mg twice a day of an extract standardized to contain 25% bilberry anthocyanosides. Maximum safe doses in pregnant or nursing women, young children, and individuals with severe hepatic or renal disease are not established, but pregnant women have been given bilberry at the aforementioned dose in clinical trials.

SIDE EFFECTS

Animal and human trials indicate that bilberry fruit has a low level of toxicity. Reported side effects are limited to rare allergic reactions and nonspecific GI effects.

DENTAL CONSIDERATIONS

Ask why the product is being used.

DRUG INTERACTIONS
If taken in high doses, bilberry conceivably could potentiate anticoagulant or antiplatelet agents, but no such interactions have been reported.

bistort
(Polygonum bistorta)

OTHER NAMES:
Adder wort, dragonwort, Easter mangiant, English serpentary, oderwort, osterick, passions, patience dock, snakeweed, sweet dock, twice writhen

Class: Herbal remedy

MAJOR INGREDIENTS
Tannins.

CLAIMED ACTIONS
Astringent, antidote for selected poisons or venoms, antidiarrheal, and antiinflammatory.

USES
Uses have included treatment of all forms of diarrhea and cholera. It has been used in a mouth rinse for gum disease, canker sores, and stomatitis. External uses include treatment of sores, wounds, and hemorrhage. It was used traditionally to treat insect bites, snake bites, gonorrhea, smallpox, measles, and intestinal worms.

ADMINISTRATION
The leaves, roots, and rhizomes can be used to form a powder; also used as a tea, tincture, infusion, or ointment.

SIDE EFFECTS
Increase in mucous production, irritation of the GI tract, and possible hepatic damage.

DENTAL CONSIDERATIONS
Be aware of patient use of product for sore throat or mouth rinse.

DRUG INTERACTIONS
Tinctures contain alcohol and should not be used with disulfiram.

black cohosh
(Cimicifuga racemosa, Cimicifuga racemosa rhizoma)

OTHER NAMES:
Black snakeroot, baneberry

Class: Herbal remedy

MAJOR INGREDIENTS
The active chemicals are described as triterpene glycosides (acetin, 27-deoxyacetin, cimigoside, cimicifugoside, and racemoside), along with phytosterin and flavone derivatives. Other constituents include ferulic acids, isoflavones, fatty acids, and a volatile oil. The fresh and dried rhizomes are the portions of the plant used.

CLAIMED ACTIONS
Black cohosh is not a typical phytoestrogen (plant-based substance with estrogenic actions) because none of its constituents bind to estrogen receptors. It has been hypothesized, though, that some unknown constituent(s) of black cohosh undergo metabolic activation and acquire selective estrogen receptor modifier activity. Effects have been noted on estrogen

receptors in bone (possibly reducing bone breakdown), brain/hypothalamus (altering luteinizing hormone release and reducing vasomotor symptoms), and vaginal cell wall (partially reversing atrophy). Uterus and breast estrogen receptors appear to be relatively unaffected.

USES
Black cohosh is primarily used to treat menopausal syndrome. Limited evidence from placebo-controlled randomized controlled trials (RCTs) suggests that it can reduce hot flashes and vaginal dryness, without causing uterine hypertrophy. Black cohosh is sometimes recommended for treatment of PMS and dysmenorrhea disorders, but no meaningful evidence supports these uses.

ADMINISTRATION
The typical dosage of black cohosh is 1 or 2 tablets twice daily of a standardized extract manufactured to contain 1 mg of 27-deoxyaceteine per tablet. It has been suggested that black cohosh should not be used for more than 6 mo except under the supervision of a physician.

CONTRAINDICATIONS
Not recommended for use by pregnant or nursing women.

SIDE EFFECTS
Use of black cohosh in clinical trials has not been associated with any significant side effects other than occasional allergic reactions or nonspecific GI distress. However, there is one case report of autoimmune hepatitis apparently induced by the use of black cohosh. Overdosage may cause vomiting,

headache, hypotension, and other symptoms.

DENTAL CONSIDERATIONS
Ask why the product is being used.

DRUG INTERACTIONS
Weak evidence hints that black cohosh can potentiate antihypertensive drugs.

boswellia
(Boswellia serrata)

OTHER NAMES:
Frankincense, salai guggul

Class: Herbal remedy

MAJOR INGREDIENTS
Boswellia is the dried oleores made from the sap of the *Boswellia serrata* tree. Its major ingredients include boswellic acids and volatile oils.

CLAIMED ACTIONS
Whole boswellia, as well as isolated boswellic acids, have shown antiinflammatory effects in vitro and in animal and preliminary human trials.

USES
Preliminary randomized controlled trials (RCTs) suggest that boswellia might reduce symptoms of asthma, osteoarthritis, and inflammatory bowel disease, presumably through antiinflammatory effects. RCTs on boswellia for rheumatoid arthritis were of low quality and produced inconsistent results. Boswellic acids are undergoing study for palliative treatment of malignant glioma, in which they may reduce cerebral

edema and possibly slow tumor growth.

ADMINISTRATION
In most clinical trials, boswellia was taken at a dose of 300–400 mg 3 times a day, in the form of an extract standardized to contain 37.5% boswellic acids. Higher doses have been tried. Safety in pregnant or nursing women, young children, and individuals with severe hepatic or renal disease is not established.

SIDE EFFECTS
Use of boswellia in clinical trials has not been associated with any significant side effects other than rare allergic reactions and nonspecific GI distress. However, these trials generally used a pharmaceutical-grade extract of the herb boswellia or simply purified boswellic acids. Preparations made from the whole herb or use under less careful supervision might present additional risks.

DENTAL CONSIDERATIONS
Ask why the product is being used.

DRUG INTERACTIONS
No dental drug interactions have been reported.

butterbur
(Petasites hybridus, P. albus, P. vulgaris)

OTHER NAMES:
Petasin, blatterdock, butterfly dock, capdockin, flapperdock, umbrella leaves

Class: Herbal remedy

MAJOR INGREDIENTS
The entire plant is used medically. The major active ingredients are thought to be the sesquiterpene alcohol esters petasin and isopetasin. Hepatotoxic pyrrolizidine alkaloids are present in the crude herb but are removed during the manufacturing process for standardized products.

CLAIMED ACTIONS
Preliminary evidence suggests that butterbur, presumably through its petasin and isopetasin content, has antiinflammatory, antispasmodic, and antihistaminic properties. Its proposed antiinflammatory effect appears to be mediated through peptido-leukotrienes rather than prostaglandins.

USES
Standardized butterbur extract is widely used for prophylaxis of migraine headaches, but only one randomized controlled trial (RCT) supports this use. A double-blind comparative study without a placebo group found weak evidence that butterbur extract might have utility in allergic rhinitis. Another RCT failed to find butterbur to be effective for allergic skin disease. Other proposed uses based on the apparent actions of butterbur but lacking meaningful supporting evidence include asthma, bladder spasms, gallbladder pain, irritable bowel syndrome, musculoskeletal pain, and tension headaches.

ADMINISTRATION
The typical dosage of butterbur is 50 mg twice daily of an extract standardized to contain 7.5 mg of petasin and isopetasin. Only products

that are certified free from pyrrolizidine alkaloids should be used.

CONTRAINDICATIONS
Until further safety studies are performed, butterbur extract is not recommended for use by pregnant or nursing women, young children, or those with liver disease.

SIDE EFFECTS
Use of pharmaceutical-grade standardized butterbur extract in clinical trials has not been associated with any significant side effects other than occasional allergic reactions and nonspecific GI distress. However, there is one case report of cholestatic hepatitis apparently linked to use of butterbur extract. Unprocessed butterbur contains toxic pyrrolizidine alkaloids and should not be used at all.

DENTAL CONSIDERATIONS
Ask why the product is being used.

DRUG INTERACTIONS
No dental drug interactions have been reported.

chamomile
(Matricaria chamomilla, Matricaria recutita, Anthemis nobilis, Matricaria flos)

OTHER NAMES:
Roman chamomile, common chamomile, German chamomile

Class: Herbal remedy

MAJOR INGREDIENTS
Volatile oil containing α-bisabolol and other bisabolol derivatives (chamazulene, apigenin), various flavonoids, umbelliferone (coumarin-like ingredient), and many other components. The portion of the plant used is the dried flower.

CLAIMED ACTIONS
Antiinflammatory, antispasmodic, antibacterial, carminative, and to promote wound healing.

USES
Chamomile cream is widely used to treat eczema and minor wounds, but only scant preliminary evidence supports this use. One randomized controlled trial (RCT) failed to find chamomile cream helpful for treatment of radiation therapy-induced skin damage; another failed to find benefit for aphthous ulcers caused by 5-fluorouracil chemotherapy. One RCT did find evidence that inhalation of chamomile essential oil can reduce common cold symptoms. Oral chamomile has been used to treat inflammation and spasm in the GI tract, but this indication has no reliable supporting evidence.

ADMINISTRATION
Available in a variety of dose forms including teas, infusions (external use), mouth rinse, and oral dose forms.

SIDE EFFECTS
Slight risk of contact dermatitis; possible cross allergies with ragweed.

DENTAL CONSIDERATIONS
Ask why the product is being used. Inquire about bleeding history in patients taking warfarin or other oral anticoagulant. Inquire about unusual bleeding episodes following dental treatment.

DRUG INTERACTIONS

Evidence is lacking, but theoretically patients taking oral anticoagulants could show increased bleeding times. Possible risk of increased sedation with CNS depressants. Black cohosh may inhibit CYP3A4 activity, potentially changing serum levels of numerous drugs, but case reports are lacking.

chaste tree, chasteberry

(Vitex agnus-castus, Agni casti fructus)

OTHER NAMES:
Chaste tree fruit, monk's pepper, chaste tree

Class: Herbal remedy

MAJOR INGREDIENTS

Iridoid glycosides (agnuide and aucubin), flavonoids, progestins, testosterone, and multiple essential oils. The portion of the plant used is the dried, ripe fruit.

CLAIMED ACTIONS

Chasteberry is thought to inhibit the release of prolactin through action on dopamine receptors, although the evidence for this effect remains incomplete. It does not have a direct estrogen-like or progesterone-like effect.

USES

Chasteberry is primarily used for treatment of cyclic breast pain, a use supported by several randomized controlled trials (RCTs). It may produce benefits in PMS, although the evidence for this indication is largely limited to one well-designed RCT.

Other proposed uses, all based on its prolactin-related actions and lacking significant clinical trial support, include amenorrhea, luteal phase defect, and infertility. No evidence or rationale indicates that chasteberry is helpful for menopausal syndrome, but it is sometimes recommended for that purpose.

ADMINISTRATION

The typical dosage of chasteberry extract is 20–40 mg daily, usually in one morning dose.

CONTRAINDICATIONS

Because of its effect on prolactin, chasteberry should not be used by pregnant or nursing women. Possible risk of increased ovulation and pregnancy in some women.

SIDE EFFECTS

Chasteberry was well tolerated in clinical trials, producing no more than nonspecific reactions. There is one case report of ovarian hyperstimulation apparently caused by chasteberry.

DENTAL CONSIDERATIONS

Ask why the product is being used.

DRUG INTERACTIONS

Based on its presumed mechanism of action, chasteberry might potentiate the action of bromocriptine. Dopamine receptor antagonists theoretically could block some herbal effects.

chondroitin sulfate

OTHER NAMES:
Chondroitin

Class: Nonherbal remedy

MAJOR INGREDIENTS

Chondroitin sulfate is a mucopolysaccharide, that is, a glycosaminoglycan (GAG). It is found in mammalian cartilaginous tissue and is believed to play a role in flexibility. It is highly viscous and related chemically to sodium hyaluronate.

CLAIMED ACTIONS

It has useful viscoelastic properties suitable for use in selected types of ocular surgery, usually in combination with sodium hyaluronate. Orally administered GAGs are believed to concentrate in cartilage. Chondrocytes use GAGs to form a new cartilage matrix. It may inhibit leukocyte elastase when high concentrations are associated with rheumatoid arthritis. Other properties may include bringing synovial fluid into the joint. All of these may contribute to reduced inflammatory activity in joints. Serum lipid-lowering and antithrombogenic effects have been suggested.

USES

The primary use of chondroitin as a dietary supplement is for treatment of osteoarthritis, often in combination with glucosamine. The results of several randomized controlled trials (RCTs) of varying quality indicate that chondroitin can reduce symptoms to approximately the same extent as NSAIDs. Weaker evidence supports a possible disease-modifying effect (slowing progressive joint damage). Chondroitin in an ophthalmic solution has been used to treat dry eyes. In combination with sodium hyaluronate it is used to support ocular surgery during cataract removal and lens implantation

surgery. Its use in cardiovascular diseases remains in doubt.

ADMINISTRATION

A variety of oral dose forms are available, many in combination with glucosamine. Professionally used ophthalmic preparations are available.

SIDE EFFECTS

Long-term side effects are unknown. GI complaints are reported occasionally.

DENTAL CONSIDERATIONS

Ask why the product is being used. Arthritic patients may also be taking aspirin, NSAIDs, or arthritic disease-modifying drugs in addition to chondroitin. Question the patient about other antiarthritic drugs used including OTC drugs.

DRUG INTERACTIONS

None reported with dental drugs.

coenzyme Q10

OTHER NAMES:
CoQ10, ubiquinone

Class: Nonherbal remedy

MAJOR INGREDIENTS

Coenzyme Q10 is a cofactor found in all animal and plant cells. There are currently no specific dietary intake recommendations for coenzyme Q10.

CLAIMED ACTIONS

CoQ10 is an essential cofactor in the Krebs cycle, playing a role in the aerobic production of adenosine triphosphate (ATP). Because heart muscle depends entirely on aerobic energy production, CoQ10 supplementation has been suggested as a way to enhance myocardial function. Further support for this treatment approach comes from evidence of reduced myocardial CoQ10 in people with CHF. In addition, certain medications often taken by individuals with heart disease, most notably statins, are thought to either suppress the endogenous production of CoQ10 or interfere with its function. This suggests a need for repletion; however, little evidence as yet indicates that exogenous CoQ10 provides any objective or subjective benefit for people using such medications (other than restoring normal CoQ10 levels). Other proposed uses of CoQ10 are based on its antioxidant properties or other unknown mechanisms.

USES

Incomplete and somewhat inconsistent evidence from double-blind trials suggests that CoQ10 may offers benefit as adjuvant therapy for CHF, enhancing cardiac performance. Weaker and again inconsistent evidence suggests possible benefits in cardiomyopathy, hypertension, cardiac reperfusion injury, and diabetes. Weak evidence hints that CoQ10 might reduce doxorubicin cardiotoxicity, improve renal function in chronic renal failure, enhance antibody response to hepatitis B vaccine, aid recovery from periodontal disease, reduce symptoms of muscular dystrophy and neurogenic atrophy, and slow the progression of Parkinson's disease. CoQ10 does not appear to be helpful as a sports supplement. See Drug Interactions for a list of the medications for which CoQ10 has

been recommended as a repletion agent.

ADMINISTRATION

The typical dosage of CoQ10 is 30–150 mg taken 2 or 3 times a day. Maximum safe doses in pregnant or nursing women, young children, and individuals with severe hepatic or renal disease are not established.

SIDE EFFECTS

CoQ10 appears to offer little to no toxic risk. Use of CoQ10 in human trials continuing for up to 6 yr has shown no serious side effects. Mild, nonspecific GI distress may occur. There have been a few questionable case reports of a CoQ10 withdrawal syndrome in individuals using the supplement for CHF.

DENTAL CONSIDERATIONS

Patients who believe that CoQ10 offers benefit for periodontal disease may be advised that the evidence for benefits with this expensive supplement is exceedingly weak.

DRUG INTERACTIONS

CoQ10 has a molecular similarity to vitamin K, which has led to concerns that CoQ10 use might antagonize the effects of warfarin. However, one study designed to evaluate this possibility found that use of CoQ10 caused no change in international normalized ratio or warfarin dosage. Drugs thought to interfere with the production or action of CoQ10, and therefore to potentially benefit from repletion, include the following: β-blocking agents (alprenolol, metoprolol, and propranolol to a greater extent than timolol), clonidine, hydrochlorothiazide, methyldopa, oral hypoglycemics (acetohexamide [Dymelor], glyburide, phenformin, and tolazamide to a greater extent than chlorpropamide, glipizide, and tolbutamide), phenothiazines, statins, and tricyclic antidepressants. The best evidence for tangible benefit with exogenous CoQ10 supplementation exists for statins and tricyclics, but the evidence is not strong.

conjugated linoleic acids

OTHER NAMES:
CLAs

Class: Nonherbal remedy

MAJOR INGREDIENTS
Conjugated linoleic acids are mixed isomers of the essential ω-6 fatty acid linoleic acid.

CLAIMED ACTIONS
The essential fatty acids in CLAs are hypothesized to affect fat metabolism. Limited and inconsistent evidence suggests that CLA supplements increase fat metabolism while retaining lean muscle mass. CLA has functional similarities to thiazolidinedione, which led to investigation of potential hypoglycemic effects; however, the limited evidence available suggests a possible hyperglycemic effect instead. Chemopreventive and hypolipidemic effects have also been hypothesized.

USES
The most common use of CLA is as an aid to enhancing body composition, said to "burn fat" while helping to increase muscle mass.

However, the clinical evidence for this effect is limited to small randomized controlled trials (RCTs) with inconsistent results. CLA does not appear to aid weight loss per se.

ADMINISTRATION
The typical dose is 3–5 g daily.

CONTRAINDICATIONS
At this time, CLA should not be used by nursing mothers because one clinical trial found that CLA supplements reduced the fat content of breast milk.

SIDE EFFECTS
CLA generally causes no side effects other than nonspecific GI distress. Safety in pregnant women, young children, and individuals with liver disease is not established.

DENTAL CONSIDERATIONS
Ask why the product is being used.

DRUG INTERACTIONS
One study found potential hyperglycemic effects with CLA, suggesting antagonistic interactions with hypoglycemic agents. However, no such interactions have been reported.

cranberry
(Vaccinium macrocarpon)

Class: Herbal remedy

MAJOR INGREDIENTS
The berries are the medicinal part used. Cranberries contain a variety of proanthocyanidins, which are its presumed active ingredients. Other constituents include fructose and

various plant acids, such as citric acid and malic acid.

CLAIMED ACTIONS

Proanthocyanidin complexes in cranberry are thought to reduce bacterial adhesion to uroepithelial cells by impairing the action of bacterial adhesins, thus interfering with the early stages of infection. This proposed mechanism does not tend to suggest benefits for infections that are already under way.

USES

Limited evidence from randomized controlled trials (RCTs) indicates that regular use of cranberry juice concentrate can reduce the incidence of acute UTIs in women. There is no evidence of benefit once an acute infection has begun. Effectiveness for treatment of chronic bacteriuria/ pyuria is unclear. One small study suggests that cranberry juice might increase insulin secretion in individuals with Type 2 diabetes, but the clinical significance of this finding is unclear.

ADMINISTRATION

Dry cranberry juice extract often is taken at a dose of 500–2000 mg, 3 times a day, depending on the product's concentration. Cranberry juice itself is very bad tasting, and palatable cranberry beverages contain little cranberry. Maximum safe doses in pregnant or nursing women, young children, and individuals with severe hepatic or renal disease are not established.

SIDE EFFECTS

Use of cranberry concentrate is not associated with side effects other than occasional allergic reactions and nonspecific, mild GI distress.

Some concerns have been expressed about possible lithogenic actions of cranberry, but it appears that balance intake is more likely to reduce risk of urolithiasis than to increase it.

DENTAL CONSIDERATIONS

Weak evidence hints that the proanthocyanidins in cranberry might offer dental benefits by impairing aggregation of the bacteria involved in plaque formation. However, because the taste of pure cranberry is difficult to tolerate unless sweetener is added, this finding will not have practical use unless an artificial sweetener can be used.

DRUG INTERACTIONS

On the basis of case reports, it appears that high intake of cranberry can increase the action of warfarin, leading to excess anticoagulation. In addition, because cranberries reduce urinary pH, excretion of various drugs might be increased, including opiates, antidepressants, antipsychotics, and some antibiotics. However, there are no actual case reports of such interactions.

creatine

OTHER NAMES:
Creatine monohydrate

Class: Nonherbal remedy

MAJOR INGREDIENTS

Creatine is manufactured in the body from arginine, glycine, and methionine. There is no dietary requirement for creatine.

CLAIMED ACTIONS

Exogenous creatine is thought to increase muscle supplies of phosphocreatine, enabling more rapid restoration of ATP levels after a short, high-intensity burst of exertion. Increased creatine levels may also enhance nerve function. These two effects combined are the basis for use of creatine in neuromuscular disorders. In mitochondrial disorders, exogenous creatine is thought to stabilize mitochondrial creatine kinase, decreasing demand on the damaged mitochondria. Creatine may also reduce lipid levels through an as-yet-unidentified mechanism.

USES

Numerous small randomized controlled trials (RCTs) indicate that creatine may slightly increase performance in high-intensity repetitive burst exercise. However, the evidence is not entirely consistent, and rather specific parameters of duration and rest appear to be necessary for benefit. Creatine is not helpful in endurance exercise, and it may or may not enhance resistance exercise capacity. Other small RCTs suggest possible benefit in CHF (increasing exercise tolerance) and hyperlipidemia. Results of studies on creatine as an aid to recovery of muscle strength after limb immobilization or as treatment for a variety of neuromuscular and mitochondrial disorders have been mixed.

ADMINISTRATION

Typical daily dose of creatine is 2–5 g/day. Athletes typically begin with a loading dose of 15–30 g/day for several days, but there is no evidence that this offers additional value.

SIDE EFFECTS

Creatine has a low level of toxicity, but long-term safety studies have not been performed. Common side effects of creatine supplementation include weight gain, mostly from water retention, as well as mild GI distress, and possibly muscle cramping and dehydration. Contrary to some reports, there is no evidence that creatine diminishes the body's ability to tolerate increased environmental temperatures. Maximum safe doses in pregnant or nursing women, young children, and individuals with severe hepatic or renal disease are not established.

DENTAL CONSIDERATIONS

Ask why the product is being used.

DRUG INTERACTIONS

No dental drug interactions have been reported.

dong quai
(Angelica sinensis)

OTHER NAMES:
Chinese angelica, dang-gui

Class: Herbal remedy

MAJOR INGREDIENTS

Active constituents of dong quai may include butylidene phthalide, ferulic acid, β-sitosterol, a variety of coumarins (oxypeucedanin, osthol, and others), an essential oil, polysaccharides, lactones, and vitamins E and B_{12}. The portion of the plant used is the root.

CLAIMED ACTIONS

Vasodilation, antispasmodic in blood vessels, CNS stimulation, and immunosuppressant and antiinflammatory properties. The mechanism of action of these effects is unclear. Contrary to some reports, dong quai does not appear to have phytoestrogen constituents.

USES

Used in Chinese herbal medicine in combination with other herbs. Uses include treatment of dysmenorrhea, other menstrual problems, and menopausal symptoms. Other uses include treatment of arthritis, hypertension, and ulcers. However, significant clinical studies are lacking. One randomized controlled trial (RCT) failed to find dong quai helpful for menopausal symptoms. The remedy does not appear in the German Commission E monographs.

ADMINISTRATION

Administered orally as an infusion, a tincture, or a chewable root.

CONTRAINDICATIONS

Women who have had breast cancer should not use dong quai. Despite a lack of estrogenic action, dong quai may stimulate breast cancer cell growth (in vitro evidence only).

SIDE EFFECTS

In clinical trials, dong quai has been generally well tolerated. Photosensitization is possible on theoretic grounds. Safety for pregnant or nursing women, young children, and individuals with severe liver or kidney disease is not established.

DENTAL CONSIDERATIONS

Ask why the product is being used. Inquire about bleeding history in patients taking warfarin or other oral anticoagulants. Inquire about unusual

bleeding episodes following dental treatment. Caution suggested for combination treatment with photosensitizing drugs.

DRUG INTERACTIONS

Dong quai may interact adversely with anticoagulants or antiplatelet agents.

echinacea
(Echinacea angustifolia, Echinacea purpurea, Echinacea pallida)

OTHER NAMES:
American cone flower, Kansas snakeroot, purple cone flower

Class: Herbal remedy

MAJOR INGREDIENTS

Caffeic acid glycoside (echinacoside), alkylamides (echinacein and others), essential oils (humulene and others), a variety of flavonoids, and many other components. As with any plant, the contents vary with the species, the parts of the plant used, and whether the plant is dried or fresh. The portions of the plant used are the flower, other aboveground parts, and even the roots. Most studies finding benefit for the common cold involved preparations made from the aboveground portion of the *E. purpurea* species.

CLAIMED ACTIONS

Stimulation of the immune system (some laboratory data suggest an increase in macrophage phagocytic activity and numbers of neutrophils); possible antibacterial, antiviral, and antiinflammatory activity lack strong support.

USES

Considerable (but not entirely consistent) evidence from randomized controlled trials (RCTs) indicates that acute use of echinacea may reduce the symptoms and duration of the common cold and influenza. Chronic use of echinacea does not appear to offer prophylactic benefits against colds. Other uses proposed but lacking meaningful supporting evidence include wound healing, *Candida* infections, supportive therapy for lower UTIs, rheumatoid arthritis, and supportive use in colon cancer.

ADMINISTRATION

Available in a variety of preparations for internal (oral administration) and external use.

CONTRAINDICATIONS

On theoretical grounds, echinacea should not be used in patients with autoimmune diseases or progressive infectious diseases, including tuberculosis, multiple sclerosis, leukocytosis, and collagen diseases, or individuals taking immunosuppressive medications.

SIDE EFFECTS

Generally limited to parenteral doses only. Fatigue, headache, and dizziness were reported with oral doses. Possible risk of cross-allergic reaction with chamomile or ragweed.

DENTAL CONSIDERATIONS

Ask why it is being used. Avoid use during immunosuppression. Use with caution in asthma, atopy, or allergic rhinitis because of potential for allergic reactions.

DRUG INTERACTIONS

May decrease effectiveness of immunosuppressants. Discontinue before use of general anesthetics.

eleutherococcus
(Eleutherococcus senticosus, Acanthopanax senticosus)

OTHER NAMES:
Siberian ginseng, Russian ginseng, eleutheroginseng

Class: Herbal remedy

MAJOR INGREDIENTS

Major constituents include a variety of unrelated lignans, setoids, phenylacrylic acid derivatives, polysaccharides, steroid glycosides, and triterpene saponins, all somewhat misleadingly named eleutherosides (eleutheroside A, B, etc.). The root and rhizome are the parts used medicinally. Note that despite the common name "Russian ginseng," *Eleutherococcus* has no botanic or biochemical similarity to true ginseng, Panax ginseng.

CLAIMED ACTIONS

Eleutherococcus is said to act as an "adaptogen," a substance that enhances an organism's general ability to adapt to stress of all kinds. However, the supporting evidence that eleutherococcus (or any other substance) has adaptogenic properties is limited to human and animal trials of substandard methodology. Some evidence indicates that eleutherococcus may increase maximal oxygen intake during intense exercise. Immunomodulatory effects have been seen in some studies, specifically increases in helper and inducer T lymphocytes.

USES

One randomized controlled trial (RCT) found evidence that regular use of eleutherococcus by individuals with chronic recurrent genital herpes reduced the rate of flare ups. One RCT failed to find eleutherococcus helpful for chronic fatigue syndrome. The majority of RCTs evaluating eleutherococcus for possible sports performance enhancement effects have failed to find benefit.

ADMINISTRATION

Typical dose of eleutherococcus is 2–3 g daily of the whole herb or 300–400 mg of a standardized extract. Maximum safe doses in pregnant or nursing women, young children, and individuals with severe hepatic or renal disease are not established.

SIDE EFFECTS

Eleutherococcus is thought to have a low level of toxicity; however, most safety studies were performed in the former Soviet Union, and whether the results can be fully relied upon is not clear. Use of eleutherococcus in clinical trials has not been associated with any significant side effects.

DENTAL CONSIDERATIONS

Ask why the product is being used.

DRUG INTERACTIONS

There is one case report in which use of eleutherococcus appears to have interfered with a laboratory test for serum digoxin levels, causing the test to falsely report an elevation that did not exist. On the basis of its possible immunomodulatory actions, eleutherococcus conceivably could interfere with the action of

immunosuppressive drugs, but no such interactions have been reported.

evening primrose oil
(Oenothera biennis)

OTHER NAMES:
Evening primrose

Class: Herbal remedy

MAJOR INGREDIENTS

The oil is a mixture of fatty acids, including linoleic acid (50%–80%), γ-linolenic acid (GLA, 6%–11%), and smaller amounts of other fatty acids, including palmitic acid, oleic acid, and stearic acid. Other ingredients include tannins, sitosterol, and trace minerals. The portion of the plant used is the seed.

CLAIMED ACTIONS

Antiatherosclerotic, relief of premenstrual tension, relief of mastalgia, and antiinflammatory actions for arthritis and dermatologic conditions. The fatty acids contained in the oil may function like essential oils and act as precursors of prostaglandins that help regulate metabolic functions.

USES

Evening primrose is primarily used as a source of GLA. Some randomized controlled trial (RCT) evidence suggests that evening primrose or GLA can reduce symptoms of diabetic neuropathy after many months of use. Weak RCT evidence hints that GLA from borage oil may help adult periodontitis. Other potential indications of GLA or evening primrose oil, with weak supporting evidence at best, include hyperlipidemia, PMS, rheumatoid arthritis, and weight loss. Claims are also made that GLA is effective in controlling symptoms of atopic dermatitis, but the most recent and best-designed RCTs failed to find benefit. The same can be said of GLA for treatment of cyclic mastitis. One RCT failed to find evening primrose oil effective for attention deficit hyperactivity disorder. This herb is not listed in the German Commission E monographs.

ADMINISTRATION
Available as capsules for oral administration.

SIDE EFFECTS
Side effects are few and occur only occasionally. They generally include digestive complaints such as GI distress and nausea.

DENTAL CONSIDERATIONS
Ask why the product is being used. As noted previously, has shown some promise for periodontitis.

DRUG INTERACTIONS
No dental drug interactions have been reported.

feverfew
(Tanacetum parthenium, Chrysanthemum parthenium)

OTHER NAMES:
Featherfew, feverfew leaf, bachelor's button

Class: Herbal remedy

MAJOR INGREDIENTS
Sesquiterpene lactones, especially parthenolide 85%, once were considered the active ingredients in feverfew. However, studies using parthenolide-rich extracts found no benefit, and attention now is focused elsewhere. One bioactive candidate is tanetin, a lipophilic avonol (6-hydroxykaempferol 3,7,4′-trimethyl ether) that inhibits proinflammatory eicosanoids. Other constituents include volatile oils (camphor, trans-chrysanthylacetate), flavonoids (luteolin, apigenin), and many other constituents. The portion of the plant used is the leaf.

CLAIMED ACTIONS
Inhibition of proinflammatory eicosanoids resulting in antiinflammatory actions. May decrease platelet aggregation and serotonin release (laboratory studies). It is not listed in the German Commission E monographs.

USES
A few small randomized controlled trials (RCTs) have found that regular use of feverfew leaf can reduce the severity, duration, or incidence of migraines. Studies using feverfew extracts standardized to parthenolide content, however, have failed to find benefits. Other proposed uses, including osteoarthritis, rheumatoid arthritis, and stimulation of menstruation, lack RCT support.

ADMINISTRATION
Available in many oral dose forms or used to make an infusion. Safety in nursing women or individuals with severe hepatic or renal disease is not established.

CONTRAINDICATIONS
Because of its history of use as an abortifacient, feverfew should not be used by pregnant women.

SIDE EFFECTS
Oral products produce few complaints; chewing the leaves may lead to oral ulcerations and swelling of circumoral tissues. Potential risk for increased bleeding time.

DENTAL CONSIDERATIONS
Ask why the product is being used. Inquire about bleeding history in patients taking warfarin or other oral anticoagulant. Inquire about unusual bleeding episodes following dental treatment.

DRUG INTERACTIONS
On a theoretic basis, feverfew might potentiate the effects of antiplatelet agents and increase gastric side effects of NSAIDs. However, no such interactions have been reported. Advise patients not to take this herb for 2–3 wk before surgery.

garlic
(Allium sativum)

OTHER NAMES:
Allium, poor man's treacle

Class: Herbal remedy

MAJOR INGREDIENTS
A volatile oil containing several sulfur compounds, a sulfur-containing amino acid identified as alliin. With grinding, alliin is converted to allicin, which is responsible for the typical odor of garlic, as well as much of its bioactivity. Ajoene and S-allylcysteine are other active compounds. The portions of the plant used are whole (fresh or dried) garlic clove and oil of garlic.

CLAIMED ACTIONS
With oral use, actions claimed for garlic include hypolipidemic, antiplatelet aggregation, antihypertensive, antioxidant, antiatherosclerotic, and immune stimulant activity. In vitro studies have found topical antibiotic, antifungal, and antiviral actions. Antithrombotic effects have been documented in vitro and in vivo.

USES
Despite widespread use for hyperlipidemia, current evidence from well-designed randomized controlled trials (RCTs) suggests that garlic does not improve lipid levels to more than a minimal extent. Some evidence from preliminary RCTs indicates that regular use of standardized garlic extracts may reduce the incidence of the common cold in adults and children. Weak RCT evidence indicates possible antihypertensive and antiatherosclerotic actions. One RCT suggests that oral use of garlic can decrease insect (tick) bites. Topically, garlic has been used to treat a wide array of bacterial, fungal, and viral infections, but there are no rigorous supporting data. Oral antibiotic effectiveness is unlikely. Use in GI fungal infections remains in doubt. Long-term effects are unknown.

ADMINISTRATION
Available in a variety of oral dose forms. The best-studied form of garlic is garlic powder specially stabilized to provide alliin, which can be converted to allicin. Raw garlic

also provides alliin/allicin, but other forms of garlic, such as cooked garlic, garlic oil, and aged garlic products, do not provide alliin. (Nonetheless, some pharmacologic effects have been seen with these other forms, presumably from other constituents.)

SIDE EFFECTS

The taste and odor of garlic are by far the most common complaints. Rarely GI symptoms occur with larger doses. Halitosis and burning of the mouth have been reported. There is one case report of spontaneous spinal epidural hematoma attributed to use of garlic products. Note that standardized garlic is more similar to raw garlic than to cooked garlic; therefore the common food use of cooked garlic cannot be taken as evidence of safety.

DENTAL CONSIDERATIONS

Ask why the product is being used. Inquire about unusual bleeding episodes following dental treatment.

DRUG INTERACTIONS

Garlic might potentiate antiplatelet or anticoagulant agents. Because of increased risk of bleeding, advise patients not to take this herb for 2–3 wk before surgery. Garlic has been found to reduce plasma concentrations of saquinavir and possibly increase the GI toxicity of ritonavir (drugs used for HIV).

ginger
(Zingiber officinale, Zingiberis rhizoma)

OTHER NAMES:
Ginger root

Class: Herbal remedy

MAJOR INGREDIENTS

The root contains a volatile oil and other chemicals termed pungent principals. These latter compounds are collectively known as gingerols, shogaols, and gingerdiols. The portion of the plant used is the root.

CLAIMED ACTIONS

Motion sickness prevention, promotion of salivary and gastric secretions, positive inotropic action, and antiplatelet and antiinflammatory effects have all been claimed for this herb. Gluonolactone, an active ingredient, has been reported to have serotonin (5-HT) antagonist activity, and gingerols may have a positive inotropic effect.

USES

Incomplete and somewhat inconsistent evidence from multiple randomized controlled trials (RCTs) of varying quality suggests that ginger can reduce motion sickness symptoms. Other RCTs suggest benefits for nausea and vomiting of pregnancy (morning sickness). Results on benefits for postsurgical anesthesia are contradictory. Ginger has been used for control of nausea from chemotherapy, but supporting evidence is weak. RCTs have shown equivocal results regarding efficacy in osteoarthritis.

ADMINISTRATION

Only the rhizome (rootlike stalk) of the plant is used. The German Commission E monographs list the dose at 2–4 g/day. Despite ginger's medical use in nausea and vomiting of pregnancy, safety during pregnancy and lactation is not established.

SIDE EFFECTS
Generally not reported except for toxic doses that could include CNS depression and arrhythmia.

DENTAL CONSIDERATIONS
Ask why the product is being used.

DRUG INTERACTIONS
Although ginger has shown antiplatelet rather than anticoagulant effects, there is one case report in which use of ginger apparently potentiated phenprocoumon. Interactions with other anticoagulants or antiplatelet agents are possible.

ginkgo
(Ginkgo biloba, Ginkgo folium)

OTHER NAMES:
Maidenhair tree, ginkyo

Class: Herbal remedy

MAJOR INGREDIENTS
Common ingredients with claimed pharmacologic activity include multiple flavonoids (biobetin, ginkgetin), flavone glycosides (quercetin), bioflavones, terpenoids (ginkgolides A, B, and C), and bilobalide. The only portion of the plant used is the leaf, made in a specific 50:1 extract. Thus the commonly tested treatment is more properly called ginkgo biloba extract (GBE) rather than ginkgo. The seeds are toxic.

CLAIMED ACTIONS
Improvement in blood flow in the microcirculation, inhibition of development of trauma-induced or toxin-induced cerebral edema,

improved hypoxic tolerance in cerebral tissues, reduction in retinal edema, increased memory performance, inhibition of age-related reduction in muscarinic receptors, and antagonism of platelet-activating factor (PAF). It may have MAOI properties.

USES
Significant, but not entirely consistent, evidence from multiple randomized controlled trials (RCTs) supports use in Alzheimer's dementia and other forms of dementia. Significant evidence also exists for benefit in intermittent claudication. Weaker evidence from RCTs supports use in normal age-related memory impairment, PMS, Raynaud's phenomenon, and vertiginous syndromes. Other potential uses with limited support include idiopathic sudden hearing loss, glaucoma, macular degeneration, and diabetic microvascular disease. Contrary to earlier reports, ginkgo does not appear to be effective for sexual dysfunction (in men or women), tinnitus, or mountain sickness.

ADMINISTRATION
Capsules and tablets of leaf extracts are available for use. Doses range from 120 to 240 mg of 50:1 dry extract for 8 wk for chronic diseases. Use for longer than 3 mo requires reevaluation of benefits.

CONTRAINDICATIONS
Not recommended for use by pregnant or nursing women. Individuals with seizure disorders should not use ginkgo.

SIDE EFFECTS
In clinical trials, ginkgo has been well tolerated, producing no more

than occasional mild allergies and nonspecific GI distress. There are several reports of internal bleeding attributable to use of ginkgo, including bleeding episodes during surgery. Seizures have been reported. One report of oral ulcerations is noted.

DENTAL CONSIDERATIONS

Ask why the product is being used. Inquire about unusual bleeding episodes following dental treatment.

DRUG INTERACTIONS

There is considerable evidence for anticoagulant and antiplatelet activity with ginkgo; do not combine with other anticoagulant or antiplatelet agents except under close supervision. Discontinue ginkgo use 2 wk before surgery and general anesthesia. Ginkgo might decrease effectiveness of calcium channel blockers and increase ototoxicity of aminoglycosides. Possible interaction between ginkgo and trazodone (Desyrel) may cause excess stimulation of gamma-aminobutyric acid (GABA) receptors leading to CNS depression and possible coma.

ginseng

(*Panax quinquefolius,* American; *Panax ginseng,* Korean)

Class: Herbal remedy

MAJOR INGREDIENTS

Constituents vary with the species of ginseng used. Contains steroid-like compounds called ginsenosides or panaxosides. Other ingredients include a volatile oil and flavonoids, along with smaller quantities of other substances.

CLAIMED ACTIONS

Panax ginseng is said to act as an "adaptogen," a substance that enhances an organism's general ability to adapt to stress of all kinds. However, the supporting evidence that ginseng (or any other substance) has adaptogenic properties is limited to animal studies and a few human trials of substandard methodology. Despite earlier reports, ginseng itself does not appear to have estrogenic effects.

USES

Preliminary randomized controlled trials (RCTs) suggest that American ginseng but not Panax ginseng may improve glucose control in Type 2 diabetes. Other uses with limited and in some cases inconsistent RCT support include increasing immune response to influenza vaccine, enhancing mental function, improving blood sugar control in diabetes, correcting erectile dysfunction, and enhancing sports performance.

ADMINISTRATION

The root is used for teas and various other oral preparations.

CONTRAINDICATIONS

Worrisome data from animal studies suggest possible teratogenic effects. Not recommended for use by pregnant women.

SIDE EFFECTS

Ginseng appears to have a low level of toxicity. Use of ginseng in clinical trials was associated with few side effects other than occasional allergic reactions and nonspecific GI distress. However, adulterants included with ginseng products may increase risk for other side effects.

DENTAL CONSIDERATIONS

Ask why the product is being used.

DRUG INTERACTIONS

No specific dental drug interactions have been reported, but ginseng may interact with MAOIs. Interactions with warfarin are unclear. Discontinue 7 days before general anesthesia and general surgical procedures.

glucosamine sulfate

OTHER NAMES:
Chitosamine, glucosamine

Class: Nonherbal remedy

MAJOR INGREDIENTS

Glucosamine sulfate, an aminomonosaccharide (2-amino-2-deoxyglucose), is a component of mucopolysaccharides and mucoproteins. Other salt forms may also be used.

CLAIMED ACTIONS

Glucosamine is used in the synthesis of glycoproteins and GAGs. It is formed in the body from glucose through intermediary metabolic steps to be incorporated into GAGs, which are essential for cartilage function in joints. Exogenous glucosamine is thought to enhance joint proteoglycan content, thereby improving the function of the failing joint.

USES

Most published randomized controlled trials (RCTs) indicate that glucosamine is superior to placebo and equally effective (though slower acting) than standard NSAIDs for treatment of osteoarthritis. Incomplete RCT evidence also points toward a possible disease-modifying effect (retarding progressive joint damage). Other proposed uses include prevention and treatment of tendon and other soft tissue injuries, but no meaningful evidence supports these indications.

ADMINISTRATION

Usual dose is 500 mg 3 times a day.

SIDE EFFECTS

Side effects are uncommon but can include GI effects such as nausea, heartburn, diarrhea, and epigastric pain. CNS side effects are rarely observed and may include headache, insomnia, and drowsiness. Contrary to earlier reports, glucosamine does not appear to be harmful for patients with diabetes. However, arthritic patients may be taking aspirin, NSAIDs, or disease-modifying osteoarthritis drugs in addition to glucosamine and chondroitin. Question the patient about other antiarthritic drugs used, including OTC drugs.

DENTAL CONSIDERATIONS

Ask why the product is being used.

DRUG INTERACTIONS

No dental drug interactions have been reported.

goldenseal
(Hydrastis canadensis)

OTHER NAMES:
Eye root, yellow root, turmeric root

Class: Herbal remedy

MAJOR INGREDIENTS

Contains the isoquinoline alkaloids hydrastine and berberine, other related alkaloids, and a volatile oil.

CLAIMED ACTIONS

Astringent and antiseptic. May stimulate bile and may have laxative action. Hydrastine has been shown to cause vasoconstriction in peripheral vessels. Berberine may have some antibacterial actions. This herb is not included in the German Commission E monographs.

USES

No proposed uses of goldenseal are supported by randomized controlled trials (RCTs). Goldenseal is frequently added to preparations designed to treat the common cold, but no evidence (or traditional history) suggests that it is effective for this purpose. Goldenseal is widely used topically for minor skin wounds and mucous membrane irritation, again without supporting evidence. Its constituent, berberine, may have some action against intestinal infections, but unrealistically high doses of goldenseal would be required to match the dose of berberine used in studies. Berberine (not goldenseal) has been used for treatment of eye infections. Numerous other proposed uses of goldenseal that lack evidence of efficacy include "masking" a positive drug screen, treating minor cardiac arrhythmias, and reducing crampy intestinal pain and dyspepsia.

ADMINISTRATION

Typical dosages for oral use are 500 mg 3 times a day, often in combination with other herbs.

Topical goldenseal preparations vary in concentration.

CONTRAINDICATIONS

Not recommended for use by pregnant or nursing women or by individuals with hepatic disease.

SIDE EFFECTS

Safe in usual doses. Adverse effects are more often observed with toxic doses (may include hypertension, convulsions, and breathing difficulties). Photosensitivity is a theoretical possibility.

DENTAL CONSIDERATIONS

Ask why the product is being used.

DRUG INTERACTIONS

No dental drug interactions have been reported.

gotu kola
(Centella asiatica)

OTHER NAMES:

TECA (titrated extract of *Centella asiatica*), TTFCA (total triterpenic fraction of *Centella asiatica*), hydrocotyle, Indian pennywort

Class: Herbal remedy

MAJOR INGREDIENTS

The aboveground parts of the plant are used medicinally. The major constituents are the triterpene acids and esters known as asiaticosides, asiatic acid, madecassic acid, and madecassoside. (Note: *Gotu kola,* unlike the unrelated kola nut, does not contain caffeine.)

CLAIMED ACTIONS

Gotu kola, or its triterpenic extract, is said to enhance the structure and function of connective tissues, an effect possibly mediated by actions on collagen cross-linking and fibronectin production. This is the basis for most of its proposed uses. However, the supporting evidence for such an effect is generally weak. *Gotu kola* extracts may weaken the protective outer coating of Mycobacterium leprae and on that basis has been used for treatment of leprosy.

USES

Several small randomized controlled trials (RCTs) found that gotu kola can decrease pain, edema, and leg fatigue in chronic venous insufficiency of the lower extremity. There is no evidence that it can alter the appearance of visible varicosities. Other small RCTs suggest benefit in the treatment of keloids and leprosy and in reducing the startle reflex to sudden loud noises. Oral and topical gotu kola have been recommended for virtually all diseases of the skin or diseases that have skin manifestations, but no RCT evidence supports these uses.

ADMINISTRATION

The studied dose of gotu kola is 20–40 mg 3 times a day of a triterpenic extract standardized to contain 40% asiaticoside, 29%–30% asiatic acid, 29%–30% madecassic acid, and 1%–2% madecassoside. Safety in pregnant women is not established, but pregnant women have been in enrolled in clinical trials, with no harmful effects seen.

SIDE EFFECTS

Gotu kola appears to have a low level of toxicity. In clinical trials, use of gotu kola has not been associated with any significant side effects other than occasional allergic reactions and mild nonspecific GI distress. However, on the basis of a study in mice, there are some concerns that topical gotu kola might have cancer-promoting actions.

DENTAL CONSIDERATIONS

Ask why the product is being used.

DRUG INTERACTIONS

No dental drug interactions have been reported.

grape seed extract
(Vitis vinifera, Vitis coignetiae)

OTHER NAMES:
Grape seed extract, grape seed oil, muskat, de pepins de raisin

Class: Herbal remedy

MAJOR INGREDIENTS

The oil of the grape seed is one of the two major sources of oligomeric proanthocyanidin complexes (OPCs), less commonly called procyanidolic oligomers (PCOs). (The other is the bark of maritime pine.) Other constituents include essential fatty acids and tocopherols (vitamin E). Pycnogenol, a trademarked and patented herbal product and dietary supplement, contains similar but not identical OPCs from the bark of the maritime pine (Pinus maritime, sometimes called Pinus nigra var. maritime). Vitis coignetiae also contains epsilon-viniferin, oligos-tilbenes and amyelopsins, and 51-nucleotidase inhibitors. Resveratrol (3,5,41-trihydroxystilbene) is present when herbal preparations are mixed with grape skin extract. The seed and sometimes the skin of the grape are used medicinally.

CLAIMED ACTIONS

OPCs have significant free-radical scavenging actions and may protect connective tissue by inhibiting hyaluronidase, elastase, and collagenase and increasing collagen cross-linking. These and other effects may lead to decreased capillary permeability. OPCs inhibit platelet aggregation and alter prostaglandin metabolism.

USES

The best-documented use of OPCs is treatment of chronic venous insufficiency. Several randomized controlled trials (RCTs) suggest that OPC treatment can reduce lower extremity pain, edema, and fatigue. Effects on visible varicosities have not been documented. Weaker RCT evidence suggests possible benefit in reducing edema caused by surgery or minor injury. Other indications for OPCs from grape seed that have some support from small RCTs include reducing capillary fragility in liver cirrhosis and alleviating symptoms of allergic rhinitis. Related OPCs from pine bark have shown some potential benefit for periodontal disease, when used in the form of chewing gum. Grape-seed OPCs have failed to prove effective for reducing lipid levels. Supposed benefits for cardiovascular disease are entirely theoretical, on the basis of antioxidant and antiplatelet properties.

ADMINISTRATION

Administered orally in tablets or capsules. Doses range from 40–300 mg/day, with maintenance doses at 40–80 mg daily.

CONTRAINDICATIONS

OPCs are thought to have antiplatelet activity, and on this basis they should not be taken by individuals using anticoagulant or antiplatelet agents.

SIDE EFFECTS

Grape-seed OPCs have undergone extensive safety testing and appear to have a low level of toxicity.

DENTAL CONSIDERATIONS

Determine why the patient is taking botanic products. Patients should discontinue use 2 wk before surgery. As noted previously, OPCs from pine bark have shown some promise for periodontitis.

DRUG INTERACTIONS

There are theoretical concerns that OPCs could potentiate antiplatelet or anticoagulant agents, but no well-documented case reports support this concern.

green tea
(Camellia sinensis)

OTHER NAMES:

EGCG, *Camellia thea, Camellia theifera,* epigallocatechin gallate, green tea polyphenols, thea bohea, thea sinensis, thea viridis

Class: Herbal remedy

MAJOR INGREDIENTS

The major constituents of green tea include catechin polyphenols (especially epigallocatechin gallate), as well as triterpene saponins, caffeine, theobromine, theophylline, flavonoids, caffeic acid derivatives, and volatile oil. The product is made by steaming the fresh-cut leaf of the plant.

CLAIMED ACTIONS

Observational studies have inconsistently suggested that green tea might reduce cancer and heart disease risk. The polyphenols in green tea have antioxidant properties. Other reported actions of green tea with weak supporting evidence include enhanced thermogenesis, hypolipidemic effects, antiinflammatory actions in periodontal disease, hepatoprotection, and protection of skin from sun damage.

USES

Green tea or extracts made from green tea are widely used with the expectation that they will reduce the risk of heart disease and cancer. However, at present the supporting evidence for these benefits is weak, and no meaningful randomized controlled trials (RCTs) indicate benefit. One small double-blind, placebo-controlled trial did provide evidence that sugarless green tea candy chews have a favorable effect on periodontal disease, as shown by relative improvements in approximal plaque index and sulcus bleeding index. More recently, green tea has become a common ingredient in weight-loss products, based only on scant preliminary evidence. The one RCT on this proposed use failed to find benefit for preventing weight regain after weight loss. Neither topical nor oral green teas have proved to provide the same level of protection from the sun as standard sunblocks, although they may provide some protection.

ADMINISTRATION

Three cups of green tea daily, or 100–150 mg 3 times daily of a green tea extract standardized to contain 80% total polyphenols and 50% epigallocatechin gallate.

SIDE EFFECTS

Green tea contains less caffeine and related stimulants than does black tea, but caffeine-related side effects, such as agitation and insomnia, may occur.

DENTAL CONSIDERATIONS

Ask why the product is being used. Individuals who chew green tea candy for putative antiperiodontal disease actions should be cautioned not to consider it a substitute for standard care.

DRUG INTERACTIONS

Green tea contains high levels of vitamin K and therefore would be expected to decrease the effectiveness of warfarin (Coumadin) and related drugs. The caffeine in green tea could interact with MAOIs.

guggul
(Commiphora mukul)

OTHER NAMES:
False myrrh, gum guggul, gugulipid, mukul myrrh tree

Class: Herbal remedy

MAJOR INGREDIENTS

Guggul is the oleo gum resin obtained by drying the sap of the Commiphora mukul tree. Its active ingredients are thought to be ketonic steroids known as guggulsterones.

CLAIMED ACTIONS

Guggulsterones are strong antagonists of two nuclear hormone receptors involved in cholesterol metabolism, which provides a plausible basis for the use of guggul in the treatment of hyperlipidemia, its major proposed use. It is widely claimed that guggul increases thyroid activity and thereby aids weight loss, but there is no meaningful supporting evidence for either part of this claim.

USES

Although earlier randomized controlled trials (RCTs) performed by researchers in India did report hypolipidemic actions, a more recent, larger, and better-designed RCT performed in the United States failed to find benefits; in fact, guggul appeared to increase levels of low-density lipoprotein cholesterol. One RCT found guggul ineffective as a weight-loss aid. Other proposed uses of guggul that lack reliable supporting evidence include improving glucose control in diabetes, aiding weight loss, and treating acne.

ADMINISTRATION

Guggul typically is used in a standardized extract form to provide 100 mg of guggulsterones daily (especially E- and Z-guggulsterone). Safety in pregnant or nursing women and in individuals with severe hepatic or renal disease is not established.

SIDE EFFECTS

Guggul appears to have a low level of toxicity. Use of standardized guggul extract in clinical trials has not been associated with any significant side effects other than occasional allergic reactions (especially skin rash) and nonspecific GI distress.

DENTAL CONSIDERATIONS

Ask why the product is being used.

DRUG INTERACTIONS

No dental drug interactions have been reported.

hawthorn
(Crataegus oxyacantha, Crataegus folium cum flore, *C. monogyna, C. laevigata)*

OTHER NAMES:
English hawthorn, maybush

Class: Herbal remedy

MAJOR INGREDIENTS

Flavonoids (hyperoside, vitexin-rhamnose, rutin, proanthocyanidins) with vasodilating properties, as well as inhibition of vasoconstriction. Proanthocyanidins reportedly block angiotensin-converting enzyme (ACE). It also contains tyramine, a biogenic amine. The flowers, leaves, fruits, and mixtures of other plant parts are used medicinally.

CLAIMED ACTIONS

Hawthorn appears to have inotropic actions. In addition, some evidence suggests that hawthorn has antiarrhythmic actions by blocking repolarizing potassium currents in ventricular myocardium, a mechanism similar to that of class III antiarrhythmics. Other reported effects include inhibition of ACE and of cyclic adenosine monophosphate phosphodiesterase.

USES
Moderately strong evidence from multiple randomized controlled trials (RCTs) indicates that hawthorn improves signs and symptoms of class I or II CHF. However, there is no evidence that hawthorn reduces risk of morbidity and mortality (a benefit shown with ACE inhibitors). Weaker RCT support indicates benefits in angina. Other proposed indications that lack substantive support include atherosclerosis, hypertension, benign cardiac arrhythmias, and prevention of postischemic arrhythmias.

ADMINISTRATION
Available in oral dose forms as an extract and plant parts for brewing teas.

SIDE EFFECTS
No contraindications or side effects have been reported.

DENTAL CONSIDERATIONS
Ask why the product is being used. Monitor vital signs in patients with cardiovascular disease.

DRUG INTERACTIONS
There are theoretical concerns of possible adverse interactions if the herb is used with other drugs that may affect cardiac function.

horse chestnut extract
(Aesculus hippocastanum)

APPENDIX H

OTHER NAMES:
HCE; raw form: buckeye, conkers

Class: Herbal remedy

MAJOR INGREDIENTS
The major constituents of horse chestnut are triterpene saponins, especially escin (also spelled "aescin"). Other constituents include flavonoids, polysaccharides, and oligomeric proanthocyanidins. Whole horse chestnut contains the toxic coumarin glycoside esculin (also spelled "aesculin"), but the esculin has been removed from the standard horse chestnut extract product. Horse chestnut seed and leaf both are used medicinally.

CLAIMED ACTIONS
HCE is thought to reduce capillary permeability. Proposed mechanisms include venotonic, antiinflammatory, antihydrolase, and antineutrophil adherence properties.

USES
Several moderate-size randomized controlled trials (RCTs) of varying quality have found evidence that HCE can reduce symptoms of venous insufficiency in the lower extremities including edema, pain, and fatigue. Benefits (prevention or treatment) regarding visible varicosities have not been documented. One RCT suggests benefits for hemorrhoids. Weaker evidence suggests potential benefits for aiding resolution of phlebitis and reducing edema after surgery or injury. Topical horse chestnut for

bruising has similarly weak supporting evidence.

ADMINISTRATION

HCE is taken at a dose of 300 mg twice a day, in a form standardized to contain 50 mg escin per dose. Enteric-coated capsules are used to prevent otherwise predictable stomach discomfort. Safety in pregnant women is not established, but animal data are reassuring, and pregnant women have been enrolled in RCTs of horse chestnut.

SIDE EFFECTS

Whole horse chestnut, as opposed to HCE, is a toxic herb and should not be used. HCE predictably causes gastric irritation if it is not delivered in an enteric-coated capsule. Enteric-coated HCE is not associated with any significant side effects other than occasional allergic reactions.

DENTAL CONSIDERATIONS

Ask why the product is being used.

DRUG INTERACTIONS

Because of its saponin content, horse chestnut might potentiate the effects of antiplatelet or anticoagulant agents.

hydroxymethyl butyrate

OTHER NAMES:

HMB, beta-hydroxy beta-methylbutyric acid

Class: Nonherbal remedy

MAJOR INGREDIENTS

Hydroxymethyl butyrate is a naturally occurring degradation product of the amino acid leucine.

CLAIMED ACTIONS

During intense exercise, muscle tissue degradation occurs, which leads to leakage of leucine and its subsequent transformation to HMB. It has been hypothesized that increased HMB levels from exogenous sources provides a downstream feedback signal that slows muscle protein degradation.

USES

Several small randomized controlled trials (RCTs), some published only in abstract form, indicate that use of HMB may enhance response to weight training, resulting in increased muscle mass. On this basis, HMB has become a popular supplement for bodybuilders. However, the supporting evidence must be regarded as weak, and the benefits, if any, are modest. Even weaker evidence hints that HMB might have an antihypertensive or hypolipidemic effect.

ADMINISTRATION

Typical dosage of HMB is 1 g 3 times a day. Maximum safe doses in young children, pregnant or nursing women, and individuals with severe hepatic or renal disease are not established.

SIDE EFFECTS

HMB appears to have a low level of toxicity. Use of HMB in clinical trials has not been associated with any significant side effects other than occasional nonspecific GI distress.

However, long-term safety studies have not been performed.

DENTAL CONSIDERATIONS
Ask why the product is being used.

DRUG INTERACTIONS
No dental drug interactions have been reported.

kava
(Piper methysticum, Piperis methystici rhizoma)

OTHER NAMES:
Kava-kava, kew, tonga

Class: Herbal remedy

MAJOR INGREDIENTS
Kava lactones (kava α-pyrones), including methysticin, kawain, and others. The dried rhizomes are the parts used medicinally.

CLAIMED ACTIONS
These lactones have demonstrable pharmacologic activity on the CNS. Reported actions include sedation, muscle relaxation, and anticonvulsive and antispasmodic effects. Suggested mechanisms of action range from gamma-aminobutyric acid (GABA) receptor modification to dopamine antagonist activity. A local anesthetic action is also claimed.

USES
Meaningful evidence from multiple randomized controlled trials (RCTs) demonstrates significant improvement of symptoms in various anxiety disorders. Other proposed uses including relief of general tension, stress, and insomnia lack support. An intoxicating effect has been reported with use of very high doses.

ADMINISTRATION
Standardized products for oral administration are available; in some areas the kava-kava is chewed. Use should be limited to no more than 3 mo.
Warning: Kava has been taken off the market in numerous countries because of reports of severe liver injury, in some cases requiring transplantation. This appears to be a rare idiosyncratic or allergic reaction rather than ordinary liver toxicity, but it has been seen even with traditionally prepared kava, as well as with pharmaceutical-grade standardized products. Until further information is known, kava should be considered an unsafe herb.

CONTRAINDICATIONS
Reports of dystonic reactions suggest that kava should not be used by patients taking antipsychotic medications. Apparent antidopaminergic actions contraindicate use in Parkinson's disease. CNS effects and possible potentiation of alcohol toxicity contraindicate use in alcoholism. Should not be used in patients with endogenous depression. Not recommended for use by pregnant or nursing women. Whether or not the risk of liver damage (see Warning) is increased in patients with preexisting liver disease is unknown.

SIDE EFFECTS
Kava in normal doses is generally well tolerated. GI complaints occasionally accompany use. Chewing kava-kava can result in circumoral numbness. Patients using kava-kava may have reduced mental

alertness, and very high intake can cause inebriation. See Warning concerning liver damage.

DENTAL CONSIDERATIONS
Caution against use of kava in all patients, especially those with existing liver disease.

DRUG INTERACTIONS
May potentiate CNS sedation if used in combination with other CNS depressants. May increase risk of dystonic reactions if given in combination with antipsychotics. Discontinue 24 hr before general anesthesia and surgical procedures.

lemon balm
(Melissa officinalis)

OTHER NAMES:
Honey plant, Melissa, sweet Mary, balm mint

Class: Herbal remedy

MAJOR INGREDIENTS
Volatile oil extract by distillation from leaves or whole plant contains geranial, neral, citronellal, linalool, and other compounds. Other constituents include glycosides, caffeic acids, flavonoids, and titerpene acids.

CLAIMED ACTIONS
Some evidence indicates that topical lemon balm extract blocks herpes virus receptors on host cells. It also may inhibit viral-related protein synthesis by action on elongation factor eEF-2. Taken internally, lemon balm may cause sedation through CNS nicotinic and muscarinic receptor-binding properties, although this mechanism is not well established.

USES
Several randomized controlled trials (RCTs) of moderate-to-low quality found evidence that use of topical lemon balm preparations can reduce the severity of acute genital or oral herpes recurrences if applied at the beginning of symptoms. There are no meaningful data on possible prophylactic effect. For oral use, lemon balm alone or combined with valerian has shown some potential value for insomnia, but not all data are consistent. One RCT found that lemon balm extract reduced agitation in individuals with Alzheimer's disease. Other proposed uses of lemon balm lack supporting evidence. These include anxiety disorders, dry skin, headache, influenza, menstrual problems, and muscle spasms.

ADMINISTRATION
Topical lemon balm for herpes is used in the form of a 70:1 extract cream, applied twice daily, and standardized using bioassay for inhibition of viral cellular lysis. Typical oral doses are 1.5 to 4.5 g/day of dried herb, or the equivalent in a standardized extract form. Maximum safe dosages of oral lemon balm for young children, pregnant or nursing women, and individuals with severe hepatic or renal disease are not established.

SIDE EFFECTS
Use of topical lemon balm has not been associated with any significant side effects other than occasional allergic reactions. Oral lemon balm is generally regarded as safe.

However, on the basis of weak evidence indicating a possible sedative effect, people taking oral lemon balm might be at increased risk if they drive or operate heavy machinery or engage in activities that require a high level of mental alertness.

DENTAL CONSIDERATIONS
Ask why the product is being used. Pregnant women should be cautioned not to regard topical lemon balm as effective prevention against transmission of herpes to the newborn. See Drug Interactions.

DRUG INTERACTIONS
In animal studies, lemon balm extracts have produced dose-dependent potentiation of pentobarbital.

licorice
(Glycyrrhiza glabra)

OTHER NAMES:
Licorice root, liquorice, licorice, deglycyrrhizinated licorice, DGL, sweet wood, Yasti Madhu, sweet wort, Reglisse, Subholz

Class: Herbal remedy

MAJOR INGREDIENTS
Whole licorice contains as its principal presumed active ingredient a terpenoid called glycyrrhizin glycoside (glycyrrhizinic acid). Deglycyrrhizinated licorice (DGL) is a popular form of licorice from which this constituent has been removed. Other constituents include asparagine, biotin, choline, fat, gum, inositol, lecithin, glycosides, volatile oil, coumarins, estrogenic substances, sterols, saponins, manganese, para-aminobenzoic acid, pantothenic acid, various pentacyclic triterpenes, phosphorous, B vitamins (1, 2, 3, 6, and 9), vitamin E, and a yellow dye.

CLAIMED ACTIONS
Glycyrrhizin has mineralocorticoid effects when used in high doses or with prolonged use. Possibly because of its glycyrrhizin content, licorice is thought to potentiate topical or oral corticosteroids and exert an estrogen-like effect. Other claimed actions with less substantiation include demulcent, diuretic, expectorant, antitussive, laxative, emetic, emollient, antiinflammatory, tissue healing, and antiarthritic effects.

USES
There are no well-documented uses of licorice or DGL. DGL has shown some promise for peptic ulcer disease, but published studies involved combination products with other active ingredients such as antacids. Various additional claims of effectiveness have been made for whole licorice including hypoglycemia, bronchitis, colitis, cystitis, stress, colds, high cholesterol levels, fever, nausea, inflammation, coughs, laryngitis, chronic fatigue syndrome, and general debility. Externally, licorice preparations have been used for eczema, psoriasis, burns, boils, sores, ulcers, and redness of the skin. DGL lozenges have been recommended for mouth ulcers. However, there is no reliable substantiation for any of these uses.

SIDE EFFECTS

Glycyrrhizin has direct mineralocorticoid effects and increases corticosteroid activity by inhibiting metabolic inactivation of cortisol. Signs of pseudohyperaldosteronism have been seen within a few wk of usage including headache, muscle weakness, muscle cramps, hypertension, heart failure, arrhythmias, water retention, sodium retention, and potassium loss. The DGL form has not been associated with any significant side effects other than occasional allergic reactions or nonspecific GI distress.

ADMINISTRATION

Given as powder, liquid, or capsules. Topically a 2% licorice juice has been used as an antibacterial ointment. A mouthwash with 200 mg deglycyrrhizinated licorice in 200 ml warm water has been used. Snuff often contains a great deal of licorice.

CONTRAINDICATIONS

Not recommended for use by pregnant women (may cause reduced gestational age at birth), by women with a history of breast cancer (potential estrogenic effects), or by men with a history of infertility or decreased libido (may reduce testosterone levels). Because of its mineralocorticoid effects, licorice should not be used by patients taking thiazide or loop diuretics, digitalis, or potassium-sparing diuretics. However, DGL products should not interact with these medications.

DENTAL CONSIDERATIONS

Limit use of whole licorice to no more than 6 weeks. DGL lozenges have been proposed for aphthous ulcers, but no evidence supports this use.

DRUG INTERACTIONS

Tobacco may alter metabolism leading to toxicity. May potentiate corticosteroid drugs, so use in combination only with caution. May potentiate or antagonize diuretics, and increased potassium loss caused by licorice presents increased risks for individuals using digoxin or antiarrhythmic drugs.

---

myrrh
(Commiphora myrrha)

OTHER NAMES:
Bola, gum myrrh tree, mu-yao

Class: Herbal remedy

MAJOR INGREDIENTS

Volatile oil (primarily sesquiterpenes), triterpenes, and gum resin

CLAIMED ACTIONS

Analgesic, antifungal, antiseptic, astringent, carminative, emmenagogue, expectorant, antispasmodic, disinfectant, immune stimulant, circulatory stimulant, stomachic, tonic, and vulnerary.

USES

Has been used as a disinfectant, as an astringent, and to treat disorders of the female reproductive system. It has long been used for treatment of oral ulcers, gingivitis, halitosis, denture-irritated mouth, and sore teeth and gums. Other uses include nonspecified chest problems and diphtheria. Used in Chinese medicine for rheumatism, arthritis, and circulatory problems.

ADMINISTRATION
Infusion, mouthwash, tincture, incense, capsules, and dental powder.

CONTRAINDICATIONS
Not recommended for use by pregnant women because of claimed uterine stimulant effects or by individuals with diabetes because of enhancement of oral hypoglycemic agents.

SIDE EFFECTS
Because of resin content and difficult clearance from the body, myrrh may cause minor renal damage if used over an extended period of time. Avoid high dose for chronic use.

DENTAL CONSIDERATIONS
Myrrh has been approved by Commission E (Germany) for treatment of inflammation of the mouth and pharynx, but topical uses are not substantiated. A tea, prepared by placing 1–2 teaspoonfuls in one cup of boiling water and steeping for 10–15 min, has been used for oral administration 3 times a day.

DRUG INTERACTIONS
Enhancement of oral hypoglycemic agents.

nettle root
(Urtica dioica radix)

OTHER NAMES:
Stinging nettle

Class: Herbal remedy

MAJOR INGREDIENTS
The presumed active constituents of nettle root are β-sitosterol and other related sitosterols. Other possibly active constituents include lectins, lignans, polysaccharides, and hydroxycoumarins. Note that nettle leaf is an entirely different herbal product from the nettle root discussed here.

CLAIMED ACTIONS
The sitosterols in nettle root, especially β-sitosterol, have multiple actions of possible relevance to prostate disease, including reducing inflammation in the prostate and alteration of sex hormone binding properties.

USES
Several small randomized controlled trials (RCTs) indicate that nettle root can improve symptoms of benign prostatic hyperplasia (BPH).

ADMINISTRATION
When taken for BPH, the typical dose is 120 mg of the dry extract twice a day, or 4–6 g/day of the whole root. Nettle root often is sold in combination with other herbs thought to be effective for BPH including saw palmetto and pygeum, and there is some evidence of a potentiating effect with the latter. Maximum safe dosages in young children, nursing women, and individuals with severe hepatic or renal disease are not established.

CONTRAINDICATIONS
On the basis of animal studies showing uterotonic action, nettle is not recommended for use by pregnant women.

SIDE EFFECTS

Although extensive safety studies have not been reported, nettle root appears to have a low level of toxicity. In drug monitoring studies, side effects were rare and nonspecific.

DENTAL CONSIDERATIONS

Ask why the product is being used.

DRUG INTERACTIONS

None known, but there are weak theoretic concerns regarding interactions with antihypertensive, hypoglycemic, and sedative pharmaceuticals.

passionflower
(Passiflora incarnate)

OTHER NAMES:
Passion vine

Class: Herbal remedy

MAJOR INGREDIENTS

Passionflower contains harman and harmaline, alkaloids with possible MAOI activity. Other constituents include cyanogenic glycosides, flavonoids, and maltol. The aerial parts of the plant are used medicinally.

CLAIMED ACTIONS

Sedative and antispasmodic uses are claimed, based primarily on animal studies.

USES

Scant preliminary evidence from small randomized controlled trials (RCTs) found suggestive evidence that passionflower might be helpful for treatment of anxiety, as well as for withdrawal from opiate dependency. Its common use for "nervous stomach" has not been formally investigated.

ADMINISTRATION

Typical dosage of crude passionflower is 1 g 3 times a day. Concentrated extracts and tinctures are available. Maximum safe doses in nursing women, young children, and individuals with severe hepatic or renal disease are not established.

CONTRAINDICATIONS

Because of the uterotropic actions of harman and harmaline, passionflower is not recommended for use by pregnant women.

SIDE EFFECTS

Passionflower is generally well tolerated when taken in usual doses.

DENTAL CONSIDERATIONS

Ask why the product is being used.

DRUG INTERACTIONS

Passionflower might potentiate the action of sedative drugs, including those used for dental anesthesia. Interactions with MAOI drugs are possible.

peppermint
(Mentha piperita)

OTHER NAMES:
Peppermint oil, essential oil of peppermint, mint, brandy mint, menthol

Class: Herbal remedy

MAJOR INGREDIENTS

The primary active constituent in peppermint is assumed to be menthol. Other constituents of the essential oil include menthone, menthofurane, menthyl acetate, neomenthol, and isomenthone. The whole leaf additionally contains caffeic acids and flavonoids. The leaf and flowers are the parts used medicinally. Most tested uses of peppermint involved preparations of the essential oil rather than whole leaf.

CLAIMED ACTIONS

Some evidence indicates that menthol relaxes GI smooth muscle. Peppermint oil has a cooling effect on the skin. It may have cholagogue properties.

USES

Several preliminary randomized controlled trials (RCTs) inconsistently suggest that peppermint oil can alleviate symptoms of irritable bowel syndrome. Other RCTs suggest that peppermint oil can decrease intestinal spasm during a barium enema. Other uses of peppermint oil with only minimal supporting evidence include functional dyspepsia and dissolution of gallstones. Inhaled peppermint oil has shown some promise for upper respiratory infections. Peppermint oil applied to the temples may produce a subjective decrease in headache sensation. There are no well-documented uses of peppermint leaf.

ADMINISTRATION

In clinical trials, peppermint oil was given in enteric-coated form at a dose of 0.2–0.4 ml 3 times a day.

Whole peppermint leaf is taken in tea form.

CONTRAINDICATIONS

Because of the potential toxicity of excessive peppermint oil, peppermint is not recommended for use by pregnant or nursing women or by individuals with severe hepatic or renal disease.

SIDE EFFECTS

Peppermint leaf has a low level of toxicity and is generally regarded as safe. At normal doses, peppermint oil generally causes few side effects. However, even at normal doses, peppermint oil can cause esophageal reflux, which is the reason for usage of enteric-coated capsules. Excessive intake of peppermint oil can cause CNS and renal damage. Inhalation occasionally causes hypersensitivity reactions.

DENTAL CONSIDERATIONS

Ask why the product is being used.

DRUG INTERACTIONS

Animal studies suggest that oral peppermint oil can increase cyclosporine bioavailability. This could cause cyclosporine levels to rise to toxic levels; conversely, if cyclosporine levels are adjusted while an individual is taking peppermint oil, discontinuation could cause a fall to subtherapeutic levels.

probiotics

OTHER NAMES:
Friendly bacteria, *Acidophilus*

Class: Nonherbal remedy

MAJOR INGREDIENTS

Probiotics in common use include *Lactobacillus acidophilus, Lactobacillus GG,* and other lactobacilli; *Bifidobacterium bifidum; Saccharomyces boulardii* (a yeast); *Streptococcus thermophilus;* and *Streptococcus salivarius.*

CLAIMED ACTIONS

Probiotics are microorganisms (usually bacteria, but also yeasts) that colonize the digestive tract and other tissues and exist in healthy symbiosis with the body. They compete with and potentially inhibit pathogenic organisms, and they may aid digestion and assist in the formation of vitamin K. Altered bowel flora may cause immunomodulatory effects.

USES

Numerous randomized controlled trials (RCTs) have evaluated the use of probiotics for preventing or treating various forms of diarrhea, including acute viral diarrhea, traveler's diarrhea, antibiotic-associated diarrhea, and chemotherapy- or radiation-induced diarrhea. In general, the results have been supportive. Probiotics may help prevent caries. One large RCT found that use of Lactobacillus GG in milk given to children ages 1–6 yr reduced incidence of caries as compared with unfortified milk. Other RCTs suggest benefits for inflammatory bowel disease, irritable bowel syndrome, and eczema. Weaker or mixed evidence has been presented regarding usefulness for urinary tract infection prophylaxis, hyperlipidemia, and prevention of upper respiratory tract infections.

ADMINISTRATION

Typical dose of bacterial probiotics supplies approximately five billion live organisms daily. *S. boulardii* yeast is taken at a dose of 500 mg twice a day. Surveys of products on the market have shown wide variations in quality.

SIDE EFFECTS

Use of probiotics by healthy people has not been associated with any significant side effects other than a short-term increase in intestinal gas production. However, immunocompromised individuals may be at risk for invasive infection by the probiotic.

DENTAL CONSIDERATIONS

Ask why the product is being used. As noted previously, some evidence indicates potential benefit for caries prophylaxis in children.

DRUG INTERACTIONS

No dental drug interactions have been reported. Use of probiotics during and for a short while after antibiotic usage may prevent antibiotic-associated diarrhea and restore normal bowel flora.

proteolytic enzymes

OTHER NAMES:
Pancreatic enzymes, digestive enzymes

Class: Nonherbal remedy

MAJOR INGREDIENTS

Commercial products generally include one or more of the following proteolytic enzymes: bromelain, chymotrypsin, pancreatin, papain, or trypsin.

CLAIMED ACTIONS

Although the primary physiologic use of proteolytic enzymes is protein digestion, some portion of exogenously delivered proteolytic enzymes appears to enter systemic circulation and exerts an antiinflammatory effect.

USES

Results of numerous reported randomized controlled trials (RCTs) on the use of proteolytic enzyme mixtures for reducing pain and edema following surgery have been mixed. Other RCTs suggest possible benefits for sports injuries and other minor injuries, again reducing pain and edema. Proteolytic enzymes have shown some promise for osteoarthritis and herpes zoster. Other claimed uses that lack RCT support include treatment of food allergies and rheumatoid arthritis.

ADMINISTRATION

Proteolytic enzymes are delivered orally in a variety of enteric-coated or non–enteric-coated forms. Dosage depends on the particular product. Maximum safe doses for pregnant or nursing women, young children, and individuals with severe hepatic or renal disease are not established.

SIDE EFFECTS

Use of proteolytic enzymes in clinical trials has not been associated with any significant side effects other than occasional allergic reactions or nonspecific GI distress.

DENTAL CONSIDERATIONS

Ask why the product is being used.

DRUG INTERACTIONS

Papain might potentiate anticoagulant and antiplatelet agents. Pancreatin could interfere with absorption of folic acid supplements.

pyruvate

OTHER NAMES:
Dihydroxyacetone pyruvate, DHAP

Class: Nonherbal remedy

MAJOR INGREDIENTS

Pyruvate is a product of aerobic glycolysis. It enters the mitochondria to form acetyl-coenzyme A (CoA) by oxidative decarboxylation. There is little pyruvate in the diet; it is synthesized endogenously.

CLAIMED ACTIONS

Some evidence suggests that exogenous pyruvate has a feedback-inhibition effect on lipid synthesis. Weaker evidence hints that an increased supply of pyruvate might enable a higher rate of ATP synthesis during exercise.

USES

Limited evidence from small randomized controlled trials (RCTs) indicates that pyruvate supplements may aid weight loss or body composition (fat/muscle proportion). In general, evidence from clinical trials does not support use of pyruvate as a sports performance-enhancing agent.

ADMINISTRATION

Typical dose is 30 g daily, taken in divided doses. It often is sold in combination with dihydroxyacetone, under the name DHAP (dihydroxyacetone pyruvate). Maximum safe doses for pregnant or nursing women, young children, and individuals with severe hepatic or renal disease are not established.

SIDE EFFECTS

Use of pyruvate in clinical trials has not been associated with any significant side effects other than occasional allergic reactions and nonspecific GI distress.

DENTAL CONSIDERATIONS

Ask why the product is being used.

DRUG INTERACTIONS

No dental drug interactions have been reported.

quercetin

OTHER NAMES:
Quercetin chalcone

Class: Nonherbal remedy

MAJOR INGREDIENTS

Quercetin is a bioflavonoid found in many foods, particularly apples, black tea, grapefruit, onions, and red wine.

CLAIMED ACTIONS

Some evidence suggests that exogenous quercetin has antiinflammatory effects and inhibits nitric oxide and tyrosine kinase. Quercetin, like many bioflavonoids, has antioxidant and chemopreventive properties in vitro. It is said to have the cromolyn-like effect of stabilizing mast cells, but the supporting evidence for this claim is weak, and no randomized controlled trials (RCTs) show actual clinical effect on allergies.

USES

One small RCT found limited evidence that quercetin may be effective for treatment of chronic prostatitis. Another small RCT hints at benefits for interstitial cystitis. Other proposed uses that lack RCT substantiation include allergies (eczema, asthma, allergic rhinitis), viral infections, and prevention of cataracts, cancer, and heart disease.

ADMINISTRATION

Quercetin usually is taken orally at a dose of 500 mg 2 times a day. Quercetin chalcone is marketed as having better oral absorption than quercetin, but this claim has not been reliably substantiated. Maximum safe doses in young children and in individuals with severe hepatic or renal disease are not established.

CONTRAINDICATIONS

Weak evidence hints that use of quercetin by pregnant or nursing women might increase the risk of infant leukemia.

SIDE EFFECTS

Use of quercetin in clinical trials has not been associated with any significant side effects other than occasional allergic reactions and nonspecific GI distress. However, despite in vitro evidence of chemoprevention, there are some indications that quercetin could have a carcinogenic effect under certain circumstances that are not yet well defined.

DENTAL CONSIDERATIONS
Ask why the product is being used.

DRUG INTERACTIONS
No dental drug interactions have been reported.

---

sage
(Salvia officinalis)

OTHER NAMES:
Broad-leaf sage, common sage, Dalmatian sage, garden sage, true sage

Class: Herbal remedy

MAJOR INGREDIENTS
Volatile oils, phenolic acids, tannins, diterpene bitter principles, triterpenes, steroids, flavones, and flavonoid glycosides.

CLAIMED ACTIONS
Antibacterial, fungistatic, virustatic, astringent, carminative, secretion promotion, and perspiration inhibition.

USES
From the earliest of times, uses have included treatment of open sores and wounds, sore throat, and fertility problems. Sage is also used to treat gum disease, canker sores, and halitosis. Other uses include antioxidant effects, menstrual pain, menopausal symptoms, and muscle spasms. Orally ingested sage reportedly reduces perspiration and encourages appetite. Other uses include stomatitis, gingivitis, pharyngitis, and hyperhidrosis. It has

been used topically to treat itching associated with insect bites, along with herpes lesions, shingles, and psoriasis.

ADMINISTRATION
Dried leaves, extract, tincture, and essential oil.

CONTRAINDICATIONS
Not recommended for use by pregnant women.

SIDE EFFECTS
Reported side effects include vertigo; tachycardia; and, for patients prone to seizures, a risk of seizures.

DENTAL CONSIDERATIONS
Efficacy for use of sage gargle for gum disease is not established.

DRUG INTERACTIONS
Interactions with insulin, oral hypoglycemics, and seizure medications. Some sage products may contain alcohol (tincture) and should not be used with disulfiram.

SAMe

OTHER NAMES:
Ademethionine, adenosylmethionine, *S*-adenosyl-methionine, *S*-adenosyl-L-methionine

Class: Nonherbal remedy

MAJOR INGREDIENTS
S-adenosyl-methionine.

CLAIMED ACTIONS
A naturally occurring molecule found in most body tissues, SAMe (pronounced "Sammy") is an active methyl carrier playing an essential

role in transmethylation. It is involved in the synthesis, metabolism, and activation of hormones, neurotransmitters, phospholipids, proteins, nucleic acids, and some natural medications. SAMe is intimately linked to vitamin B_{12} and folic acid metabolism. When these vitamins are absent, reduced levels of SAMe can result, such that SAMe affects serotonin and many body tissues, including cartilage and membranes. It functions as an antidepressant via an unknown mechanism but is associated with increased levels of serotonin, dopamine, and norepinephrine.

USES
Moderate evidence from placebo-controlled and comparative randomized controlled trials (RCTs) indicates that oral SAMe can reduce symptoms of osteoarthritis, to approximately the same extent as low doses of NSAIDs. Weaker RCT evidence supports efficacy in depression, fibromyalgia, and cholestasis. In highly preliminary studies, SAMe has shown promise for treatment of Gilbert's disease and other liver disorders.

ADMINISTRATION
Oral dose forms have variable bioavailability; doses used in clinical trials were generally 1200–1600 mg/day daily, taken in divided doses.

CONTRAINDICATIONS
None reported; however, there is a possible risk of hypomania in patients with bipolar disorder.

SIDE EFFECTS
GI complaints such as diarrhea, nausea, and vomiting, and CNS effects such as hypomania in bipolar disorder and anxiety.

DENTAL CONSIDERATIONS
Determine why the patient is taking the drug.

DRUG INTERACTIONS
SAMe might interfere with the effectiveness of L-dopa, which is used for treatment of Parkinson's disease. Based on a case report of a toxic interaction with clomipramine, combination of SAMe with standard antidepressants should be used only with caution.

saw palmetto
(Serenoa repens, Sabal fructus)

OTHER NAMES:
Sabal, cabbage palm, saw palmetto berry

Class: Herbal remedy

MAJOR INGREDIENTS
Contains various sitosterols (phytosterols) such as β-sitosterol and other sitosterol compounds, flavonoids, polysaccharides, and free fatty acids. The ripe, dried fruit of the plant is used medicinally.

CLAIMED ACTIONS
Reported to be antiandrogenic and antiinflammatory. May have some low-level estrogenic activity. The antiandrogenic activity is suggested to occur by inhibition of the enzyme testosterone-5-α-reductase. This action prevents the conversion of testosterone to dihydrotestosterone, the active androgenic hormone. Some data support blockade of dihydrotestosterone to receptors in

the cell nucleus. Limited data seem to support the estrogenic effects. The antiinflammatory effects remain doubtful. Use of saw palmetto does not affect prostate-specific antigen levels.

USES
This herbal product has been used for treatment of symptoms associated with BPH, particularly urinary difficulties. Clinical trials show better results than placebo and apparent comparative results to finasteride (Proscar) and other pharmaceuticals for BPH. Saw palmetto appears to cause some reduction in prostate gland size, although not to the same extent as finasteride. (Note: Several effective pharmaceuticals for BPH cause no change in prostate gland size.) Use in prostatitis and baldness remains speculative.

ADMINISTRATION
Saw palmetto is taken at a dose of 160 mg twice a day of an extract standardized to contain 85%–95% fatty acids and sterols.

CONTRAINDICATIONS
Not recommended for use by pregnant women or by women of childbearing age because of unclear influence of saw palmetto on other androgens and possible estrogenic effects.

SIDE EFFECTS
Use of saw palmetto in clinical trials was associated with a few, nonspecific side effects. There is one case report of saw palmetto apparently causing increased bleeding during surgery; for this reason, use of saw palmetto

should be discontinued 2 wk before surgery.

DENTAL CONSIDERATIONS
Ask why the product is being used.

DRUG INTERACTIONS
No dental drug interactions have been reported.

St. John's wort
(Hypericum perforatum, Hyperici herba)

OTHER NAMES:
Hypericum, kaimath weed, John's wort

Class: Herbal remedy

MAJOR INGREDIENTS
Contains quinoids (hypericin, pseudohypericin), anthraquinones, flavonoids (hyperoside, quercitin, rutin), bioflavonoids, and a volatile oil. One of the pharmacologically active components is hyperforin; another, hypericin, has photosensitizing properties. Flavonoids, including amentoflavone, may contribute to the pharmacologic action of the herb. The aboveground parts of the plant harvested during the flowering season are used medicinally.

CLAIMED ACTIONS
The primary actions are antidepressant, antiinflammatory, and antimicrobial. The constituent hyperforin appears to inhibit uptake of serotonin, dopamine, and norepinephrine.

USES

Used for treatment of mild to moderate major depression. According to most of the many randomized controlled trials (RCTs) performed, it is more effective than placebo and, except in severe major depression, is as effective as tricyclics or selective serotonin reuptake inhibitors. The volatile oil seems to increase the healing of burns. Hypericin has shown in vitro activity against HIV, but human trials indicate that hypericin must be taken in toxic doses in order to produce any clinical effect. One RCT failed to find St. John's wort helpful for polyneuropathy. Topical St. John's wort has shown some promise for treatment of eczema.

ADMINISTRATION

A variety of oral preparations are available, standardized to either hypericin or hyperforin.

SIDE EFFECTS

In the extensive clinical trial experience with St. John's wort, side effects have been limited and generally nonspecific. Photosensitization may occur at higher doses or with topical use. Like all antidepressants, St. John's wort can cause episodes of mania in people with bipolar disorder. There are some reports that use of St. John's wort by individuals with Alzheimer's disease may increase agitation. Safety during pregnancy and lactation is not established.

DENTAL CONSIDERATIONS

Ask why the product is being used.

DRUG INTERACTIONS

St. John's wort affects a variety of cytochromes, as well as the transport protein P-glycoprotein, and can reduce levels and thereby activity of numerous medications to a clinically significant extent. Interacting drugs include oral contraceptives (leading to unwanted pregnancy), protease inhibitors and nonnucleoside reverse transcriptase inhibitors (leading to reduced anti-HIV effectiveness), cyclosporine (leading to organ rejection), clozapine, digoxin, losartan, metronidazole, olanzapine, omeprazole, statins, warfarin, and various chemotherapy drugs. Note that if blood levels of a drug are stabilized while a patient is taking St. John's wort, discontinuation of the herb may cause a dangerous rise in levels. In addition, St. John's wort should be used only with caution, if at all, in patients taking other antidepressive medications, including MAOIs, tricyclic antidepressants, and selective serotonin reuptake inhibitors, because case reports suggest a risk of serotonin syndrome. Combined use with tramadol might present a similar risk. Although St. John's wort does not appear to have MAOI actions at normal doses, there is one case report of an MAO-like interaction between St. John's wort and tyramine-containing foods. Discontinue use 2 wk before general anesthesia. Avoid dental (or other) drugs with a potential for photosensitivity.

stevia
(Stevia rebaudiana)

OTHER NAMES:
Caa'inhem, Paraguayan sweet herb, sweet herb, sweet leaf of Paraguay, sweetleaf

Class: Herbal remedy

MAJOR INGREDIENTS

Major active constituents include diterpene steviosides and rebaudioside. Flavonoids and volatile oil are present as well. The leaves of the plant are used medicinally.

CLAIMED ACTIONS

Steviosides are sweeter than sucrose by weight, producing a taste said to be preferable to saccharine, though not entirely without aftertaste. Steviosides have shown an antihypertensive effect, but only at much higher doses than reasonable for intake as a sugar substitute.

USES

Stevia enjoys wide use as a noncaloric sweetening agent in Japan and several other countries. However, stevia has not received approval for use under this designation in the United States; nonetheless, it is used widely as a sweetener without claiming it as such. Concentrated steviosides at far higher doses are beginning to be used by people with hypertension; such use may be expected to increase in the future.

ADMINISTRATION

Approximately $^1/_6$ teaspoon of ground stevia (or 2–4 drops of stevia liquid extract) equals the sweetness of 1 teaspoon of ordinary sugar. This supplies approximately 30 mg steviosides. For hypertension, the dose used in clinical trials was 250–500 mg concentrated steviosides 3 times a day. Maximum safe doses in pregnant or nursing women, young children, and individuals with severe hepatic or renal disease are not established.

SIDE EFFECTS

Stevia is generally regarded as a safe herb, but animal studies suggest that high doses may have antifertility actions in both males and females. The widespread use of stevia in Japan suggests reasonable safety in children and pregnant women.

DENTAL CONSIDERATIONS

Patients may be using stevioside-sweetened products to avoid caries, a use that may be reasonable.

DRUG INTERACTIONS

If a person is accustomed to consuming 25 teaspoons of sugar per day, the equivalent in stevia might produce an antihypertensive effect. Certain more susceptible people might respond at a lower dose. This suggests the possibility of potentiation interactions with antihypertensives, but no such interactions have yet been reported.

valerian
(Valeriana officinalis, Valerianae radix)

OTHER NAMES:
Valerian root, Indian valerian

Class: Herbal remedy

MAJOR INGREDIENTS

Valepotriates (isovaltrate and others), a volatile oil (bornyl isovalerenate and isovalerenic acid), sesquiterpenes, and multiple other substances. Pharmacologically active components are not identified with any certainty but may be isovaleric acid and related derivatives. The fresh underground parts and roots are used medicinally.

CLAIMED ACTIONS

Sedation, reduction in nervousness, sleep promoting, and antispasmodic. Laboratory data suggest valerian may increase gamma-aminobutyric acid (GABA) levels at synapses.

USES

Evidence from several randomized controlled trials (RCTs) suggests that valerian can improve sleep, especially with continued use. Other proposed uses of valerian lacking meaningful supporting evidence include treatment of restlessness, reduction in nervousness (anxiolytic), agitation associated with menstruation, colic, stomach cramps, and uterine spasticity. Antispasmodic properties are not well defined. It has been used externally by adding it to bath water.

ADMINISTRATION

Available for oral use as a variety of products, including tinctures, infusions, and extracts.

SIDE EFFECTS

Generally not observed in usual doses. GI complaints, headache, sleeplessness, mydriasis, excitability, and cardiac disturbances may occur with long-term use.

DENTAL CONSIDERATIONS

Ask why the product is being used.

DRUG INTERACTIONS

Although no interactions have been reported, monitor patients for increased sedation when using other CNS depressants. May potentiate CNS depressants.

xylitol

Class: Nonherbal remedy

MAJOR INGREDIENTS

Xylitol is a polyol with the same intensity of sweetness as sucrose, but it cannot serve as a metabolic base for oral microbes.

CLAIMED ACTIONS

Xylitol inhibits the growth of Streptococcus mutans and on this basis has been proposed as a prophylactic agent against dental caries. Xylitol may also inhibit growth of *Streptococcus pneumoniae* and thereby reduce the risk of respiratory infections caused by this organism.

USES

In several large randomized controlled trials (RCTs), children who used gums, lozenges, syrups, toothpastes, or candies containing xylitol experienced a reduced incidence of caries compared with control groups. Use of xylitol by nursing mothers may confer some protection to the child, presumably because infants receive their initial *S. mutans* colonization from their mothers. Other RCTs suggest that xylitol use by children may reduce the incidence of otitis media. Xylitol has been suggested as a prophylactic for periodontal disease, but this use has not yet undergone significant study.

ADMINISTRATION

A typical dose of xylitol used in clinical trials for caries prevention was 4.3–10 g/day. Higher doses appear to be more effective than lower doses.

SIDE EFFECTS

High consumption of xylitol can cause mild GI distress and possibly diarrhea, especially in children.

DENTAL CONSIDERATIONS

Patients should be reminded that xylitol gum and related products should be used in addition to standard dental hygiene recommendations, not as a substitute for them.

DRUG INTERACTIONS

No dental drug interactions have been reported.

---

yohimbe bark
(Pausinystalia yohimbe)

OTHER NAMES:
Yohimbe cortex

Class: Herbal remedy

MAJOR INGREDIENTS

The principal alkaloid is yohimbine (quebrachine), with lesser amounts of stereoisomers of yohimbine along with other indole alkaloids, including corynantheidine and allo-yohimbine. It also contains a variety of plant tannins. The dried bark of the trunk and branches of the tree are the parts used medicinally.

CLAIMED ACTIONS

The major effects of this drug are due to yohimbine. Do not confuse the prescription drug yohimbine with yohimbe. Yohimbine has α_2-adrenergic antagonist activity. Presynaptic α_2-adrenergic receptors regulate norepinephrine release. In a feedback-type action, antagonism of these receptors is associated with greater norepinephrine release. It may also dilate blood vessels; claims are made for a calcium channel blocking action and inhibition of MAO enzymes.

USES

Has been used to treat erectile dysfunction, as an aphrodisiac, for exhaustion, and even for orthostatic hypotension. Limited data concern yohimbine and not yohimbe. Yohimbine has not been approved for this application. According to the German Commission E monographs, yohimbe's effectiveness is not documented, and it is not recommended.

ADMINISTRATION

Limited products are available and usually in combination with other ingredients.

CONTRAINDICATIONS

Not recommended for use by patients with hepatic or renal impairment or with psychiatric disorders.

SIDE EFFECTS

Usual doses produce few side effects. However, significant adverse effects are reported with large doses and include increased salivation, anxiety, hallucinations, exanthema, nervousness, irritability, tachycardia, and sweating. Other effects also are possible. Cardiac failure, possibly fatal, has been reported.

DENTAL CONSIDERATIONS

Ask why the product is being used.

DRUG INTERACTIONS

No specific dental drug interactions have been reported, but it may have MAOI action. Avoid use of indirect-acting sympathomimetics and tricyclic antidepressants.

Bibliography

Blake S: Alternative remedies CD-ROM, St. Louis, 2001, Mosby.

Blumenthal M, et al: The complete German Commission E monographs, Austin, 1998, American Botanical Council.

Miller LG: Herbal medicinals: selected clinical considerations focusing on known or potential drug-herb interactions, Arch Intern Med 158:2200–2211, 1998.

Mosby's drug consult 2004: the comprehensive reference for generic and brand name drugs, ed 14, St. Louis, 2004, Mosby.

Mosby's handbook of herbs and supplements and their therapeutic uses, St. Louis, 2003, Mosby.

Natural medicines comprehensive database, Stockton, CA, 2004, Pharmacist's Letter/Prescriber's Letter, Therapeutic Research Faculty.

Nonherbal dietary supplements, Pharmacist's Letter 98(4), 1998.

O'Hara MA, et al: A review of 12 commonly used medicinal herbs, Arch Fam Med 7:523–536, 1998.

PDR for herbal remedies, Montvale, NJ, 1998, Medical Economics.

Therapeutic use of herbs, continuing education booklets part 1 and part 2, Stockton, CA, 1998, Pharmacist's Letter.

Appendix I Pregnancy and Pediatrics

TABLE I-1
FDA Drug Pregnancy Risk Category Descriptions

Pregnancy Risk Category	Description	Application in Dentistry
A	Drug has been studied in humans. Evidence supports its safe use. Remote possibility of fetal harm.	Can be appropriately administered during pregnancy.
B	Animal studies demonstrate no fetal risk. Inadequate studies in pregnant women Slightly increased fetal risk.	Can be appropriately administered during pregnancy.
C	Teratogenic risk cannot be ruled out. Animal studies show potential adverse fetal effects. Potential benefits may outweigh risks.	Can be used with caution.
D	Drug demonstrates risk in humans. Potential benefits may outweigh risks.	Should be avoided.
X	Drug demonstrates harm in mother or fetus. Risk clearly outweighs benefit.	Contraindicated.

From Hupp JR, Williams TP, Firriolo FJ: Dental clinical advisor, ed 1, St Louis, 2006, Elsevier.

TABLE I-2
FDA Drug Pregnancy Risk Category and Use during Breast-feeding

Generic Name	Brand Name	FDA Pregnancy Risk Category	Use during Breast-feeding
Antimicrobials			
Amoxicillin	Amoxil, Polymox	B	Yes
Amoxicillin + clavulanic acid	Augmentin	B	Yes
Azithromycin	Zithromax	B	Yes
Cephalexin	Keflex	B	Yes
Chlorhexidine	Peridex	B	Yes
Clindamycin	Cleocin	B	Yes
Doxycycline	Doryx, Vibramycin, Atridox, Periostat	D	No
Erythromycin[†]	Ery-Tab, E-Mycin, E.E.S., PCE	B	Yes
Fluconazole	Diflucan	C	No
Ketoconazole	Nizoral	C	No
Metronidazole	Flagyl	B	Caution
Nystatin	Mycostatin	B	Yes
Penicillin V Potassium	V-Cillin K, V-Pen	B	Yes
Tetracycline	Actisite, Achromycin	D	No

Continued

TABLE I-2

FDA Drug Pregnancy Risk Category and Use during Breast-feeding—cont'd

Generic Name	Brand Name	FDA Pregnancy Risk Category	Use during Breast-feeding
Analgesics			
Acetaminophen	Tylenol	B	Yes
Aspirin	Bayer	C/D3	No
Celecoxib/Valdecoxib	Celebrex/Bextra	C/D3	Unknown
Codeine	Various combinations	C/D*	Yes
Hydrocodone	Various combinations	C/D*	Caution
Ibuprofen	Advil, Motrin	B/D3	Yes
Naproxen	Aleve, Anaprox	B/D3	Unknown
Oxycodone	Various combinations	C/D*	Caution
Sedatives			
Chloral hydrate	Somnote	C	Yes
Diazepam	Valium	D	No
Hydroxyzine	Atarax/Vistaril	C	Unknown
Lorazepam	Ativan	D	No
Midazolam	Versed	D	No
Nitrous oxide	N/A	None†	Controversial
Triazolam	Halcion	X	No
Local Anesthetics			
Articaine	Septocaine	C	Unknown
Bupivacaine	Marcaine	C	Yes
Etidocaine	Duranest	B	Yes
Lidocaine	Xylocaine	B	Yes
Mepivacaine	Carbocaine	C	Yes
Prilocaine	Citanest	B	Yes
Vasoconstrictors			
Epinephrine 1:100,000; 1:200,000	N/A	C*	Yes
Levonordefrin 1:20,000	Neo-Cobefrin	None	Yes
Topical Anesthetics			
Benzocaine	Anbesol, Hurricaine	C	Yes
Lidocaine	Xylocaine, DentiPatch	B	Yes
Tetracaine	Pontocaine	C	Yes

C/D3, Pregnancy risk category D during the third trimester.
C/D*, Pregnancy risk category D in high doses at term or with prolonged use.
C*, Pregnancy risk category C in high doses.
†Avoid estolate form.
‡Best used in the second and third trimesters and for less than 30 min with at least 50% O_2; consult physician.
Modified from Hilgers K, Douglass J, Mathieu G: Pediatr Dent 25:459–467, 2003.

TABLE I-3
Drug Usage in Pediatric Dentistry

Drug	Route	Dose	Frequency	Notes
Antibiotics				
Amoxicillin	PO	25–50 mg/kg/day	3 times a day	Syrup or chewable tablets for young children
	IV	100–400 mg/kg/day	3 times a day	
	PO, IV	50 mg/kg up to adult dose 3 g	30 min–1 hr before procedure	Endocarditis prophylaxis. For highly susceptible patients, half dose 6 hr later
Amoxicillin + clavulanic acid	PO	20–40 mg/kg/day	3 times a day	For β-lactam resistant organisms only
Ampicillin	IV	50–100 mg/kg/day	4 times a day	Endocarditis prophylaxis
	IV	50 mg/kg	stat	
Benzylpenicillin	IV	15–350 mg/kg/day	4 times a day	First IV drug of choice for odontogenic infections
		20,000–500,000 Units/kg/day		
Penicillin VK	PO	Younger than 5 yr 500 mg/day	4 times a day	Give 1 hr before meals
		Older than 5 yr 1–2 g/day		
Cephalexin	PO	25–50 mg/kg/day	4 times a day	
Cephalothin IV	IV	40–80 mg/kg/day	4 times a day	Not in pregnancy
Cephazolin	IV	25–50 mg/kg/day		
Erythromycin	PO	25–40 mg/kg/day	4 times a day	Ethylsuccinate is readily absorbed
Metronidazole	IV	22.5 mg/kg/day	3 times a day	Not in pregnancy
	PO	10–15 mg/kg/day	3 times a day	
Gentamicin	IV	2.5 mg/kg (children) up to 80 mg maximum	stat	Endocarditis prophylaxis, highly susceptible patients. In conjunction with ampicillin. Follow-up dose of ampicillin or amoxicillin required 6 hr later.

Continued

TABLE I-3
Drug Usage in Pediatric Dentistry—cont'd

Drug	Route	Dose	Frequency	Notes
Antibiotics				
Clindamycin	PO, IV	15–40 mg/kg/day	4 times a day	Risk of pseudomem-branous colitis
	PO, IV	10 mg/kg up to adult dose 600 mg	PO: 1 hr before, IV: stat	Endocarditis prophylaxis, susceptible patients Follow-up dose half initial dose, 6 hr later (5 mg/kg up to 300 mg)
Vancomycin	IV	20 mg/kg up to adult dose 1 g	infused over 1 hr	Endocarditis prophylaxis, susceptible patients allergic to penicillin
Antifungals				
Nystatin	Tablets	500,000 Units	tds	
	Mixture	100,000 Units/mL	every 6 hr	Apply to affected area
Amphotericin B	Lozenges	10 mg	every 6 hr	Apply to affected area
	Suspension	100 mg/mL	every 6 hr	Apply to affected area
	Ointment	3%	every 6 hr	Apply to affected area
Analgesics and Sedatives				
Aspirin	PO	325–650 mg	every 4 hr	Should not be used in children younger than 12 yr because of the risk of Reye's syndrome
Paracetamol	PO, PR	15 mg/kg	every 4 hr	Hepatotoxic if overdose

TABLE I-3

Drug Usage in Pediatric Dentistry—cont'd

Drug	Route	Dose	Frequency	Notes
Codeine phosphate	PO	1–1.5 mg/kg single dose 1–3 mg/kg/day	4–6 divided doses	Similar side effects to narcotics, including nausea and constipation
Pethidine	IV, IM	1 mg/kg	every 3–4 hr	Maximum 100 mg
Morphine	IV, IM	0.1–0.2 mg/kg	every 6 hr	Should only be used in admitted patients
Naloxone	IM, IV	1–10 mcg/kg	stat	May be repeated at 2–3 min intervals if necessary
Midazolam	IV, IM	0.1–0.2 mg/kg	single dose	Sedation, may be given intranasally
Chloral hydrate	PO	30–50 mg/kg/day, 15–20 mg/kg single dose	every 4–6 hr	Sedation
Trimeprazine	PO	3–4 mg/kg	single dose	Valergen, sedation
Metoclopramide	PO, IM	3–5 yr: 2 mg 5–9 yr: 2.5 mg 9–14 yr: 5 mg 15–19 yr: 10 mg	single dose	Single dose after narcotic if vomiting or nausea Maxolon. Dystonic reactions may occur
Other Medications				
Kenalog in Orabase	Ointment	Triamcinolone 0.1%	every 4–6 hr	Recurrent severe oral ulceration in children, apply to ulcer but do not rub ointment in
ε aminocaproic acid	IV	30 mg/kg		Antifibrinolytic, loading dose of 100 mg/kg
Tranexamic acid	PO	15–20 mg/kg	4 times a day	Antifibrinolytic
DDAVP	IV	0.3 mcg/kg		Infused over 1 hr before surgery
Heparin	IV	50–100 Units/kg	every 4–6 hr	Anticoagulant

Continued

TABLE I-3
Drug Usage in Pediatric Dentistry—cont'd

Drug	Route	Dose	Frequency	Notes
Tetanus toxoid	IM	0.5 mL	single dose	If immunization protocol not complete, course should be given. Otherwise, a booster may be required for tetanus-prone wounds if longer than 2 yr since last booster

From Cameron AC, Widmer RP: Handbook of pediatric dentistry, ed 2, London, 2003, Mosby.

The table that forms Table K–2 is a guide to the administration of commonly used drugs in pediatric dentistry. Medications for children should always be prescribed in relation to weight. It is of utmost importance that clinicians understand the contraindications and precautions relevant to the drugs they are prescribing, and should consult prescribing information supplied by the pharmaceutical manufacturers and relevant pharmacopeia.
PR = per rectum; stat = immediately.

Appendix J   Preventing Medication Errors and Improving Medication Safety

Medication safety is a high priority for the health care professional. Prevention of medication errors and improved safety for the patient are important, especially in today's health care environment, when today's patient is older and sometimes sicker and the drug therapy regimen can be more sophisticated and complex.

A medication error is defined by the National Coordinating Council for Medication Error Reporting and Prevention (NCC MERP) as "any preventable event that may cause or lead to inappropriate medication use or patient harm while the medication is in the control of the health care professional, patient, or consumer." Most medication errors occur as a result of multiple compounding events as opposed to a single act by a single individual.

Use of the wrong medication, strength, or dose; confusion over sound-alike or look-alike drugs; administration of medications by the wrong route; miscalculations (especially when used in pediatric patients or when administering medications intravenously); and errors in prescribing and transcription all can contribute to compromising the safety of the patient. The potential for adverse events and medication errors is definitely a reality and is potentially tragic and costly in both human and economic terms.

Health care professionals must take the initiative to create and implement procedures to reduce, and hopefully prevent, medication errors. The first priority in preventing medication errors is to establish a multidisciplinary team to improve medication use. The goal for this team would be to assess medication safety and implement changes that would make it difficult or impossible for mistakes to reach the patient. Some important criteria in making improved medication safety successful include the following:

• Promote a nonpunitive approach to reducing medication errors.
• Increase the detection and the reporting of medication errors, near misses, and potentially hazardous situations that may result in medication errors.
• Determine root causes of medication errors.
• Educate about the causes of medication errors and ways to prevent these errors.
• Make recommendations to allow organization-wide, system-based changes to prevent medication errors.
• Learn from errors that occur in other organizations and take measures to prevent similar errors.

Some common causes and ways to prevent medication errors and improve safety include the following:

Communicating Prescription Information

Poor handwriting can make it difficult to distinguish between two medications with similar names. Also, many drug names sound similar, especially when the names are spoken over the telephone, poorly enunciated, or mispronounced.

• Take time to write legibly.
• Keep phone or verbal orders to a minimum to prevent misinterpretation.
• Repeat back orders taken over the telephone.
• When ordering a new or rarely used medication, print the name.
• Always specify the drug strength, even if only one strength exists.

• Print generic and brand names of look-alike or sound-alike medications.

Zeros and Decimal Points

Hastily written orders can present problems even if the name of the medication is clear.

• Never leave a decimal point "naked." Place a zero before a decimal point when the number is less than a whole unit (e.g., use 0.25 mg or 250 mcg, not .25 mg).

• Never have a trailing zero following a decimal point (e.g., use 2 mg, not 2.0 mg).

Abbreviations

Errors can occur because of a failure to standardize abbreviations. Establishing a list of abbreviations that should never be used is recommended.

• Never abbreviate unit as "U," spell out "unit."

• Do not abbreviate "once daily" as od or qd, or "every other day" as qod; spell it out.

• Do not use DC, because it may be misinterpreted as either discharge or discontinue.

• Do not abbreviate drug names; spell out the generic and/or brand names.

Ambiguous or incomplete orders:

These types of orders can cause confusion or misinterpretation of the writer's intention. Examples include situations in which the route of administration, dose, or dosage form has not been specified.

• Do not use slash marks—they are read as the number one (1).

• When reviewing an unusual order, verify the order with the person writing the order to prevent any misunderstanding.

• Read over orders after writing.

• Encourage that the drug's indication for use be provided on medication orders.

• Provide complete medication orders—do not use "resume preop" or "continue previous meds."

High-alert medications:

Medications in this category have an increased risk of causing significant patient harm when used in error. Mistakes with these medications may or may not be more common but may be more devastating to the patient if an error occurs. A list of high-alert medications can be obtained from the Institute for Safe Medication Practices (ISMP) at *www.ismp.org*. Technologies available today that can be used to address and help to solve potential medication problems or errors include the following:

• Electronic prescribing systems— This refers to computerized prescriber order entry systems. Within these systems is the capability to incorporate medication safety alerts (e.g., maximum dose alerts, allergy screening). Additionally, these systems should be integrated or interfaced with pharmacy and laboratory systems to provide drug–drug and drug–disease interaction alerts and include clinical order screening capability.

• Bar codes—These systems are designed to use bar-code scanning devices to validate identity of patients, verify medications administered, document administration, and provide safety alerts.

• "Smart" infusion pumps—These pumps allow users to enter drug infusion protocols into a drug library along with predefined dosage limits. If a dosage is outside the limits established, an alarm is sounded and drug delivery is halted, informing the clinician that the dose is outside the recommended range.

• Automated dispensing systems/ point-of-use dispensing systems— These systems should be integrated with information systems, especially pharmacy systems.

• Pharmacy order entry system— This should be fully integrated with an electronic prescribing system with

the capability of producing medication safety alerts. Additionally, the system should generate a computerized medication administration record (MAR), which would be used by a nursing staff while administering medications.

From Mosby's 2006 drug consult for nurses, St. Louis, 2006, Mosby.

Generic and Trade Name Index

Entries can be identified as follows: generic name, Trade Name/Trade Name[Region], DRUG CATEGORY, *Combination Product*

Mini CD-ROM to Accompany *Mosby's Dental Drug Reference,*
Eighth Edition

MINIMUM SYSTEM REQUIREMENTS
This CD will run on both PC and Mac.

Microsoft Windows Users
To function properly, your computer should support at least an 800 × 600 pixels
screen resolution, 256 colors, 128 MB RAM, and operate on the Windows 98
SE, 2000, or XP operating system. Additionally, be sure your browser has
"Show pictures" enabled. For Internet Explorer users, you will find the "Show
pictures" option by selecting the following from your menu: Tools > Internet
Options > Advanced > Multimedia. If the "Show pictures" box is not checked,
do so.

This software is designed to run with Internet Explorer 6.0, Netscape 7 or
later, and Firefox 1.x.

Use MS PowerPoint to view the ".ppt" files. These files can also be viewed
using MS PowerPoint file viewer.

Use MS Word to view the ".rtf" files. These files can also be viewed using
MS Word file viewer.

Macintosh Users
Your computer should meet the following minimum requirements:
800 × 600 pixels screen resolution, 256 colors, 128 MB RAM, and operate
on the MAC OS 10.2 or later operating system.

Use MS PowerPoint to view the ".ppt" files and MS Word to view the ".rtf"
files. Microsoft currently does not offer an OS X-native version of the
PowerPoint viewer and MS Word viewer. You need a full version of PowerPoint
to view the PowerPoint presentations and MS Word to view the .rtf files.

This software is designed to run with Safari 1.3 or later and Firefox 1.x.
Refer to the help files for problems specific to the browser.

INSTALLATION INSTRUCTIONS
Windows
1. If your system does not support Autorun, click on MDDR.exe to begin.
2. To use the Search feature, install the Java Runtime Environment, version
   1.4.1 (available in the software folder). You should have administrator
   privileges for this installation. After installation, start the application by
   clicking MDDR.exe.
3. For Windows 98 users, the Visual Basic 6.0 Service Pack 5 Run-Time
   Redistribution Pack (VBRun60sp5.exe) is provided on the CD. Install it
   from the software folder.
4. PowerPoint viewer ("ppviewer2003.exe") can be installed from the
   software folder of the CD.
5. MSWord Viewer ("wdviewer2003.exe") can be installed from the software
   folder of the CD.

Macintosh

1. Click on the CD icon that appears on your desktop; then select MDDR to open the application.
2. The CD requires the installation of MRJ 2.2.5 in order to use the Search feature (available in the software folder). If manually installed, start the application by clicking on MDDR.
3. If the browser does not launch after clicking on the "I Agree" button from the MDDR application or by clicking on the "Start" button on the MServerX applet, open Index.htm to launch the Home page.

KNOWN ISSUES

1. To get the program to launch in your default browser,

Windows Users

Shift-Right-click the Home.htm file, select "Open With," and then select the default browser from the "Choose Program..." menu.

Macintosh Users

Control-click the Home.htm file, select "Get Info," and then select the default browser from the "Opens With" drop-down menu.

2. If Active Content warning is displayed while running the product, please do the following:

  On Tools > Internet Options > Advanced tab > Security >Select "Allow active content from CDs to run on my Computer."
3. While using Netscape 8, ensure that "Open requested Pop-ups in New Tab" option is deselected. If not, select the Site Controls icon on the tab and deselect this option.

TECHNICAL SUPPORT

Technical support for this product is available between 7:30 AM and 7 PM CST, Monday through Friday. Before calling, be sure that your computer meets the minimum system requirements to run this software. Inside the United States, call 1-800-692-9010. Outside the United States, call 314-872-8370. You may also fax your questions to 314-523-4932.

  You may also contact Technical Support via e-mail at: technical.support@ elsevier.com.

  For access to a list of Frequently Asked Questions (FAQ), as well as troubleshooting tips, please visit our website at http://www.us.elsevier.health. com/TechSupport

  Part number: 9996048055

  Pentium, Windows, Adobe, and Macintosh are registered trademarks.

  Copyright © 2008, 2007 by Mosby, Inc., an affiliate of Elsevier Inc. All rights reserved.

Weights and Equivalents

Metric System

Weight

kilogram	kg	1000 grams
gram	g	1 gram
milligram	mg	0.001 gram
microgram	μg	0.001 milligram

Volume

liter	L	1000 milliliters
milliliter	ml	0.001 liter

Weight Conversion, Pounds to Kilograms

Kilograms (kg)	_Pounds (lb)_
1	2.2
10	22
15	33
20	44
40	88
60	132
80	176

Household Equivalents—Approximate

Utensil	_Volume_
1 teaspoonful	5 ml
1 tablespoonful	15 ml
1 teacupful	120 ml
1 tumbler glassful	240 ml
1 pint	480 ml